FETAL, NEONATAL AND PEDIATRIC NEURORADIOLOGY

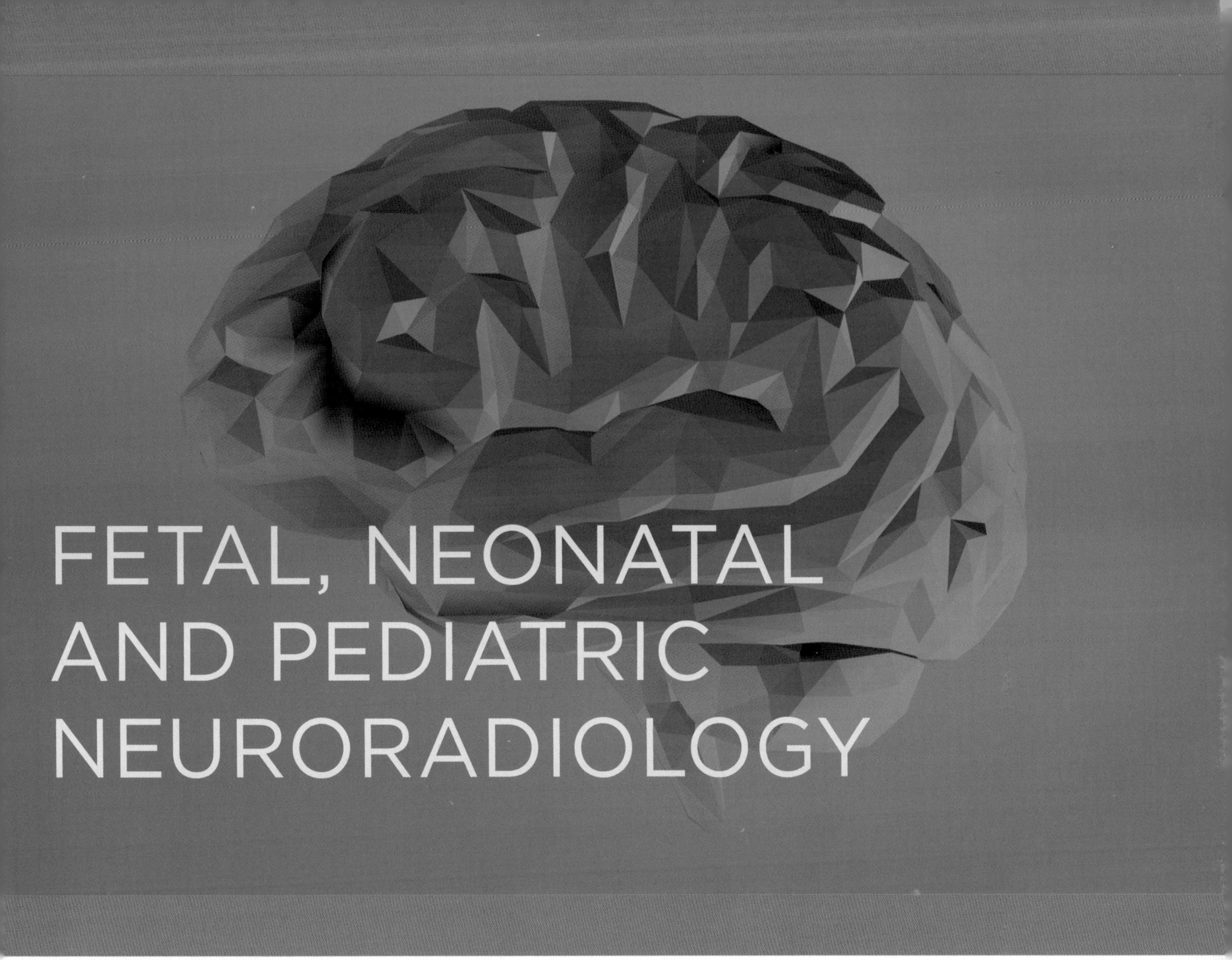

FETAL, NEONATAL AND PEDIATRIC NEURORADIOLOGY

STEPHEN F. KRALIK, MD
Associate Professor of Radiology
Edward B. Singleton Department of Radiology
Texas Children's Hospital
Baylor College of Medicine
Houston, Texas

NILESH K. DESAI, MD
Associate Professor of Radiology
Edward B. Singleton Department of Radiology
Texas Children's Hospital
Baylor College of Medicine
Houston, Texas

AVNER MEODED, MD
Pediatric Neuroradiologist
Associate Professor of Radiology
Edward B. Singleton Department of Radiology
Texas Children's Hospital
Baylor College of Medicine
Houston, Texas

THIERRY A.G.M. HUISMAN, MD
Radiologist-in-Chief and Edward B. Singleton Chair of Radiology
Professor of Radiology, Pediatrics, Neurosurgery, Neurology and OBGYN
Edward B. Singleton Department of Radiology
Texas Children's Hospital
Baylor College of Medicine
Houston, Texas

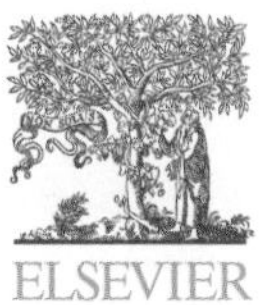

ELSEVIER

Elsevier
3251 Riverport Lane
St. Louis, Missouri 63043

FETAL, NEONATAL AND PEDIATRIC NEURORADIOLOGY ISBN: 978-0-323-79695-8

Senior Content Strategist: Melanie Tucker
Director, Content Development: Ellen Wurm-Cutter
Content Development Specialist: John Tomedi
Marketing Manager: Kate Bresnahan
Publishing Services Manager: Deena Burgess
Project Manager: Anne Collett
Design Direction: Brian Salisbury

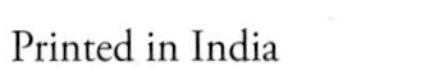

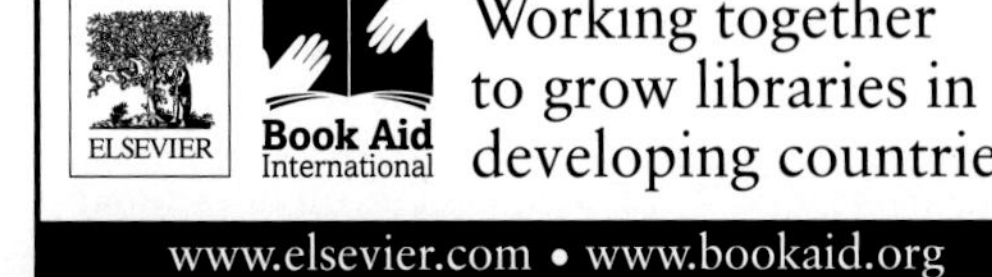

Printed in India

Last digit is the print number: 9 8 7 6 5 4 3 2 1

This book is dedicated to my beautiful wife, Veronica, and our precious baby boy, Leo—for their love, patience and support which were essential to the success of this book. I would also like to acknowledge my parents, who taught me the value of education and hard work, my siblings, who made growing up together a joy, and the many teachers and trainees over the years who helped me craft my abilities. Finally, I thank Christ our Lord, who gave me all of these blessings and more, without which this book would not have been possible.

Stephen F. Kralik, MD

To my incredible wife, Erica, the mother of our children, always a pinnacle of strength, keeping me grounded and alive. To Shefali and Maya, my curious daughters, life is a chance to make change. The world needs you. To my father, Kundan and my mother, Kalpana. I only now realize what you gave me. Mom, I will miss you forever. To my sister, Ami, love forever.

Nilesh K. Desai, MD

To my parents, Michal and Abraham, and my wife, Maria Grazia, and children, Emily and Jonathan, for their endless love and support.

Avner Meoded, MD

I would like to dedicate this book to my wife Charlotte, my children Max, Laura and Emily as well as the many fabulous colleagues, mentors and friends who have always been there to assist and guide me on my academic journey over the past three decades.

Thierry A.G.M. Huisman, MD

PREFACE

This text was first discussed more than 6 years ago by Drs. Thierry Huisman and Andrea Poretti, at the time envisioned to be a consummate amalgamation of in-depth neuroimaging and clinical neurology. The book was meant to embolden the radiologic reader with clinical context and conversely fortify the neurologic reader with radiologic context. The first two chapters were completed in short order, however, tragedy struck with the untimely death of Andrea Poretti in 2017. The first two chapters fell permanently silent and the vision seemingly ended.

In 2020, Drs. Huisman and Kralik reimagined writing a comprehensive fetal, neonatal, and pediatric neuroimaging textbook. The goal was to create a textbook that would appeal to a broad audience by finding a middle ground on the amount of imaging and text that was currently lacking in available publications. Our goal became to provide the reader with information of every day importance, enough content expertise for clinical confidence, and finer details for continued education. Drs. Desai and Meoded joined us and brought diverse training and teaching backgrounds and expertise into the authorship of this textbook.

To accomplish this vision for the textbook we offer the following: a 50-50 balance of imaging and text, and most topics to be covered in one page. Second, succinct text and key points to allow the reader to rapidly understand topics. Most chapters have a short introductory page which briefly discusses the chapter's content, followed by pages with individual topics. The topic-based text allows for critical reading in sustained bursts. Third, we cover brain, spine, and head and neck diseases seen in clinical practice to ensure this book can be relied upon for *all* of pediatric neuroimaging. Fourth, we include imaging of fetal, neonatal, and pediatric patients to ensure the reader has the appropriate and full spectrum of example cases. Fifth, we include handy bonus material and quick tools, including useful references for each topic, chapter summary pages with major topics broken down into manageable groupings, and a differential diagnosis chapter (Chapter 20) that can be called upon in daily practice. This chapter is meant to bring the book topics together and may assist the reader in clinical practice in when a diagnosis is unknown. Chapter 20 synthesizes yet discriminates the most commonly encountered cases in pediatric neuroradiology. Finally, the eBook offers the reader necessary access at their fingertips on a variety of electronic devices, and contains additional chapters covering normal anatomy and imaging techniques.

A major focal point of this text is the high-quality images used for each case. Common and uncommon entities were included, ensuring that both the novice and experienced reader benefit from each presentation. Cases were carefully selected, with all images and content vetted by the author group for quality and relevance.

We hope the reader enjoys and relies on this text for both personal knowledge building, and, importantly, for assisting in patient care.

STEPHEN F. KRALIK
NILESH K. DESAI
AVNER MEODED
THIERRY A.G.M. HUISMAN

ACKNOWLEDGMENTS

The authors wish to acknowledge Joseph C. Swisher and Dr. Maria Grazia Sacco Casamassima, MD, for their excellent artistic contributions to this book, and Dr. Isaac C. Wu, MD, for his insight and advice on the text's content and organization.

FOREWORD

Fetal, Neonatal and Pediatric Neuroradiology starts with a section on normal CNS development, and from then on it springs forward to malformations—18 chapters dealing not only with brain disorders, but also with head and neck and spine abnormalities and lesions. The breadth of the entities it addresses is impressive.

There are two types of thinking: verbal and visual. I like to think of most radiologists as visual thinkers, but I accept that, among us, many are verbal thinkers. This book satisfies both types. The text-based information is complete, approachable, and easy to digest and remember, while the illustrations are superb. Not only is there an abundance of beautiful diagrams, but the diagnostic images shown (which include conventional methods and advanced ones) are superb and use two-tone and full-color formats. Make no mistake, this is a gorgeously illustrated tome bound to satisfy even the most demanding radiologists. Tables also abound, making it easier to remember differential diagnoses and other key components of each entity. All in all, it is a wonderful learning experience.

Unlike other case books which tend to be single-authored, this one benefits from the expertise of four seasoned pediatric neuroradiologists, all of them practicing at the prestigious Texas Children's Hospital in Houston, Texas. All four should be congratulated for this outstanding work which should be helpful to all involved in the care of children with brain, neck, and spine conditions.

Whenever I buy a book and read its reviews, I am wary of those that only have "5-star" ratings. But with this one, that should not be the case. It should get only 5 stars reviews because that is what it deserves. I hope you enjoy reading it as much as I did and I am sure that once you have done so, you will keep it at hand's reach for many years to come.

MAURICIO CASTILLO MD, FACR
Distinguished Professor of Radiology,
UNC Chapel Hill
Past President and Gold Medal,
ASNR and ARRS
Emeritus Editor, AJNR

BRIEF CONTENTS

CONTENTS

PART I NORMAL DEVELOPMENT

CHAPTER 1 Normal Development 1

PART II BRAIN

CHAPTER 2 Brain Malformations 61

PART III NECK, FACE, ORBIT, AND TEMPORAL BONE

CHAPTER 12 Orbital and Craniofacial Malformations 525

CHAPTER 13 Temporal Bone Malformations 551

CHAPTER 14 Neck, Face, Orbit, and Temporal Bone Masses 567

CHAPTER 15 Infectious and Inflammatory Disorders of the Head and Neck 633

1 Normal Development

INTRODUCTION

The human brain is a fascinating and essentially miraculous structure with layers upon layers of complexity in its anatomic organization, microscopic connectivity, biochemical workings, and functions. No human can grasp all of the complexity that allows the brain to function, but that doesn't stop us from trying! Learning about the brain's development is particularly exciting, daunting, and exhausting. Understanding even just a small fraction of the necessary processes that allow the brain to develop from the moment of conception to birth and from birth to adulthood can be rewarding and bring a great sense of wonder.

Understanding normal development of the central nervous system begins with a basic understanding of embryology of the brain and spine; however, by the time at which imaging is routinely performed in clinical care of patients, a significant degree of brain and spine development has already occurred. Abnormalities in early brain development account for many of the malformations seen on imaging. As such, this chapter will primarily focus on the imaging appearances seen during normal development and provide a basic overview of embryology.

A general approach for evaluating normal brain development on imaging begins with knowledge of the age of the patient and then determination of normal formation of major structures. A pattern approach is most useful to ensure one does not overlook an important structure. Major intracranial structures that should be evaluated include the size, sulcation, gyration, and myelination of the cerebral hemispheres; size, formation, and proportions of the cerebellum, brainstem, and posterior fossa; presence of the septum pellucidum and formation and size of the corpus callosum; presence of the olfactory bulbs and sulci; formation and size of the basal ganglia and thalami; rotation of the hippocampi; and formation and size of the ventricles. The appearance of these structures will be discussed in this chapter, and useful biometric data will be provided. Importantly, assessment of extracranial structures, including the eyes, ears, and facial bones, should be performed because anomalies in these structures have associated brain anomalies.

In addition to the imaging patterns of normal brain development on conventional imaging, advanced magnetic resonance imaging (MRI) techniques that are not routinely clinically performed, including diffusion tensor imaging, spectroscopy, and functional MRI, will be discussed. These techniques provide additional insight into normal brain development. Last, the formation of the anterior cranial fossa, paranasal sinus development, and spine development will be discussed.

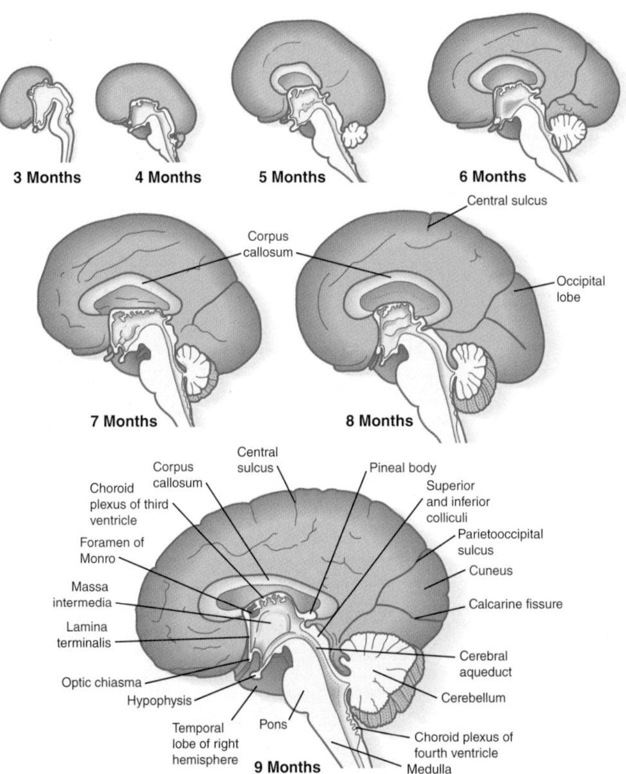

Medial Views of the Developing Brain. (From Carlson BM. *Human Embryology and Developmental Biology.* 6th ed. Elsevier; 2019.)

BRAIN DEVELOPMENT

The central nervous system develops through the process of primary neurulation during week 3–4, when notochord induces the ectoderm to become neuroectoderm and develop into the neural plate. The neural plate folds and becomes the neural tube and separates from the ectoderm (disjunction). The cranial end of the neural tube is the anterior/rostral neuropore, and the caudal opening is the posterior/caudal neuropore. Prior to neural tube closure, the anterior neural tube forms three primary brain vesicles or pouches referred to as the prosencephalon (forebrain), mesencephalon (midbrain), and rhombencephalon (hindbrain). Abnormalities in development occurring at these stages lead to malformations, including anencephaly and many of the spine malformations discussed in Chapter 6.

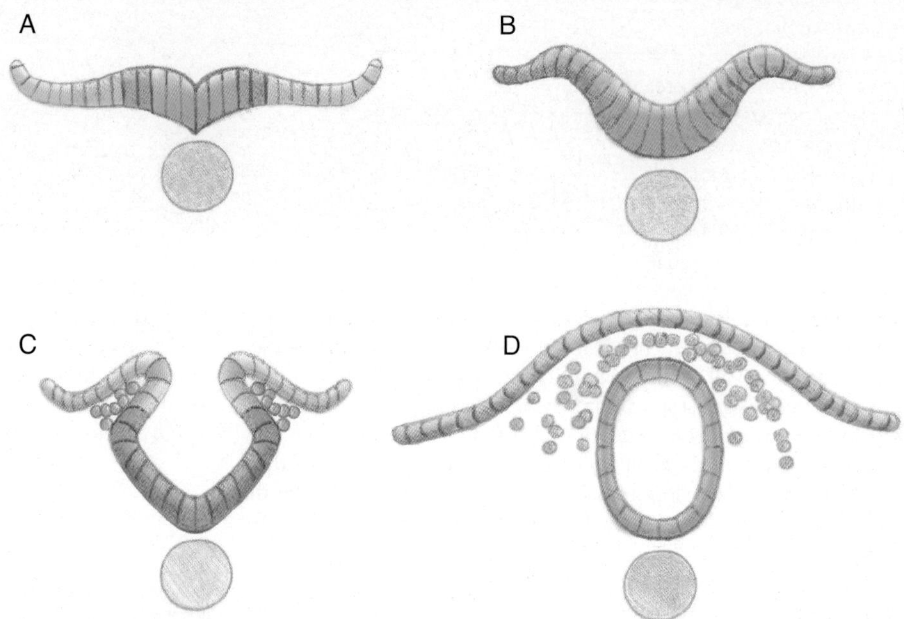

Primary Neurulation (Weeks 3–4). The notochord interacts with the overlying ectoderm to form the neural plate (A). The neural plate then bends to begin formation of the neural tube (B). Continued infolding of neural plate (C). Disjunction is the separation of the neural tube from the ectoderm (D).

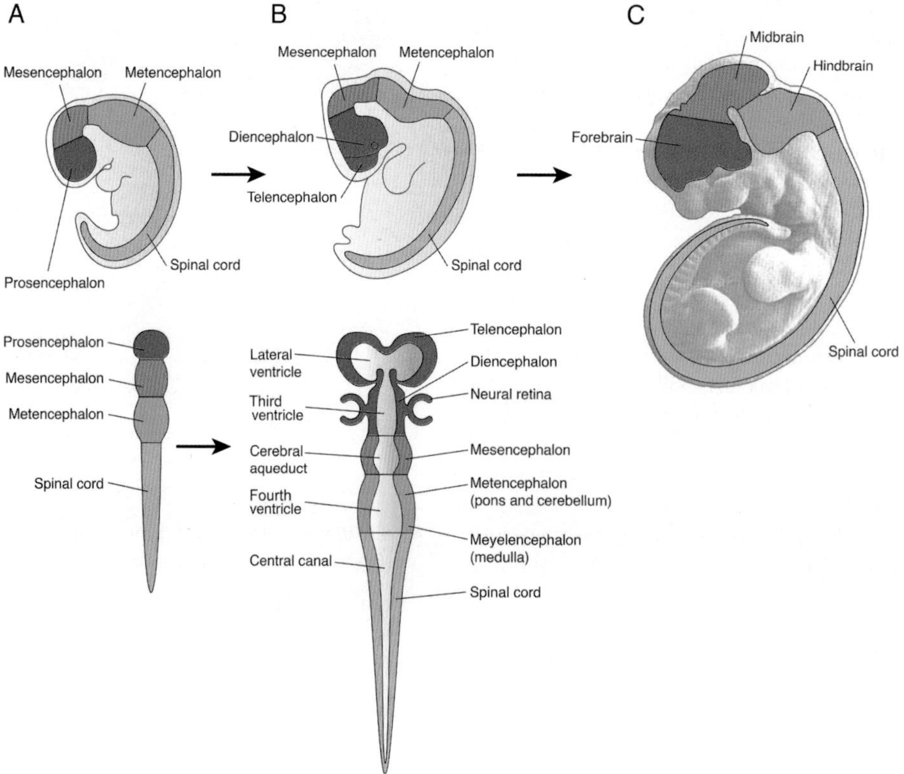

Embryology of the brain and spinal cord. The primary three divisions of the brain occur as three brain vesicles or swellings of the neural tube: the forebrain (prosencephalon), midbrain (mesencephalon), and hindbrain (rhombencephalon) (A). The next stage features further subdivisions–the forebrain vesicle subdivides into the paired telencephalic vesicles and the diencephalon, and the rhombencephalon subdivides into the metencephalon and the myelencephalon (B). These basic brain divisions can be related to the overall anatomical organization of the brain (C). (From Sanes DH, Reh TA, Harris WA, Landgraf M. *Development of the Nervous System*, 4th ed. Academic Press; 2019.)

CEREBRAL HEMISPHERE DEVELOPMENT

At approximately 35 days of gestation, the prosencephalon divides into the telencephalon and diencephalon. The telencephalon, which forms the cerebral hemispheres (also the caudate and putamen), separates as outpouchings in the region of the foramen of Monro from the diencephalon (which forms the thalami, hypothalamus, and globus pallidi). The thin-walled cerebral hemisphere vesicles expand and cover the diencephalon; cerebral hemispheres will separate in the midline along the roof of the telencephalon. The germinal matrix, which contains the cells that will form the cortex, will develop then within the walls of the telencephalon.

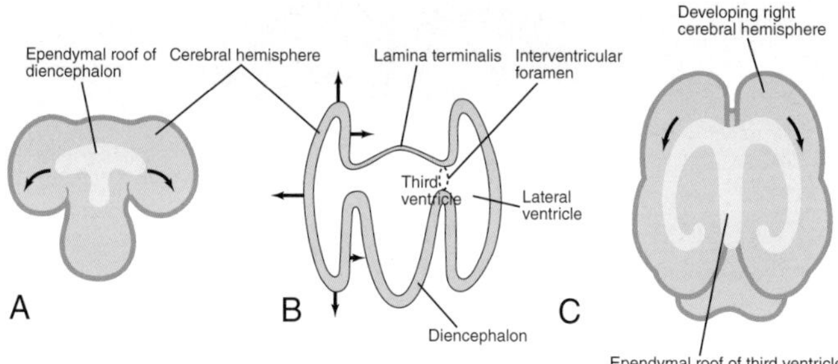

Ventricle Embryology. (A) Sketch of the dorsal surface of the forebrain. Arrows indicate how the ependymal roof of the diencephalon is carried out to the dorsomedial surface of the cerebral hemispheres. (B) Diagrammatic section of the forebrain showing how the developing cerebral hemispheres grow from the lateral walls of the forebrain and expand in all directions until they cover the diencephalon. The rostral wall of the forebrain, the lamina terminalis, is very thin. (C) Sketch of the forebrain showing how the ependymal roof is finally carried into the temporal lobes as a result of the C-shaped growth pattern of the cerebral hemispheres carry the ependymal roof into the temporal lobes. The *arrows* indicate some of the directions in which the hemispheres expand. (From Moore, Keith L, TVN Persaud, Torchia MG. *Before We Are Born: Essentials of Embryology and Birth Defects*. 10th ed. Elsevier; 2020.)

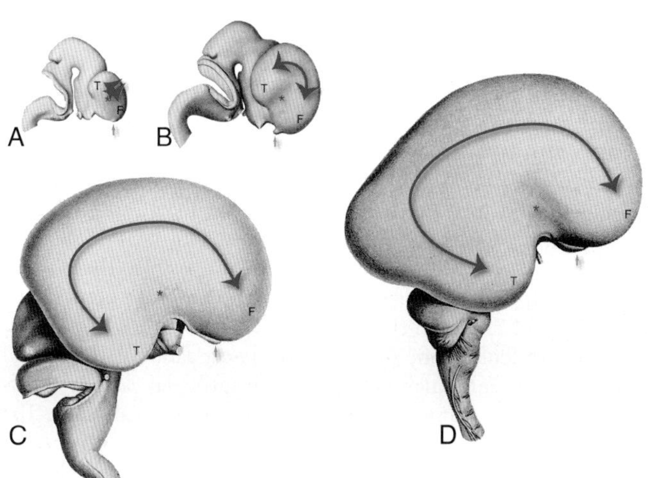

"Rotation" of the Cerebral Hemispheres Into a C shape. Although commonly described as a rotation, the change in shape is actually caused by disproportionate growth of cortex above the location of the future insula (*). The frontal *(F)* and temporal *(T)* poles actually move little, but expansion of the cortex between them causes development of the C shape during the second (A and B), third (C), and fourth (D) months. The olfactory bulb is indicated by *green arrows*. (From Hochstetter F. *Beiträge zur Entwicklungsgeschichte des menschlichen Gehirns*. I. Teil, Vienna, 1919, Franz Deuticke. In: Vanderah TW, Gould DJ, Nolte J, eds. *Nolte's The Human Brain: An Introduction to its Functional Anatomy.* 8th ed. Elsevier; 2021.)

REFERENCES

1. Garel C, Chantrel E, Brisse H, et al. Fetal cerebral cortex: normal gestational landmarks identified using prenatal MR imaging. *AJNR Am J Neuroradiol.* 2001 Jan;22(1):184–189.
2. Stiles J, Jernigan TL. The basics of brain development. *Neuropsychol Rev.* 2010 Dec;20(4):327–348.

CEREBRAL HEMISPHERE DEVELOPMENT

The cerebral cortex, basal ganglia, thalami, and hypothalamic are initially continuous with each but will eventually separate and reach their final positions as the cerebral hemispheres enlarge. The germinal matrix develops in the walls of the telencephalon, and areas known as the ganglionic eminences develop as larger regions of the germinal matrix. As the neurons from the germinal matrix proliferate and migrate to the outer cortex, they also form permanent and transient axonal connections. During this stage of development, zones in the telencephalon are visible. These zones change in appearance during development and peak between 15 and 24 weeks' gestation (Fig. 1.1).

The ventricular zone gives rise to descendants of the neural plate and subventricular zone. The periventricular zone is a cell-sparse layer with axons that give rise to the corpus callosum. The subventricular zone is the source of cortical and striatal neurons, astrocytes, and glial cells. The intermediate zone is a region of axonal connections. The subplate contains maturing neurons and connections important for cortical layer organization. The subplate reaches maximum thickness at 22 weeks' gestation and disappears at 30 weeks. The cortical plate is the final destination of migrating neurons and will develop into a six-layered neocortex with the innermost layer (layer VI) forming first and, as neurons continue to migrate, will progressively form the more outer layers. Proliferation and migration of glial progenitors continue in the postnatal period into adulthood.

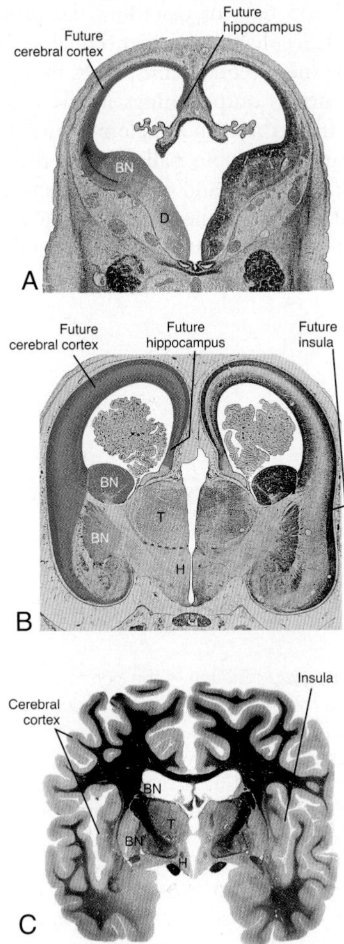

Fusion between the diencephalon and telencephalon as the cerebral hemispheres enlarge. (A) During the second month, the telencephalic vesicles, including zones that will become the cerebral cortex and basal nuclei *(BN)*, are separate from but continuous with the diencephalon (D) and its cavity. As a result of subsequent rapid telencephalic growth, the basal nuclei portion folds down toward the diencephalon. At the end of the third month (B), the telencephalon and diencephalon have fused. After further rapid growth, the insula, overlying the point of fusion, becomes overgrown by other cerebral cortex in the adult brain (C). *H*, Hypothalamus; *T*, thalamus. (A and B from Hochstetter F. *Beiträge zur Entwicklungsgeschichte des menschlichen Gehirns*. I. Teil, Vienna, 1919, Franz Deuticke. C from Vanderah TW, Gould DJ, Nolte J, eds. *Nolte's The Human Brain: An Introduction to Its Functional Anatomy.* 8th ed. Elsevier; 2021.)

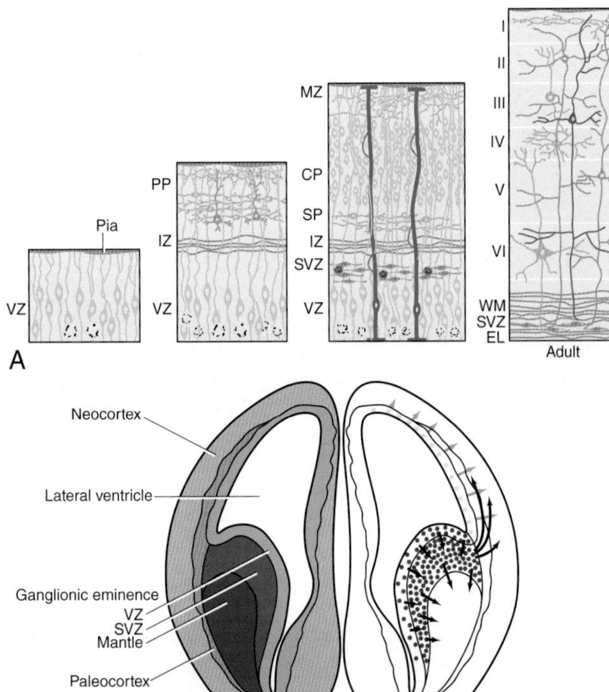

Fig. 1.1 Cytodifferentiation and Lamination of the Neocortex. (A) A series of four stages of development of the neocortex in section. The green cells in the marginal zone *(MZ)* are the Cajal-Retzius cells. *CP*, Cortical plate; *EL*, ependymal layer; *IZ*, intermediate zone; *PP*, preplate; *SP*, subplate; *WM*, white matter; *I–VI*, numbered layers of neocortex. (B) Migration of interneurons (nonpyramidal cells) from their origin in the ventricular and subventricular zones (VZ, SVZ) of the ganglionic eminences via tangential pathways *(arrows on right side)* to the neocortex. A small minority of cortical interneurons arise from the cortical germinative zones *(yellow)*. The germinative zones of the ganglionic eminences also produce the neurons of the corpus striatum and the globus pallidus (basal ganglia). (From Schoenwolf GC, Bleyl SB, Brauer PR, Francis-West PH. *Larsen's Human Embryology.* 5th ed. Elsevier; 2015.)

IMAGING OF CEREBRAL HEMISPHERE DEVELOPMENT

On ultrasound between 17 and 28 weeks, the cortex and subplate are hypoechoic and indistinguishable, and the intermediate zone is mildly hyperechoic.

On MRI between 16 and 20 weeks, the brain has a three-layered pattern on T2W imaging consisting of the:

- Germinal matrix (hypointense)
- Intermediate zone (hyperintense)
- Cortex (hypointense)

On MRI from 20 to 28 weeks, the brain has a five-layered pattern on T2W imaging consisting of the:

- Germinal matrix/ventricular zone (hypointense)
- Periventricular zone (hyperintense)
- Subventricular and intermediate zones (hypointense)
- Subplate (hyperintense)
- Cortical plate/cortex (hypointense)

Understanding the normal development of the cortex allows one to understand how abnormalities affecting the germinal matrix and neuronal migration can result in heterotopia, polymicrogyria, and cortical dysplasias.

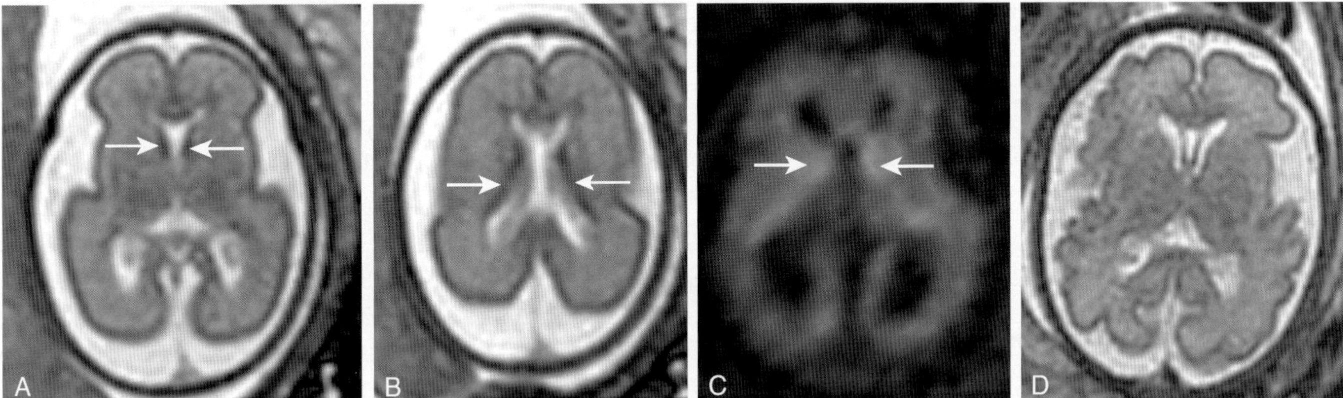

Fig. 1.2 Normal Germinal Matrix. (A and B) Axial T2W and (C) axial DWI fetal MRI images at 20 weeks' gestation show the germinal matrix as T2 hypointense areas with DWI hyperintensity along the ventricles (*arrows*), which decrease in prominence with increasing gestational age as seen on (D) axial T2W fetal MRI at 30 weeks' gestation.

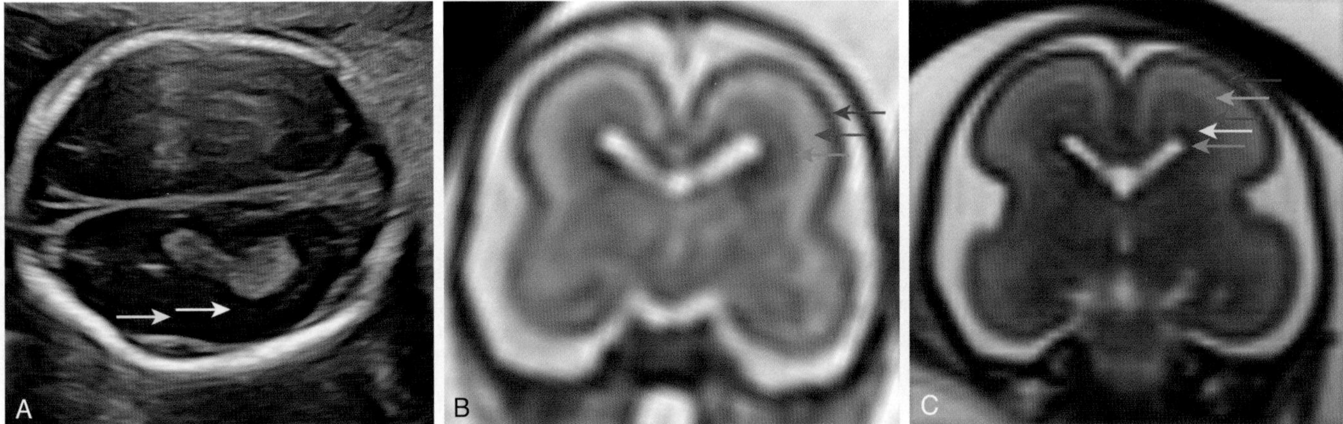

Fig. 1.3 Normal Fetal Parenchyma. (A) Ultrasound axial image at 18 weeks' gestation shows the hypoechoic cortex and subplate and mild hyperechoic intermediate zone. (B) Coronal T2W fetal MRI at 20 weeks shows a three-layered pattern (germinal matrix—orange; intermediate zone—purple; cortex—red). (C) Coronal T2W fetal MRI at 23 weeks' multilayered pattern (germinal matrix—orange; periventricular zone—yellow; subventricular and intermediate zones—purple; subplate—green; cortex—red).

CEREBRAL HEMISPHERE SULCATION

The formation of the brain also requires formation of the gyri and sulci. The fetal brain has a relatively smooth contour until approximately 16 weeks' gestation, when the sylvian fissure first appears. The primary and secondary sulci will appear in an orderly fashion (Table 1.1). Analysis of normal brain development on fetal MRI requires an understanding of the normal gyration/sulcation pattern of the brain for the gestational age of the fetus. Overgyration and undergyration of the fetal brain may both be signs of a pathologic process. The following pages will illustrate the changing sulcation pattern, major time points for sulci, and reference images of the brain for each gestational week from 24 to 35 weeks. Reference images for sulcation are often useful in routine clinical care when assessing appropriate sulcation with respect to fetal age.

■ TABLE 1.1 Chronology of Sulcation

	Gestational Age (wk)		
	Neuropathologic Appearance[a]	**Detectable in 25% to 75% of Brains in Present MR Study**	**Present in More Than 75% of Brains in Present MR Study**
Sulci of the Medial Cerebral Surface			
Interhemispheric fissure	10		22–23
Callosal sulcus	14		22–23
Parietooccipital fissure	16		22–23
Cingular sulcus	18	22–23	24–25
Secondary cingular sulci	32	31	33
Marginal sulcus		22–23	27
Calcarine fissure	16	22–23	24–25
Secondary occipital sulci	34	32	34
Sulci of the Ventral Cerebral Surface			
Hippocampic fissure			22–23
Collateral sulcus	23	24–25	27
Occipitotemporal sulcus	30	29	33
Sulci of the Lateral Cerebral Surface			
Superior frontal sulcus	25	24–25	29
Inferior frontal sulcus	28	26	29
Superior temporal sulcus (posterior part)	23	26	27
Superior temporal sulcus (anterior part)		30	32
Inferior temporal sulcus	30	30	33
Intraparietal sulcus	26	27	28
Insular sulci	34–35	33	34
Sulci of the vertex			
Central sulcus	20	24–25	27
Precentral sulcus	24	26	27
Postcentral sulcus	25	27	28

[a]According to Chi et al., sulci observed in 25% to 50% of the brains. (Chi JG, Dooling EC, Gilles FH. Gyral development of the human brain. *Ann Neurol.* 1977;1:86–93.)

From Garel C, Chantrel E, Brisse H, et al. Fetal cerebral cortex: normal gestational landmarks identified using prenatal MR imaging. *AJNR Am J Neuroradiol.* 2001 Jan;22(1):184–189. PMID: 11158907.

REFERENCE

1. Garel C, Chantrel E, Brisse H, et al. Fetal cerebral cortex: normal gestational landmarks identified using prenatal MR imaging. *AJNR Am J Neuroradiol.* 2001 Jan;22(1):184–189. PMID11158907.

EXPECTED GESTATIONAL AGE OF MAJOR SULCI ON FETAL MRI

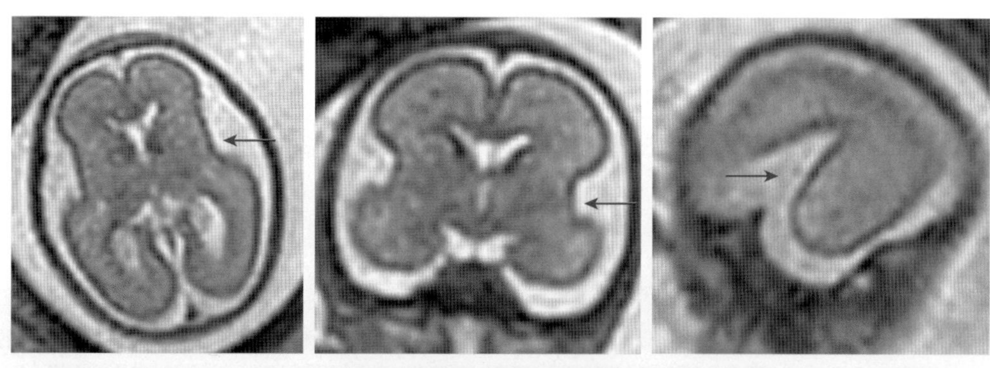

16-20 weeks: Sylvian fissure

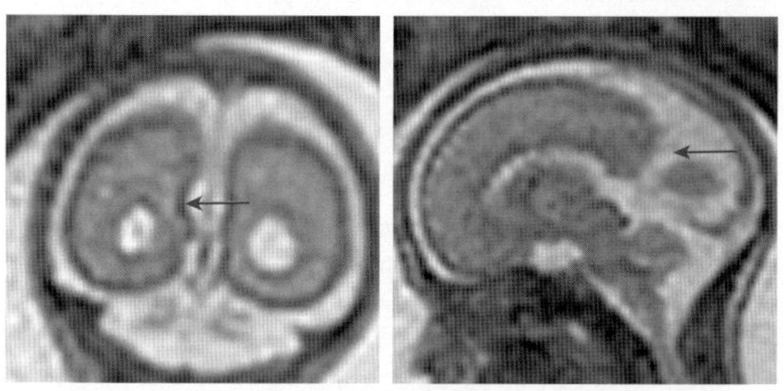

20-22 weeks: Parieto-occipital sulcus

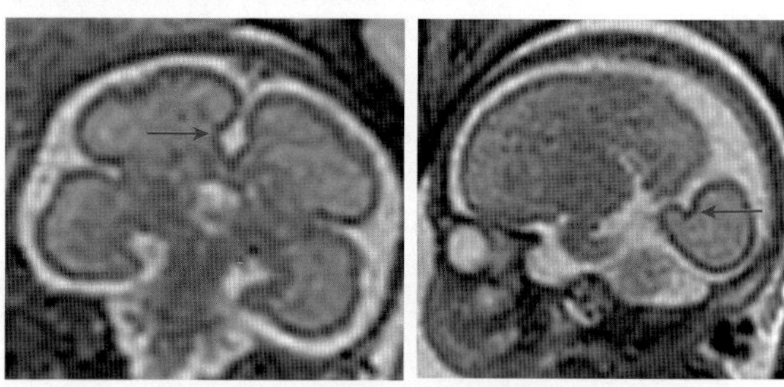

24 weeks: Calcarine and cingulate sulcus

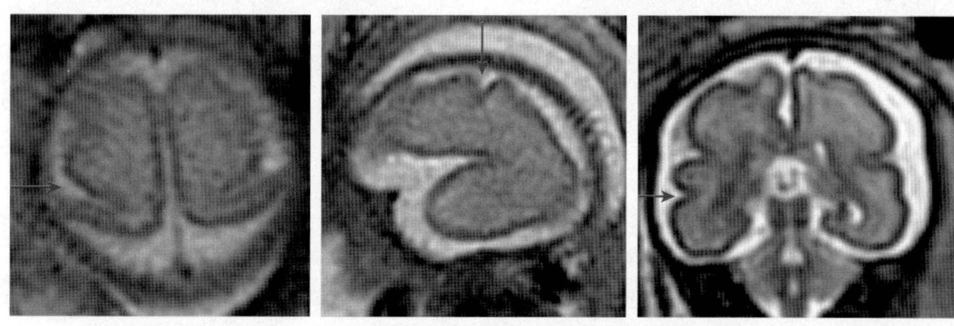

27 weeks: central sulcus, interparietal sulcus,
superior temporal sulcus, superior frontal sulcus, and precentral sulcus

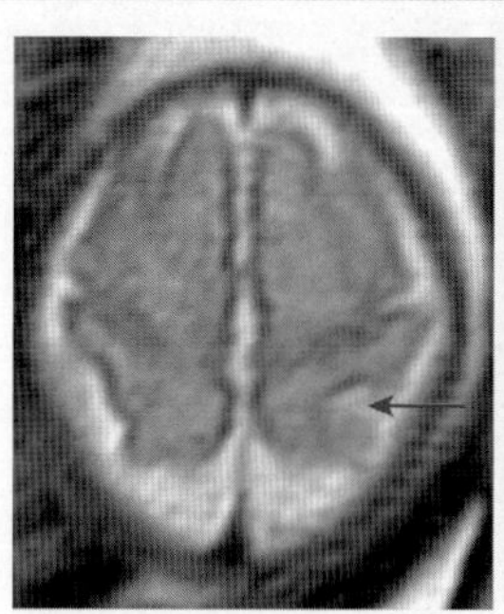

28 weeks: Post central sulcus

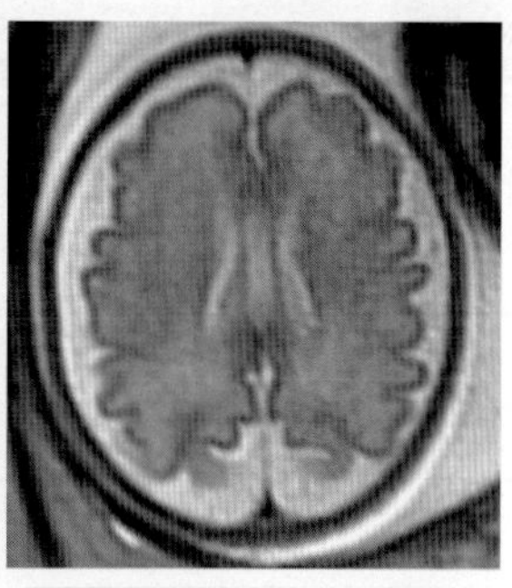

32 weeks: Secondary sulcus

PROGRESSION OF SULCATION: WEEKS 24–29

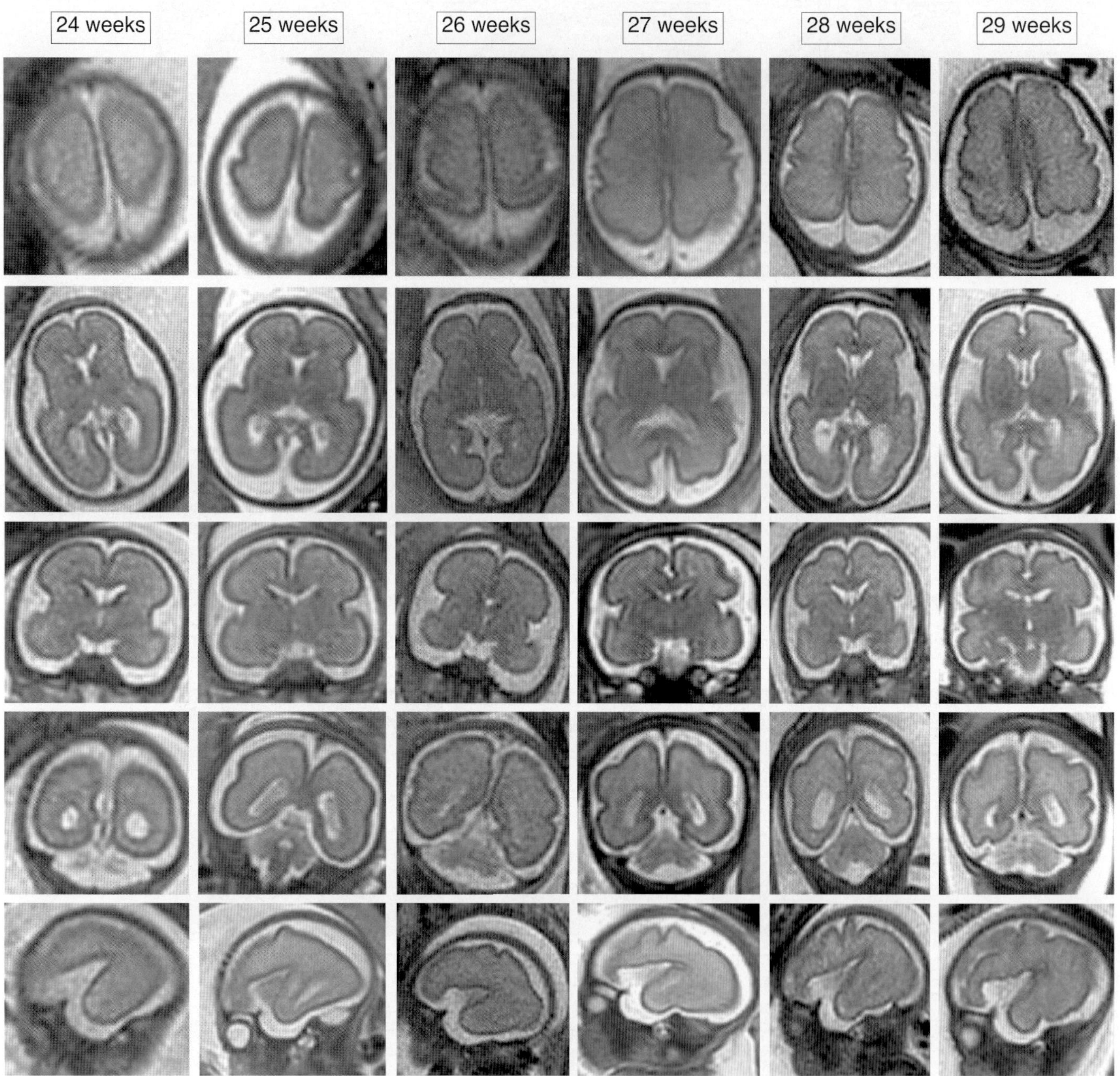

PROGRESSION OF SULCATION: WEEKS 30–35

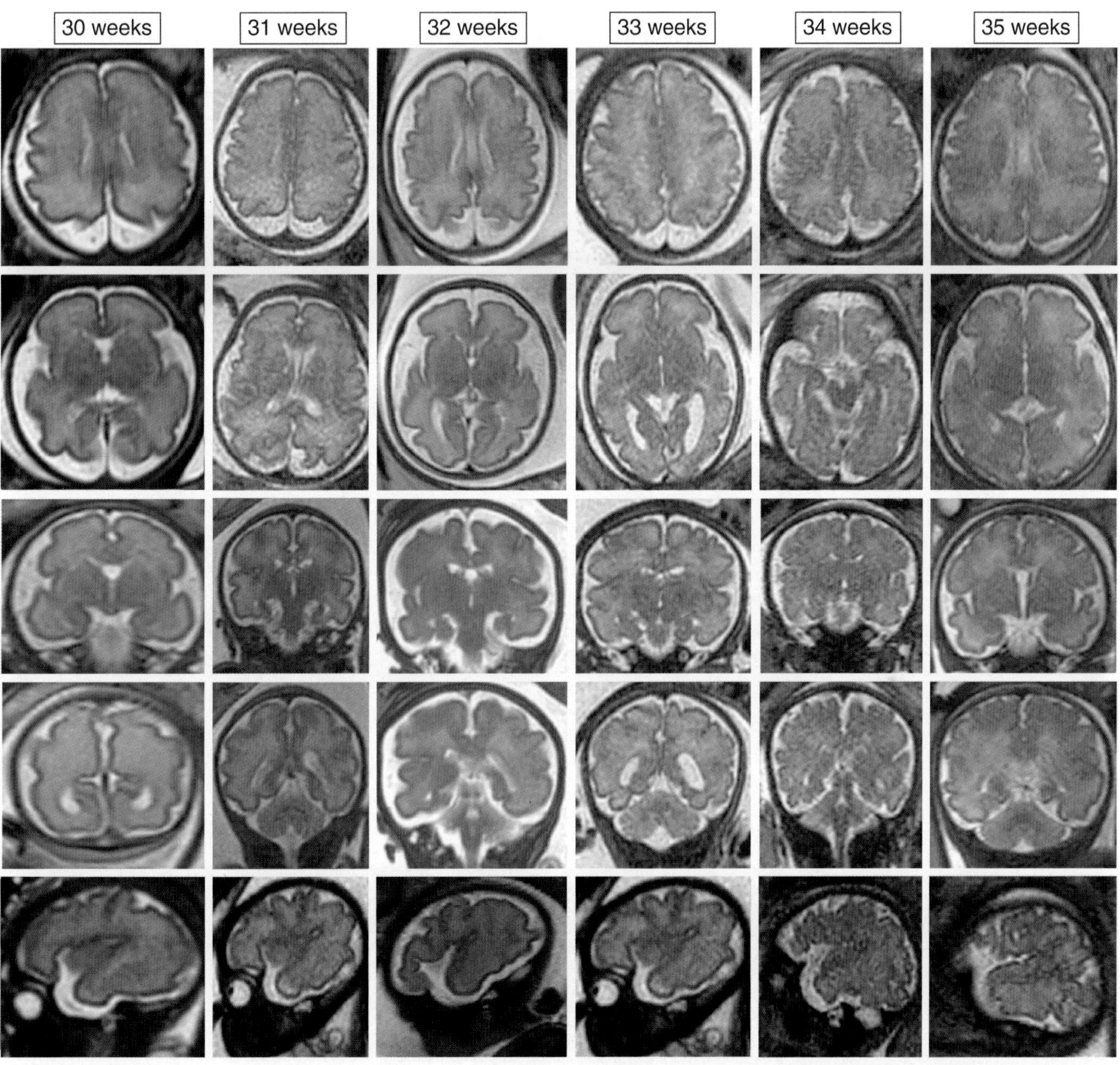

NORMAL SULCATION: 19–23 WEEKS

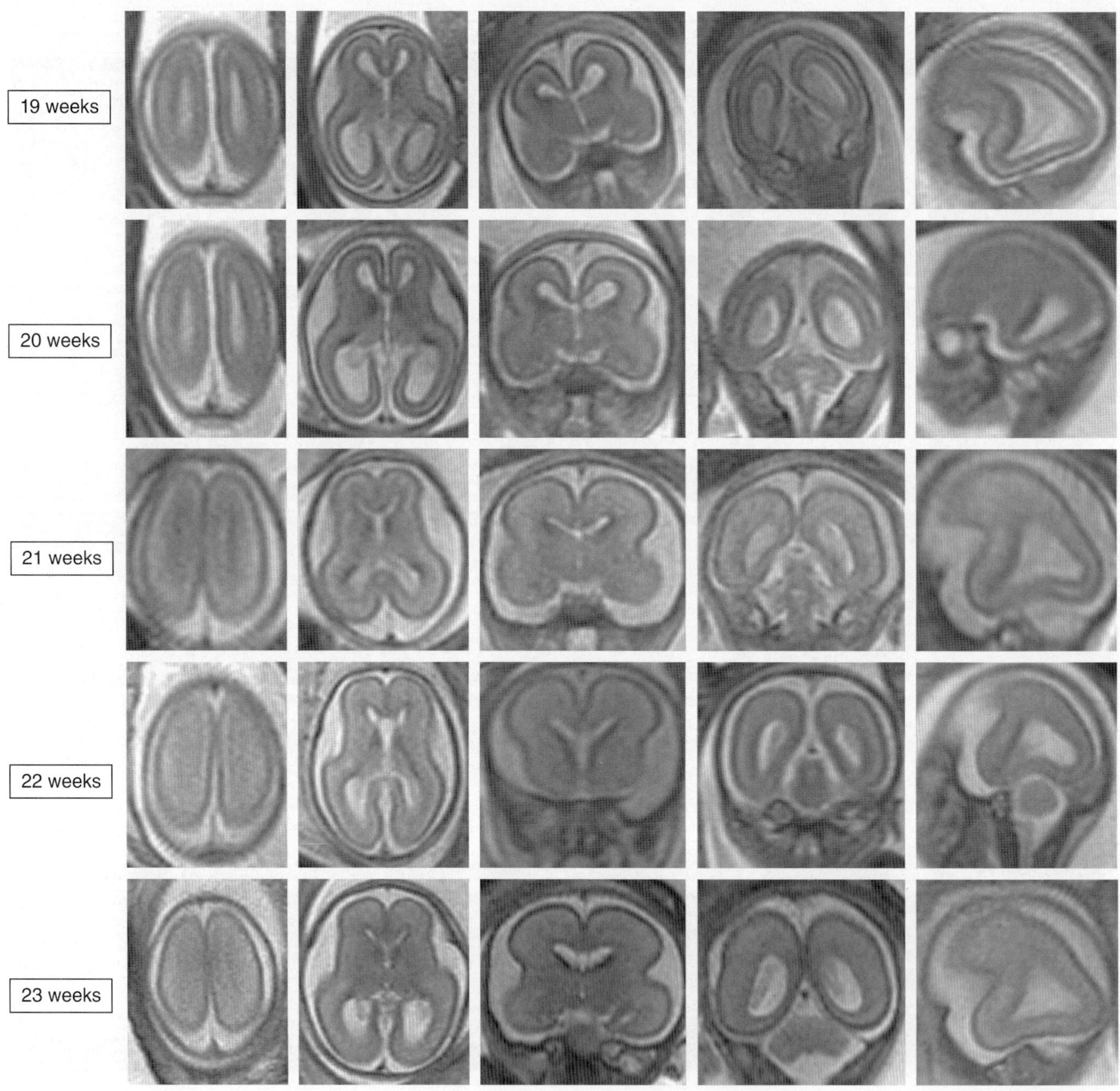

Sulci present: Sylvian fissures. Minimal differences in the sulcation between 19 and 23 weeks
Sulci developing: Parietooccipital sulcus

NORMAL SULCATION: 24 WEEKS

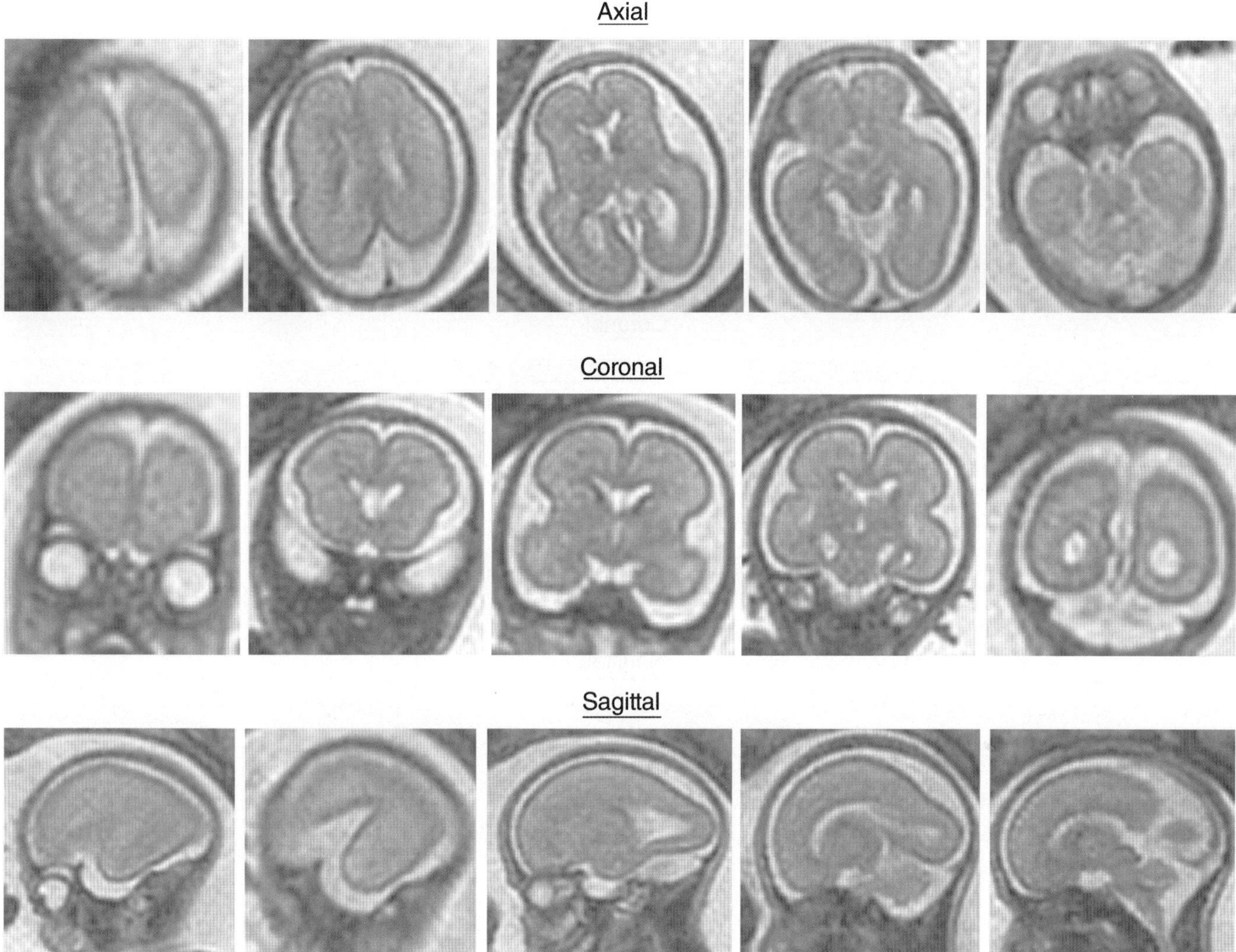

Sulci present: Sylvian, parietooccipital
Sulci developing: Calcarine, cingulate

NORMAL SULCATION: 25 WEEKS

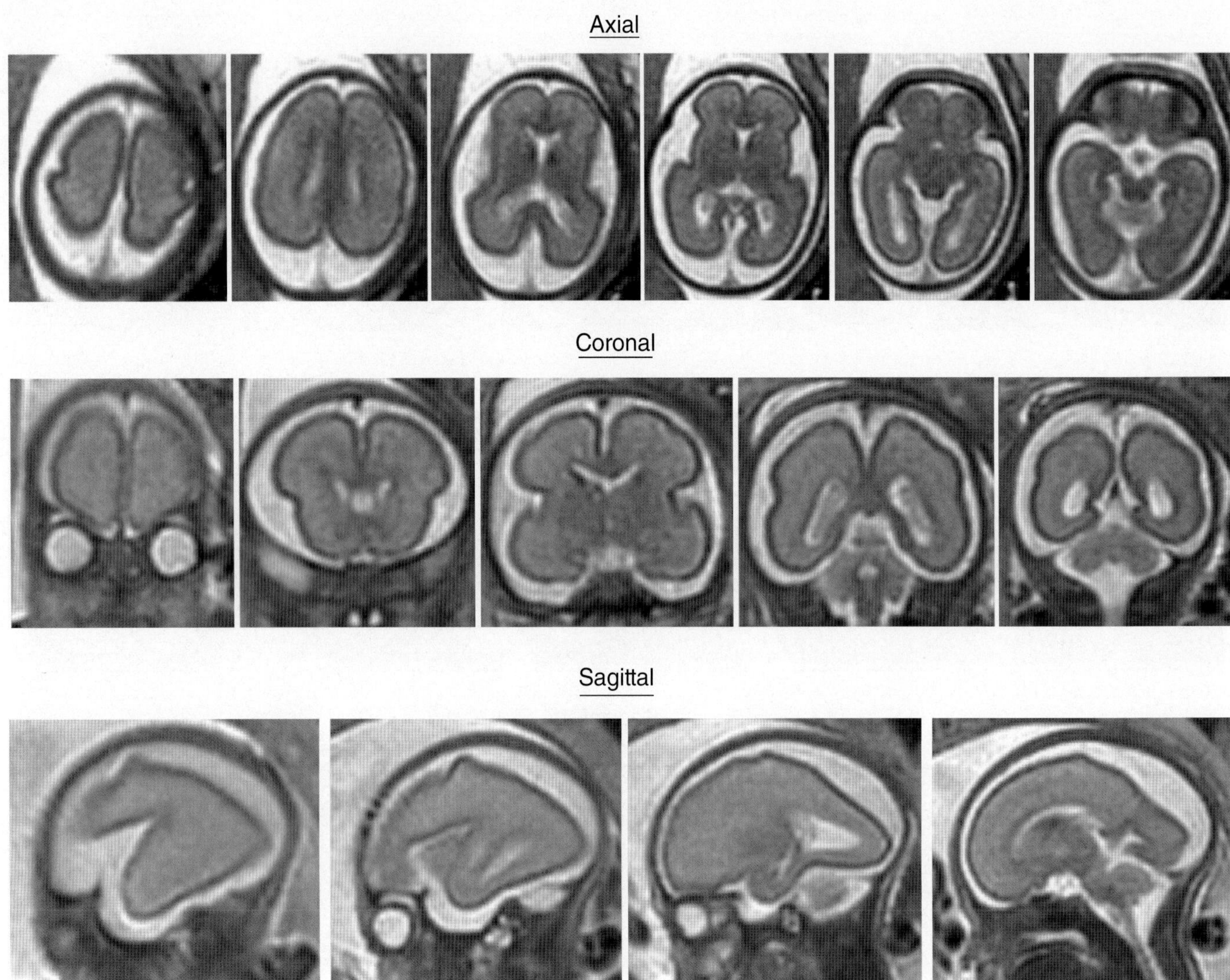

Sulci present: Sylvian, parietooccipital
Sulci developing: Calcarine, cingulate

NORMAL SULCATION: 26 WEEKS

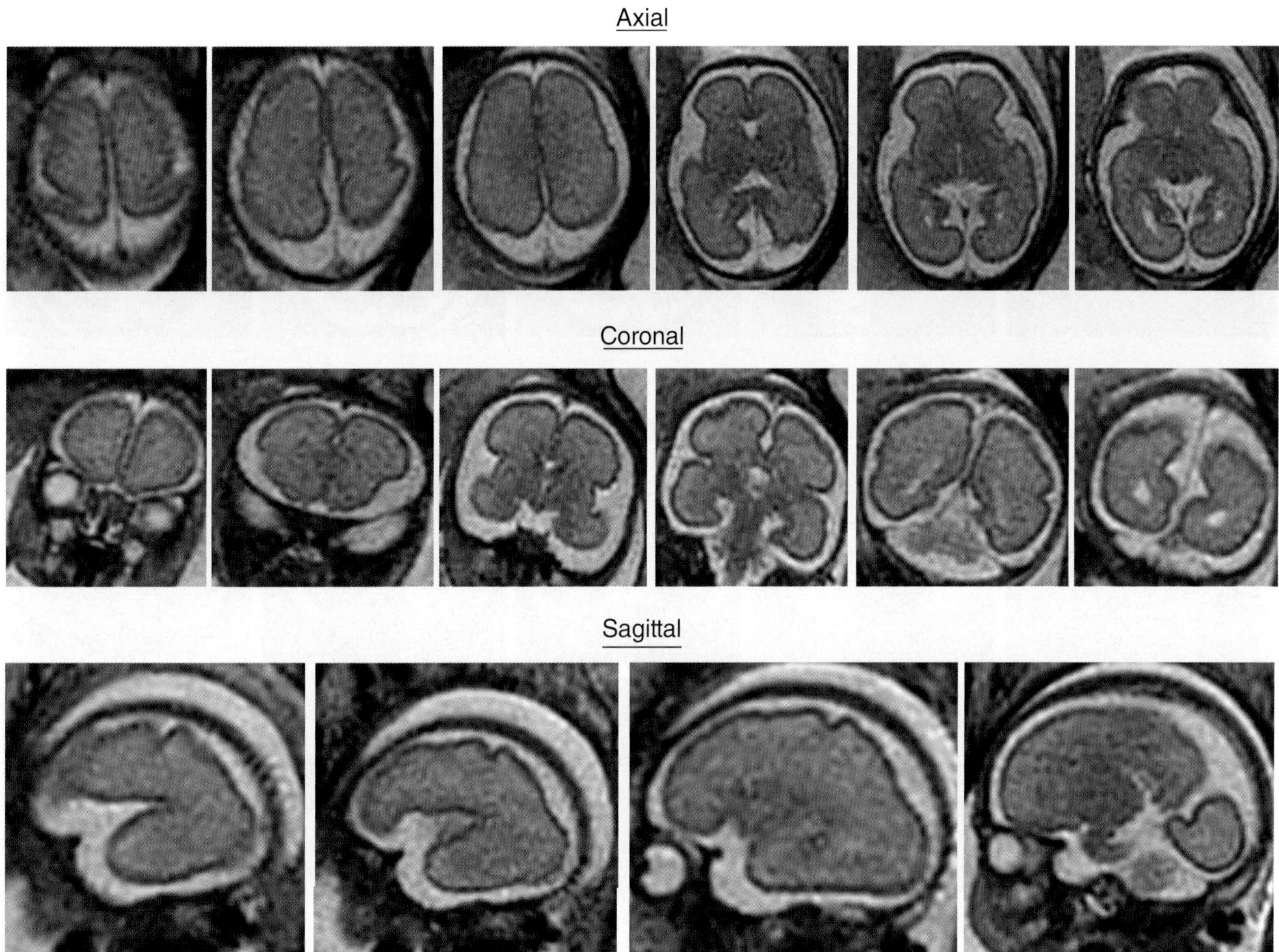

Sulci present: Sylvian, parietooccipital
Sulci developing: Calcarine, cingulate

NORMAL SULCATION: 27 WEEKS

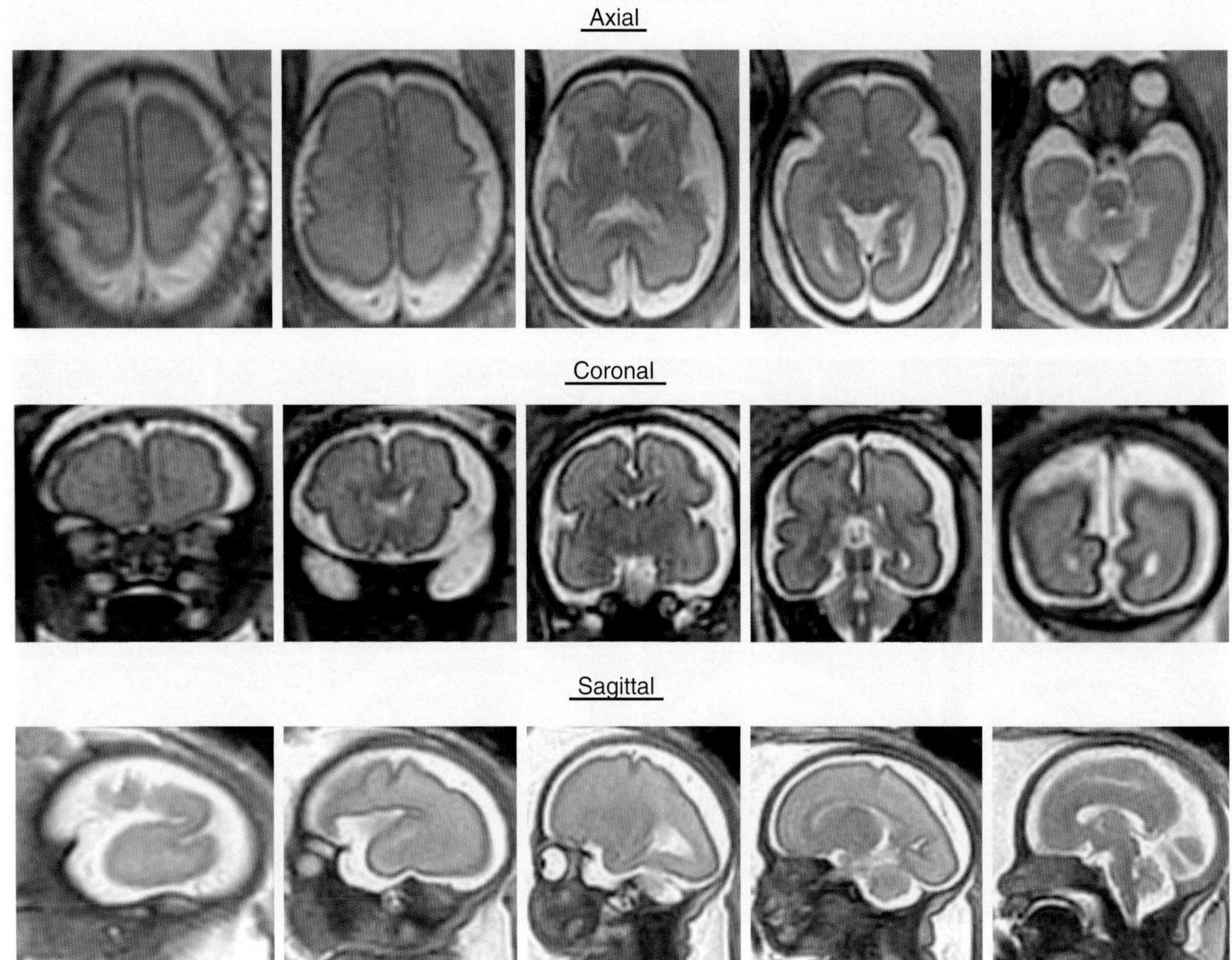

Sulci present: Sylvian, parietooccipital, calcarine, cingulate
Sulci developing: Central, interparietal, superior temporal, superior frontal, precentral

NORMAL SULCATION: 28 WEEKS

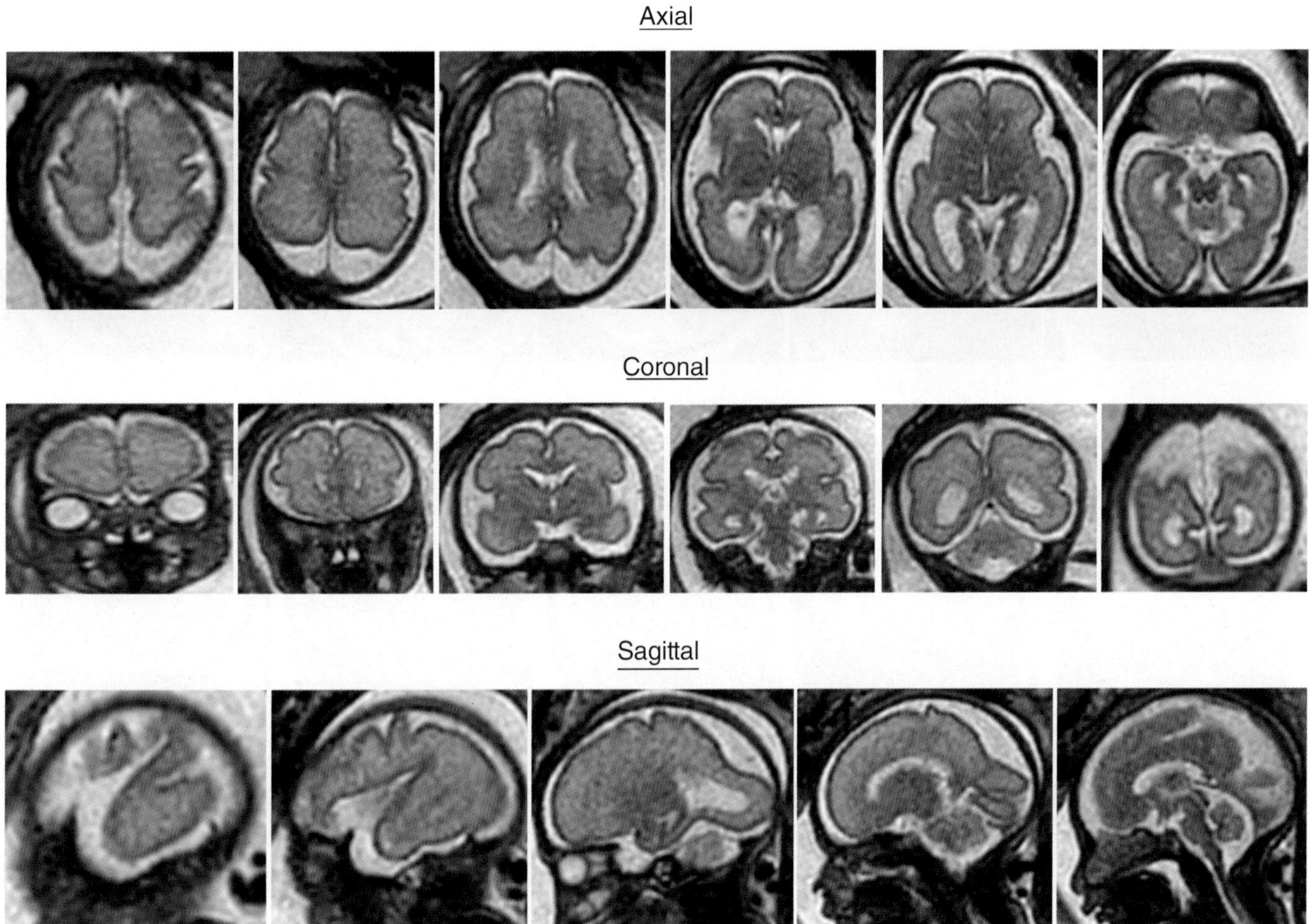

Sulci present: Sylvian, parietooccipital, calcarine, cingulate, central, interparietal, superior temporal, superior frontal, precentral
Sulci developing: Postcentral sulci

NORMAL SULCATION: 29 WEEKS

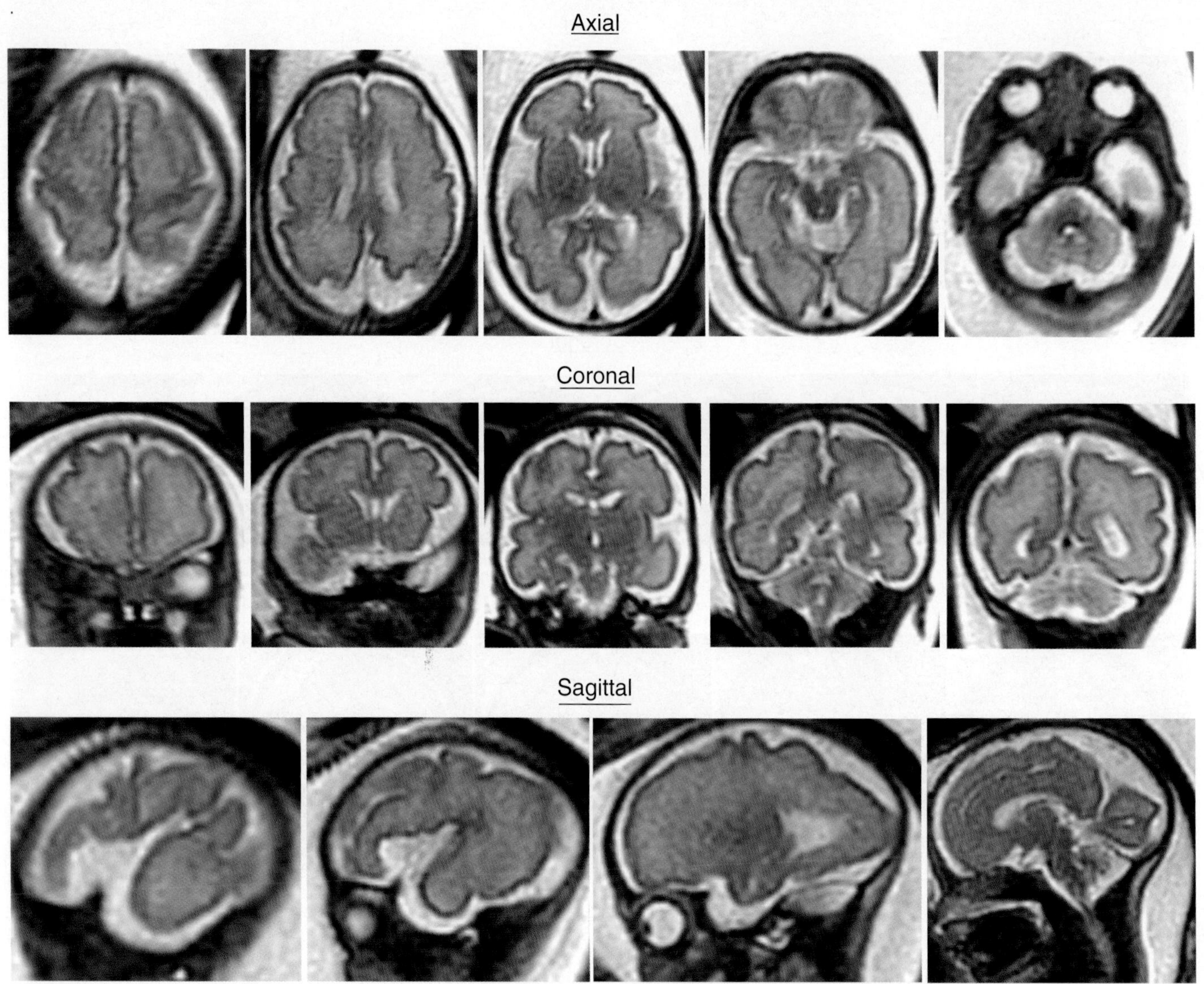

Sulci present: Sylvian, parietooccipital, calcarine, cingulate, central, interparietal, superior temporal, superior frontal, precentral
Sulci developing: Postcentral sulci

NORMAL SULCATION: 30 WEEKS

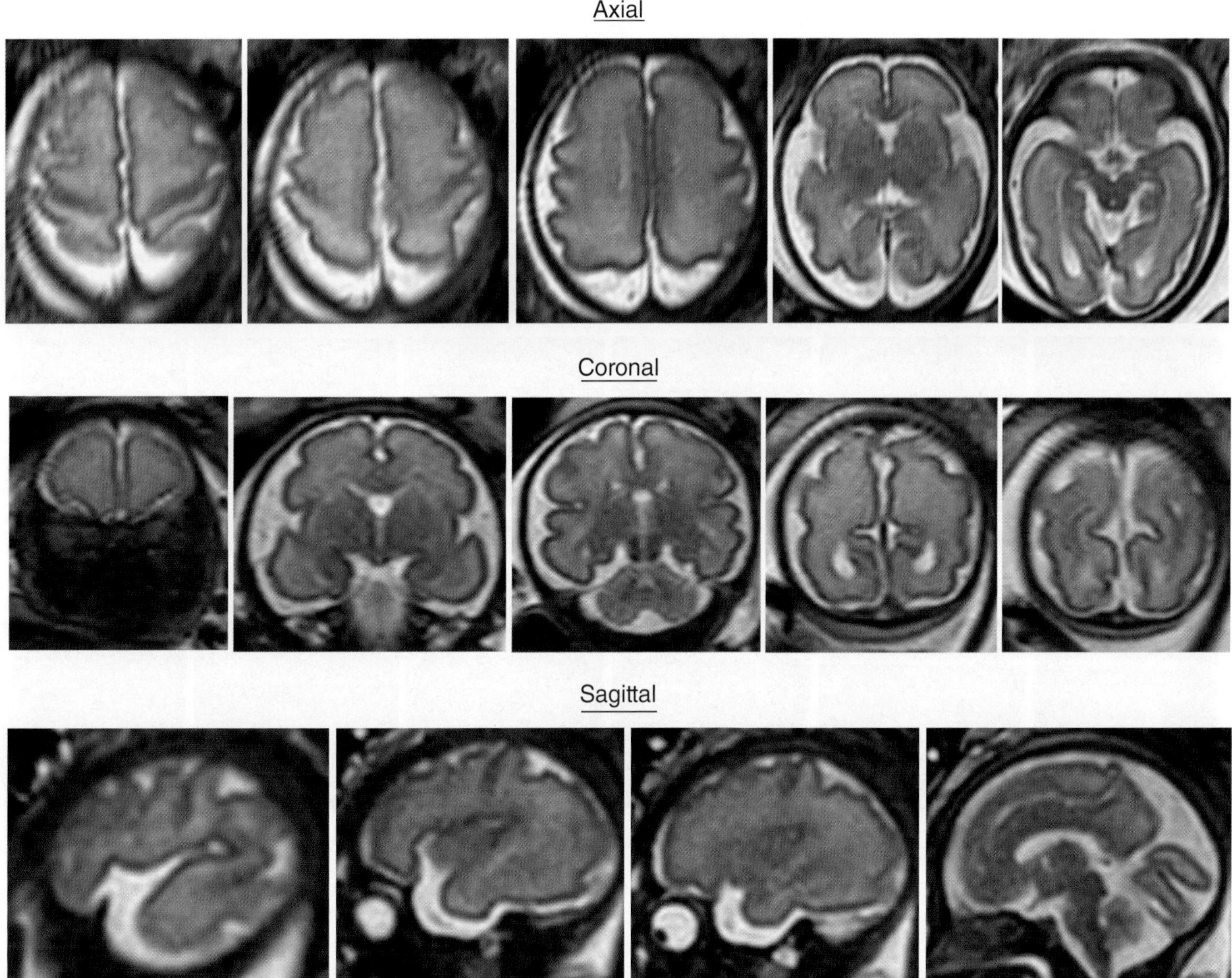

Sulci present: Primary sulci
Sulci developing: Secondary sulci

NORMAL SULCATION: 31 WEEKS

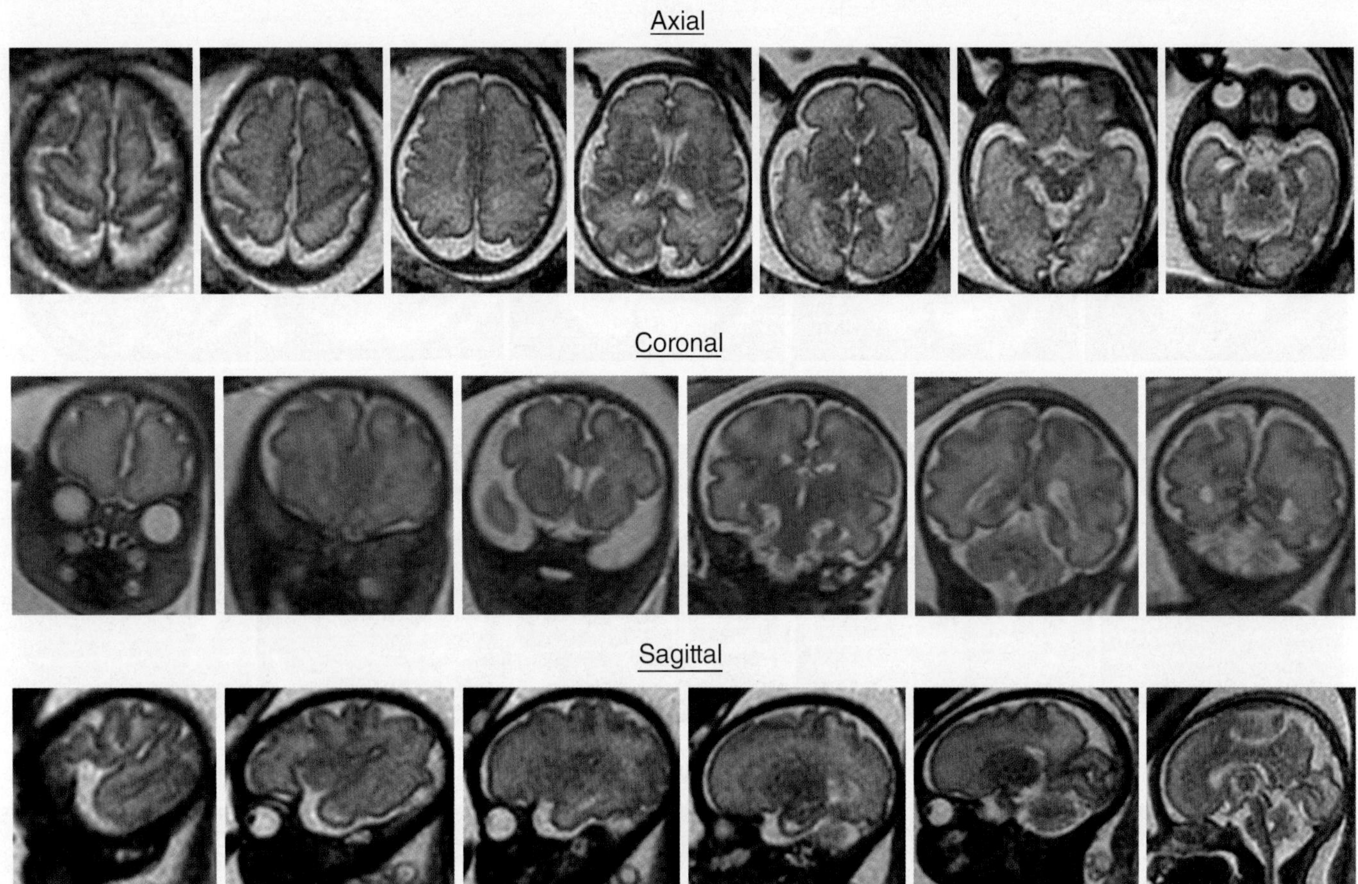

Sulci present: Primary sulci
Sulci developing: Secondary sulci

NORMAL SULCATION: 32 WEEKS

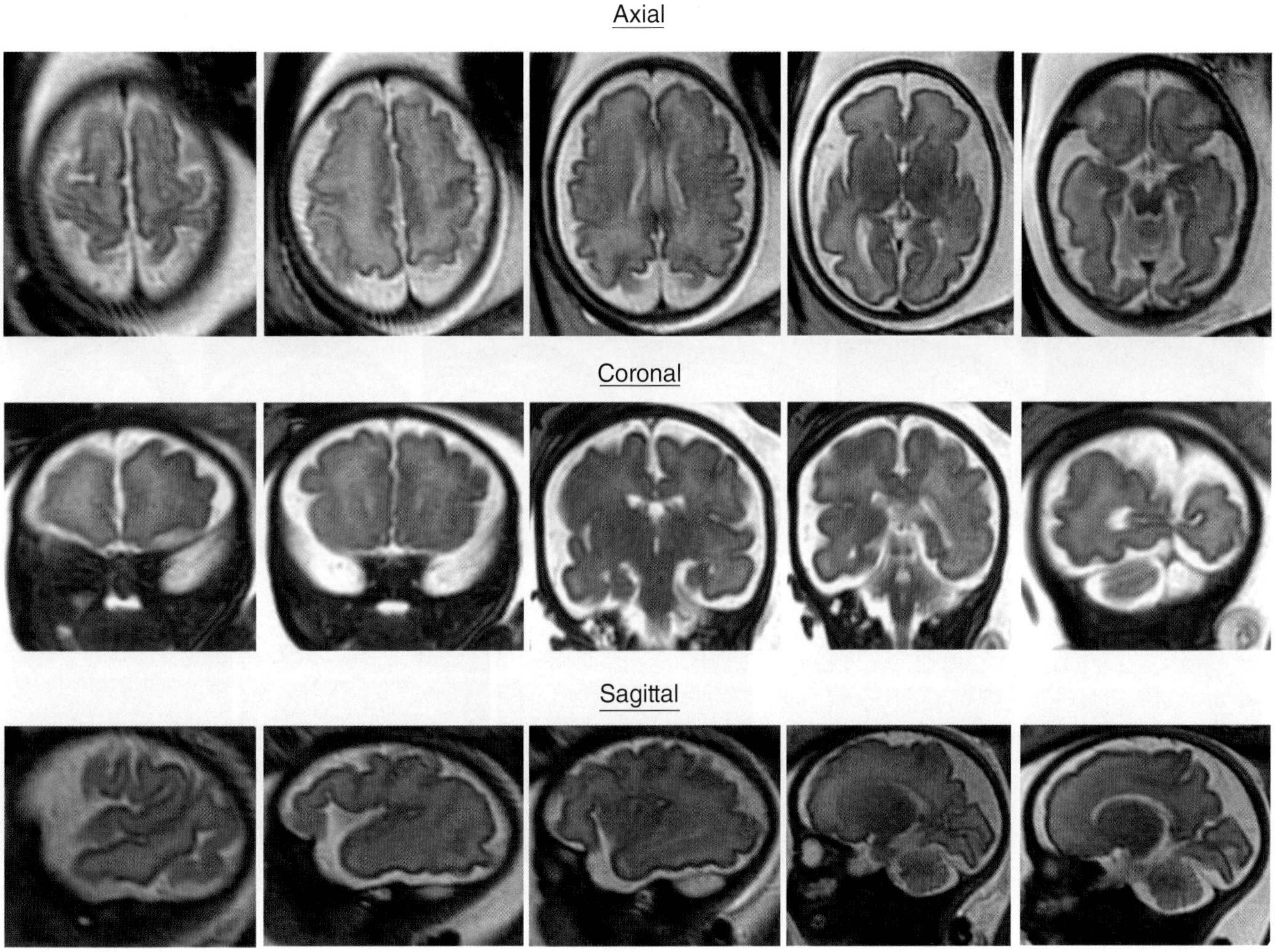

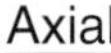

Axial

Coronal

Sagittal

Sulci present: Primary sulci
Sulci developing: Secondary sulci

NORMAL SULCATION: 33 WEEKS

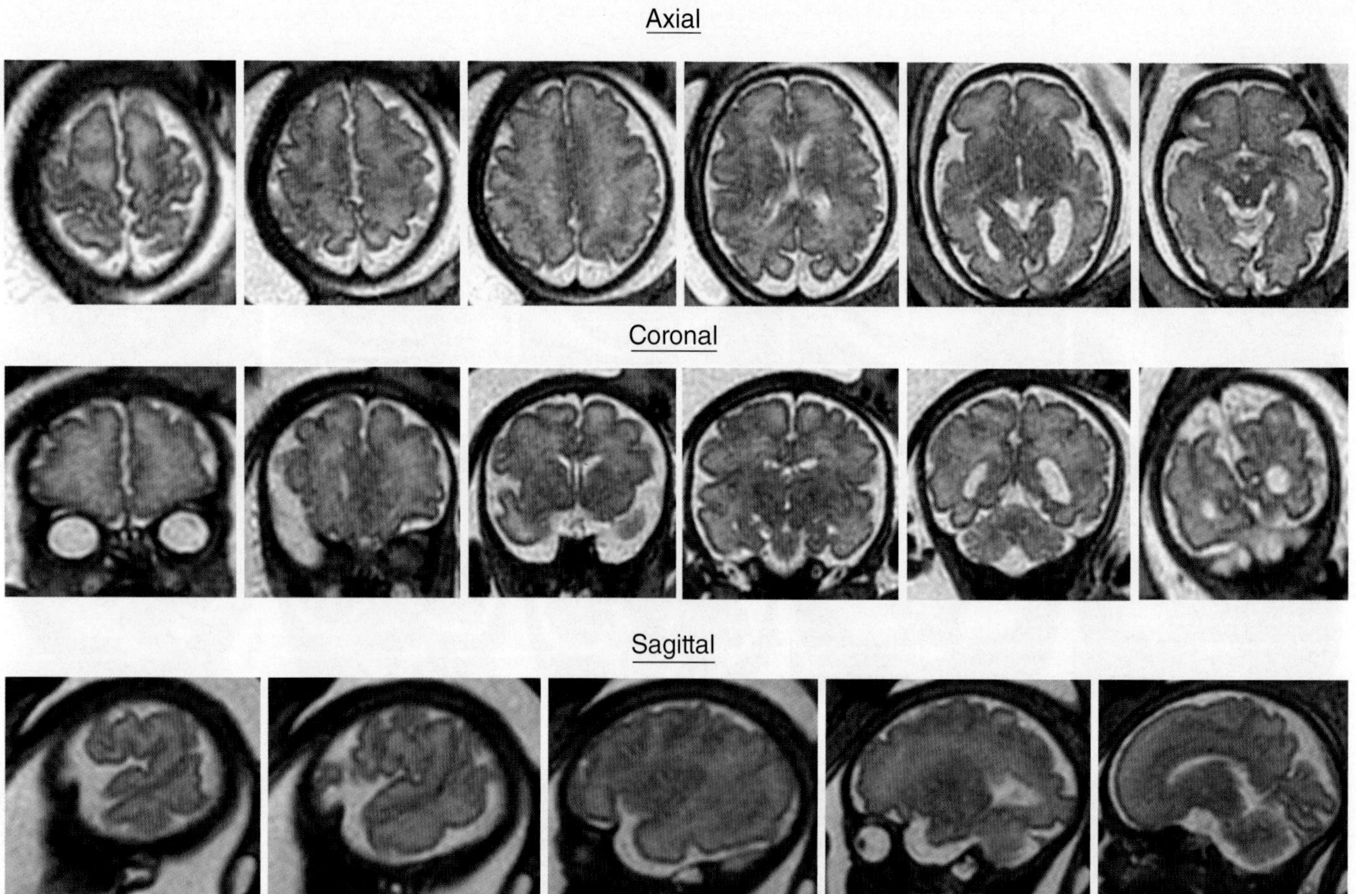

Sulci present: Primary sulci
Sulci developing: Secondary sulci

NORMAL SULCATION: 34 WEEKS

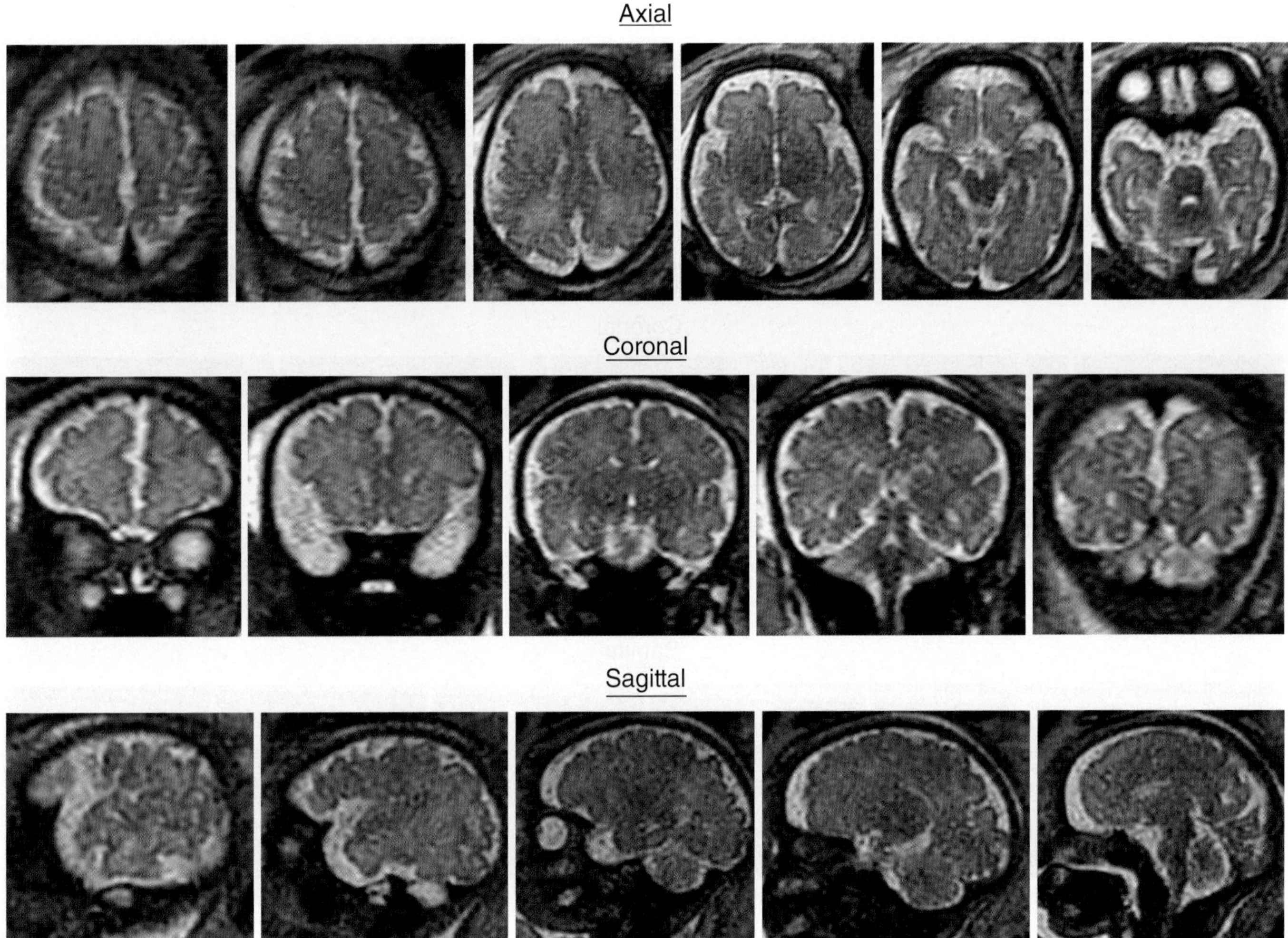

Sulci present: Primary sulci
Sulci developing: Secondary sulci

NORMAL SULCATION: 35 WEEKS

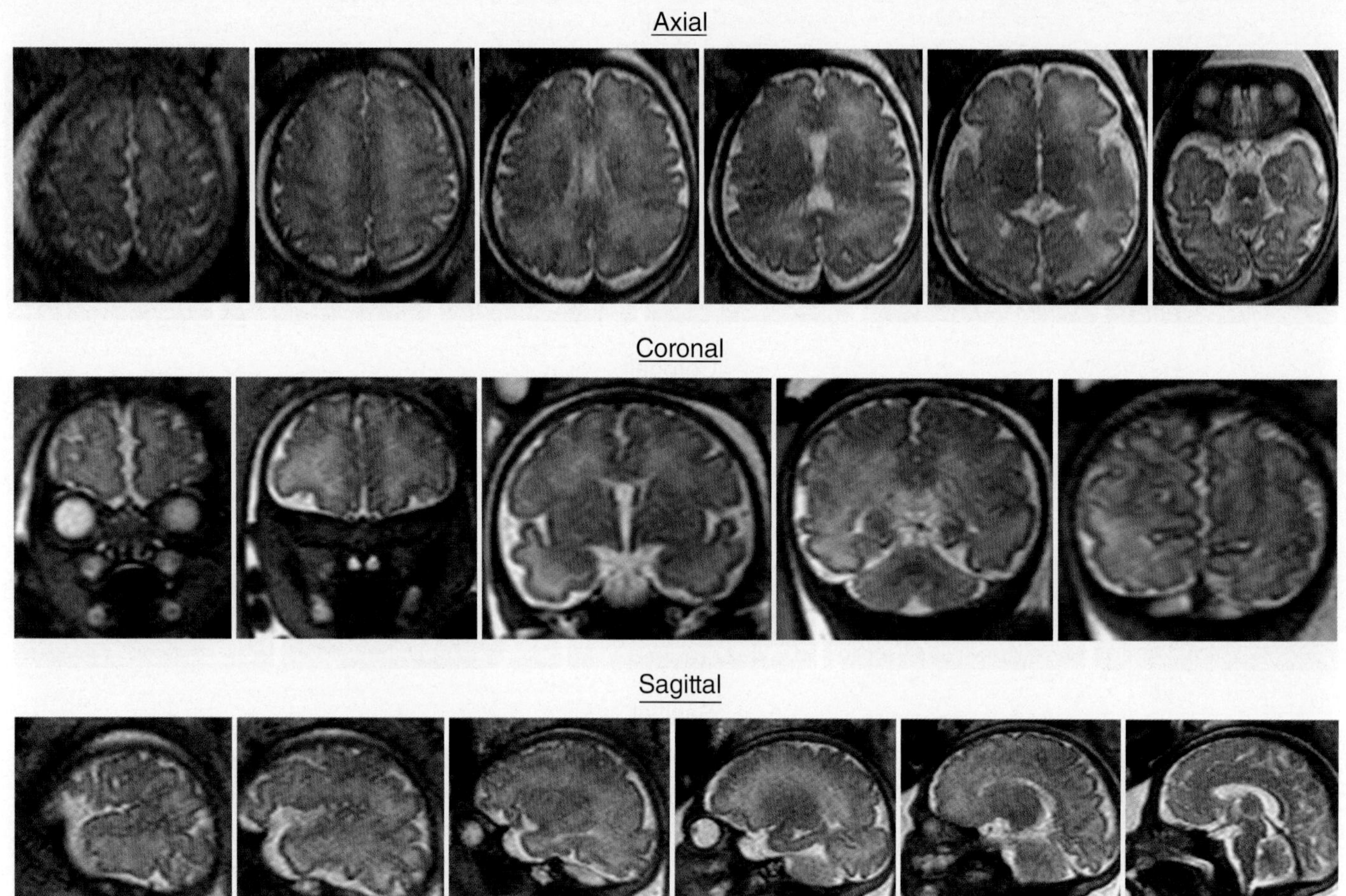

Sulci present: Primary sulci
Sulci developing: Secondary sulci

FETAL BRAIN BIOMETRY

■ TABLE 1.3 Fetal Brain Measurements

	AP Vermis			Height of Vermis			Transcerebellar Diameter			AP Pons			Frontooccipital Diameter (FOD)		
GA	#	Avg.	SD	#	Avg.	SD	#	Avg.	SD	#	Avg.	SD	#	Avg.	SD
16	15	3.51	0.31	15	4.73	0.43	15	14.73	0.70	15	5.02	0.34	15	35.38	1.72
17	12	4.15	0.32	12	5.65	0.39	12	15.94	0.60	12	5.44	0.26	12	38.39	2.00
18	17	4.87	0.43	17	6.70	0.63	18	17.16	1.35	15	6.14	0.43	18	44.02	2.28
19	17	5.45	0.54	17	7.19	0.80	18	17.92	1.30	15	6.18	0.61	19	47.75	2.74
20	24	6.17	0.65	24	8.11	1.07	24	19.32	1.45	23	6.29	0.64	25	51.57	2.62
21	16	6.49	0.76	17	8.96	1.45	17	20.39	1.38	13	6.39	0.58	19	57.41	2.53
22	12	7.41	0.44	13	9.97	1.00	14	21.91	1.81	12	6.48	0.72	13	59.59	3.00
23	10	8.21	1.12	12	11.23	1.32	13	24.32	1.40	12	7.77	0.39	13	64.92	1.93
24	15	8.57	0.58	15	11.84	0.83	15	25.33	1.83	15	7.78	0.46	16	66.90	1.60
25	13	9.65	1.24	13	12.05	0.84	13	27.42	2.75	13	8.11	0.83	13	69.98	3.44
26	14	9.71	0.96	14	13.54	1.19	13	28.12	1.31	13	8.99	0.65	14	74.99	2.92
27	14	10.45	1.15	14	14.87	0.88	13	30.25	1.95	13	9.19	1.14	13	77.56	3.45
28	15	11.09	1.08	15	15.38	1.46	15	32.68	1.21	15	10.08	1.05	15	79.36	3.50
29	14	11.82	1.03	14	15.87	0.98	15	34.92	1.40	14	10.85	0.84	14	84.94	2.21
30	13	12.00	0.68	13	16.64	1.55	13	35.94	2.23	12	11.22	0.53	13	87.35	3.58
31	12	12.83	0.96	12	17.51	0.82	12	38.06	1.77	12	11.57	0.73	12	91.10	4.37
32	12	12.93	1.50	12	18.31	1.58	11	40.33	2.57	12	11.97	1.47	11	92.22	1.57
33	13	13.89	1.12	13	19.12	0.97	12	40.98	1.85	13	12.28	1.31	13	92.73	4.13
34	12	14.90	0.60	13	19.79	1.30	14	44.34	3.31	13	12.75	0.81	14	99.18	3.74
35	14	14.90	0.88	15	20.09	1.29	17	45.78	2.19	15	13.25	0.83	16	101.60	5.21
36	13	16.48	0.91	13	22.32	3.10	13	48.12	3.82	13	13.54	1.74	13	102.56	4.15
>37	14	16.96	2.18	14	22.33	1.97	14	49.83	3.44	14	13.86	1.39	14	104.96	4.22

Data from Kline-Fath BM, Bulas DI, Bahado-Singh R. *Fundamentals and advanced fetal imaging: ultrasound and MRI*, Philadelphia, 2020, Wolters Kluwer.

FETAL BRAIN BIOMETRY

	Cerebral Biparietal Diameter (C-BPD)		Bone Biparietal Diameter (B-BPD)		Length of Corpus Callosum (LCC)	
GA	**#**	**Avg.**	**SD**	**#**	**Avg.**	**SD**
16	15	29.06	0.94	15	32.93	1.46
17	12	31.29	1.12	12	35.25	1.39
18	18	34.42	1.98	18	39.20	2.43
19	18	36.23	1.77	18	42.50	1.92
20	24	38.85	2.33	24	45.64	2.44
21	18	42.04	2.85	19	50.45	3.00
22	14	44.61	1.89	14	51.39	4.19
23	13	47.80	1.07	13	56.88	2.59
24	16	49.23	1.79	15	57.18	2.44
25	13	51.07	4.87	13	60.86	4.91
26	14	55.41	2.66	14	64.31	4.01
27	14	59.05	3.81	13	67.26	3.55
28	15	60.43	2.20	14	68.22	2.46
29	15	65.23	2.03	15	73.25	2.48
30	13	67.16	2.25	13	75.04	3.66
31	12	69.72	3.01	12	78.16	4.07
32	11	74.09	3.42	11	81.56	4.04
33	13	74.91	2.27	13	83.29	2.31
34	14	79.33	3.90	13	85.64	3.46
35	18	79.45	4.60	18	86.60	5.45
36	13	82.50	4.57	13	90.75	7.23
>37	14	83.90	5.86	14	90.88	7.07

Data from Kline-Fath BM, Bulas DI, Bahado-Singh R. *Fundamentals and Advanced Fetal Imaging: Ultrasound and MRI.* Wolters Kluwer; 2020.

SULCATION ON POSTNATAL ULTRASOUND

26 weeks

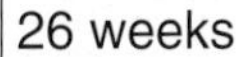

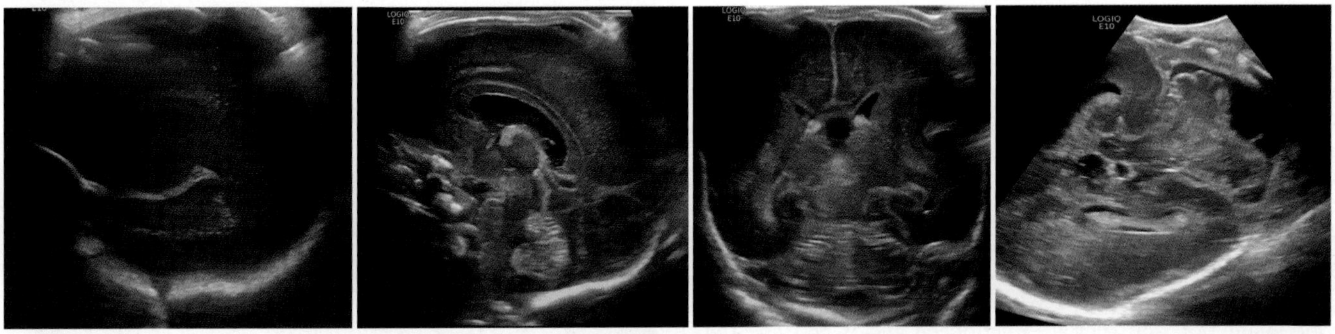

30 weeks

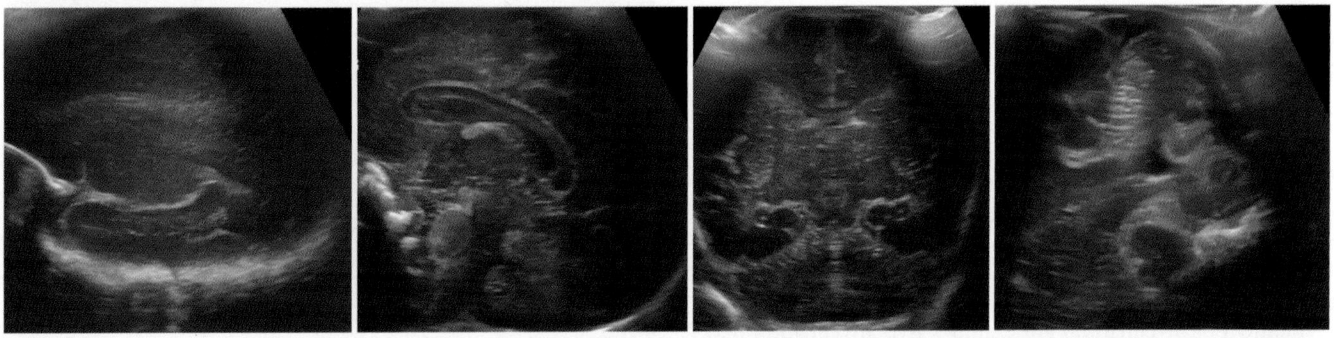

34 weeks

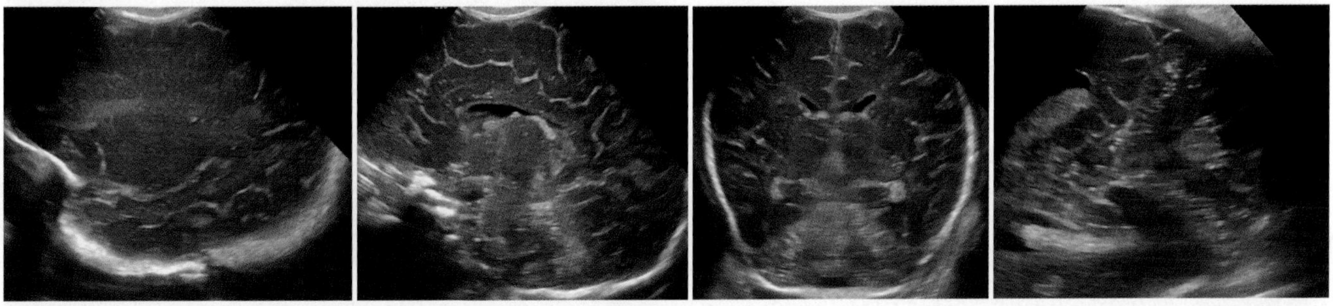

38 weeks

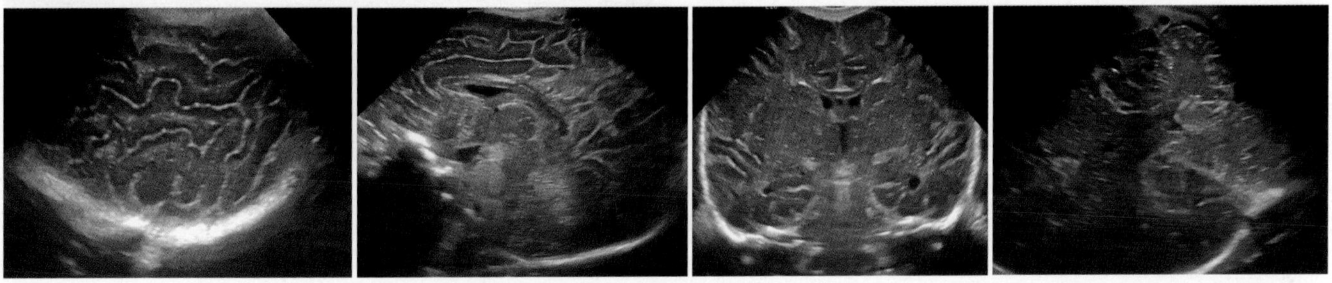

MYELINATION

Myelination increases the transmission of an action potential 10–100× that of an unmyelinated axon. Myelination is important for normal brain development as it allows efficient transmission of nearly an infinite number of transmissions between neurons. Myelination also aids in axonal integrity and regulation of ion composition and fluid around the axon. Myelin consists of a lipid bilayer formed by an extension of the oligodendrocyte cell process, and multiple sheaths wrap around an axon. Myelin is composed of ~70% lipid and 30% protein. Lipids in myelin include cholesterol, phospholipids, and glycosphingolipids. The main proteins in myelin include proteolipid protein (50%), myelin basic protein (30%), and phosphodiesterase (4%).

Myelination generally proceeds from inferior → superior, posterior → anterior, and central → peripheral and is best assessed using T1W and T2W imaging. Myelination can be seen on fetal MRI; however, because obtaining high-quality fetal MRI T1W imaging can be difficult, most of the changes are seen on T2W. In the postnatal brain, high-quality T1W and T2W brain imaging can be obtained. The T1W hyperintensity progresses faster than T2W hypointensity such that after the first year of life the brain will appear completely myelinated on T1W images but will only appear complete on T2W images between 3 and 4 years of age. This delay in T2 signal is due to the immature myelin containing greater water content than mature myelin. Histologically, the brain continues to myelinate up to approximately age 30.

Understanding the normal myelination pattern for age is necessary for detecting abnormalities that may manifest with abnormal development of myelination. For example, hypomyelination may indicate a metabolic disorder. Some disorders cause accelerated myelination, such as focal cortical dysplasia, hemimegalencephaly, and Sturge-Weber syndrome. Acute and subacute ischemic injuries can result in loss of normal myelin signal in areas in newborns such as in the posterior limb of the internal capsule. Last, age adjustment for weeks of prematurity should be performed when determining appropriate myelination in a premature infant.

The following section will illustrate the imaging appearance of the brain as myelination progresses to completion.

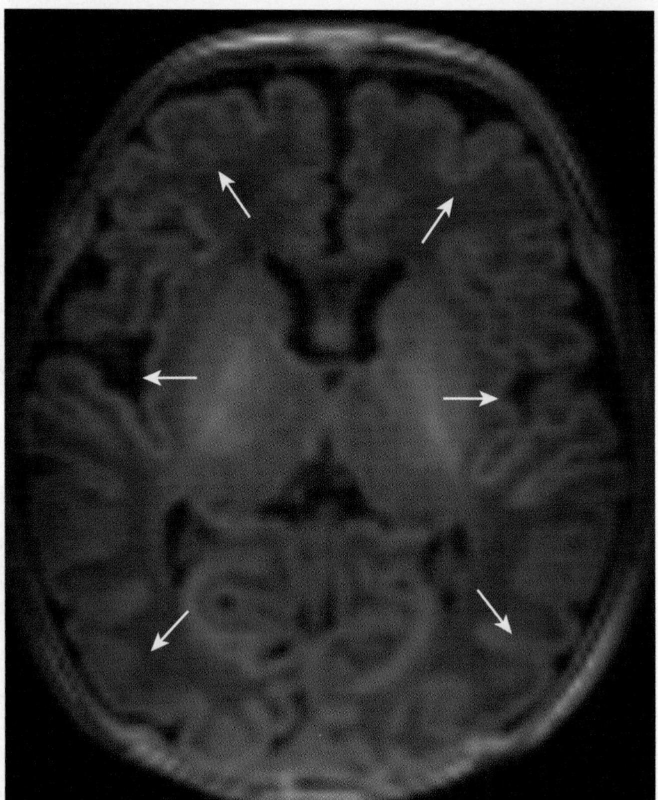

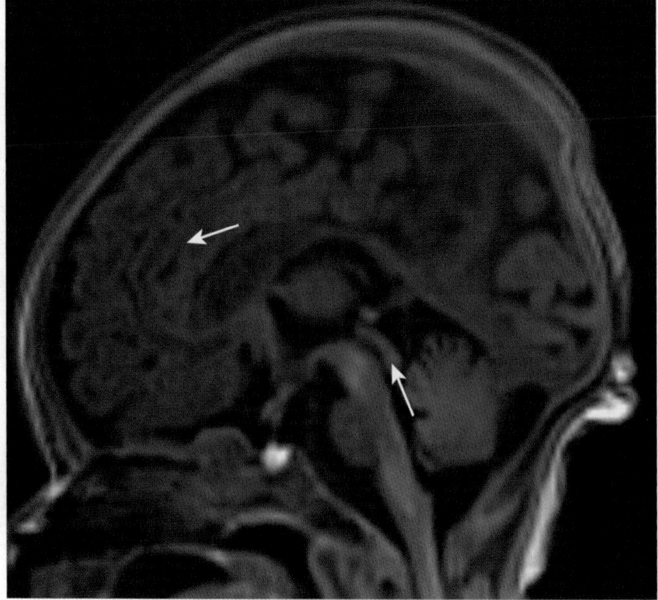

REFERENCE

1. Branson HM. Normal myelination: a practical pictorial review. *Neuroimaging Clin N Am*. 2013 May;23(2):183–195.

MYELINATION: FETAL MRI

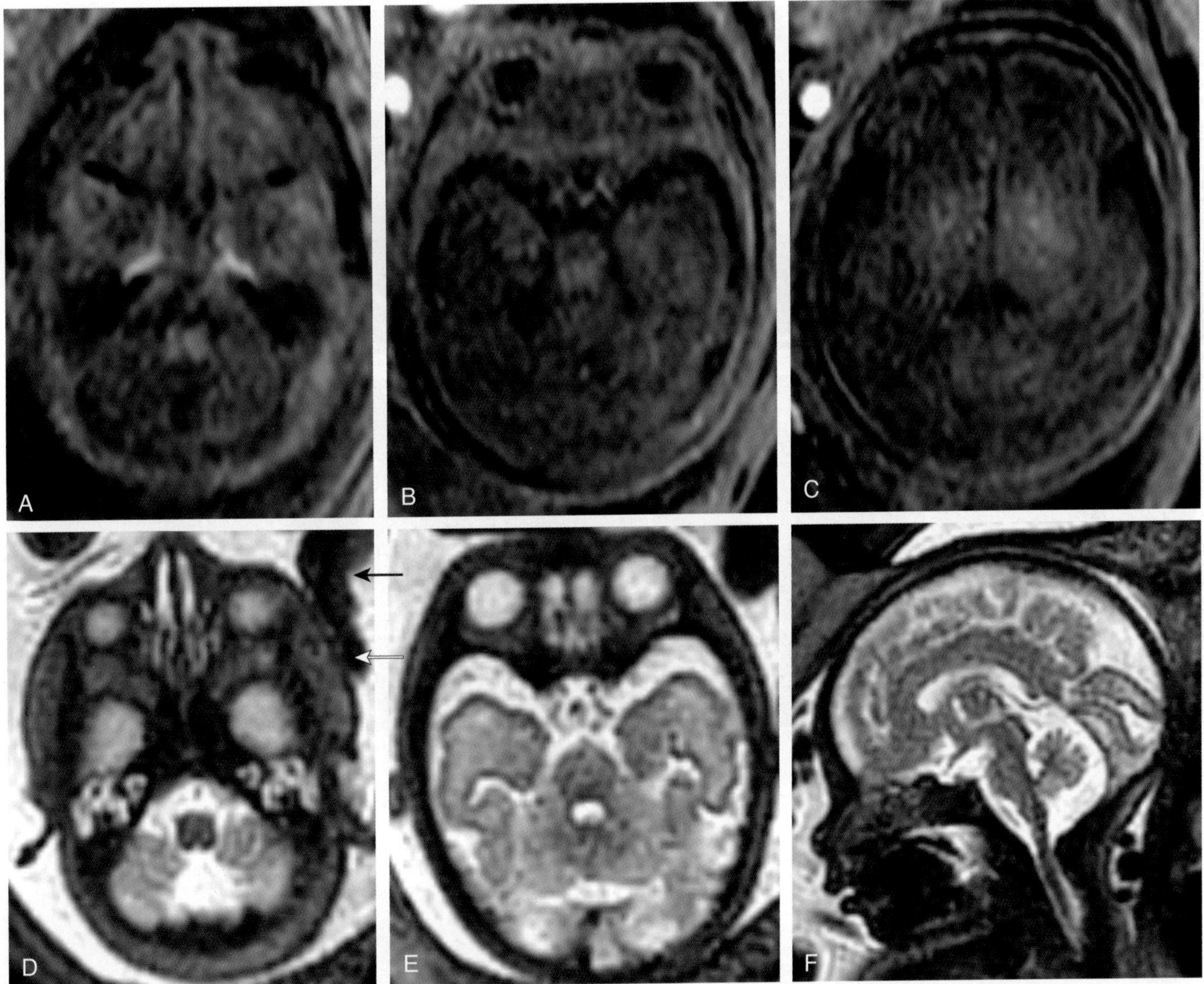

Fig. 1.4 Myelination on Fetal MRI at 34 Weeks' Gestation. (A to C) Axial T1W and (D to F) axial and sagittal T2W images demonstrate T1 hyperintense, T2 hypointense signal in the medulla, dorsal pons, basal ganglia, and ventral lateral thalami.

Myelination can be detected on fetal MRI. Myelination first occurs in the medulla at 18 weeks followed by the dorsal pons between 20 and 30 weeks and the midbrain at 32 weeks. After 32 weeks, myelination can be seen in the putamen, ventral lateral thalami, and posterior limb of the internal capsule.

Between 15 and 28 weeks' gestation, the fetal cerebral hemisphere have predominantly a tangential organization and prominent crossroads of projection, association, and commissural fibers.

NORMAL MYELINATION: NEWBORN

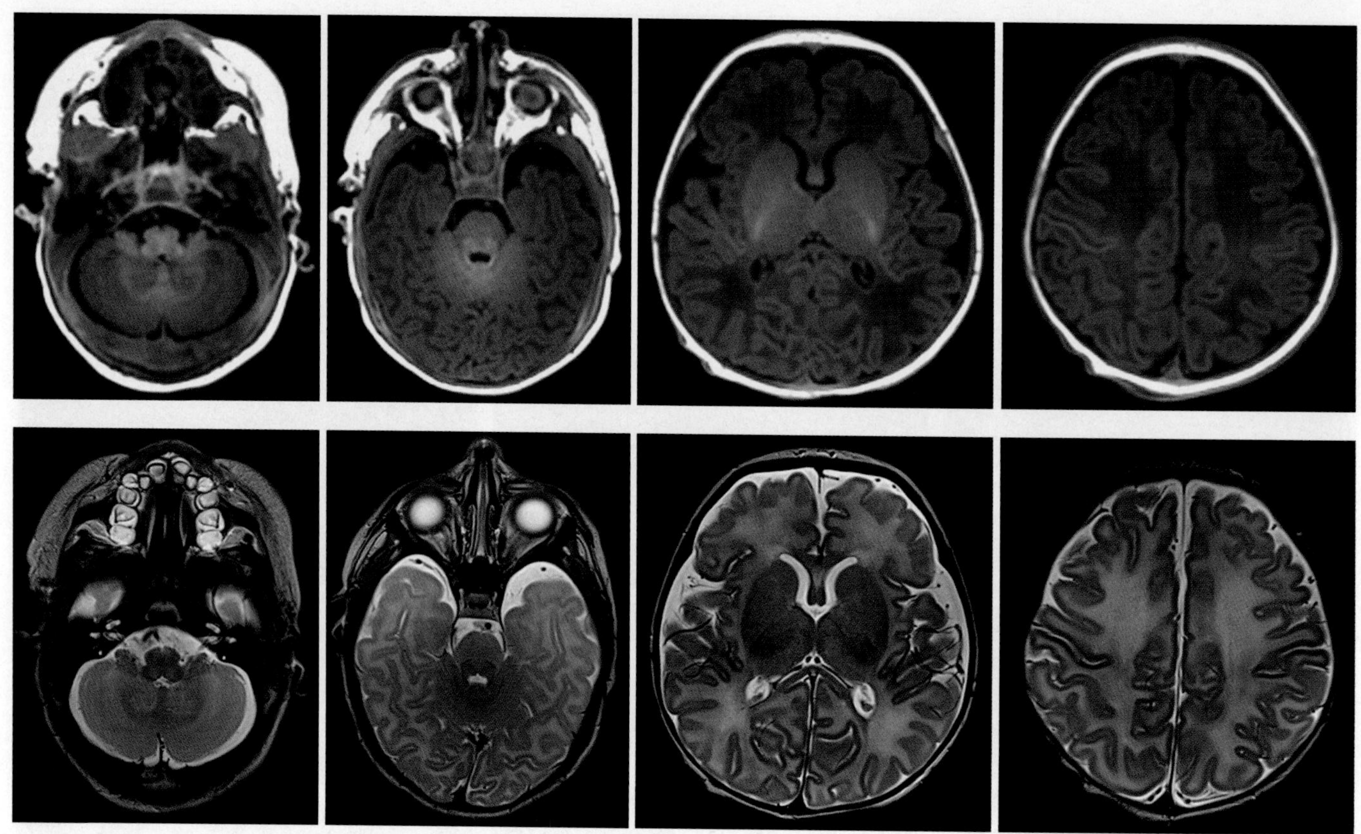

Myelination Pattern

- T1: Medulla, dorsal pons, VL thalamus, dorsal posterior limb internal capsule, corticospinal tract, perirolandic cortices
- T2: Same

NORMAL MYELINATION: 3 MONTHS

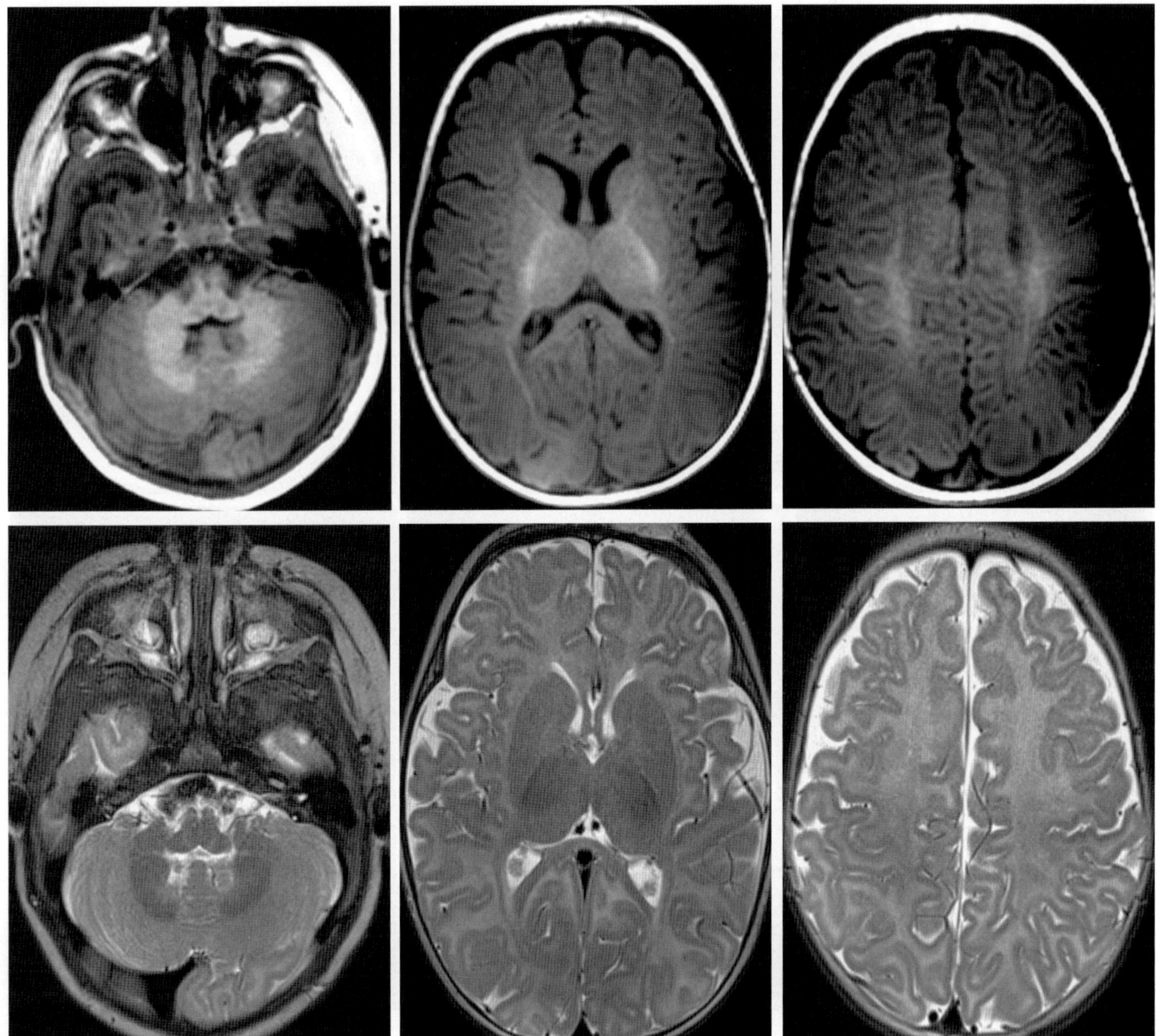

Myelination Pattern

- T1: Deep cerebellar white matter myelinates
- T2: Same

NORMAL MYELINATION: 4 MONTHS

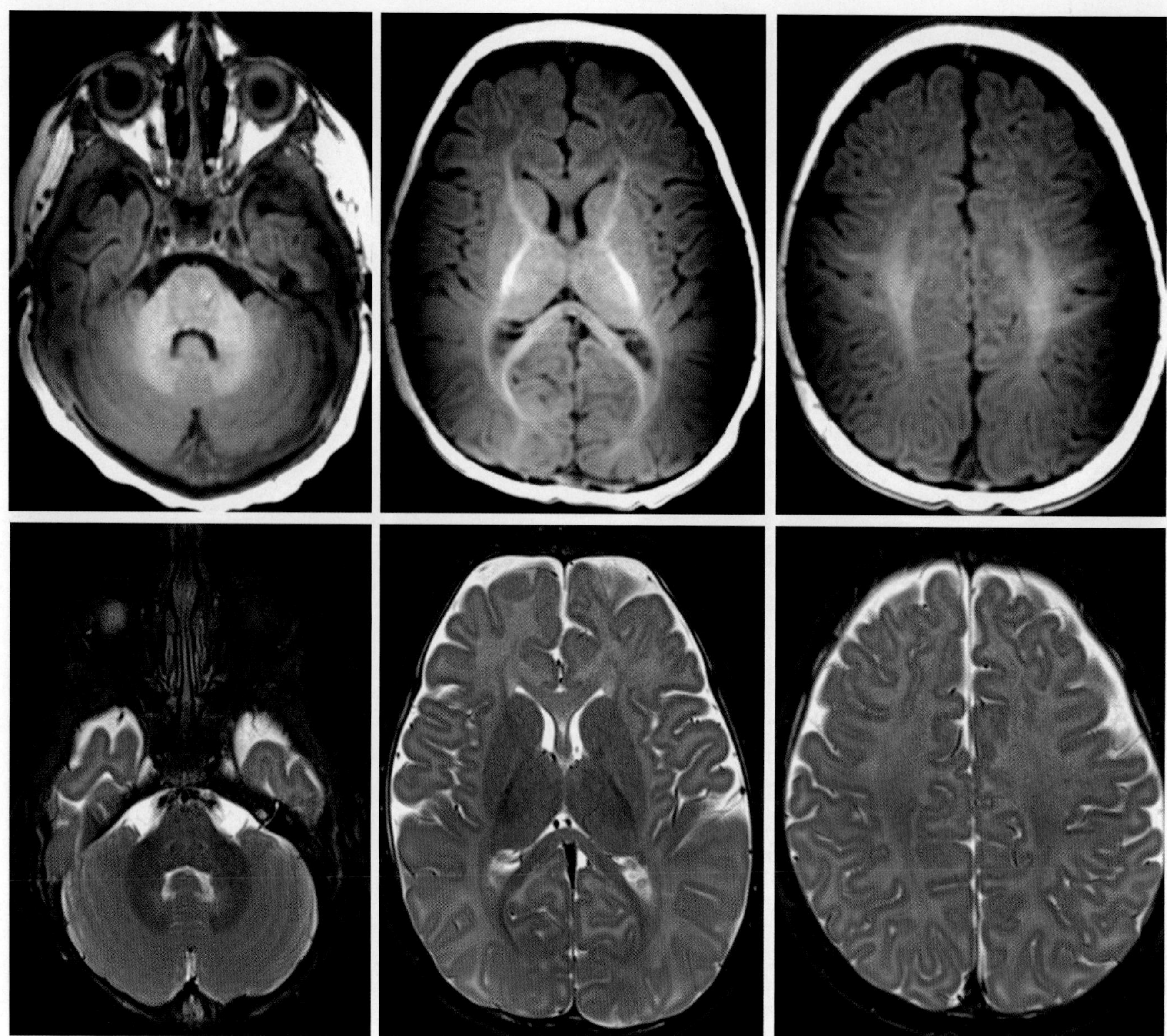

Myelination Pattern

- T1: Anterior limb internal capsule, and splenium of corpus callosum myelinate
- T2: No new areas

NORMAL MYELINATION: 6 MONTHS

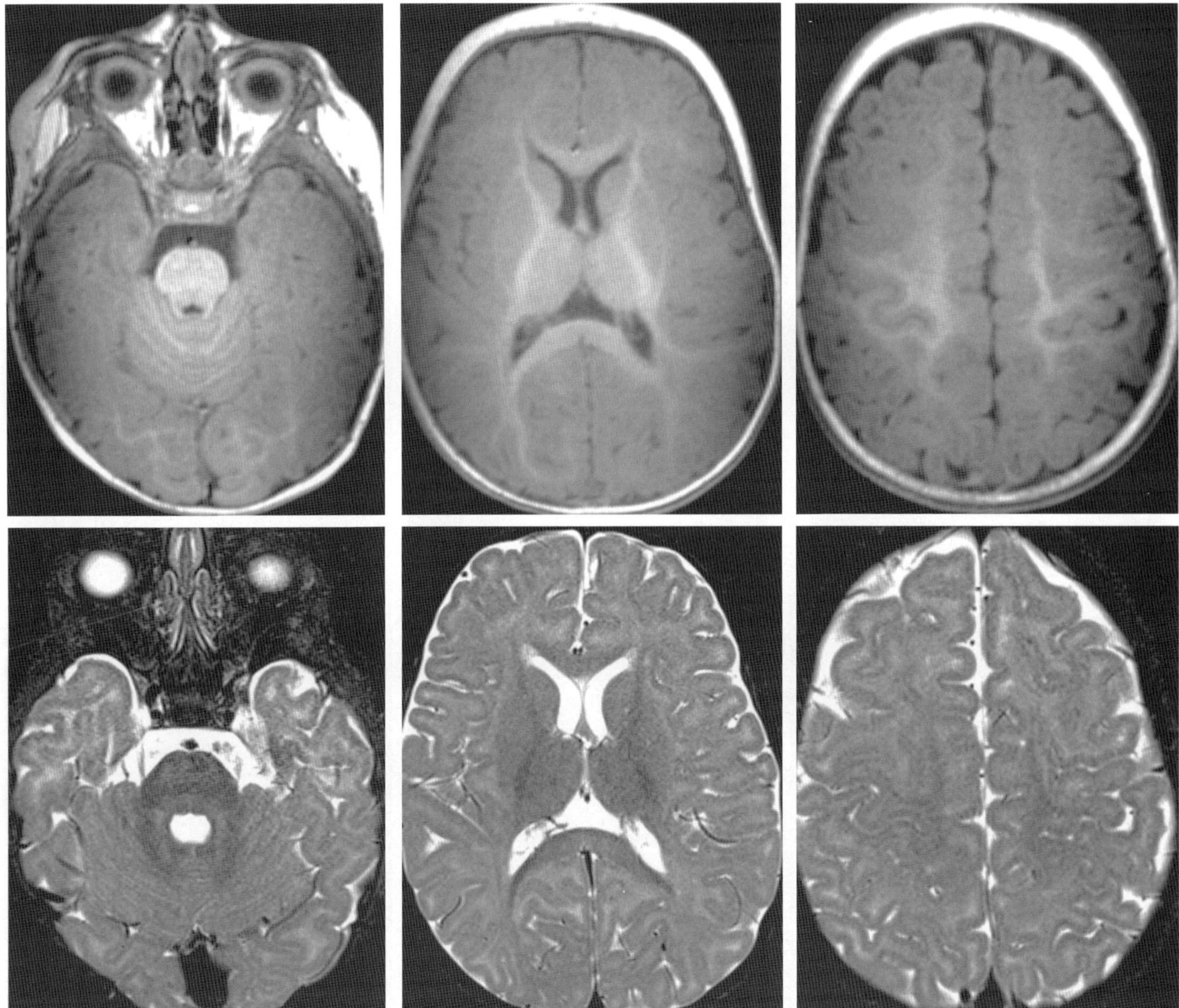

Myelination Pattern

- T1: Genu of corpus callosum myelinates
- T2: Splenium of corpus callosum myelinates

NORMAL MYELINATION: 9 MONTHS

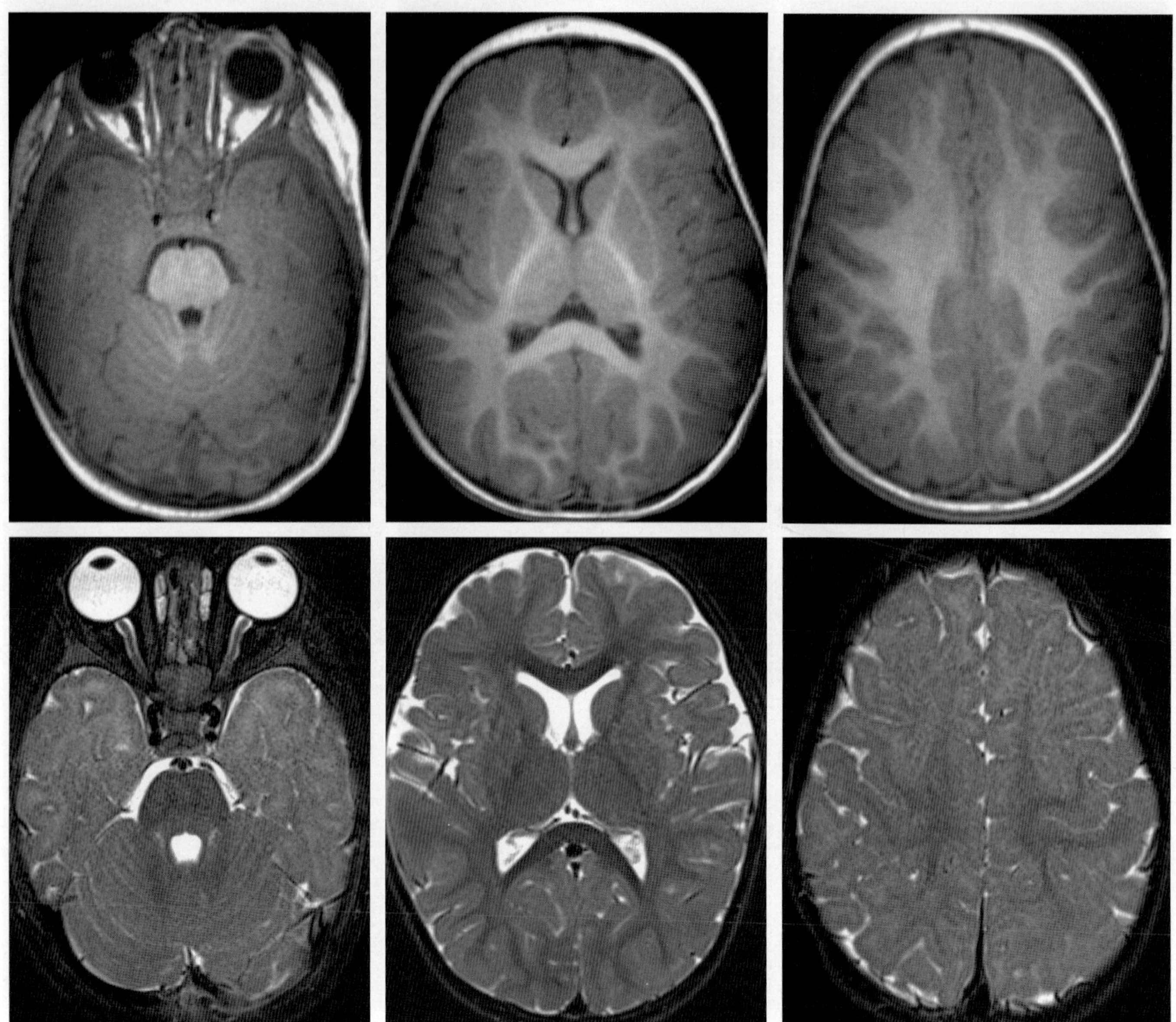

Myelination Pattern

- T1: Near complete myelination except anterior temporal lobe subcortical white matter
- T2: Genu of the corpus callosum, and anterior limb internal capsule myelinate

NORMAL MYELINATION: 12 MONTHS

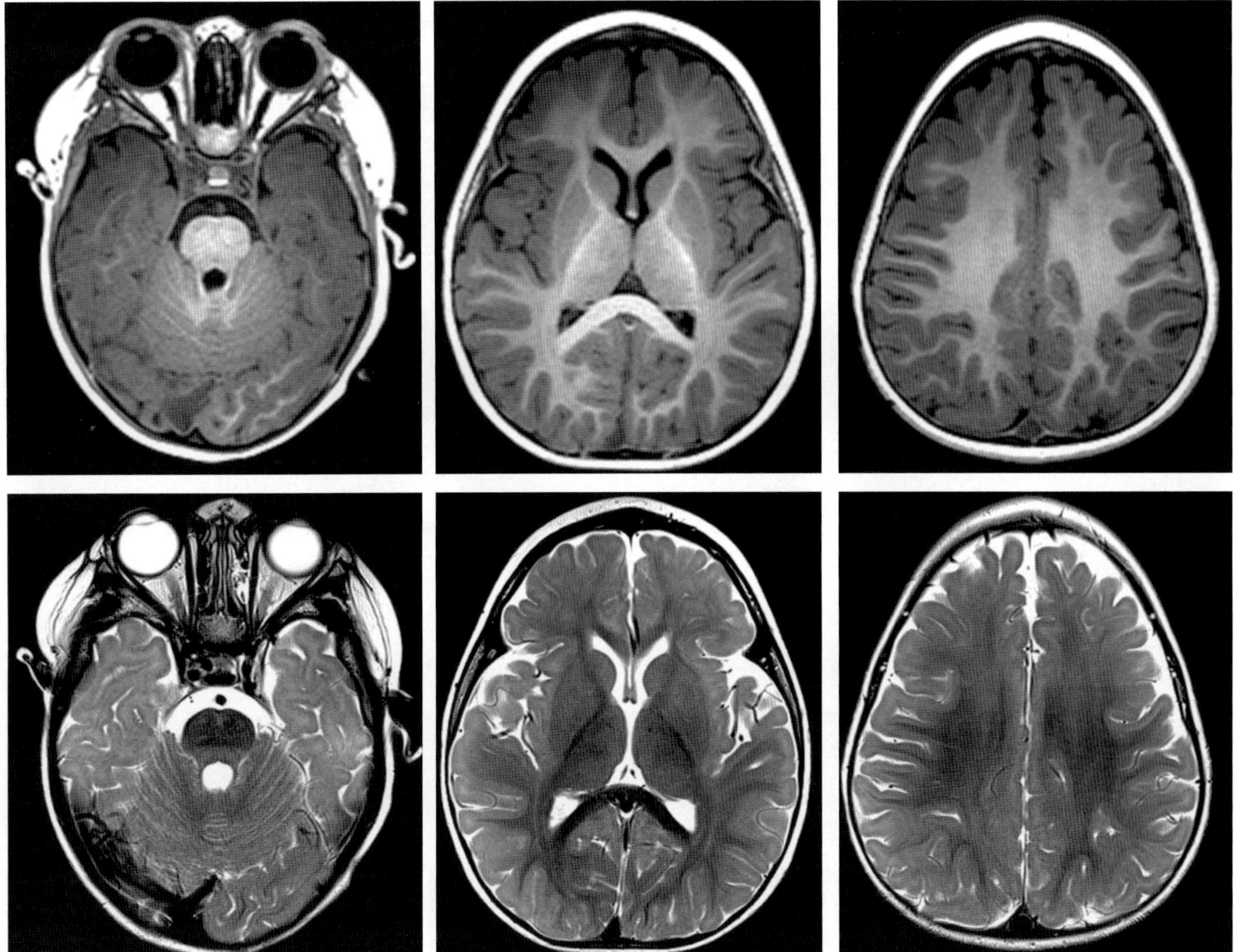

Myelination Pattern

- T1: Complete myelination
- T2: Occipital subcortical white matter myelinates

NORMAL MYELINATION: 14 MONTHS

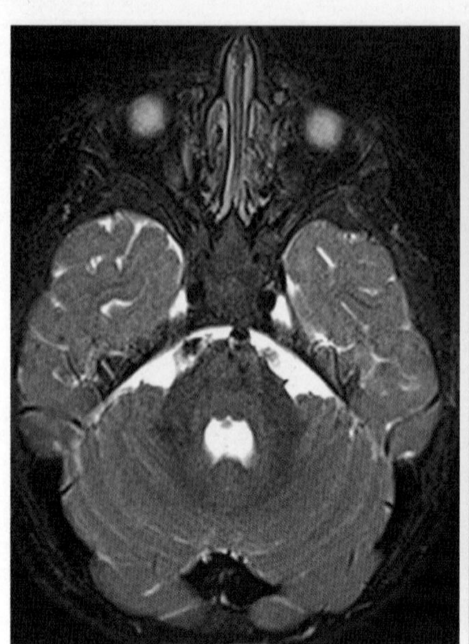
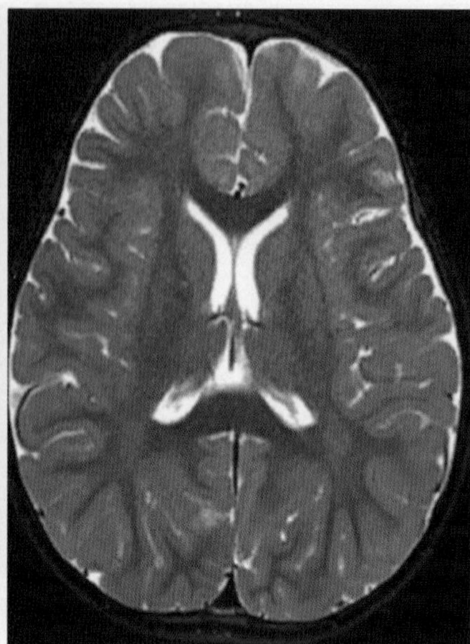
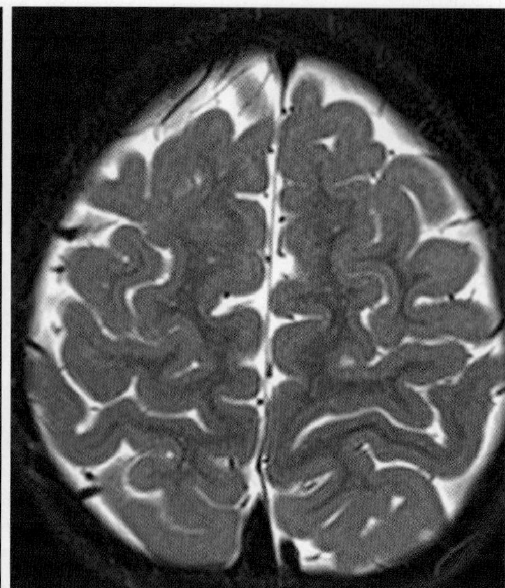

Myelination Pattern

- T1: Complete myelination
- T2: Frontal subcortical white matter myelinates

NORMAL MYELINATION: 18 MONTHS

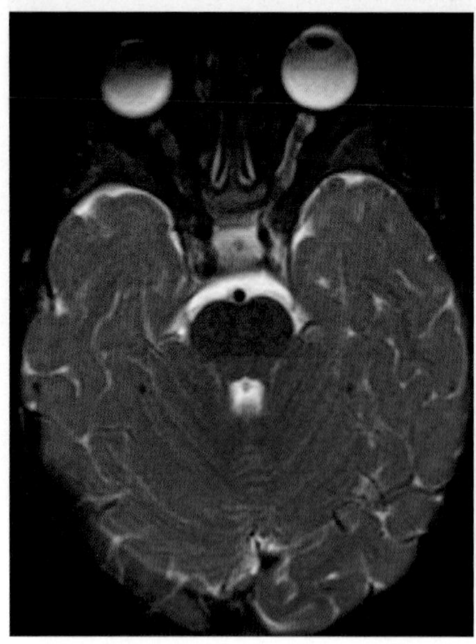
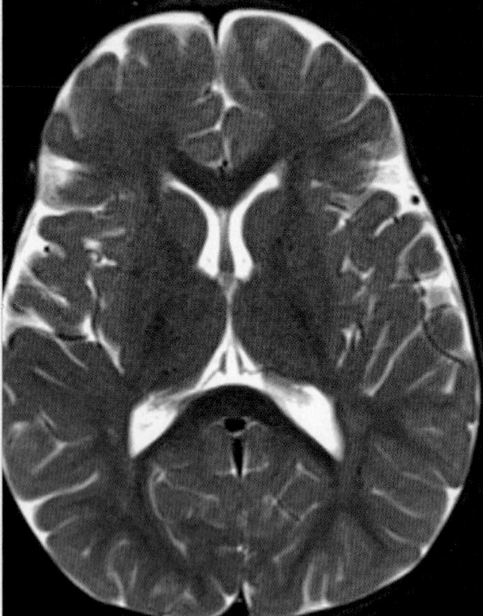
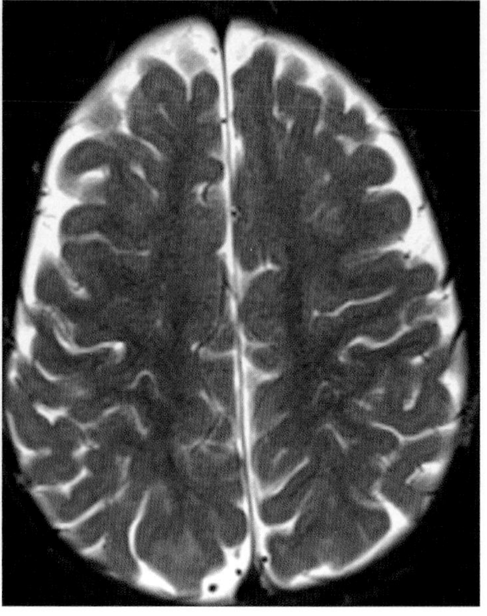

Myelination Pattern

- T1: Complete myelination
- T2: Frontal subcortical white matter myelinates

NORMAL MYELINATION: 24 MONTHS

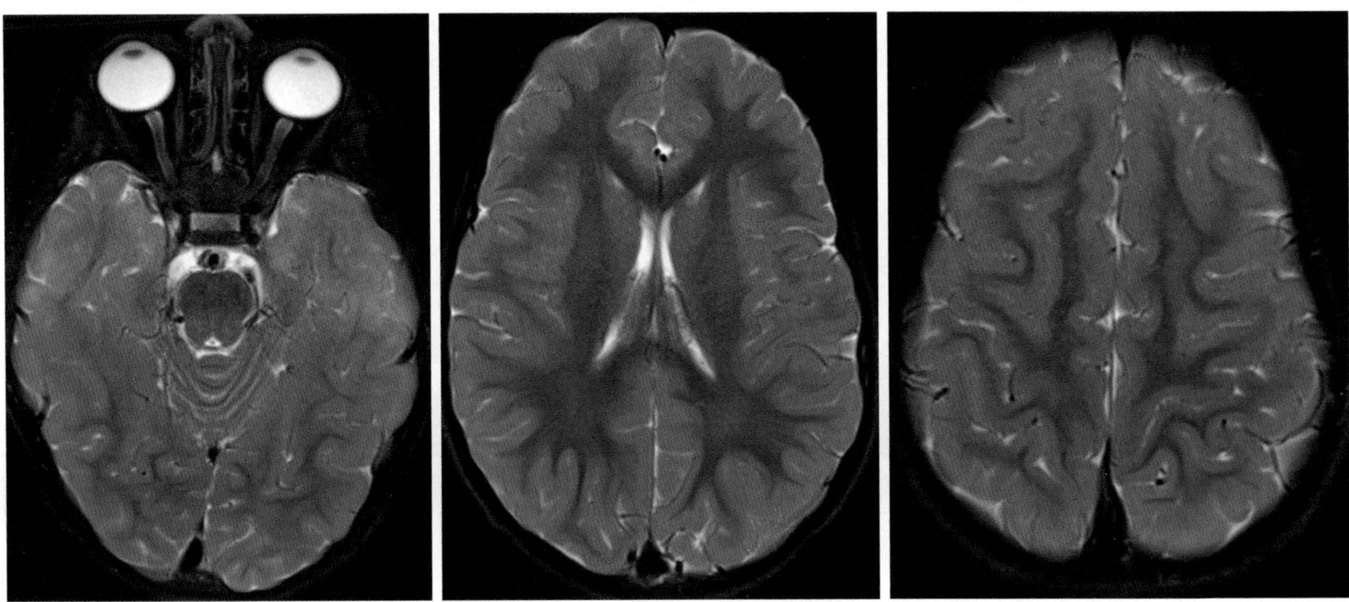

Myelination Pattern

- T1: Complete myelination
- T2: Complete except for terminal zones in the periatrial white matter and anterior temporal subcortical white matter

NORMAL MYELINATION: 36 MONTHS

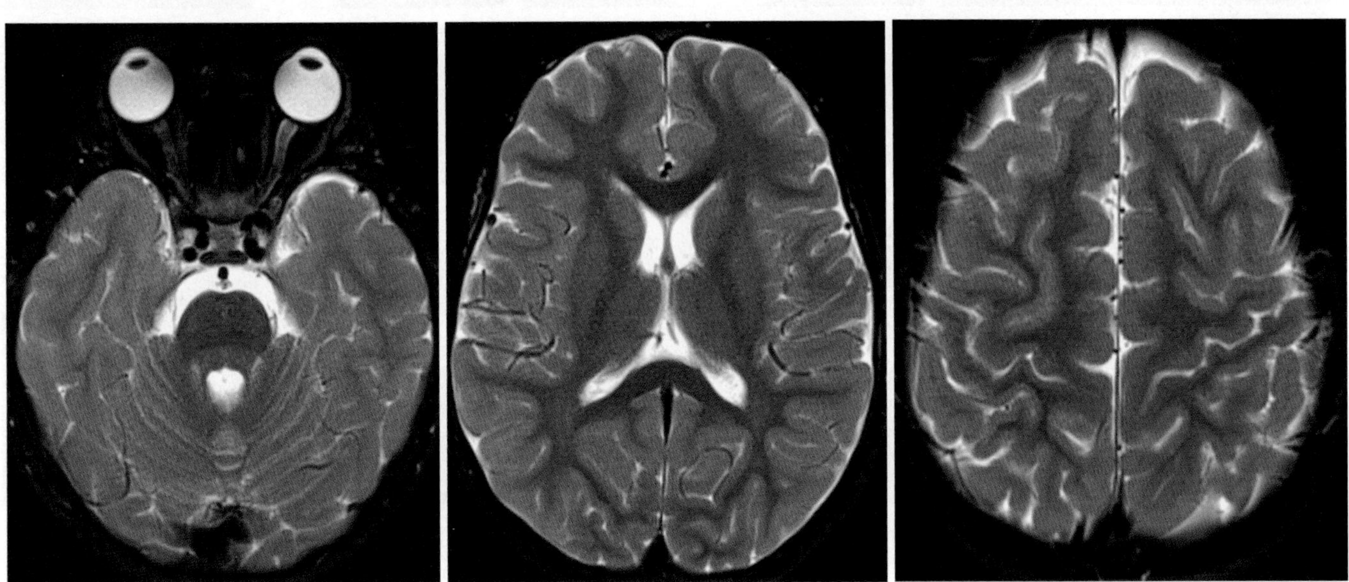

Myelination Pattern

- T1: Complete myelination
- T2: Complete myelination

POSTNATAL HEAD CT DEVELOPMENT

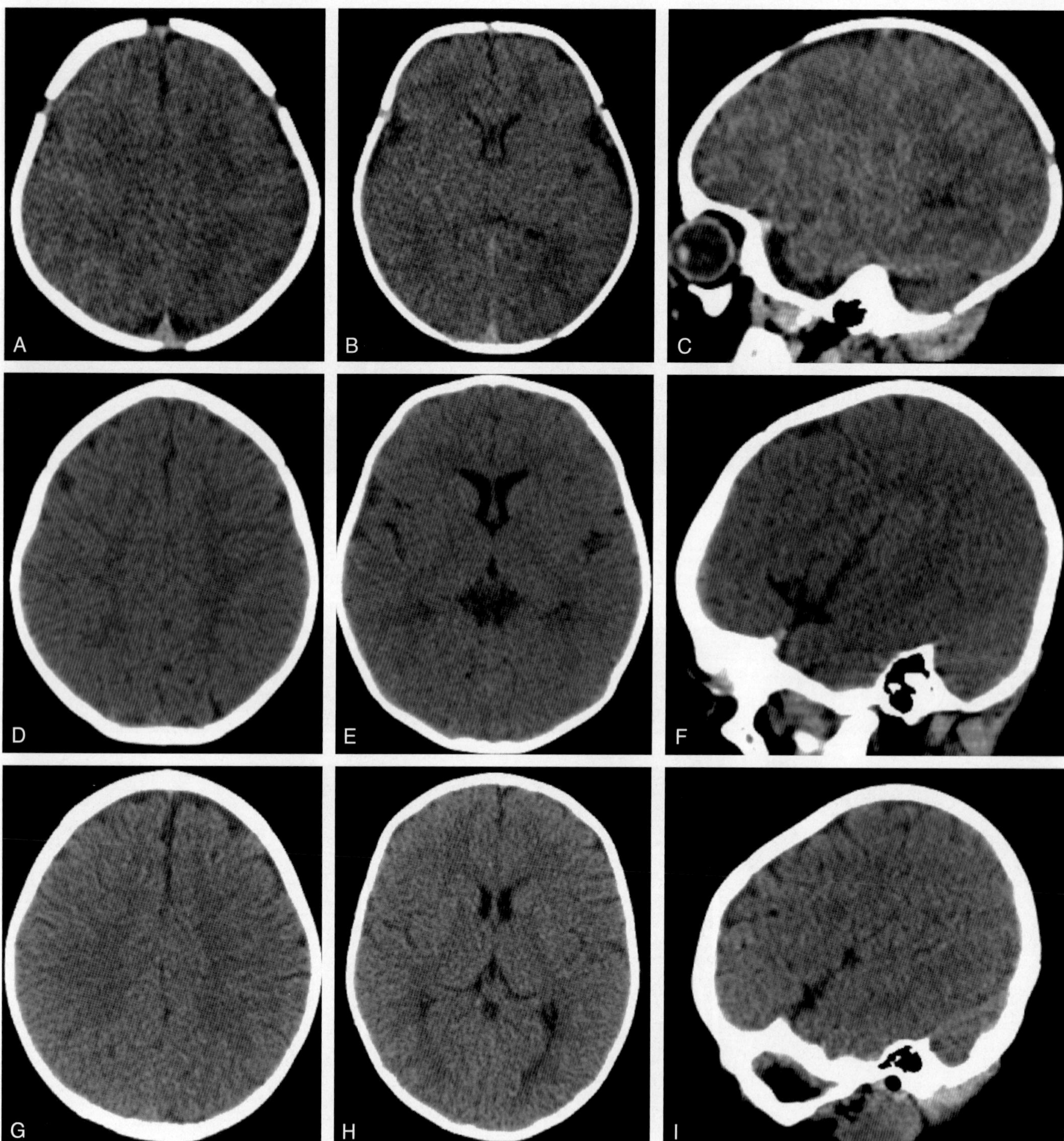

Head CT during postnatal development. Axial and sagittal head CT imaging in a (A to C) full-term newborn, (D to F) 6-month infant, and (G to H) 1-year-old infant demonstrate the changes in density and contrast in gray and white matter that occur with progressive myelination. The 1-year-old head CT contrast of brain structures is similar to that of adults.

CORPUS CALLOSUM EMBRYOLOGY

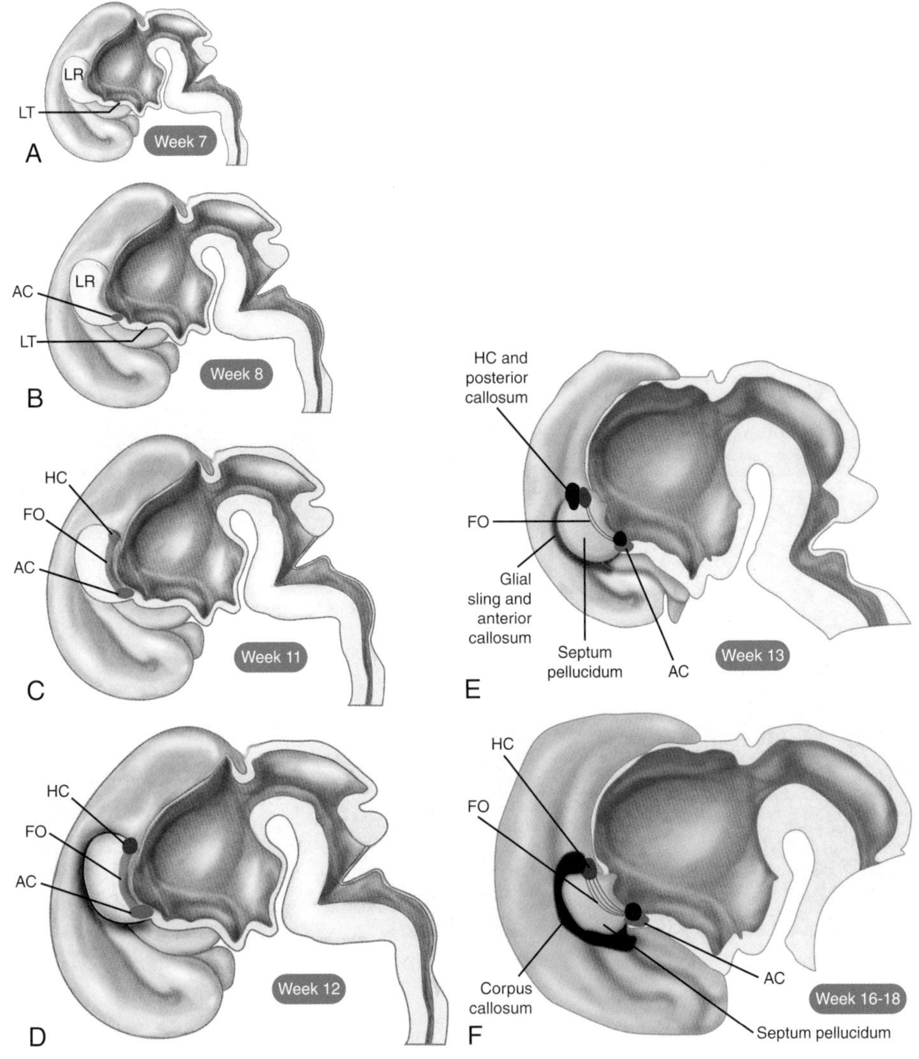

Fig. 1.5 Development of the Lamina Reuniens and of the Corpus Callosum, Sagittal Midline. (In Volpe JJ. *Volpe's Neurology of the Newborn*. 6th ed. Elsevier; 2018. Modified from Barkovich AJ, Raybaud C. *Pediatric Neuroimaging*. 5th ed. LWW; 2012:371–372.)

The corpus callosum is by far the largest commissure in the brain and is a major structure that should be evaluated when evaluating brain development. As the corpus callosum is a major midline structure, malformations of the corpus callosum can be isolated or in conjunction with other cerebral malformations.

As shown in Fig. 1.5, (A) during week 7, the upper portion of the lamina terminalis *(LT)*, which connects the hemispheres across the midline, thickens and forms the lamina reuniens *(LR)* of His (A).

(B) In the following week, olfactory commissural fibers cross the midline through the ventral aspect of the LR to form the anterior commissure *(AC)*.

(C) In the following weeks, fibers develop between the anterior mediobasal cortex (septal nuclei) and the future hippocampus to form the ipsilateral fornix *(FO)*; about week 11, some forniceal fibers cross the midline in the dorsal portion of the lamina reuniens and form the hippocampal commissure *(HC)*.

(D) During week 12, the corticoseptal boundary becomes defined at the medial edge of the future neocortex, and a glial sling forms along this boundary.

(E) By week 13, three commissural sites have been established: anterior commissure, hippocampal commissure, and glial sling. Depending on their origin, early neocortical commissural fibers cross the midline along the anterior commissure (temporooccipital fibers), the glial sling (frontal fibers), or the hippocampal commissure (parietooccipitotemporal fibers).

(F) The corpus callosum grows by adding further commissural fibers and forms a single continuous structure stretched between the anterior commissure and the hippocampal commissure; it circumscribes the future septum pellucidum. Later, the prominent development of the frontal lobes results in posterior growth of the anterior corpus callosum, which displaces the hippocampal commissure and the splenium backward above the velum interpositum (roof above the third ventricle), stretching the body of the fornix. The corpus callosum becomes longer and thicker in development.

CORPUS CALLOSUM DEVELOPMENT

The corpus callosum should be present on imaging at 18 weeks' gestation. Because ultrasound is usually routinely performed in the second trimester, the cavum septum pellucidum has been an important structure when determining normal formation of the corpus callosum. The cavum septum pellucidum is closely associated with formation of the corpus callosum and should be visible by 18 weeks on ultrasound. Absence of the cavum septum pellucidum raises concern for a malformation of the corpus callosum and is an indication for fetal MRI to confirm dysgenesis or agenesis of the corpus callosum and to assess for associated malformations. Multiplanar fetal MRI T2W images reliably can determine whether a fully formed corpus callosum is present. Sagittal T2W imaging is typically the best plane for visualizing the entire corpus callosum (Fig. 1.6).

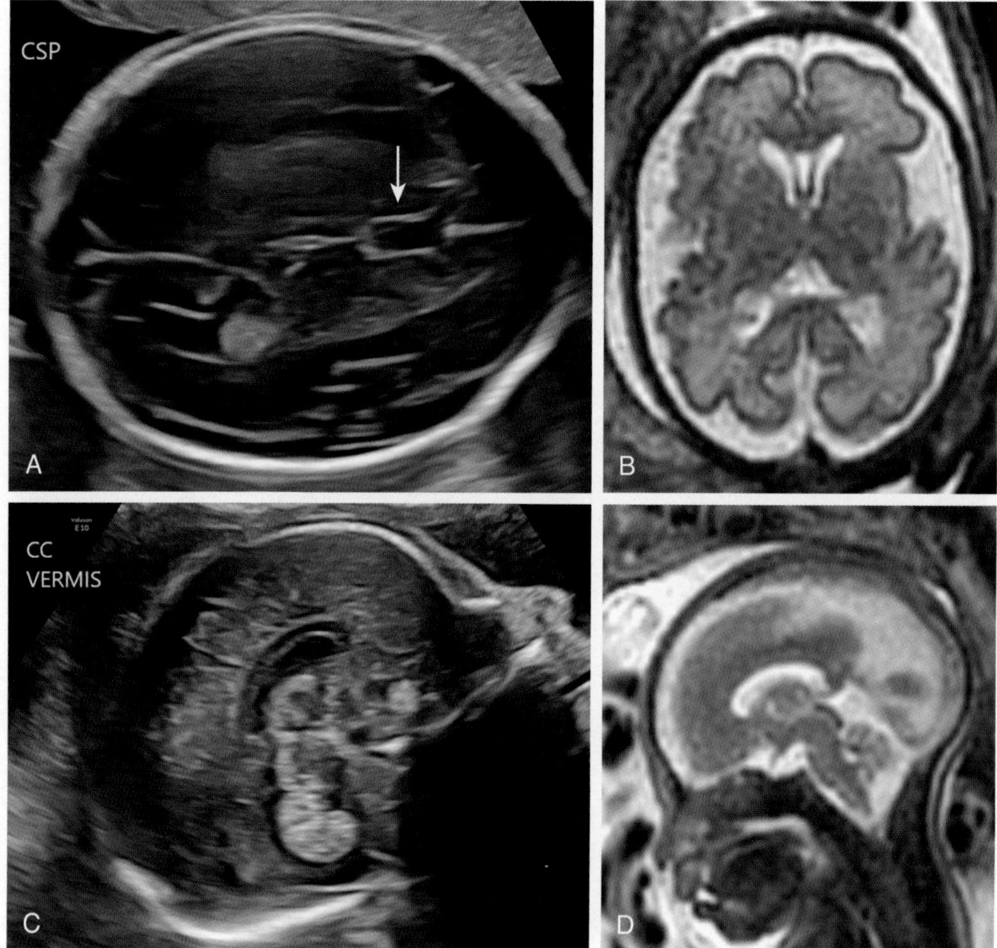

Fig. 1.6 Corpus Callosum. (A and B) Normal septum pellucidum and (C and D) normal corpus callosum on ultrasound and fetal MRI.

CORPUS CALLOSUM DEVELOPMENT

As the brain develops, the corpus callosum becomes longer and thicker. Biometric data of the corpus callosum (with measurement details shown in the figure) indicate most of the postnatal enlargement of the corpus callosum occurs in the first 4 years of life, after which the size is essentially stable. While subjective assessment of callosal length and thickness is usually done in routine clinical care, biometric data can be useful for some patients and are provided as a reference in Table 1.2.

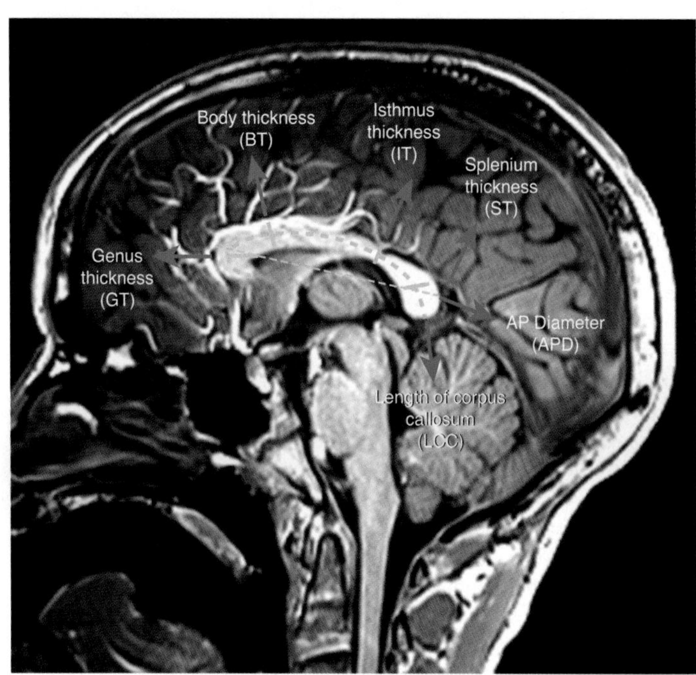

REFERENCE

1. Garel C, Cont I, Alberti C, et al. Biometry of the corpus callosum in children: MR imaging reference data. *AJNR Am J Neuroradiol.* 2011 Sep;32(8):1436–1443.

TABLE 1.2 Corpus Callosum Biometery. Median, 3rd, and 97th Percentiles for the Different Measurements as a Function of Age

	Age (yr)																		
Percentile	**0**	**0.5**	**1**	**1.5**	**2**	**2.5**	**3**	**4**	**5**	**6**	**7**	**8**	**9**	**10**	**11**	**12**	**13**	**14**	**15**
APD																			
3rd	36.8	43.7	47.9	50.6	52.4	53.6	54.4	55.5	56.2	56.8	57.4	57.9	58.5	59.1	59.7	60.4	61	61.7	62.5
Median	43.6	50.9	55.6	58.6	60.6	61.9	62.9	64.1	64.8	65.5	66	66.6	67.2	67.9	68.6	69.3	70.1	71	72
97th	62	63.9	66.8	69.1	70.6	71.7	72.5	73.5	74.2	74.8	75.4	76	76.6	77.3	78.1	79	79.9	81.1	82.3
LCC																			
3rd	47.6	60	66.9	70.7	72.7	73.8	74.4	75	75.3	75.6	76	76.5	77.1	77.7	78.4	79.2	80.1	81	82
Median	56.3	70.2	78.3	82.9	85.5	87	87.9	88.7	89.2	89.7	90.2	90.8	91.5	92.3	93.3	94.4	95.7	97.2	99
97th	81.7	89.1	95.3	99.1	101.3	102.6	103.3	104.1	104.5	105	105.6	106.3	107.1	108.2	109.4	110.9	112.7	114.8	117.5
GT																			
3rd	2.5	3.7	4.6	5.2	5.7	6	6.3	6.7	6.9	7	7.1	7.2	7.3	7.3	7.4	7.5	7.5	7.6	7.6
Median	4.3	5.8	6.9	7.7	8.3	8.8	9.1	9.6	9.9	10.1	10.2	10.3	10.4	10.5	10.6	10.6	10.7	10.8	10.8
97th	8.3	8.9	9.7	10.4	11	11.4	11.8	12.3	12.6	12.9	13	13.1	13.2	13.3	13.4	13.5	13.5	13.6	13.7
BT																			
3rd	1.3	1.8	2.2	2.6	2.9	3.1	3.3	3.5	3.7	3.8	3.9	3.9	4	4	4	4	3.9	3.9	3.7
Median	2.3	3	3.6	4.1	4.5	4.8	5	5.3	5.5	5.7	5.8	5.8	5.8	5.9	5.9	5.9	5.9	5.9	5.9
97th	5	5.3	5.7	6.1	6.5	6.8	7	7.4	7.6	7.7	7.8	7.9	7.9	8	8	8	8.1	8.2	8.4
IT																			
3rd	1.2	1.4	1.5	1.6	1.7	1.7	1.8	1.9	2	2.1	2.2	2.2	2.3	2.4	2.4	2.4	2.5	2.5	2.5
Median	1.9	2.2	2.5	2.7	2.8	3	3.1	3.2	3.4	3.5	3.6	3.7	3.8	3.8	3.9	4	4	4	4.1
97th	3.9	4.1	4.3	4.5	4.6	4.8	4.9	5.1	5.3	5.5	5.6	5.7	5.8	5.9	6	6	6.1	6.2	6.2
ST																			
3rd	1.9	3.4	4.4	5.1	5.6	6	6.2	6.7	6.9	7.2	7.4	7.5	7.6	7.7	7.7	7.7	7.5	7.1	6.3
Median	3.9	5.6	6.7	7.5	8.1	8.5	8.8	9.2	9.5	9.8	10	10.1	10.3	10.4	10.5	10.5	10.6	10.6	10.5
97th	9	9.2	9.9	10.5	10.9	11.3	11.5	11.9	12.2	12.5	12.7	12.8	13	13.1	13.3	13.5	13.7	14.1	14.8

From Garel C, Cont I, Alberti C, et al. Biometry of the corpus callosum in children: MR imaging reference data. *AJNR Am J Neuroradiol.* 2011 Sep;32(8):1436–1443.

POSTERIOR FOSSA DEVELOPMENT

Posterior fossa embryology is complex and still incompletely understood. Some knowledge of normal development of the posterior fossa helps to understand malformations that occur in the posterior fossa, including brainstem malformations, Dandy-Walker malformations, and Chiari malformations.

As previously discussed, the neural tube forms three vesicles: the prosencephalon (forebrain), mesencephalon (midbrain), and rhombencephalon (hindbrain) (Fig. 1.7). The mesencephalon forms the midbrain, and the rhombencephalon forms the pons and medulla. The cavity in the hindbrain will become the fourth ventricle. The upper portion of the rhombencephalon develops a constriction known as the isthmus rhombencephali, which separates it from the mesencephalon. Due to unequal growth of the primary vesicles, three flexures develop, known as the cephalic flexure, pontine flexure, and cervical flexure, resulting in an M shape. The rhombencephalon divides into two secondary vesicles, known as the metencephalon and myelencephalon. The pons develops from thickening of the floors and lateral walls of the metencephalon, while thickening of the floor and lateral walls of the myelencephalon forms the medulla. A complex balance of biochemical signaling is required for normal development of the brainstem and cerebellum. The isthmic organizer controls patterning of the future midbrain and pons through several genes and molecules (OTX2, GBX2, FGF8, WNT1, EN1, EN2, Pax, Lmx 1b). Alteration in these molecules leads to anomalies in this region, often detected by abnormal craniocaudal proportions of the brainstem segments.

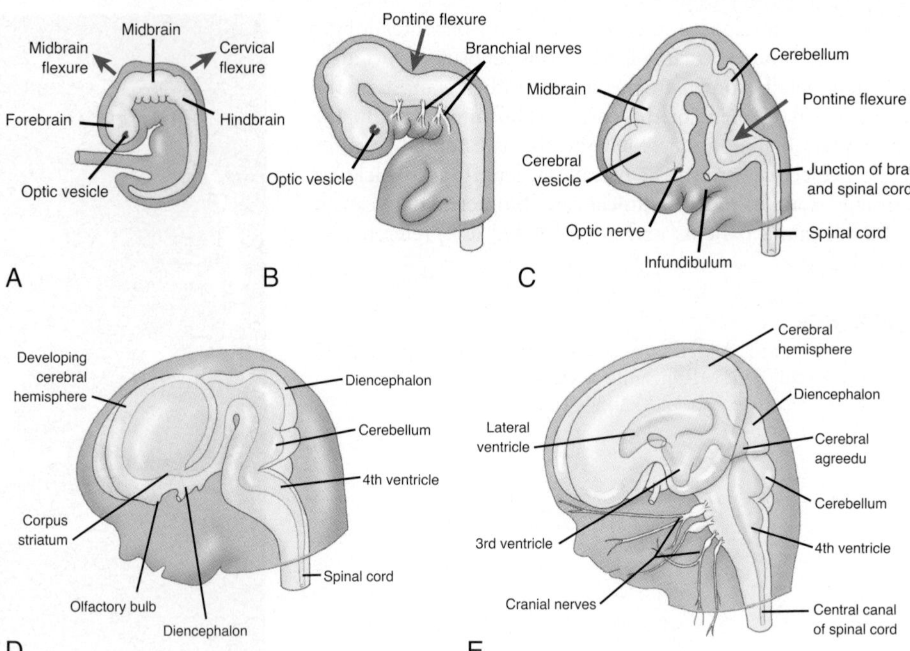

Fig. 1.7 Development of the Brain and the Ventricular System. Note how the brain flexures affect the shape of the brain, enabling it to be accommodated in the head. The cerebral hemispheres expand and gradually cover the diencephalon and midbrain. The nerves of the branchial arches become the cranial nerves. (A) 28 days. (B) 35 days. (C) 56 days. (D) 10 weeks. (E) 14 weeks. (From Hagen-Ansert SL. *Textbook of Diagnostic Ultrasonography.* 6th ed. Elsevier; 2006.)

POSTERIOR FOSSA DEVELOPMENT

At the fifth gestational week the cerebellar hemispheres appear, followed by the vermis at 9 weeks, which grows to cover the fourth ventricle by the 20th week. The alar plates of the caudal third of the mesencephalon form the vermis, and the alar plates of the metencephalon form the cerebellar hemispheres. The cerebellum forms from two germinal matrixes: the ventricular zone along the roof of the fourth ventricle and the rhombic lips laterally at the junction of the roof plate and neural tube. The ventricular zone gives rise to the deep cerebellar nuclei, Purkinje cells, and interneurons. The rhombic lips give rise to the granule cell precursors and precerebellar nuclei in the brainstem. The cerebellum continues to develop postnatally into a three-layered cortex with an external gray molecular layer, an intermediate Purkinje layer, and an internal granule layer.

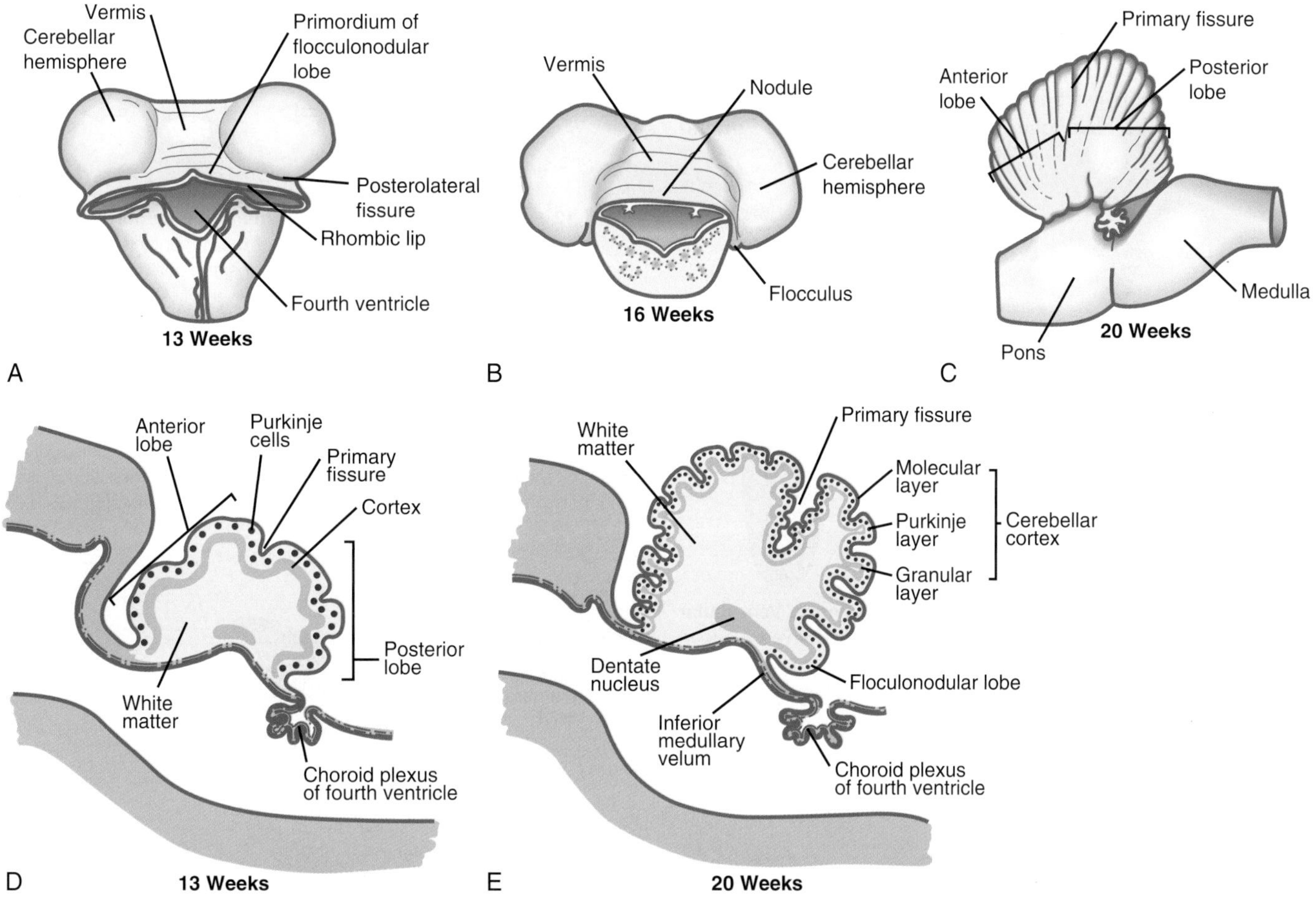

Fig. 1.8 Development of the Cerebellum. (A and B) Dorsal views. (C) Lateral view. (D and E) Sagittal sections. (From Carlson BM. *Human Embryology and Developmental Biology.* 6th ed. Elsevier; 2019.)

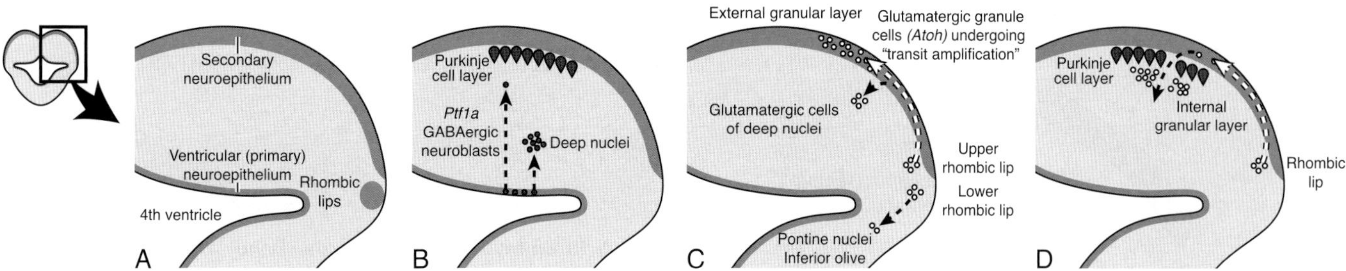

Fig. 1.9 (A) Cerebellar primary and secondary neuroproliferative sites. (B) Neuronal migration of GABAergic cells from the primary ventricular neuroepithelium. (C) Neuronal proliferation and migration of glutamatergic neuronal precursors from the rhombic lips into the secondary neuroproliferative zone of the external granular layer. (D) Internal migration of the granule cells from the external granular layer through the Purkinje cell layer to form the internal granular layer. (From Volpe JJ. *Volpe's Neurology of the Newborn.* 6th ed. Elsevier; 2018.)

POSTERIOR FOSSA DEVELOPMENT

Because of the pontine flexure, the fourth ventricle becomes shorter craniocaudally and wider transversely. The roof of the fourth ventricle has an anterior membranous area (AMA) and a posterior membranous area (PMA), which are separated by the choroidal fold/choroid plexus. Neuroblastic proliferation causes the anterior membranous area to thicken and form two lateral plates called rhombic lips, which approach each other and fuse in the midline and will constitute the cerebellum. The growth of the rhombic lips causes the anterior membranous area to regress. Growth and backward extension of the cerebellum pushes the choroid plexus inferiorly; the PMA decreases in size and causes a caudal protrusion of the fourth ventricle, known as the Blake pouch, at 7 weeks. The choroid plexus extends into the roof of the pouch caudal to the vermis. The Blake pouch perforates between the 9th and 10th week to form the foramen of Magendie. Delayed perforation (usually by 24–26 weeks) or persistence of the Blake pouch is an abnormality of the posterior membranous area and as such should have a normal vermis because the posterior membranous area does not contribute to vermis formation, and the choroid plexus should be located below the vermis. The Dandy-Walker malformation conversely is a malformation of the anterior membranous area. Ultimately, the vermis is completely formed by the 15th week of gestation.

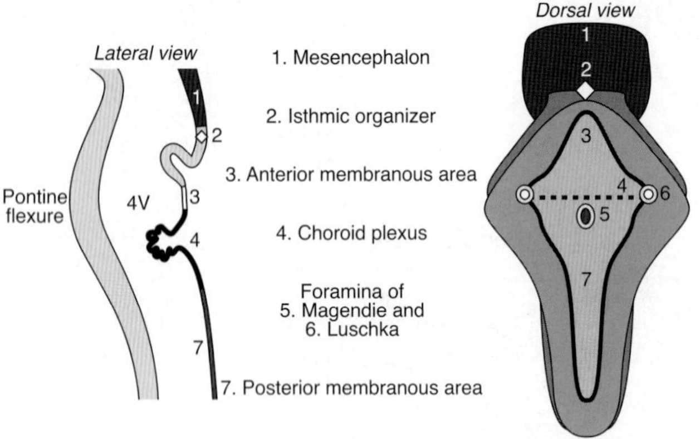

Fig. 1.10 Normal Landmarks of the Developing Fourth Ventricular Roof. (From Volpe JJ. *Volpe's Neurology of the Newborn.* 6th ed. Elsevier; 2018.)

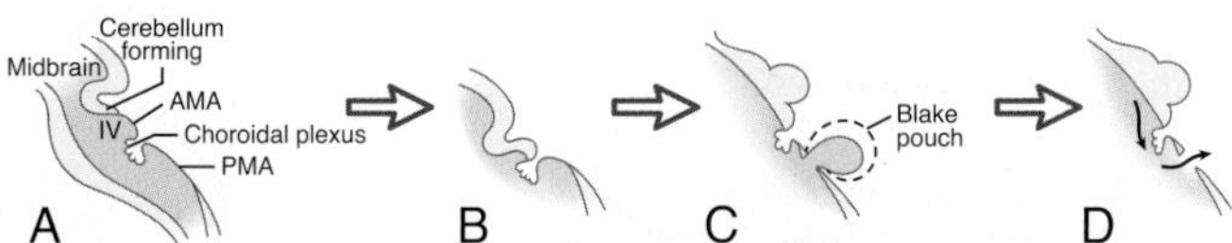

Fig. 1.12 Normal Steps in the Development of the Fourth Ventricle. In the early stages of gestation, the roof of the IV ventricle is divided by the rudimental choroid plexus into two portions: the anterior membranous area (AMA) and the posterior membranous area (PMA) (A). In normal individuals, the AMA is incorporated within the developing choroid glomus (B). Shortly after, the PMA shows a finger-like posterior expansion called a Blake pouch (C), which later disappears, leaving a median opening named Blake metapore, which corresponds to the future foramen of Magendie (D). (Modified from Tortori-Donati P, Fondelli MP, Rossi A, Carini S. Cystic malformations of the posterior cranial fossa originating from a defect of the posterior membranous area. Mega cisterna magna and persisting Blake's pouch: two separate entities. *Childs Nerv Syst.* 1996 Jun;12[6]:303–308. PMID: 8816293. doi:10.1007/BF00301017).

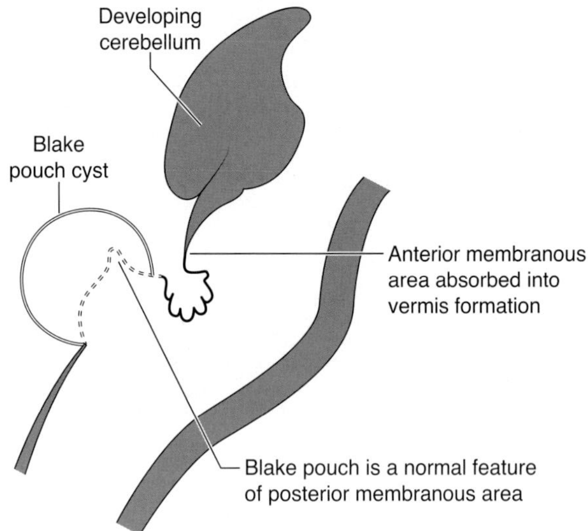

Fig. 1.11 Blake Pouch. Blake pouch is a normal feature of posterior membranous area. Failure or delay of the foramen Magendie to open leads to cyst formation. (From Volpe JJ. *Volpe's Neurology of the Newborn.* 6th ed. Elsevier; 2018.)

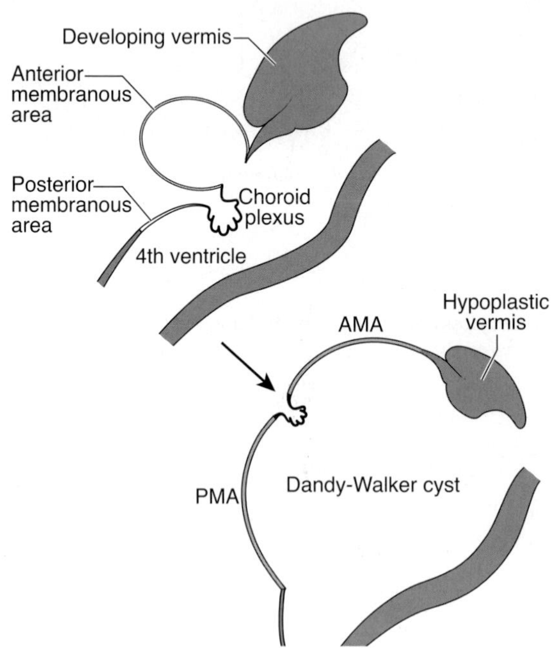

Fig. 1.13 Embryologic Basis of the Dandy-Walker Malformation. Diagram showing how the Dandy-Walker malformation involves the anterior membranous area which leads to hypoplastic and rotated vermis. (From Volpe JJ. *Volpe's Neurology of the Newborn.* 6th ed. Elsevier; 2018.)

IMAGING OF POSTERIOR FOSSA DEVELOPMENT

Typical imaging assessment of normal posterior fossa development includes evaluating the size of the posterior fossa, the craniocervical junction, position of the tentorium, proportions and morphology of the brainstem, appearance and size of the fourth ventricle, size of the cisterna magna, size and separation of the cerebellar hemispheres, and normal size and appearance of the vermis. The evaluation of the vermis requires additional assessment of its size and rotation, detection of the primary fissure, determining the tegmentovermian angle, and the detection and position of the fastigial point. Ultimately, four important questions must be answered: (1) Is the posterior fossa normal in size? (2) Is the fourth ventricle normal in size and shape? (3) Are the vermis, cerebellar hemispheres, and brainstem normal? (4) Are there any other anomalies, including hydrocephalus?

The posterior fossa is routinely evaluated on prenatal ultrasound; however, the accuracy for detection of an isolated posterior fossa abnormality is only 65% compared to 88% with fetal MRI. On ultrasound, the ventral pons demonstrates increased echogenicity compared to the dorsal pons due to higher cellularity and crossing fibers. The cerebellar folia are more echogenic than the remainder of the cerebellar hemispheres, and the vermis is more echogenic than the cerebellar hemispheres. The cisterna magna represents the fluid space posterior to the cerebellum and should measure <10 mm.

On fetal MRI, the vermis is well seen on axial, coronal, and sagittal images but best assessed on sagittal images, which allow determination of the fastigial point, tegmentovermian angle (TVA), and the vermis AP and craniocaudal size. The fastigium declive line can be used to assess whether the superior and inferior portions are relatively equal. The fastigial point is visible at 18–20 weeks. Abnormal fastigial points are present in malformations of the brainstem as well as rhombencephalosynapsis and Joubert syndrome. The tegmentovermian angle (TVA) which is an angle formed along the posterior pons with the anterior vermis on sagittal images should be <10 degrees. A TVA between 10 and 40 degrees raises concern for a Blake pouch cyst or vermian hypoplasia and requires follow-up to ensure complete vermis rotation as the inferior vermis can remain open to the fourth ventricle and cisterna magna until 18 weeks. A TVA >40 degrees raises concern for a Dandy-Walker malformation. TVA between 10 and 40 degrees can be seen in midgestation and requires follow up MRI to assess if the vermis rotates to a normal position. During the second trimester, the transverse cerebellar diameter in millimeters should be equal to the gestational age. The AP diameter of a cerebellar hemisphere should be approximately half the transverse cerebellar diameter. Lastly, between 20 and 30 weeks the pons is more hypointense.

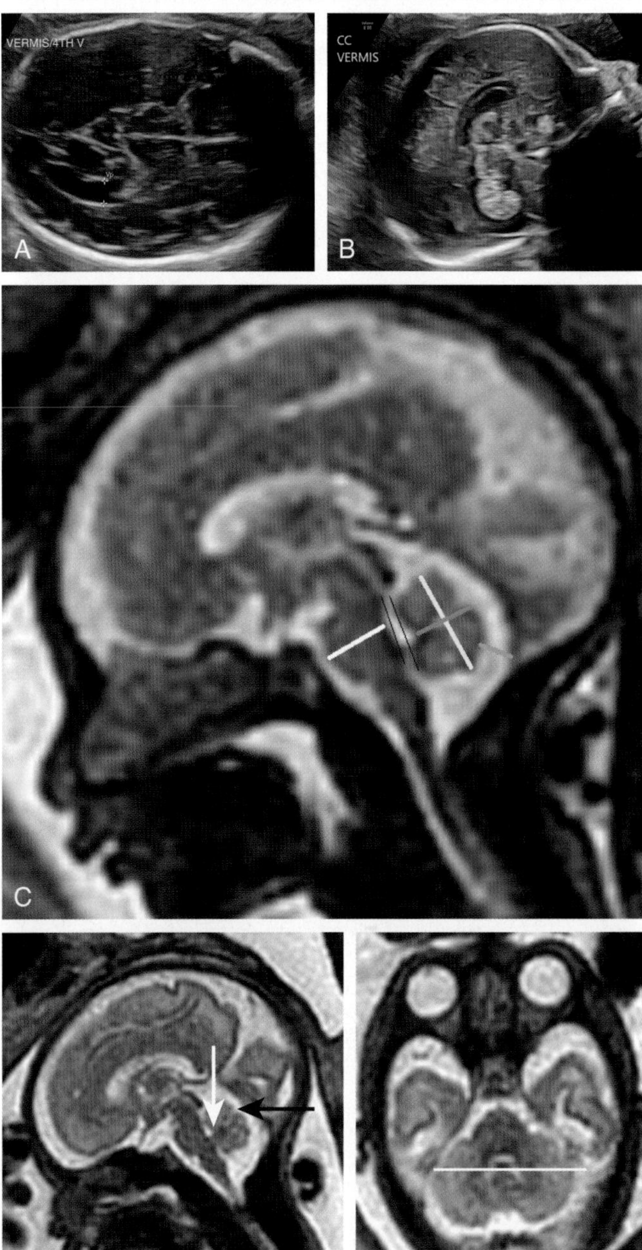

Fig. 1.14 Fetal Posterior Fossa. (A and B) Axial and sagittal ultrasound images demonstrate the cerebellar hemispheres, cisterna magna, echogenic vermis, and ventral pons. (C through E) Axial and sagittal T2W images demonstrate the transverse cerebellar diameter *(white)*, AP pons *(white)*, AP and craniocaudal vermis *(yellow and orange)*, cisterna magna *(green)*, TVA *(black)*, fastigial point *(white arrow)*, and primary fissure *(black arrow)*.

VENTRICLES

Ventricular size assessment is a major component of evaluation of normal brain development. The lateral ventricles are relatively constant in size from 14 to 40 weeks of gestation and measure less than 10 mm on ultrasound and MRI at the level of the atria on coronal imaging and this measurement. A 1- to 2-mm measurement discrepancy can occur between ultrasound and MRI. Mild ventriculomegaly occurs when the lateral ventricles measure 10 to 12 mm, moderate ventriculomegaly when the lateral ventricles measure 13 to 15 mm, and severe ventriculomegaly occurs when the ventricles measure >15 mm. The normal third ventricle measures less than 4 mm, and the normal fourth ventricle less than 6 mm.

Although ventricle size is important in assessing brain development, the degree of ventriculomegaly is not consistently correlated with a child's outcome. Fetal ventriculomegaly can be isolated as well as associated with additional anomalies. Fetal MRI can detect sonographically occult abnormalities in up to 40% to 50% of patients with ventriculomegaly, and the presence of associated anomalies with ventriculomegaly is associated with abnormal outcomes in 40% to 50% of patients.

Attention to the normal ventricular configuration and contour is also important as it is altered in abnormalities including agenesis of the corpus callosum, periventricular heterotopia, and injuries such as periventricular hemorrhage can lead to abnormal contour of the ventricles.

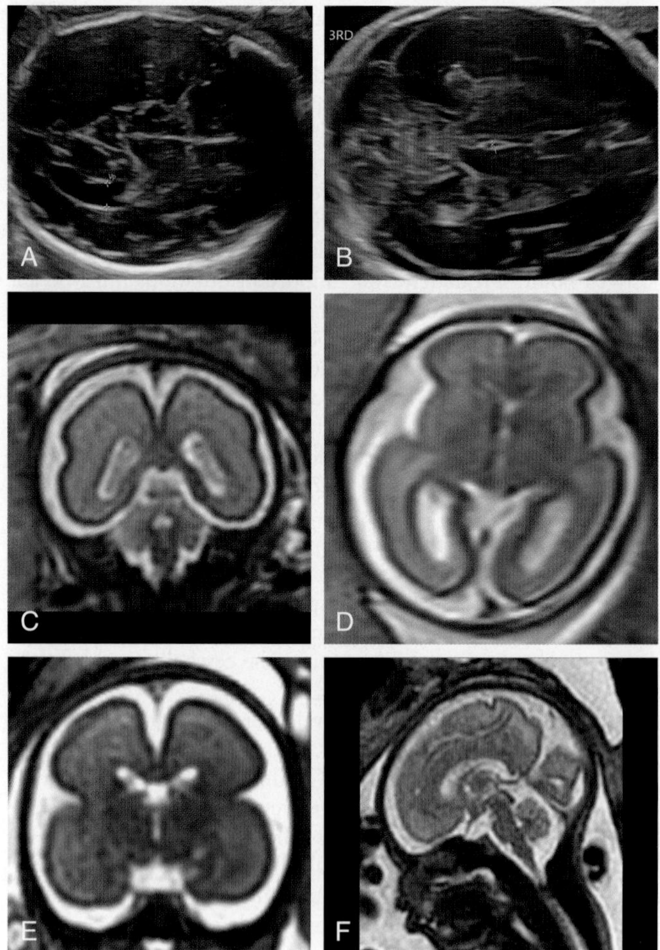

Fig. 1.15 Normal Fetal Ultrasound and MRI of the Ventricles. (A and B) Axial ultrasound images of the lateral ventricles and third ventricle. (C to F) Multiplanar T2W fetal MRI images of the ventricles.

BRAIN DEVELOPMENT: DIFFUSION IMAGING

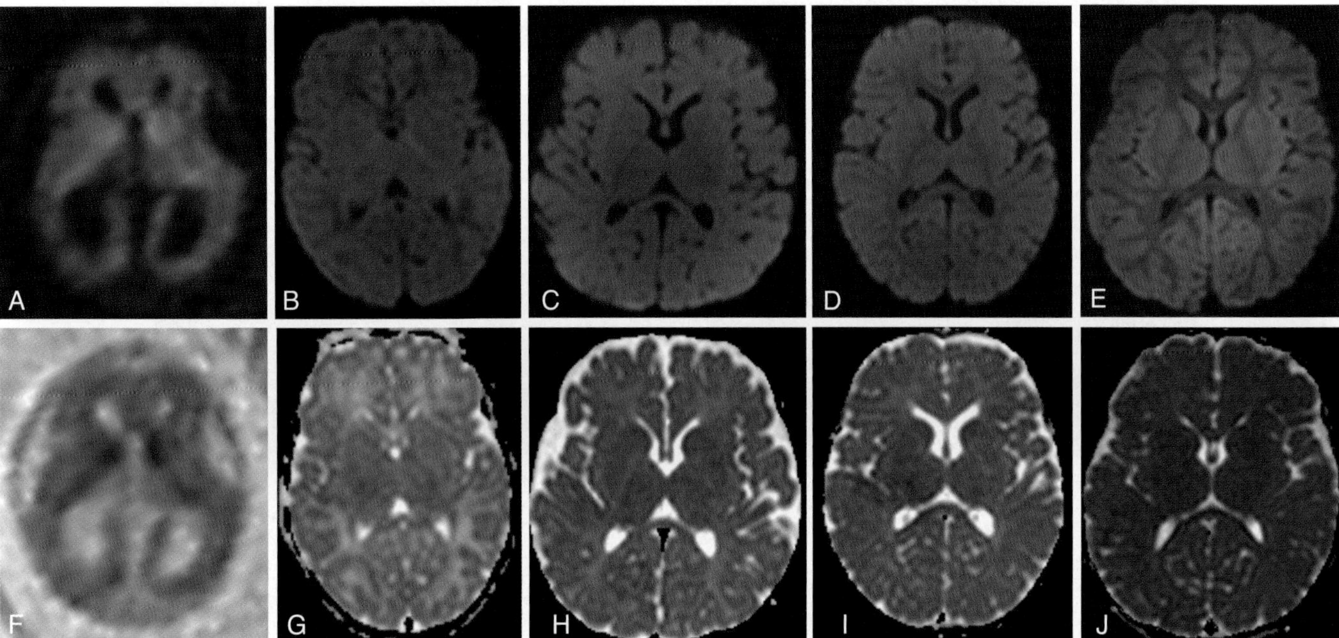

Fig. 1.16 Changes in DWI and ADC Appearance of the Brain. (A and F) A 20-week fetus. (B and G) A 6-day-old neonate. (C and H) A 4-month-old infant. (D and I) A 9-month-old infant. (E and J) A 2-year-old child.

Diffusion-weighted imaging (DWI) and diffusion tensor imaging are able to indirectly demonstrate changes occurring in the brain's microstructure during development. Structural organization and myelination result in increases in fractional anisotropy and decreases in ADC values. Postnatally, ADC values have been shown to decrease logarithmically with postnatal age, with most of the changes occurring within the first year of life. Visually on DWI and ADC images, the fetal and neonatal brain demonstrates significant contrast between the gray matter and the white matter due to the significantly higher ADC values (hyperintensity) of the white matter compared to gray matter. The contrast between these structures decreases during the first year of life until they are relatively symmetrically isointense at 9 months of age. Early myelinating structures such as the corticospinal tract will demonstrate lower ADC values (more hypointense) compared to white matter tracts that later are myelinated.

REFERENCES

1. Khan S, Vasung L, Marami B, Rollins CK, Afacan O, Ortinau CM, Yang E, Warfield SK, Gholipour A. Fetal brain growth portrayed by a spatiotemporal diffusion tensor MRI atlas computed from in utero images. *Neuroimage*. 2019 Jan 15;185:593–608.
2. Forbes KP, Pipe JG, Bird CR. Changes in brain water diffusion during the 1st year of life. *Radiology*. 2002 Feb;222(2):405–409.

BRAIN DEVELOPMENT: DIFFUSION IMAGING

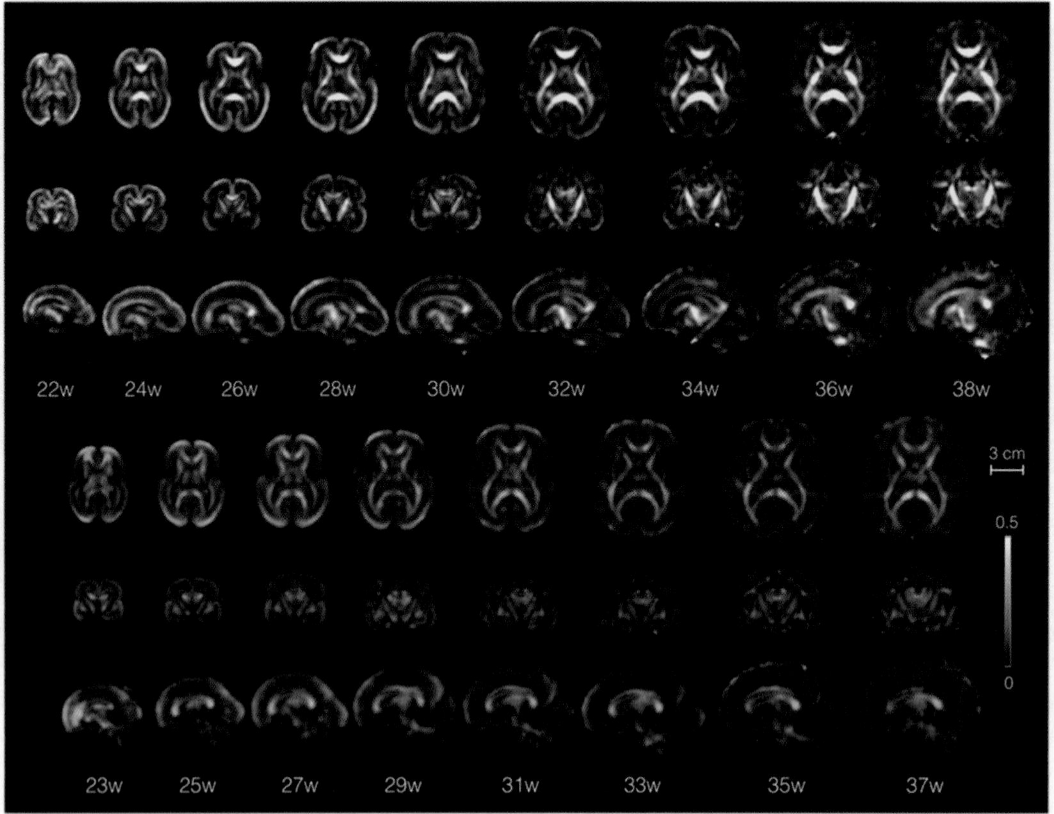

Fig. 1.17 Axial, coronal, and sagittal views of fractional anisotropy *(grayscale)* and color fractional anisotropy templates from the in utero DTI atlas. Gestational age in weeks is mentioned below the images. (From Khan S, Vasung L, Marami B, et al. Fetal brain growth portrayed by a spatiotemporal diffusion tensor MRI atlas computed from in utero images. Neuroimage. 2019;185:593–608.)

Diffusion tensor imaging fractional anisotropy maps are able to demonstrate changes in the fetal and postnatal brain during development. Myelination of the white matter leads to increases in FA (hyperintense). However, even prior to myelination, increases in FA are visible, indicative of structural organization. Highly organized structures like the corpus callosum and internal capsules readily stand out on FA maps. Interestingly, the fetal cerebral cortex undergoes a change from high FA, presumed to be due to radial organization, to lower FA presumed to be due to subsequent laminar organization.

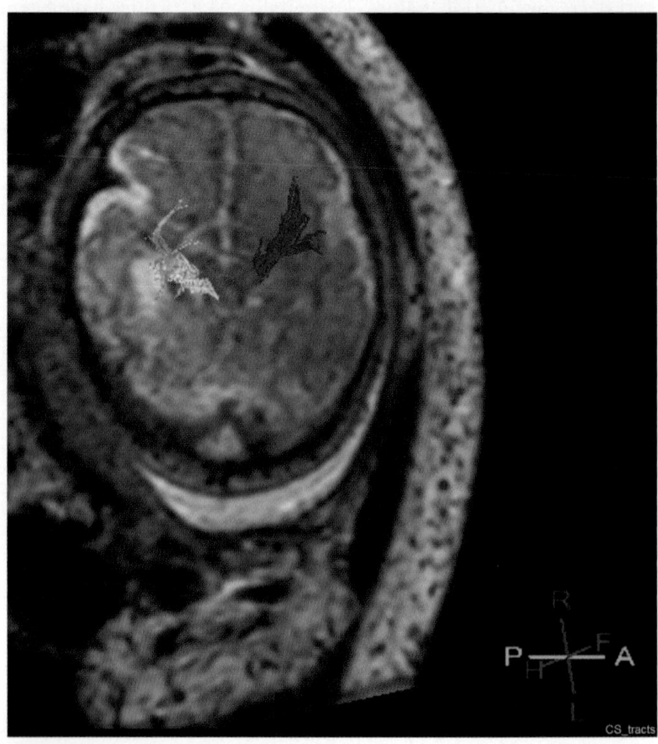

Fig. 1.18 Tractography image from a fetal MRI DTI demonstrating the corticospinal tracts.

BRAIN DEVELOPMENT: MR SPECTROSCOPY

H^1 MR spectroscopy (MRS) demonstrates changes in the metabolites with brain development. The majority of the descriptions of changes in MRS with brain development come from spectra from the basal ganglia or the anterior or posterior cerebral white matter. In the basal ganglia, at birth the choline peak is the dominant peak followed by NAA and then creatine, forming a "reverse checkmark" pattern. The NAA peak increases after birth and becomes the dominant peak at 6 months of age. The choline/creatine ratio decreases postnatally until approximately 3 years of age. A small lactate peak can be detected in neonates but otherwise is considered abnormal when detected. Myo-inositol is detected on short echo MRS and decreases rapidly to adult levels at approximately 2 months of age. Last, it is important to realize that spectroscopy patterns will differ between regions of the brain. For example, in term infants the basal ganglia and thalamic NAA and creatine concentrations are higher than that of the frontal lobe.

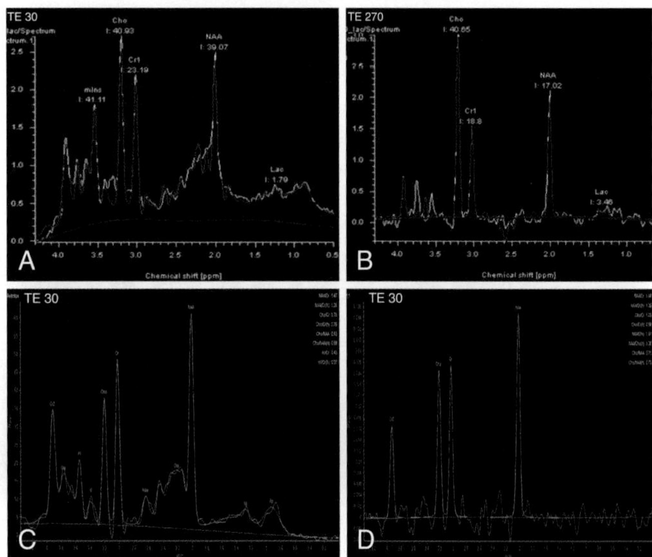

Fig. 1.19 Normal 1H MR Spectroscopy Patterns in Development. 1H MR spectroscopy from the basal ganglia in a full-term 5-day-old neonate with (A) short TE (30 ms) and (B) long TE (270 ms) and from a 7-month-old infant with (C) short TE (30 ms) and (D) long TE (270 ms). The NAA peak should be greater than the creatine peak at birth and increase to become the dominant peak after 6 months of age.

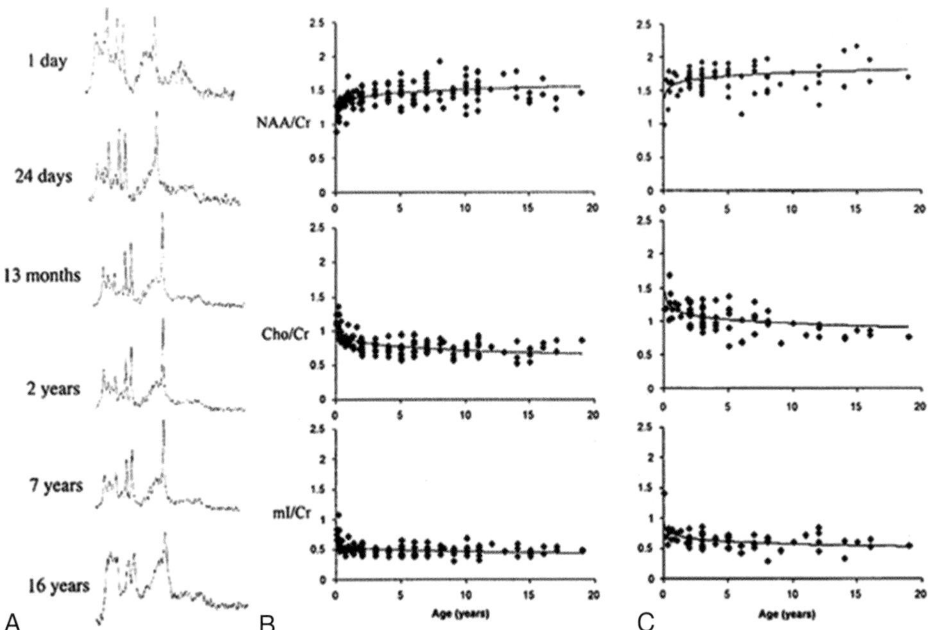

Fig. 1.20 Representative spectra (A) acquired at short echo within the basal ganglia reflect the progression of gray matter metabolite signal intensities with age. The metabolite signal dependence upon age is graphically illustrated with the metabolite ratio curves plotted against age for the basal ganglia (B) and frontal white matter (C). These values were obtained using the PROBE-PRESS (GE Medical Systems, Milwaukee, WI) technique with TE 35 ms and TR 2,000 ms. (From Cecil KM, Jones BV. Magnetic resonance spectroscopy of the pediatric brain. *Top Magn Reson Imaging*. 2001 Dec;12[6]:435–452.)

REFERENCE

1. Cecil KM, Jones BV. Magnetic resonance spectroscopy of the pediatric brain. *Top Magn Reson Imaging*. 2001 Dec;12(6):435–452.

BRAIN DEVELOPMENT: FUNCTIONAL MRI

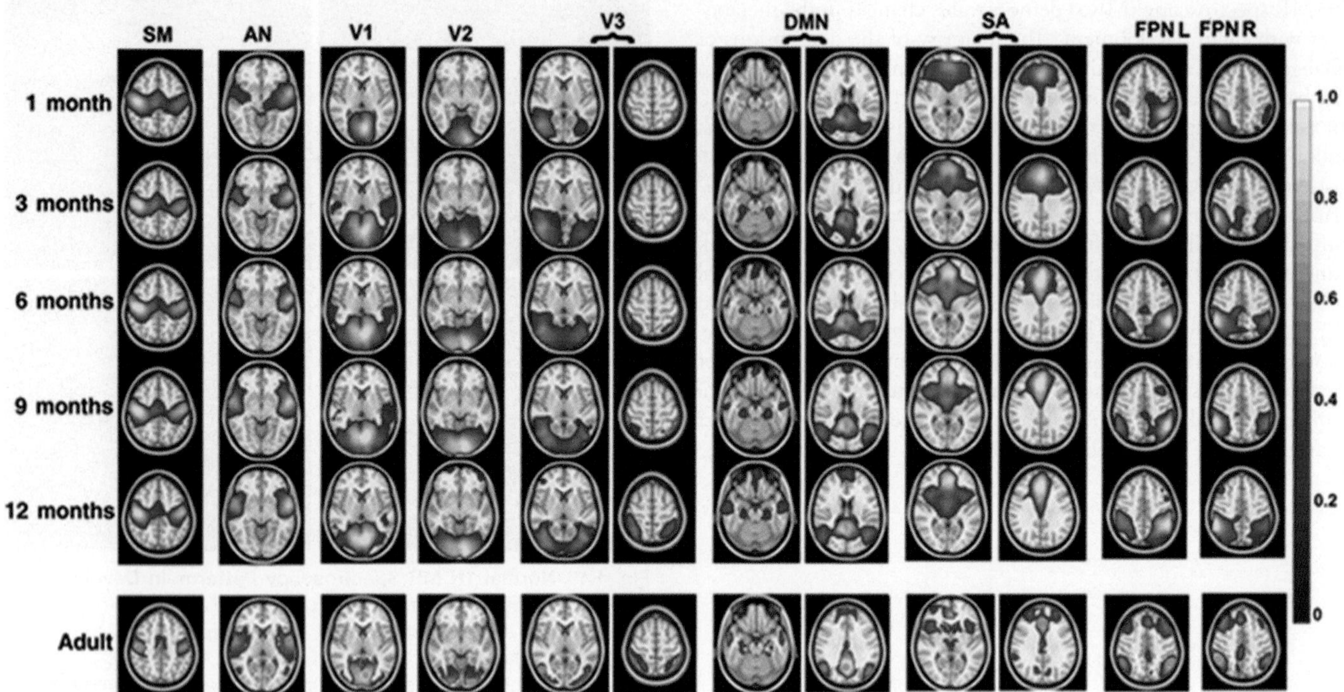

Fig. 1.21 Development during the first year of life comparison to the adult network patterns of nine brain cortical functional networks: sensorimotor *(SM)*, auditory network *(AN)*, medial occipital visual network *(V1)*, occipital pole visual network *(V2)*, lateral visual/parietal network *(V3)*, default mode network *(DMN)*, salience network *(SA)*, and frontoparietal networks *(FPN)*. *Color bar* indicates correlation strength. (From Gao W, Alcauter S, Elton A, et al. Functional network development during the first year: relative sequence and socioeconomic correlations. *Cereb Cortex*. 2015 Sep;25[9]:2919–2928.)

Using resting state functional MRI, network connectivity can be demonstrated in the fetal and neonatal brain. The sensorimotor *(SM)*, auditory network *(AN)*, and two primary visual networks (*V1* and *V2*) demonstrate connectivity patterns at birth that undergo minimal changes in the first year of life and resemble adult patterns, suggesting these networks are the earliest developing functional networks. Meanwhile, the default mode network *(DMN)*, salience network *(SA)*, lateral visual/parietal network *(V3)*, and frontoparietal networks *(FPN)* undergo significant changes in connectivity in the first year of life. The V3 and DMN networks more closely resemble adult network patterns at the end of the first year of life compared to SA and FPN.

CRANIUM AND SKULL BASE DEVELOPMENT

The mesenchyme surrounding the cranial end of the notochord and neural tube forms the facial bones, calvarium, and skull base. The notochord terminates at the inferior border of the dorsum sella, and a remnant remains visible at 10 weeks of gestation and could explain the predilection of chordomas for the central skull base. The calvarium begins to ossify at the eighth to ninth week of gestation. The frontal and supraoccipital bones are the first to ossify followed by the parietal bones. The frontal bones, parietal bones, interparietal portion of the occipital bone, and medial pterygoid plates of the sphenoid bone ossify by membranous ossification, the greater wings of the sphenoid are unique in that they ossify by both membranous and enchondral ossification, and the remainder of the bone ossify by enchondral ossification. The sphenooccipital synchondrosis persists until age 15 to 18 years and allows the skull base to continue to grow. Many skeletal disorders such as achondroplasia will have premature closure of the sphenooccipital suture and a small central skull base and narrow foramen magnum.

Fibroblast growth factors (FGFs) and the FGF receptors (FGFRs) are important in keeping a balance between proliferation of osteoprogenitor cells and differentiation of new bone of the membranous portions of the calvarium. Suture closure occurs when the balance shifts to bone production. Many genetic disorders of FGFRs, such as Apert syndrome, result in craniosynostosis.

During the first three years of life the diploic space of the calvarium is thin and the bone is primarily hypointense on T1W. From ages 3 to 7 years the diploic space increases and the marrow space between the inner and outer cortical bone widens and becomes hyperintense on T1W MRI.

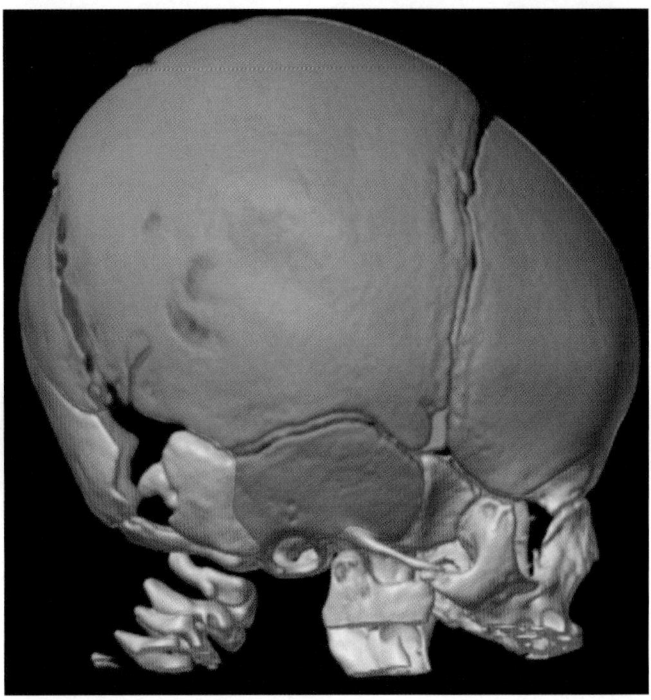

Fig. 1.22 Skull Development. Membranous ossification occurs in areas in *purple*, while the remainder ossifies by enchondral ossification.

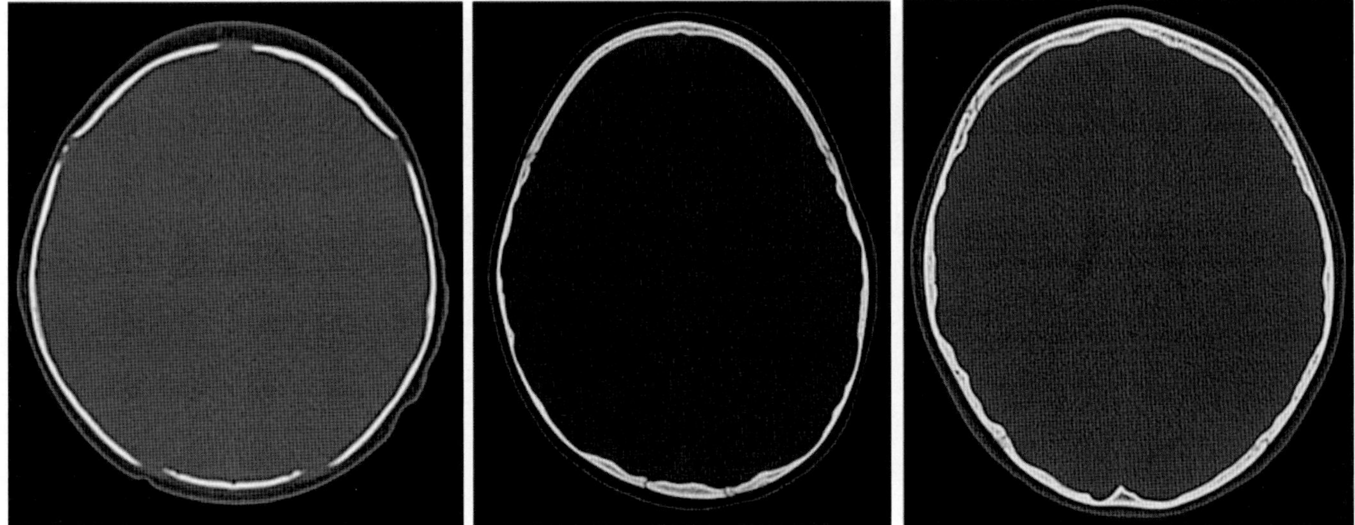

Fig. 1.23 Representative axial CT demonstrate the progressive thickening that occurs in the (A) neonate, (B) 3-year-old toddler, and (C) 10-year-old child.

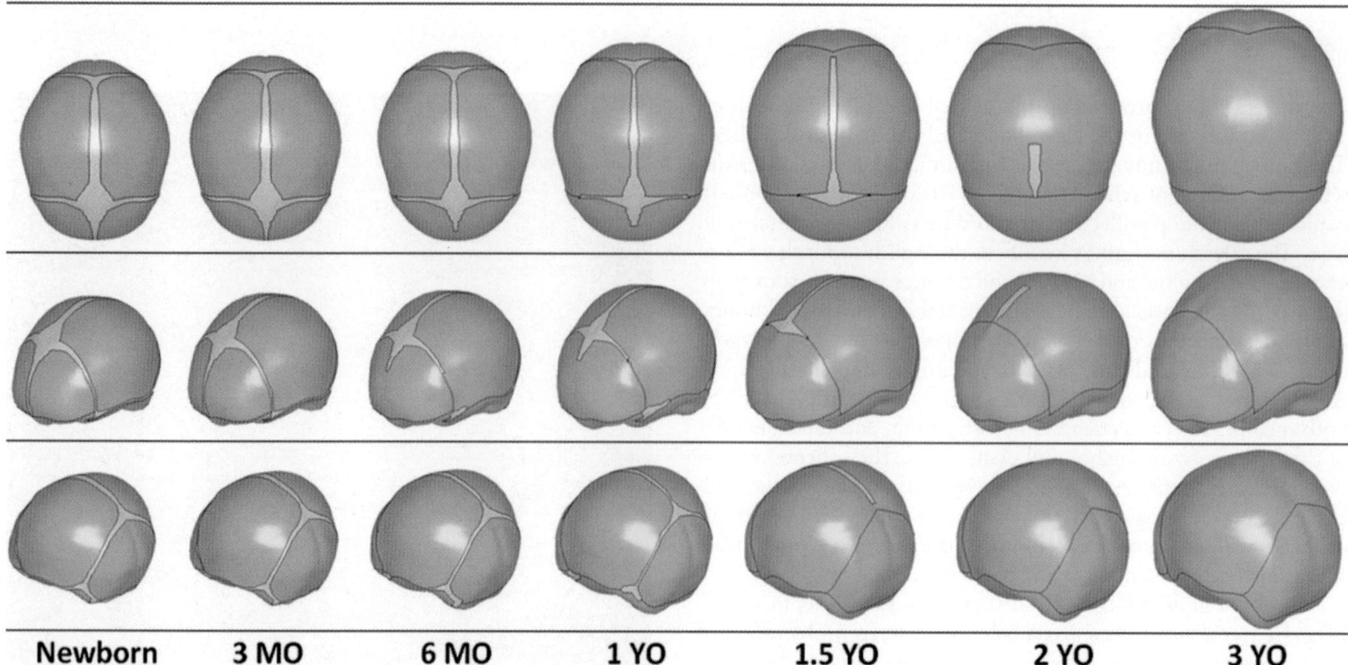

Fig. 1.24 Skull Development. Skull size/shape and suture changes by age. (From Li Z, Park BK, Liu W, Zhang J, Reed MP, Rupp JD, Hoff CN, Hu J. A statistical skull geometry model for children 0-3 years old. *PLoS One*. 2015 May 18;10[5]:e0127322.)

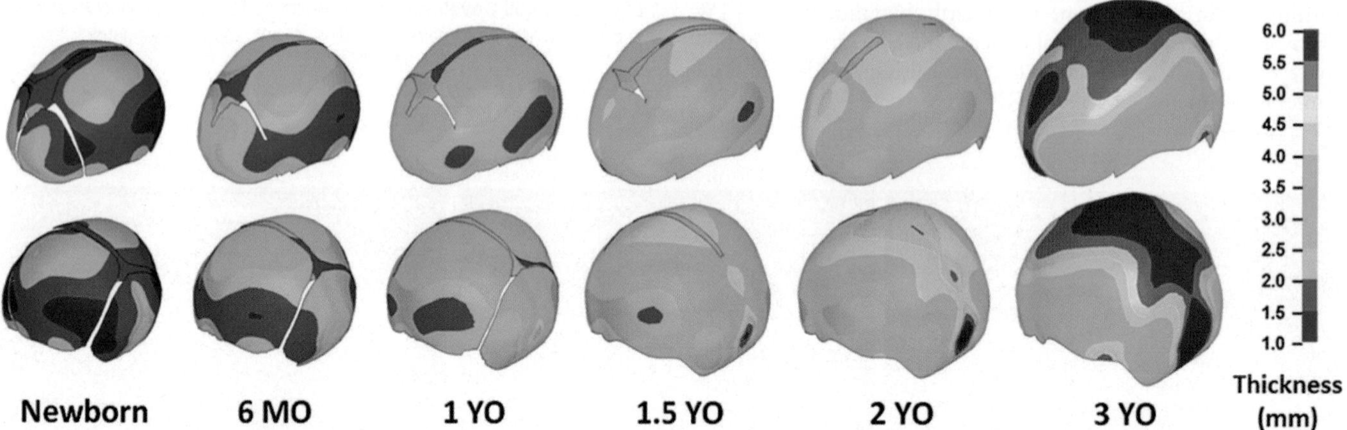

Fig. 1.25 Skull Development. Skull thickness distribution by age. (From Li Z, Park BK, Liu W, Zhang J, Reed MP, Rupp JD, Hoff CN, Hu J. A statistical skull geometry model for children 0-3 years old. *PLoS One*. 2015 May 18;10[5]:e0127322.)

SKULL SUTURE VARIANTS

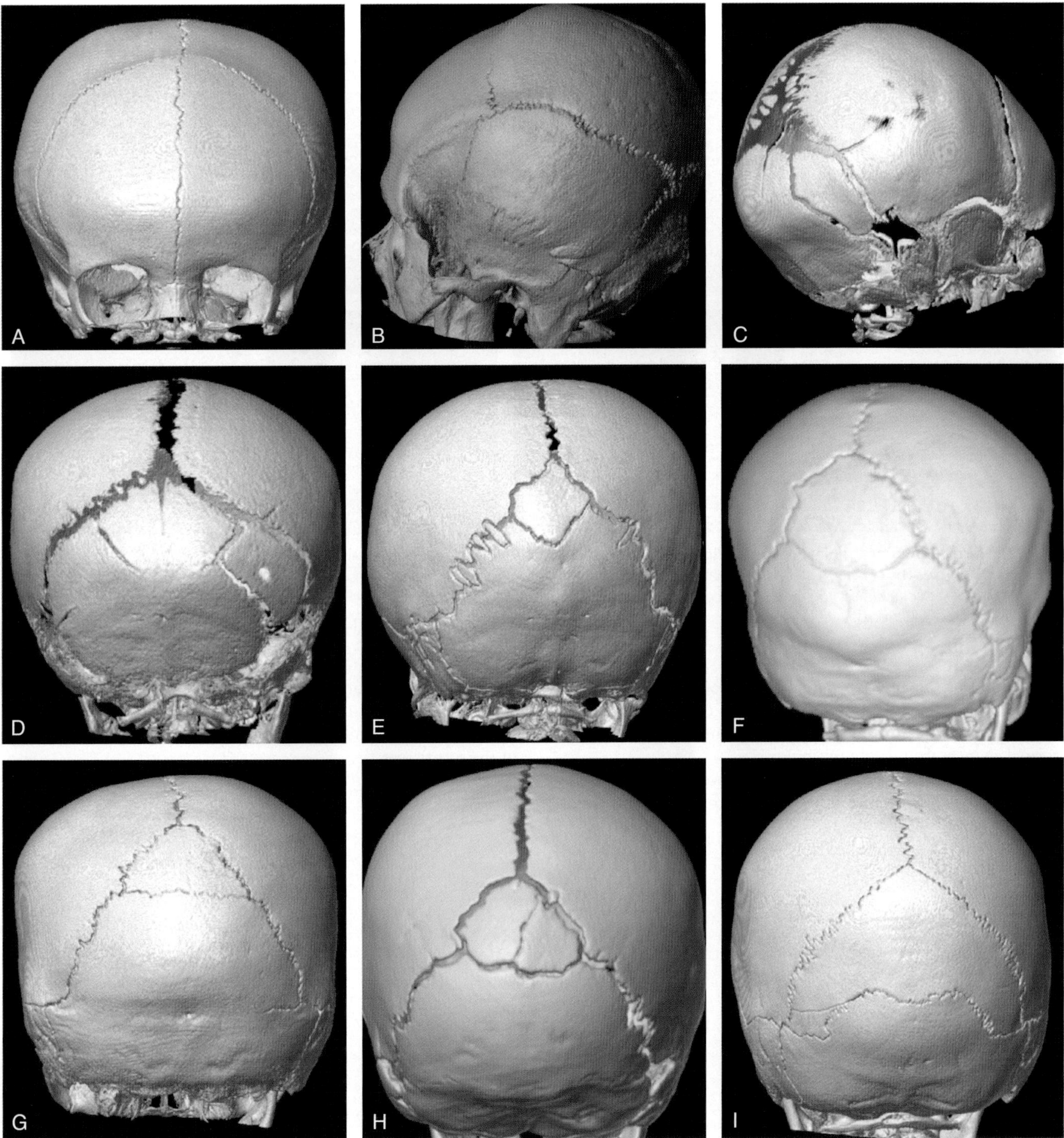

Fig. 1.26 Skull Suture Variants. 3D volumetric reconstructions are useful for recognizing an anatomic variant of the sutures which on 2D CT images may mimic a fracture. (A) Persistent metopic suture. (B) Accessory parietal suture. (C) Remnant of an accessory parietal suture, a midline and lateral occipital suture, and lateral accessory occipital ossification center. (D) Small remnants of accessory parietal sutures and midline and lateral occipital sutures with a lateral accessory ossification center. (E to H) Accessory occipital sutures forming a midline superior occipital ossification center. (I) Transversely oriented persistent mendosal suture. A fracture extends laterally from the right side of the accessory suture.

NORMAL ANTERIOR CRANIAL FOSSA DEVELOPMENT

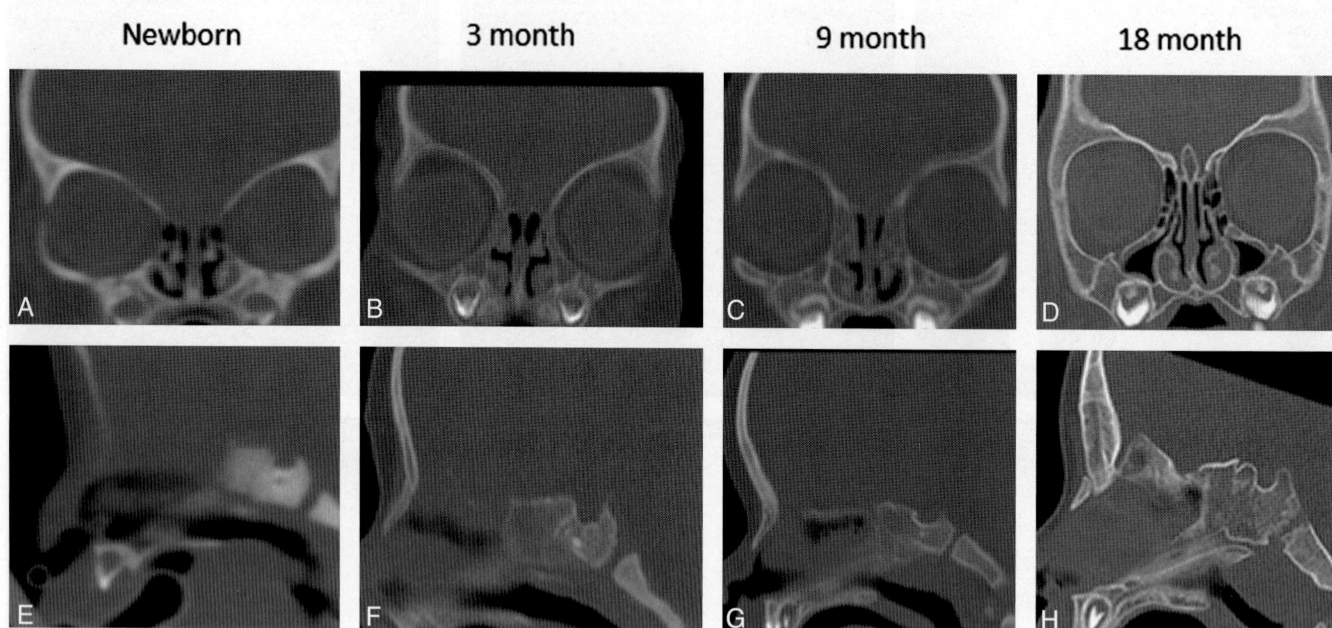

Fig. 1.27 Normal Anterior Cranial Fossa Ossification. Coronal and sagittal CT imaging in (A, E) newborn, (B, F) 3-month-old, (C, G) 9-month-old, and (D, H) 18-month-old. The cribriform plate ossifies lateral to medial beginning at 6 to 8 months and is complete by 12 to 14 months. The crista galli ossification begins at 6 to 8 months, progresses posterior to anterior, and is complete by 18 months. A bifid crista galli (not seen here) should raise suspicions for the presence of a dermoid.

Ossification of the anterior cranial fossa occurs in neonates and infants and leads to changes in appearance on imaging. Understanding the normal imaging appearance can help prevent these normal changes from being misinterpreted.

Dedicated imaging and evaluation of the anterior cranial fossa are generally not performed unless there is concern for an abnormality of the anterior cranial fossa, such as in the setting of a potential nasal dermoid or encephalocele. CT best depicts the ossification changes, while MRI provides complementary assessment of the soft tissues.

NORMAL SINUS DEVELOPMENT

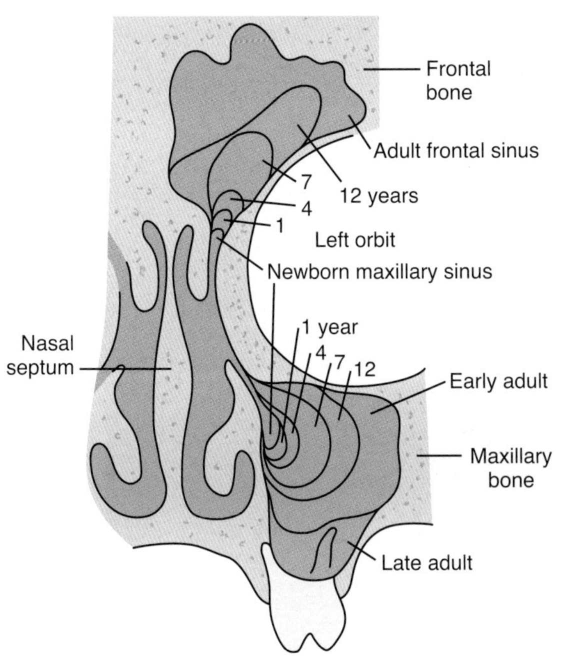

Fig. 1.28 Development of paranasal sinuses from newborn to adult. (From Davis PJ, Cladis FP, Motoyama EK. *Smith's Anesthesia for Infants and Children.* 8th ed. Mosby; 2011.)

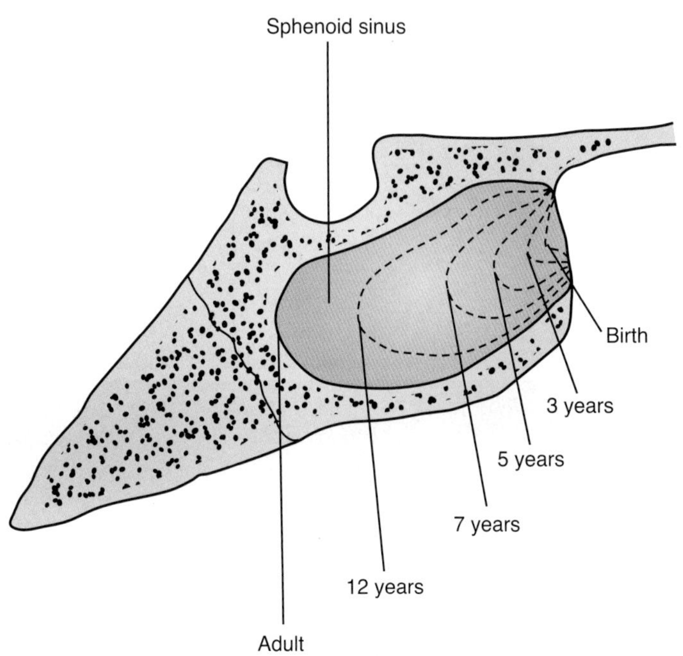

Fig. 1.29 The sphenoid sinus contains red marrow at birth. Development is complete by age 14. (From Zitelli BJ, McIntire SC, Nowalk A. *Zitelli and Davis' Atlas of Pediatric Physical Diagnosis.* 7th ed. Elsevier; 2018.)

Sinus Development

Ethmoid sinus: Present at birth. Progresses posteriorly and lateral walls become convex.

Maxillary sinus: Present at birth with only a small portion beneath the orbit. Extends past the infraorbital canal by age 4. Reaches the maxillary bone and hard palate by age 9. Pneumatizes the alveolar ridge after the permanent teeth erupt.

Sphenoid sinus: Contains red marrow at birth. Pneumatization proceeds in an inferior, posterior, and lateral direction. Complete by age 14.

Frontal sinus: Not present at birth. Last sinus to develop. Pneumatizes at age 2. Reaches half the orbital height by age 4 and reaches top of the orbit by age 8. Extends into frontal bone by age 10. Reaches full size after puberty.

NORMAL SINUS DEVELOPMENT

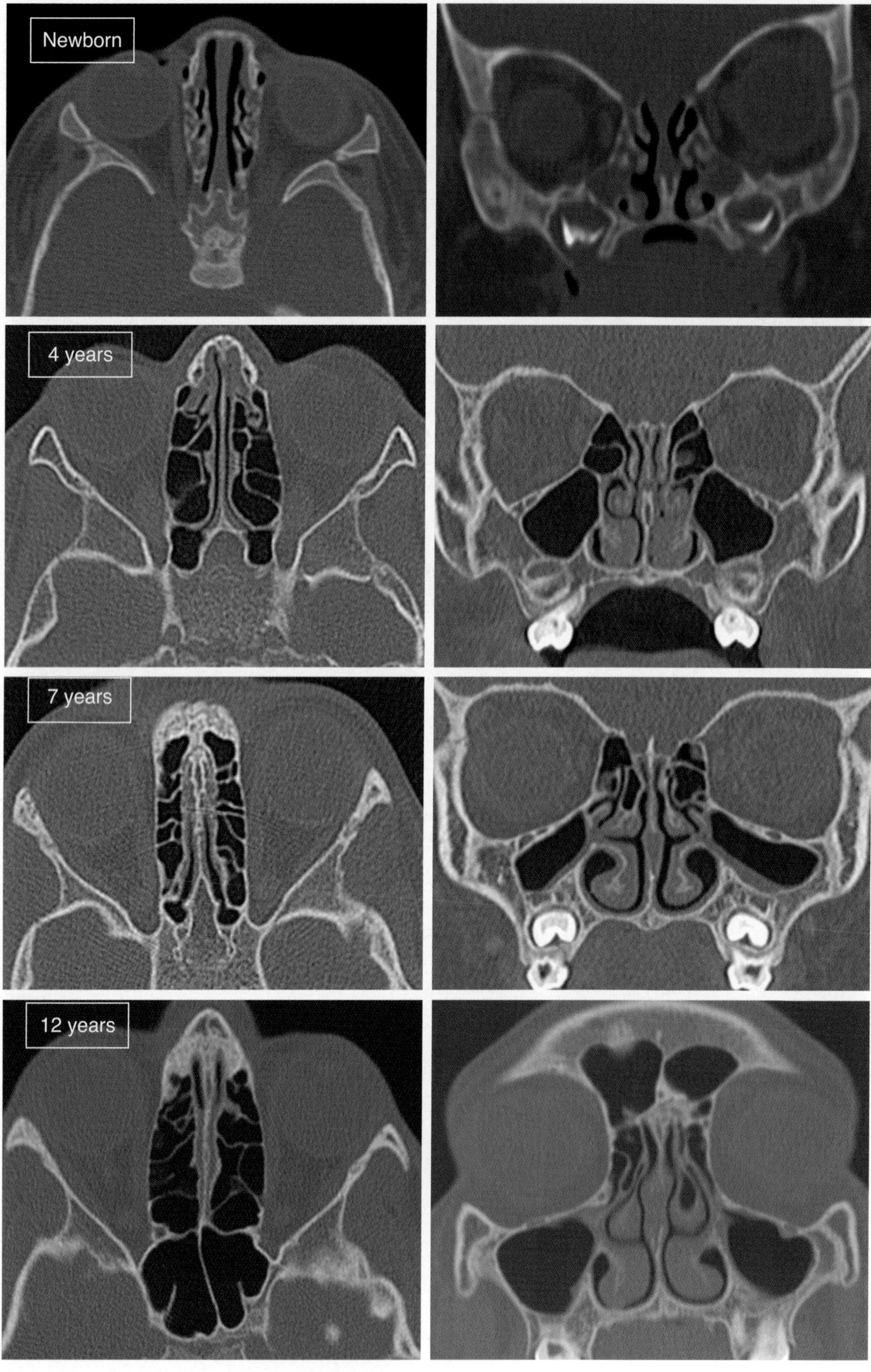

FACE AND NECK EMBRYOLOGY

The face is formed by cell streams after migration of neural crest cells. Rostrally the neural crest cells cover the forebrain and are divided by the optic vesicle. The medial stream forms the frontonasal process. Caudally the cells migrate to the first branchial arches. The face forms from the frontonasal process, two maxillary processes, and two mandibular processes. The branchial arches lead to development of the neck.

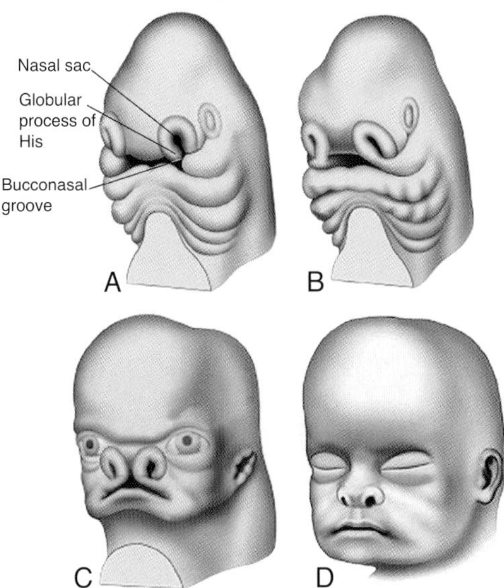

Fig. 1.30 Anterior oblique drawing of a 5-week embryo (A) shows the further growth of the medial and lateral nasal processes and the development of the nasal sac. The bucconasal groove is shown. (B) Anterior oblique drawing of a 6-week embryo shows closure of bucconasal groove completing the floor of the nasal cavity and progressive flattening of the nasal sac openings, mainly as a result of ventrolateral growth of the medial nasal processes. The nasal sacs are also pushed toward the midline as the maxillary processes grow. Anterior oblique drawing of a 7-week embryo (C) and a 10-week (D) embryo shows the progressive medial movement of the nasal sacs and the resulting progressive pushing upward of the frontonasal process. (Som PM, Naidich TP. Illustrated review of the embryology and development of the facial region, part 1: Early face and lateral nasal cavities. *AJNR Am J Neuroradiol*. 2013 Dec;34[12]:2233–2240. doi:10.3174/ajnr.A3415. Epub 2013 Mar 14. PMID: 23493891; PMCID: PMC7965203. Copyright © 2013 by American Journal of Neuroradiology.)

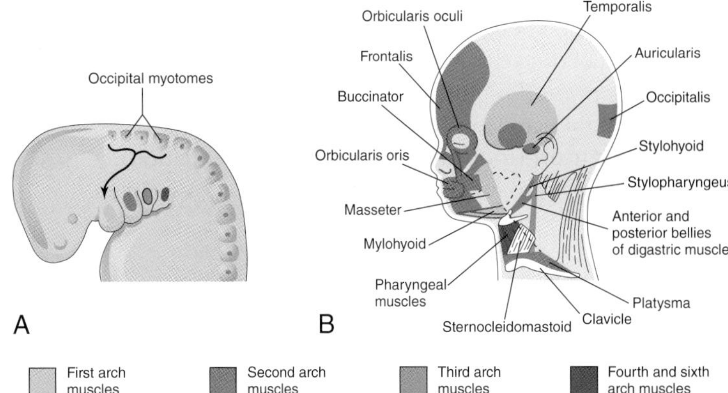

Fig. 1.31 (A) Lateral view of the head, neck, and thoracic regions of a 4-week embryo showing the muscles derived from the pharyngeal arches. The *arrow* shows the pathway taken by myoblasts from the occipital myotomes to form the tongue musculature. (B) The head and neck regions of a 20-week fetus, showing the muscles derived from the pharyngeal arches. Parts of the platysma and sternocleidomastoid muscles have been removed to show the deeper muscles. Note that myoblasts from the second arch migrate from the neck to the head, where they give rise to the muscles of facial expression. These muscles are supplied by the facial nerve (cranial nerve VII), the nerve of the second pharyngeal arch. (From Moore, Keith L, TVN Persaud, Torchia MG. *Before We Are Born: Essentials of Embryology and Birth Defects.* 10th ed. Elsevier; 2020.)

TABLE 1.4 Derivatives of the Branchial Complex

Derivative	Cleft (Ectoderm)	Arch (Mesoderm)	Pouch (Endoderm)
First	External auditory canal	Mandible	Eustachian tube
		Muscles of mastication	
Second	Sinus of His	Muscles of facial expression	Palantine tonsil
		Malleus and incus	Supratonsillar fossa
		Hyoid bone	
Third	Sinus of His	Hyoid bone Stylopharyngeus muscle	Inferior parathyroid glands
			Thymus
Fourth	Sinus of His	Epiglottis Thyroid cartilage Pharyngeal muscles Aortic arch	Superior parathyroid glands
Fifth/Sixth		Cartilage of neck	

From Babyn PS. *Teaching Atlas of Pediatric Imaging.* Thieme Medical Publishers; 2006.

REFERENCE

1. Som PM, Naidich TP. Illustrated review of the embryology and development of the facial region, part 1: Early face and lateral nasal cavities. *AJNR Am J Neuroradiol.* 2013 Dec;34(12):2233–2240.

SPINE EMBRYOLOGY

Spine Embryology

The formation of the spine occurs during the second through sixth weeks of gestation through:

- Gastrulation (weeks 2–3): Conversion of a bilaminar to trilaminar layer with the middle layer the mesoderm.
- Primary neurulation (weeks 3–4): The notochord interacts with the overlying ectoderm to form the neural plate (Fig. 1.32, A). The neural plate then bends to begin formation of the neural tube (B). Continued infolding of neural plate (C). Disjunction is the separation of the neural tube from the ectoderm (D).
- Secondary neurulation and retrogressive differentiation.
- Spinal dysraphisms occur when these processes are disrupted.

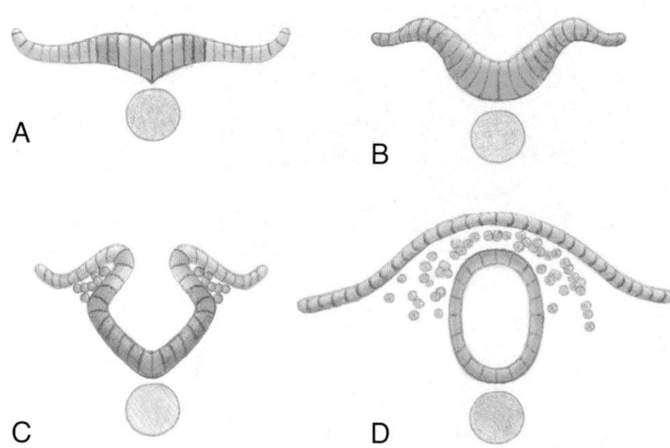

Fig. 1.32 Spine Formation, Second Through Sixth Weeks.

Classification of Spinal Dysraphisms and Imaging Approach

Spinal dysraphisms can be classified by embryologic anomaly (Fig. 1.33). This classification is important; however, an imaging algorithm, as follows, is more clinically useful:

- Determine whether the malformation is exposed to the skin to determine whether the malformation is a closed or open defect.
- Determine whether there is a subcutaneous mass.
- Determine the necessary imaging features for final diagnosis.

REFERENCE

1. Huisman TA, Rossi A, Tortori-Donati P. MR imaging of neonatal spinal dysraphia: what to consider? *Magn Reson Imaging Clin N Am.* 2012 Feb;20(1):45–61.

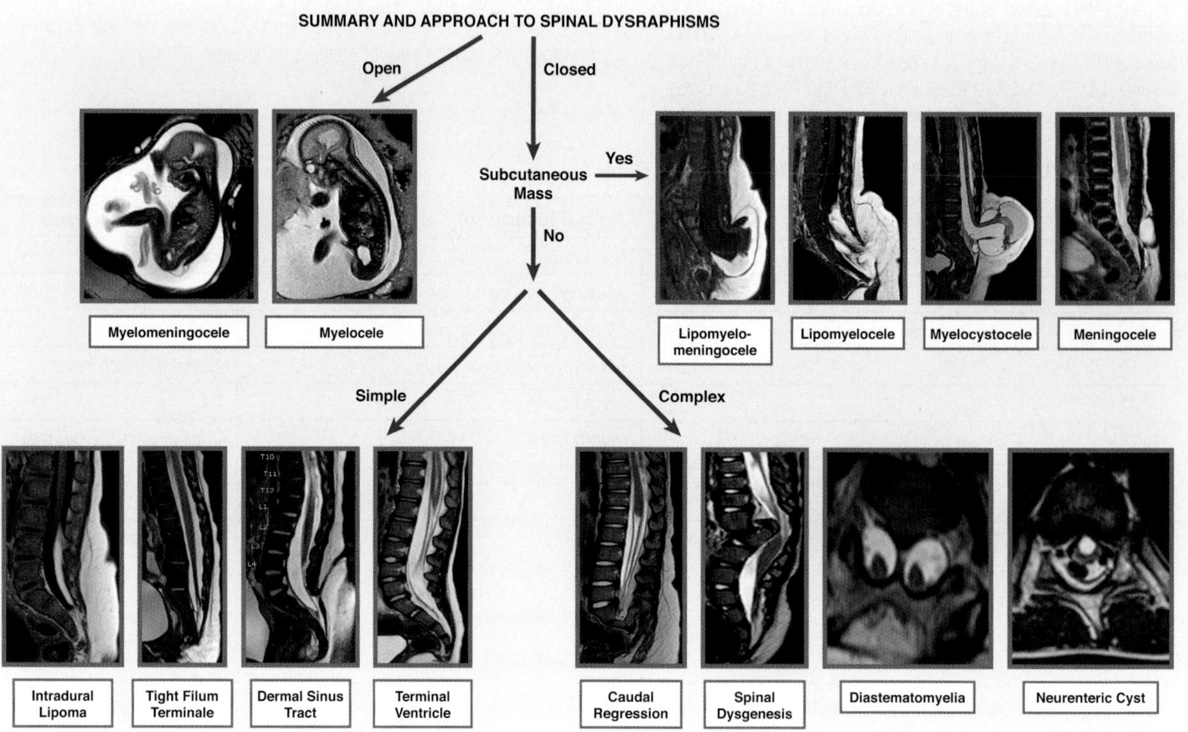

Fig. 1.33 Imaging Approach to Spinal Dysraphisms.

SPINE EMBRYOLOGY

Notochord and somites are the primary structures responsible for the vertebral column. Each somite develops into a sclerotome (spine) and a dermomyotome (muscle and overlying dermis of the spine). Fusion of adjacent sclerotomes eventually forms each vertebral body.

Formation of the vertebrae and anomalies of vertebral formation can be understood through embryology. The notochord induces the mesoderm to condense into pairs of somites. The somites will develop into myotomes, which form the muscle, skin, and sclerotomes, which, in turn, form the cartilage, bones, and ligaments. At the fourth or fifth gestational week, each sclerotome will undergo segmentation into a cranial and caudal half. The caudal half of one sclerotome combines with the cranial half of the next sclerotome. This leads to the intersegmental artery trapped in the center of the vertebral body. Simultaneously portions of the notochord will disintegrate, and small portions will remain as the nucleus pulposis. Between days 40 and 60, the vertebral mesenchyme will undergo chondrification. All vertebrae develop from three primary ossification centers, except the C2 vertebrae.

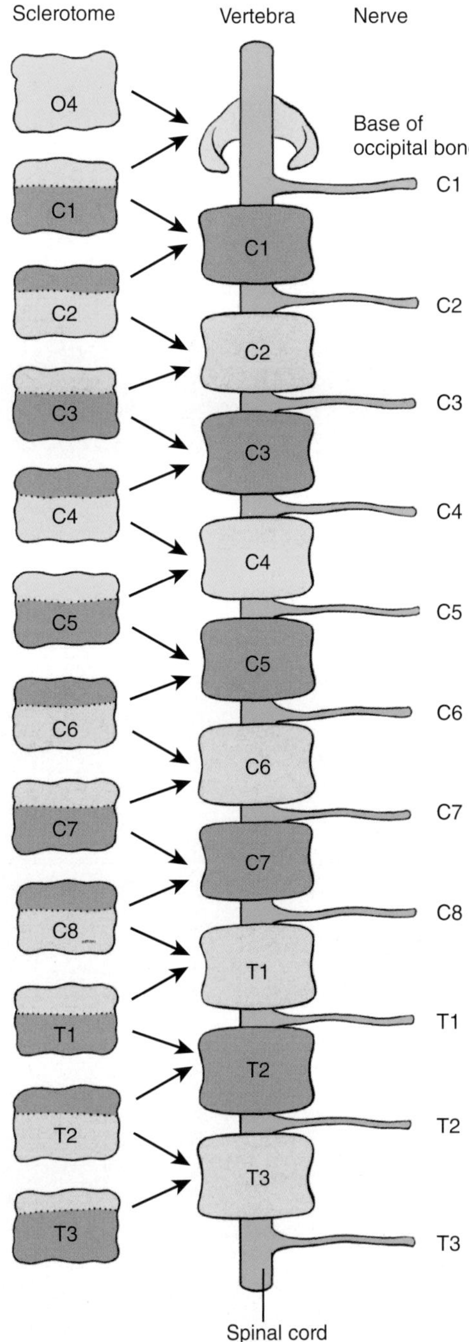

Fig. 1.34 The mechanism by which the cervical region develops eight cervical nerves but only seven cervical vertebrae. The ventral roots of spinal nerves grow out from the spinal cord toward the sclerotome. With resegmentation of the sclerotomes, the cranial half of the first cervical sclerotome fuses with the occipital bone of the skull. As a result, the nerve projecting to the first cervical somite is now located cranial to the first cervical vertebrae. In the thoracic, lumbar, and sacral regions, the number of spinal nerves matches the number of vertebrae. (From Schoenwolf GC, Bleyl SB, Brauer PR, Francis-West PH. *Larsen's Human Embryology.* 6th ed. Elsevier; 2022.)

SPINE OSSIFICATION CENTERS

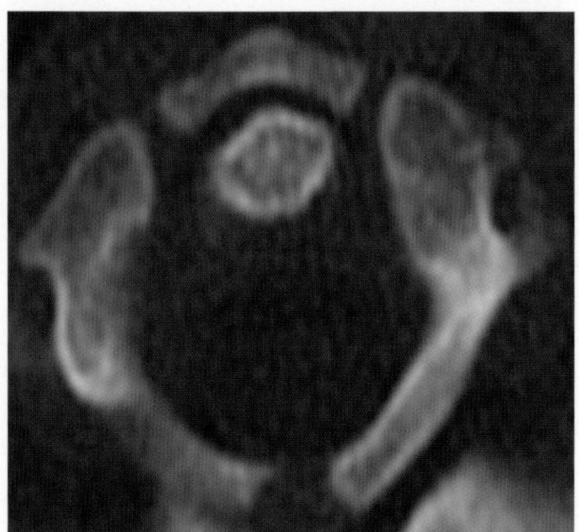

C1 Vertebrae

3 ossification centers:

1. Anterior arch: Ossifies at 1 year; complete ossification and fusion in 80% of children by 12 years
2. Two neural arches: Fuse posteriorly in 80% by 5 years

Many ossification variants of C1 exist, including no anterior ossification center, multiple anterior ossification centers, and a central posterior arch ossification center.

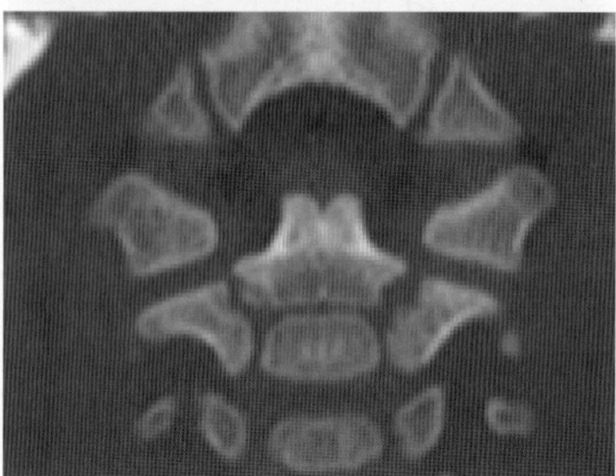

C2 Vertebrae

6 ossification centers:

1. Odontoid tip: Fusion at the apicodental synchondrosis occurs in 80% by 10½ years
2. Odontoid: Two ossification centers fused in the midline at birth
3. Body: Fusion at the subdental synchondrosis (between the dens and body), and neurocentral synchondroses (between the body and neurocentral arches) occurs in 80% by 9 years
4. Neural arches: Two ossification centers that fuse posteriorly at 2 to 3 years

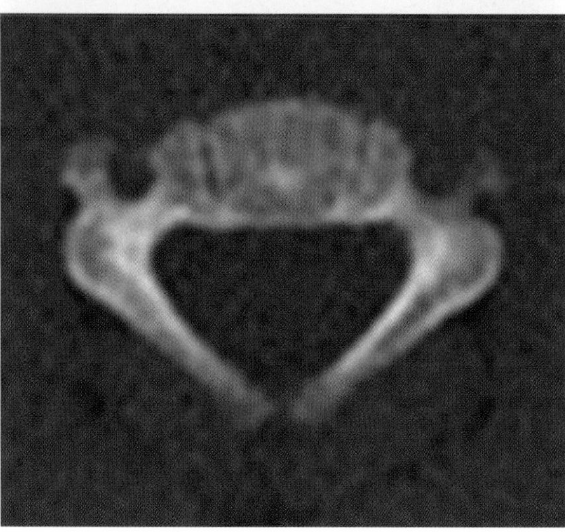

C3-C7 Vertebrae

3 ossification centers:

1. Body: Fuses with neural arches by 3 to 6 years
2. Two neural arches: Fuse posteriorly at 2 to 3 years

Secondary ossification centers at the tips of transverse processes, and spinous processes may persist to the third decade.

REFERENCE

1. Karwacki GM, Schneider JF. Normal ossification patterns of atlas and axis: a CT study. *AJNR Am J Neuroradiol.* 2012 Nov;33(10):1882–1887.

SPINE OSSIFICATION VARIANTS

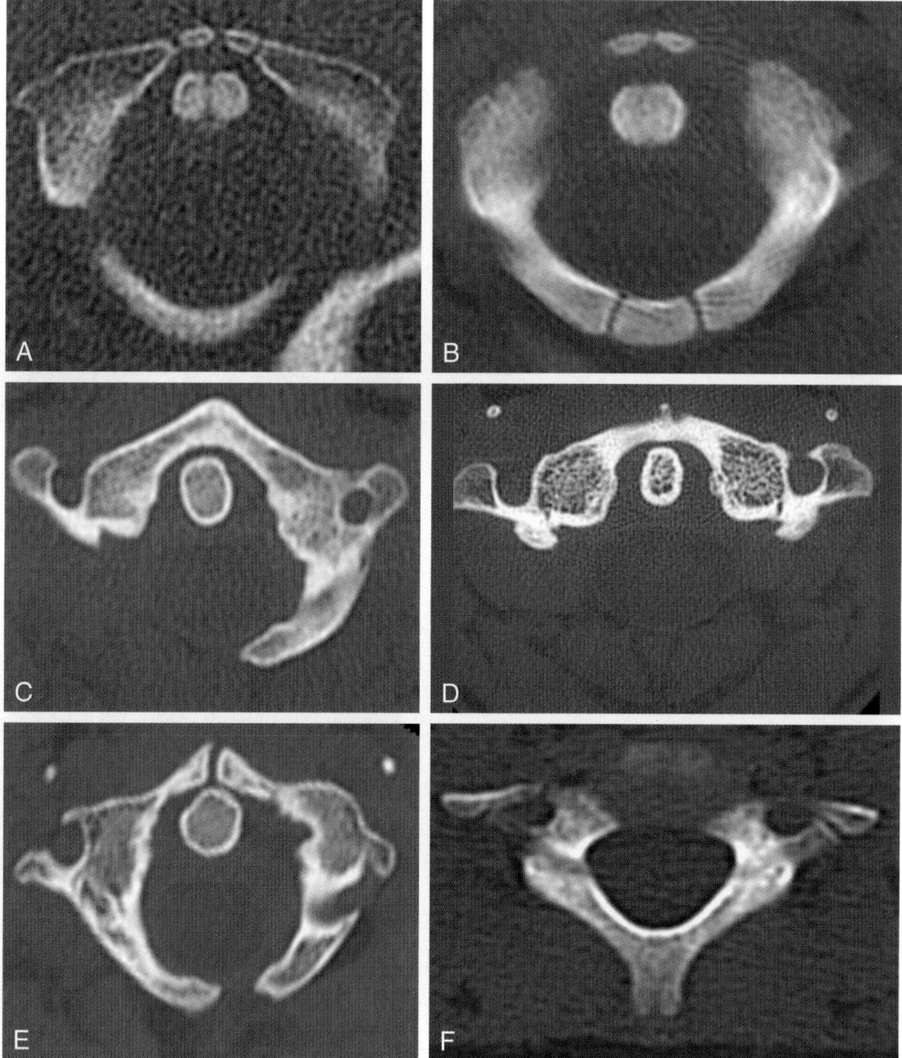

Fig. 1.35 Spine Ossification Variants. (A) Two ossification centers in the anterior arch of C1. (B) Central ossification center in the posterior arch of C1. (C) Absent right posterior arch of C1. (D) Absence of both posterior arches of C1. (E) Incomplete fusion of the anterior and posterior arches of C1. (F) Incomplete fusion of the transverse processes of C7.

REFERENCE

1. Hyun G, Allam E, Sander P, et al. The prevalence of congenital C1 arch anomalies. *Eur Spine J.* 2018 Jun;27(6):1266–1271.

MRI OF SPINE DEVELOPMENT

Three patterns are identified on MRI with spine development that are due to changes in the hematopoietic-to-fatty marrow ratio and ossification of the bone. Individual time frames are an approximation and not meant to categorize an individual as skeletally mature or immature.

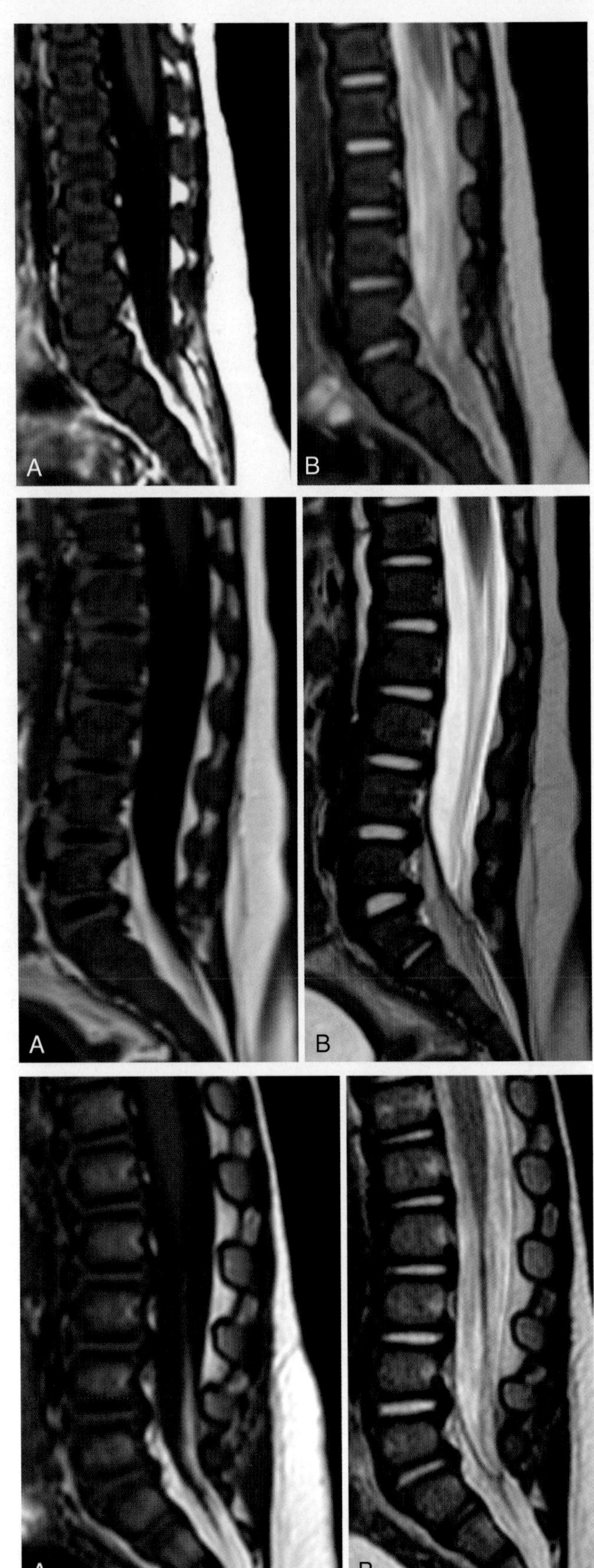

Stage 1: Approximately Age < 1 Month

T1W: Center of vertebral body is smaller and less intense relative to the cartilage endplates; cartilage endplates are hyperintense and create a bowtie appearance; intervertebral disc is isointense.

T2W: Endplates are slightly less intense than the vertebral body; intervertebral disc is hyperintense.

Stage 2: Approximately Age 1–6 Months

T1W: Center of vertebral body appears larger relative to the cartilage endplates; cartilage endplates are hyperintense; intervertebral disc is isointense.

T2W: Endplates are more hypointense and contrasting to the vertebral body; intervertebral disc is hyperintense.

Stage 3: Approximately Age > 7 Months

T1W: Vertebral bodies are hyperintense to muscle and become rectangular by 2 years of age with exception of the corners, which are still cartilaginous; endplates are primarily hypointense, except the corners, which will gradually become hypointense; intervertebral disc is isointense.

T2W: Hypointense endplates and mild hyperintensity of the vertebral body; intervertebral disc is hyperintense.

REFERENCE

1. Sze G, Baierl P, Bravo S. Evolution of the infant spinal column: evaluation with MR imaging. *Radiology*. 1991 Dec;181(3):819–827.

2 Brain Malformations

INTRODUCTION

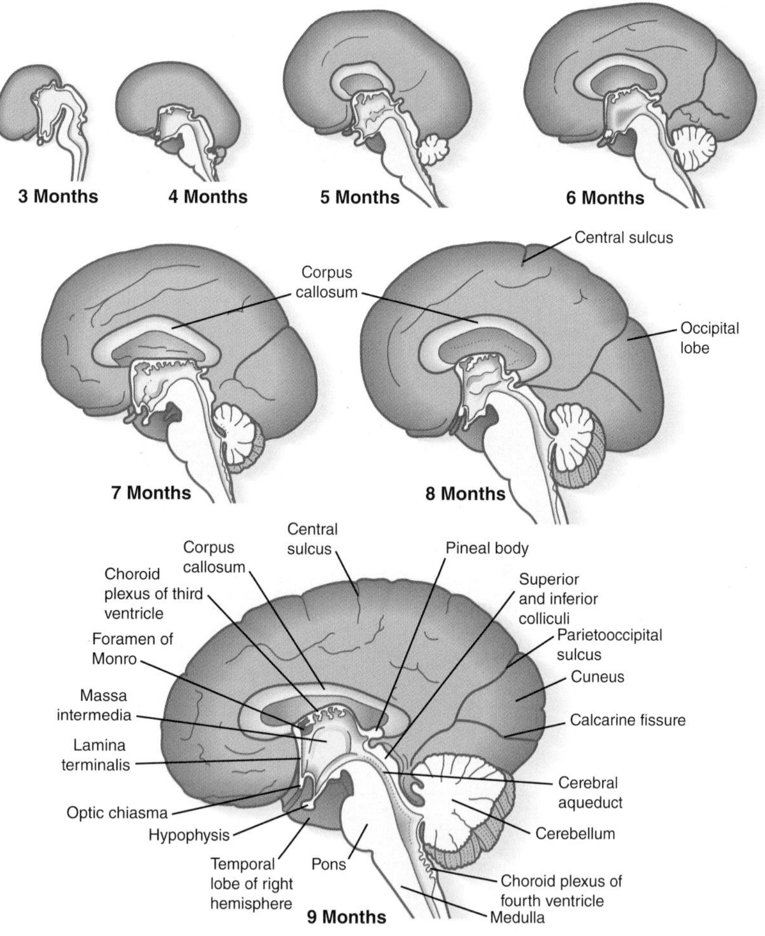

Fig. 2.1 Medial Views of the Developing Brain. (From Carlson BM. *Human Embryology and Developmental Biology*. 6th ed. Elsevier; 2019.)

Brain malformations represent a disruption of normal development and can be caused by genetic, infectious, ischemic, and hemorrhagic factors. As seen in Table 2.1, the time at which the insult occurs during development will determine the malformation. Because the majority of brain malformations occur early in development, the majority of malformations will be present when imaging is performed. Brain malformations are often first encountered on ultrasound and magnetic resonance imaging (MRI). In general, MRI provides the best assessment of brain malformation.

A pattern approach is necessary to detect malformations; more than one structure can be malformed. Major intracranial structures that should be evaluated include the following:

- Size, sulcation, gyration, and myelination of the cerebral hemispheres
- Size, formation, and proportions of the cerebellum, brainstem, and posterior fossa
- Presence of the septum pellucidum and formation and size of the corpus callosum
- Presence of the olfactory bulbs and sulci
- Formation and size of the basal ganglia and thalami
- Rotation of the hippocampi
- Formation and size of the ventricles

Importantly, assessment of extracranial structures should include the eyes, ears, and facial bones as anomalies in these structures have associated brain anomalies. This chapter will focus on the imaging appearance of brain malformations and provide basic embryology underlying the malformation.

■ TABLE 2.1 Timing of Developmental Events

Week	Major Developments	Appearance	Malformations
3	Neural groove and folds Three primary vesicles visible Cervical and cephalic flexures Motor neurons appear	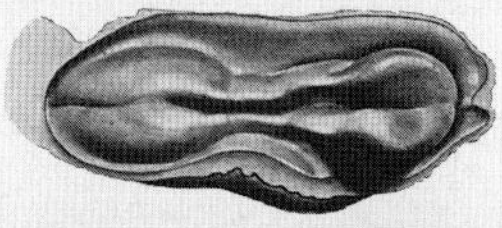	Neural tube defects
4	Neural tube starts to close (day 22) Rostral end of neural tube closes (day 24) Caudal end of neural tube closes (day 26) Neural crest cells begin to migrate Secondary neurulation starts Motor nerves emerge	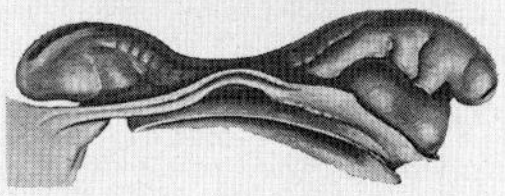	Neural tube defects, holoprosencephaly
5	Optic vesicle, pontine flexure Five secondary vesicles visible Sulcus limitans, sensory ganglia Sensory nerves grow into CNS Rhombic lips Basal nuclei begin Thalamus, hypothalamus begin Autonomic ganglia, lens, cochlea start	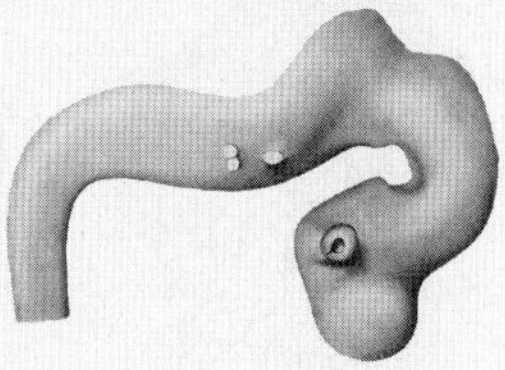	Holoprosencephaly, sacral cord abnormalities
6–7	Telencephalon enlarged Basal nuclei prominent Secondary neurulation complete Cerebellum and optic nerve begin Choroid plexus Insula	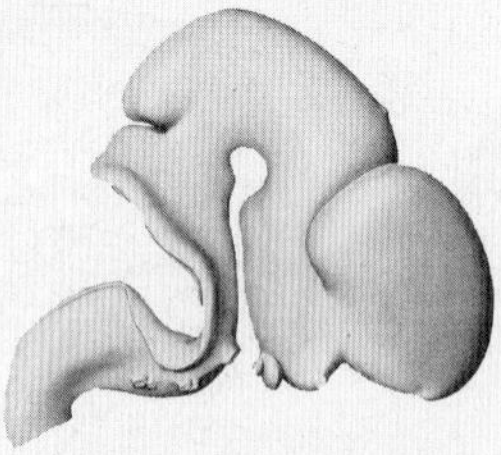	
8–12	Neuronal proliferation Cerebral and cerebellar cortex begin Anterior commissure, optic chiasm Internal capsule Reflexes appear	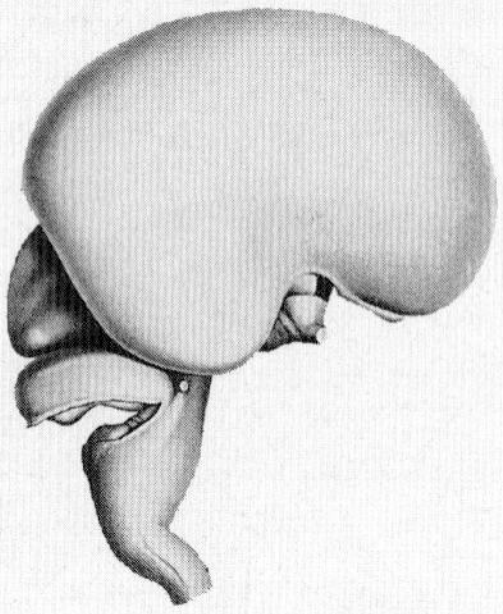	Migration/proliferation problems (e.g., abnormal cortex or gyri)
12–16	Neuronal proliferation and migration Glial differentiation Corpus callosum	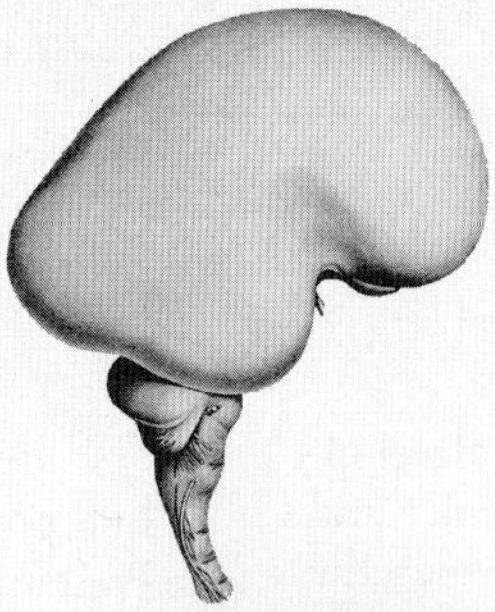	Migration/proliferation problems (e.g., abnormal cortex or gyri)
16–40	Neuronal migration Cortical sulci Glial proliferation Some myelination (mostly postnatal) Synapse formation	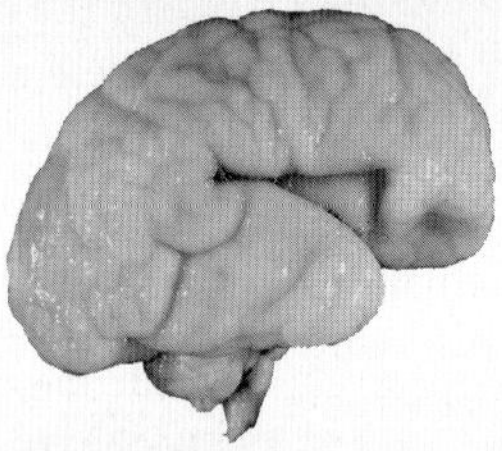	Hemorrhage, other destructive events

Table from Vanderah TW, Gould DJ, Nolte J. *Nolte's The Human Brain: An Introduction to Its Functional Anatomy.* 8th ed. Elsevier; 2021. Top two illustrations from Arey LB. *Developmental Anatomy.* 4th ed. WB Saunders; 1941. Bottom illustration courtesy Dr. Naomi Rance, University of Arizona College of Medicine; all others from Hochstetter F. *Beiträge zur Entwicklungsgeschichte des menschlichen Gehirns.* I. Teil, Franz Deuticke; 1919.

CORPUS CALLOSUM: DEVELOPMENT

Development

The corpus callosum is by far the largest commissure of the three telencephalic commissures and the principal anatomic and neurophysiologic connection pathway between the two hemispheres. The anterior commissure and hippocampal commissure represent the other two smaller telencephalic commissures and are closely related to the formation of the corpus callosum. The anterior commissure connects the olfactory cortex and crosses along the lamina terminalis. The hippocampal commissure is present but indistinguishable from the inferior margin of the posterior corpus callosum and connects the hippocampi. Formation of the corpus callosum is shown in Fig. 2.2.

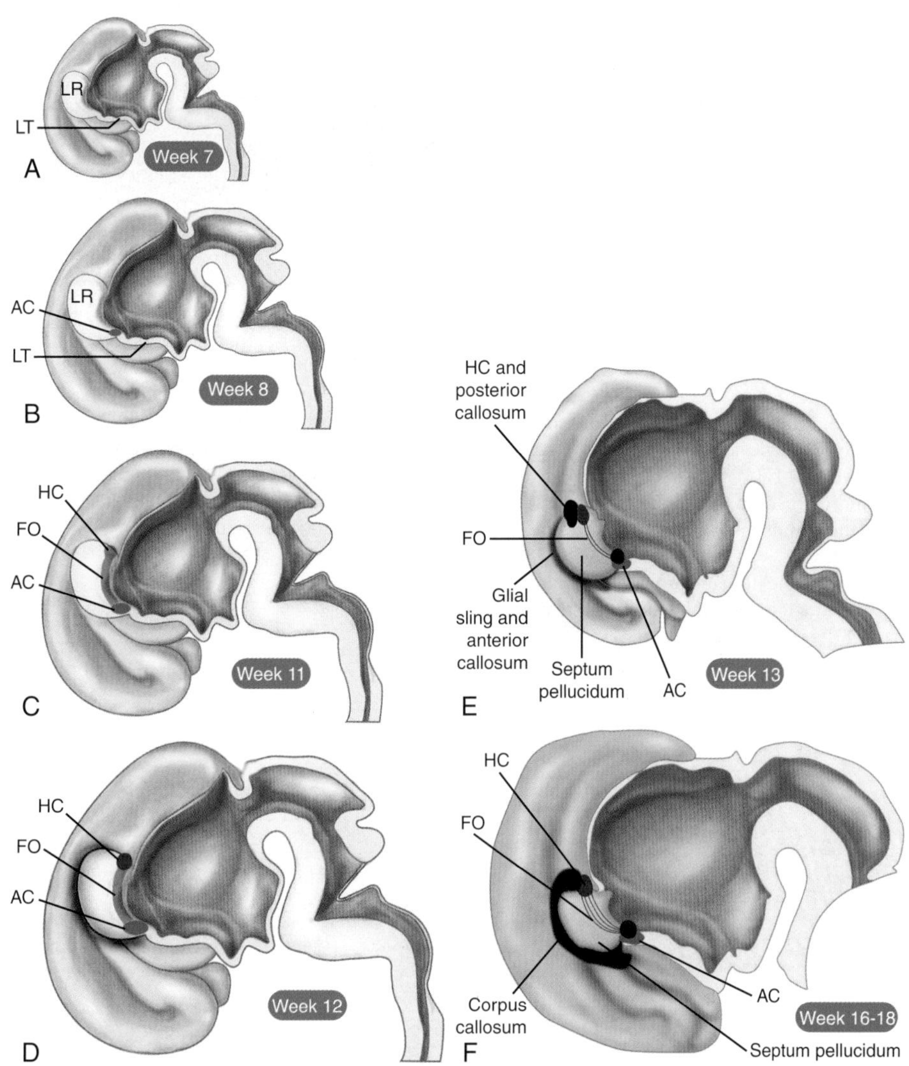

Fig. 2.2 Formation of the Corpus Callosum. (A) During week 7, the upper portion of the lamina terminalis *(LT)*, which connects the hemispheres across the midline, thickens and forms the lamina reuniens *(LR)* of His. (B) In the following week, olfactory commissural fibers cross the midline through the ventral aspect of the LR to form the anterior commissure *(AC)*. (C) In the following weeks, fibers develop between the anterior mediobasal cortex (septal nuclei) and the future hippocampus to form the ipsilateral fornix *(FO)*; about week 11, some forniceal fibers cross the midline in the dorsal portion of the lamina reuniens and form the hippocampal commissure *(HC)*. (D) During week 12, the corticoseptal boundary becomes defined at the medial edge of the future neocortex, and a glial sling forms along this boundary. (E) By week 13, three commissural sites have been established: anterior commissure, hippocampal commissure, and glial sling. Depending on their origin, early neocortical commissural fibers cross the midline along the anterior commissure (temporo-occipital fibers), the glial sling (frontal fibers), or the hippocampal commissure (parieto-occipitotemporal fibers). (F) The corpus callosum enlarges by adding further commissural fibers and forms a single continuous structure stretched between the anterior commissure and the hippocampal commissure. Later, the prominent development of the frontal lobes results in posterior growth of the anterior corpus callosum, which displaces the hippocampal commissure and the splenium backward above the velum interpositum (roof above the third ventricle), stretching the body of the fornix. The corpus callosum becomes longer and thicker in development and reaches its final shape between 18 and 20 weeks' gestation. (From Volpe J, Inder TE, Darras BT, et al. *Volpe's Neurology of the Newborn*. 6th ed. Elsevier; 2018. As modified from Barkovich AJ, Raybaud C. *Pediatric Neuroimaging*. 5th ed. LWW; 2012:371–372.)

Imaging

- The anterior to posterior segmentation of corpus callosum includes the rostrum, genu, body, isthmus, and splenium.
- The majority of callosal fibers join symmetric areas of the cerebral cortex.
- The corpus callosum should be present on imaging at 18 weeks' gestation. The cavum septum pellucidum is closely associated with formation of the corpus callosum and should be visible by 18 weeks on ultrasound. Absence of the cavum septum pellucidum raises concern for a malformation of the corpus callosum. Sagittal T2W imaging is typically the best plane for visualizing the entire corpus callosum.
- As the brain develops, the corpus callosum becomes longer and thicker. Biometry data of the corpus callosum indicate most of the postnatal enlargement of the corpus callosum occurs in the first 4 years of life, after which the size is essentially stable. While subjective assessment of callosal length and thickness is usually done in routine clinical care, biometry data can be useful for in some patients and are provided in Chapter 1.
- The following examples will demonstrate malformations of the corpus callosum on imaging.

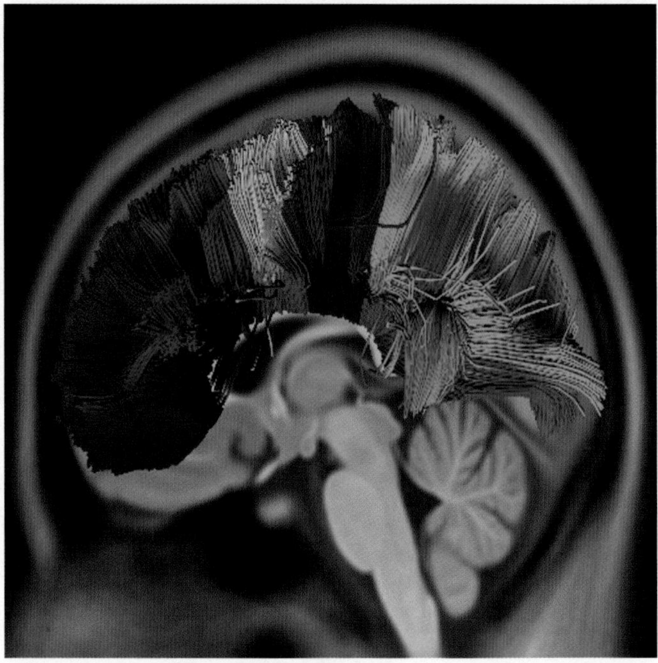

Corpus Callosum Crossing Fibers. Diffusion tensor imaging fiber tracking of anatomic segments of the corpus callosum demonstrates the following: 1) Rostrum and genu (red fibers) connect with the prefrontal and orbitofrontal cortices; 2) Anterior mid body of the corpus callosum (blue fibers) connect with the premotor and supplementary motor areas; 3) Posterior mid body of the corpus callosum (yellow fibers) connect with the primary motor areas; 4) Isthmus (purple fibers) connect with the primary sensory area; 5) Splenium (green fibers) connect with the parietal and temporal lobes and the visual cortex.

REFERENCES

1. Kier EL, Truwit CL. The normal and abnormal genu of the corpus callosum: an evolutionary, embryologic, anatomic, and MR analysis. *AJNR Am J Neuroradiol.* 1996 Oct;17(9):1631–1641.
2. Richards LJ. Axonal pathfinding mechanisms at the cortical midline and in the development of the corpus callosum. *Braz J Med Biol Res.* 2002 Dec;35(12):1431–1439.
3. Hofer S, Frahm J. Topography of the human corpus callosum revisited–comprehensive fiber tractography using diffusion tensor magnetic resonance imaging. *Neuroimage.* 2006 Sep;32(3):989–994.

AGENESIS, HYPOGENESIS, AND DYSGENESIS OF THE CORPUS CALLOSUM

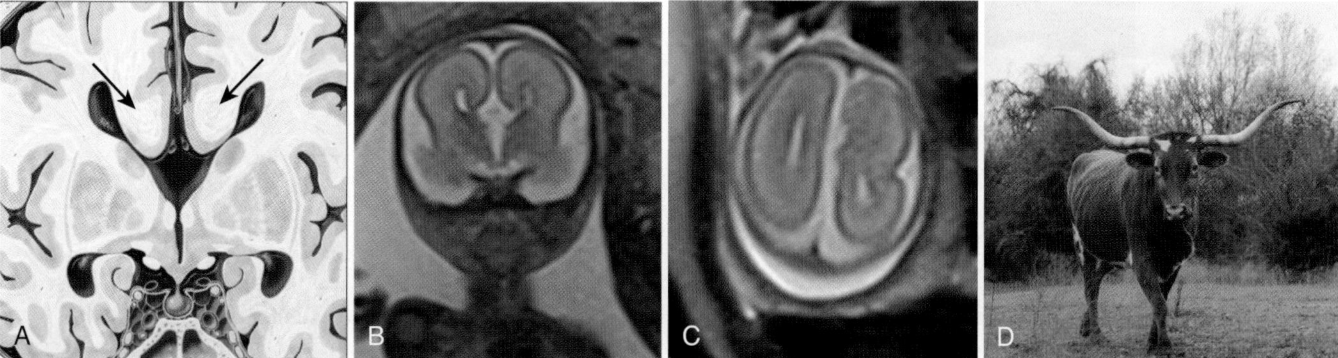

Fig. 2.3 Agenesis of the Corpus Callosum. (A) Illustration of agenesis of the corpus callosum with Probst bundles (*arrows*). (B and C) Coronal and axial T2W fetal MRI demonstrate complete absence of the corpus callosum, widened interhemispheric fissure, high riding third ventricle, incomplete inversion of the cingulate gyrus, and lateral ventricles resembling a longhorn (D). (A from StatDX, Copyright © 2022 Elsevier. D from istock.com/Candice Estep.)

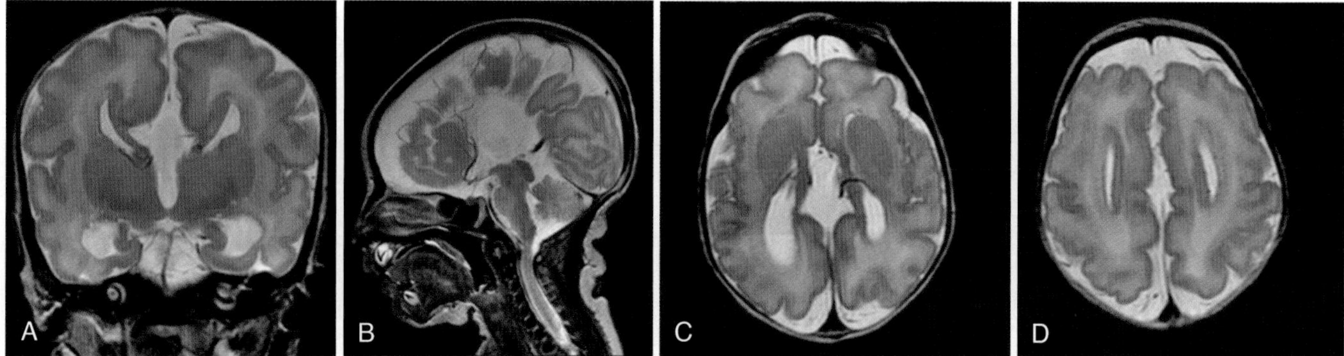

Fig. 2.4 Agenesis of the Corpus Callosum. (A to D) Multiplanar T2W MRI in a child with characteristic imaging findings compatible with complete corpus callosum agenesis. On midsagittal imaging (B) there is no visible corpus callosum. On coronal imaging (A) there is a high riding roof of the third ventricle, mild widening of the interhemispheric fissure, under rotation of the hippocampi, incomplete inversion of the cingulate gyrus, absent septum pellucidum, and T2 hypointense white matter bundles known as Probst bundles along the medial contour of the lateral ventricles. Axial imaging (C and D) demonstrate the parallel lateral ventricles and mild colpocephaly of the atria of the lateral ventricles.

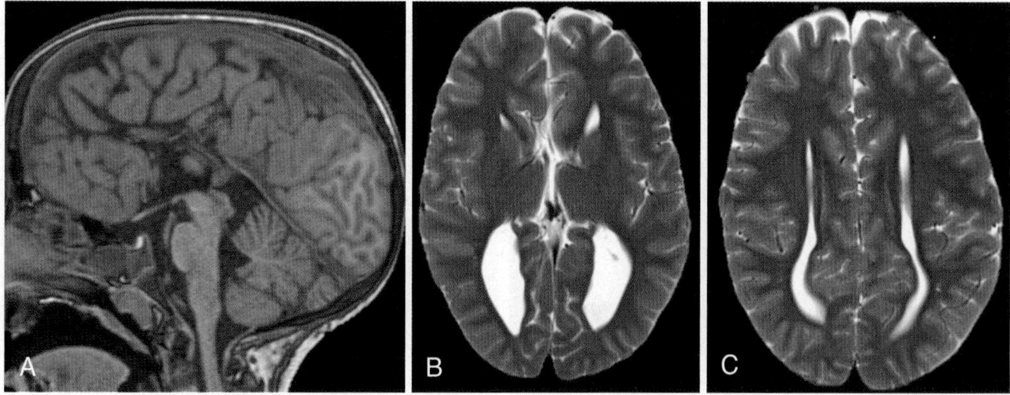

Fig. 2.5 Agenesis of the Corpus Callosum. (A) Sagittal T1W and (B and C) axial T2W images demonstrate absence of the corpus callosum, colpocephaly, and parallel ventricles. The anterior commissure is small but present.

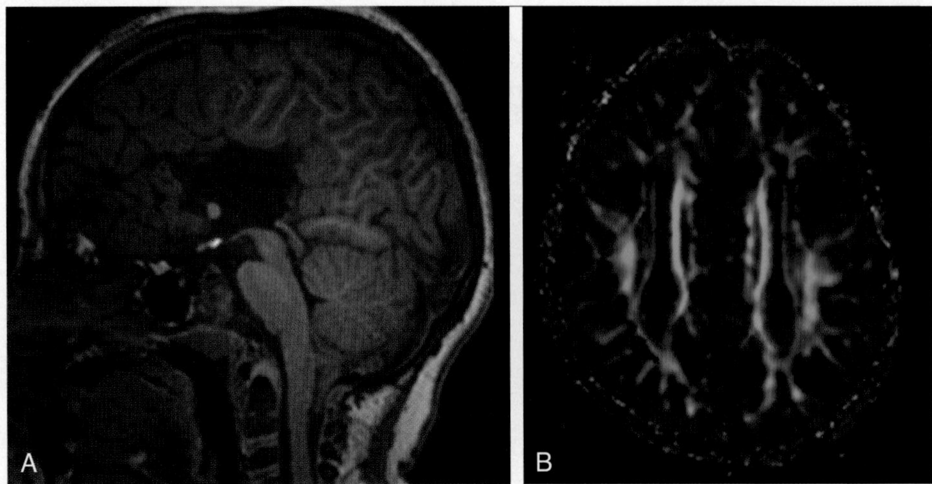

Fig. 2.6 Agenesis of the Corpus Callosum. (A) Sagittal T1W and (B) axial color-coded fractional anisotropy maps of a child with complete corpus callosum agenesis show the characteristic lack of the corpus callosum on midsagittal imaging, absent cingulate gyrus, and radiating appearance of the mesial sulci toward the mildly widened third ventricle. The anterior commissure is mildly enlarged. On color-coded fractional anisotropy maps the aberrant course of the Probst bundles are noted as green encoded fibers along the medial contour of the lateral ventricles. Incidental note is made of a Chiari I malformation with low positioning of the cerebellar tonsils and ectopic posterior pituitary gland.

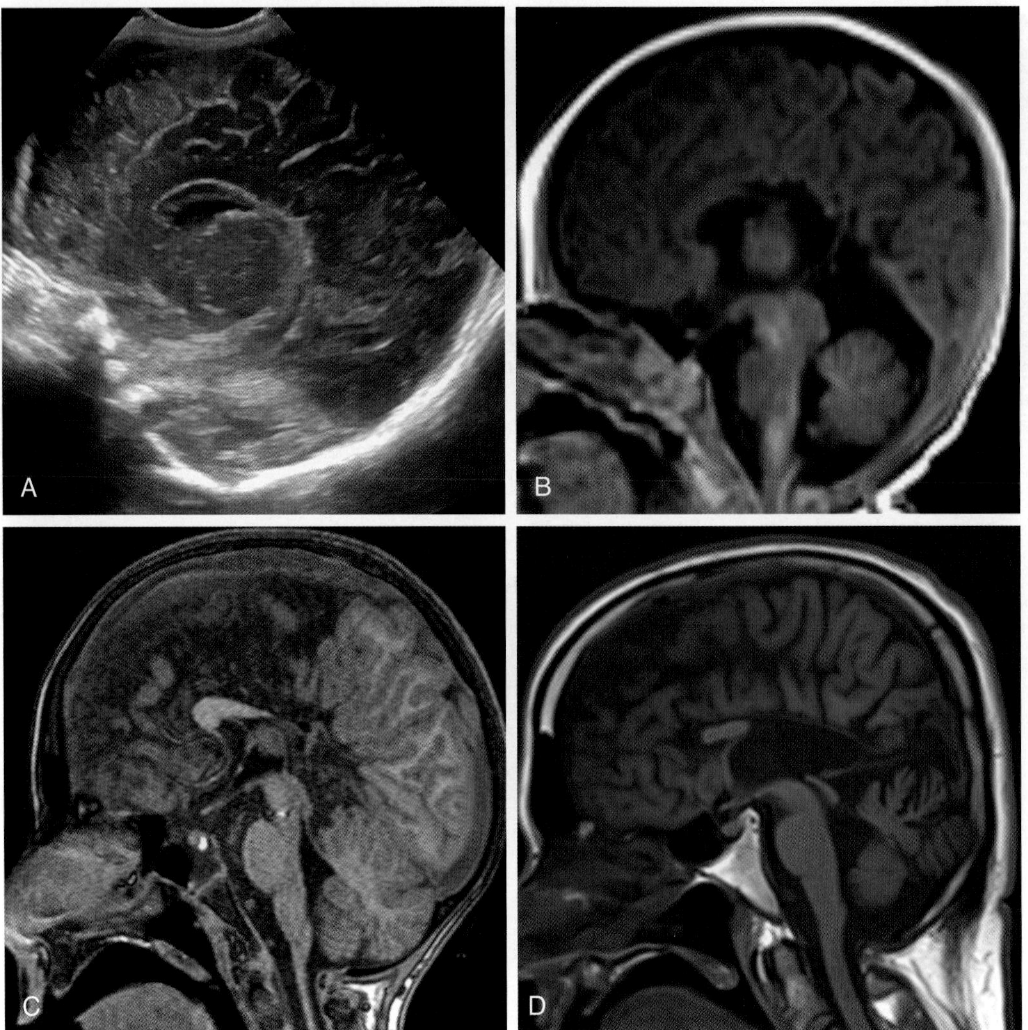

Fig. 2.7 Hypogenesis of the Corpus Callosum. Multiple patients. (A) Sagittal ultrasound and (B) sagittal T1W images demonstrate hypogenesis of the corpus callosum with formation of approximately the anterior half of the corpus callosum. (C and D) Sagittal T1W images in two additional patients demonstrating varying degrees of hypogenesis of the corpus callosum. The anterior commissure is small but present.

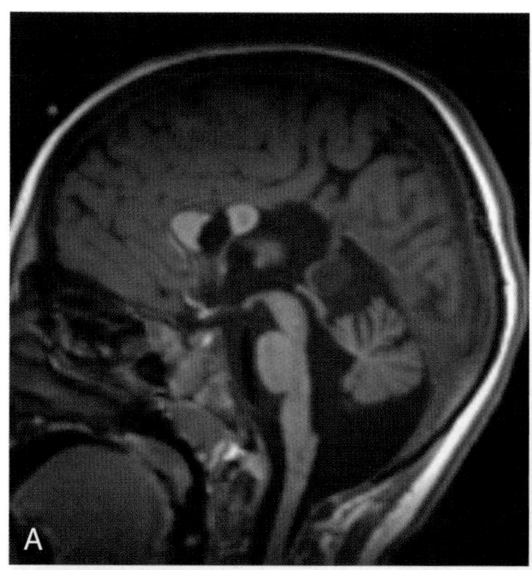

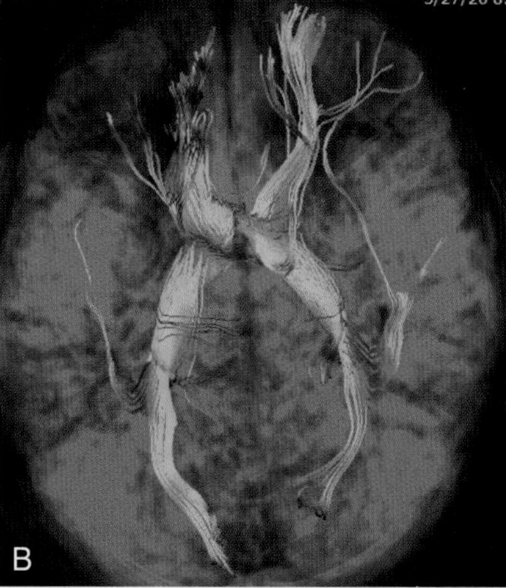

Fig. 2.8 Dysgenesis of the Corpus Callosum. (A) Sagittal T1W and (B) DTI tractography images demonstrate dysgenesis of the corpus callosum with aberrant crossing fibers connecting heterotopic areas of the brain. The anterior commissure is small but present.

Key Points

Background

- Agenesis, hypogenesis, and dysgenesis are malformations of the corpus callosum occurring from 8–20 weeks' gestation. Agenesis refers to complete absence of the corpus callosum. Hypogenesis refers to partial formation of the corpus callosum. Dysgenesis refers to abnormal formation of the corpus callosum.
- Prevalence is ~1:10,000 live births.
- Etiologies include genetic, infectious, and teratogenic causes. Corpus callosum malformations should be differentiated from destructive lesions (e.g., adjacent white matter ischemic lesion), which are discussed later in this chapter, or high-grade thinning (e.g., high-grade obstructive hydrocephalus).
- Malformations of the corpus callosum can be isolated or associated with cerebral anomalies (~50% of patients) and extracerebral anomalies (~60% of patients).
- Over 80 chromosomal, genetic, and sporadic syndromes are associated with malformation of the corpus callosum. Approximately 50% to 80% of patients have an associated syndrome and malformation, and chromosomal anomalies are found in 15% to 20% of patients.
- Prognosis is variable for callosal malformations and ranges from normal to developmental delay, epilepsy, and behavioral disorders. Prognosis is influenced by the presence of additional anomalies. Outcomes in isolated agenesis of the corpus callosum are normal in ~75%, borderline or moderate disability in 14%, and severe disability in 11% of patients. Outcomes in partial agenesis of the corpus callosum are normal in ~66%, borderline or moderate disability in 7%, and severe disability in 27% of patients.

Imaging

- In agenesis of the corpus callosum, the corpus callosum and hippocampal commissure are absent, and the anterior commissure is absent in about half of patients.
- In hypogenesis of the corpus callosum, a variable amount of corpus callosum is present from anterior to posterior, the hippocampal commissure may be absent depending on the degree of dysgenesis, but the anterior commissure is always present.
- Imaging findings include the following:
  - Partial or complete absence of the corpus callosum
  - Absent cingulate gyri and sulci
  - Perpendicular radiation of midline gyri from the third ventricle to the periphery
  - Widened interhemispheric fissure
  - Parallel orientation of the lateral ventricles and widened atria of the lateral ventricles (colpocephaly)
  - White matter bundles known as the Probst bundles course along the superomedial border of the lateral ventricles
  - Elevated third ventricle and lateral ventricles mimic a Texas longhorn configuration on coronal imaging
  - Absent septum pellucidum
  - Absent or hypoplastic anterior and hippocampal commissures
  - Malrotated, vertically oriented ventral hippocampi
  - Diffusion tensor imaging show a lack of fibers crossing the midline matching the area of the missing corpus callosum.
- Postnatal MRI is recommended in patients as ~15% of prenatally diagnosed isolated agenesis of the corpus callosum are found to have additional anomalies on postnatal imaging.
- Additional malformations, such as pituitary gland anomalies, migrational abnormalities (most commonly gray matter heterotopia), or bilateral schizencephaly, should be excluded.
- Corpus callosum malformations may also be part of complex brain malformations, including Aicardi syndrome, Chiari II malformation, or Dandy-Walker syndrome.

REFERENCES

1. Raybaud C. The corpus callosum, the other great forebrain commissures, and the septum pellucidum: anatomy, development, and malformation. *Neuroradiology*. 2010;52:447–477.
2. Huisman TA, Bosemani T, Poretti A. Diffusion tensor imaging for brain malformations: does it help? *Neuroimaging Clin N Am*. 2014;24:619–637.

CORPUS CALLOSUM AGENESIS WITH INTERHEMISPHERIC CYST

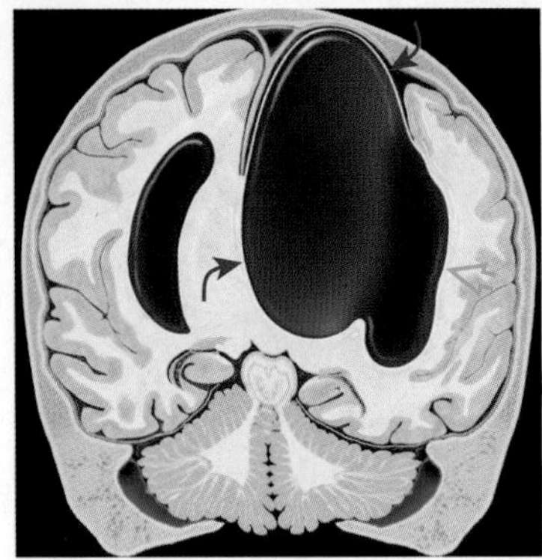

Fig. 2.9 Illustration of callosal agenesis with a type 1 interhemispheric cyst (*red arrows*) communicating with the ventricle (*straight arrow*). (From StatDX, Copyright © 2022 Elsevier.)

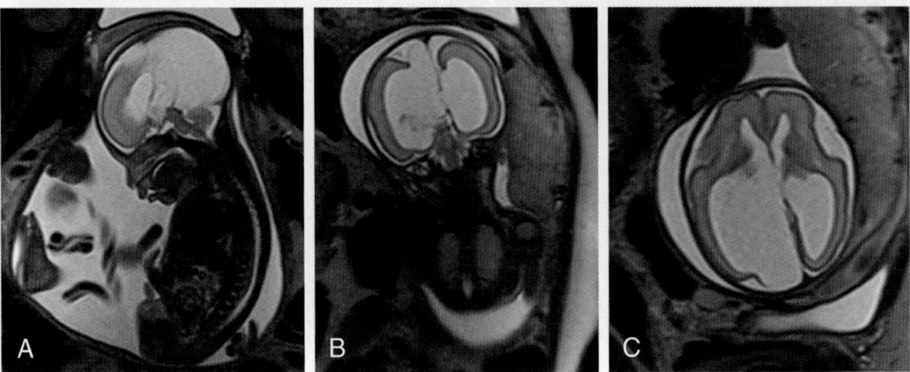

Fig. 2.10 Callosal Agenesis With Type 1 Interhemispheric Cyst. Sagittal (A), coronal (B), and axial (C) T2W fetal MRI demonstrate corpus callosum agenesis, moderate bilateral supratentorial ventriculomegaly, and type 1 interhemispheric cyst seen as asymmetric dilatation of the right lateral ventricle protruding posteriorly and superiorly.

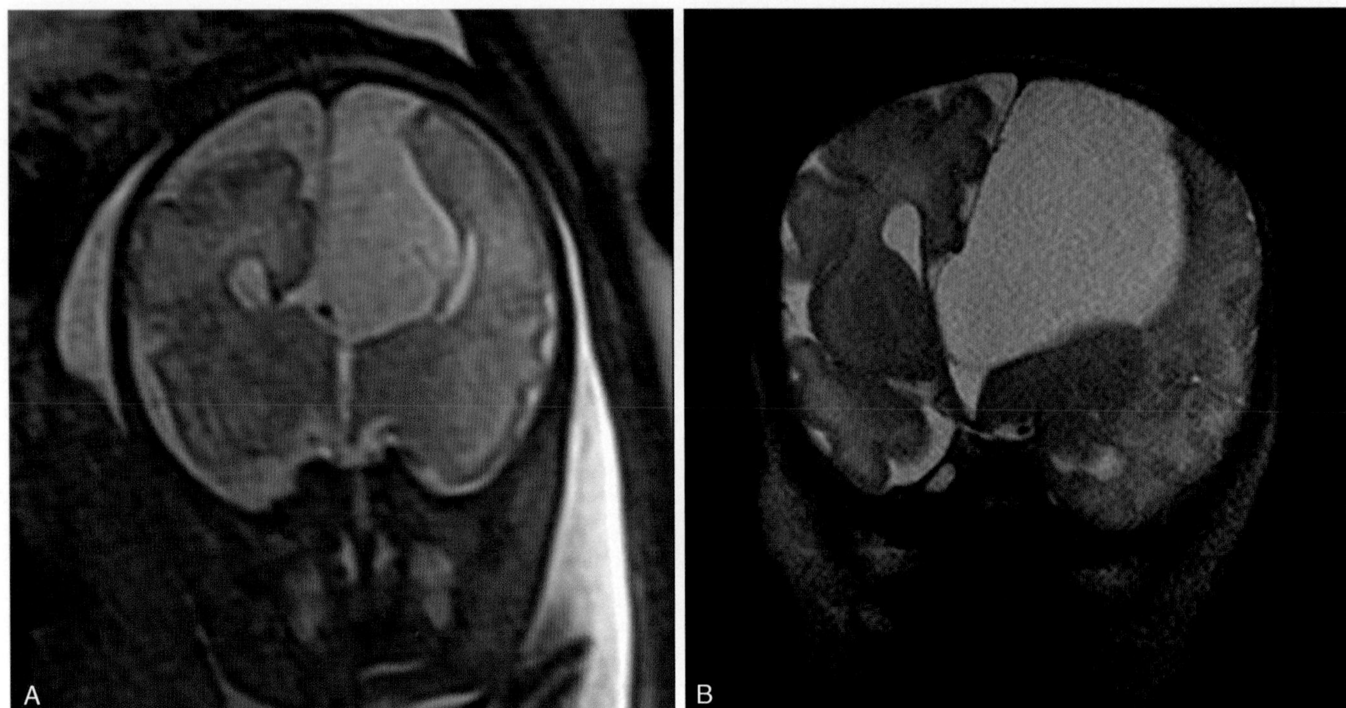

Fig. 2.11 Callosal Agenesis With Type 1 Interhemispheric Cyst. (A and B) Coronal fetal and matching postnatal T2W MRI demonstrate corpus callosum agenesis and large interhemispheric cyst to the left of the midline. The left lateral ventricle is displaced and compressed laterally. There is malrotation of the right cingulate gyrus and compression of the left cingulate gyrus.

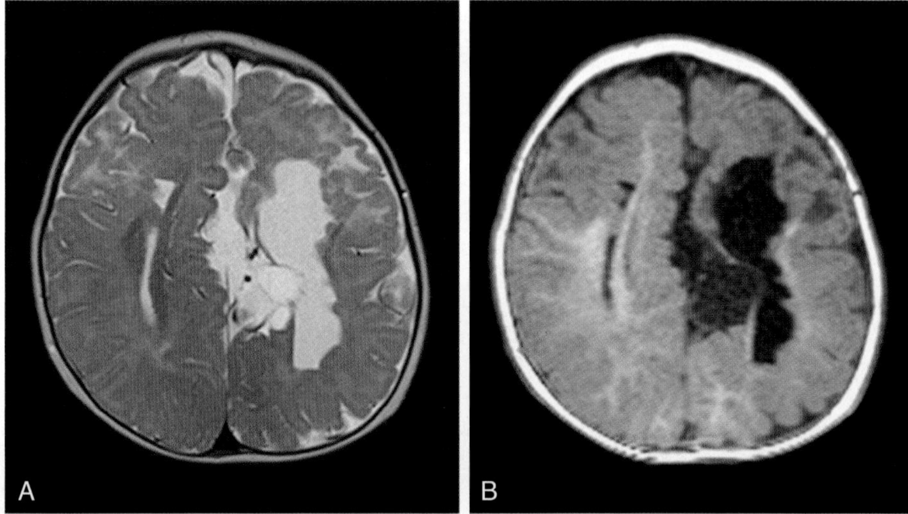

Fig. 2.12 Callosal Agenesis With Type 2 Interhemispheric Cyst. (A) Axial T2W and (B) T1W MRI demonstrate corpus callosum agenesis, parallel course of the lateral ventricles, Probst bundles along the medial contour of the lateral ventricles, a multilobulated left paramedian interhemispheric cyst, multifocal subependymal heterotopias, and polymicrogyria with delayed subcortical myelination in the lateral frontal lobes.

Key Points

Background

- Corpus callosum malformations may be associated with interhemispheric cysts, also known as cystic meningeal dysplasia.
- This malformation is believed to be secondary to a disruption of the normal development of the commissural plate and adjacent cortex. The cysts can occur from expansion of the roof of the third ventricle due to lack of an overlying corpus callosum or multiple cysts due to abnormal differentiation of the primitive meninges.
- Often presents early with macrocephaly.
- Prognosis is variable, ranging from normal development to epilepsy, developmental delay, and neurologic deficits.
- In a series of 40 patients with asymmetric ventriculomegaly, interhemispheric cyst and agenesis or dysgenesis of the corpus callosum (known as AVID), 26 (65%) survived more than 2 years of age and of these 26, 12 (46%) had epilepsy, 14 (54%) could sit independently, 4 (16%) were in mainstream schools, 16 (62%) had expressive language problems, and 7 (28%) had near normal development without seizures.
- Often requires ventricular shunting.

Imaging

- Callosal agenesis or dysgenesis, absent septum pellucidum, and an interhemispheric cyst are the hallmark imaging findings. Often seen as asymmetric ventriculomegaly as the cyst communicates with one ventricle. Diencephalic-mesencephalic junction dysplasia and aqueductal stenosis can be associated with agenesis of the corpus callosum with interhemispheric cyst.
- Based upon their morphology they can be classified in two types:
  - Type 1: The *cyst is communicating with the ventricle*, likely represents a diverticulum of the ventricles, and is T1- and T2-isointense to CSF.
  - Type 2: The *cyst is not communicating with the ventricle*. Typically multiple cysts are present and the cysts are T1-hyperintense relative to CSF. Type 2 cysts are often associated with migrational abnormalities, including heterotopias and cortical malformations like polymicrogyria, or may be part of syndromes. Type 2 cysts often require ventricular shunting. Aicardi syndrome can have this appearance.
- Differential diagnosis:
  - Porencephaly: Should have normal head size, associated gliosis or hemorrhage, and no mass effect
  - Schizencephaly: Gray matter lined cleft without mass effect
  - Arachnoid cyst: Located over the convexity rather than midline

REFERENCES

1. Barkovich AJ, Simon EM, Walsh CA. callosal agenesis with cyst: a better understanding and new classification. *Neurology*. 2001;56:220–227.
2. Huisman TA, Poretti A. Chapter 7. Disorders of brain development. In: Magnetic Resonance Imaging of the Brain and Spine, 5th ed. Edited by Scott Atlas, MD. Wolters Kluwer: Lippincott Williams & Wilkins.
3. Limoges N, Ostrander B, Kennedy A, Woodward PJ, Bollo RJ. Neurological and clinical outcomes in infants and children with a fetal diagnosis of asymmetric ventriculomegaly, interhemispheric cyst, and dysgenesis of the corpus callosum. *J Neurosurg Pediatr*. 2021 Nov 19:1–5.

CORPUS CALLOSUM LIPOMA

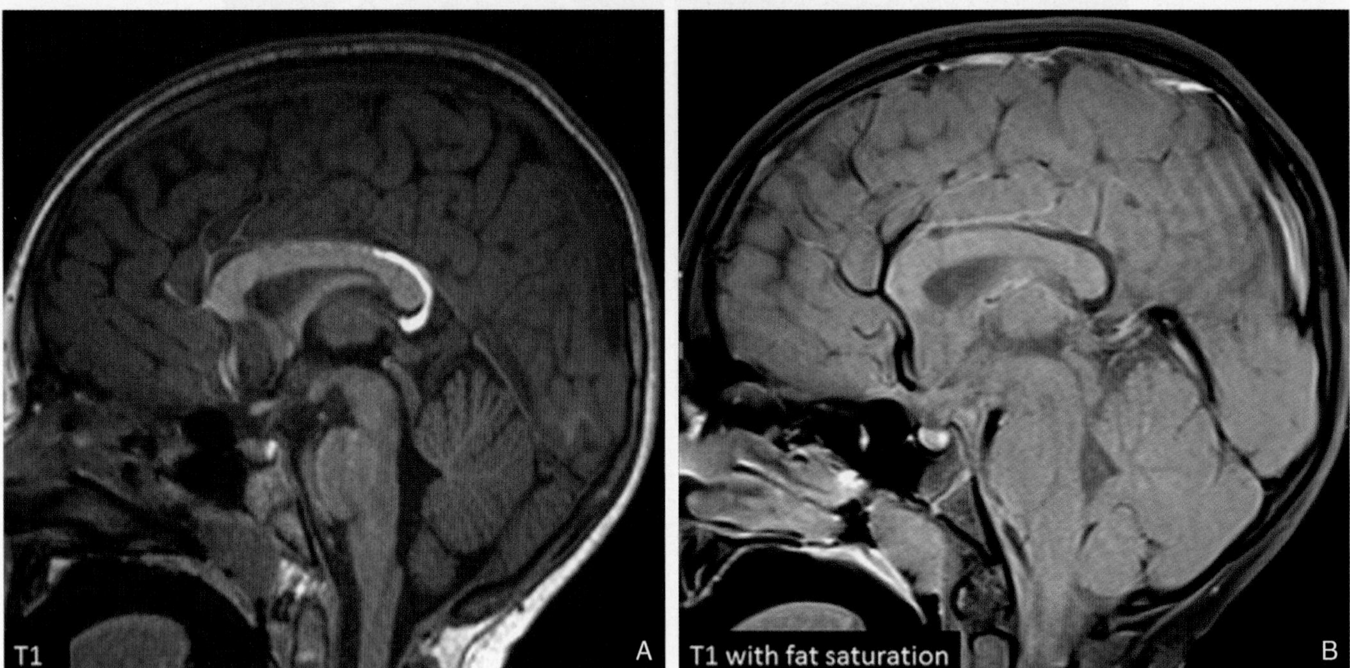

Fig. 2.13 Curvilinear Callosal Lipoma. (A) Sagittal T1W MRI of the brain without and (B) with fat saturation demonstate a T1 hyperintense curvilinear lipoma following the contour of the splenium of the corpus callosum. T fat-saturated sequence confirms the diagnosis of a corpus callosum lipoma as evidenced by signal suppression on fat-saturated imaging.

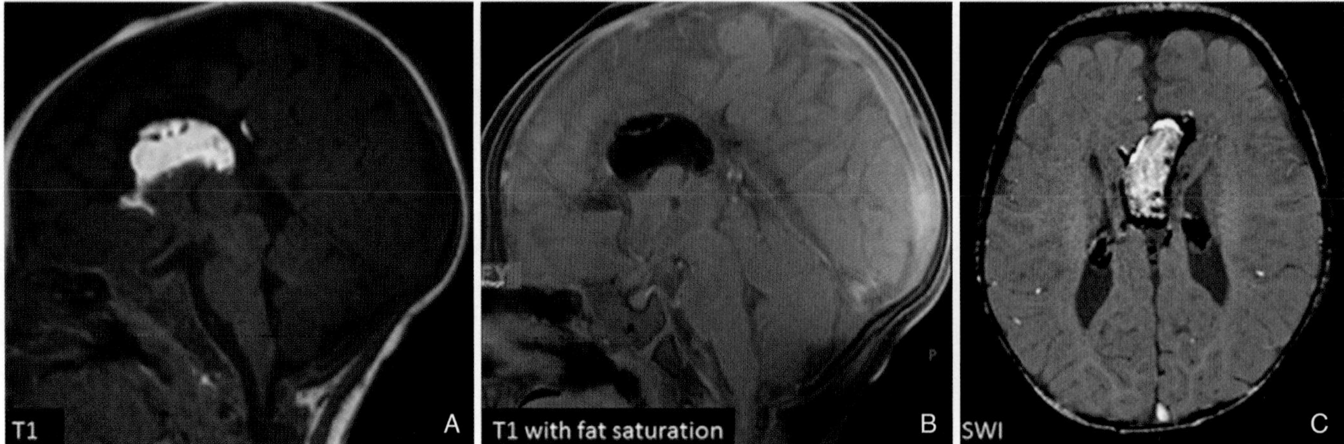

Fig. 2.14 Lobular Callosal Lipoma. (A, B) Sagittal T1W imaging without and with fat suppression as well as (C) axial SWI imaging reveal a large globular interhemispheric T1 hyperintense lipoma in the expected location of the anterior corpus callosum. Fat saturation confirms the lipoma as evidenced by the signal suppression. On axial SWI imaging peripheral SWI hypointensity is noted due to chemical shift artifact.

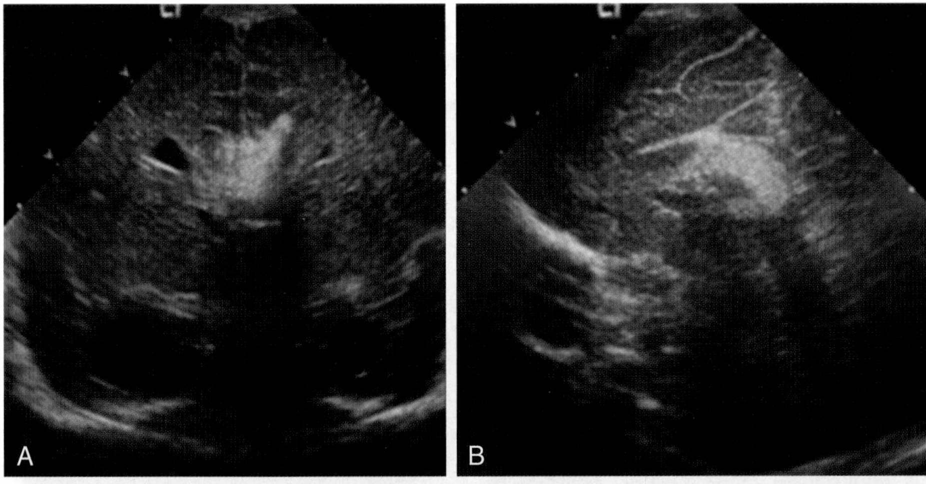

Fig. 2.15 Callosal Lipoma. (A) Coronal and (B) sagittal ultrasound of the brain reveal a focal hyperechogenic mass lesion in the midline, respectively within the expected region of the corpus callosum. The lateral ventricles appear slightly lateralized. These findings are compatible with corpus callosum lipoma respectively interhemispheric lipoma.

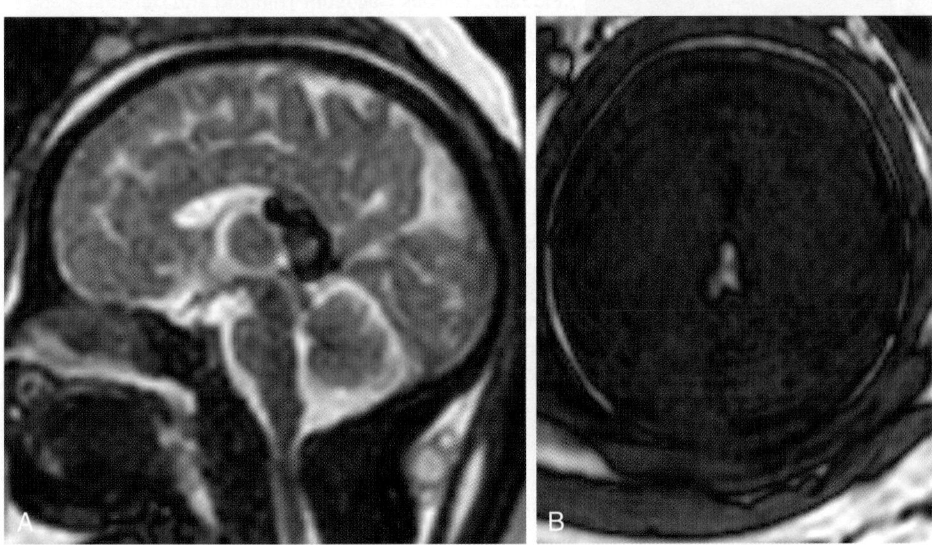

Fig. 2.16 Callosal Lipoma. (A) Sagittal T2W and (B) axial T1W fetal MRI demonstrate a curvilinear T2 hypointense, T1 hyperintense callosal lipoma.

Key Points

Background

- Midline lipomas are believed to be secondary to an abnormal differentiation of the meninx primitive. The meninx primitive can disrupt the development of the corpus callosum and adjacent cortex.
- Larger lipomas associated with callosal malformations are more likely to be associated with neurologic disability compared to thin, curvilinear lipomas.
- Lipomas may grow as the child grows.

Imaging

- A pericallosal or interhemispheric lipoma appears hyperechogenic on ultrasound and hyperintense on T1-weighted MRI; the MRI signal is suppressed on fat-saturated MR sequences. Uncommonly, on fetal MRI the lipoma can sometimes lack the T1W hyperintensity due to immature fat cells.
- On gradient echo MR imaging, marked fat-related chemical shift signal loss may be seen along the periphery of the lesion along the direction of the frequency encoding gradient.
- The lipomas may be of various sizes and typically follow the course of the corpus callosum.
  - *Lobular*, mass-like focal lipomas are usually associated with callosal malformations.
  - *Thin, curvilinear* lipomas are less likely associated with callosal malformations.

REFERENCES

1. Raybaud C. The corpus callosum, the other great forebrain commissures, and the septum pellucidum: anatomy, development, and malformation. *Neuroradiology*. 2010;52:447–477.
2. Huisman TA, Poretti A. Chapter 7. Disorders of brain development. In: Magnetic Resonance Imaging of the Brain and Spine, 5th ed. Edited by Scott Atlas, MD. Wolters Kluwer, Lippincott Williams & Wilkins.

CORPUS CALLOSUM THINNING AND DEFECTS

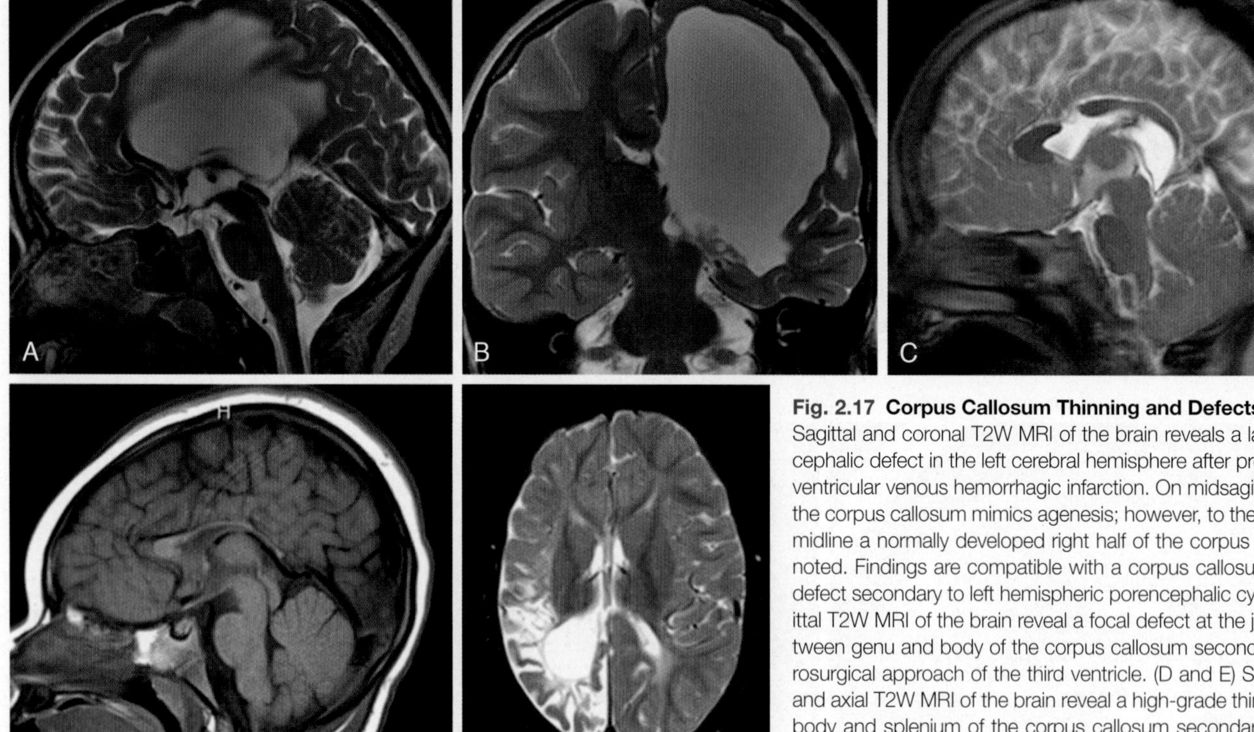

Fig. 2.17 Corpus Callosum Thinning and Defects. (A and B) Sagittal and coronal T2W MRI of the brain reveals a large porencephalic defect in the left cerebral hemisphere after previous periventricular venous hemorrhagic infarction. On midsagittal imaging the corpus callosum mimics agenesis; however, to the right of the midline a normally developed right half of the corpus callosum is noted. Findings are compatible with a corpus callosum thinning/defect secondary to left hemispheric porencephalic cyst. (C) Sagittal T2W MRI of the brain reveal a focal defect at the junction between genu and body of the corpus callosum secondary to neurosurgical approach of the third ventricle. (D and E) Sagittal T1W and axial T2W MRI of the brain reveal a high-grade thinning of the body and splenium of the corpus callosum secondary to an old injury as confirmed by the axial T2W imaging with extensive defect predominantly in the right parieto-occipital region.

Key Points

- Corpus callosum may appear "dysplastic" on a midsagittal image secondary to a remote injury. Examples include the following:
  - Chronic porencephalic cyst after neonatal periventricular hemorrhagic infarction
  - Neurosurgical interhemispheric transcallosal approach to the third ventricle
  - Periventricular white matter injury due to a neonatal hypoxic ischemic event
- Differentiation from a true malformation is essential for prognosis.
- Depending on the timing of injury (prenatal versus postnatal), differentiation must be made between malformation, disruption, and destruction.

REFERENCES

1. Huisman TA, Bosemani T, Poretti A. Diffusion tensor imaging for brain malformations: does it help? *Neuroimaging Clin N Am.* 2014;24:619–637.
2. Huisman TA, Poretti A. Chapter 7. Disorders of brain development. In: Magnetic Resonance Imaging of the Brain and Spine, 5th ed. Edited by Scott Atlas, MD. Wolters Kluwer, Lippincott Williams & Wilkins.

AICARDI SYNDROME

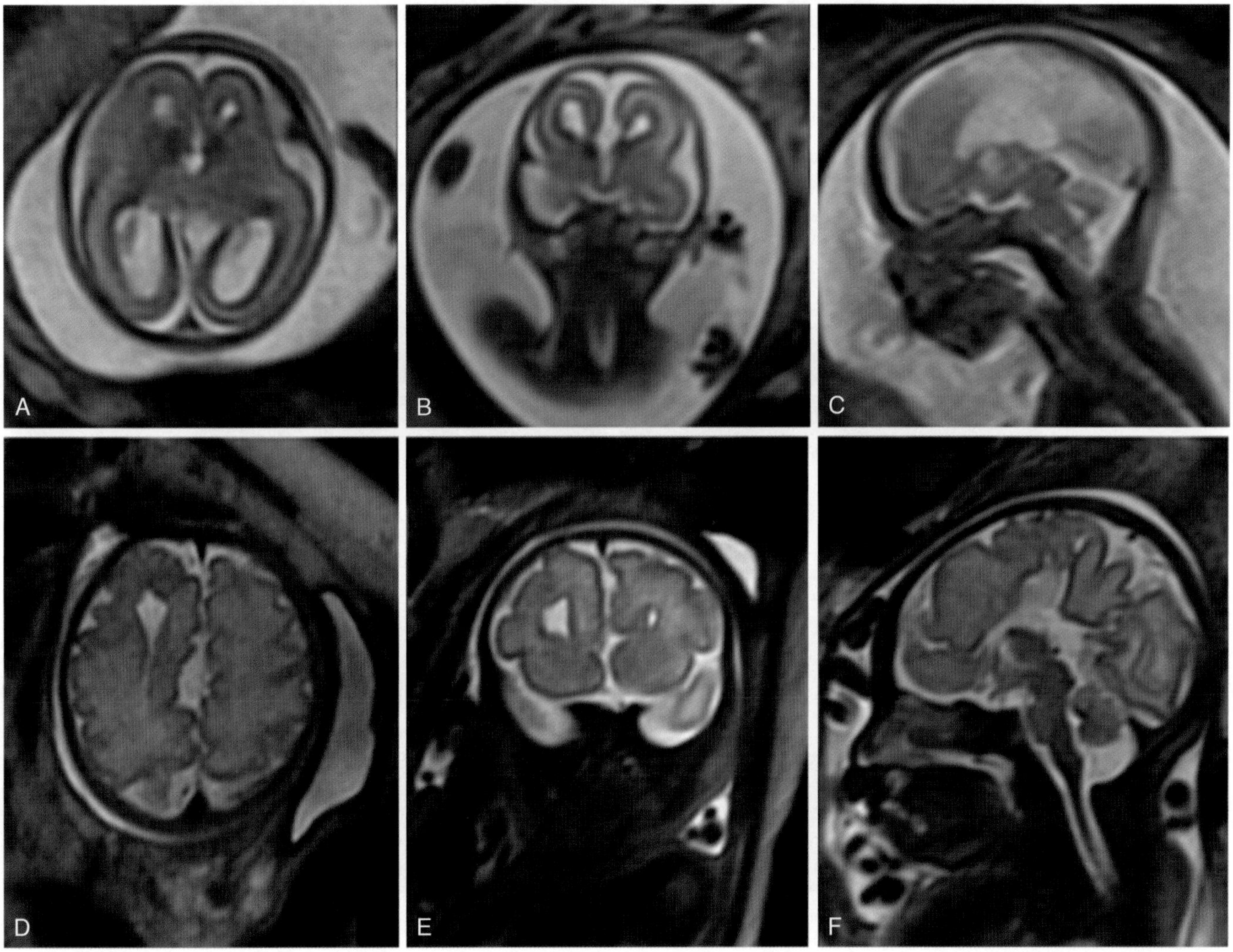

Fig. 2.18 Aicardi Syndrome. (A to C) Initial T2W fetal MRI images demonstrate agenesis of the corpus callosum, widened interhemispheric fissure, high-riding third ventricle, asymmetry in the shape of the mildly widened anterior horns of the lateral ventricles, and box-like configuration of the right anterior horn. (D to F) Follow-up T2W fetal MRI images redemonstrate agenesis of the corpus callosum and now identification of schizencephaly lined by T2 hypointense gray matter within the right frontal lobe.

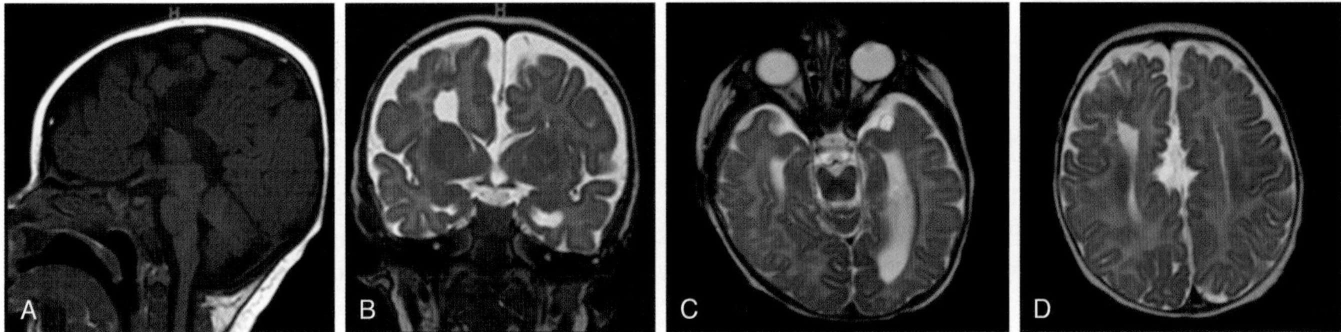

Fig. 2.19 Aicardi Syndrome. MRI from the same patient in Fig. 2.18 with (A) sagittal T1W and (B to D) coronal and axial T2W images confirm agenesis of the corpus callosum, right frontal lobe schizencephaly, polymicrogyria, and subependymal heterotopia, as well as a subtle left-sided coloboma.

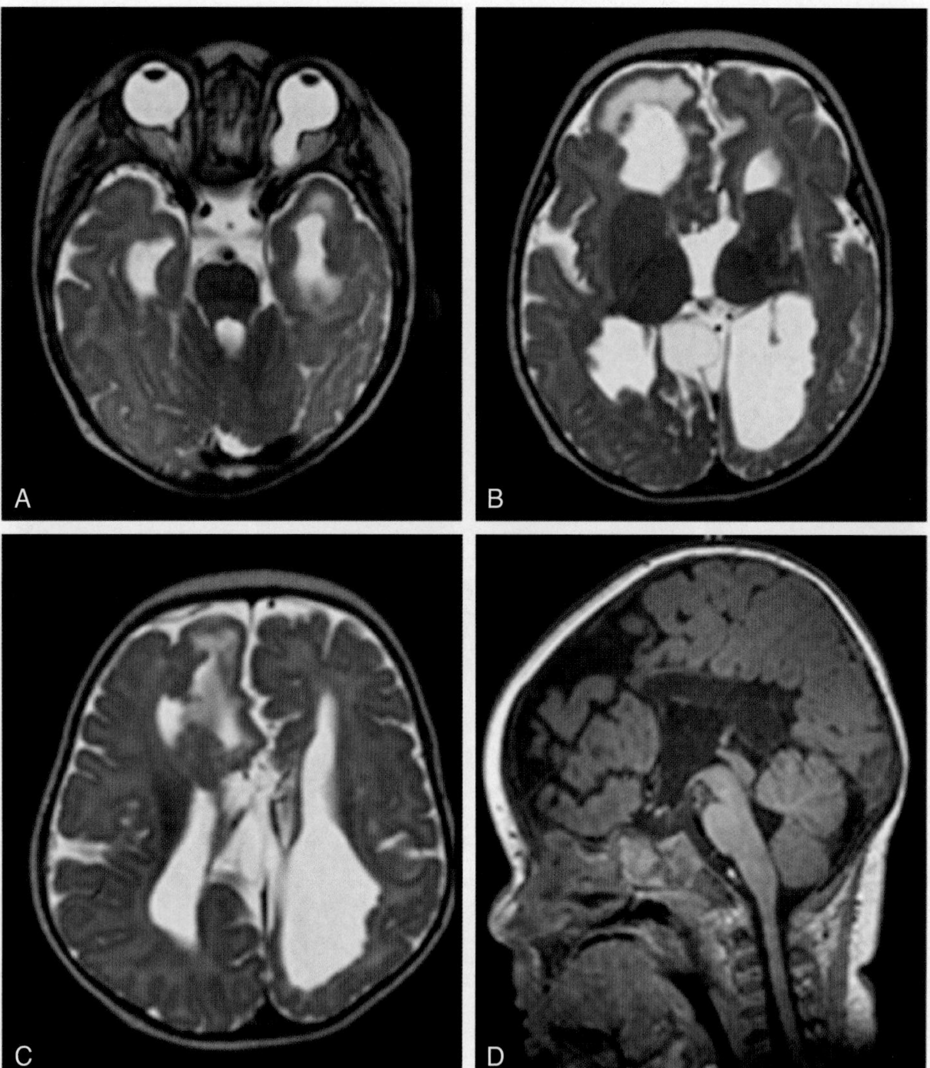

Fig. 2.20 Aicardi Syndrome. (A to C) Axial T2W and (D) sagittal T1W MRI of a child with confirmed Aicardi syndrome demonstrates complete corpus callosum agenesis, parallel course of the lateral ventricles, moderate ventriculomegaly, extensive subependymal heterotopias, migrational abnormality involving the right frontal lobe with hypomyelination of the frontal white matter is seen in combination with bilateral, left greater than right colobomas extending into the optic nerves.

Key Points

Background

- Defined by Dr. Jean Aicardi as an association of infantile spasms, agenesis of the corpus callosum, and chorioretinal lacunae in infant girls.
- Aicardi syndrome is an *X-linked dominant disorder and lethal in 46 XY males*. Consequently, Aicardi syndrome is seen in females. The gene causing Aicardi syndrome, however, is unknown.
- *Poor prognosis* with severe neurologic and cognitive impairments, epilepsy, and reduced life span, on average ranging from 8 to 18 years.
- Infants with Aicardi usually have infantile spasms, which are characterized as single jerks of the body that occur usually while awake. Children typically grow out of infantile spasms and have generalized tonic-clonic seizures or other types of seizures.

Imaging

- Findings include *agenesis of the corpus callosum, migrational abnormalities*, including gray matter heterotopia, polymicrogyria or pachygyria, choroid plexus cysts or papillomas, and *optic nerve colobomas* or *microphthalmia.*
- White matter dysmyelination may also be seen.
- Vertebral (block or hemivertebrae) and rib abnormalities may coexist.
- Interhemispheric cyst when present is usually multilocular.
- With exception of the corpus callosum agenesis, imaging findings may be subtle on early fetal MR imaging and become more obvious on follow-up MR imaging.

REFERENCES

1. Huisman TA, Poretti A. Chapter 7. Disorders of brain development. In: Magnetic Resonance Imaging of the Brain and Spine, 5th ed. Edited by Scott Atlas, MD. Wolters Kluwer, Lippincott Williams & Wilkins.
2. Hopkins B, Sutton VR, Lewis RA, et al. Neuroimaging aspects of Aicardi syndrome. A. *J Med genet A*. 2008;146A(22):2871–2878.

CORTICAL MALFORMATIONS

Understanding cortical malformations requires an understanding of basic cortical development.

The germinal matrix develops in the walls of the telencephalon. Areas known as the ganglionic eminences develop as larger regions of the germinal matrix. As the neurons from the germinal matrix proliferate and migrate to the outer cortex, they form permanent and transient axonal connections, and the zones in the telencephalon are visible during this stage of development. These zones change in appearance during development and peak between 15 and 24 weeks of gestation (Fig. 2.21).

The ventricular zone gives rise to descendants of the neural plate and subventricular zone. The periventricular zone is a cell sparse layer with axons that give rise to the corpus callosum. The subventricular zone is the source of cortical and striatal neurons, astrocytes, and glial cells. The intermediate zone is a region of axonal connections. The subplate contains maturing neurons and connections important for cortical layer organization. The subplate reaches maximum thickness at 22 weeks' gestation and disappears at 30 weeks. The cortical plate is the final destination of migrating neurons and will develop into a six-layered neocortex with the innermost layer (layer VI) forming first, and, as neurons continue to migrate, will progressively form the more outer layers. Proliferation and migration of glial progenitors continues in the postnatal period into adulthood.

Cortical malformations can be categorized as malformations due to abnormal neuronal or glial proliferation, abnormal neuronal migration, or abnormal postmigrational development (Box 2.1). This section will illustrate the common cortical malformations and disorders in which these are common findings. Cortical dysplasias, which are cortical malformations resulting from abnormal neuronal/glial proliferation and postmigrational development, are discussed in Chapter 8, Epilepsy.

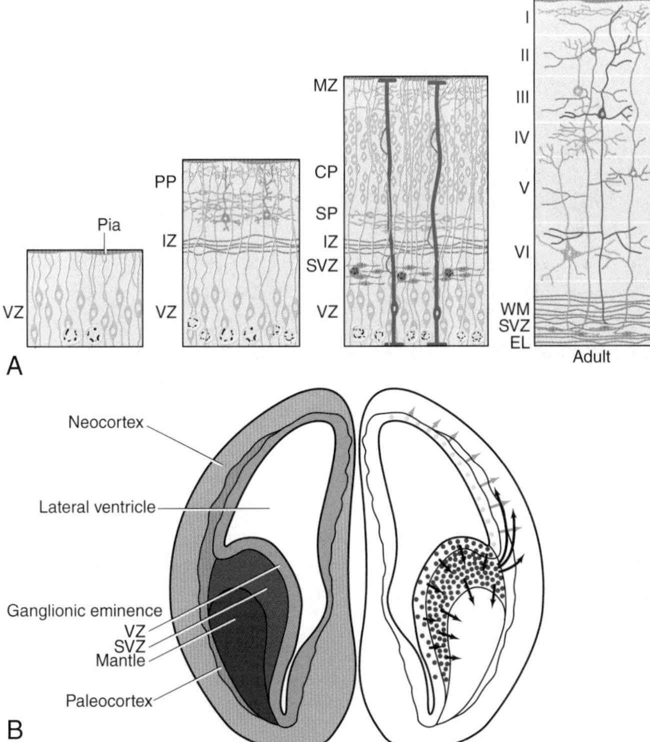

Fig. 2.21 Cytodifferentiation and Lamination of the Neocortex. (A) Appearance of the lamination of the neoncortex at different stages of development shown in cross section. The green cells in the marginal zone (MZ) are the Cajal-Retzius cells. *CP*, Cortical plate; *EL*, ependymal layer; *IZ*, intermediate zone; *PP*, preplate; *SP*, subplate; *WM*, white matter; *I–VI*, numbered layers of neocortex. (B) Migration of interneurons (nonpyramidal cells) from their origin in the ventricular and subventricular zones (VZ, SVZ) of the ganglionic eminences via tangential pathways (*arrows on right side*) to the neocortex. A small minority of cortical interneurons arise from the cortical germinative zones *(yellow)*. The germinative zones of the ganglionic eminences also produce the neurons of the corpus striatum and the globus pallidus (basal ganglia). (From Schoenwolf GC, Bleyl SB, Brauer PR, Francis-West PH. *Larsen's Human Embryology*. 5th ed. Elsevier; 2015.)

BOX 2.1

Classification of Congenital Cortical Malformations

Group I. Malformations Secondary to Abnormal Neuronal and Glial Proliferation or Apoptosis
I.A. Microcephaly
I.B. Megalencephalies and Hemimegalencephaly
I.C. Cortical dysgenesis with abnormal cell proliferation (FCD type 2)

Group II. Malformations due to Abnormal Neuronal Migration
II.A Heterotopia
II.B. Lissencephaly
II.C. Subcortical heterotopia and sublobar dysplasia
II.D. Cobblestone malformations

Group III. Malformations Secondary to Abnormal Postmigrational Development
III.A. Polymicrogyria and schizencephaly
III.B. Polymicrogyria without schizencephalic clefts
III.C. Focal cortical dysplasias (FCD type 1)
III.D. Postmigrational microcephaly

From Barkovich AJ, Guerrini R, Kuzniecky RI, Jackson GD, Dobyns WB. A developmental and genetic classification for malformations of cortical development: Update 2012. *Brain*. 2012;135(5):1348–1369. doi:10.1093/brain/aws019

MICROCEPHALY

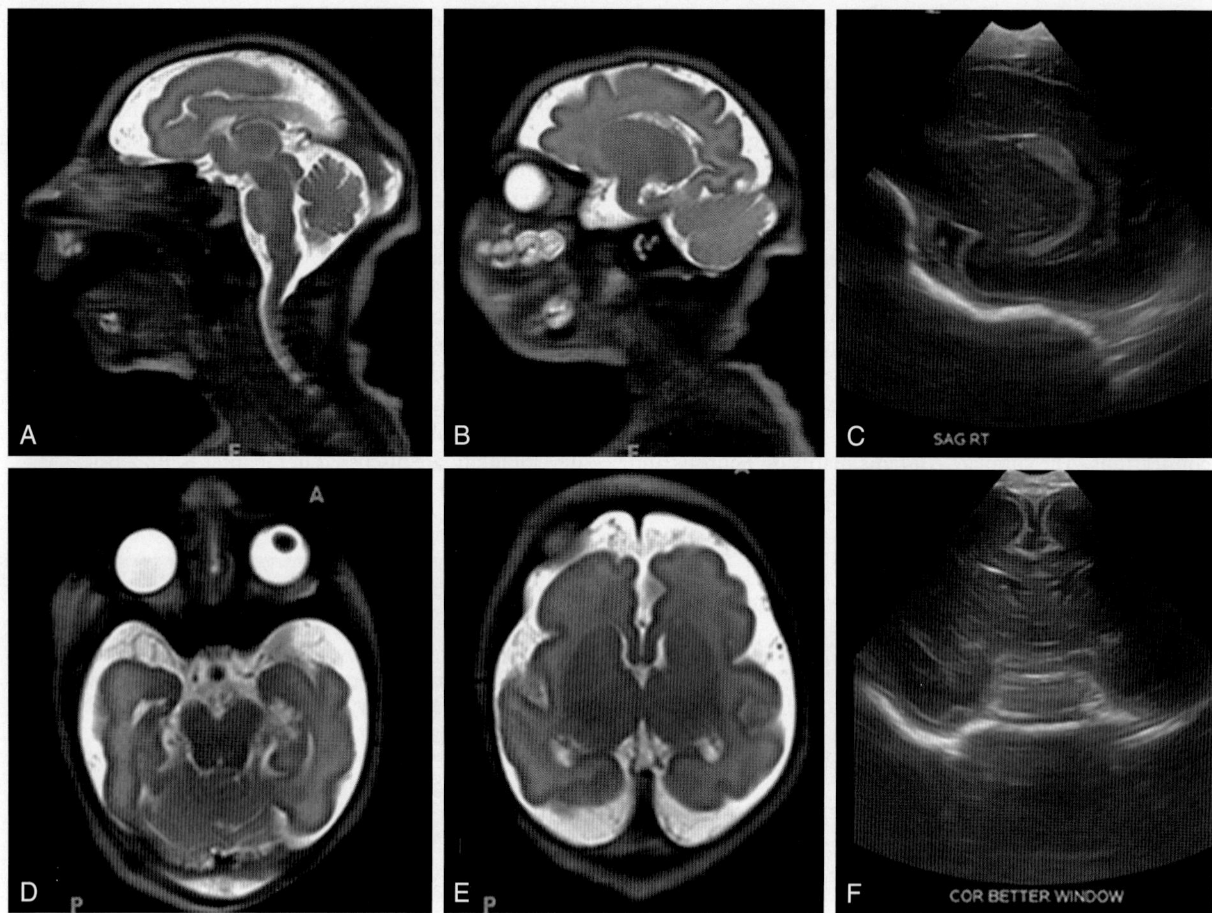

Fig. 2.22 Microcephaly With Simplified Gyral Pattern. (A and B) Sagittal and (D and E) axial T2W MR imaging and matching (C and F) sagittal and coronal ultrasound imaging show significant global microcephaly with high-grade simplified gyral pattern indicated by lack of tertiary sulcation and shallow sulci, and moderate widening of the subarachnoid space.

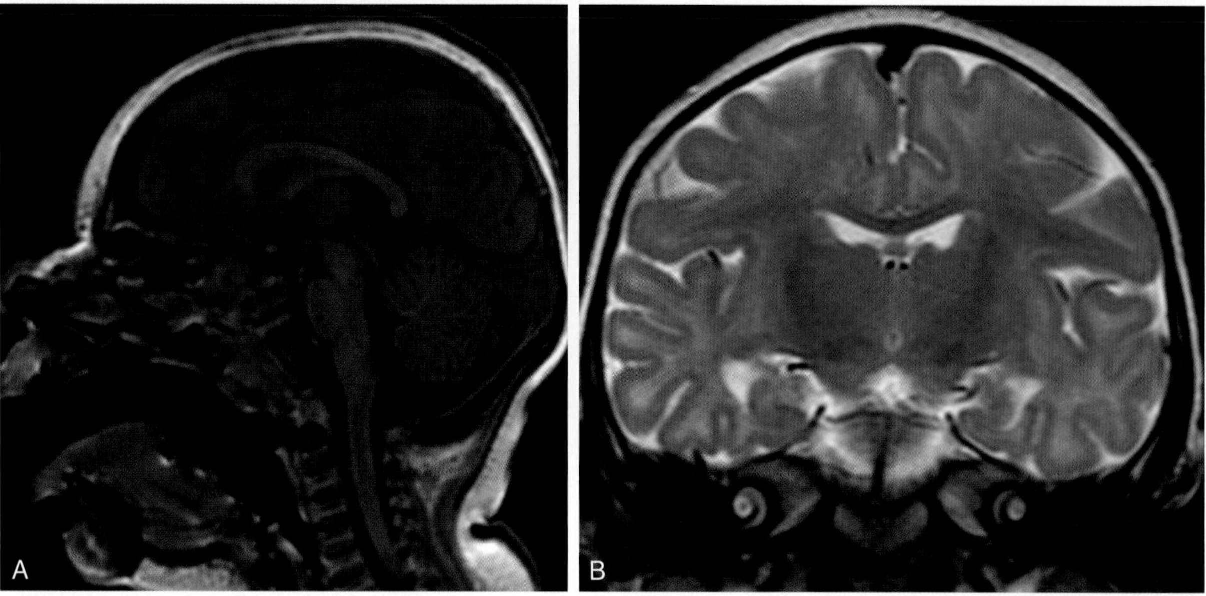

Fig. 2.23 Microcephaly Primary Hereditary. (A) Sagittal T1W and (B) coronal T2W images demonstrate global microcephaly with normal cortical thickness and sulcation.

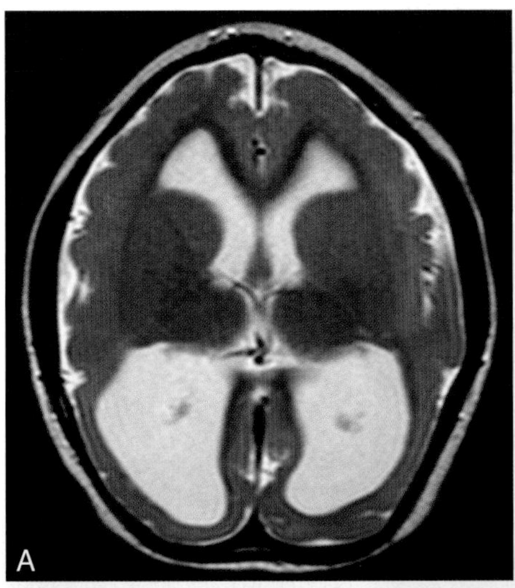
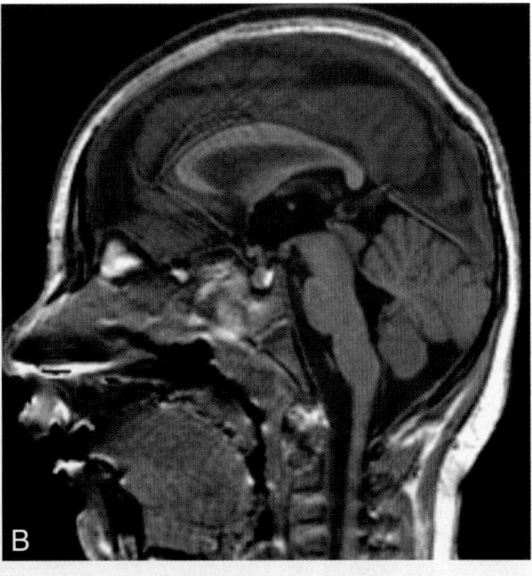

Fig. 2.24 Microcephaly With Polymicrogyria. (A) Axial T2W and (B) sagittal T1W images demonstrate microcephaly, polymicrogyria, reduced white matter volume, ventriculomegaly, and fully formed but thinned corpus callosum. The brainstem and cerebellum are normal.

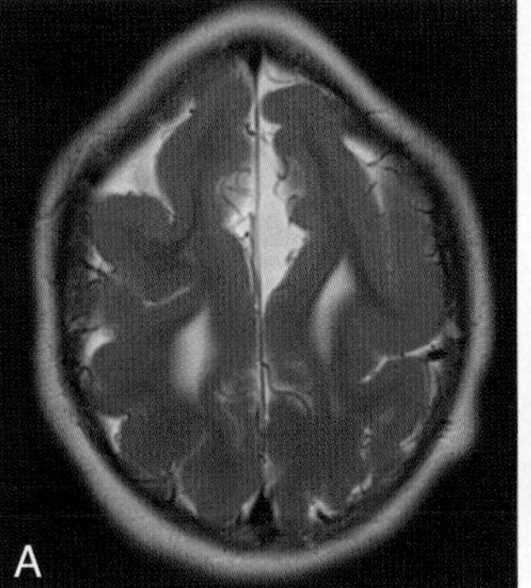
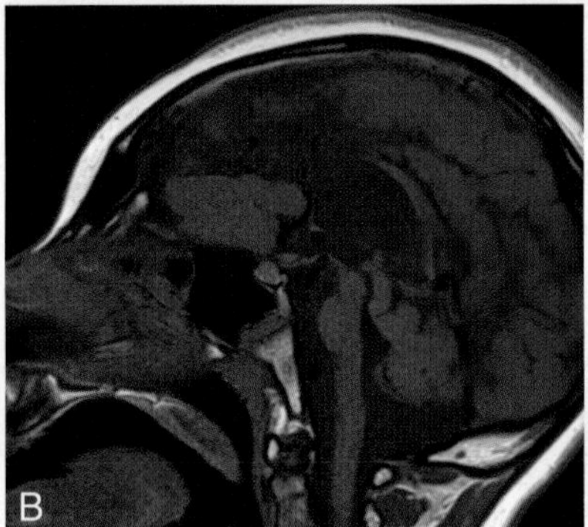
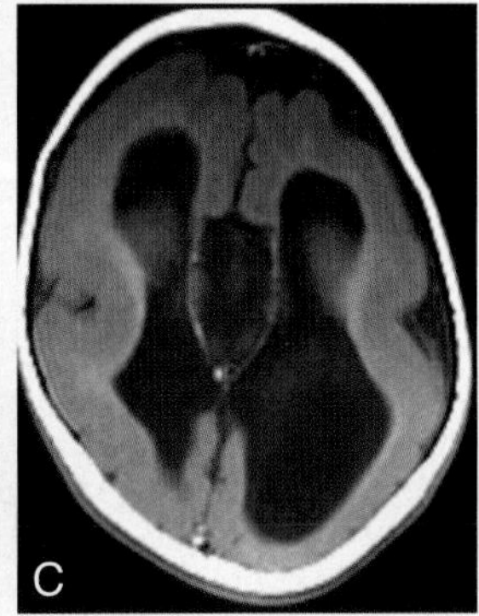
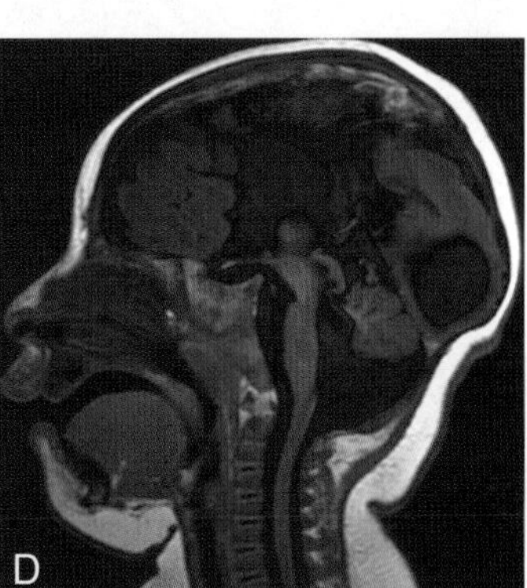

Fig. 2.25 Microlissencephaly. Two patients. (A and B) Axial T2W and sagittal T1W images demonstrate global microcephaly, pachygyria, cortical thickening, callosal dysgenesis with interhemispheric cyst, and hypoplastic brainstem and cerebellum. (C and D) Axial and sagittal T1W images demonstrate lissencephalic appearance of the brain, cortical thickening, agenesis of the corpus callosum, and hypoplasia of the brainstem and cerebellum.

Key Points

Background

- Microcephaly is defined as a head circumference at least 3 standard deviations below age-matched normative values.
- Primary or genetic mediated microcephaly is believed to result from early exhaustion of the neuronal precursors or accelerated neuronal apoptosis.
- Primary microcephaly must be differentiated from secondary, acquired microcephaly due to brain injury (e.g., after a hypoxic ischemic injury or TORCH infection).
- Multiple classifications are available of which the significance is being debated.
- Prognosis varies but often is associated with epilepsy, motor deficits, and intellectual disability. Patients with microcephaly primary hereditary typically have mild to moderate intellectual disability and speech and motor delay. Patients with microlissencephaly often have severe hypertonia or hypotonia, seizures, and early death.

Imaging

- On sagittal imaging the cranial vault/brain appears disproportionally small compared to the maxillofacial skeleton.
- Microcephaly may be associated with several patterns of the cerebral cortex and remainder of the brain:
  - Microcephaly primary hereditary (MCPH) demonstrates microcephaly with architecturally normal cortical thickness and folding.
  - Microcephaly with simplified gyral pattern (MSG) demonstrates absent tertiary sulcation, shallow sulci, delayed/impaired myelination, and normal cortical thickness. The corpus callosum may be thin but is typically completely formed from anterior to posterior.
  - Microlissencephaly with increased cerebral cortical thickness, agenesis or dysgenesis of the corpus callosum, and hypoplasia of the brainstem and cerebellum.
  - Microcephaly with polymicrogyria or cortical dysplasia.

REFERENCES

1. Raybaud C, Widjaja E. Development and dysgenesis of the cerebral cortex: malformations of cortical development. *Neuroimaging Clin N Am*. 2011;21(3):483–543.
2. Huisman TA, Poretti A. Chapter 7. Disorders of brain development. In: Magnetic Resonance Imaging of the Brain and Spine, 5th ed. Edited by Scott Atlas, MD. Wolters Kluwer, Lippincott Williams & Wilkins.
3. Barkovich AJames, Guerrini Renzo, Kuzniecky Ruben I, Jackson Graeme D, William B. Dobyns, A developmental and genetic classification for malformations of cortical development: update 2012. *Brain*. May 2012;135(5):1348–1369.

HEMIMEGALENCEPHALY

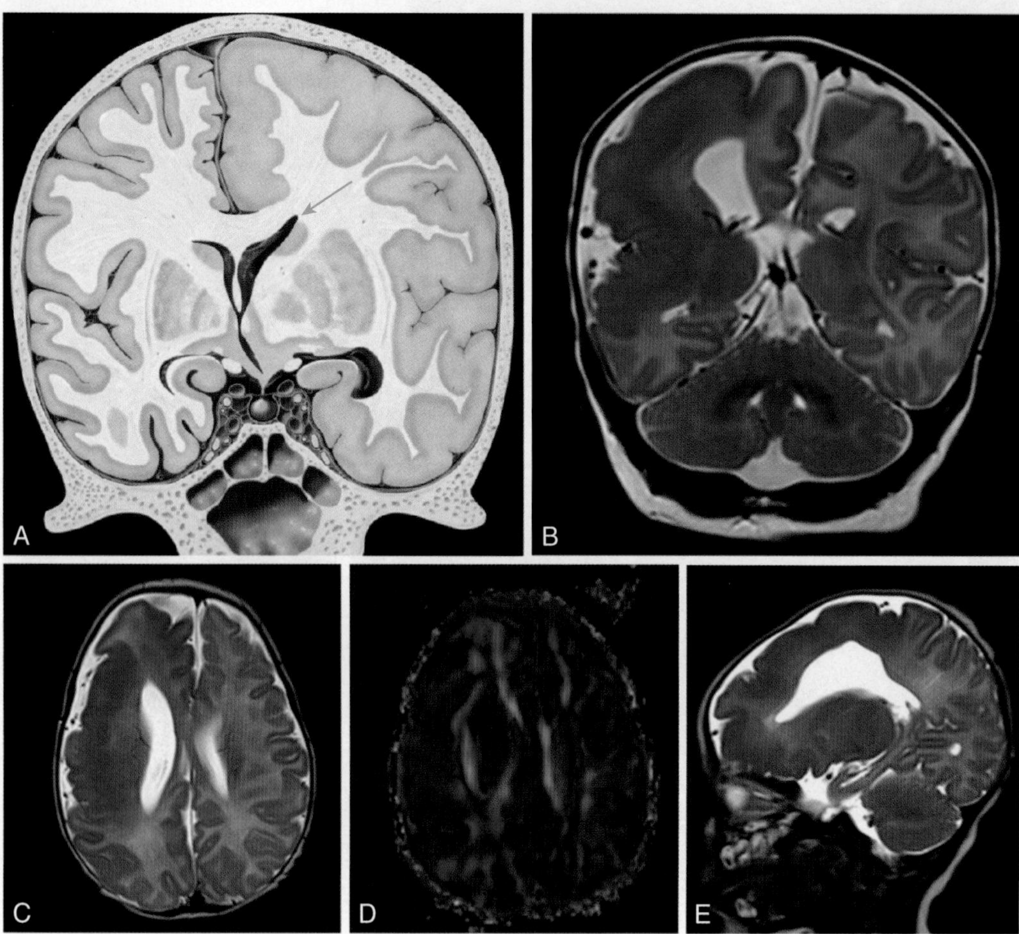

Fig. 2.26 Hemimegalencephaly. (A) Illustration of hemimegalencephaly with enlarged left cerebral hemispheres with diffuse pachygyria, and enlarged ipsilateral lateral ventricle. (B to E) axial, coronal, and sagittal T2W MRI of the brain, including color-coded fractional anisotropy maps in a child with right supratentorial hemimegalencephaly, show a mild overall enlargement of the right cerebral hemisphere with malformed and thickened cortical ribbon as well as enlarged ipsilateral lateral ventricle. On the color-coded fractional anisotropy maps, significant disorganization of the cortical ribbon and subcortical white matter is noted. (A from Stat-DX. Copyright © 2022 Elsevier.)

Key Points

Background

- Hemimegalencephaly is characterized by a diffuse hamartomatous overgrowth of part or entirety of a cerebral hemisphere. The ipsilateral cerebellum may also be enlarged (total hemimegalencephaly).
- The exact etiology remains unclear, but this severe congenital malformation is presumed to be secondary to a combination of an accelerated, *excessive neuronal proliferation and impaired apoptosis*.
- Most children present with intractable seizures, developmental delay, and hemiplegia.
- Hemimegalencephaly is seen as an isolated finding but may also be part of various syndromes including PIK3/akt/mTOR disorders, hypomelanosis of Ito, neurofibromatosis type 1, Klippel-Trenaunay syndrome, and Proteus syndrome.

Imaging

- The *enlarged cerebral hemisphere* shows a *thickened, dysmorphic cortical ribbon* with simplified gyration and shallow sulci. The adjacent white matter is abnormal with features consistent with dysmyelination.
- Color-coded fractional anisotropy maps confirm the disorganization of the cortical ribbon and the subcortical, hemispheric white matter.
- Characteristically, the *ipsilateral lateral ventricle is enlarged* compared to the contralateral side, often commensurate with the enlarged affected hemisphere. In addition, the shape of the enlarged ventricle is abnormal. The midline is in most cases preserved.
- The hemicranium containing the enlarged hemisphere is typically enlarged, resulting in an increased head circumference/macrocephaly.

REFERENCE

1. Huisman TA, Poretti A. Chapter 7. Disorders of brain development. In: Magnetic Resonance Imaging of the Brain and Spine, 5th ed. Edited by Scott Atlas, MD. Wolters Kluwer, Lippincott Williams & Wilkins.

LISSENCEPHALY AND PACHYGYRIA

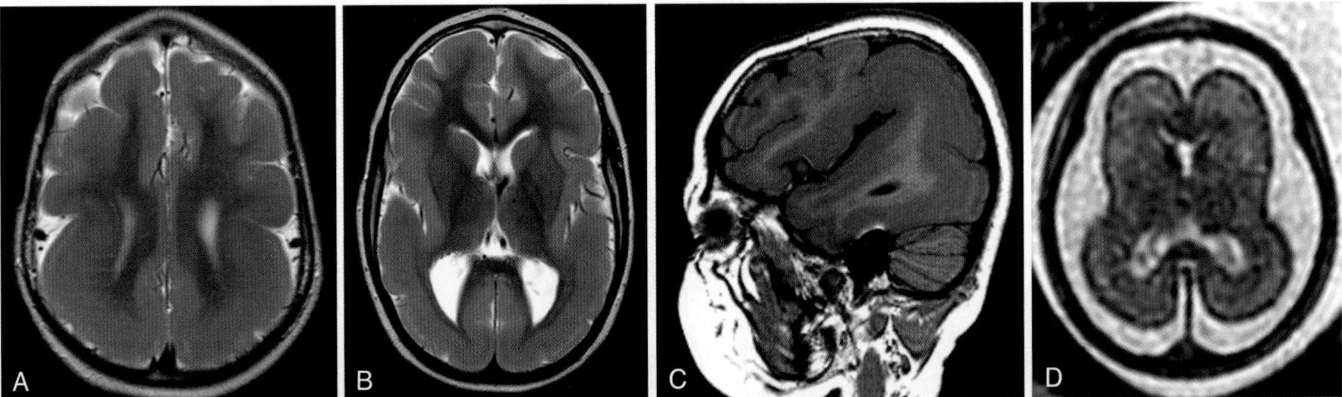

Fig. 2.27 Lissencephaly and Pachygyria due to LIS1 Mutation. (A to C) Axial T2W and sagittal T1W images demonstrate lissencephaly with more agyria posteriorly compared to anterior pachygyria. (D) Axial T2W fetal MRI of a 28-week fetus demonstrate lack of sulcation and figure-8 pattern consistent with lissencephaly.

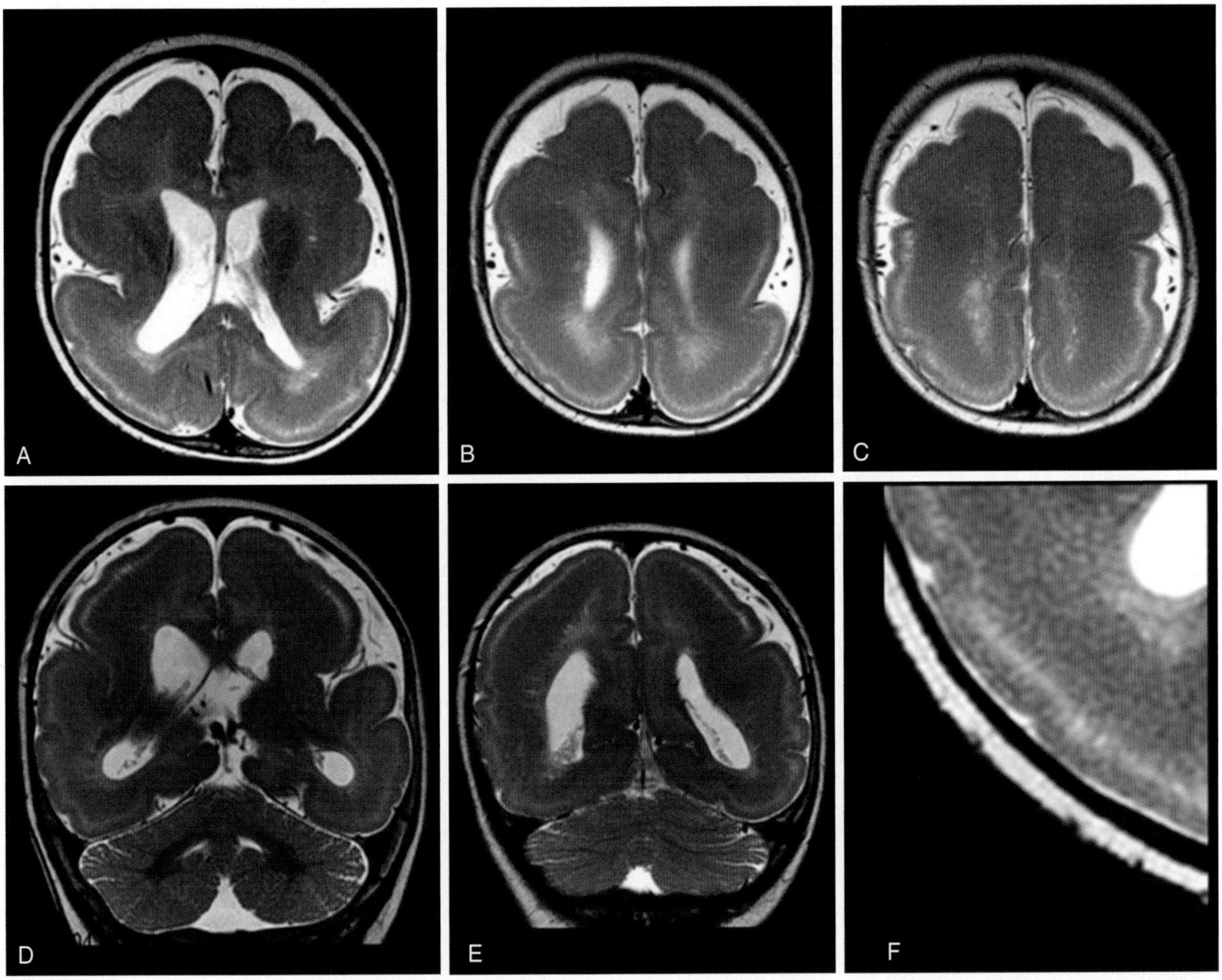

Fig. 2.28 Lissencephaly and Pachygyria due to LIS1 Mutation. (A to C) Axial, and (D and E) coronal T2W MRIs of a child with marked lissencephaly, with smooth brain surface, T2 hyperintense cell sparse zone in between of the thin cortical ribbon, and wide band of arrested neurons within the region of the cerebral hemispheres. (F) Magnified T2W image showing the thin cortical ribbon, hyperintense cell sparse zone, and isointense arrested neuronal layer.

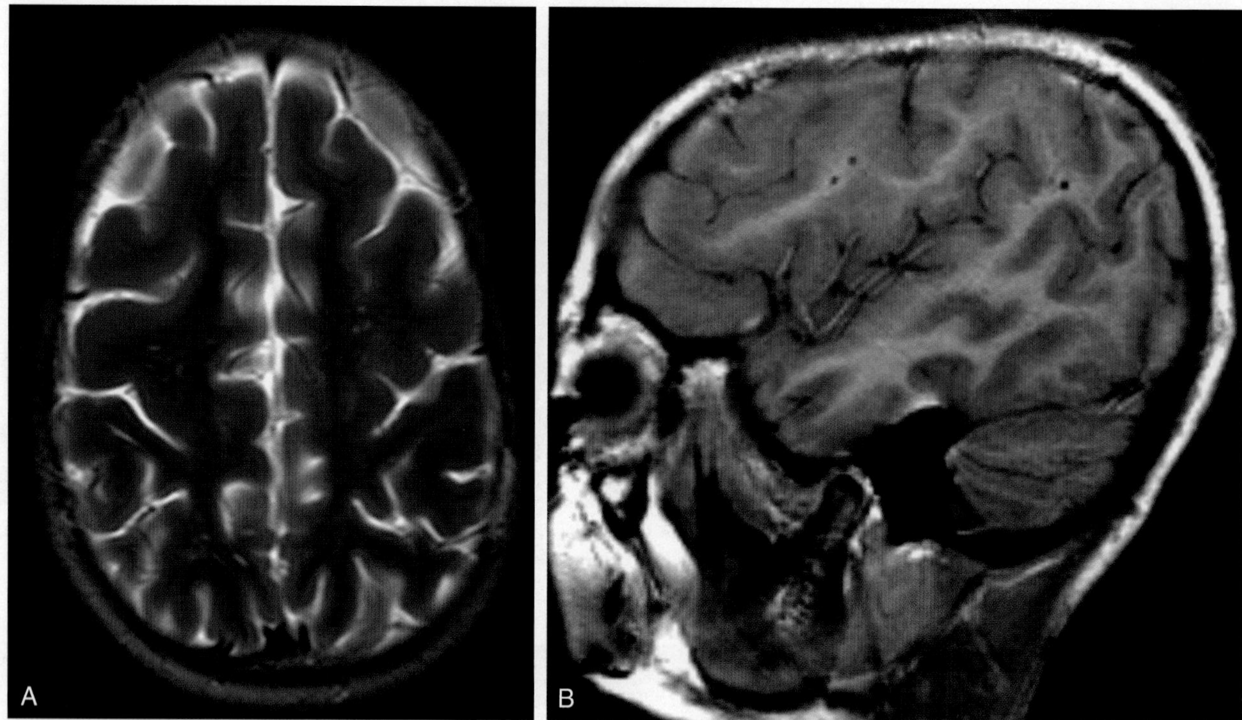

FIG. 2.29 Pachygyria From DCX Mutation. (A) Axial T2W and (B) sagittal T1W images demonstrate broad frontal gyri consistent with pachygyria and more normal posterior gyri. Genetic evaluation confirmed a DCX gene mutation.

Key Points

Background

- Lissencephaly and pachygyria are cortical malformations due to *abnormal neuronal migration* often occurring as a spectrum in patients.
- Lissencephaly results from an arrested neuronal migration resulting in a four-layer cortical ribbon.
- Lissencephaly may be secondary to a LIS1 mutation (classic lissencephaly), DCX mutation also known as X-linked (XLIS), TUBA1A gene mutation, or secondary to infections (cytomegalovirus). LIS1 and DCX mutations account for 40% to 75% of patients with classic lissencephaly.
- Pachygyria is likely caused by abnormal regulation of microtubule activities.
- Pachygyria can be caused by infections or be part of overgrowth syndromes, including hemimegalencephaly.

Imaging

- Lissencephaly is characterized by the appearance of a smooth brain surface with little or no gyri (agyria) and sulci generally resembling a *figure-8 shape*. Pachygyria is characterized by broad/wide gyri, shallow or absent sulci, and abnormal thickened cortical ribbon with a smooth inner and outer contour of the cortex. Many cases of occurring as a spectrum in patients have a combination of agyria and pachygyria.
- Pattern of agyria-pachygyria can indicate underlying genetic mutation:
  - LIS1 mutations often have greater agyria of the parietal and occipital lobes and pachygyria of the frontal lobes.
  - DCX mutations have more severe involvement of the frontal lobes compared to the occipital lobes.
  - TUBA1A gene mutations often demonstrate classic lissencephaly as well as malformation of the corpus callosum, rounded hippocampi, and pontocerebellar hypoplasia.

REFERENCES

1. Raybaud C, Widjaja E. Development and dysgenesis of the cerebral cortex: malformations of cortical development. *Neuroimaging Clin N Am.* 2011;21(3):483–543.
2. Huisman TA, Poretti A. Chapter 7. Disorders of brain development. In: Magnetic Resonance Imaging of the Brain and Spine, 5th ed. Edited by Scott Atlas, MD. Wolters Kluwer, Lippincott Williams & Wilkins.

GRAY MATTER HETEROTOPIA

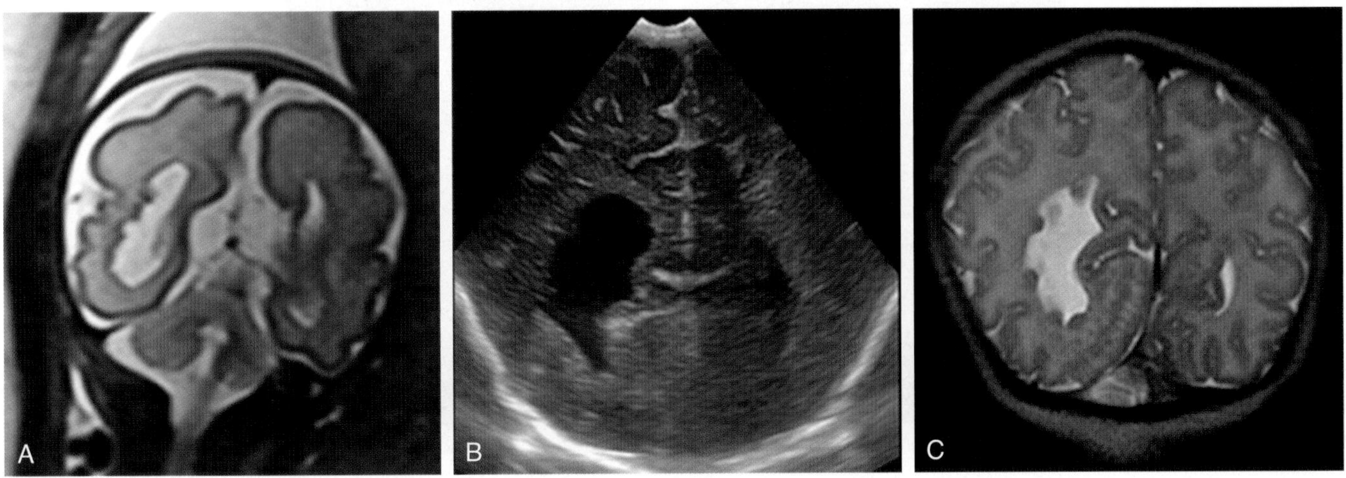

Fig. 2.30 Gray Matter Heterotopia. (A) Coronal T2W fetal MRI, and postnatal (B) coronal ultrasound and (C) coronal T2W MRI demonstrate right periventricular nodular gray matter heterotopia. Additional findings of polymicrogyria in the lateral right occipital lobe on fetal MRI seen as abnormal sulcation, and also present in the medial occipital lobes seen on postnatal MRI.

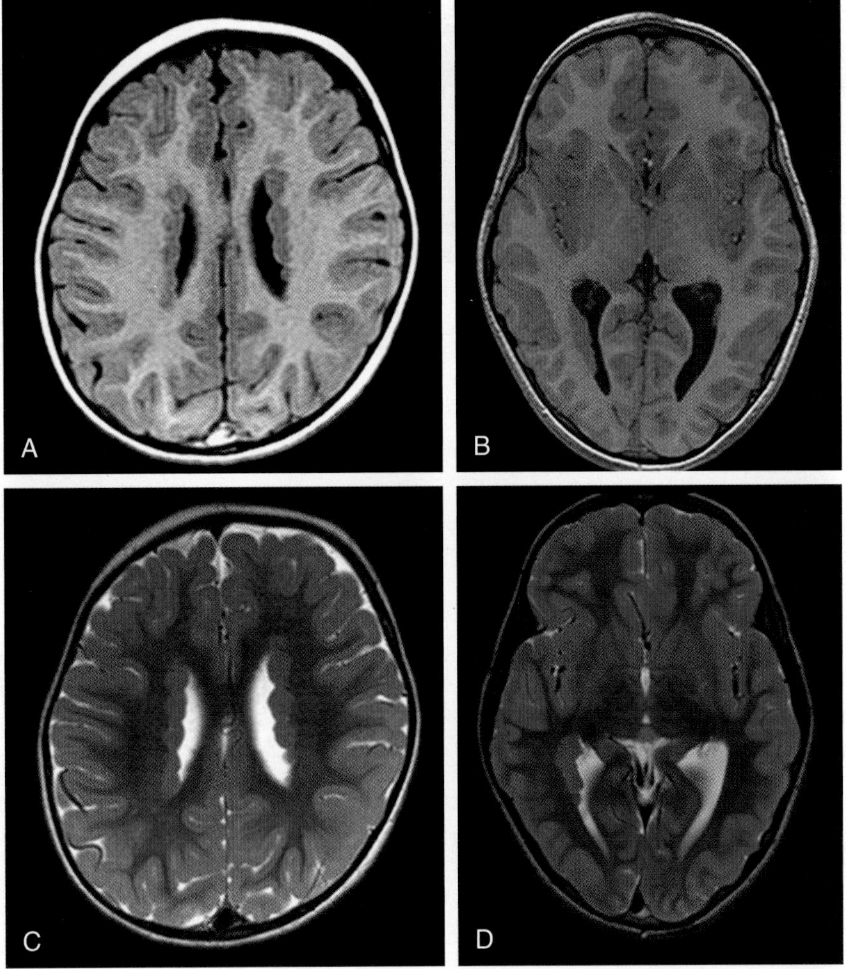

Fig. 2.31 Gray Matter Heterotopia. (A and B) Axial T1W and (C and D) axial T2W MRI of a child with bilateral isointense periventricular gray matter heterotopias lining the lateral ventricles.

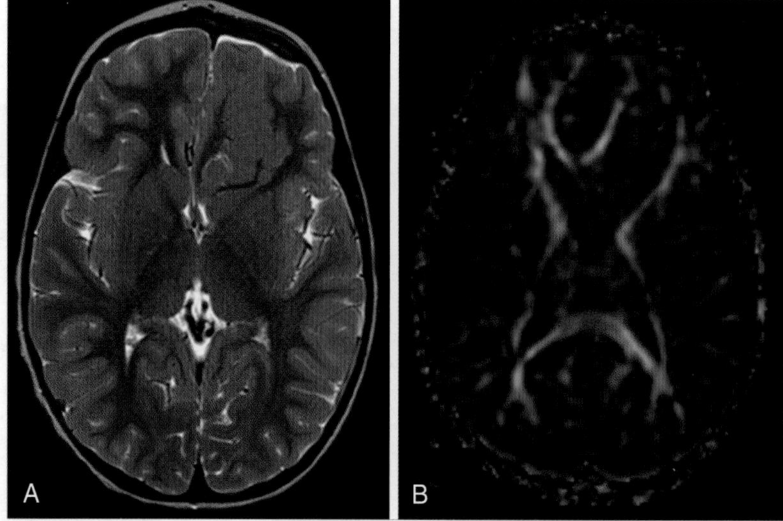

Fig. 2.32 Gray Matter Heterotopia. (A) Axial T2W and (B) fractional anisotropy maps of a child with extensive isointense transmantle gray matter heterotopia within the left frontal lobe extending from the surface of the left frontal lobe up to the level of the left frontal horn. Matching low anisotropic diffusion on fractional anisotropy maps.

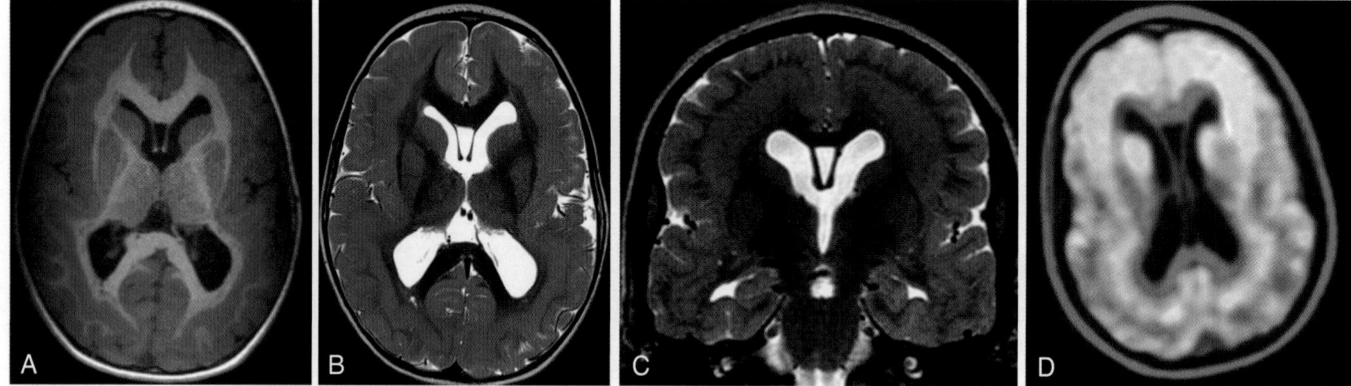

Fig. 2.33 Gray Matter Band Heterotopia in DCX Mutation. (A and B) Axial T1W and axial T2W images demonstrate T1 and T2 isointense subcortical band heterotopia in a 2-year-old female found to have DCX gene mutation. (C and D) Coronal T2W and axial FDG PET CT images in a 10-year-old female with DCX gene mutation demonstrates band heterotopia with increased FDG uptake in the heterotopia greater than the cortex.

Key Points

Background

- Heterotopia refers to an abnormal collection of neurons in an anomalous location other than the cortical gray matter.
- Heterotopia is believed to be secondary to an *arrested migration of neurons* from the germinal matrix toward the cortical ribbon along the radial glial path.
- Heterotopia may occur isolated or be part of complex brain malformations or syndromes including Chiari II malformation, commissural anomalies, Joubert syndrome, fragile X syndrome, and FLNA gene mutation.
- Clinical symptoms are variable. Mild degrees of periventricular heterotopia may be incidentally identified. Other patients may have developmental delay, seizures, and motor dysfunction.

Imaging

- Heterotopias are isointense to cortical gray matter on all MRI sequences and do not show contrast enhancement.
- On (color-coded) fractional anisotropy maps, heterotopia have low FA values due to the high degree of isotropic diffusion, similar to cortical and central gray matter.
- Heterotopia may be subcortical or periventricular.
- Heterotopia may be focal/nodular, multifocal, linear/band-like, unilateral, or bilateral. Band heterotopia is typically seen in females with LIS1 or DCX mutation.
- Large heterotopia may exert a mass effect on adjacent structures.
- Overlying cortical ribbon may be affected/malformed.

REFERENCES

1. Raybaud C, Widjaja E. Development and dysgenesis of the cerebral cortex: malformations of cortical development. *Neuroimaging Clin N Am.* 2011;21(3):483–543.
2. Huisman TA, Poretti A. Chapter 7. Disorders of brain development. In: Magnetic Resonance Imaging of the Brain and Spine, 5th ed. Edited by Scott Atlas, MD. Wolters Kluwer, Lippincott Williams & Wilkins.

GLIONEURONAL HETEROTOPIA

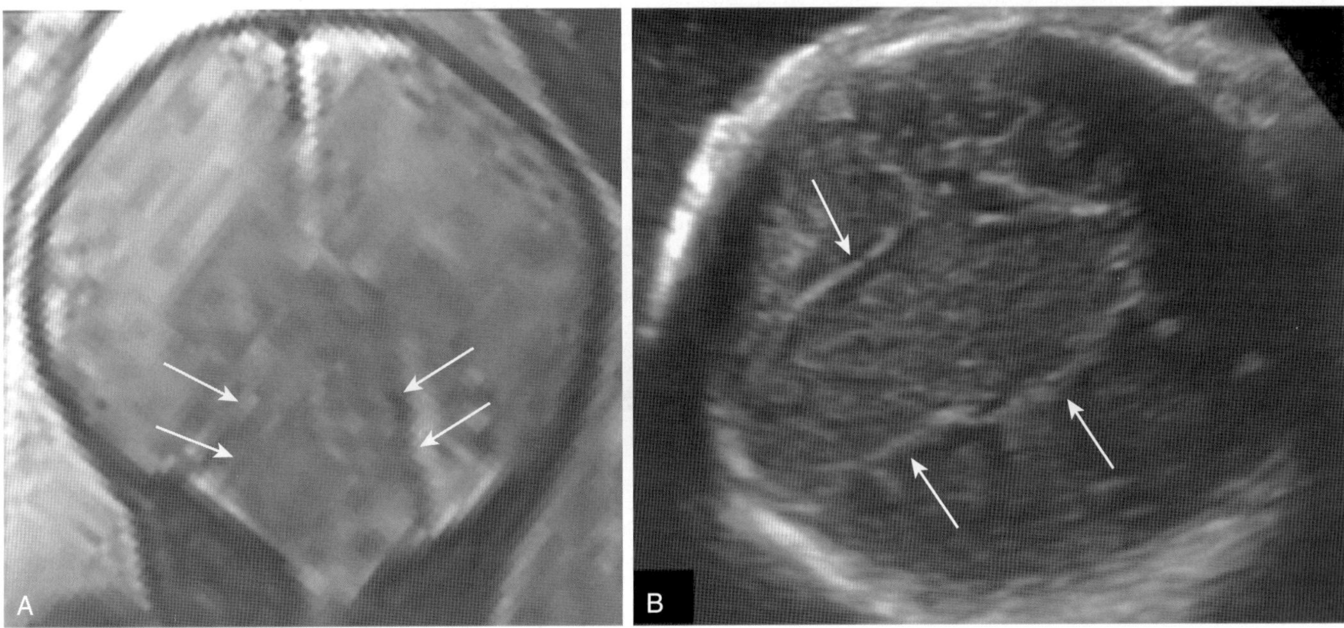

Fig. 2.34 Glioneuronal Heterotopia. (A) Coronal T2W fetal MRI and (B) matching prenatal axial ultrasound image of a fetus with a large T2 hypointense malformative mass lesion within the right posterior fossa outlined by *white arrows*. This significant displacement of the adjacent cerebellum and brainstem. Diagnosis would be difficult to make and requires postnatal follow up MRI.

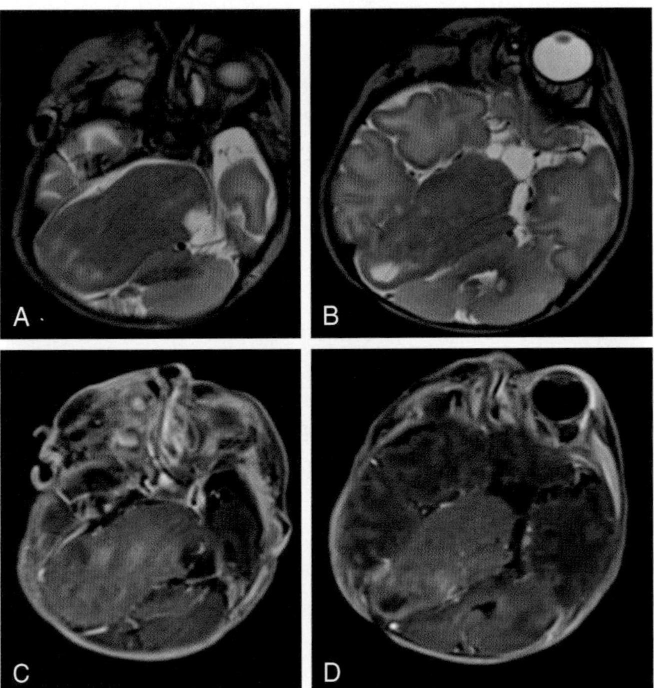

Fig. 2.35 Glioneuronal Heterotopia. (A and B) Postnatal T2W and (C and D) T1W+C MRI (same child as seen in Fig. 2.34) with well-circumscribed mass lesion in the right posterior fossa, signal intensities matching a mixture of cortical gray matter and white matter; within the lesion small amount of fluid, likely cerebral spinal fluid, is noted. No matching contrast enhancement. Significant mass effect exerted on the adjacent brainstem and right cerebellum. The right orbit is hypoplastic; the right globe is lacking. The diagnosis of a rare extra-axial glioneuronal heterotopia is challenging but can be made when all the findings are considered.

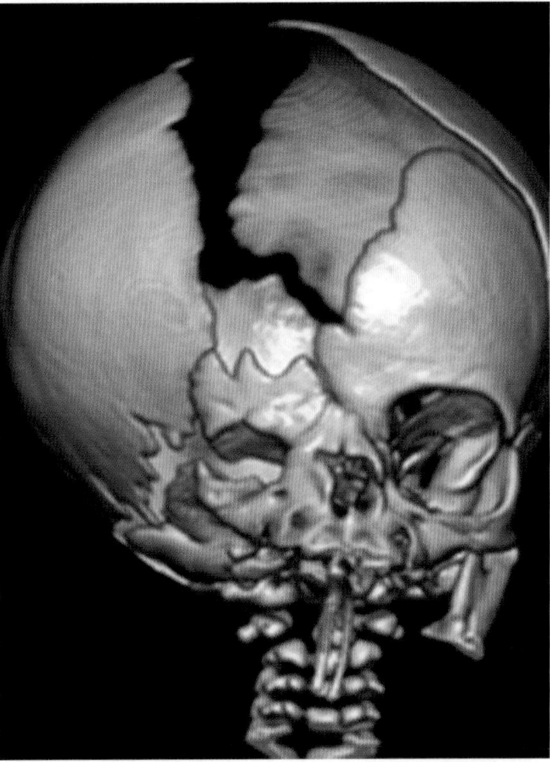

Fig. 2.36 Glioneuronal Heterotopia. 3D volumetric reconstruction (CT) of the skull of the same child as shown in Figs. 2.34 and 2.35, confirming the hypoplastic right orbit and significant deformity of the skull with wide open metopic suture and anterior fontanelle.

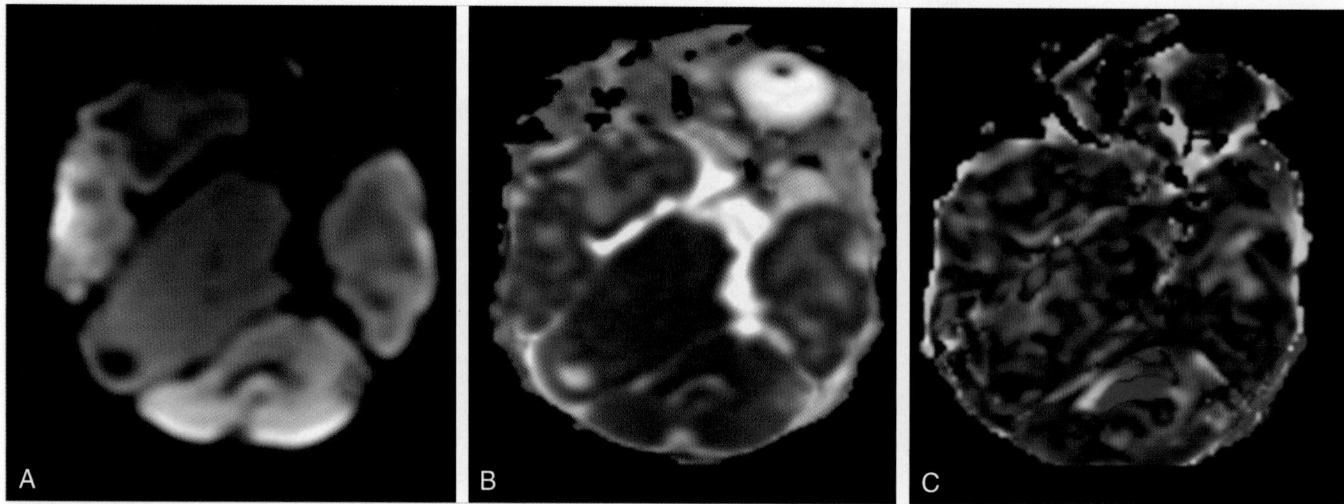

Fig. 2.37 Glioneuronal Heterotopia. (A) Axial DWI image, (B) ADC and (C) FA maps of the same child as shown in Figs. 2.34 to 2.36, confirming the glioneuronal nature of the lesion.

Key Points

Background

- Also known as neuroglial hamartoma. A focal mass lesion/malformation composed of differentiated derivatives of neuroectodermal tissue, including disorganized mature neuronal and glial cells.
- Occurs between the fifth and sixth week of gestation, when the forebrain vesicle is divided into the telencephalon and diencephalon.
- Most are large at presentation, supporting that the etiologic event occurs early in gestation.
- Glioneuronal heterotopia is clinically and pathologically benign and must be differentiated from true neoplasms.

Imaging

- On neuroimaging the lesions are typically extraaxial with lack of infiltration of adjacent brain structures. The CT and MRI characteristics follow gray and white matter densities/signal intensities on all sequences. No directional diffusion seen on fractional anisotropy maps. Faint or absent contrast enhancement. Lack of growth on serial imaging supports diagnosis.
- Glioneuronal heterotopias are typically located extracranially, including the orbit, pharynx, middle ear, neck, and thorax. The nasal cavity represents the most common location.
- Rarely, glioneuronal heterotopias may be located intracranially. Intracranial glioneuronal heterotopias are frequently associated with congenital craniofacial anomalies.
- Prenatal ultrasound or fetal MRI allows diagnosis of the lesion but is challenging.

REFERENCES

1. Huisman TA, Brehmer U, Zeilinger G, et al. Parapharyngeal neuroglial heterotopia extending through the skull base in a neonate with airway obstruction. *J Pediatr Surg*. 2007 Oct; 42(10):1764–1767.
2. Meoded A, Turan S, Harman C, et al. Pre- and postnatal ultrasound and magnetic resonance imaging of intracranial extra-axial glioneuronal heterotopia. *Fetal Diagn Ther*. 2011;30(4):314–316.

COBBLESTONE MALFORMATIONS

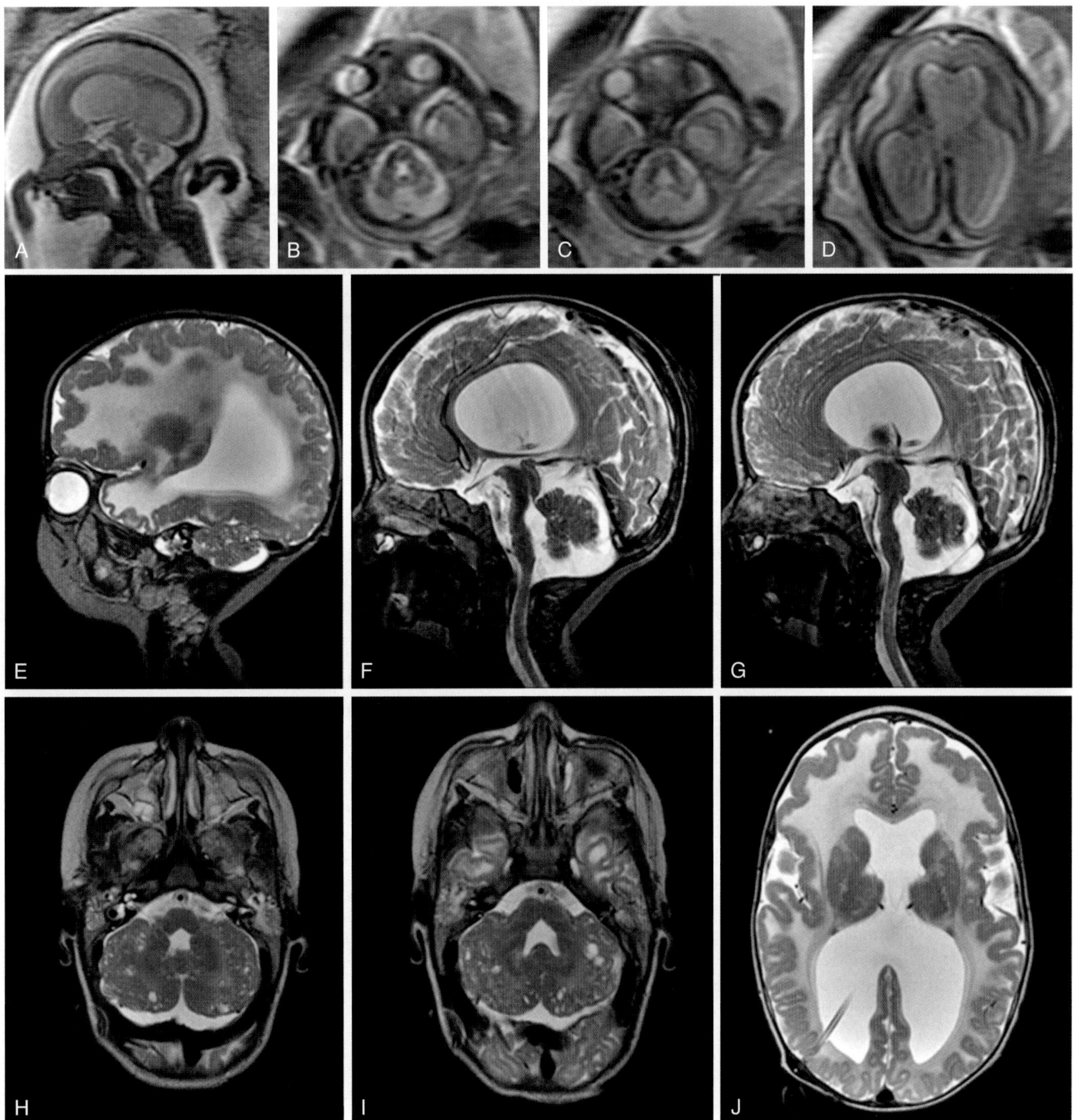

Fig. 2.38 Congenital Muscular Dysplasia. (A to D) Sagittal and axial T2W fetal MRI demonstrating characteristic elongation and mild kinking of the brainstem, hypoplastic pontine belly, elongated and malformed tectal plate, subtle cysts within the cerebellar fissures, and moderate supratentorial ventriculomegaly. (E to J) Sagittal and axial T2W postnatal MRI of the same patient confirm the prenatal imaging findings of elongation and mild kinking of the brainstem, lack of the pontine belly, multiple cysts within the cerebellar fissures, deformed and elongated tectal plate, aqueductal stenosis, extensive cobblestone cortical malformation resembling polymicrogyria, white matter edema/hypomyelination, and moderate ventriculomegaly.

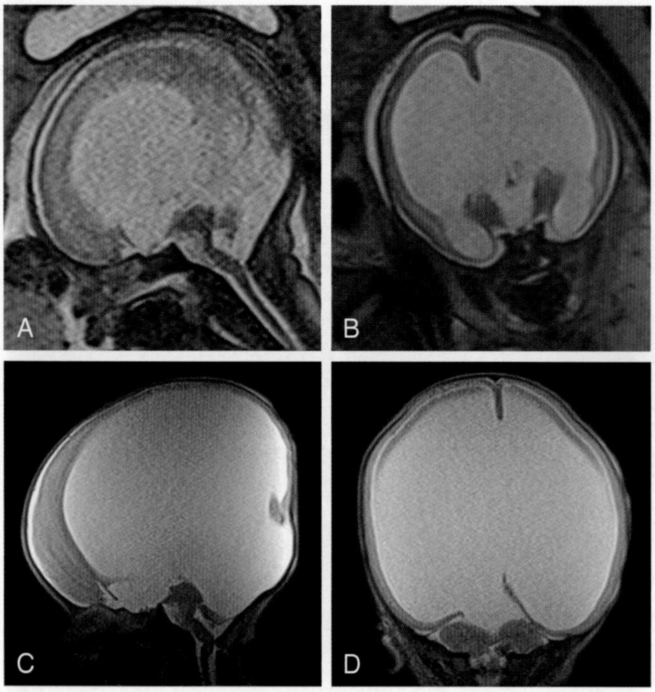

A B C D

Fig. 2.39 Walker-Warburg. (A and B) Sagittal, and coronal T2W fetal MRI and (C and D) postnatal sagittal and coronal T2W MRI demonstrate kinking and elongation of the brainstem, diffuse cobblestone cortical malformation and high-grade supratentorial ventriculomegaly.

Key Points

Background

- Cobblestone malformations are *malformations of neuronal migration.*
- Multiple genes (autosomal recessive inheritance) have been identified linked to alpha-dystroglycan mutations. Consequently, these disorders are also known as alpha-dystroglycanopathies.
- Abnormal glycosylation of the cell-surface glycoprotein alpha-dystroglycan results in a deficient binding of extracellular matrix proteins containing laminin domains. This binding is essential for muscle fibers to attach to the muscle basal lamina, and deficiency prevents normal muscle contraction (*muscular dystrophy*). Proper function of glycosylated alpha-dystroglycan is also relevant for the linkage of radial glial cells to the basement membrane during development of the cortical ribbon, and for the glial guide cells to the retinal limiting membrane. The lack of a proper attachment of the radial glial cells to the pial basement membrane allows for *overmigration of neurons* through the pial basement membrane into the subpial and subarachnoid space, resulting in the typical cobblestone appearance. Consequently, in dystroglycanopathies additional neuronal cerebral and cerebellar migrational abnormalities and *retinal abnormalities* including colobomas may accompany the muscular dystrophy.
- Clinically, they are subclassified into merosin-positive or -negative muscular dystrophy (CMD1), Fukuyama congenital muscular dystrophy (CMD2), muscle eye brain disease (CMD3), and Walker-Warburg syndrome (CMD4).
- Muscle biopsy typically confirms diagnosis.
- Neonates present at birth with hypotonia, early onset progressive muscular weakness, delayed motor development, impaired vision, and seizures.

Imaging

- Cortical anomalies, including cobblestone lissencephaly, polymicrogyria, and/or pachygyria
- Z-shaped or kinked, thin brainstem, and cervicomedullary kinking
- Cortical/subcortical cerebellar inclusion cysts, hypoplastic vermis and cerebellum, and tectal plate deformities
- Abnormal myelination
- Ventriculomegaly
- Malformed corpus callosum
- Retinal abnormalities as well as colobomas
- Occipital encephaloceles may be seen in CMD4
- Imaging findings typically become more prominent on postnatal imaging, in particular the dysmyelination and cortical anomalies

REFERENCES

1. Bosemani T, Orman G, Boltshauser E, Tekes A, Huisman TA, Poretti A. Congenital abnormalities of the posterior fossa. *Radiographics.* 2015;35(1):200–220.
2. Tali A, Poretti A, Boltshauser E, Huisman TA. Differential diagnosis of ventriculomegaly and brainstem kinking on fetal MRI. *Brain Dev.* 2016;38(1):103–108.
3. Huisman TA. Fetal MRI of the Central Nervous System and Abdomen. *Semin Roentgenol.* 2008;43(4):314–336.

POLYMICROGYRIA

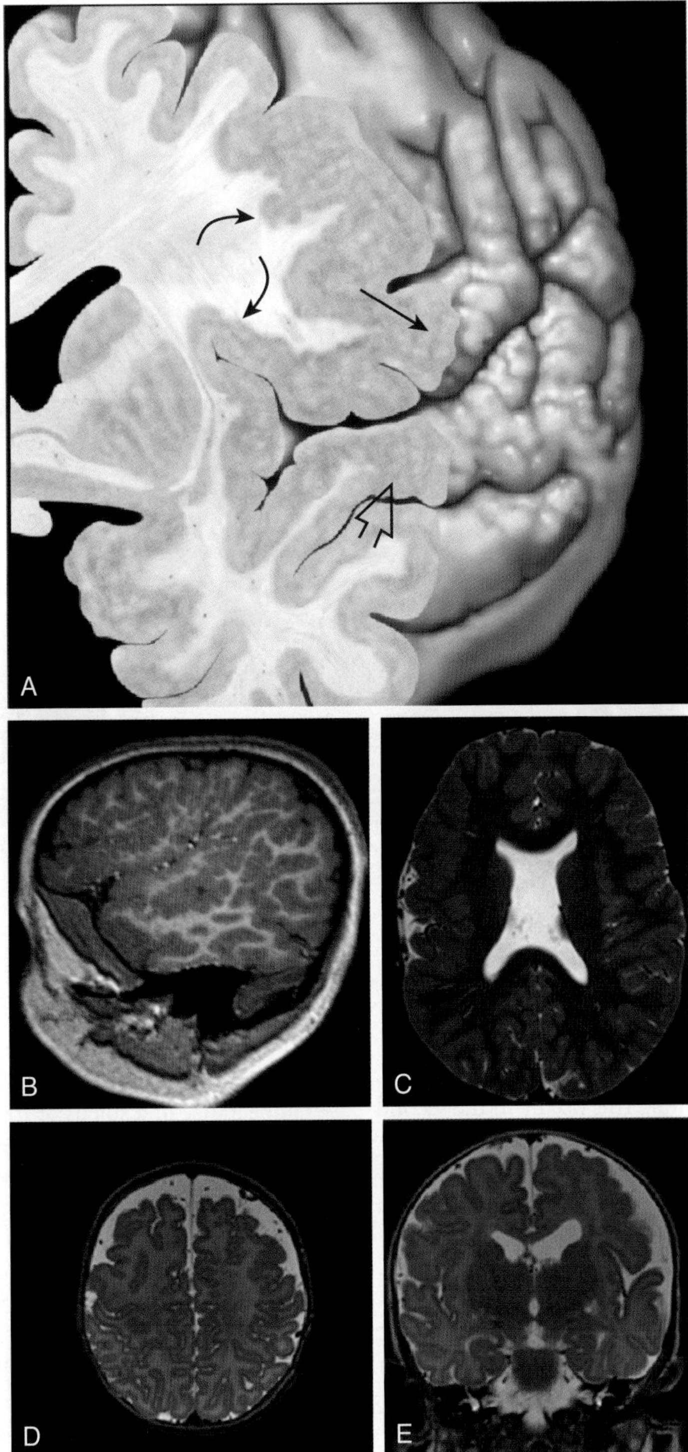

Fig. 2.40 Polymicrogyria. (A) Illustration of polymicrogyria. (B and C) Sagittal T1W and axial T2W MRI of a child with septo-optic dysplasia and extensive right perirolandic thickening of the cortical ribbon compatible with polymicrogyria. (D and E) Axial and coronal T2W MRI of a child with left lateral frontal polymicrogyria characterized by multiple small gyri, additional mild left ventriculomegaly. (A from StatDX. Copyright © 2022 Elsevier.)

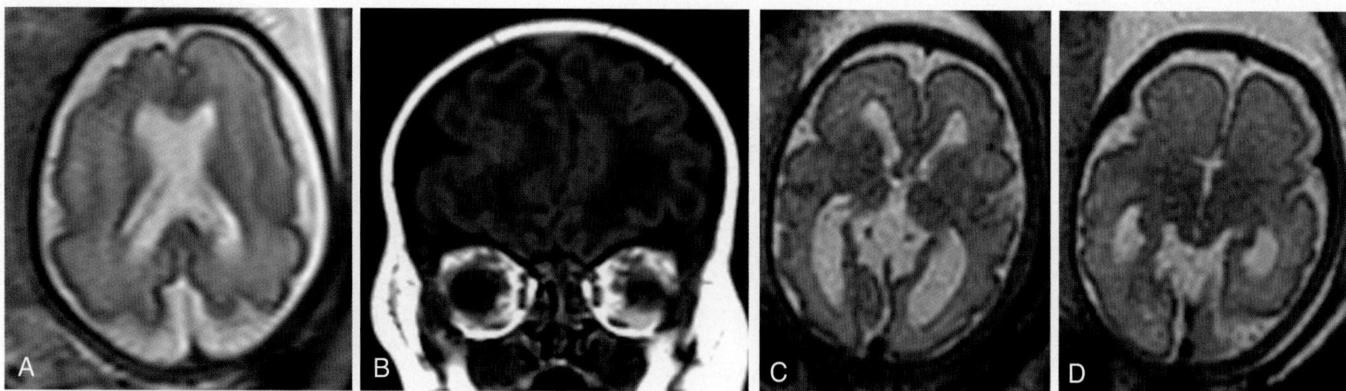

Fig. 2.41 Polymicrogyria. (A and B) Axial T2W fetal MRI and postnatal coronal T1W MRI demonstrate right frontal lobe polymicrogyria. (C and D) Axial T2W fetal MRI in a fetus with TUBA1A gene mutation demonstrates bilateral perisylvian polymicrogyria characterized by abnormal sulcation of bilateral sylvian fissures.

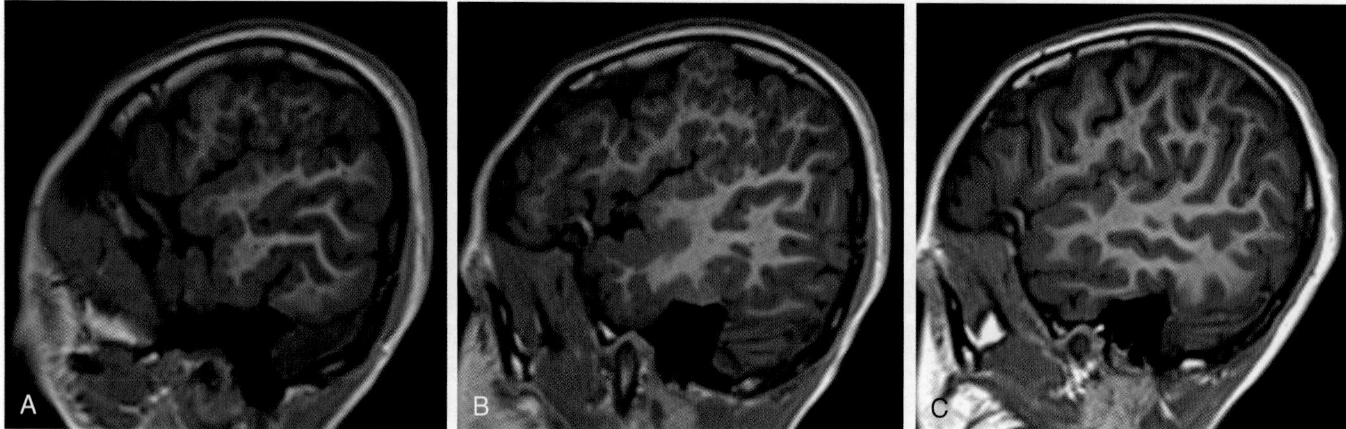

Fig. 2.42 Polymicrogyria. (A and B) Sagittal T1W images demonstrate right lateral perisylvian polymicrogyria. (C) Sagittal T1W image of the normal left sylvian fissure for comparison.

Key Points

Background

- Polymicrogyria results from abnormal *late neuronal migration/early cortical organization* impairing the normal lamination of the cortical ribbon. This occurs in the second half of the second trimester.
- Polymicrogyria may be secondary to intrauterine infections, ischemia, toxins (e.g., alcohol) or genetic/ syndrome related (e.g. Aicardi syndrome, Zellweger syndrome, tubulinopathy, mTORopathy).
- Polymicrogyria may be focal or multifocal, unilateral or bilateral.
- If the polymicrogyria is bilateral and symmetrical, evaluation for a genetic disorder or syndrome should be performed.
- Prognosis is variable and depends on extent and location, associated anomalies. Unilateral polymicrogyria can be found in otherwise healthy children who present in the first or second decade with seizures.

Imaging

- Abnormal cortical ribbon characterized by multiple small and irregular-shaped gyri with small, shallow or fused intervening sulci.
- The surface of the brain may appear "smooth" due to the obliterated or fused sulci.
- Dysplastic, abnormal leptomeningeal vessels may overlay the abnormal cortical ribbon.
- On fetal MRI, polymicrogyria can appear as either early appearance of a sulcus or irregular cortical sulcation.
- Polymicrogyria typically lines a schizencephalic cleft.
- Associations: CMV infection, septo-optic dysplasia, callosal anomalies, gray matter heterotopia, MPPH syndrome (macrocephaly, polymicrogyria, polydactyly, hydrocephalus), tubulinopathy, Zellweger syndrome.

REFERENCES

1. Raybaud C, Widjaja E. Development and dysgenesis of the cerebral cortex: malformations of cortical development. *Neuroimaging Clin N Am*. 2011;21(3):483–543.
2. Huisman TA, Poretti A. Chapter 7. Disorders of brain development. In: Magnetic Resonance Imaging of the Brain and Spine, 5th ed. Edited by Scott Atlas, MD. Wolters Kluwer, Lippincott Williams & Wilkins.

SCHIZENCEPHALY

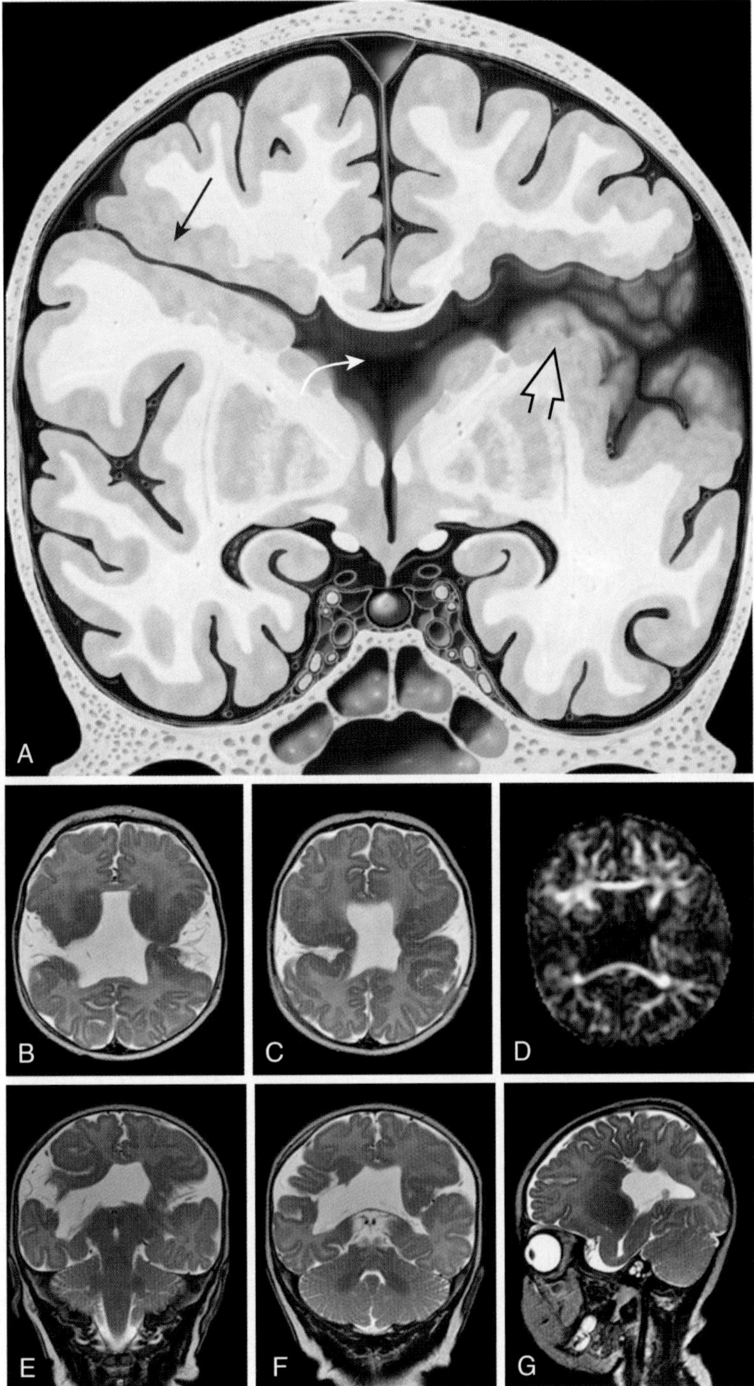

Fig. 2.43 Schizencephaly. (A) Illustration of a right sided closed lip schizencephaly and left-sided open lip schizencephaly lined by polymicrogyria (thin black arrow on the right and wide black arrow on the left) communicating with the ventricle (curved arrow). (B to G) Axial, coronal, and sagittal T2W MRI, including fractional anisotropy maps of a child with bilateral schizencephaly and absent septum pellucidum. On the right, cerebral spinal fluid is noted in between of the lips of the schizencephaly compatible with open-lip schizencephaly, On the left, the lips are approaching each other compatible with closed-lip schizencephaly. Thickened and dysmorphic gray matter is lining the clefts. Dysplastic vessels extending into the region of the clefts. The leaves of the septum pellucidum are lacking. On fractional anisotropy the schizencephaly is clearly depicted. (A from StatDX. Copyright 2022 Elsevier.)

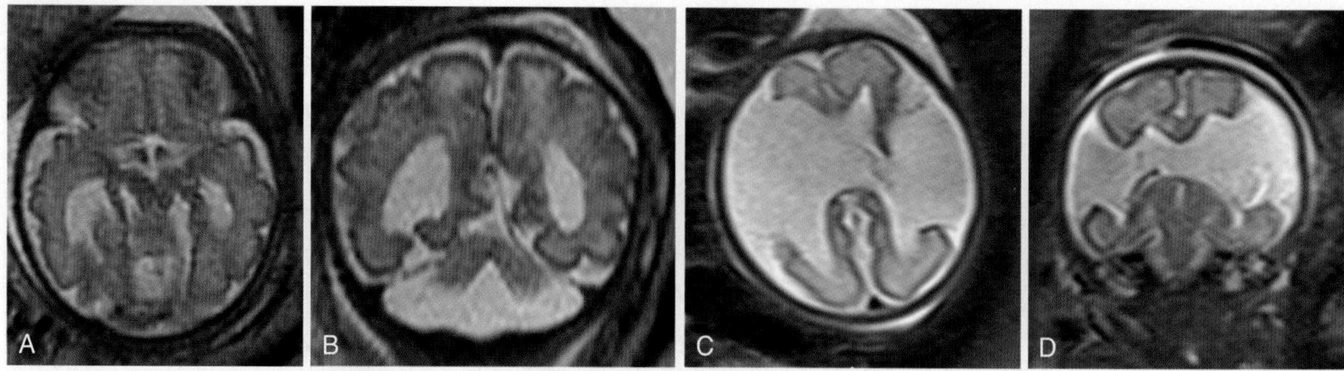

Fig. 2.44 Schizencephaly. Two patients. (A and B) Axial and coronal T2W fetal MRI displaying a right temporal occipital closed lip schizencephaly. (C and D) Axial and coronal T2W fetal MRI demonstrate large bilateral frontal temporal parietal open-lip schizencephaly.

Key Points

Background

- Schizencephaly is a *malformation of cortical migration* resulting in a gray matter–lined cleft in the cerebral hemisphere communicating from the subpial space to the ventricle.
- The most likely etiology of a schizencephaly is an early, intrauterine vascular insult during neuronal migration and cortical organization occurring at ~16 to 21 weeks' gestation, similar to polymicrogyria.
- Open-lip schizencephaly is more frequently symptomatic compared to closed-lip schizencephaly. Bilateral schizencephaly is associated with more severe neurocognitive impairment compared to unilateral. 90% of patients have motor dysfunction, 78% have cognitive dysfunction, and 68% have seizures.

Imaging

- Schizencephaly is defined as a cleft extending from the surface of the brain toward the ventricle lined by malformed gray matter (transmantle clefting). The cortical gray matter lining the cleft is dysplastic with abnormal lamination and may include areas of pachygyria and polymicrogyria.
- Schizencephaly is subdivided into open-lip and closed-lip schizencephaly.
- In open-lip schizencephaly, the lips/borders of the cleft are separated by cerebrospinal fluid, while in closed-lip schizencephaly the lips/borders of the cleft are "touching" each other with minimal or no cerebrospinal fluid within the cleft.
- In closed-lip schizencephaly, a focal dimple may be seen along the ventricular wall at the "insertion site" of the cleft.
- Dysplastic vessels may extend into the cleft.
- Schizencephaly may be unilateral (~60%) or bilateral (~40%). In bilateral schizencephaly the leaves of the septum pellucidum are nearly always absent; in unilateral schizencephaly they are absent in most cases.
- On (color-coded) fractional anisotropy maps the aberrant course or lack of affected white matter tracts are easily identified.
- Schizencephaly can be diagnosed on fetal MRI in most cases.
- Additional findings include: agenesis or hypogenesis of the corpus callosum (38%), septo-optic dysplasia (17%), hydrocephalus (24%), and microcephaly (42%).

REFERENCES

1. Raybaud C, Widjaja E. Development and dysgenesis of the cerebral cortex: malformations of cortical development. *Neuroimaging Clin N Am*. 2011;21(3):483–543.
2. Huisman TA, Poretti A. Chapter 7. Disorders of brain development. In: Magnetic Resonance Imaging of the Brain and Spine, 5th ed. Edited by Scott Atlas, MD. Wolters Kluwer, Lippincott Williams & Wilkins.
3. Braga VL, da Costa MDS, Riera R, Dos Santos Rocha LP, de Oliveira Santos BF, Matsumura Hondo TT, de Oliveira Chagas M, Schizencephaly Cavalheiro S. A Review of 734 Patients. *Pediatr Neurol*. 2018 Oct;87:23–29.

PORENCEPHALIC CYST

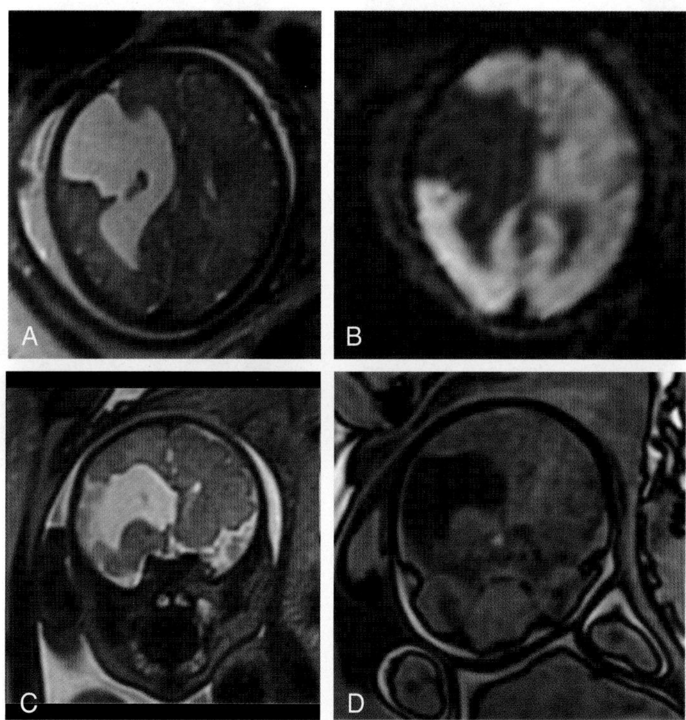

Fig. 2.45 Porencephalic Cyst. Fetal MRI (A) axial T2W, (B) axial DWI, (C) coronal T2W, and (D) coronal T1W images of a child with a CSF isointense porencephalic cyst within the right frontal lobe.

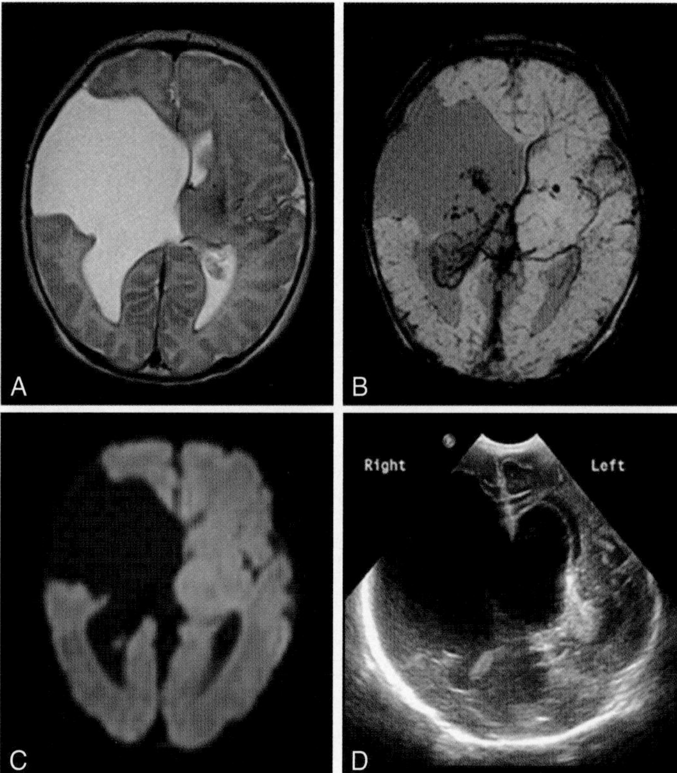

Fig. 2.46 Porencephalic Cyst. (A) Axial T2W, (B) axial SWI, and (C) axial DWI postnatal MRI including (D) coronal ultrasound study of the same patient as shown in Fig. 2.45 confirm a large right frontal porencephalic cyst filled with cerebrospinal fluid. On SWI hypointense blood products are noted within the area of the porencephalic cyst. On ultrasound the defect appears well circumscribed and isoechoic with cerebrospinal fluid.

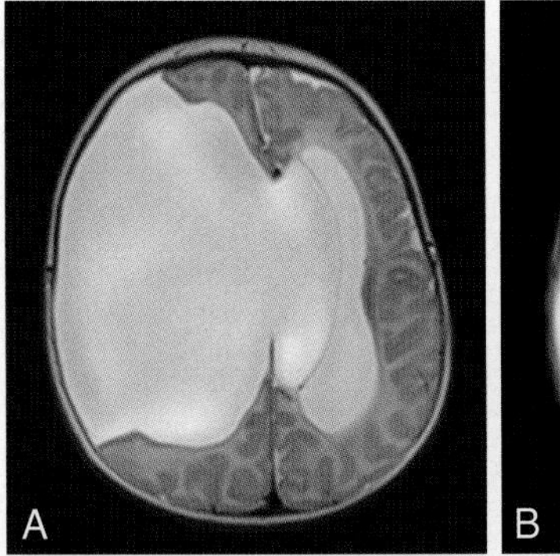

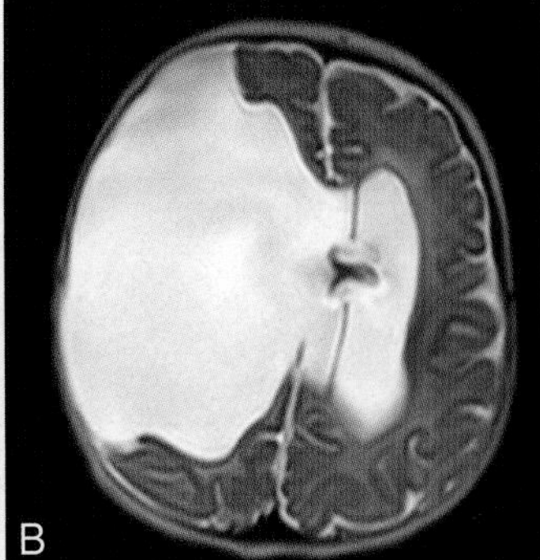

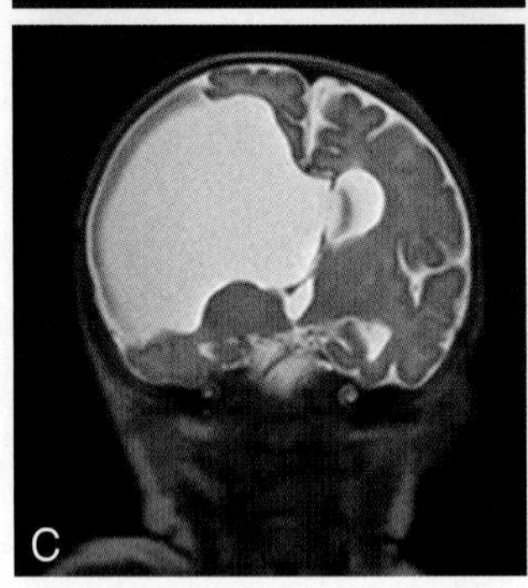

Fig. 2.47 Porencephalic Cyst. (A) Axial T2W and subsequent follow-up (B and C) axial and coronal T2W MRI of a child with a large right-sided porencephalic cyst. On the initial study the left leaf of the septum pellucidum is bowing toward the left lateral ventricle, after subsequent surgical fenestration CSF flow-related signal void is noted across the left leaf of the septum pellucidum, which has returned to a more normal nondisplaced location.

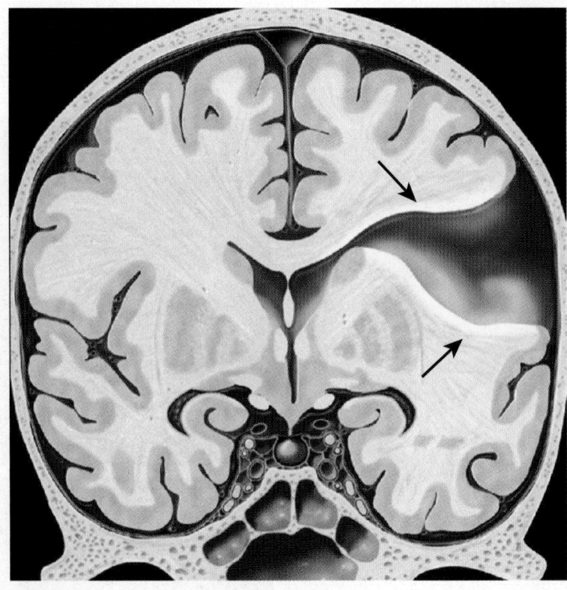

Fig. 2.48 Porencephalic Cyst. Illustration of a porencephalic cyst which is lined by gliotic white matter (arrows) and the communication to the ventricle. (From StatDX. Copyright © 2022 Elsevier.)

Key Points

Background

- Porencephalic cysts are focal brain defects filled with cerebrospinal fluid. These are not *classified as malformations due to the destructive etiology* but are presented here in this section because of the imaging pattern.
- In most cases they are chronic sequelae of remote injury, which may include a focal arterial or venous stroke, focal intraparenchymal hemorrhage, trauma, surgery, or infection.
- Porencephalic cysts are frequent complications of hemorrhagic periventricular venous infarctions secondary to a germinal matrix hemorrhage.
- Depending on the timing of the injury, prenatal versus postnatal, additional malformations (e.g., cortical dysplasia) may coexist secondary to a disruption of normal intrauterine brain development.
- May be isolated within the white matter or may communicate with the adjacent ventricular system or subarachnoid space.
- Depending on the etiology, timing of injury, size, and location of the cyst in relation to functional centers, symptoms may vary, including minimal to severe functional deficits, motor and cognitive developmental delays, and seizure activity.

Imaging

- Unilateral large focal porencephalic cysts are often accompanied with hemiatrophy of the brainstem, including Wallerian degeneration, in particular if the corona radiata or perirolandic area is involved.
- Typically, marginated by white matter with or without adjacent white matter gliosis; the overlying cortical ribbon may be thinned.
- On color-coded fractional anisotropy maps, a reduction in size or occasional complete lack of white matter tracts may be observed.
- Prenatal or early postnatal destructive lesions typically show little to no gliosis on follow-up because of the immature response of the brain to injury.
- Occasionally porencephalic cysts may exert mass effect on adjacent brain tissue, even when communicating with ventricular system, and may require fenestration or drainage.
- On imaging the cysts follow the imaging characteristics of cerebrospinal fluid. If the cyst is not communicating with the ventricular system or subarachnoid space an increased protein content within the cyst may result in an increased signal intensity on T1W/FLAIR imaging.

REFERENCE

1. Huisman TA, Poretti A. Chapter 7. Disorders of brain development. In: Magnetic Resonance Imaging of the Brain and Spine, 5th ed. Edited by Scott Atlas, MD. Wolters Kluwer, Lippincott Williams & Wilkins.

HYDRANENCEPHALY

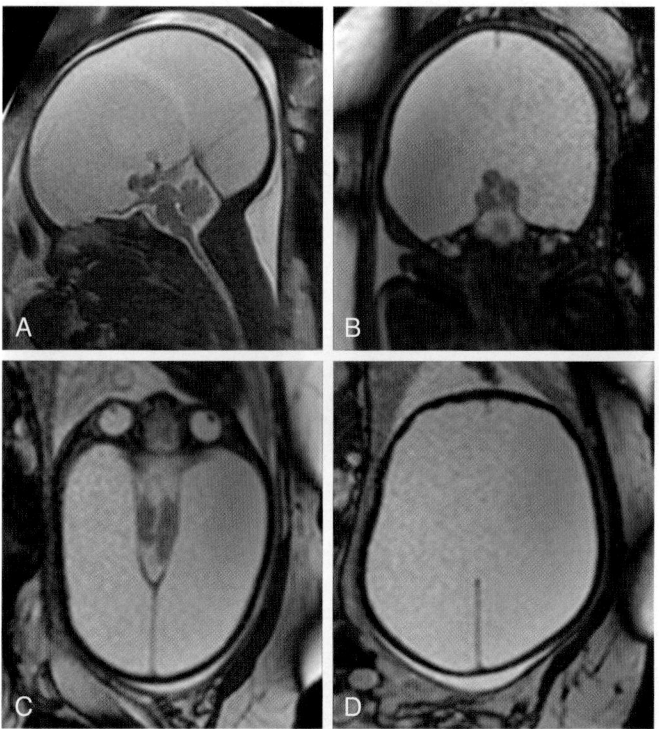

Fig. 2.49 Hydranencephaly. (A to D) Sagittal, coronal, and axial T2W fetal MRI of a child with hydranencephaly. Complete absence of the supratentorial cerebral hemispheres, small residual central gray matter in the midline, normal-appearing brainstem and cerebellum and presence of the falx. The cranial vault is completely filled with cerebrospinal fluid contained by the remnant of the walls of the lateral ventricles.

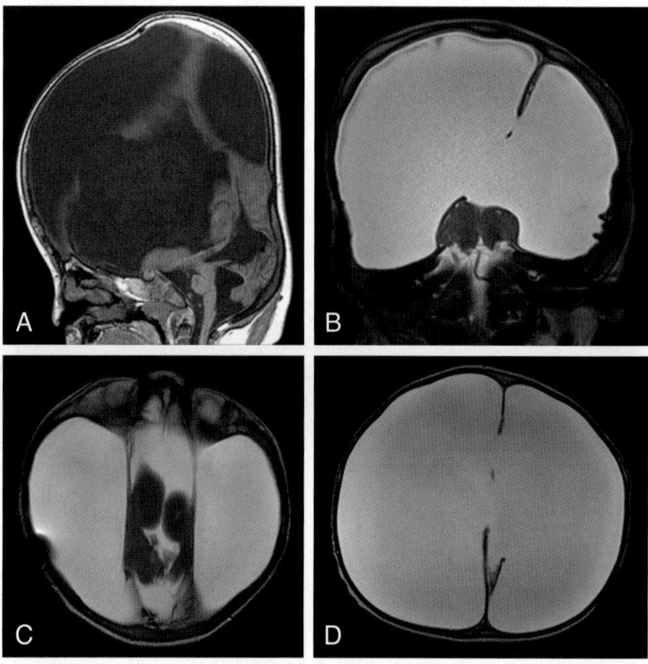

Fig. 2.50 Hydranencephaly. (A) Sagittal T1W, (B) coronal, and (C and D) axial T2W postnatal MRI demonstrate the cranial vault is completely filled with cerebral spinal fluid contained by the remnants of the walls of the lateral ventricles. There is fusion of the residual central gray matter in the midline, the leaves of the septum pellucidum are ruptured, distal internal carotid arteries are absent, and there is macrocephaly.

Key Points

Background

- Complete or near complete absence of the supratentorial brain (hemispheric white matter and cortical gray matter) likely secondary to occlusion or atresia of the supraclinoid internal carotid arteries occurring in the second trimester. Causes can include in utero TORCH infections, twin-twin transfusion, maternal toxins, thrombotic causes, and COL4A1 mutation.
- Hydranencephaly is *not a malformation* because it is a destructive process, but it is presented in this section due to the imaging pattern.
- Initially infants have microcephaly that progresses to macrocephaly due to poor CSF regulation. Shunting of the supratentorial CSF may be indicated to assist management of macrocephaly.
- Prognosis is poor, with function limited to the brainstem.

Imaging

- *Absent cerebral hemispheres* (some remaining medial temporal and occipital lobes can be seen) and CSF-filled cranium.
- Brainstem, cerebellum, thalami, and choroid plexus, which are supplied by the vertebral arteries, are typically intact. Parts of the basal ganglia and medial occipital lobes may also be present. The preserved tissue survives via an intact posterior circulation.
- The *falx cerebri is present.*
- Residual leptomeninges may be seen following the inner table of the skull.
- No circle of Willis is seen; no supraclinoid internal carotid arteries visible.
- Differential Diagnosis:
  - Alobar holoprosencephaly: absent falx
  - Severe hydrocephalus: thin mantle of cortex present

REFERENCE

1. Huisman TA, Poretti A. Chapter 7. Disorders of brain development. In: Magnetic Resonance Imaging of the Brain and Spine, 5th ed. Edited by Scott Atlas, MD. Wolters Kluwer, Lippincott Williams & Wilkins.

ZELLWEGER SYNDROME

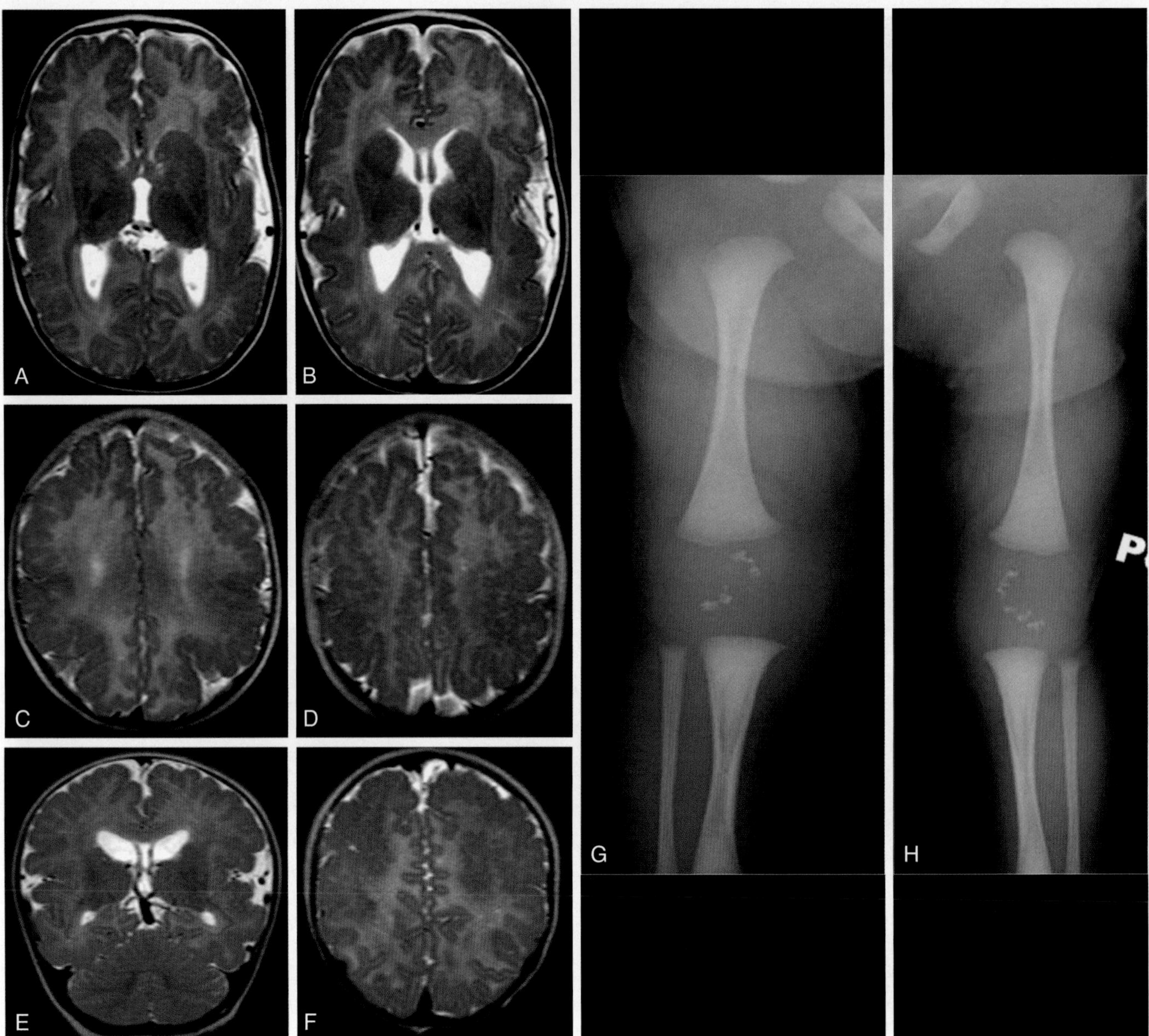

Fig. 2.51 Zellweger Syndrome. (A to F) Axial and coronal T2W images, demonstrate bilateral frontoparietal and perisylvian polymicrogyria. (G and H) AP radiographs of the legs demonstrate stippled growth plates.

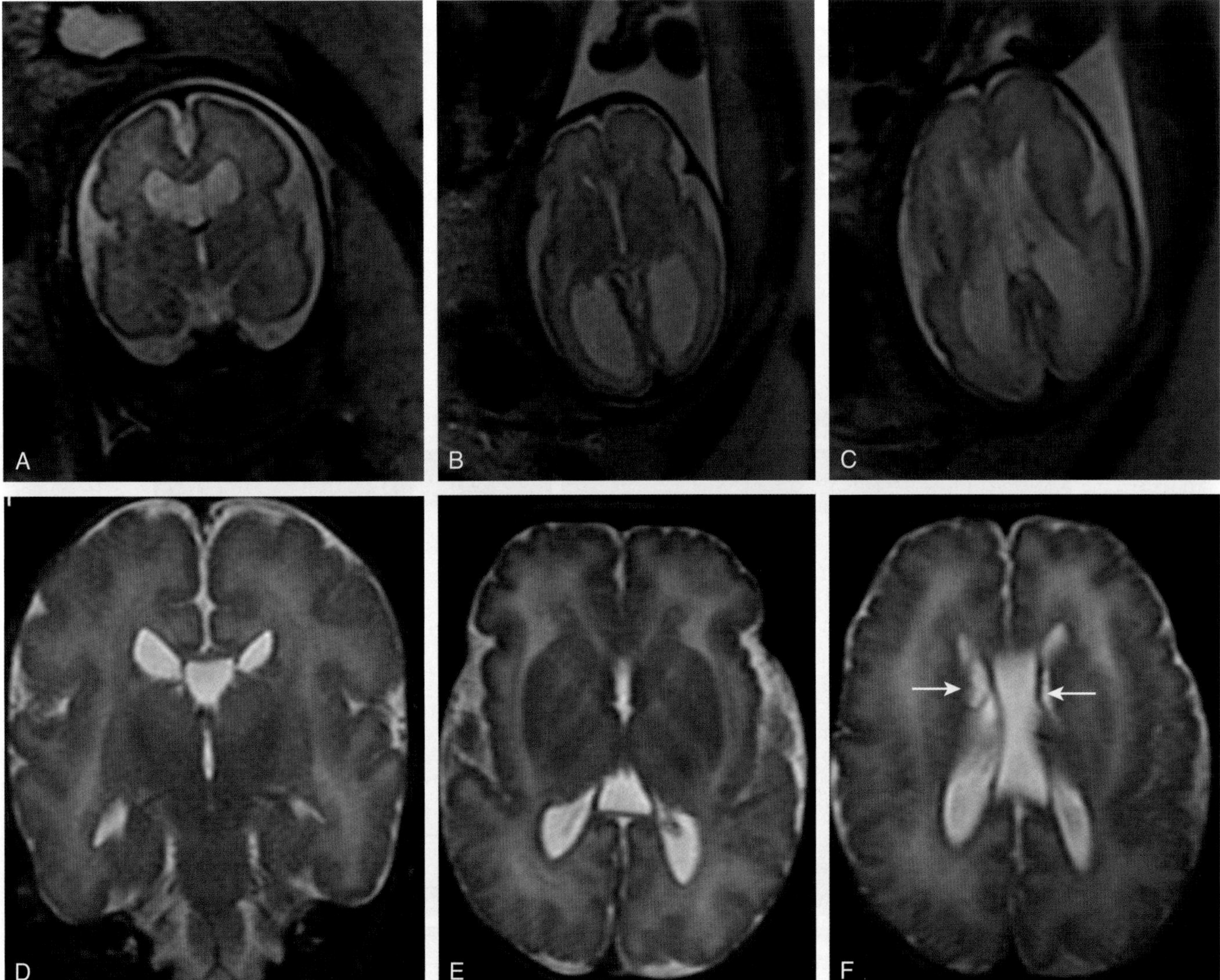

Fig. 2.52 Zellweger Syndrome. (A to C) Fetal MR axial T2W images and (D to F) corresponding postnatal coronal and axial T2W images demonstrate bilateral perisylvian polymicrogyria and germinolytic cysts at the caudothalamic grooves (*arrows*).

Key Points

Background

- Autosomal recessive *peroxisome disorder* that can result from multiple gene mutations
- Congenital anomalies (craniofacial, eyes, liver, bone, brain), hypotonia, psychomotor retardation, facial dysmorphism, seizures, periarticular calcifications, and hepatomegaly; death frequently within 1 year

Imaging

- Bilateral *perisylvian polymicrogyria*; small gyri in the anterior frontal and temporal lobes
- *Caudothalamic groove germinolytic cysts*
- Hypomyelination
- MRS: elevated lipid and lactate on short echo

REFERENCE

1. Barkovich AJ, Raybaud C. *Pediatric Neuroradiology*. 6th edition Philadelphia: Wolters-Kluwer; 2019.

PI3K-MTOR-AKT DISORDERS

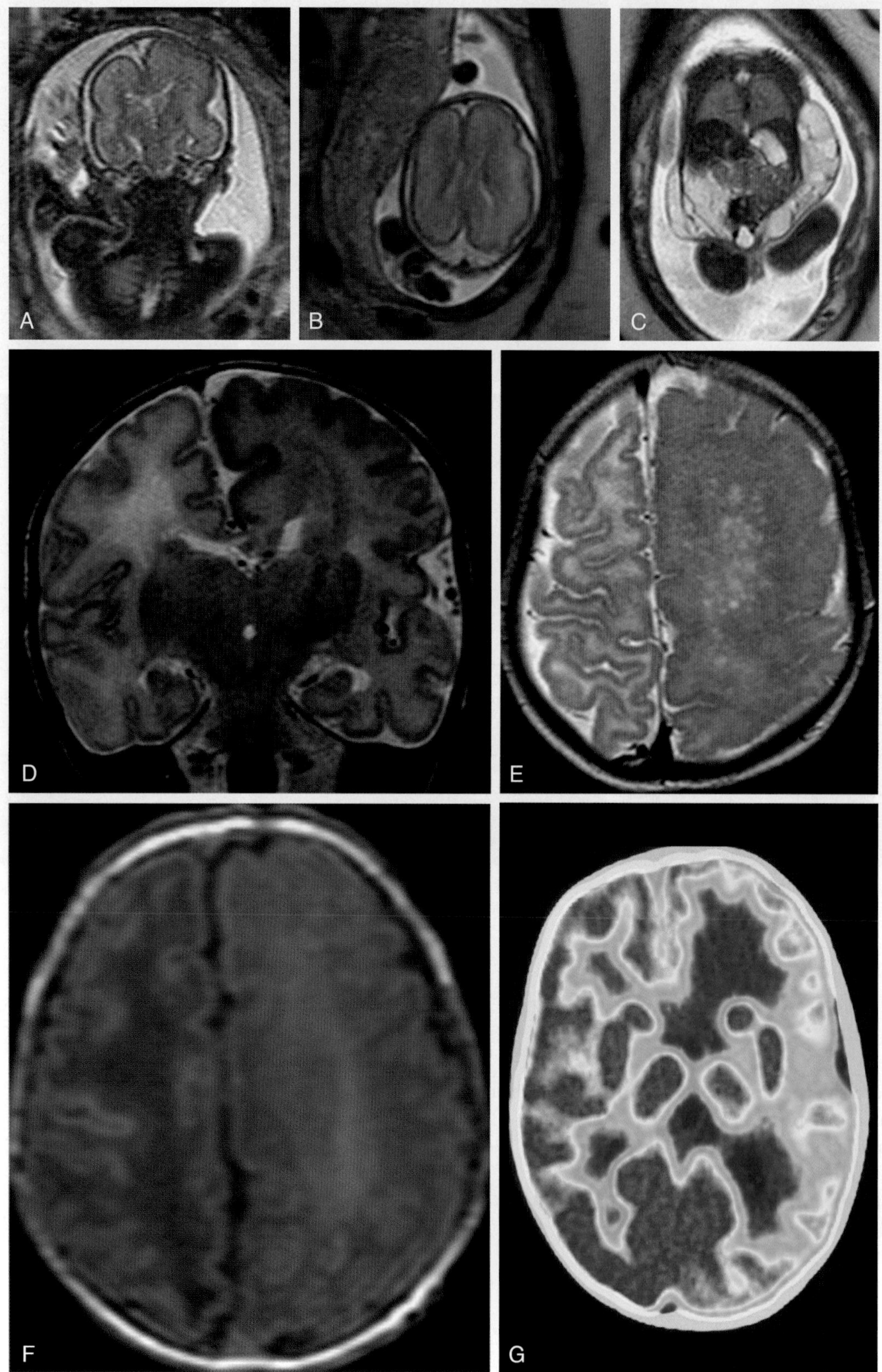

Fig. 2.53 PIK3CA-Overgrowth Syndrome. (A to C) Coronal, and axial T2W fetal MR images demonstrate a hemimegalencephaly with a large abdominal lymphatic malformation. (D to F) Coronal and axial T2W and axial T1W images demonstrate the postnatal appearance of left hemimegalencephaly with enlarged left cerebral hemisphere, diffuse polymicrogyria, and accelerated myelination. (G) Axial FDG PET CT image demonstrates hypometabolism of the enlarged left hemisphere.

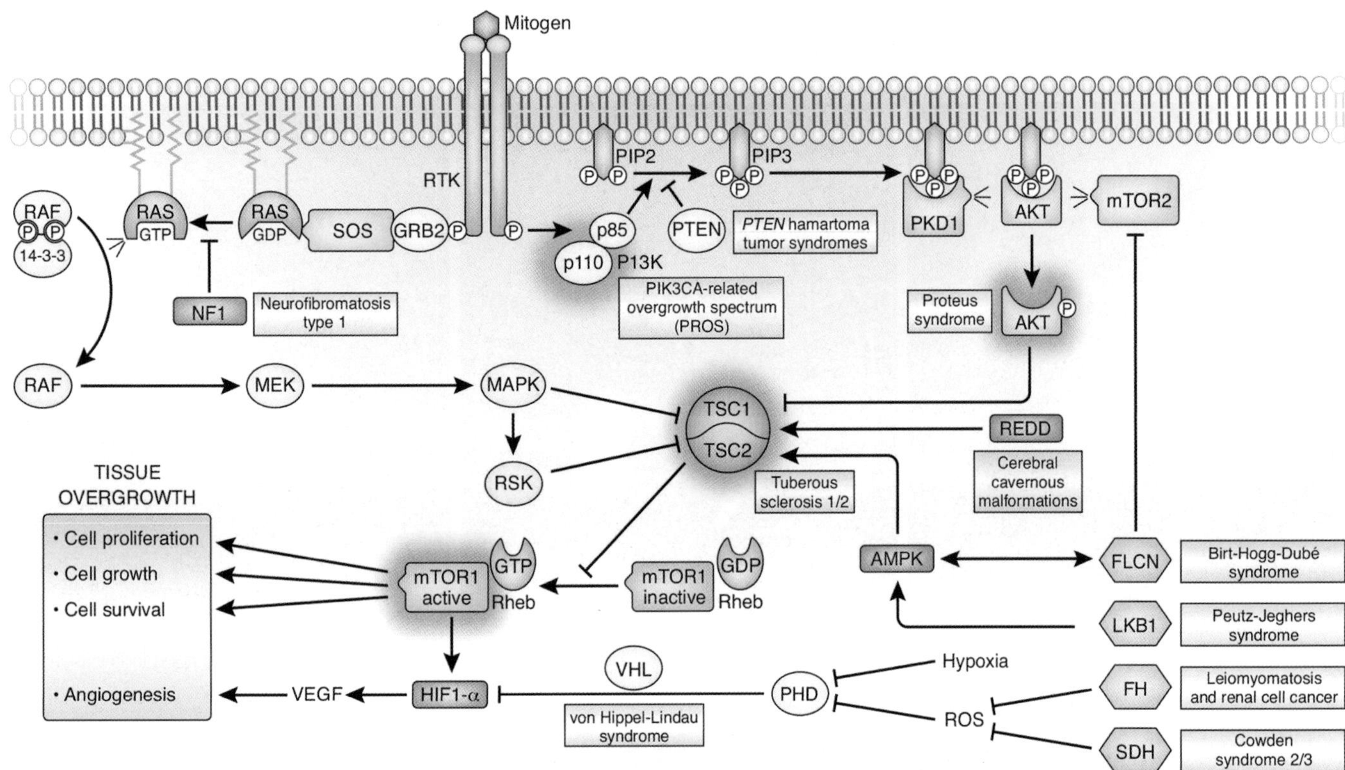

Fig. 2.54 PI3K-AKT-mTOR and Interacting Signaling Pathways With Associated Heritable Diseases. (From Vahidnezhad H, Youssean L, Uitto J. Molecular genetics of the PI3K-akt-mtor pathway in genodermatoses: diagnostic implications and treatment opportunities. *J Invest Dermatol.* 2016;136[1]:15–23. doi:10.1038/jid.2015.331)

Key Points

Background

- PI3K/AKT/mTOR signaling pathway (Fig. 2.54) involved in multiple disorders.
- Tuberous sclerosis: *TSC1* and *TSC2* genes result in dysregulation of mammalian target of rapamycin (mTOR) and lead to cortical dysplasias.
- PTEN hamartoma tumor syndrome (also known as Cowden and Bannayan-Riley-Ruvalcaba syndromes): the PTEN mutation leads to dysregulated AKT activity and the PIK3CA-related overgrowth spectrum, which includes epidermal nevi, CLOVES syndrome, megalencephaly-capillary-malformation, congenital lipomatous overgrowth, fibroadipose hyperplasia, and hemihyperplasia multiple lipomatosis.

Imaging

- Brain and extracranial findings in PI3K3CA-related overgrowth spectrum include the following:
  - Hemimegalencephaly, megalencephaly, and polymicrogyria
  - Focal cortical dysplasia
  - Ventriculomegaly
  - Tonsillar ectopia/Chiari I malformation
  - Large, isolated lymphatic malformation

REFERENCES

1. Jansen LA, Mirzaa GM, Ishak GE, et al. PI3K/Akt pathway mutations cause a spectrum of brain malformations from megalencephaly to focal cortical dysplasia. *Brain*. 2015;138:1613–1628.
2. Keppler-Noreuil KM, Rios JJ, Parker VER, et al. PIK3CA-related overgrowth spectrum (PROS): Diagnostic and testing eligibility criteria, differential diagnosis, and evaluation. *Am J Med Genet A*. 2015 Feb;0(2):287–295.

TUBULINOPATHY

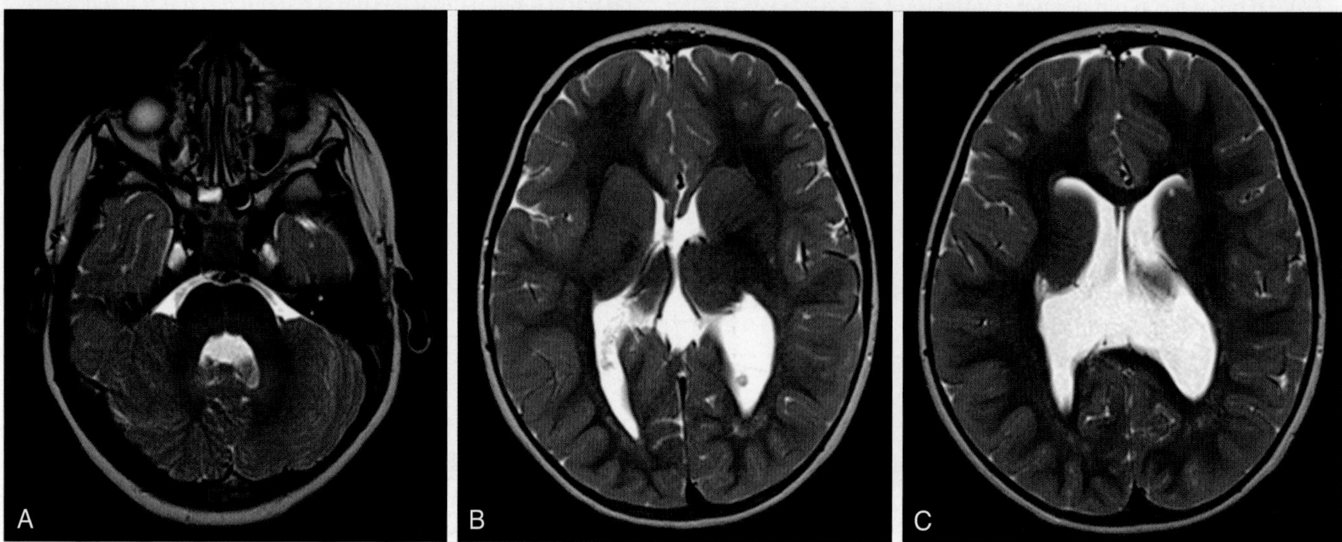

Fig. 2.55 Tubulinopathy. (A to C) Axial T2W images in child with confirmed tubulinopathy with round/malrotated and dysmorphic appearing basal ganglia, hypoplasia of the anterior limbs of the internal capsule, and slight clefting of the ventral pons.

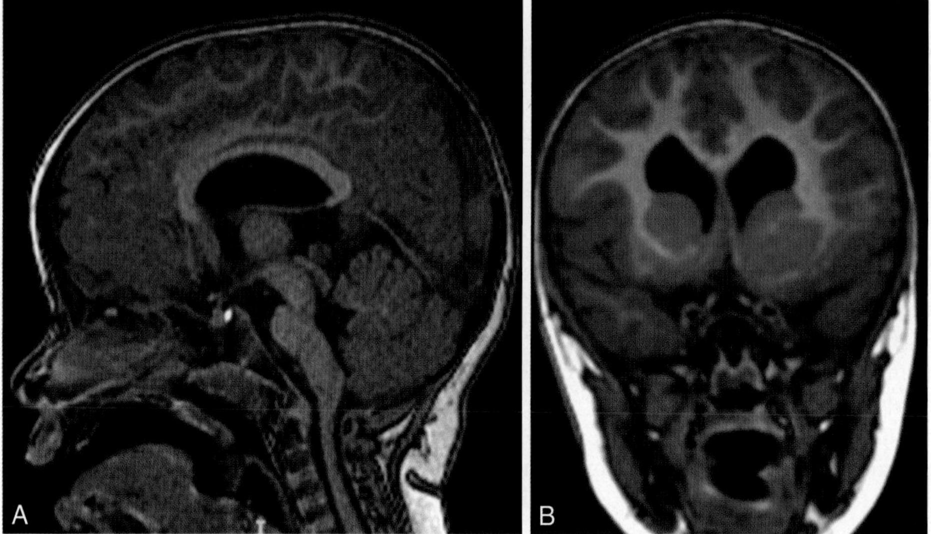

Fig. 2.56 Tubulinopathy. (A and B) Sagittal and coronal T1W images in a child with confirmed tubulinopathy show dysmorphic/malrotated basal ganglia in combination with elongation of the mesencephalon.

Key Points

Background

- Tubulinopathies result from mutations of the genes *TUBA*, *TUBB*, or *TUBG* encoding for the different isotypes of alpha-, beta- or gamma-tubulin, proteins that form the components of microtubules. The isotypes are the basis for the microtubule cytoskeleton that are assembled from the polymers of these tubulin heterodimers. The microtubule cytoskeleton is essential for the normal nervous system development.
- Mutations of these essential genes consequently result in complex malformations affecting the neuronal proliferation, migration, and axonal pathfinding.

Imaging

- Depending on the genetic mutation, various brain malformations are present, including the following:
  - Basal ganglia malformation: A relatively characteristic imaging findings is that the b*asal ganglia may appear malrotated*, in particular the caudate nucleus, putamen, and globus pallidus are difficult to separate from

each other on imaging. This is partially secondary to hypoplasia of the anterior limbs of the internal capsule (absence of the ALIC sign).

- Cortical malformations: lissencephaly, pachygyria, polymicrogyria-like cortical dysplasia, simplified gyral pattern, and microlissencephaly
- Cerebellar hypoplasia
- Brainstem malformation: Pontine thinning or clefting, asymmetric cerebral peduncles
- Malformation of the corpus callosum

REFERENCES

1. Mutch CA, Sahin PM, Barry B, et al. Disorders of microtubule function in neurons: Imaging correlates. *AJNR, Am Journal of Neuroradiol.* 2016;37(3):528–535.
2. Bosemani T, Orman G, Boltshauser E, et al. Congenital abnormalities of the posterior fossa. *Radiographics.* 2015;35(1):200–220.
3. Huisman TA, Poretti A. Chapter 7. Disorders of brain development. In: Magnetic Resonance Imaging of the Brain and Spine, 5th ed. Edited by Scott Atlas, MD. Wolters Kluwer, Lippincott Williams & Wilkins.

OTHER DISORDERS WITH CORTICAL MALFORMATIONS

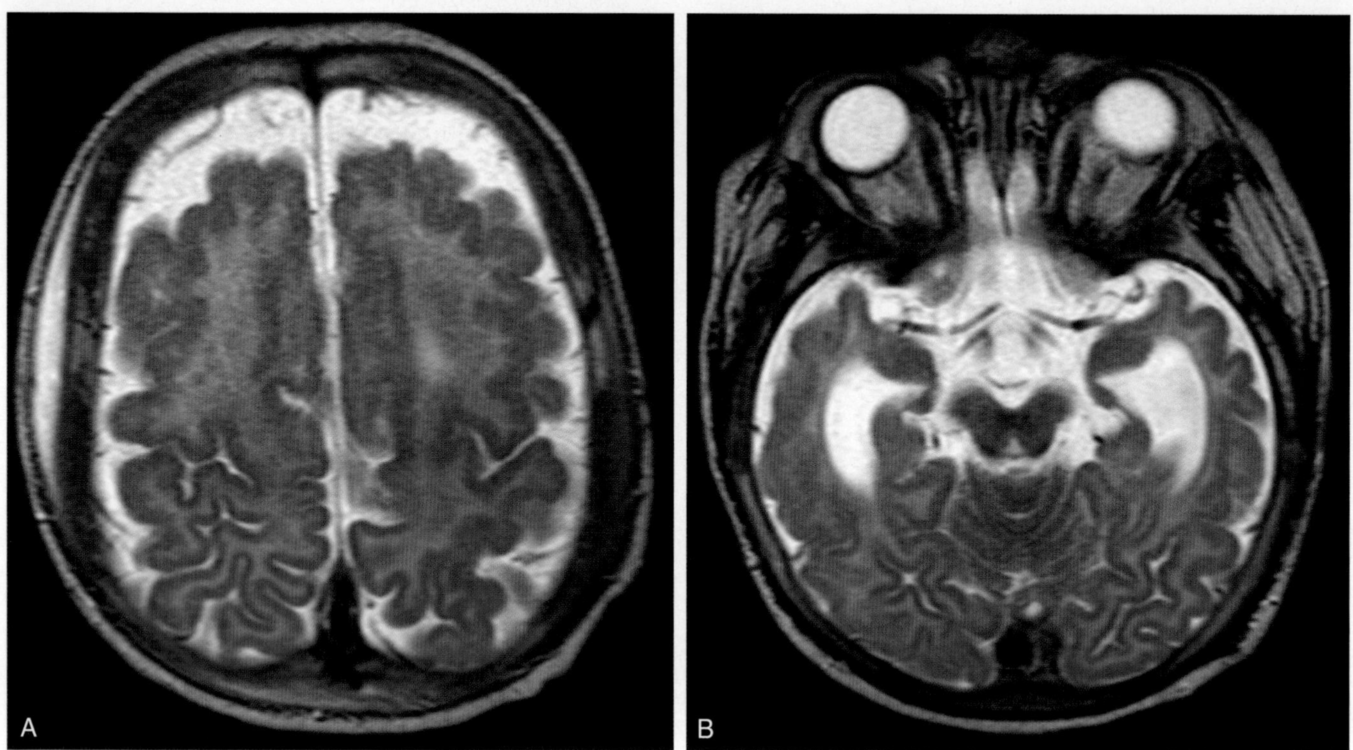

Fig. 2.57 GPR56 Mutation. (A and B) Axial T2W images demonstrate bilateral frontal polymicrogyria, midbrain hypoplasia, and cerebral volume loss.

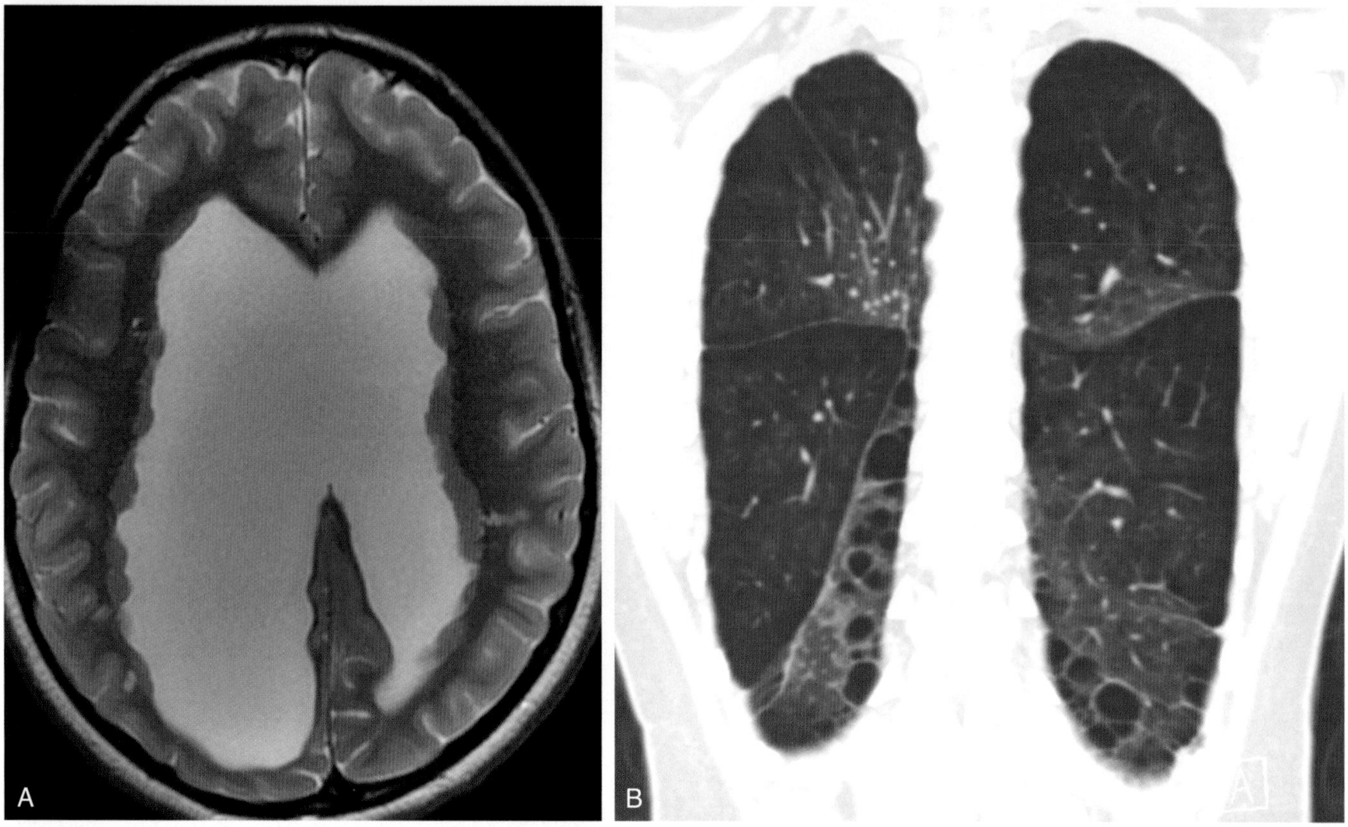

Fig. 2.58 Filamin A Deficiency. (A) Axial T2W image demonstrates extensive periventricular gray matter heterotopia and hydrocephalus. (B) Coronal reformat CT image demonstrates bilateral inferior lung emphysema.

Key Points

- GPR56: Autosomal recessive disorder; involves a protein involved in cell-cell and cell-extracellular matrix interactions; clinically manifests with developmental delay, seizures, dysconjugate gaze, pyramidal and cerebellar signs. Imaging: *bilateral frontoparietal polymicrogyria* with *decreasing anterior-posterior gradient of severity*, cerebellar cysts, thick corpus callosum, hypoplastic pons, and diffusion tensor imaging (DTI) demonstrate reduced transverse pontine fibers and middle cerebellar peduncle fibers and some patients with aberrant fibers from the corticospinal tract crossing the corpus callosum.
- Filamin A deficiency: X-linked disorder; filamin A is an actin-binding protein that regulates cell shape and migration. Imaging demonstrates *gray matter heterotopia*, cerebellar hypoplasia, bilateral perisylvian or temporo-parieto-occipital polymicrogyria, and hydrocephalus. Lungs demonstrate *emphysema*, which manifests with respiratory distress in infancy.
- Chudley-McCullough syndrome (GPSM2): autosomal recessive; clinical features include severe to profound sensorineural hearing loss; imaging findings include *frontal polymicrogyria*, heterotopia, callosal hypogenesis, dysplastic inferior cerebellar fissures.
- Reelin mutation: Imaging findings include *pachygyria/lissencephaly* and bilateral cerebellar hypoplasia.
- VLDRL: Imaging findings include *pachygyria/lissencephaly and bilateral cerebellar hypoplasia.*
- CASK: Imaging findings include *simplified gyral pattern and cerebellar hypoplasia.*
- MPPH syndrome: Macrocephaly, polymicrogyria, polydactyly, hydrocephalus.

REFERENCES

1. Poretti A, Bolthauser E, Huisman TAGM. Cerebellar and brainstem malformations. *Neuroimaging Clin N Am.* 2016 Aug;26(3):341–357.
2. Quattrocchi CC, Zanni G, Napolitano A, et al. Conventional magnetic resonance imaging and diffusion tensor imaging studies in children with novel GPR56 mutations: further delineation of a cobblestone-like phenotype. *Neurogenetics.* 2013;14:77–83.
3. Ozdemir M, Dilli A. Chudley-McCullough syndrome. *J Clin Imaging Sci.* 2018 Nov 15;8:45.

HOLOPROSENCEPHALY SPECTRUM

At approximately 35 days of gestation, the prosencephalon divides into the telencephalon and diencephalon. The telencephalon, which forms the cerebral hemispheres, separates as outpouchings in the region of the foramen of Monro. The thin-walled cerebral hemisphere vesicles expand and cover the diencephalon. The telencephalon vesicle will partition in the midline along the roof of the telencephalon, leading to the interhemispheric fissure and differentiation of the falx. Separation of the embryonic prosencephalic vesicle depends on a balance between ventral and dorsal midline induction. The segmentation has a posterior → anterior, caudal → rostral, and dorsal → ventral pattern, which means the inferior frontal lobes are the last region to separate.

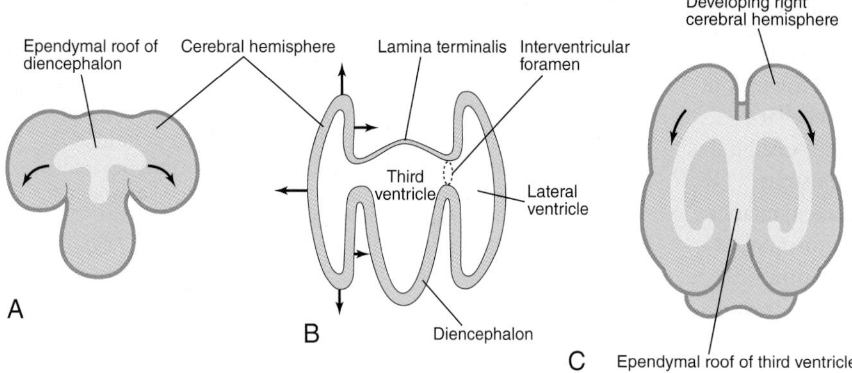

Fig. 2.59 Ventricle Embryology. (A) Sketch of the dorsal surface of the forebrain, indicating how the ependymal roof of the diencephalon is carried out to the dorsomedial surface of the cerebral hemispheres. (B) Diagrammatic section of the forebrain showing how the developing cerebral hemispheres grow from the lateral walls of the forebrain and expand in all directions until they cover the diencephalon. The rostral wall of the forebrain, the lamina terminalis, is very thin. (C) Sketch of the forebrain showing how the ependymal roof is finally carried into the temporal lobes as a result of the C-shaped growth pattern of the cerebral hemispheres. The *arrows* indicate some of the directions in which the hemispheres expand. (From Moore, Keith L, TVN Persaud, Torchia MG. *Before We Are Born: Essentials of Embryology and Birth Defects*. 10th ed. Elsevier; 2020.)

Holoprosencephalies are a result of abnormal ventral induction occurring ~fifth to sixth week of gestation. The interhemispheric fissure fails to form, and the prosencephalic vesicle is not split into the two telencephalic vesicles, resulting in varying degrees of midline fusion. Etiology of holoprosencephaly is heterogeneous and includes teratogens (alcohol, retinoic acid), environmental factors (maternal diabetes), and genetic causes (~25% to 50% of cases), including trisomy 13 and at least 14 gene mutations, of which sonic hedgehog gene (30% to 40%) and ZIC1 (5%) are the most common. Additional maxillofacial malformations may exist, including hypotelorism, midline clefts, single central incisor, absent metopic suture, and cyclopia (the face may predict the brain). Additional midline structures that may be affected include the rhinencephalon (hypoplastic olfactory bulbs), hypothalamus/pituitary gland, septum pellucidum, and corpus callosum.

Holoprosencephaly is subdivided in alobar, semilobar, and lobar forms, depending on the severity and extent of the midline anomaly (Table 2.2). Holoprosencephaly and similar malformations are discussed in this section.

TABLE 2.2 Types of Holoprosencephaly

Finding	Craniofacial Anomalies	Ventricles	Septum Pellucidum	Falx Cerebri	Interhemispheric Fissure	Thalami, Basal Ganglia
Alobar	Severe	Monoventricle	Absent	Absent	Absent	Fused
Semi-lobar	Variable	Rudimentary temporal and occipital horns	Absent	Present posteriorly	Present Posteriorly	Partial fusion
Lobar	Absent or mild	Squared-off frontal horns	Absent	Well-formed	Present	Separated

ALOBAR HOLOPROSENCEPHALY

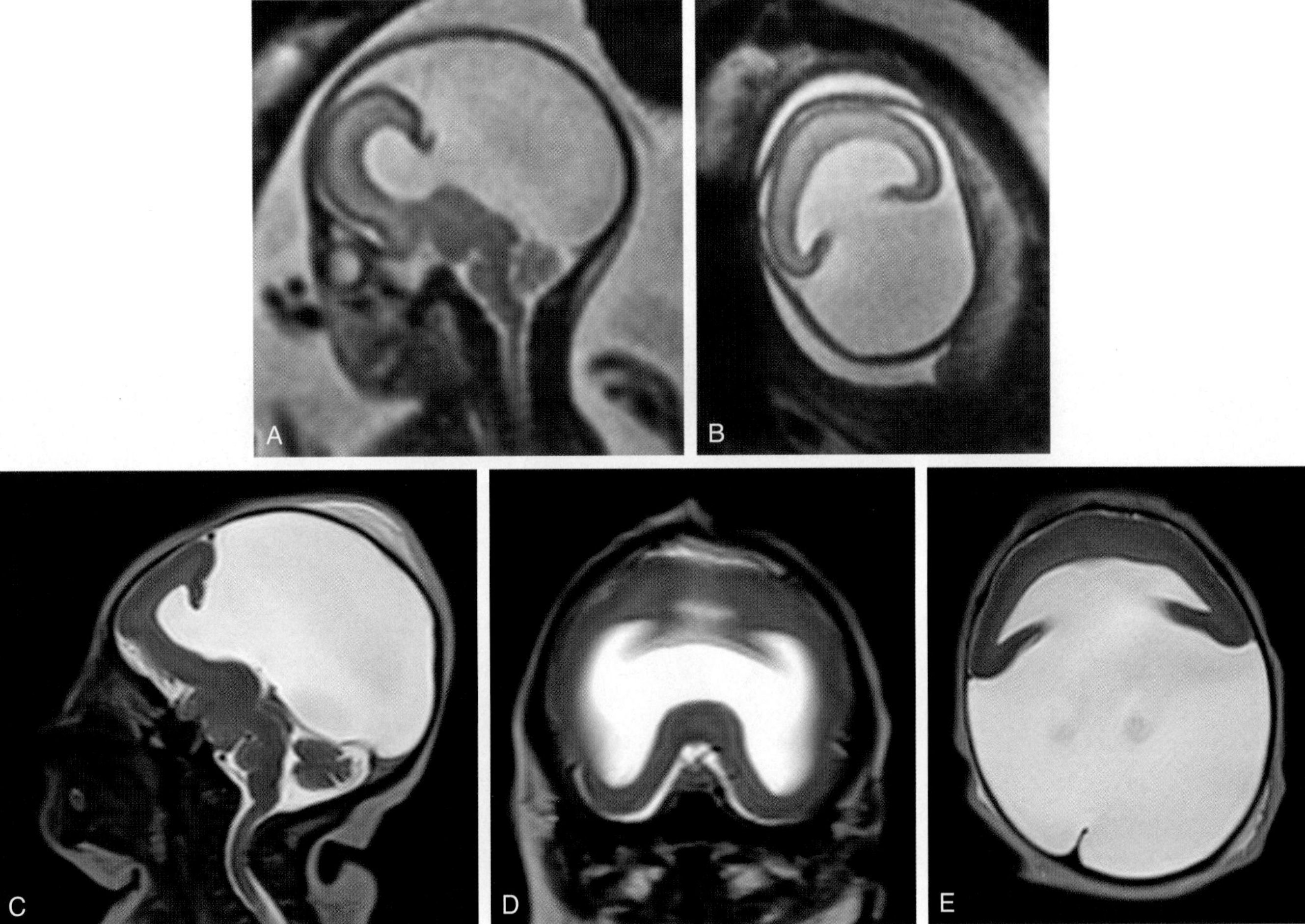

Fig. 2.60 Alobar Holoprosencephaly. (A and B) Sagittal and axial T2W fetal MRI of a child with alobar holoprosencephaly. A large monoventricle is noted with lack of splitting of the telencephalic vesicle; brain tissue is extending across the midline without interruption. (C to E) Postnatal sagittal, coronal, and axial T2W MRI of the same child with alobar holoprosencephaly characterized by a large monoventricle and frontal lobes crossing the midline without interruption as well as fusion of the basal ganglia in the midline.

Key Points

Background

- Malformation of *ventral induction* leading to complete absence of cleavage of the prosencephalon
- Severe neurologic dysfunction

Imaging

- A single "pancake-like" supratentorial brain extending across the midline
- Crescent-shaped *monoventricle*, absence of the temporal horns and third ventricle. The monoventricle extends posteriorly (also known as dorsal cyst)
- *Absence of the interhemispheric fissure* and falx cerebri
- *Absent septum pellucidum*
- Absent corpus callosum
- Fused thalami, hypothalamus, and basal ganglia
- Absent sylvian fissure
- Absent or hypoplastic optic nerves and olfactory bulbs
- Migrational abnormalities and a delayed myelination of the white matter may be seen
- *Maxillofacial malformations* may exist, including hypotelorism, midline clefts, single central incisor, absent metopic suture, and cyclopia (the face may predict the brain)

REFERENCE

1. Huisman TA, Poretti A. Chapter 7. Disorders of brain development. In: Magnetic Resonance Imaging of the Brain and Spine, 5th ed. Edited by Scott Atlas, MD. Wolters Kluwer, Lippincott Williams & Wilkins.

SEMILOBAR HOLOPROSENCEPHALY

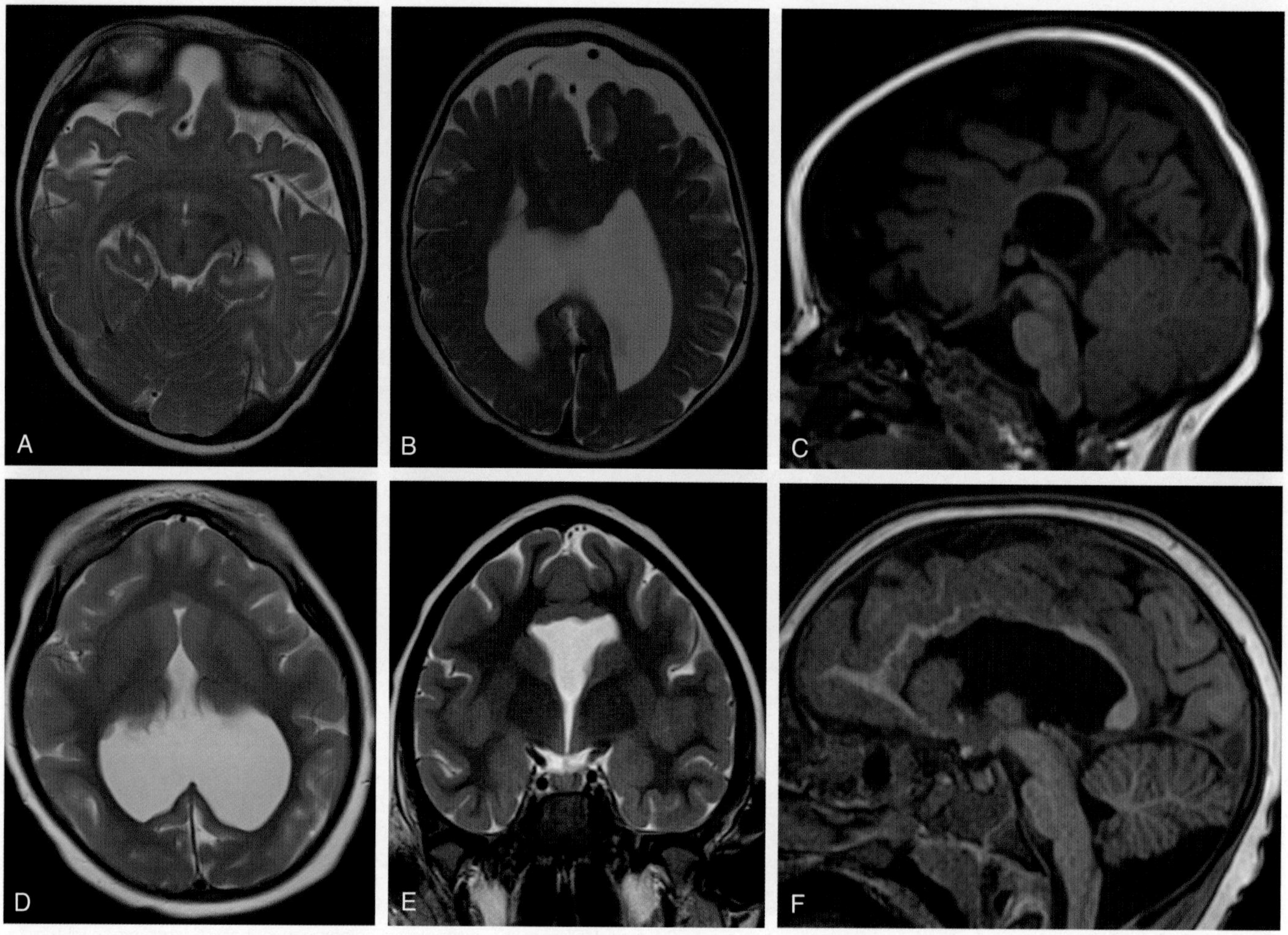

Fig. 2.61 **Semilobar Holoprosencephaly**. (A and B) Axial T2W and (C) sagittal T1W images demonstrate fusion of the frontal lobes, absent anterior falx, absent septum pellucidum, separated posterior cerebral hemispheres, presence of the posterior falx, azygous ACA, and malformed corpus callosum with presence of the splenium and posterior body but absent remaining corpus callosum. (D and E) Axial and coronal T2W and (F) sagittal T1W images in another patient with similar findings of semi lobar holoprosencephaly with additional gray matter heterotopia in the midline.

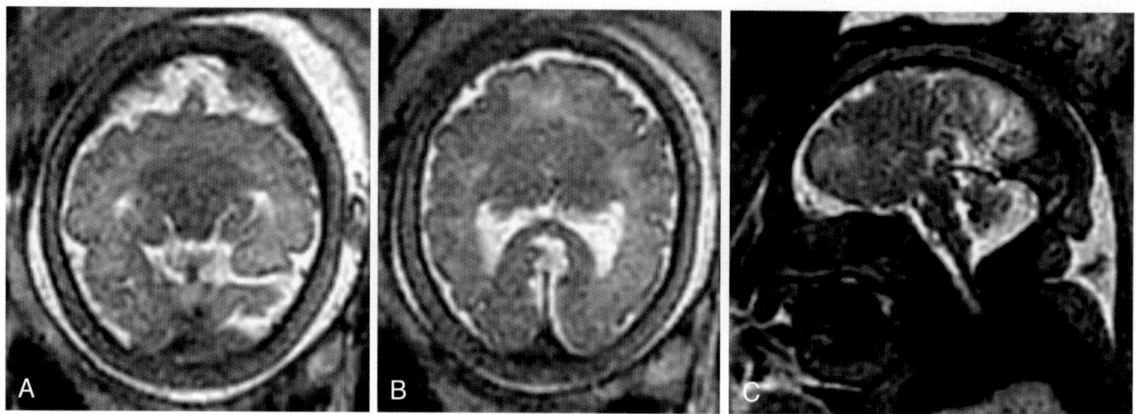

Fig. 2.62 **Semilobar Holoprosencephaly**. (A to C) Axial, and sagittal T2W fetal MRI demonstrate fusion of the frontal lobes, absent anterior interhemispheric flax while the posterior half of the brain is however divided in 2 halves an interhemispheric falx. The temporal horns are present and a small posterior corpus callosum is present.

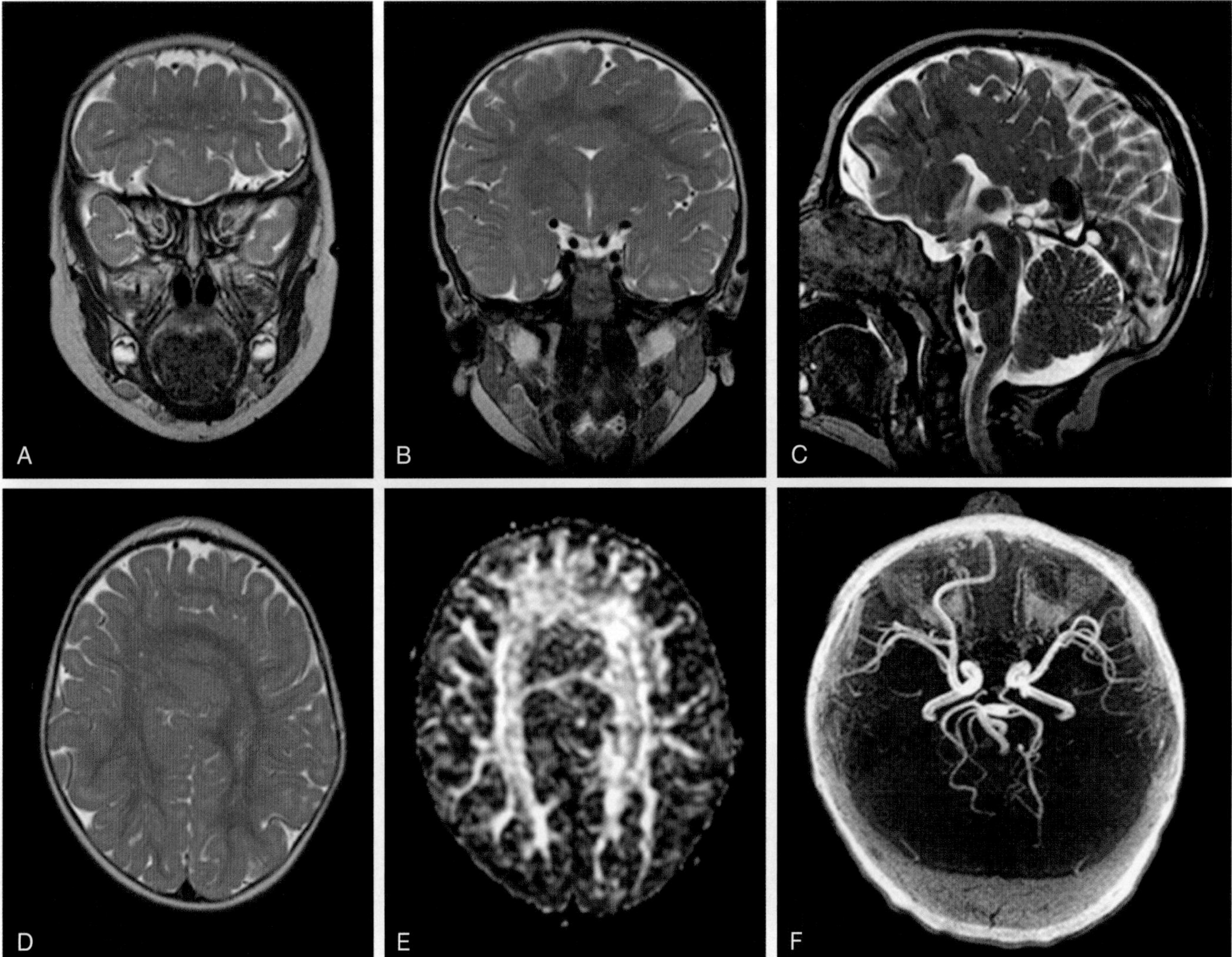

Fig. 2.63 Semilobar Holoprosencephaly. (A to D) Coronal, sagittal, and axial T2W MRI, (E) axial DTI FA map and (F) axial MRA in a child with semilobar holoprosencephaly show both frontal lobes and anterior horns of the lateral ventricles extending across the midline without interruption. The genu and body of the corpus callosum are lacking, the splenium of the corpus callosum is developed, matching the division of the parietal and occipital lobes. Fractional anisotropy maps showed the uninterrupted extension of white matter across the midline in the frontal region. MRA shows a single azygos artery on the right.

Key Points

Background

- Malformation due to abnormal *ventral induction*, leading to partial cleavage of the prosencephalon.
- Patients have developmental delay and spasticity.

Imaging

- *Anteriorly the brain is fused*; the hemispheric white matter extends uninterrupted across the midline.
- The interhemispheric fissure and falx cerebri is posteriorly formed, dividing the adjacent brain.
- The *anterior corpus calcium is missing*; the posterior corpus callosum, in particular the splenium, is developed. This is because presence of the interhemispheric fissure is necessary for callosal formation.

Absent septum pellucidum:

- Partial formation of the occipital and temporal horns.
- Thalami and basal ganglia are partially fused.
- Absent or hypoplastic olfactory bulbs and tracts.
- Maxillofacial anomalies are uncommon and may include hypotelorism and cleft lip.
- The circle of Willis is anomalous with a single anterior azygos artery supplying the anterior brain.

REFERENCE

1. Huisman TA, Poretti A. Chapter 7. Disorders of brain development. In: Magnetic Resonance Imaging of the Brain and Spine, 5th ed. Edited by Scott Atlas, MD. Wolters Kluwer, Lippincott Williams & Wilkins.

LOBAR HOLOPROSENCEPHALY

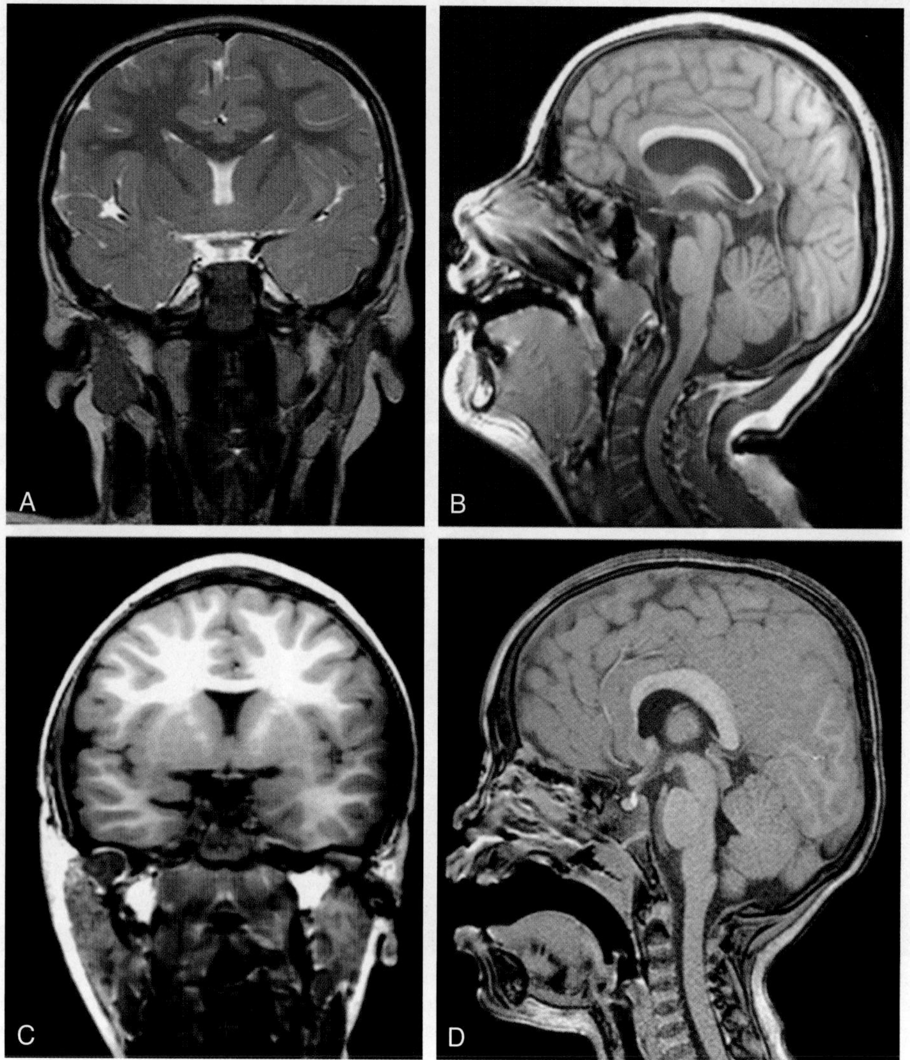

Fig. 2.64 Lobar Holoprosencephaly. (A) Coronal T2W and (B) sagittal T1W images *(top row)* and (C and D) coronal and sagittal T1W images *(lower row)* of 2 children with lobar holoprosencephaly. In both children fusion of the caudal frontal lobes, in particular hypothalami is noted, the genu and rostrum of the corpus callosum hypoplastic, the leaves of the septum pellucidum are lacking, and the remainder of the brain is separated. In addition, the second child has a cleft palate.

Key Points

Background

- Malformation due to abnormal *ventral induction.*
- Mildest form of holoprosencephaly with continuity of the anterior, caudal frontal lobes across the midline, while the remainder of the brain is separated in two hemispheres.
- Patients have mild developmental delay, hypothalamic/pituitary dysfunction, and vision problems.

Imaging

- Fusion of the anterior, caudal frontal lobes across the midline.
- *Absent septum pellucidum.*
- Lateral ventricles are split, but the anterior horns may appear small and hypoplastic. The third ventricle is normally developed.
- The interhemispheric fissure is fully formed.
- *The genu and rostrum of the corpus callosum are hypoplastic, poorly developed.*
- The thalami and basal ganglia are separated.
- The anterior circle of Willis is anomalous with a single azygous artery present.
- Rarely maxillofacial anomalies can be present.

REFERENCE

1. Huisman TA, Poretti A. Chapter 7. Disorders of brain development. In: Magnetic Resonance Imaging of the Brain and Spine, 5th ed. Edited by Scott Atlas, MD. Wolters Kluwer, Lippincott Williams & Wilkins.

SYNTELENCEPHALY

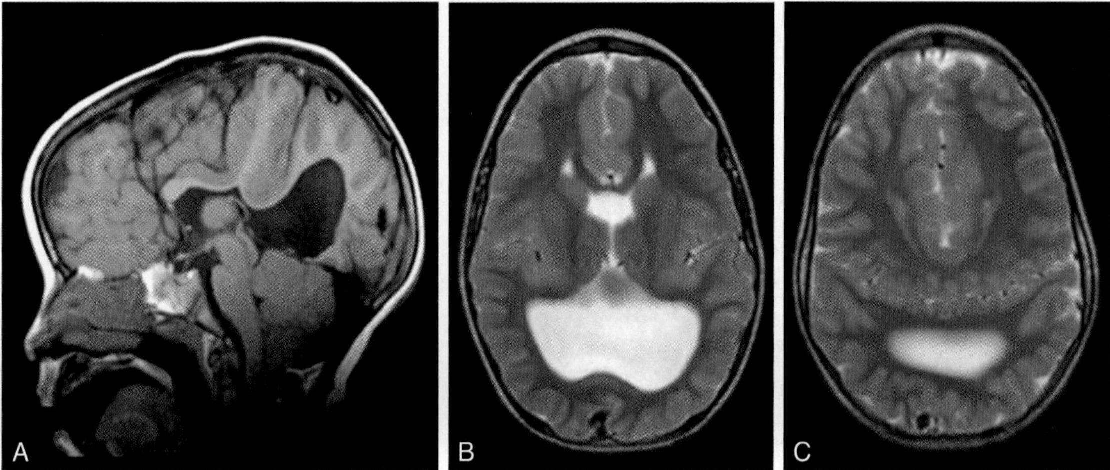

Fig. 2.65 Syntelencephaly. (A) Sagittal T1W and (B and C) axial T2W MRI child with syntelencephaly with characteristic separation of both frontal lobes and fusion of the parieto-occipital lobes, matching malformation of the corpus callosum. Fusion of the posterior lateral ventricles.

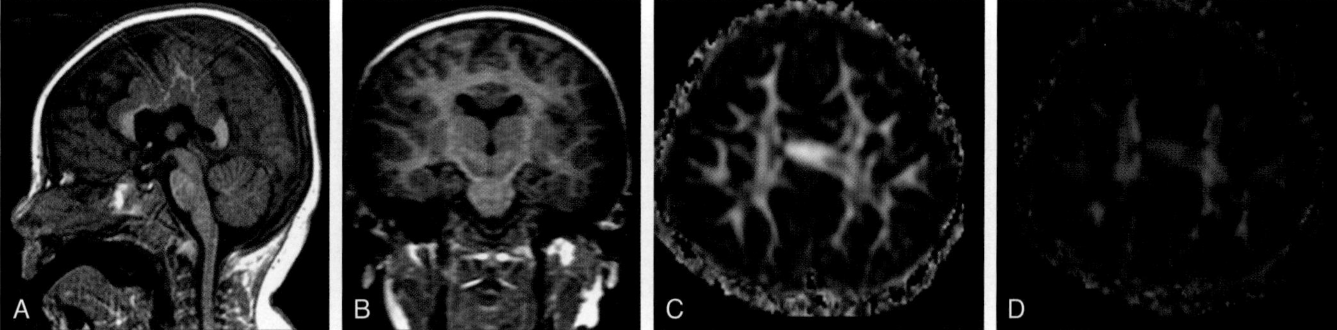

Fig. 2.66 Syntelencephaly. (A and B) Sagittal and coronal T1W MRI and (C and D) axial FA maps, including color coding in a child with syntelencephaly, normally developed genu and splenium of the corpus callosum, and fusion of the cerebral hemispheres in the midline. Confirmation of the midline fusion is noted on the fractional anisotropy maps with white matter bundles crossing the midline, color coded in the red.

Key Points

Background

- Variant form of holoprosencephaly, also known as middle interhemispheric variant of holoprosencephaly (MIH).
- Etiology is *abnormal dorsal midline induction.*
- High occurrence in babies born to mothers with diabetes. ZIC2 gene mutation is associated.
- Neurologic symptoms include spasticity (86%), hypotonia (57%), dystonia (50%), seizures (40%), and developmental delay. Often present in infancy and are microcephalic.

Imaging

- *Fusion of the posterior frontal and parietal regions* of both cerebral hemispheres.
- More vertical orientation of the sylvian fissures.
- Gray matter is typically noted along the superior contour of the nonseparated segment of the lateral ventricles.
- Anterior and posterior interhemispheric fissure and cerebral falx are present.
- Basal forebrain, anterior frontal lobes, and occipital lobes are well separated.
- Callosal dysgenesis with normally developed genu and splenium of the corpus callosum, while the body is partially absent.
- *Absent septum pellucidum*
- Normal midline separation of the basal ganglia, thalami, and hypothalamus.
- Additional malformations, including Chiari I or II malformations, have been reported.
- Azygous ACA

REFERENCES

1. Huisman TA, Poretti A. Chapter 7. Disorders of brain development. In: Magnetic Resonance Imaging of the Brain and Spine, 5th ed. Edited by Scott Atlas, MD. Wolters Kluwer, Lippincott Williams & Wilkins.
2. Verschuuren S, Poretti A, Meoded A, Izbudak I, Huisman TA. Diffusion tensor imaging and fiber tractography in syntelencephaly. *Neurographics*. 2013;3(4):164–168.

SEPTO-OPTIC DYSPLASIA

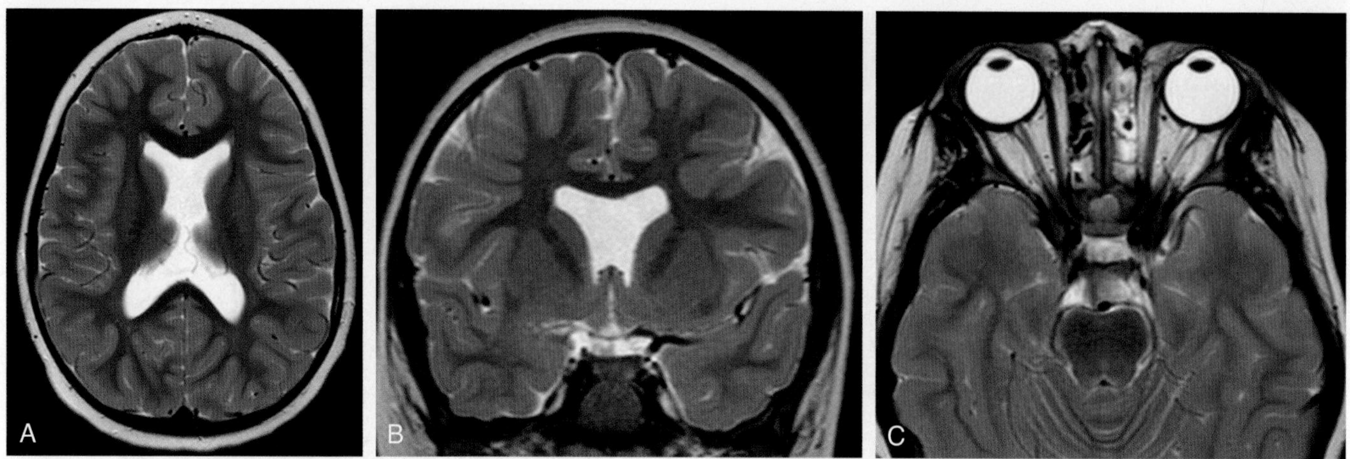

Fig. 2.67 Septo-optic Dysplasia. (A to C) Axial and coronal T2W images demonstrate absent septum pellucidum, and bilateral optic nerve hypoplasia. The pituitary gland was normal (not shown).

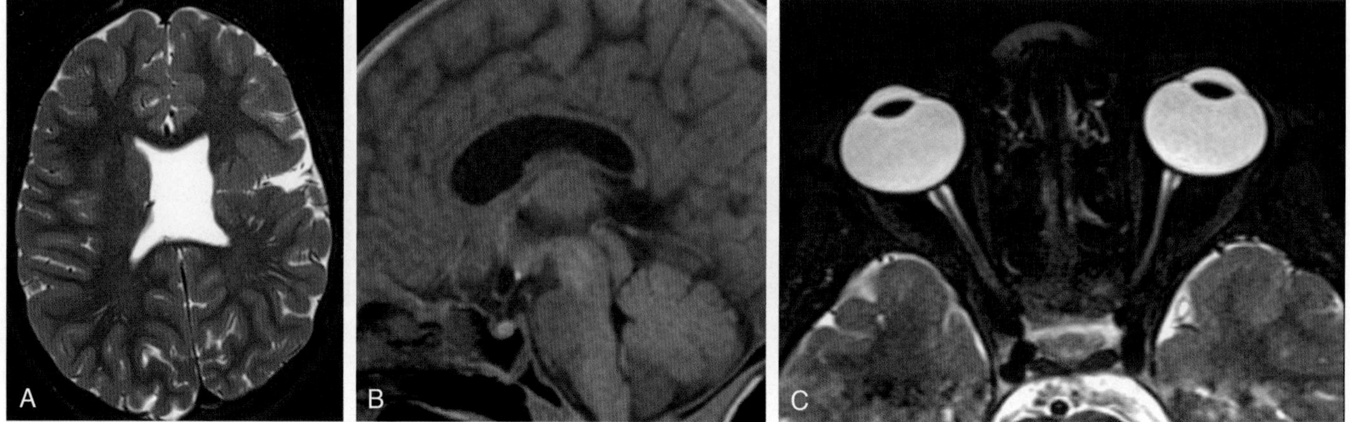

Fig. 2.68 Septo-optic Dysplasia. (A) Axial T2W, (B) sagittal T1W, and (C) axial T2W images demonstrate absent septum pellucidum, ectopic posterior pituitary gland, and bilateral optic nerve hypoplasia as well as a left posterior frontal closed-lip schizencephaly.

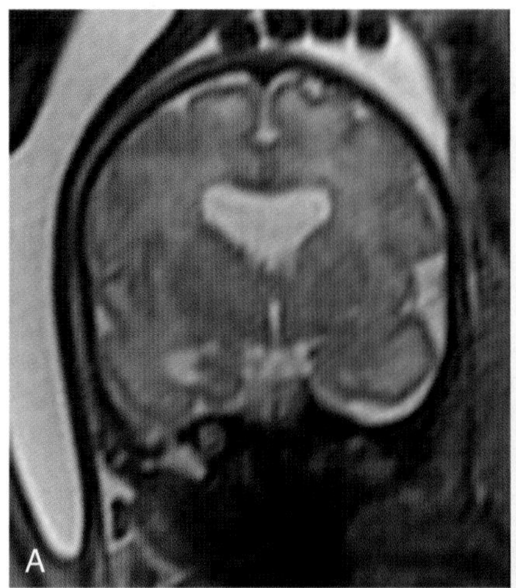

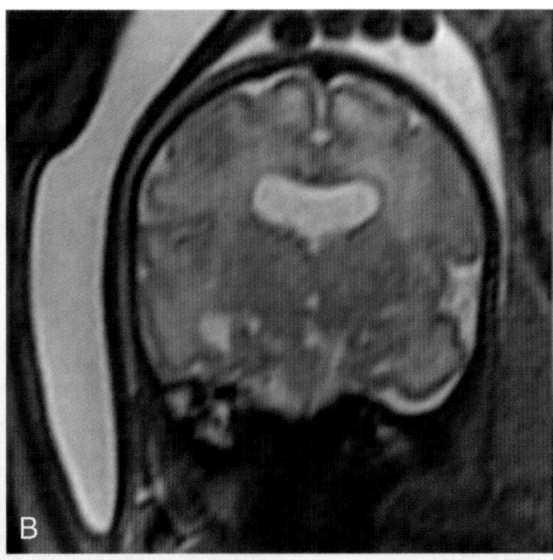

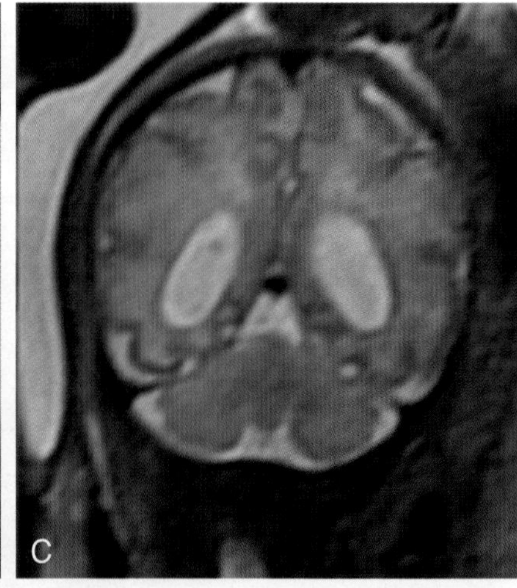

Fig. 2.69 Septo-optic Dysplasia. (A to C) Coronal T2W fetal MRI in a child with septo-optic dysplasia demonstrating box-like configuration of the anterior horns of the lateral ventricles, absent septum pellucidum, and small-appearing optic nerves/optic chiasm. Fetal MRI diagnosis is challenging, particularly because determination of hypoplastic optic nerves is difficult to confirm on fetal MRI. In the setting of an absent septum pellucidum without additional findings, a postnatal MRI should be performed.

Key Points

Background

- Septo-optic dysplasia (SOD) is characterized by any combination of optic nerve hypoplasia, pituitary hypofunction, and midline brain anomaly, typically absent septum pellucidum, and less commonly agenesis of the corpus callosum, or hypoplasia of the pons, vermis, and/or medulla. 30% of patients have all three anomalies.
- SOD is considered, by some experts, the mildest form of holoprosencephaly.
- SOD is a disorder of *ventral induction* secondary to genetic, environmental factors (maternal diabetes, alcohol, antiepileptic drugs) and CMV infection. HESX1, OTX2, SOX2 and PAX6 mutations have been linked to SOD.
- Variable neurologic prognosis from normal development and cognition to developmental delay, autism, and epilepsy. Presence of schizencephaly impacts prognosis.
- Pituitary endocrine dysfunction, hypothyroidism, hypogonadism, and adrenal insufficiency can lead to severe hypoglycemia, adrenal crisis, seizures, and sudden death.
- The degree of visual impairment is variable and ranges from normal vision to complete blindness.

Imaging

- *Absent septum pellucidum* resulting in a typical box-like configuration of the anterior lateral ventricles on coronal imaging.
- *Optic nerves including optic chiasm appear hypoplastic.* The hypoplastic optic nerves are usually beyond the spatial resolution of fetal MRI. Similarly, transfontanelle ultrasound may identify the box-like anterior lateral ventricles but fails to depict the optic nerve hypoplasia.
- *Pituitary gland anomalies* include anterior pituitary hypoplasia, ectopic posterior pituitary, and thin or absent pituitary infundibulum.
- Schizencephaly may be unilateral or bilateral.
- Anterior corpus callosum hypoplasia.
- Hypoplasia of the midbrain, pons, and/or medulla.
- Differential diagnosis includes rupture of the leaves of the septum pellucidum secondary to hydrocephalus, isolated absent septum pellucidum, and holoprosencephaly.

REFERENCES

1. Huisman TA, Poretti A. Chapter 7. Disorders of brain development. In: Magnetic Resonance Imaging of the Brain and Spine, 5th ed. Edited by Scott Atlas, MD. Wolters Kluwer, Lippincott Williams & Wilkins.
2. Orman G, Benson JE, Kweldam CF, Bosemani T, Tekes A, de Jong MR, Seyfert D, Northington FJ, Poretti A, Huisman TA. Neonatal head ultrasonography today: a powerful imaging tool!. *J Neuroimaging*. 2015 Jan-Feb;25(1):31–55.

SEPTOPREOPTIC HOLOPROSENCEPHALY

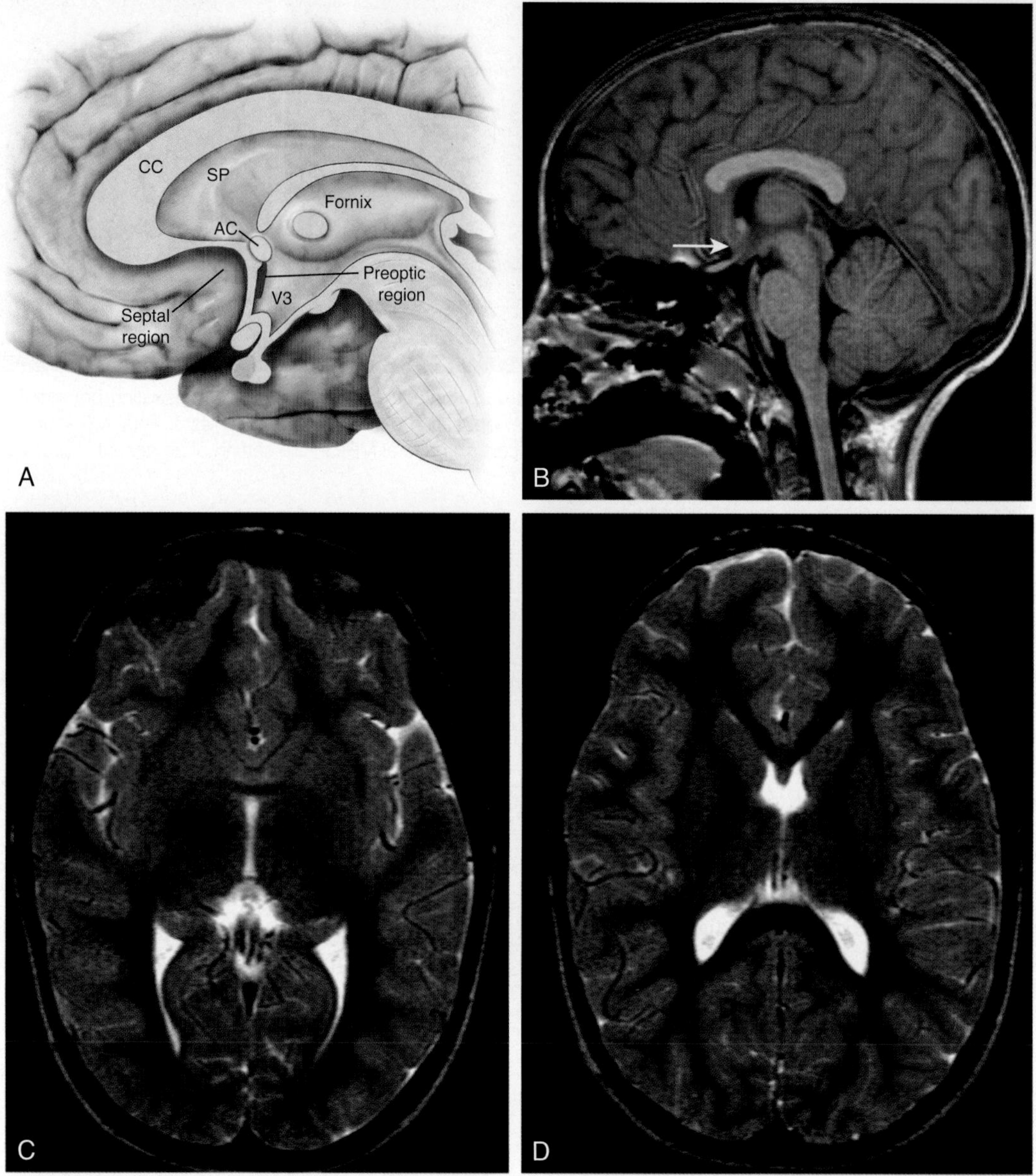

Fig. 2.70 Septopreoptic Holoprosencephaly. (A) Illustration of the septal and preoptic regions. *AC*, anterior commisure; *CC*, corpus callosum; *SP*, septum pellucidum; *V3*, third ventricle. (B) Sagittal T1W and (C and D) axial T2W images demonstrate absent rostrum and hypoplastic genu of the corpus callosum, thickening and fusion at the subcallosal and preoptic regions *(arrow)*, and absent septum pellucidum. (A from Volpe JJ. *Volpe's Neurology of the Newborn*. 6th ed. Elsevier; 2018.)

Key Points

Background

- Septopreoptic dysplasia is a controversial mild form of holoprosencephaly in which there is fusion in the septal/subcallosal and/or preoptic regions
- Associated with language delay, learning disability, and abnormal behavior but normal motor function

Imaging

- Fusion/thickening in the subcallosal frontal lobe anterior to the third ventricle. Lobar holoprosencephaly is differentiated by basal frontal lobe fusion
- Variable absence of the septum pellucidum
- Absent or hypoplastic anterior corpus callosum
- Thickened or dysplastic fornix
- Azygous ACA
- Mild midline craniofacial anomalies: piriform aperture stenosis and single maxillary central incisor

REFERENCE

1. Hahn JS, Barnes PD, Clegg NJ, Stashinko EE. Septopreoptic holoprosencephaly: a mild subtype associated with midline craniofacial anomalies. *AJNR Am J Neuroradiol*. 2010 Oct;31(9):1596–1601.

ABSENT SEPTUM PELLUCIDUM: OTHER CAUSES

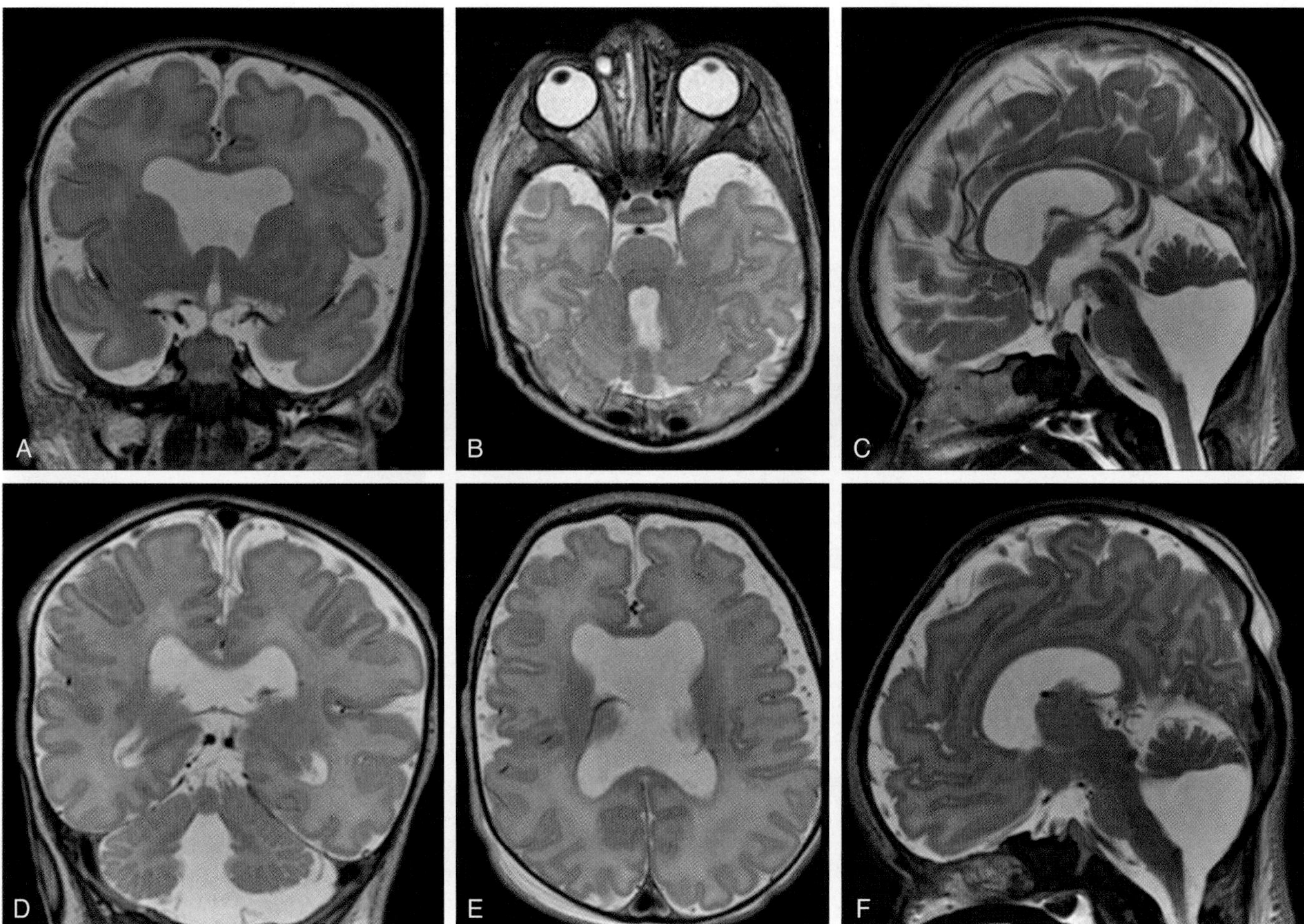

Fig. 2.71 Absent Septum Pellucidum. (A and D) Coronal, (B and E) axial, and (C and F) sagittal T2W MRI of a child with nonvisualization of the leaves of the septum pellucidum associated with a Dandy-Walker malformation with cystic widening of the fourth ventricle and hypoplasia of the vermis.

Key Points

- In addition to holoprosencephaly and septo-optic dysplasia, absent septum pellucidum can be seen with the following:
  - Dandy-Walker malformation
  - Callosal malformations
  - Hydrocephalus: The leaves of the septum pellucidum may rupture after a long-standing high-grade supratentorial hydrocephalus mimicking a septo-optic dysplasia. The chiasm and optic nerves are of normal size.
  - Isolated

REFERENCE

1. Huisman TA, Poretti A. Chapter 7. Disorders of brain development. In: Magnetic Resonance Imaging of the Brain and Spine, 5th ed. Edited by Scott Atlas, MD. Wolters Kluwer, Lippincott Williams & Wilkins.

ENCEPHALOCELES AND CRANIUM ANOMALIES

Meningoencephaloceles are defects in the skull and dura associated with extracranial herniation of meninges. These occur with an incidence of 1 per 4000 live births. A meningocele is a herniation of CSF lined by meninges. A meningoencephalocele is a herniation of meninges and brain. The etiology is unknown, but a defect in the anterior/rostral neural tube closure is suspected. The occipital meningoencephalocele is the most common location in Europe and North America, and frontoethmoidal meningoencephalocele is the most common in southeast Asia. Prognosis is affected by the amount and location of herniated brain tissue, hydrocephalus, and additional malformations.

In addition to meningoencephaloceles, anencephaly and related disorders are illustrated in this section (Fig. 2.72). These are rare lethal malformations that may be encountered on fetal imaging. Craniofacial disorders are discussed in the craniofacial malformation chapter.

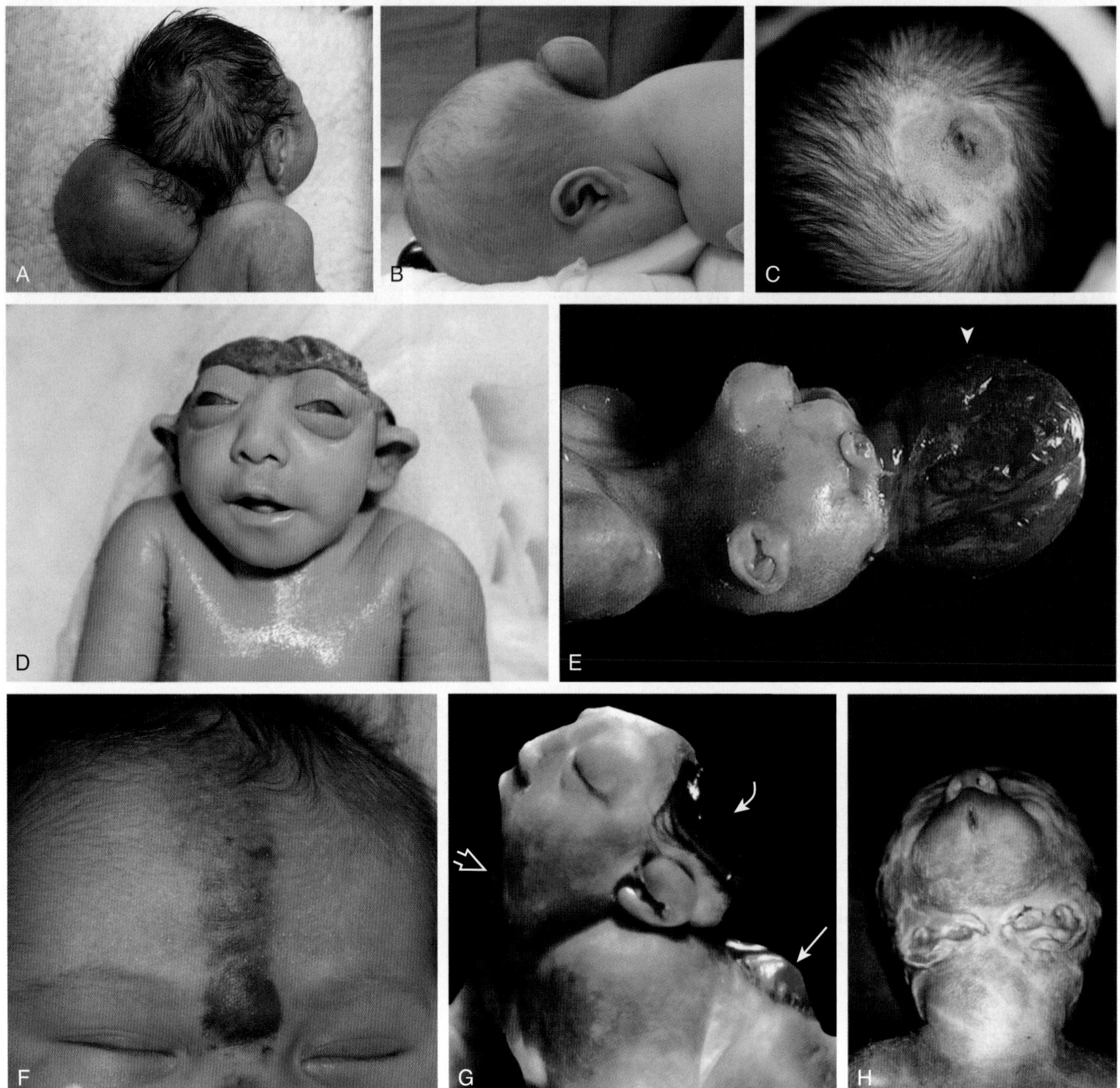

Fig. 2.72 Selected Encephaloceles and Cranium Anomalies. (A) Meningoencephalocele of the occipital region. (B) Occipital encephalocele. (C) Atretic encephalocele with a surrounding hemangioma. (D) Anencephaly. (E) Exencephaly. (F) Sinus pericrania. (G) Iniencephaly. (H) Otocephaly. (A, H from Gilbert-Barness E. *Potter's Pathology of the Fetus, Infant and Child.* 2nd ed. Mosby; 2007. B, C from Winn HR. *Youmans and Winn Neurological Surgery.* 8th ed. Elsevier; 2023. D from Gangane SD. *Human Genetics.* 6th ed. Elsevier; 2023. E from Klatt EC. *Robbins and Cotran Atlas of Pathology.* 4th ed. Elsevier; 2021. F from Bolognia JL, Schaffer JV, Duncan KO, Ko CJ. *Dermatology Essentials.* 2nd ed. Elsevier; 2022. G from Woodward PJ. *Diagnostic Imaging.* 4th ed. Elsevier; 2021.)

CONGENITAL MENINGOENCEPHALOCELE

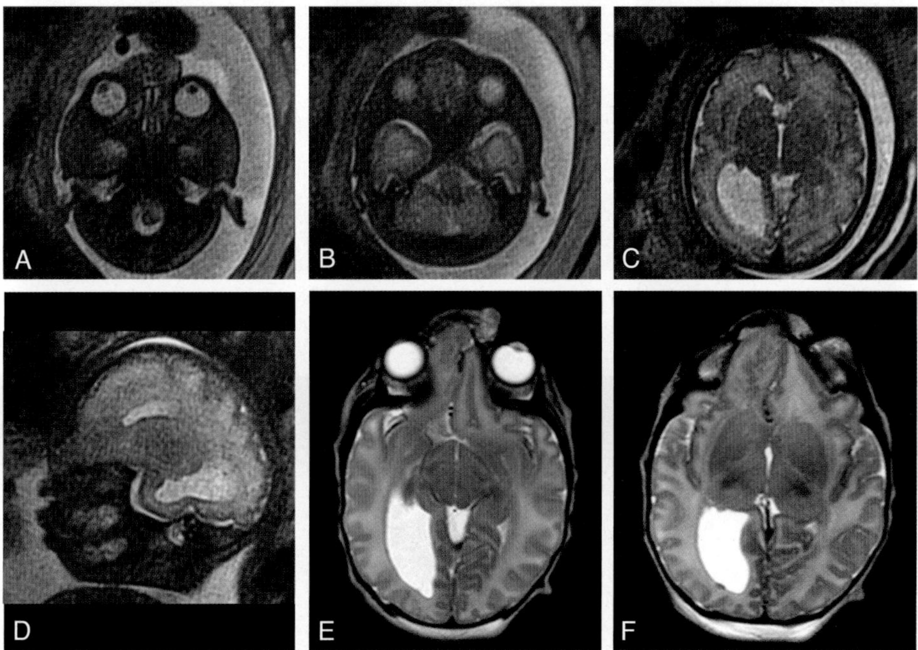

Fig. 2.73 Meningoencephalocele. (A to D) Axial and sagittal T2W fetal MRI images in a child with a right frontal basal meningoencephalocele extending into the nasal cavity. Significant widening of the anterior skull base is noted, including herniation of the frontal basal brain through the osseous defect, well seen on the sagittal imaging. In addition, moderate right-sided ventriculomegaly and nodular contour of the bordering of the right lateral ventricle compatible with subependymal heterotopia. (E and F) Axial T2W postnatal MR confirms a frontal basal meningoencephalocele with malformed/dysplastic right frontal basal gyri, right-sided ventriculomegaly, and subependymal heterotopia along the occipital horn of the right lateral ventricle.

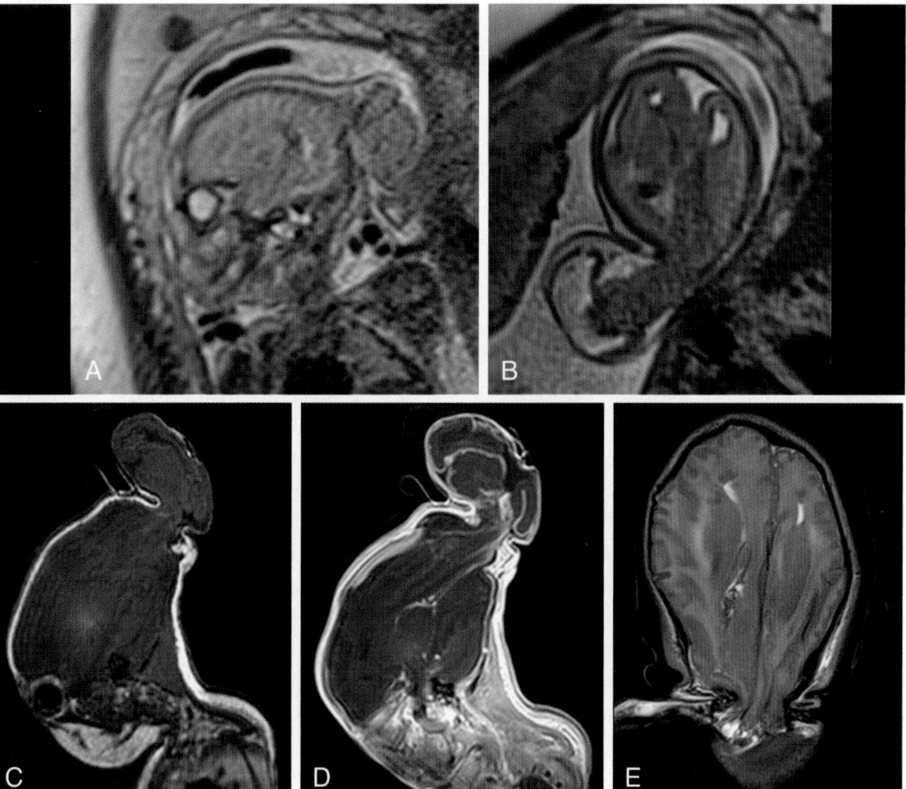

Fig. 2.74 Meningoencephalocele. (A and B) Sagittal and axial T2W the fetal MRI in child with a large occipital meningoencephalocele, and mild microcephaly. (C to E) Sagittal T1W, sagittal T1W+C, and axial T2W postnatal MRI confirm the large occipital meningoencephalocele. Part of the brain vasculature is herniating into the meningoencephalocele. Additional T2 hypointense heterotopic gray matter is seen within both frontal lobes.

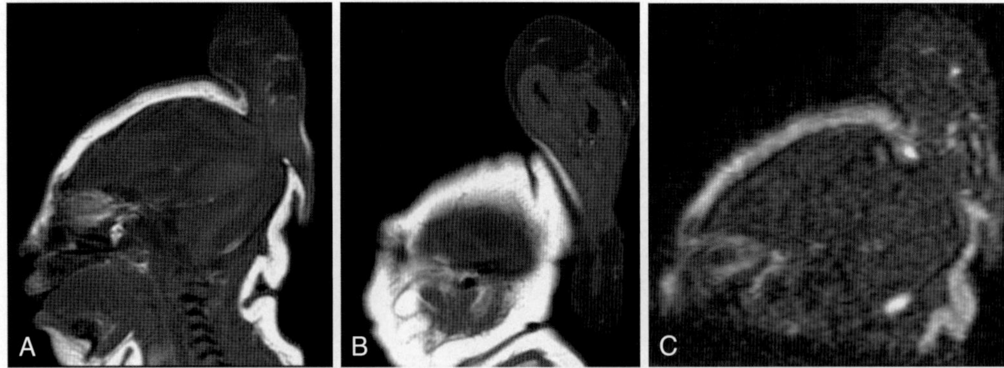

Fig. 2.75 Meningoencephalocele. (A and B) Sagittal T1W and (C) sagittal noncontrast MR venogram demonstrate a large occipital meningoencephalocele, which also contains herniated lateral ventricles and multiple vessels. There is associated severe microcephaly.

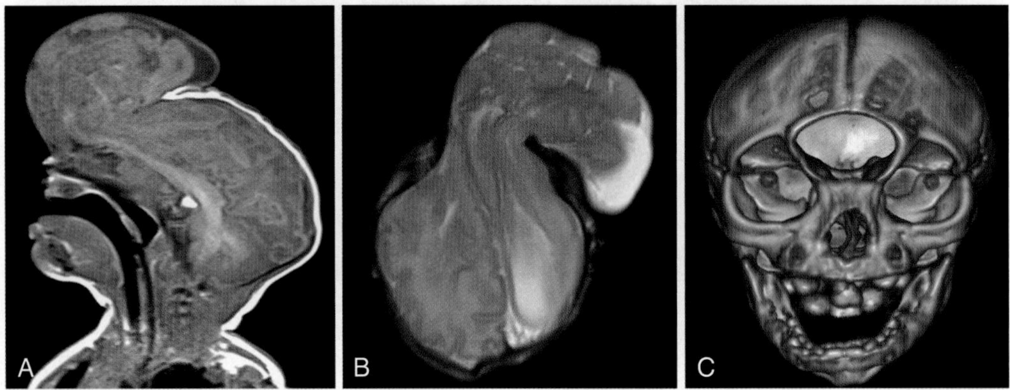

Fig. 2.76 Meningoencephalocele. (A) Sagittal T1W, (B) axial T2W, and (C) 3D volumetric CT images demonstrate a large frontal bone defect with herniation of the bilateral frontal lobes.

Key Points

Background

- Encephaloceles are the congenital or developmental herniation of parts of the brain through a focal skull defect.
- Etiology is still uncertain. Possibly secondary to a defective closure of the primary neural tube versus a postneurulation event in which initially correctly developed brain tissue herniates through an early mesenchymal defect that will eventually progress into a "hole" of the dura and skull later during development.
- Parts of the ventricular system may "co-herniate" through the defect. On imaging it may appear as if the brain, including ventricles, is being "pulled out" of the cranial fossa.
- Prognosis depends on amount of herniated tissue, location, contents, and additional malformations. Meningoceles can have normal neurologic outcome. Encephaloceles can have epilepsy and poor outcome. Occipital encephaloceles have worse prognosis compared to skull base encephaloceles.
- Encephaloceles are usually sporadic but can occur with trisomy 13 and 18, Meckel-Gruber syndrome (occipital; encephalocele, cystic renal disease, polydactyly) and Chiari III malformation.

Imaging

- Depending on the overall amount of herniated tissue, the skull may be small and respectively microcephalic.
- If a meningoencephalocele is seen in close proximity to dural sinuses, coexistent herniation of the venous structures should be determined.
- The brain tissue within the meningoencephalocele is frequently dysplastic and disorganized; in addition the adjacent intracranial brain has a high incidence of additional migrational abnormalities, including corpus callosum anomalies.
- Locations:
  - Occipital (80%): Most common location. Associated with Meckel-Gruber syndrome, Chiari III, Dandy-Walker malformation, cortical malformations, and callosal malformations
  - Frontoethmoidal (15%): Nasofrontal, nasoethmoidal, naso-orbital, and ethmoidal. Associated callosal malformations, schizencephaly, and interhemispheric lipoma
  - Parietal: uncommon
  - Skull base and nasopharyngeal: Sphenoethmoidal, and sphenonasopharyngeal. Associated with facial clefts, and morning glory disc anomaly
- Associated anomalies: Heterotopia, polymicrogyria, and callosal malformations

REFERENCE

1. Huisman TA, Poretti A. Chapter 7. Disorders of brain development. In: Magnetic Resonance Imaging of the Brain and Spine, 5th ed. Edited by Scott Atlas, MD. Wolters Kluwer, Lippincott Williams & Wilkins.

SECONDARY OR ACQUIRED MENINGOENCEPHALOCELE

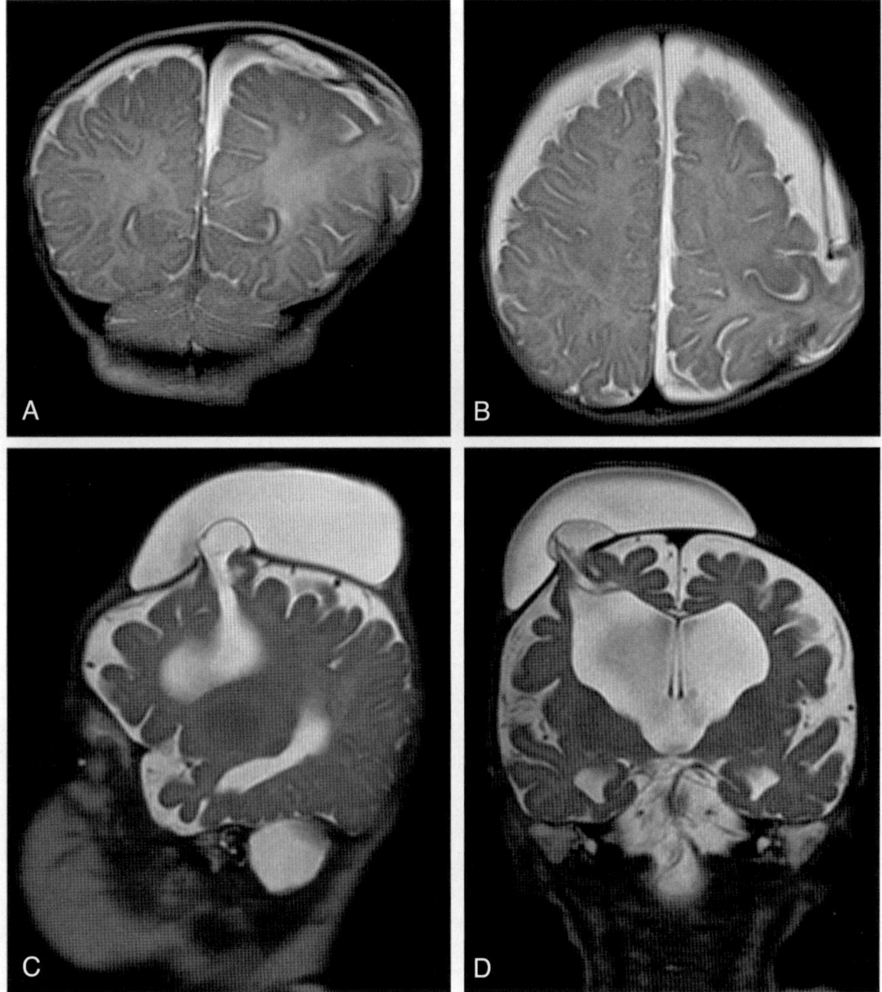

Fig. 2.77 Meningoencephalocele. (A and B) Coronal and axial T2W MRI of the brain in a child with a posttraumatic left parietal meningoencephalocele, in which brain tissue is herniating through a persistent skull defect resulting in a growing fracture. (C and D) Sagittal and coronal T2W MRI of a child with a secondary meningoencephalocele in which meningeal and cerebral structures are herniating through an old burr hole for a previous ventriculoperitoneal shunt. A large subcutaneous CSF isointense fluid collection has developed.

Key Points

Background

- "Secondary" or "acquired" meningoencephaloceles are not true malformations and may be seen after a traumatic brain injury with a skull fracture or after a neurosurgical procedure with persistent skull defects.
- In young children, dura may get trapped within the skull fracture site, allowing for chronic cerebrospinal fluid pulsations to prevent fracture healing with resultant appearance of a growing fracture. Brain tissue may subsequently herniate through the growing defect.
- Brain tissue may also directly herniate through a fracture site or through a neurosurgical burr hole after, for example, previous shunt placement or decompression of an epidural hematoma.
- The herniated brain tissue frequently involutes or scars (as seen on follow-up).
- Because these kind of meningoencephaloceles are not malformative, no associated intracranial developmental anomalies are to be expected.

Imaging

- Similar to "true" or congenital meningoencephaloceles, various degrees of herniation of meninges and/or brain issue may be encountered.

REFERENCES

1. Pinto PS, Poretti A, Meoded A, Tekes A, Huisman TA. The unique features of traumatic brain injury in children. Review of the characteristics of the pediatric skull and brain, mechanisms of trauma, patterns of injury, complications and their imaging findings – part 1. *J Neuroimaging*. 2012 Apr;22(2):e1–e17.
2. Pinto PS, Poretti A, Meoded A, Tekes A, Huisman TA. The unique features of traumatic brain injury in children. Review of the characteristics of the pediatric skull and brain, mechanisms of trauma, patterns of injury, complications and their imaging findings – part 2. *J Neuroimaging*. 2012 Apr;22(2):e18–e41.

ATRETIC ENCEPHALOCELE

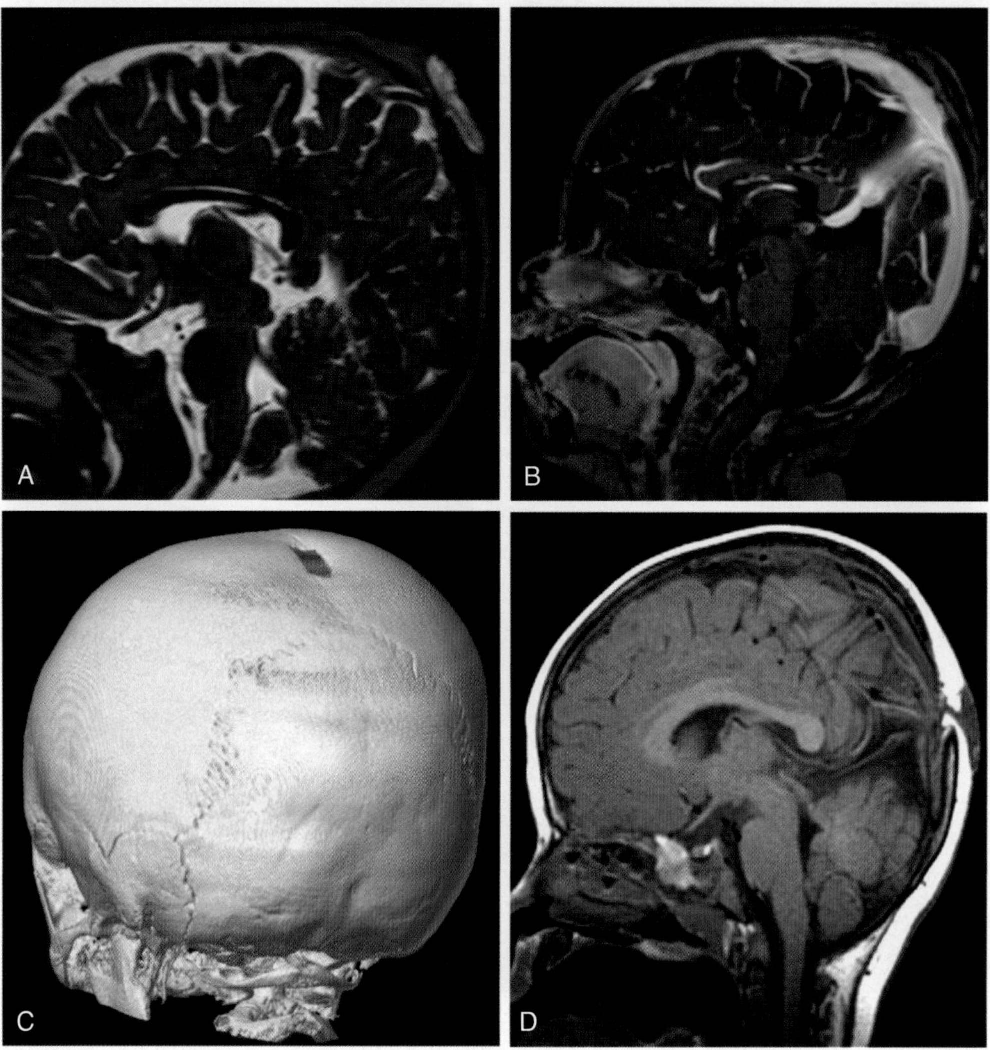

Fig. 2.78 Atretic Encephalocele. (A) Sagittal T2W, (B) sagittal T1W+C, and (C) 3D volumetric CT images demonstrate an atretic parietal encephalocele with T2 hyperintense tissue in the scalp, a persistent falcine sinus, and midline parietal bone defect. Different patient with (D) sagittal T1W image of an atretic parietal occipital encephalocele with thin fibrous tract extending from the brain through the bone and into the scalp.

Key Points

Background

- Atretic meningoencephaloceles are variants of the congenital meningoencephaloceles, in which degenerated herniated brain tissue is present in combination with included dura and fibrous strands.
- Prognosis is good with typically normal neurologic outcome.

Imaging

- Most frequently seen in the midline along the course of the sagittal suture in the parieto-occipital region.
- The skull defect may be miniature; the underlying superior sagittal sinus is often fenestrated allowing the atretic meningoencephalocele to herniate in the midline.
- There is an increased incidence of additional venous anomalies, including an interhemispheric ascending falcine sinus or persistent falcine sinus.
- The tentorium cerebelli may be elevated pointing toward the atretic meningoencephalocele.

REFERENCE

1. Huisman TA, Poretti A. Chapter 7. Disorders of brain development. In: Magnetic Resonance Imaging of the Brain and Spine, 5th ed. Edited by Scott Atlas, MD. Wolters Kluwer, Lippincott Williams & Wilkins.

ANENCEPHALY

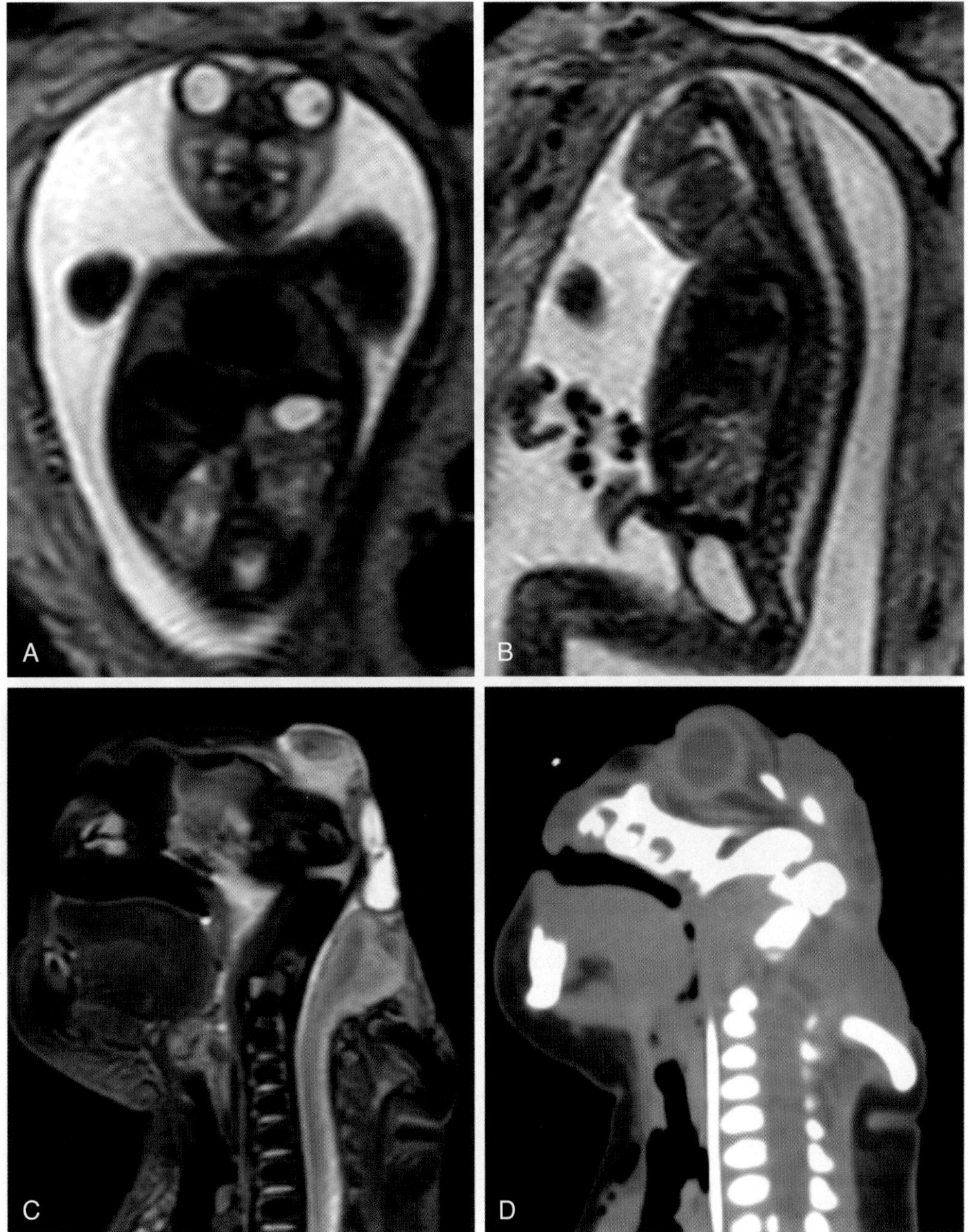

Fig. 2.79 Anencephaly. (A and B) Coronal and sagittal T2W fetal MR images. (C) Postnatal autopsy sagittal T2W image and (D) postnatal autopsy sagittal reformat CT image demonstrate absence of the calvarium and cerebral and cerebellar hemispheres.

Key Points

Background

- Rare lethal malformation due to a neural tube defect.
- Part of the acrania-exencephaly-anencephaly sequence.
- Begins at fourth week of gestation when the rostral neural tube is closing. There is failure of migration of mesenchyme, leading to lack of formation of the calvarium and scalp. The unprotected brain undergoes progressive destruction due to mechanical trauma and amniotic fluid exposure.
- With acrania, the calvarium and skull base are absent but the cerebral and cerebellar hemispheres are present.

Imaging

- Absent cerebral and cerebellar hemispheres
- Remnant of disorganized forebrain tissue covered by angiomatous stroma
- Absent calvarium above the orbits
- Normal skull base
- Deformed facial structures

REFERENCE

1. Sharif A, Zhou Y. Fetal MRI characteristics of exencephaly: A case report and literature review. *Case reports in Radiology*. 2016(4):1–4.

EXENCEPHALY

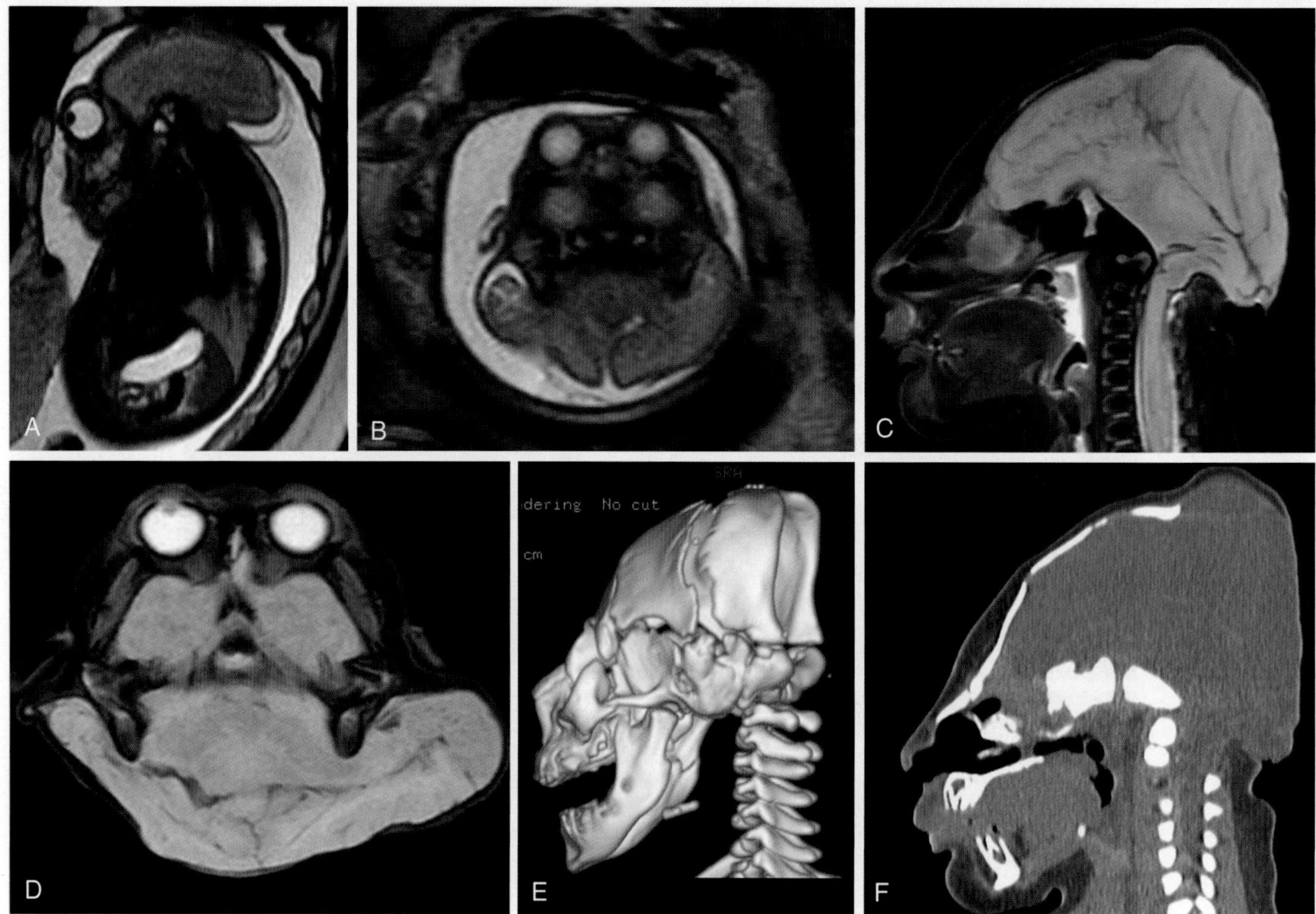

Fig. 2.80 Exencephaly. (A and B) Sagittal and axial T2W fetal MR images. (C and D) Postnatal autopsy sagittal and axial T2W images. (E and F) Postnatal autopsy sagittal reformat CT and 3D volumetric CT images demonstrate poorly formed calvarium with large posterior defect, allowing for herniation of dysplastic brain.

Key Points

Background

- Rare lethal malformation with controversial etiology, possibly within the group of neural tube defects
- Considered an embryologic precursor to anencephaly as the vascular layer of epithelium covering the brain slowly degrades due to presence of the amniotic fluid
- Along a spectrum of a large encephalocele
- Part of the acrania-exencephaly-anencephaly sequence

Imaging

- Calvarium is absent or poorly formed and brain tissue herniates into the amniotic fluid
- Cerebral and cerebellar hemispheres present but dysplastic and covered by vascular layer of endothelium
- Calvarium usually absent above the orbits
- Skull base normal
- Facial structures are normal

REFERENCE

1. Sharif A, Zhou Y. Fetal MRI characteristics of exencephaly: A case report and literature review. *Case Rep Radiol.* 2016(4):1–4.

APROSENCEPHALY-ATELENCEPHALY

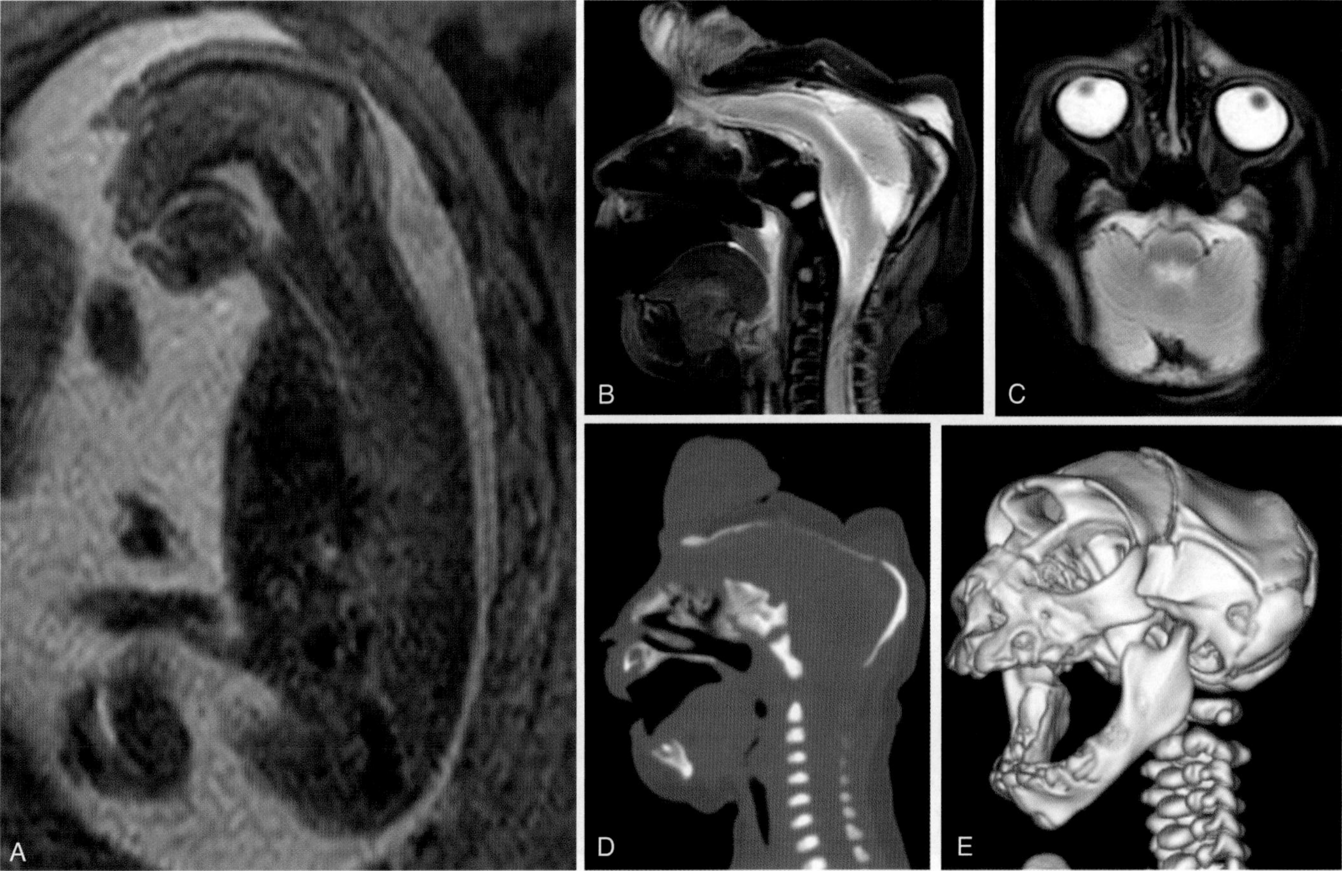

Fig. 2.81 Aprosencephaly-Atelencephaly. (A) Sagittal T2W fetal MR image, (B and C) postnatal autopsy sagittal and axial T2W images, and (D and E) postnatal autopsy sagittal reformat CT and 3D volumetric CT images demonstrate microcephaly flattened but formed calvarium and largely absent telencephalon with anterior encephalocele of the dysplastic remnant through an anterior calvarial defect.

Key Points

Background

- Rare lethal fetal malformation with a spectrum of varying degrees of absence of the telencephalon and diencephalon.
- Both the telencephalon, which the cerebrum develops from, and the diencephalon, which the thalami develop from, are absent in aprosencephaly while the cerebral hemispheres are absent in atelencephaly.
- The prosencephalon gives rise to the telencephalon and diencephalon during the fifth week of gestation. In aprosencephaly-atelencephaly there is absent or abnormal formation of the prosencephalon.
- Many similar features of aprosencephaly are shared with holoprosencephaly, including midline facial anomalies of cyclopia and cleft lip/palate; however, they are considered distinct entities and in the anencephaly-aprosencephaly-holoprosencephaly continuum.
- The XK aprosencephaly syndrome described in 1979 by Lurie et al includes the triad of aprosencephaly, limb anomalies, and genital anomalies.

Imaging

- Severe microcephaly with absent supratentorial cerebral structures and dysplastic rudimentary prosencephalon.
- The scalp and calvarium are present, which differentiates it from anencephaly.
- Cerebellum is normal or dysplastic.
- Midline facial anomalies: micro-ophthalmia, hypertelorism, cyclopia, anophthalmia, cleft lip/palate, micrognathia.

REFERENCE

1. Nagaraj UD, Lawrence A, Vezina LG, et al. Prenatal evaluation of atelencephaly. *Pediatr Radiol.* 2016(46):145–147.

SINUS PERICRANII

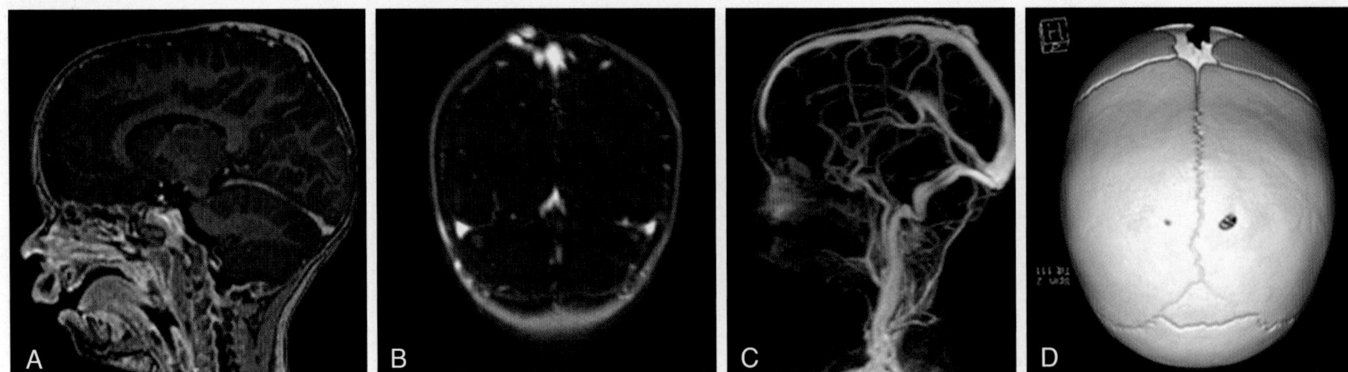

Fig. 2.82 Sinus Pericranii. (A) Sagittal T1W+C, (B) coronal source MR venography, (C) sagittal MPR, and (D) 3D volumetric CT reconstruction of the skull in a child with a sinus pericranii show a direct connection of the superficial venous system via emissary veins to subcutaneous calvarial veins. On the 3D CT reconstruction prominent parietal osseous vascular channel is well depicted.

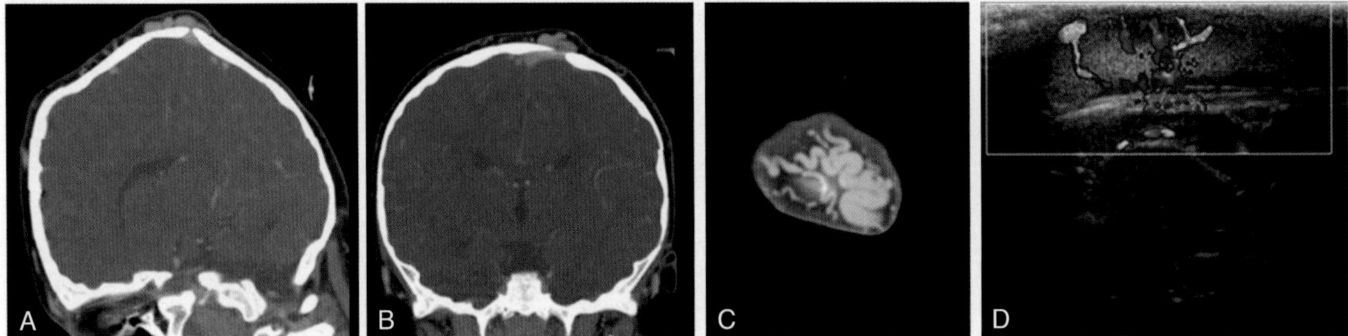

Fig. 2.83 Sinus Pericranii. (A) Sagittal, (B) coronal, and (C) axial contrast-enhanced CT study in a child with a sinus pericranii identifies multiple varicose subcutaneous calvarial veins that communicate over a left paramedian skull defect with the superficial venous system just adjacent to the superior sagittal sinus. (D) On ultrasound the direct connection of the emissary veins is well noted, in addition to mild venous edema in the adjacent soft tissues.

Key Points

Background

- Sinus pericranii are varicose subcutaneous calvarial veins that communicate with intracranial dural venous sinuses via the emissary veins.
- The concomitant dilatation of the emissary veins may result in a focal widening of the calvarial venous vascular channel; focal remodeling of the external or internal table may be observed.
- These low-pressure, slow-flow venous vascular lesions are typically midline or paramedian along the course of the superior sagittal sinus.
- They present clinically as a soft focal scalp swelling that can easily be compressed.

Imaging

- Ultrasound examination with Doppler interrogation are diagnostic to confirm the vascular nature of the lesion.
- Contrast-enhanced CT or MRI with CT or MR venography allows study of the full extent of the malformation. Occasionally an adjacent developmental venous anomaly (DVA) may coexist.

REFERENCE

1. Huisman TA, Poretti A. Chapter 7. Disorders of brain development. In: Magnetic Resonance Imaging of the Brain and Spine, 5th ed. Edited by Scott Atlas, MD. Wolters Kluwer, Lippincott Williams & Wilkins.

CEREBRAL AQUEDUCT ABNORMALITIES

Abnormalities resulting in obstruction of CSF flow through the cerebral aqueduct result in obstructive hydrocephalus, affecting the lateral and third ventricles. Congenital aqueductal stenosis is a common cause of fetal and neonatal hydrocephalus. The stenosis can be intrinsic or extrinsic due to external compression. Aqueductal stenosis can also be acquired due to hemorrhage or infectious material causing arachnoid webs or gliosis that obstruct the aqueduct. This section will illustrate common causes of aqueductal stenosis.

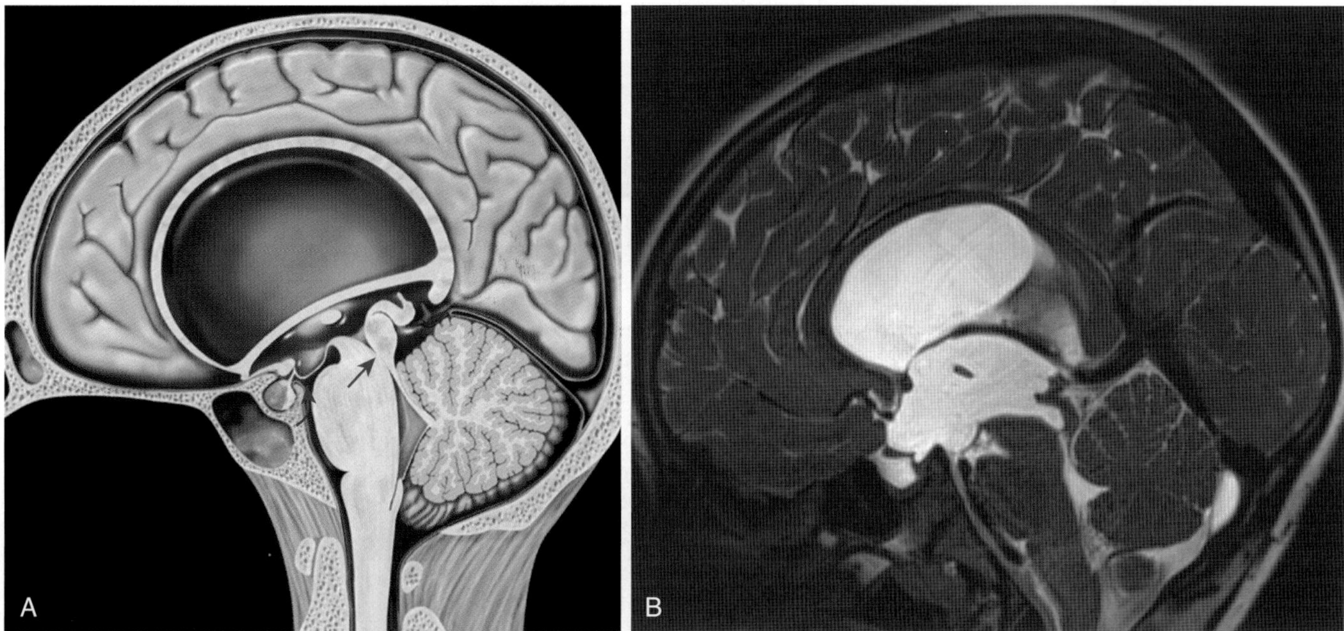

Fig. 2.84 Aqueductal Stenosis. (A) Sagittal graphic shows obstructive hydrocephalus with markedly enlarged lateral and third ventricles, a stretched (thinned) corpus callosum, and a funnel-shaped cerebral aqueduct *(red arrow)* related to distal obstruction. Note the normal size of the 4th ventricle and depression of the floor of the 3rd ventricle *(curved red arrow)* from the hydrocephalus. (B) Sagittal T2W image demonstrating similar findings of aqueductal stenosis. (Image A From StatDX. Copyright © 2022 Elsevier.)

CONGENITAL AQUEDUCTAL STENOSIS

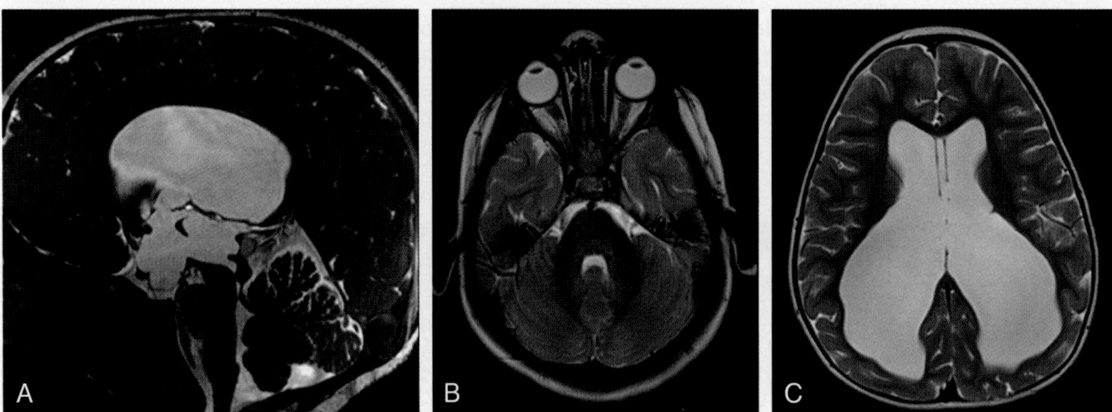

Fig. 2.85 Aqueductal Stenosis. (A) High-resolution T2W sagittal MRI and (B and C) axial T2W images of a child with high-grade supratentorial ventriculomegaly, significant widening of the third ventricle with inferior bowing and displacement of the floor of the third ventricle, normal-size fourth ventricle is normal in size, and widening of the upper part of the Sylvian aqueduct proximal to a focal stenosis within the lower third of the Sylvian aqueduct.

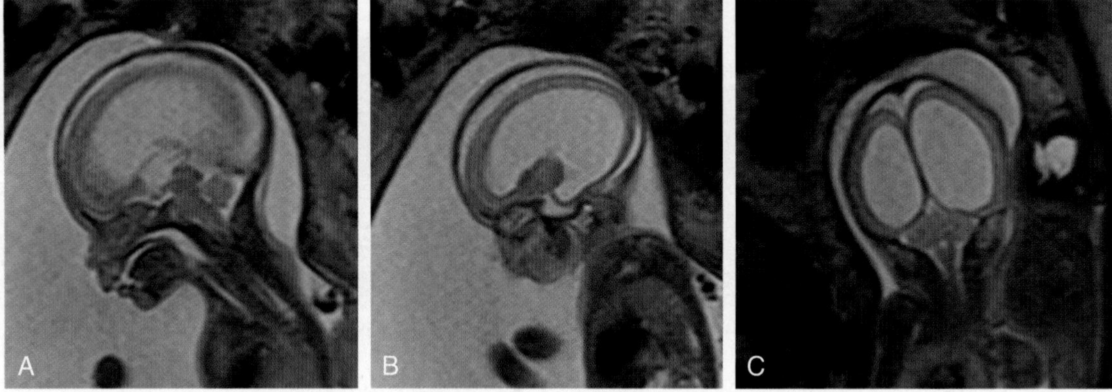

Fig. 2.86 Aqueductal Stenosis. (A to C) Sagittal and coronal T2W fetal MRI of a child with congenital aqueductal stenosis. High-grade widening of the lateral and third ventricles, normal-size fourth ventricle, and no cerebrospinal fluid noted within the region of the Sylvain aqueduct, confirming diagnosis of congenital aqueductal stenosis.

Key Points

Background

- Characterized by a focal stenosis of the Sylvian aqueduct with resultant moderate to severe dilatation of the third and lateral ventricles and normal-size fourth ventricle.
- The exact etiology of an isolated, intrinsic congenital aqueductal stenosis remains the focus of research. A genetic etiology known as X-linked hydrocephalus with stenosis of the Sylvian aqueduct (HSAS) is caused by mutation of L1CAM gene.
- Treated with third ventriculostomy or ventriculoperitoneal shunting.

Imaging

- The cerebral aqueduct is narrowed or occluded, often by a thickened tectum. The Sylvian aqueduct may be dilated proximal to the stenosis.
- In high-grade focal stenosis, a cerebrospinal fluid flow related signal void may be seen within and adjacent to the third ventricle. No flow is identified when the Sylvian aqueduct is completely occluded/atretic.
- The *lateral and third ventricles are enlarged and the fourth ventricle is normal in size.*
- Interstitial edema may be recognized within the supratentorial periventricular white matter, in particular along the anterior and posterior horns of the lateral ventricles.
- The corpus callosum is thinned in high-grade hydrocephalus.
- Associations: rhombencephalosynapsis, alpha-dystroglycanopathies, and CRASH syndrome (X-linked hydrocephalus, aqueductal stenosis, corpus callosum hypoplasia/agenesis, adducted thumbs, spasticity and mild to moderate intellectual disability).

REFERENCE

1. Huisman TA, Poretti A. Chapter 7. Disorders of brain development. In: Magnetic Resonance Imaging of the Brain and Spine, 5th ed. Edited by Scott Atlas, MD. Wolters Kluwer, Lippincott Williams & Wilkins.

AQUEDUCTAL STENOSIS: POSTHEMORRHAGIC

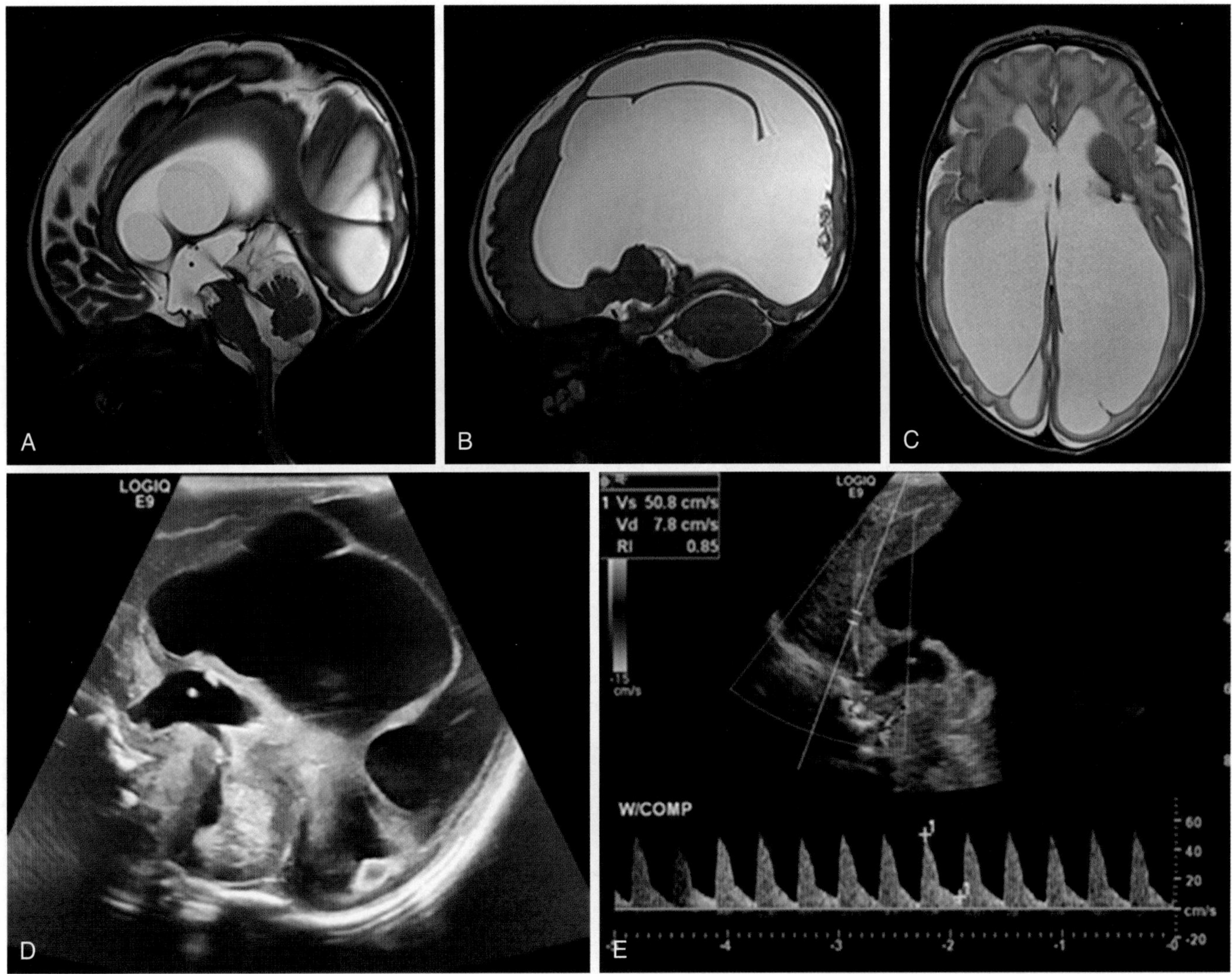

Fig. 2.87 Aqueductal Stenosis. (A to C) Sagittal and axial T2W MRI of a child with posthemorrhagic aqueductal stenosis. High-grade widening of the supratentorial ventricular system, including third ventricle, inferior bowing of the floor of the surgery ventricle, normal-size fourth ventricle. High-grade stenosis/adhesion within the lower third of the Sylvian aqueduct. Blood clots noted within the posterior dependent parts of the lateral ventricle after intraventricular spilling of blood secondary to a left-sided germinal matrix hemorrhage. (D and E) Sagittal ultrasound imaging including duplex sonography with sampling of branch of the anterior circulation in the same patient confirms a high-grade widening of the supratentorial ventricular system in combination with a normal-size fourth ventricle and focal stenosis at the level of the lower third of the Sylvian aqueduct. Resistive index value significantly elevated measuring up to 0.85.

Key Points

Background

- Intrinsic aqueductal stenosis may be secondary to adhesions after an intraventricular hemorrhage or infection.

Imaging

- Focal webs may be seen outlined by cerebrospinal fluid.
- Intraventricular blood products in neonates are often secondary to germinal matrix hemorrhages that have extended into the ventricular system.
- Focal hypoechogenic or T2-hypointesne blood products may be seen within the regions of the caudothalamic groove.
- Intraventricular blood products can accumulate in the dependent posterior horns of the lateral ventricles.
- Susceptibility weighed MR imaging is most sensitive for the blood products.
- T2- or SWI-hypointense superficial hemosiderosis can be seen along the brainstem and within the brain sulci.

REFERENCE

1. Huisman TA, Poretti A. Chapter 7. Disorders of brain development. In: Magnetic Resonance Imaging of the Brain and Spine, 5th ed. Edited by Scott Atlas, MD. Wolters Kluwer, Lippincott Williams & Wilkins.

AQUEDUCTAL STENOSIS: EXTRINSIC COMPRESSION

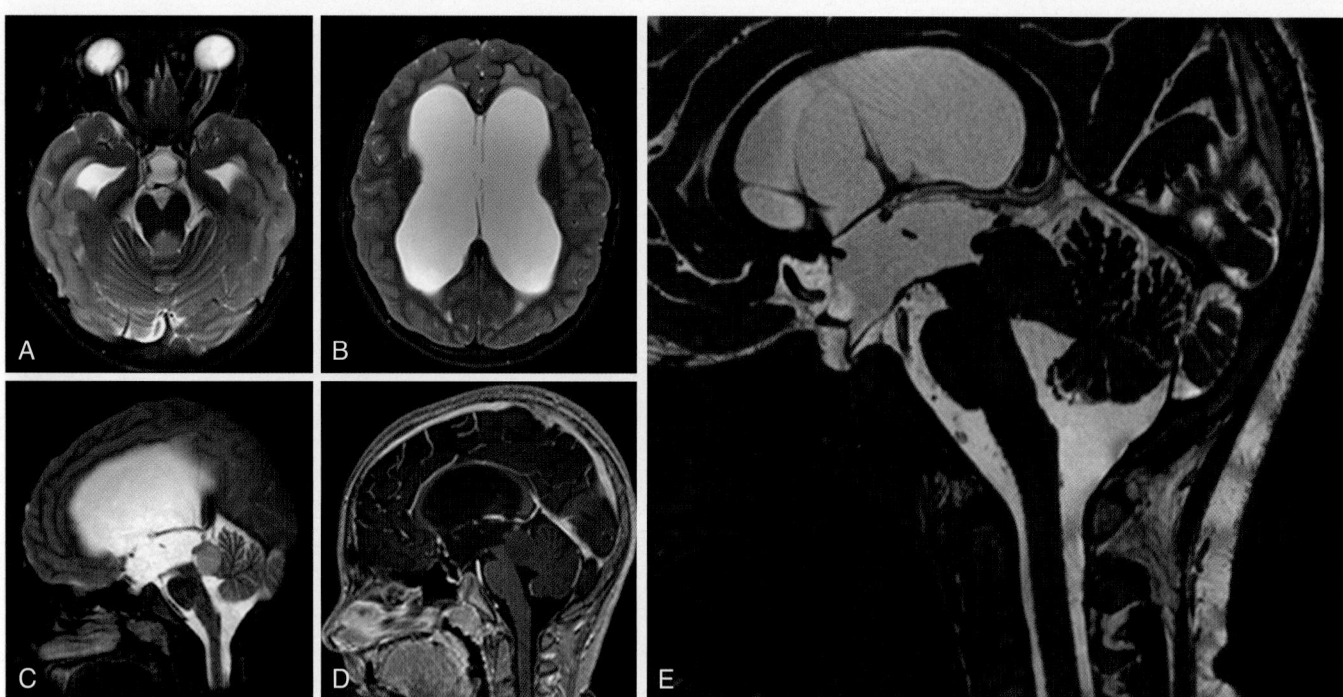

Fig. 2.88 Aqueductal Stenosis. (A, B, C, and E) Axial and sagittal T2W and (D) sagittal T1W+C MRI of a child with tectal glioma. Significant enlargement of the tectal plate secondary to the glioma, secondary high-grade stenosis of the Sylvian aqueduct with high-grade supratentorial ventriculomegaly.

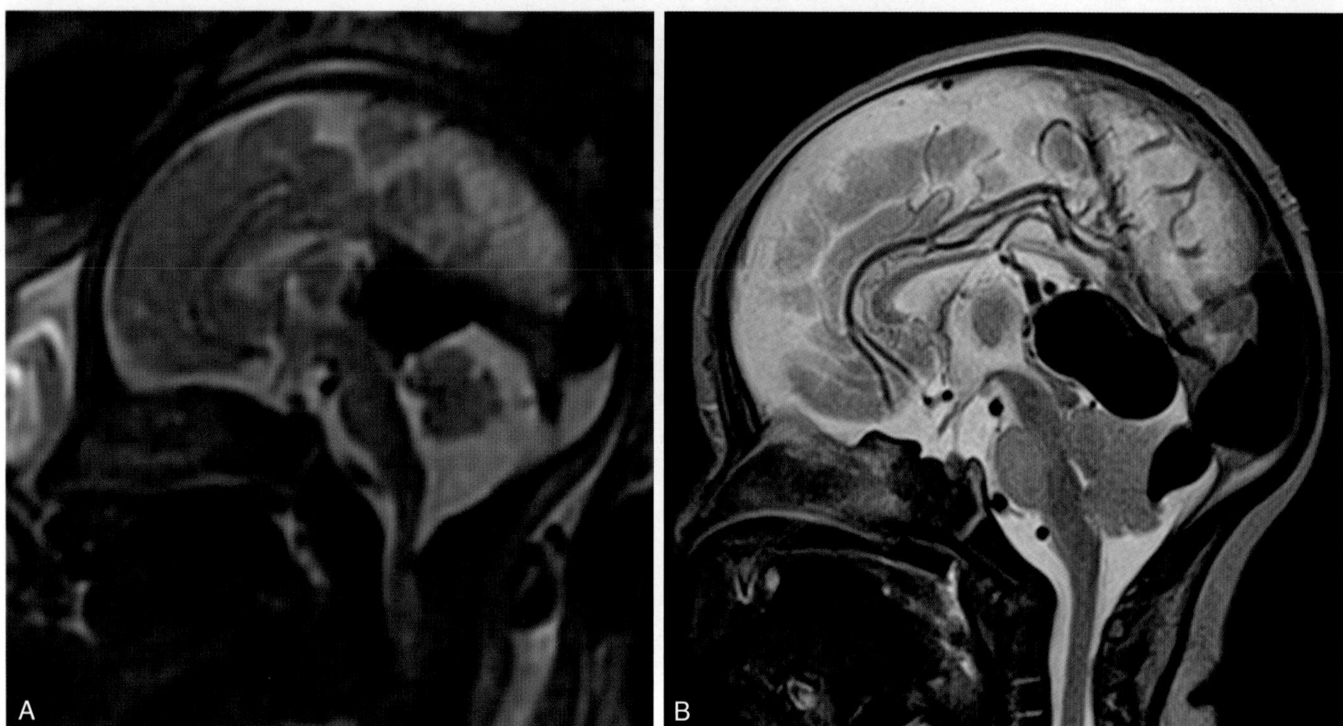

Fig. 2.89 Aqueductal Stenosis. (A) Sagittal T2W fetal MRI and (B) postnatal T2W MRI in a child with vein of Galen aneurysmal malformation. On both imaging studies a high-grade widening of the vein of Galan, straight sinus and torcular Herophili are noted fed by dilated branches of the anterior and posterior circulation. Compression of the tectal plate and Sylvian aqueduct by the aneurysmal dilated vein of Galen.

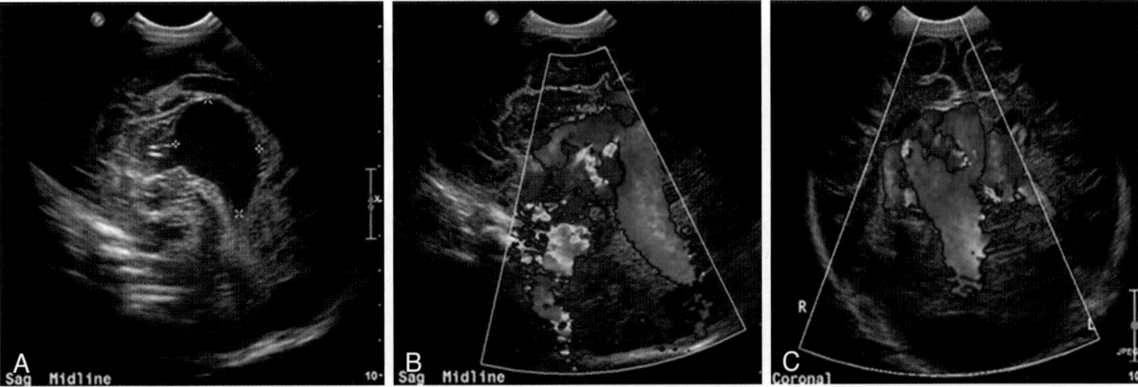

Fig. 2.90 Aqueductal Stenosis. (A to C) Sagittal ultrasound including sagittal and coronal color-coded Doppler sonography of the brain in a child with a vein of Galen aneurysmal malformation. The vein of Galen appears hypoechogenic with turbulent flow characterized by mixture of red and blue encoded flow within the vein of Galen, as well as along the drainage over the straight sinus. Massively dilated arterial feeders originating from the anterior and posterior circulation.

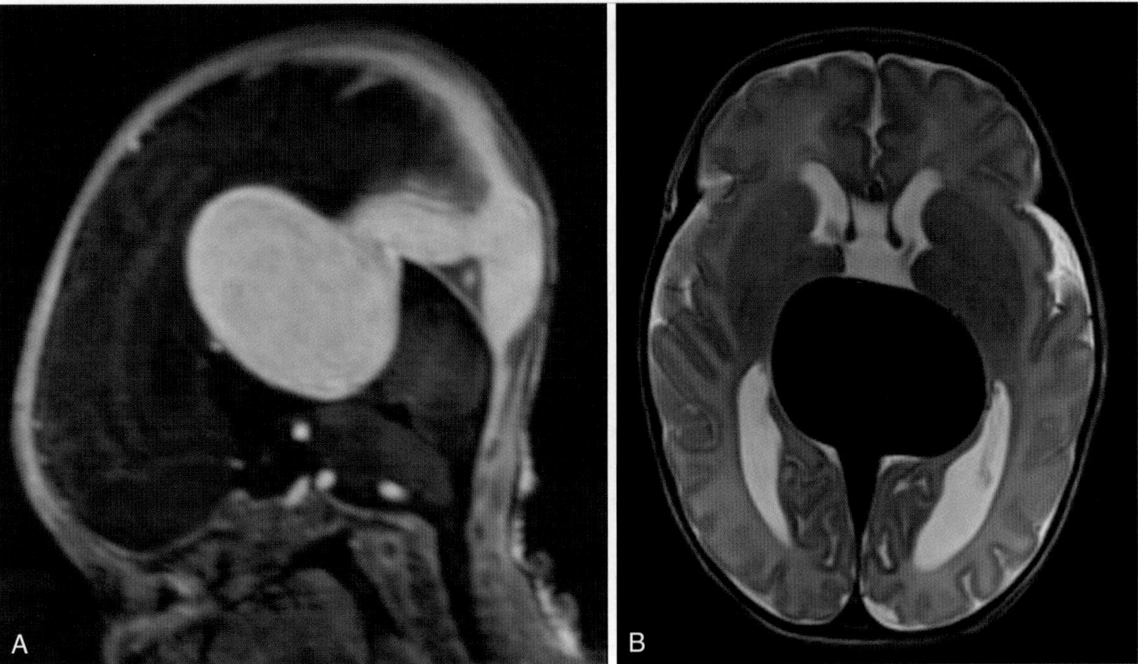

Fig. 2.91 Aqueductal Stenosis. (A) Sagittal T1W+C and (B) axial T2W MRI in a child with high-grade dilatation of the vein of Galen as well as moderate widening of the straight sinus and torcular Herophili. Significant mass effect is exerted on the Sylvian aqueduct and posterior third ventricle with resultant supratentorial ventriculomegaly.

Key Points

- Extrinsic aqueductal stenosis may be secondary to focal mass lesions in close proximity to the Sylvian aqueduct, compressing the lumen.
- Tectal gliomas are low-grade lesions that appear T2 hyperintense, have little to no contrast enhancement, and may circumvent the narrowed Sylvian aqueduct.
- Tectal gliomas may be subtle and occasionally difficult to identify if a severe supratentorial ventriculomegaly compresses and displaces the mesencephalon and brainstem. The lesion may become more apparent after adequate decompression of the supratentorial system, either by ventriculoperitoneal shunting or third ventriculostomy.
- Vein of Galen aneurysmal malformations (VGAMs) are congenital midline vascular malformations in which the arterialized, dilated vein of Galen exerts a mass effect on the tectal plate and Sylvian aqueduct.
- VGAMs are easily identified on transfontanellar ultrasound by their hypoechogenic aneurysmal sac and matching turbulent flow on color-coded Doppler sonography.
- VGAMs are also easily identified by the flow-related signal void on most MRI sequences as well as on the various MR-angiography sequences.
- In VGAMs the supratentorial ventriculomegaly is also secondary to the arteriovenous shunting, in which the arterialization of the venous system impairs the resorption of cerebrospinal fluid in the venous system.

REFERENCE

1. Huisman TA, Poretti A. Pediatric Neurovascular Imaging (CT, MRI, Ultrasound). In: Pediatric Vascular Neurosurgery: A Comprehensive Guide to Pediatric Neurosurgical Disorders and its management. Ed: Gavin W. Britz. Springer Verlag.

POSTERIOR FOSSA MALFORMATIONS

Understanding the normal development of the posterior fossa helps to understand malformations that occur in the posterior fossa, including brainstem malformations, Dandy-Walker malformations, and Chiari malformations.

As previously discussed in Chapter 1, Normal Development, the neural tube forms three vesicles: the prosencephalon (forebrain), mesencephalon (midbrain), and rhombenecephalon (hindbrain). The rhombencephalon divides into two secondary vesicles, known as the metencephalon and myelencephalon. The cavity in the hindbrain will become the fourth ventricle. The pons develops from thickening of the floors and lateral walls of the metencephalon while thickening of the floor and lateral walls of the myelencephalon forms the medulla. Complex biochemical signaling results in the normal patterning of the brainstem.

Because of the pontine flexure, the fourth ventricle becomes shorter craniocaudally and wider transversely. The roof of the fourth ventricle has an anterior membranous area and a posterior membranous area, which are separated by the choroidal fold/choroid plexus. Neuroblastic proliferation causes the anterior membranous area to thicken and form two lateral plates called rhombic lips, which approach each other, fuse in the midline, and will constitute the cerebellum. The growth of the rhombic lips causes the anterior membranous area to regress. Growth and backward extension of the cerebellum pushes the choroid plexus inferiorly; the posterior membranous area decreases in size and causes a caudal protrusion of the fourth ventricle, known as the Blake pouch, at 7 weeks. The Blake pouch perforates between the ninth and tenth week to form the foramen of Magendie.

Malformations of the posterior fossa occur due to disruption of the normal development of these structures. A general approach to posterior fossa malformations includes grouping into the following:

1. Small posterior fossa: Chiari malformations
2. Posterior fossa cystic malformation: Dandy-Walker malformation, Blake pouch cyst, vermian hypoplasia, arachnoid cyst, and mega cisterna magna
3. Brainstem and cerebellar malformation: Pontocerebellar hypoplasia, alpha-dystroglycanopathies, tubulinopathies, Joubert syndrome
4. Predominant brainstem malformation: Pontine tegmental cap dysplasia, horizontal gaze palsy with progressive scoliosis, diencephalic-mesencephalic junction dysplasia, brainstem disconnection
5. Predominant cerebellar malformation: Rhombencephalosynapsis, cerebellar dysplasia, cerebellar tubers, cerebellar cysts, and ectopic cerebellar tissue

This general approach will be used to organize the posterior malformations discussed in this section.

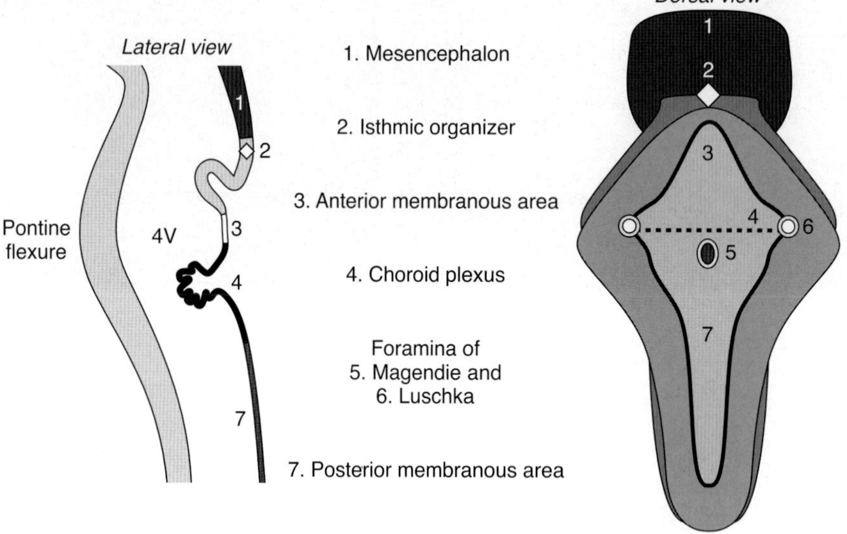

Posterior Fossa Embryology. Normal landmarks of the developing fourth ventricular roof. (From Volpe JJ. *Volpe's Neurology of the Newborn*. 6th ed. Elsevier; 2018.)

CHIARI I MALFORMATION

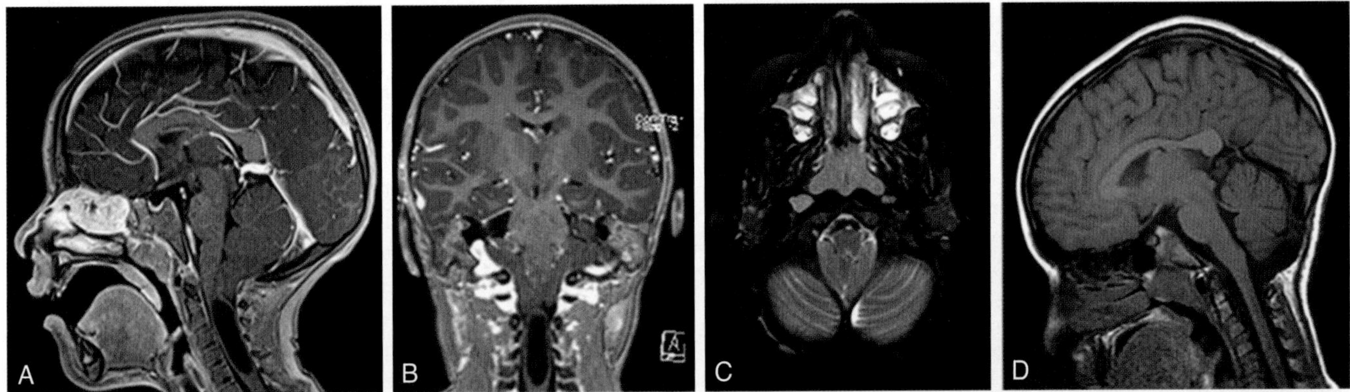

Fig. 2.92 Chiari I Malformation. (A and B) Sagittal and coronal T1W+C and (C) axial T2W MR of a child with Chiari I malformation show a low positioning of the cerebellar tonsils below the level of the foramen magnum dorsally to the upper cervical spinal cord, slightly more prominent on the right compared to the left. On axial imaging the lower brainstem and upper cervical spinal cord are embraced by the cerebellar tonsils. Furthermore, significant dilatation of the central canal of the upper cervical spinal cord. (D) On follow-up sagittal T1W MR complete resolution of the spinal cord central canal widening after posterior fossa decompression.

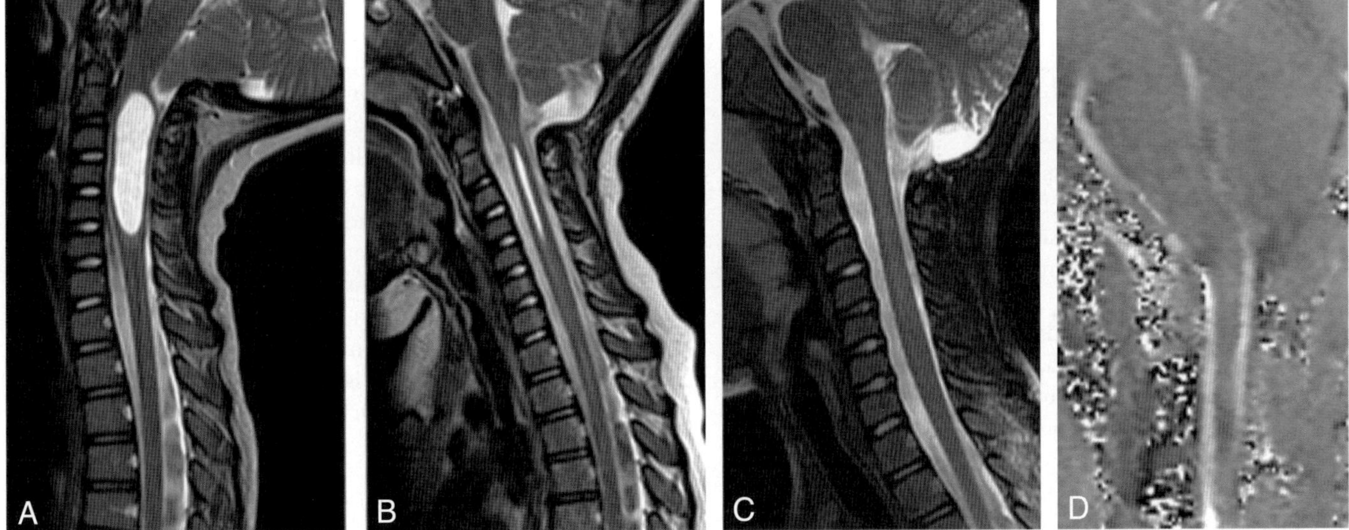

Fig. 2.93 Chiari I Malformation. (A to C) Serial sagittal T2W MRI of the craniocervical junction and matching CSF flow study in a child with Chiari I malformation and dilatation of the upper cervical spinal cord central canal. After posterior fossa decompression, complete resolution of the central canal widening and reconstituted CSF flow along the anterior and posterior contour of the lower brainstem and upper cervical spinal cord as evidenced on the (D) CSF flow study.

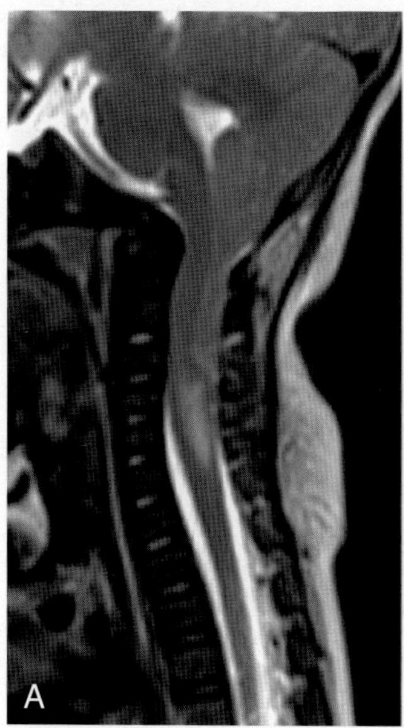

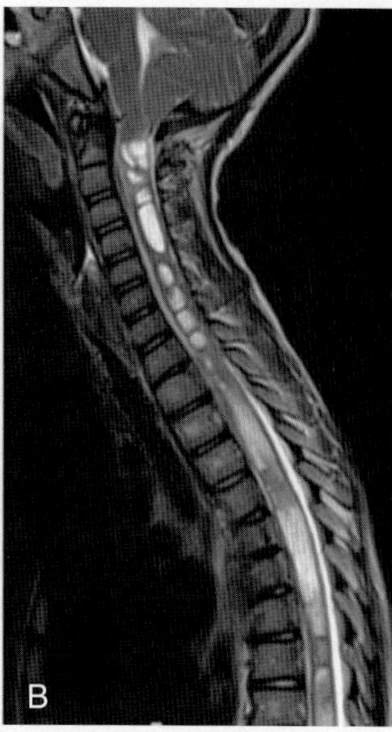

Fig. 2.94 Chiari I Malformation. (A and B) Sagittal T2W MRI of two children with Chiari I malformation. In the first child intramedullary venous stasis and edema is noted in the upper cervical spinal cord. In the second child nearly holocordal partially septated widening of the central canal is noted.

Key Points

Background

- Chiari I malformation, first described in 1891 by the Austrian pathologist Hans Chiari, is primarily characterized by a low positioning of the cerebellar tonsils, extending more than 5 mm below the level of the foramen magnum or McRae line.
- Etiology presumed to be due to occipital bone and/or skull base bone hypoplasia, leading to reduced posterior fossa volume, leading to tonsillar herniation. Most Chiari I malformations are not present at birth but develop in childhood or teenage years.
- Symptoms vary significantly. Chiari I malformations may be incidentally detected on imaging and asymptomatic in 14% to 56% of patients or be linked to a vast array of symptoms, including headache, neck pain, numbness, ataxia, and weakness, which are believed to be secondary to hindbrain compression.
- The degree of tonsillar herniation has an imperfect correlation with clinical symptoms.
- Treatment may be conservative or posterior fossa decompression with duraplasty and occipital bone resection; the posterior arch of the atlas can also be resected to increase space. Symptoms and syringohydromyelia typically improve significantly after decompression.

Imaging

- The cerebellar tonsils are peg-like, crowd the foramen magnum, and extend 6 mm or more below McRae line (the line formed from the basion to the opisthion) in children <10 years of age and 5 mm or more in children >10 years of age. Tonsillar herniation between 3 and 5 mm is termed *tonsillar ectopia*.
- Several studies have identified associations of Chiari I malformations with alterations in clivus length, occipital bone length, retroflexion of the odontoid, and narrow clival-spinal angle. Likely a complex combination of altered size of bones of the skull base, posterior fossa, and upper cervical spine leads to the small posterior fossa.
- Impairment or obstruction of the rhythmic bidirectional cerebrospinal fluid flow at the craniocervical junction may result in a syringohydromyelia in 30% to 85% of patients, typically involving the cervical more than thoracic spinal cord.
- Hydrocephalus can occur in 6% to 25% of patients due to CSF flow obstruction at the foramen magnum.
- Cerebrospinal fluid flow imaging allows study of the degree of impaired flow both qualitatively and quantitatively. Patients with Chiari I malformation demonstrate increased peak systolic and diastolic CSF velocity, and simultaneous bidirectional CSF flow and alterations in CSF flow correlate with syrinx size and outcome after surgery.
- Additional findings can include kinking of the cervicomedullary junction, and skull base malformations of platybasia and basilar invagination. Identification of skull base malformations is important to identify patients who may require posterior fusion.

REFERENCES

1. Bosemani T, Orman G, Boltshauser E, Tekes A, Huisman TA, Poretti A. Congenital abnormalities of the posterior fossa. *Radiographics*. 2015;35(1):200–220.
2. Huisman TA, Poretti A. Chapter 7. Disorders of brain development. In: Magnetic Resonance Imaging of the Brain and Spine, 5th ed. Edited by Scott Atlas, MD. Wolters Kluwer, Lippincott Williams & Wilkins.
3. Poretti A, Boltshauser E, Huisman TA. Chiari malformations and syringohydromyelia in children. *Semin Ultrasound CT MR*. 2016;37:129–142.

SECONDARY CHIARI I MALFORMATION

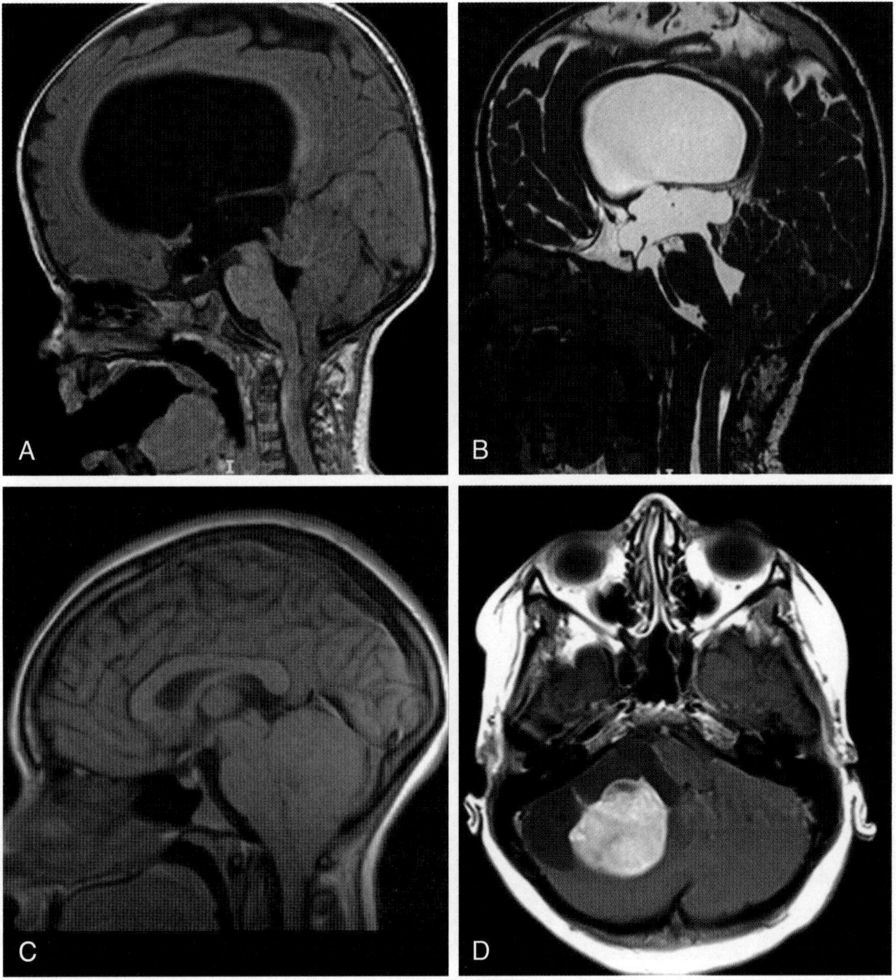

Fig. 2.95 Secondary Chiari Malformation. (A and B) Sagittal T1W and T2W MRI of a child with downward herniation of the cerebellar tonsils into the upper cervical spinal canal secondary to a high-grade supratentorial hydrocephalus. (C and D) Sagittal T1W and axial T1W+C MRI in a child with a large posterior fossa pilocytic astrocytoma. Moderate global ventriculomegaly and downward herniation of the cerebellar tonsils into the upper cervical spinal canal.

Key Points

- A downward displacement of the cerebellar tonsils, mimicking a true Chiari I malformation may be secondary to mass-occupying lesions within the posterior fossa, supra- or infratentorial hydrocephalus, CSF hypotension, and idiopathic intracranial hypertension.
- The term "secondary" Chiari I malformation should be avoided because it may result in unnecessary confusion.
- If low lying cerebellar tonsils are noted on a cervical spine study, the brain should be examined to differentiate between a Chiari I malformation and an intracranial pathology that may be causative for the tonsillar descent.
- The tonsillar descent is typically reversible when the intracranial pathology has been resolved.

REFERENCES

1. Bosemani T, Orman G, Boltshauser E, Tekes A, Huisman TA, Poretti A. Congenital abnormalities of the posterior fossa. *Radiographics*. 2015;35(1):200–220.
2. Huisman TA, Poretti A. Chapter 7. Disorders of brain development. In: Magnetic Resonance Imaging of the Brain and Spine, 5th ed. Edited by Scott Atlas, MD. Wolters Kluwer, Lippincott Williams & Wilkins.
3. Poretti A, Boltshauser E, Huisman TA. Chiari malformations and syringohydromyelia in children. *Semin Ultrasound CT MR*. 2016;37:129–142.

CHIARI II MALFORMATION

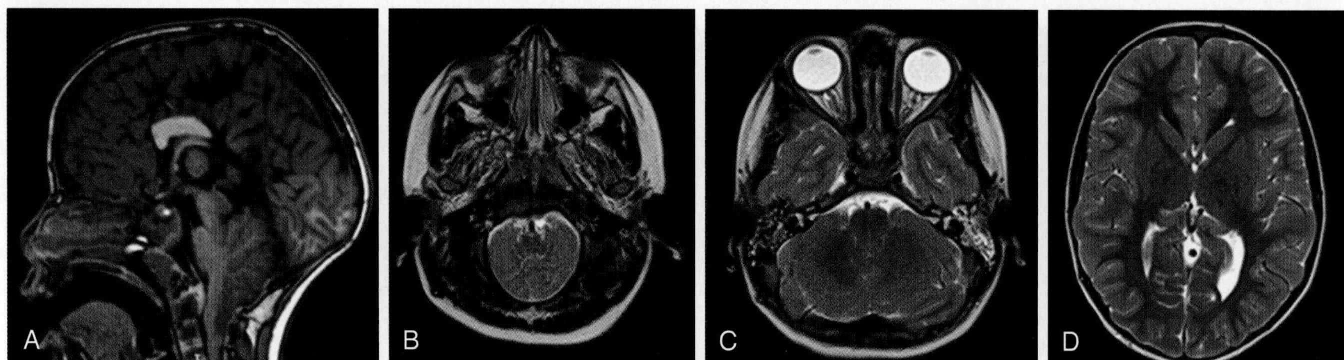

Fig. 2.96 Chiari II Malformation. (A) Sagittal T1W and (B to D) axial T2W MRI in a child with Chiari II malformation characterized by a small posterior fossa, crowding of the foramen magnum with cerebellar tonsils herniating into the upper cervical spinal canal, crowding of the brainstem by the cerebellar hemispheres, towering cerebellum, beak-like configuration of the tectal plate, prominent interthalamic adhesion, and corpus callosum hypogenesis.

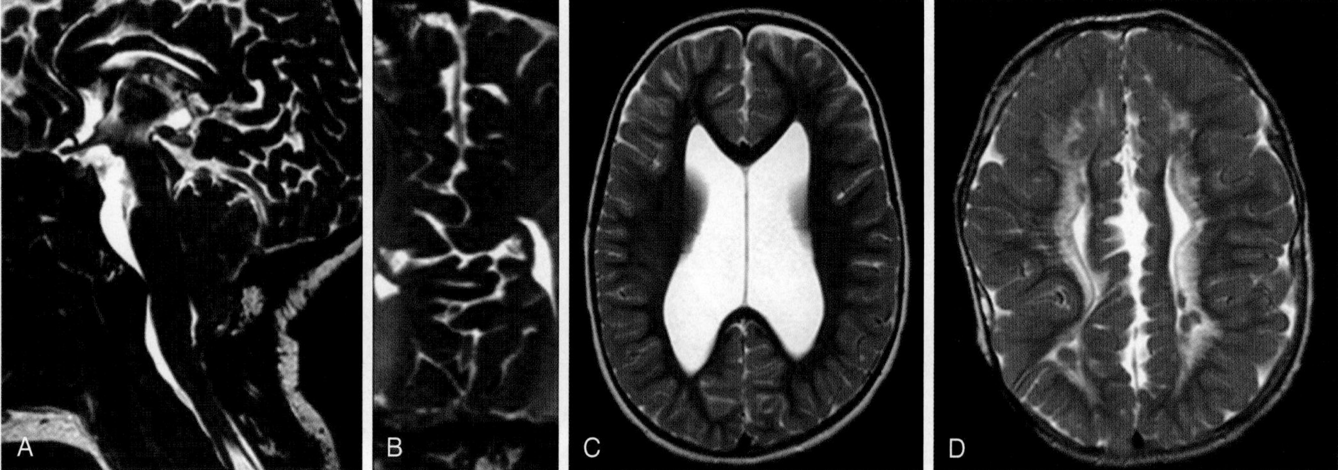

Fig. 2.97 Chiari II Malformation. (A to D) Sagittal, small field of view coronal and axial T2W MRI in a child with Chiari II malformation demonstrate small posterior fossa with herniation of cerebellar tissue and tonsils into the upper cervical spinal canal, crowded foramen magnum, dilatation of the central canal within the cervical spinal cord, beak-like configuration of the tectal plate, malformation of the corpus callosum, hypoplastic falx with resultant interdigitation of the mesial hemispheric gyri, moderate supratentorial hydrocephalus. Postventriculoperitoneal shunting collapse of the lateral ventricles with more apparent depiction of the subependymal heterotopias bilaterally and stenogyria of the cerebral cortex.

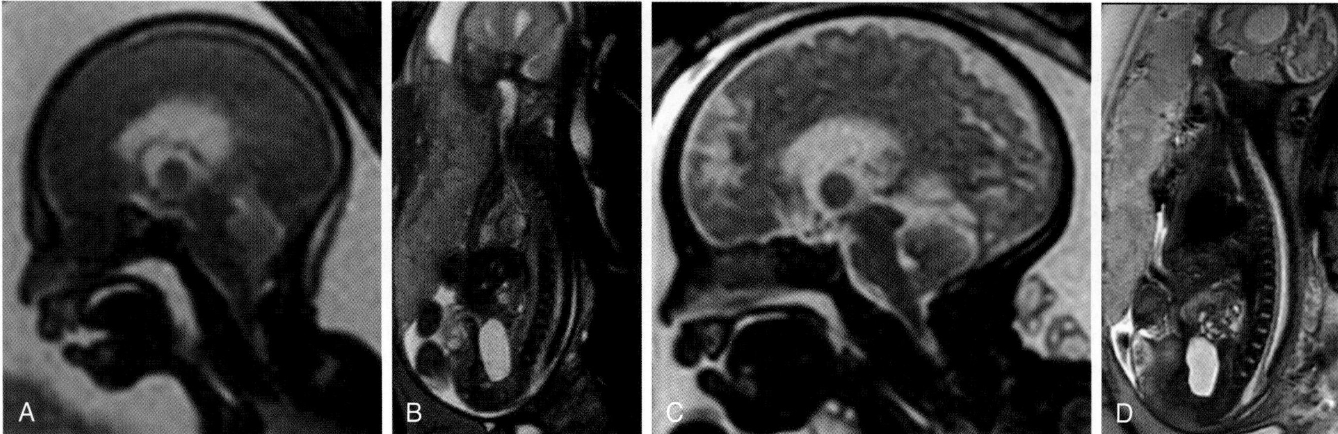

Fig. 2.98 Chiari II Malformation. (A and B) T2W fetal MR images demonstrate a lumbosacral myelomeningocele with Chiari II malformation with hindbrain herniation, small posterior fossa, and ventriculomegaly. (C and D) Post in utero repair T2W fetal MR images demonstrate resolution of hindbrain herniation, small posterior fossa, ventriculomegaly, and closure of the myelomeningocele defect.

Key Points

Background

- An Arnold-Chiari or Chiari II malformation can be described as a "congenital too small posterior fossa." Most anatomic findings seen in Chiari II are secondary to a disproportion between the size of the posterior fossa and the volume of its contents, brainstem, and cerebellum.
- Chiari II malformations are typically associated or secondary to an open neural tube defect. The "unified theory" suggests that the ongoing leakage of cerebrospinal fluid out of the open neural tube prevents adequate expansion of the posterior fossa during intrauterine development.
- In Chiari II malformations the neural tube defect is most frequently located at the lumbosacral level; however, open defects may be present at any level along the neuroaxis.
- Intrauterine fetoscopic repair of the neural tube defect early during pregnancy may reverse the degree of the associated Chiari II malformation and ventriculomegaly but are associated with increased risk of epidermoid cyst formation.
- In select cases the improved lower extremity functionality and improved ventriculomegaly/macrocephaly will also improve intrauterine fetal position from a breech presentation to a cephalic presentation.

Imaging

- In Chiari II malformation variable combinations and degrees of severity of findings can be seen. Common findings include the following:
  - Small posterior fossa with associated crowding of the posterior fossa, effacement of the basal cisterns, compressed small fourth ventricle, anterior displacement, and possible compression of the brainstem against the clivus and foramen magnum
  - Downward herniation of the cerebellar tonsils into the upper cervical canal and secondary dorsal kinking of the upper cervical spinal cord due to the downward displacement of the craniocervical junction
  - Low insertion of the tentorium close to the foramen magnum
  - Upward herniation of the superior vermis and cerebellum through the tentorial incisura, also known as towering cerebellum
  - Deformity of the quadrigeminal plate or tectal beaking
  - Supratentorial ventriculomegaly/hydrocephalus
  - Prominent interthalamic adhesion/ massa intermedia
  - Fenestration of the falx and associated interdigitation of the gyri across the midline
  - Malformations of the corpus callosum, typically dysgenesis of the splenium
  - Migrational abnormalities including heterotopias, and internal derangement of major fiber tracts in the brainstem
  - In children with a shunted previously significant ventriculomegaly, the occipital lobes may demonstrate stenogyria due to the collapse of the occipital cortex over the decompressed occipital horns of the lateral ventricle. This is not to be confused with a true cortical dysplasia such as polymicrogyria.
- Similar to Chiari I malformation, the altered CSF flow may be complicated by a focal or holocordal hydromyelia or syringomyelia.
- Color-coded fractional anisotropy maps may confirm an aberrant pyramidal decussation and anomalous or deficient transverse pontine fibers.
- Chiari II malformations should be excluded on fetal MRI if an open neural tube defect is suspected or diagnosed by prenatal ultrasound or MRI and vice versa.

REFERENCES

1. Bosemani T, Orman G, Boltshauser E, Tekes A, Huisman TA, Poretti A. Congenital abnormalities of the posterior fossa. *Radiographics*. 2015;35(1):200–220.
2. Huisman TA, Poretti A. Chapter 7. Disorders of brain development. In: Magnetic Resonance Imaging of the Brain and Spine, 5th ed. Edited by Scott Atlas, MD. Wolters Kluwer, Lippincott Williams & Wilkins.
3. Poretti A, Boltshauser E, Huisman TA. Chiari malformations and syringohydromyelia in children. *Semin Ultrasound CT MR*. 2016;37:129–142.

CHIARI III MALFORMATION

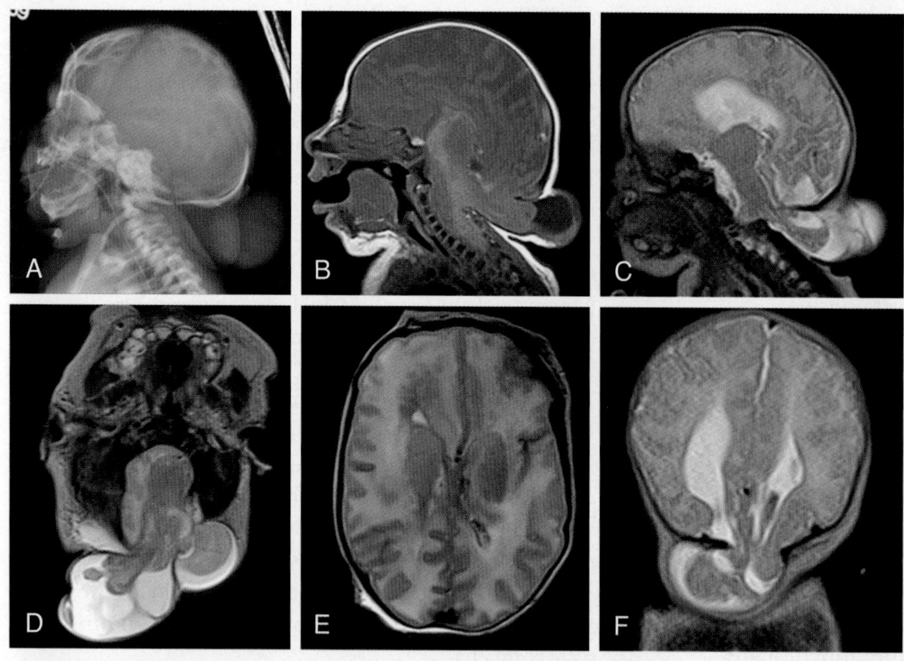

Fig. 2.99 Chiari III Malformation. (A) Lateral skull radiography, matching (B) sagittal T1W and (C to E) axial and coronal T2W fetal MRI in a child with Chiari III malformation. The lateral skull radiography shows a lobulated soft tissue mass lesion in the suboccipital region, mild microcephaly, as well as a copper-beaten appearance of the skull, indicating hydrocephalus. On the MRI, herniation of the occipital lobes as well as cerebellar hemispheres are noted through a large posterior defect at the craniocervical junction. The occipital horns of the lateral ventricles extend into the herniated brain tissue; furthermore heterotopic T2 hypointense gray matter is noted within both frontal lobes.

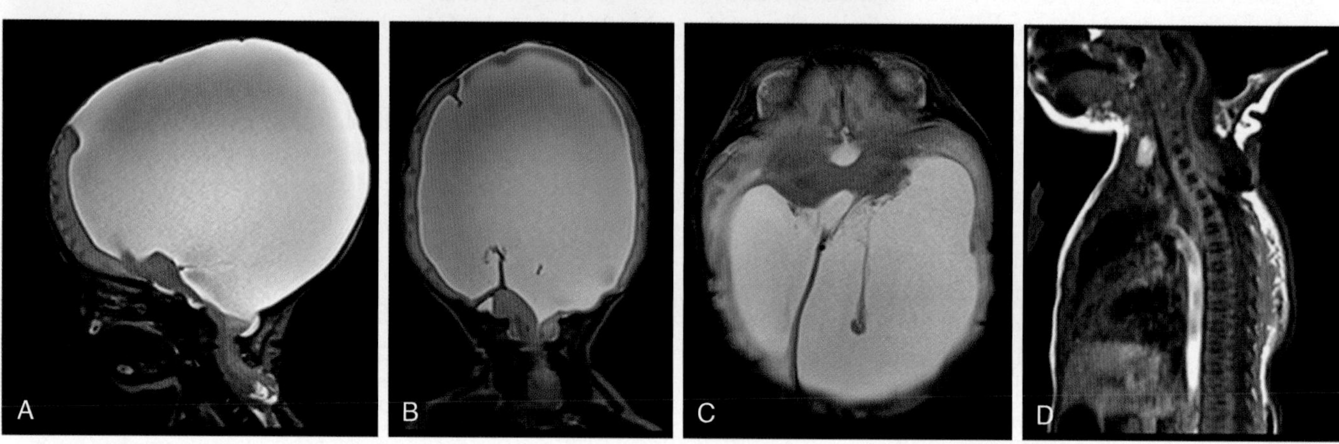

Fig. 2.100 Chiari III Malformation. (A to C) Sagittal, coronal, and axial T2W MRI of the brain, including (D) sagittal T1W MRI of the cervical spinal cord, in a child with Chiari III malformation show herniation of cerebellar tissue and tonsils through a posterior defect within the upper posterior spinal canal, extremely small posterior fossa, associated high-grade supratentorial ventriculomegaly, and midline fusion of both thalami.

Key Points

- Chiari III malformations are extremely rare and linked to a high morbidity and mortality.
- The hallmark imaging findings constitute a small posterior fossa and a low occipital and/or high cervical encephalocele with cerebellar tissue herniation. The brainstem and fourth ventricle may also be displaced.
- Additional infra- and supratentorial malformations may be observed, including migrational abnormalities, corpus callosum anomalies, and hydrocephalus.
- Associated posterior arch anomalies of the upper cervical column and hydromyelia may be present.
- The internal nuclei and wiring architecture of the brainstem has been reported to be anomalous.
- Correct nomenclature and classification remains challenging; it currently is debated if a Chiari III malformation is better classified as a high cervical myelocystocele.

REFERENCES

1. Bosemani T, Orman G, Boltshauser E, Tekes A, Huisman TA, Poretti A. Congenital abnormalities of the posterior fossa. *Radiographics*. 2015;35(1):200–220.
2. Huisman TA, Poretti A. Chapter 7. Disorders of brain development. In: Magnetic Resonance Imaging of the Brain and Spine, 5th ed. Edited by Scott Atlas, MD. Wolters Kluwer, Lippincott Williams & Wilkins.
3. Poretti A, Boltshauser E, Huisman TA. Chiari malformations and syringohydromyelia in children. *Semin Ultrasound CT MR*. 2016;37:129–142.

CHIARI IV MALFORMATION

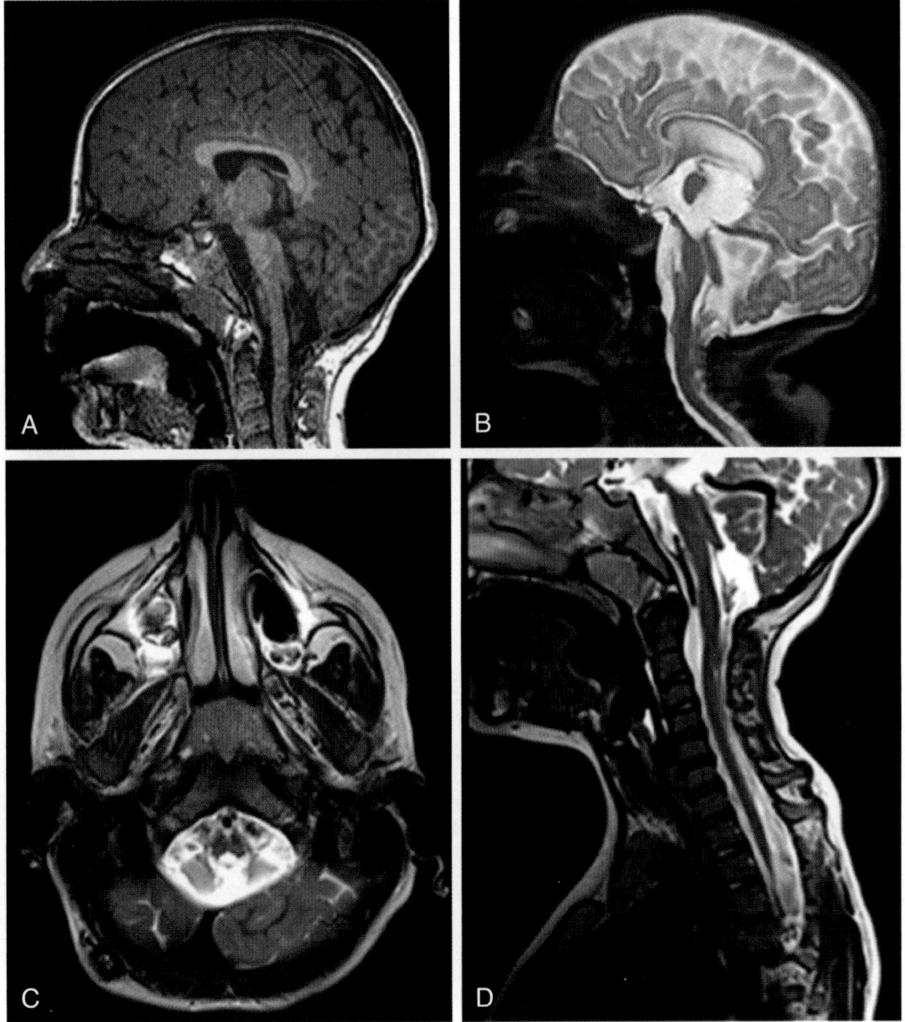

Fig. 2.101 Chiari IV Malformation. (A) Sagittal T1W, (B to D) sagittal and axial T2W MRI of the brain, and sagittal T2W MRI of the cervical spinal cord in a child with Chiari IV malformation. Findings include high-grade atrophy/hypoplasia of both cerebellar hemispheres in an extremely small posterior fossa, high-grade thinning, and volume loss of the brainstem with absent pontine belly, malformed tectal plate, and prominent interthalamic adhesion.

Key Points

- Chiari IV has been used to describe/classify cases of high-grade cerebellar hypoplasia in combination with a lack of the pontine belly located within an extremely small posterior fossa secondary to an open neural tube defect.
- The term *Chiari IV* is controversial; the author prefers to consider this an extreme variant of a Chiari II malformation. Occasionally this combination of findings is also coined "vanishing cerebellum" associated with an open neural tube defect.

REFERENCES

1. Bosemani T, Orman G, Boltshauser E, Tekes A, Huisman TA, Poretti A. Congenital abnormalities of the posterior fossa. *Radiographics*. 2015;35(1):200–220.
2. Huisman TA, Poretti A. Chapter 7. Disorders of brain development. In: Magnetic Resonance Imaging of the Brain and Spine, 5th ed. Edited by Scott Atlas, MD. Wolters Kluwer, Lippincott Williams & Wilkins.
3. Poretti A, Boltshauser E, Huisman TA. Chiari malformations and syringohydromyelia in children. *Semin Ultrasound CT MR*. 2016;37:129–142.

CYSTIC POSTERIOR FOSSA MALFORMATIONS

Cystic posterior fossa malformations include Dandy-Walker malformation, Blake pouch cyst, vermian hypoplasia, arachnoid cyst, and mega cisterna magna. Knowledge of embryology is helpful in understanding some of these malformations.

The roof of the fourth ventricle has an anterior membranous area (AMA) and a posterior membranous area (PMA), which are separated by the choroidal fold/choroid plexus (Fig. 2.102). Neuroblastic proliferation causes the AMA to thicken and form two lateral plates called rhombic lips, which approach each other and fuse in the midline and will constitute the cerebellum. The growth of the rhombic lips causes the AMA to regress. Growth and backward extension of the cerebellum pushes the choroid plexus inferiorly; the PMA decreases in size and causes a caudal protrusion of the fourth ventricle known as the Blake pouch at 7 weeks. The choroid plexus extends into the roof of the pouch caudal to the vermis. The Blake pouch perforates between the 9th and 10th week to form the foramen of Magendie. Delayed perforation (usually by 24–26 weeks) or persistence of the Blake pouch is an abnormality of the posterior membranous area and as such should have a normal vermis because the posterior membranous area does not contribute to vermis formation, and the choroid plexus should be located below the vermis (Fig. 2.103A). The Dandy-Walker malformation conversely is a malformation of the anterior membranous area (see Fig. 2.103B).

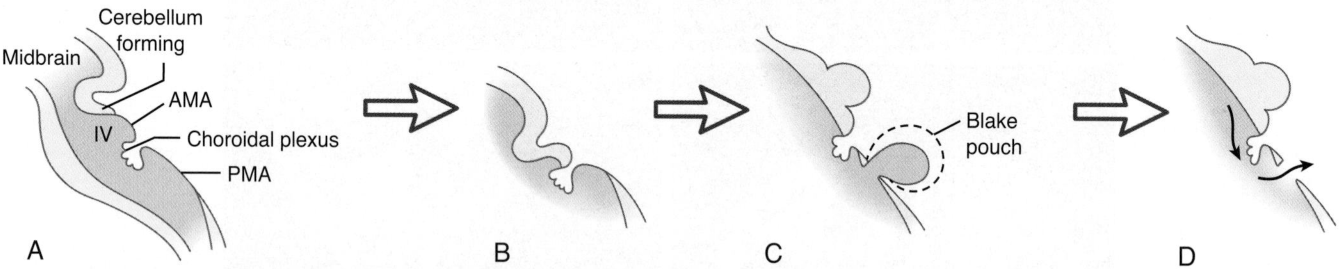

Fig. 2.102 Posterior Fossa Embryology. In the early stages of gestation, the roof of the fourth ventricle is divided by the rudimental choroid plexus into two portions: the anterior membranous area *(AMA)* and the posterior membranous area *(PMA)* (A). In normal individuals, the AMA is incorporated within the developing choroid glomus (B). Shortly after, the PMA shows a finger-like posterior expansion called Blake pouch (C), which later disappears, leaving a median opening named Blake metapore, which corresponds to the future foramen of Magendie (D). (Modified from Tortori-Donati P, Fondelli MP, Rossi A, Carini S. Cystic malformations of the posterior cranial fossa originating from a defect of the posterior membranous area. Mega cisterna magna and persisting Blake's pouch: two separate entities. *Childs Nerv Syst*. 1996 Jun;12[6]:303–308. PMID: 8816293. doi: 10.1007/BF00301017)

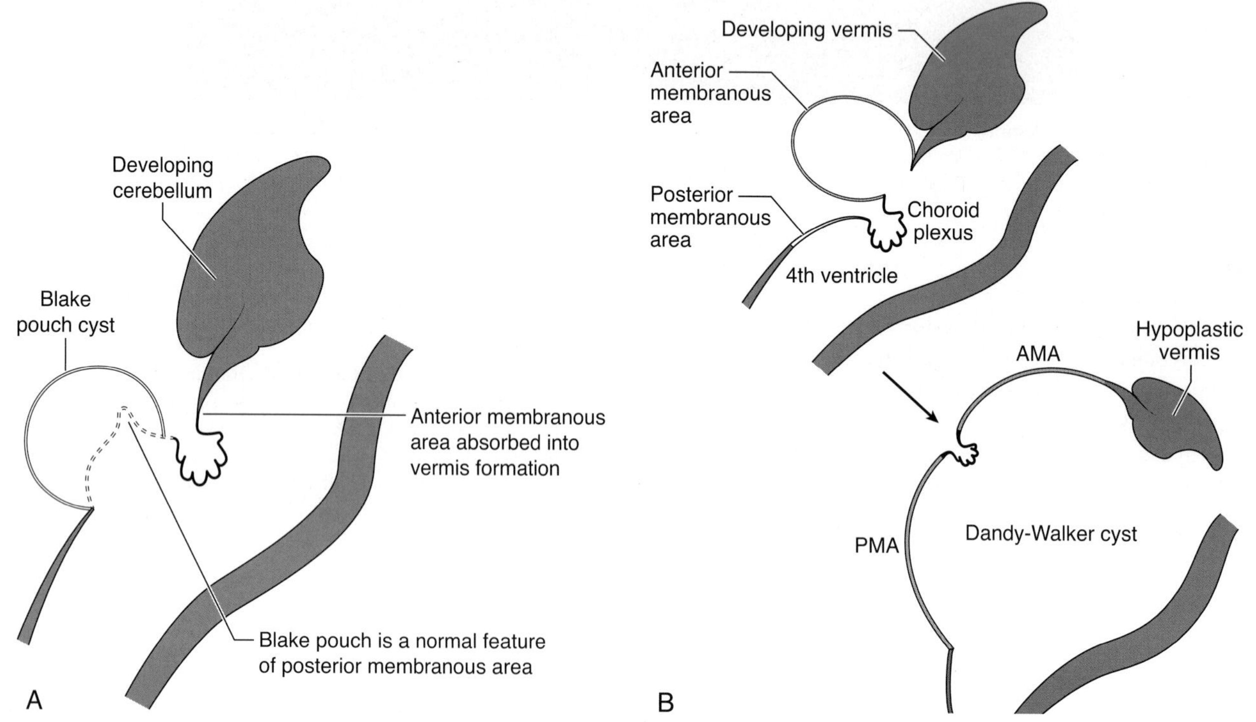

Fig. 2.103 Blake pouch and Dandy-Walker. Blake pouch (A) is a normal feature of posterior membranous area. Failure or delay of the foramen Magendie to open leads to cyst formation. (B) Development of the Dandy-Walker cyst. Diagram showing dorsal view of the rhombencephalon. (From Volpe JJ. *Volpe's Neurology of the Newborn*. 6th ed. Elsevier; 2018.)

POSTERIOR FOSSA CYSTS

■ Differential Diagnosis of Posterior Fossa Cysts

Malformation	Vermis	Fourth Ventricle	Posterior Fossa	Hydrocephalus	Occipital Scalloping
Dandy-Walker 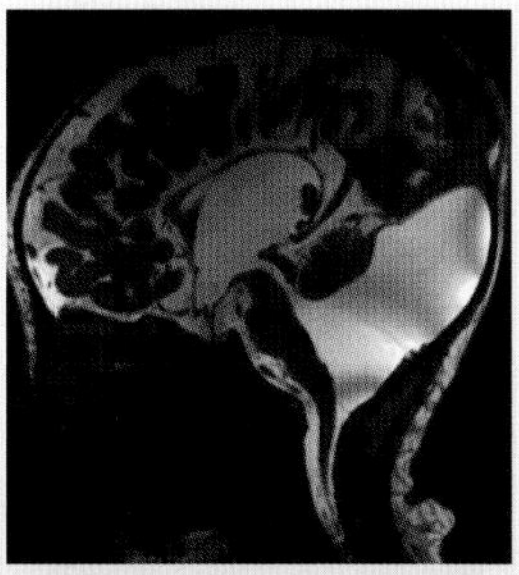	Hypoplastic, markedly rotated	Enlarged	Enlarged	Frequent	Yes
Vermian hypoplasia 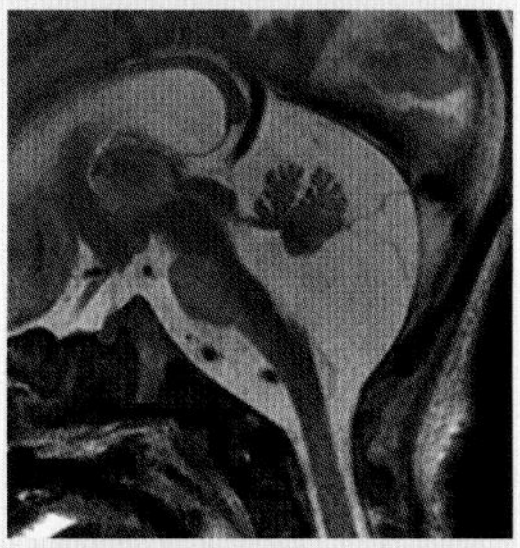	Inferior portion hypoplastic, and rotated to a lesser extent than Dandy-Walker	Enlarged	Normal or slightly enlarged	Usually absent	No
Blake pouch cyst 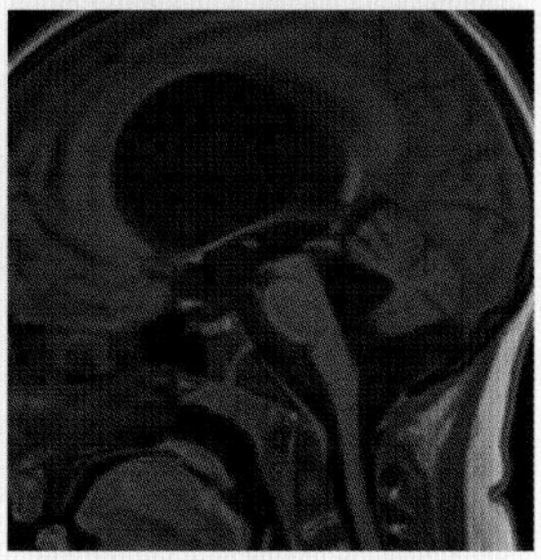	Normal, slightly upwardly rotated usually less than vermina hypoplasia	Often enlarged	Normal or slightly enlarged	Variable depending on whether the cyst perforates	Possible
Arachnoid cyst 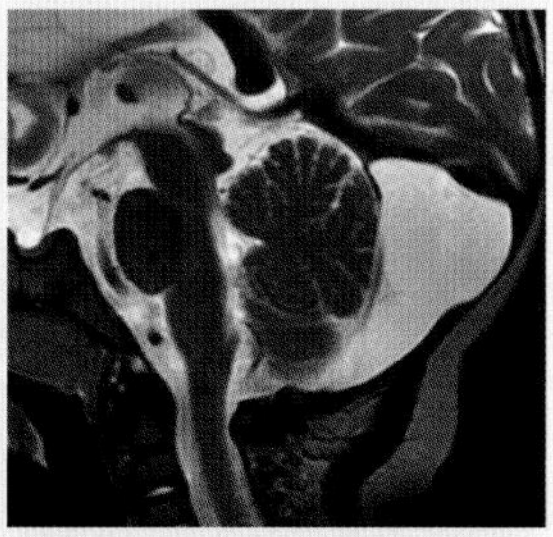	Normal, occasionally compressed, not rotated	Normal or reduced	Normal or slightly enlarged	Rare	Yes
Mega cisterna magna 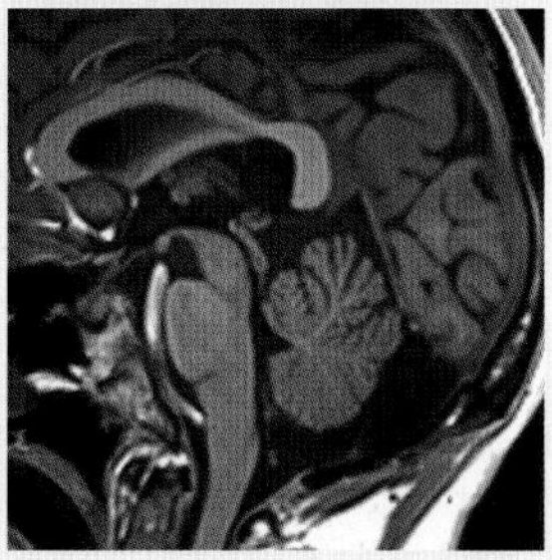	Normal and not rotated	Normal or slightly enlarged	Normal	Absent	No

DANDY-WALKER MALFORMATION

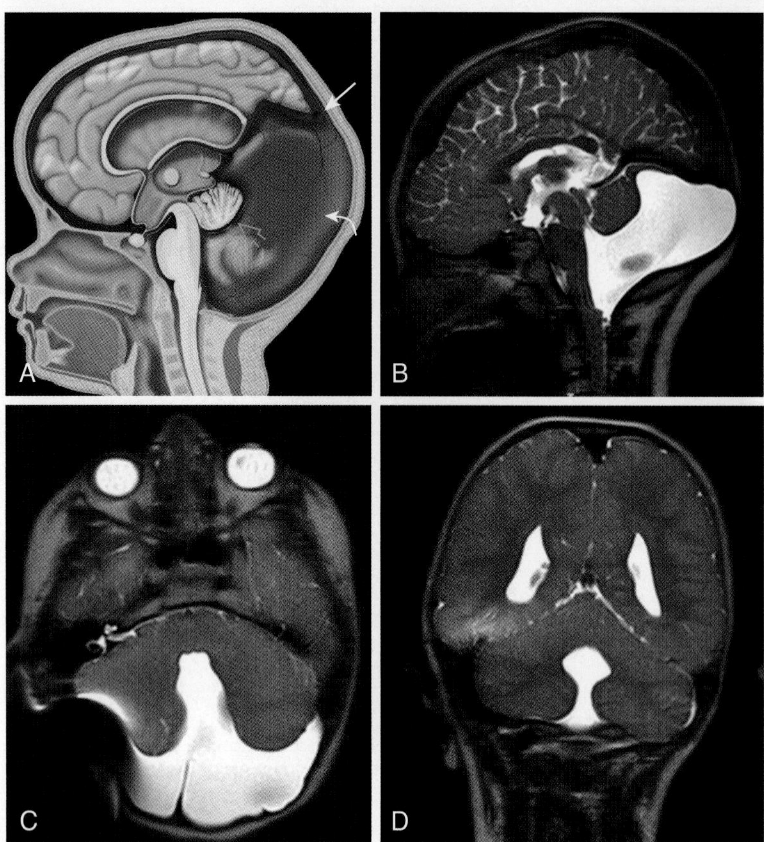

Fig. 2.104 Dandy-Walker Malformation. (A) Illustration of Dandy-Walker malformation with hypoplastic rotated vermis (*blue arrow*), enlarged posterior fossa (*curved arrow*), and elevated torcula (*straight arrow*). (B to D) Sagittal, axial, and coronal T2W fetal MRI in a child with a Dandy-Walker malformation with high-grade cystic dilatation of the fourth ventricle, expansion of the posterior fossa, elevation of the torcular Herophili, vermian hypoplasia, and supratentorial hydrocephalus. (A from StatDX. Copyright © 2022 Elsevier.)

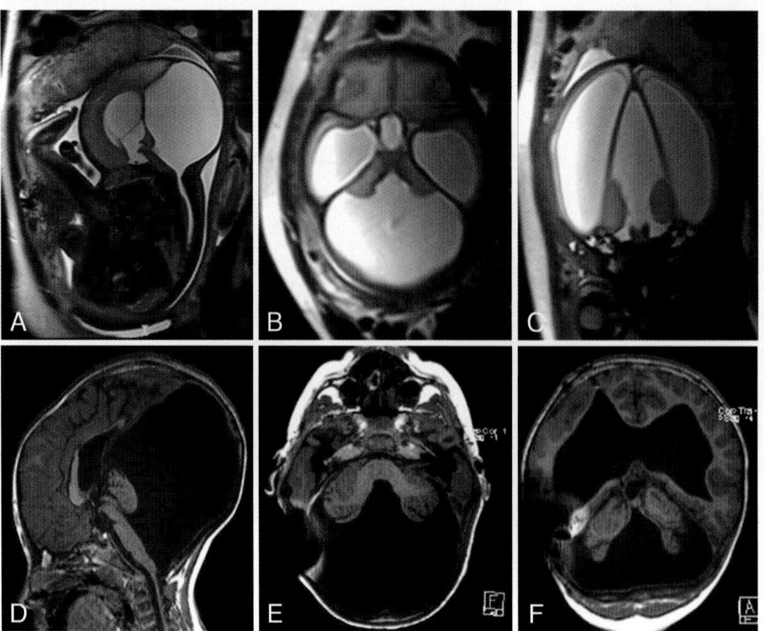

Fig. 2.105 Dandy-Walker Malformation. (A to C) Sagittal, axial, and coronal T2-weighted fetal MRI of a Dandy-Walker malformation with high-grade cystic dilatation of the fourth ventricle, expansion of the posterior fossa, elevation of the torcular Herophili, and supratentorial hydrocephalus. (D to F) Sagittal, axial, and coronal T1W postnatal MRI confirm the Dandy-Walker malformation with high-grade cystic dilatation and herniation of the fourth ventricle, high-grade enlargement of the posterior fossa, hypoplasia of the vermis with counterclockwise upward rotation. There is a small brainstem including hypoplastic pontine belly and residual high-grade supratentorial ventriculomegaly and thin posterior corpus callosum.

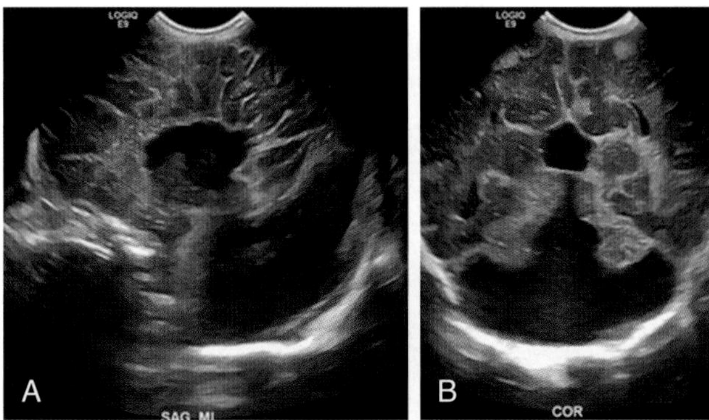

Fig. 2.106 **Dandy-Walker Malformation**. (A and B) Sagittal and coronal ultrasound of the brain in a child with Dandy-Walker malformation with hypoechogenic cystic dilatation of the fourth ventricle, lateral displacement of the cerebellar hemispheres, elevation of the tentorium cerebelli/torcular Herophili, and complete corpus callosum agenesis.

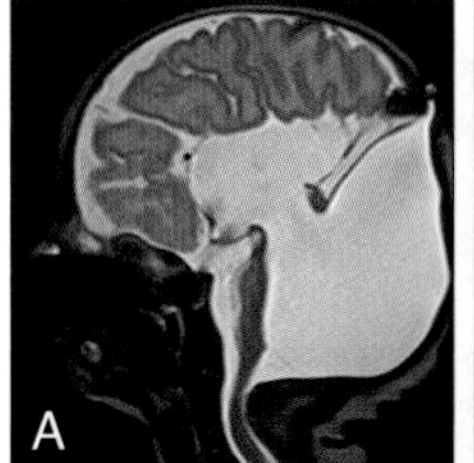

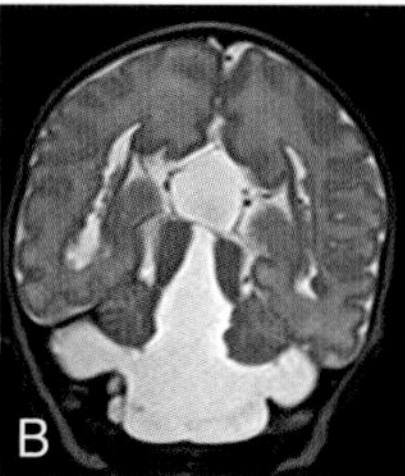

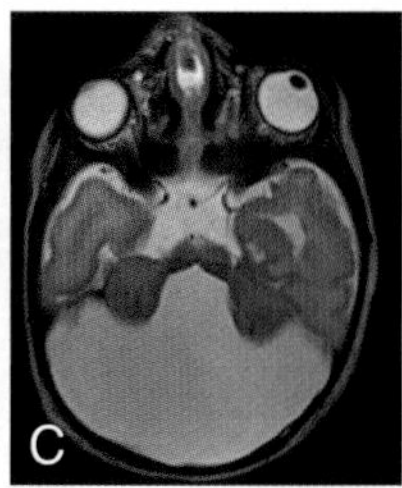

Fig. 2.107 **Dandy-Walker Malformation**. (A to C) Sagittal, coronal, and axial T2W MRI in a child with a Dandy-Walker malformation with high-grade cystic expansion of the fourth ventricle, high-grade hypoplasia of the vermis, lateral displacement of the small cerebellar hemispheres, wide Sylvian aqueduct, high-grade hypoplasia of the brainstem, significant elevation of the torcular Herophili, and supratentorial complete corpus callosum agenesis with extensive subependymal T2 hypointense heterotopias. On fetal MRI, a "tail sign" is often present which represents the hypoplastic posterior vermis.

Key Points

Background

- Complex malformation of the posterior fossa named after Drs. Walter Dandy and Arthur Walker, characterized by a hypoplasia of the inferior vermis with an enlarged, posterior extending fourth ventricle in combination with varying degrees of upward rotation of the developed parts of the vermis, lateral displacement of the cerebellar hemispheres, elevation of the torcular Herophili, and widening of the posterior fossa.
- A wide variability of Dandy-Walker malformations may be seen, resulting in a confusing, to be avoided, variation in nomenclature (e.g., Dandy-Walker variant, Dandy-Walker spectrum, Dandy-Walker syndrome).
- The exact etiology of this malformation is still not yet conclusively determined, but etiologies include a developmental defect in the anterior membranous area with insult to the rhombic lip which controls the posterior vermis leading to reduced proliferation or lack of expansion of progenitors. The posterior lobe of the cerebellum enlarges later than the anterior and central lobes. The posterior lobe does not significantly enlarge in gestational weeks 14-18, but afeter 18 weeks there is exponential growth of the posterior lobe. It is suspected in Dandy-Walker malformation that the rhombic lip is disrupted prior to 14 weeks while vermian hypoplasia occurs after 14 weeks of gestation.
- The incidence and severity of developmental delay is determined by the degree of ventriculomegaly and presence of additional findings, but the developmental outcome remains difficult to predict.
- Additional abnormalities outside of the central nervous system may include cardiac anomalies, ocular pathologies, and musculoskeletal findings.
- Dandy-Walker malformation is usually sporadic with low risk of recurrence but can be seen with some chromosomal anomalies in 16% and other gene mutations, including *ZIC1*, *ZIC4*, *FOXC1*, *FGF17*, *LAMC1*, and *NID1*.

Imaging

- The two primary imaging findings are the following:
  - Enlarged fluid filled posterior fossa with elevation of the torcular Herophili
  - Hypoplastic and counterclockwise rotation of the cerebellar vermis
- The degree of vermian hypoplasia extends from inferior to superior, meaning that middle and/or superior vermian hypoplasia is only seen when the inferior part is lacking.
- The tegmentovermian angle is usually >45 degrees.
- Lateral displacement of the cerebellar hemispheres.
- The brainstem is typically pushed against the clivus but in most cases is fully developed.
- On fetal MRI, a "tail sign" is often present which represents the hypoplastic posterior vermis.
- Additional anomalies are present in 50% to 60% of Dandy-Walker malformations. These include hydrocephalus, corpus callosum anomalies, migrational abnormalities (i.e. cortical dysplasia, polymicrogyria and heterotopia), and occipital encephalocele.

REFERENCES

1. Bosemani T, Orman G, Boltshauser E, Tekes A, Huisman TA, Poretti A. Congenital abnormalities of the posterior fossa. *Radiographics*. 2015;35(1):200–220.
2. Huisman TA, Poretti A. Chapter 7. Disorders of brain development. In: Magnetic Resonance Imaging of the Brain and Spine, 5th ed. Edited by Scott Atlas, MD. Wolters Kluwer, Lippincott Williams & Wilkins.
3. Miller E, Orman G, Huisman TAGM. Fetal MRI assessment of posterior fossa anomalies: A review. *J Neuroimaging*. 2021 Jul;31(4):620–640.

VERMIAN HYPOPLASIA

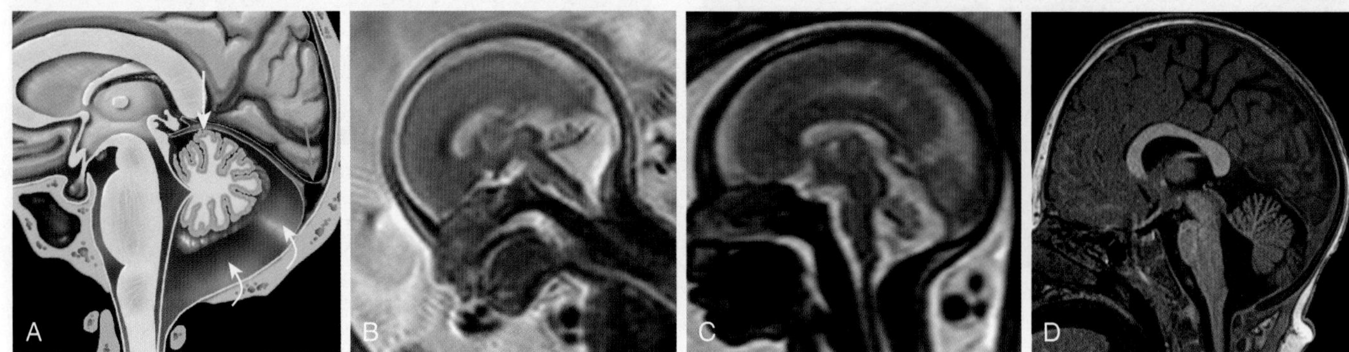

Fig. 2.108 Vermian Hypoplasia. (A) Illustration of vermian hypoplasia with small vermis (*straight arrow*) that leads to increased space in the posterior fossa (*curved arrow*) but with normal torcula position (*blue arrow*). (B) Sagittal T2W fetal MRI demonstrates hypoplasia and counterclockwise rotation of the vermis, a cerebellar tail sign, and mildly enlarged posterior fossa. (C) Sagittal T2W fetal MRI demonstrates mild hypoplasia and counterclockwise rotation of the vermis, and normal sized posterior fossa. (D) Sagittal T1W MRI demonstrates mild hypoplasia and counterclockwise rotation of the vermis, and a normal to mildly enlarged posterior fossa. (A from StatDX. Copyright © 2022 Elsevier.)

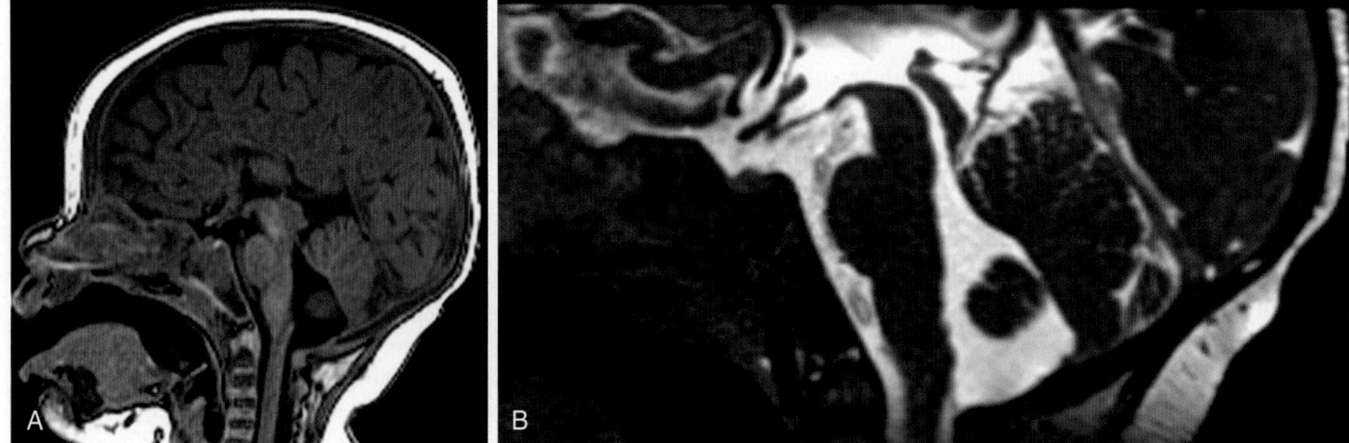

Fig. 2.109 Vermian Hypoplasia. (A) Sagittal T1W and (B) focused T2W MRI of the brain in a child with inferior vermian hypoplasia; the most inferior parts of the vermis are lacking. Posterior fossa size is normal.

Key Points

Background

- The terms *vermian hypoplasia* and *inferior vermian hypoplasia* have been increasing in usage to describe what was previously called Dandy-Walker variant.
- Etiology is uncertain but suspected to be due to disruption of the rhombic lip after 14 weeks gestation.
- Approximately 75% of cases have a favorable outcome.

Imaging

- The cerebellar vermis is small and counterclockwise rotated; the fourth ventricle is enlarged, but the posterior fossa size is normal or mildly enlarged. Torcular position is normal.
- Should be able to identify seven vermis lobules on fetal MRI by 22 weeks.
- Fastigial point is not distinct, and the tegmentovermian angle is typically 30–40 degrees.
- Postnatal imaging is recommended to confirm the diagnosis because fetal MRI can overdiagnose vermian hypoplasia. In addition, delayed rotation of the vermis can occur in which the counterclockwise-rotated vermis seen in the second trimester can return to a normal position in third trimester or postnatal imaging.
- Hydrocephalus is typically absent.
- Additional CNS anomalies occur in ~50%.

REFERENCE

1. Miller E, Orman G, Huisman TAGM. Fetal MRI assessment of posterior fossa anomalies: A review. *J Neuroimaging*. 2021 Jul;31(4):620–640.

BLAKE POUCH CYST

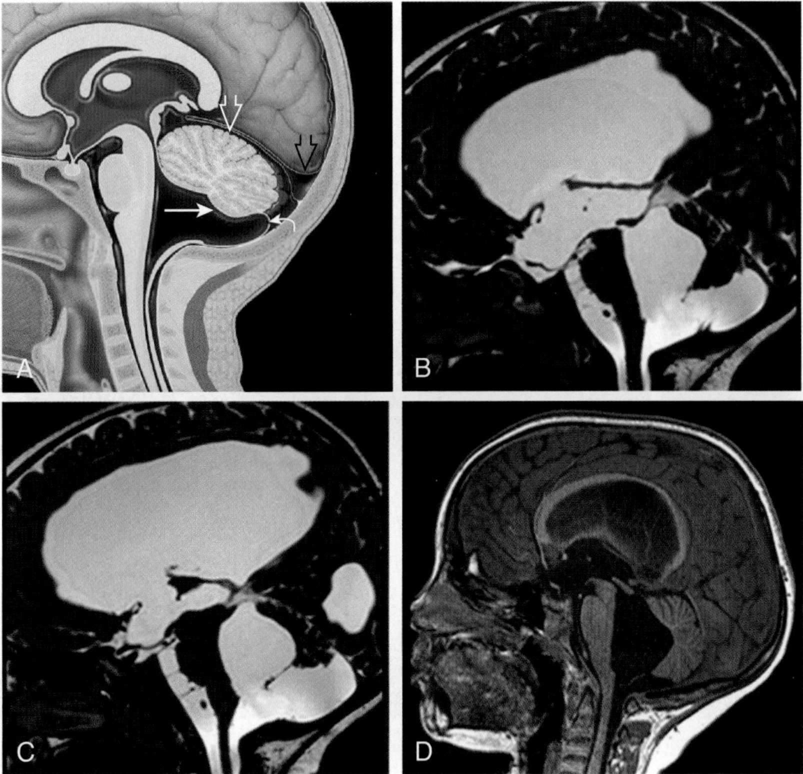

Fig. 2.110 Blake Pouch Cyst. (A) Illustration of a Blake pouch cyst. (*curved arrow*), rotation of the vermis (*wide white arrow*), posterior displaced choroid plexus (*straight white arrow*), and normal torcular position (*black arrow*). (B and C) Sagittal T2W and (D) sagittal T1W MRI in a child with Blake pouch cyst performed before and after ventriculoperitoneal shunting showing significant widening of the fourth ventricle with compression displacement of the completely developed vermis secondary to a persistent Blake pouch cyst. Choroid plexus is noted along the inferior contour of the inferior medullary velum. Scalloping of the occipital bone and high-grade supratentorial hydrocephalus, which is subsequently drained after ventriculoperitoneal shunting. (A from StatDX. Copyright © 2022 Elsevier.)

Key Points

Background

- Blake pouch cyst refers to a cerebrospinal fluid–filled cystic outpouching of the inferior fourth ventricle below the inferior vermis. The Blake pouch is a transient structure along the posterior or inferior medullary velum that regresses during the first trimester of pregnancy to form the midline cerebrospinal fluid outflow tract of the fourth ventricle, also known as the foramen of Magendie.
- A persistent or delayed fenestration of the Blake pouch cyst is a defect in the posterior membranous area and consequently should not have hypoplasia of the vermis.
- Neurosurgical fenestration of the Blake pouch typically resolves the cerebrospinal fluid circulation impairment.
- No increased incidence of additional developmental central nervous system anomalies has been reported.

Imaging

- Fluid-filled posterior fossa that is normal to mildly increased size. Torcula position is normal.
- Counterclockwise rotation of a normal-size vermis. Tegmentovermian angle is between 18 and 30 degrees.
- The choroid plexus of the fourth ventricle may herniate into the Blake pouch below the vermis facilitating differentiation from a Dandy-Walker malformation, where typically the fourth ventricle choroid plexus is absent.
- If the laterally positioned foramina of Luschka fail to adequately "drain" the fourth ventricle, possibly compressed by the Blake's pouch cyst, the fourth ventricle may enlarge; in severe cases the entire ventricular system may become obstructed.
- The cyst wall may be seen on thin-sliced heavily T2-weighted imaging and does not communicate with the cisterna magna.
- The inferior vermis may be displaced superiorly and/or posteriorly resulting in a widened fourth ventricle.

REFERENCES

1. Bosemani T, Orman G, Boltshauser E, Tekes A, Huisman TA, Poretti A. Congenital abnormalities of the posterior fossa. *Radiographics*. 2015;35(1):200–220.
2. Huisman TA, Poretti A. Chapter 7. Disorders of brain development. In: Magnetic Resonance Imaging of the Brain and Spine, 5th ed. Edited by Scott Atlas, MD. Wolters Kluwer, Lippincott Williams & Wilkins.

RETROCEREBELLAR ARACHNOID CYST

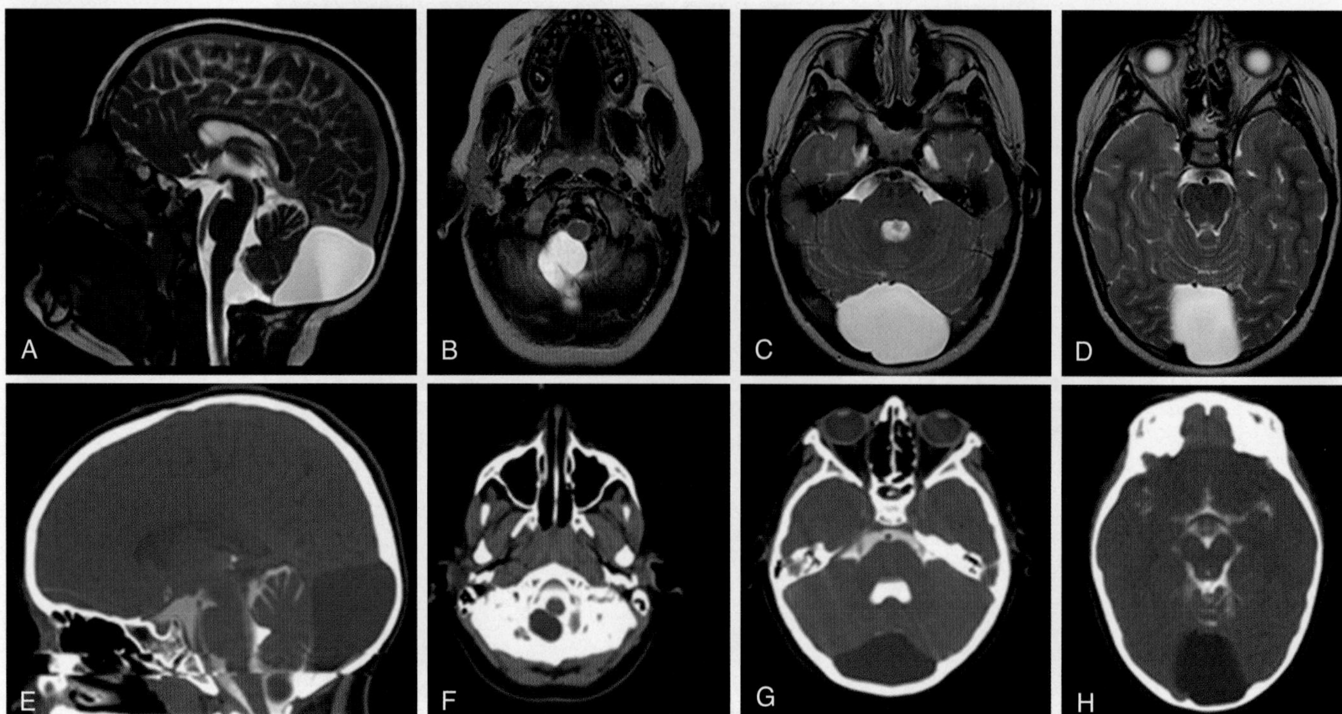

Fig. 2.111 Arachnoid Cyst. (A to D) Sagittal and axial T2W MRI of the brain in a child with a retrocerebellar arachnoid cyst. In supine position a mild sedimentation leveling is noted within the arachnoid cyst, which pushes the vermis and cerebellum anteriorly. Additionally, there is thinning and scalloping of the overlaying occipital skull. (E to H) Sagittal and axial CT study of the brain after intrathecal contrast injection of the same patient show hyperdense contrast within the basal cisterns, within the vermian fissures and fourth ventricle. No contrast is extending into the hypodense cystic lesion dorsally to the vermis confirming the contained nature of the arachnoid cyst, which is not communicating with the subarachnoid space.

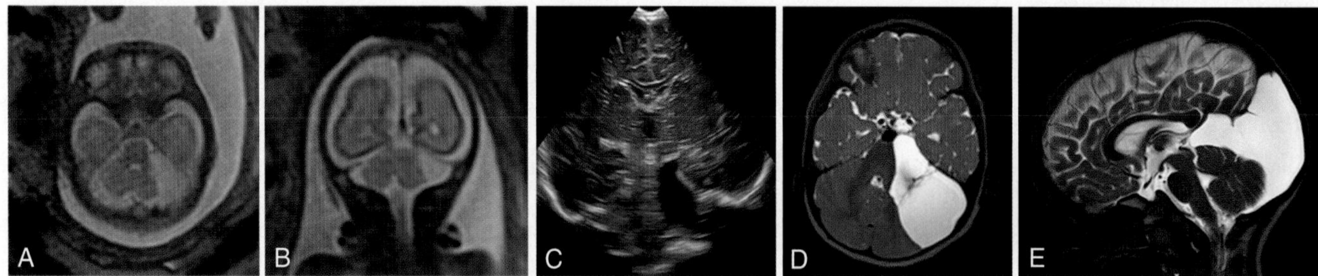

Fig. 2.112 Arachnoid Cyst. (A and B) Axial and coronal T2W fetal MRI in a fetus with a left lateral posterior fossa T2 hyperintense arachnoid cyst compressing and displacing the left cerebellar hemisphere. (C) Postnatal coronal ultrasound and (D and E) axial and sagittal T2W MRI of the same patient show a matching hypoechogenic, T2 hyperintense, well-circumscribed, partially septated arachnoid cyst in the left lateral posterior fossa, displacing the left cerebellar hemisphere and brainstem. No supratentorial ventriculomegaly is present.

Key Points

Background

- Arachnoid cysts are focal fluid collections lined by arachnoidea that do not communicate with the ventricular system or subarachnoid space.

Imaging

- Retro- or paracerebellar arachnoid cysts follow the imaging characteristics of cerebrospinal fluid.
- The cyst is typically well marginated, but the cyst wall is rarely visible on standard imaging.
- In most cases, the cyst is unilocular; however, multiple smaller cysts may be observed in close proximity to the larger cyst.
- The posterior fossa may be enlarged, the overlying occipital skull may be thinned or even remodeled due to the chronic pressure, and the torcular Herophili may be elevated.
- The adjacent vermis and cerebellar hemispheres are normal in size but may be compressed or displaced.
- Obstructive hydrocephalus is a rare complication.
- Occasionally, the signal intensity of the arachnoid cyst may be T1 and FLAIR hyperintense compared to cerebrospinal fluid due to intralesional hemorrhaging or increased protein content. A fluid-sedimentation leveling may be observed.
- The arachnoid cysts do not communicate with the subarachnoid space, and if contrast medium is injected into the subarachnoid space, the cyst will not enhance.

REFERENCE

1. Bosemani T, Orman G, Boltshauser E, Tekes A, Huisman TA, Poretti A. Congenital abnormalities of the posterior fossa. *Radiographics*. 2015;35(1):200–220.

MEGA CISTERNA MAGNA

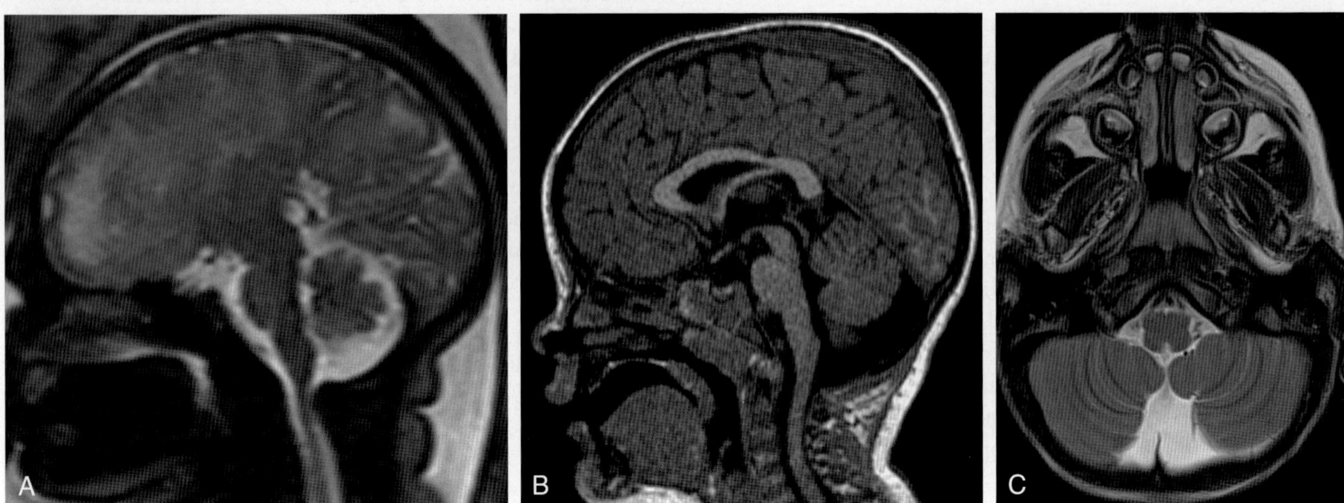

Fig. 2.113 Mega Cisterna Magna. (A) Sagittal T2W fetal MRI demonstrating a mega cisterna magna with an enlarged CSF space inferior to the vermis communicatin with the fourth ventricle without an enlarged posterior fossa, vermian hypogenesis, or abnormal rotation of the vermis, (B and C) Sagittal T1W and axial T2W images demonstrate characteristic findings of a mega cisterna magna.

Key Points

Background

- A mega cisterna magna is a large variant of the cisterna magna located in the posterior and inferior posterior fossa.
- The mega cisterna magna freely communicates with the subarachnoid space.
- Arachnoidal septae freely cross the mega cisterna magna.
- A mega cisterna magna is a frequent asymptomatic incidental finding with no clinical significance.

Imaging

- Differentiation from a posterior fossa arachnoid cyst is occasionally challenging on imaging.
- A mega cisterna magna is defined as >10 mm on midsagittal images of the posterior fossa.
- The vermis is normal in size and the tegmentovermian angle is normal.
- The posterior fossa size is usually normal or mildly enlarged.

REFERENCE

1. Bosemani T, Orman G, Boltshauser E, Tekes A, Huisman TA, Poretti A. Congenital abnormalities of the posterior fossa. *Radiographics*. 2015;35(1):200–220.

JOUBERT SYNDROME

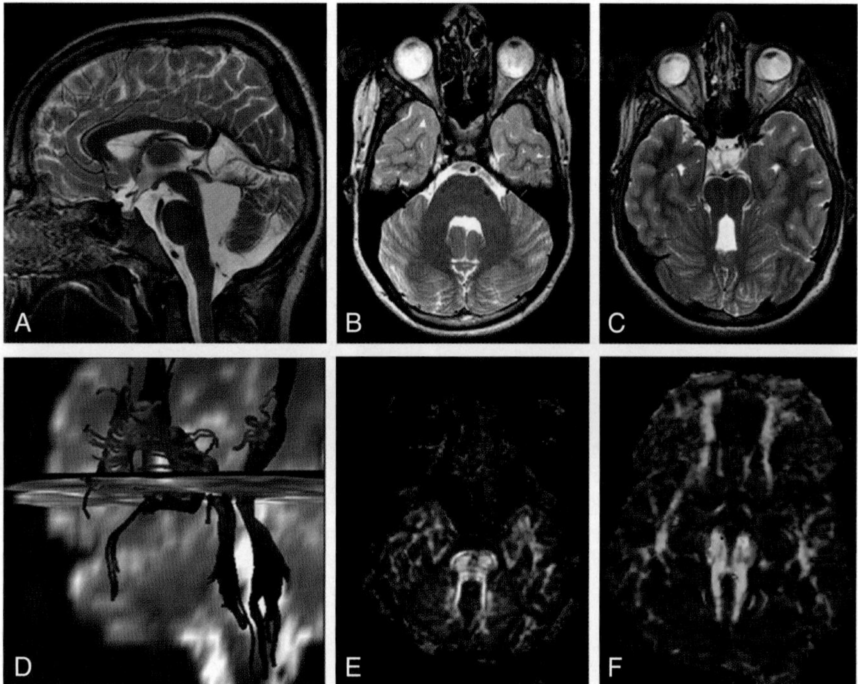

Fig. 2.114 Joubert Syndrome. (A to C) Sagittal and axial T2W MRI of the brain, (D) coronal oblique tractography, (E) fractional anisotropy maps, and (F) color-coded FA maps in Joubert syndrome. Sagittal image shows aplasia of the lower two-thirds of the vermis, a small remnant of the superior vermis, the fastigium of the mildly enlarged fourth ventricle is displaced superiorly, and the mesencephalon is elongated. Axial imaging shows the superior cerebellar peduncles are thickened and course in the axial plane, resulting in a molar tooth appearance of the pontomesencephalic junction. On tractography an aberrant course of the cortical spinal tracts is noted, and on the color-coded fractional anisotropy maps the decussation of the superior cerebellar peduncles (central red dot) is lacking.

Key Points

Background

- Joubert syndrome belongs to the group of ciliopathies in which deficient nonmotile cilia result in varying degrees of vermian hypoplasia and an aberrant course of white matter tracts and decussations in the brainstem and cerebellum.
- Joubert syndrome is an autosomal recessive disorder, and a growing number of abnormal genes have been linked to the syndrome.
- Because nonmotile cilia are present in almost any organ of the human body, multiple associated abnormalities can coexist, including ocular colobomas, retinal dysplasia, nephronophthisis, hepatic fibrosis, and polydactyly. Consequently, this syndrome has also been referred to as "oculo-cerebro-renal syndrome."

Imaging

- Malformations involve the brainstem and cerebellum.
- On axial imaging the superior cerebellar peduncles are thickened and course in a more axial plane, allowing for a molar tooth appearance of the pontomesencephalic junction, which is accentuated by the deepened interpeduncular fossa. Consequently, Joubert syndrome has also been coined as molar tooth syndrome (MTS).
- Hypoplastic vermis allows the mesial surfaces of the cerebellar hemispheres to oppose each other in the midline. On midsagittal imaging the appreciated fissures/sulci consequently do not match the normal vermian anatomy but follow the cerebellar anatomy.
- The shape of the fourth ventricle on axial imaging is also compared with a "bat wing" or "umbrella."
- On sagittal imaging the fastigium of the fourth ventricle is superiorly displaced, the mesencephalon appears elongated, the isthmus is thin, and the fourth ventricle may be enlarged.
- On color-coded fractional anisotropy maps a lack of the normal "red dot" dorsally to the interpeduncular fossa is missing due to an absence of decussating fibers in the superior cerebellar peduncles. The "horizontal" course of the superior cerebellar peduncles result in a "green" encoding per diffusion tensor color-coding convention. In addition, the normal pyramidal tract decussation in the lower brainstem is missing.
- Multiple additional central nervous system anomalies have been identified in Joubert syndrome, including interpeduncular heterotopias, suboccipital encephaloceles, migrational abnormalities, and corpus callosum anomalies.

REFERENCES

1. Bosemani T, Orman G, Boltshauser E, Tekes A, Huisman TA, Poretti A. Congenital abnormalities of the posterior fossa. *Radiographics*. 2015;35(1):200–220.
2. Poretti A, Huisman TA, Scheer I, Boltshauser E. Joubert syndrome and related disorders: spectrum of neuroimaging findings in 75 patients. *AJNR Am J Neuroradiol*. 2011 Sep;32(8):1459–1463.

PONTOCEREBELLAR HYPOPLASIA

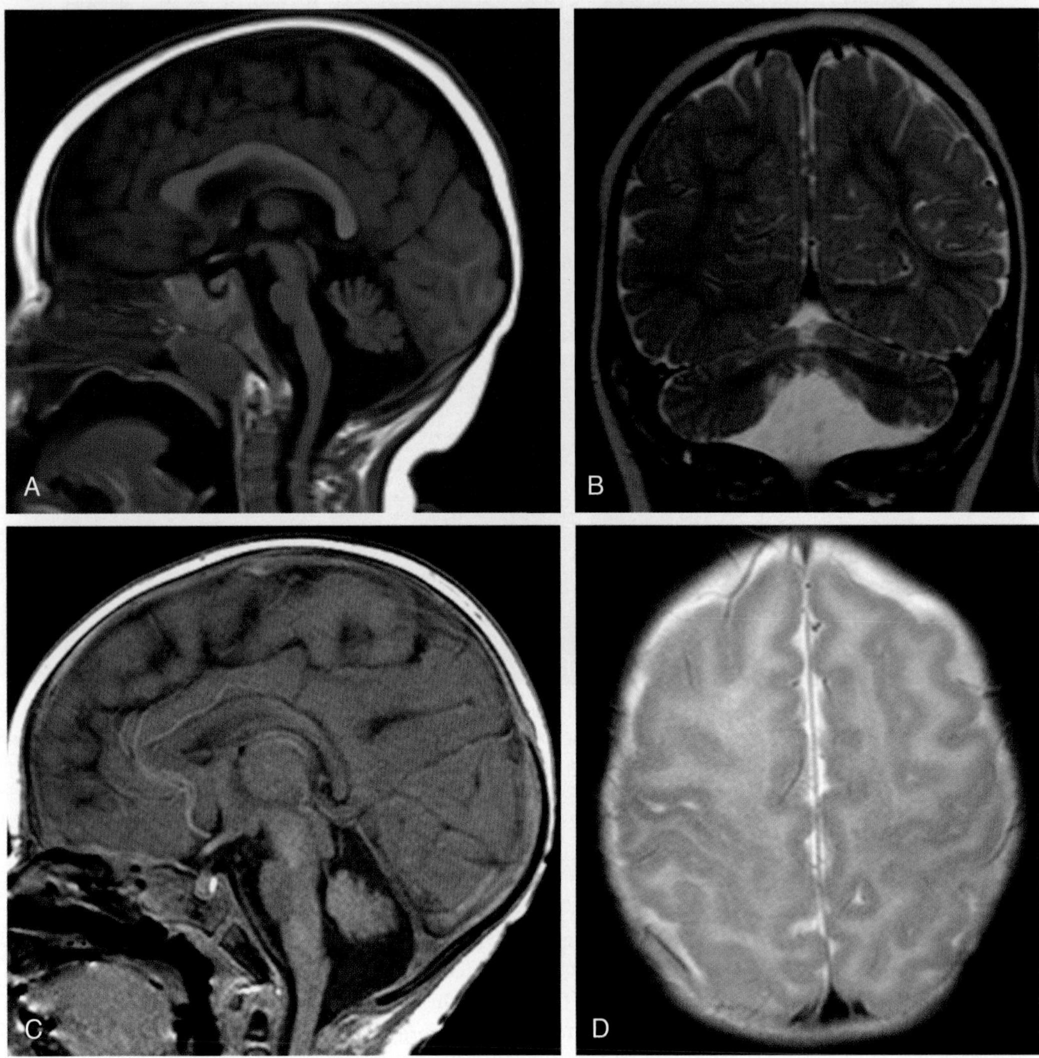

Fig. 2.115 Pontocerebellar Hypoplasia. (A and B) Sagittal T1W and coronal T2W images of a 1-year-old with microcephaly, developmental delay, and sensorineural hearing loss due to CASK mutation demonstrates hypoplasia of the cerebellum and pons. (C and D) Sagittal T1W and axial T2W images of a 3-month-old with developmental delay and microcephaly with VLDLR mutation demonstrating pontocerebellar hypoplasia with frontal pachygyria.

Key Points

Background

- Pontocerebellar hypoplasia (PCH) refers to heterogeneous group of autosomal recessive neurodegenerative disorders characterized by reduced volume of the pons and cerebellum. Eleven subtypes of PCH have been described.
- Clinical symptoms depend on the PCH subtype and can include weakness, abnormal tone, seizures, and developmental delay.
- Genetic mutations in CASK, VLDLR, and RELN can also result in pontocerebellar hypoplasia that is malformation related rather than neurodegeneration related.

Imaging

- Small cerebellar hemispheres and reduced volume of the ventral pons
- Normal or mildly reduced posterior fossa size
- Variable cerebral atrophy and delayed myelination
- CASK, VLDLR, and RELN mutations are associated with cortical malformations including pachygyria and simplified gyral pattern

REFERENCES

1. Poretti A, Boltshauser E, Huisman TA. Cerebellar and Brainstem Malformations. *Neuroimaging Clin N Am*. 2016 Aug;26(3):341–357.
2. Severino M, Huisman TAGM. Posterior Fossa Malformations. *Neuroimaging Clin N Am*. 2019 Aug;29(3):367–383.

DIENCEPHALIC-MESENCEPHALIC JUNCTION DYSPLASIA

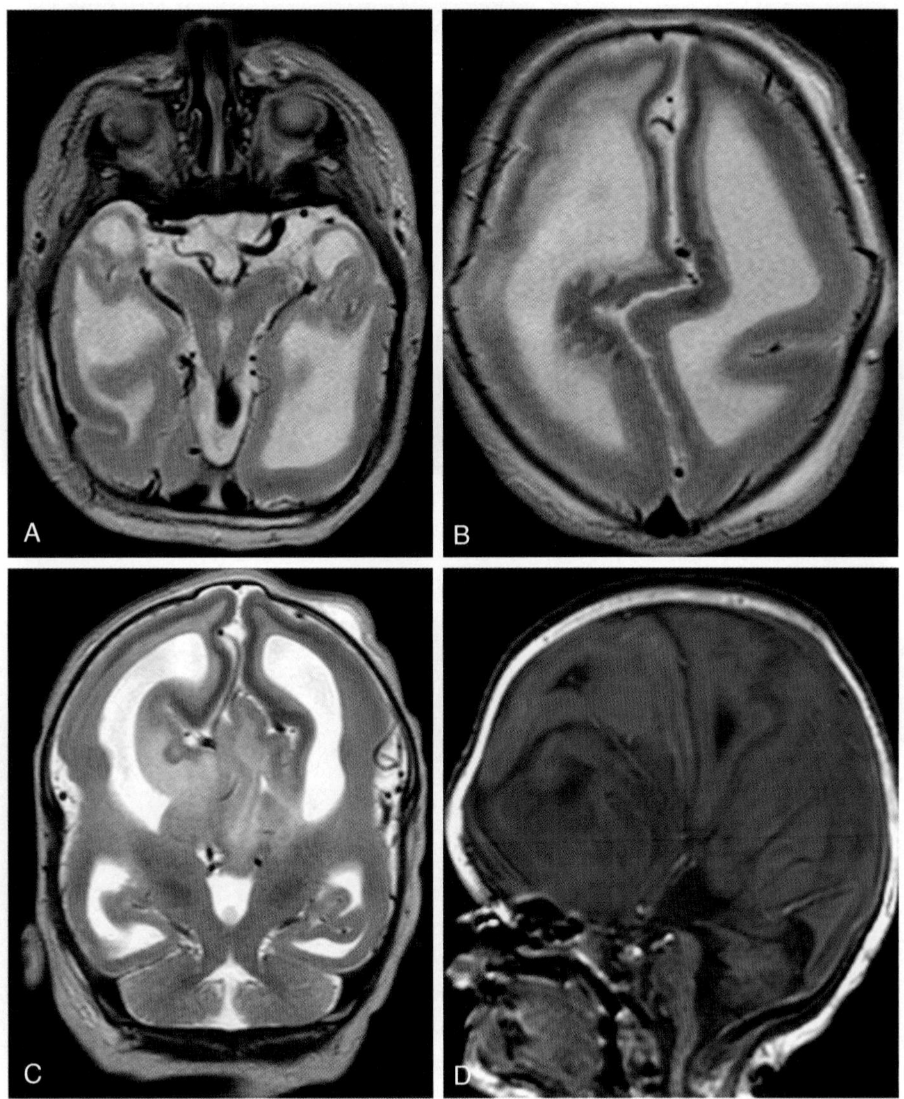

Fig. 2.116 Diencephalic Mesencephalic Junction Dysplasia. (A and B) Axial T2W, (C) coronal T2W, and (D) sagittal T1W images demonstrate butterfly appearance of the midbrain, diffuse cortical malformation with lack of sulcation with exception of areas of deep infolding, severe white matter volume loss, macrocephaly, and brainstem and cerebellar hypoplasia.

Key Points

Background

- Rare autosomal recessive brain malformation of the junction between the diencephalon and mesencephalon.
- The diencephalon-mesencephalon junction is controlled by expression of Engrailed and Paired-Box (PAX) transcription factors. More PAX-6 shifts the junction caudally, whereas more Engrailed-2 and Engrailed-3 shift the junction rostrally.

Imaging

- Butterfly appearance of the midbrain on axial plane
- Callosal agenesis or hypoplasia
- Hypomyelination
- Ventriculomegaly

REFERENCES

1. Bosemani T, Orman G, Boltshauser E, Tekes A, Huisman TA, Poretti A. Congenital abnormalities of the posterior fossa. *Radiographics.* 2015;35(1):200–220.
2. Barkovich AJ, et al. A developmental and genetic classification for midbrain-hindbrain malformations. *Brain.* 2009 Dec;132(12):3199–3230.

PONTINE TEGMENTAL CAP DYSPLASIA

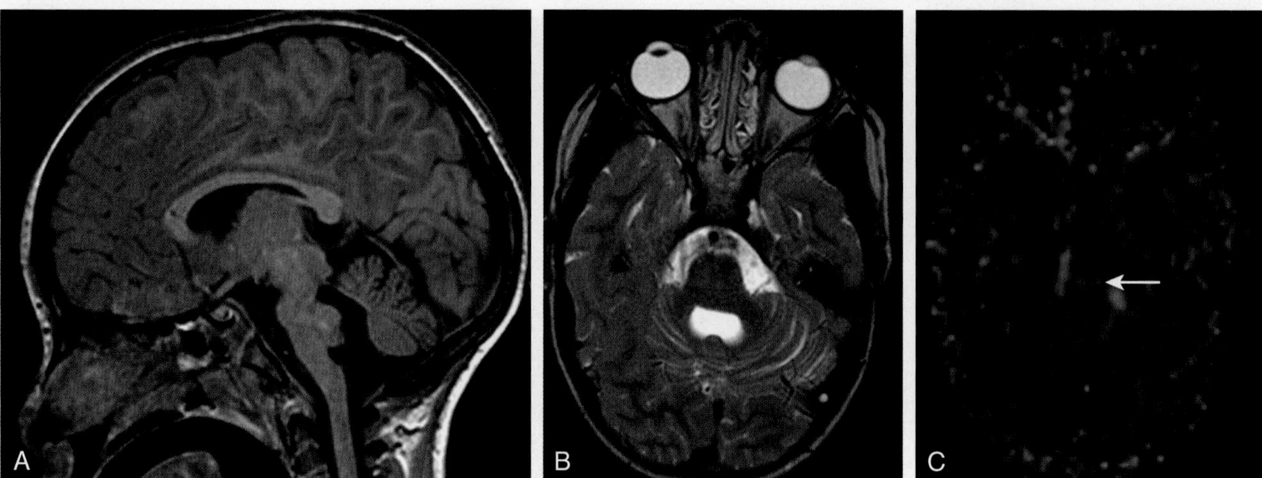

Fig. 2.117 Pontine Tegmental Cap Dysplasia. (A) Sagittal T1W, (B) axial T2W MRI of the brain, including (C) color-coded FA maps in a child with pontine tegmental cap dysplasia show a lobulated "cap" of tissue along the dorsal contour of the pons; the anterior pontine belly appears small. On axial imaging the anterior contour of the fourth ventricle is mildly flattened. On color-coded fractional anisotropy maps the "cap" represents aberrant location of transverse, red color encoded fibers (*arrow*).

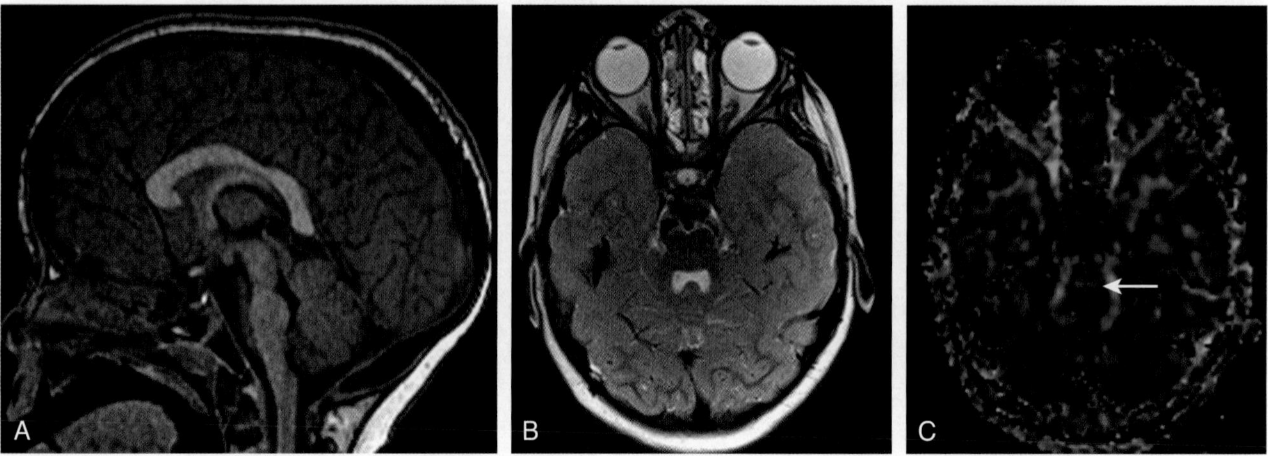

Fig. 2.118 Pontine Tegmental Cap Dysplasia. (A) Sagittal T1W, (B) axial T2W MRI of the brain including (C) color-coded FA maps in a child with pontine tegmental cap dysplasia shows a soft tissue "cap" along the dorsal contour of the pons protruding into the fourth ventricle, the pontine belly is lacking. On the color-coded fractional anisotropy map the "cap" corresponds to transverse coursing aberrant fibers (*arrow*).

Key Points

- Pontine tegmental cap dysplasia is characterized by a dorsally vaulted pontine tegmentum (cap) that protrudes into the fourth ventricle, a flattened ventral pons, partial absence or hypoplasia of the middle and/or inferior cerebellar peduncles, a molar tooth-like appearance of the midbrain on axial imaging secondary to the horizontal course of the superior cerebellar peduncles, mild to moderate vermian hypoplasia, and an absence of the inferior olivary prominence pontomesencephalic junction.
- Diffusion tensor imaging and color-coded fractional anisotropy maps confirm the absence of the transverse fibers in the middle and ventral pons, while a band of misguided transverse coursing ectopic fibers is seen within the "cap."
- Additional findings outside of the central nervous system may include vertebral formation anomalies, rib malformations, and congenital heart disease.
- The primary brainstem involvement is linked to sensorineural hearing loss, facial nerve paralysis, trigeminal anesthesia, and difficulty in swallowing.
- Depending on the severity of the malformation, various grades of neurocognitive delay may be observed.

REFERENCES

1. Bosemani T, Orman G, Boltshauser E, Tekes A, Huisman TA, Poretti A. Congenital abnormalities of the posterior fossa. *Radiographics*. 2015;35(1):200–220.
2. Chokshi FH, Poretti A, Meoded A, Huisman TA. Normal and abnormal development of the cerebellum and brainstem as depicted by diffusion tensor imaging. *Semin Ultrasound CT MR*. 2011 Dec;32(6):539–554.

HORIZONTAL GAZE PALSY AND PROGRESSIVE SCOLIOSIS

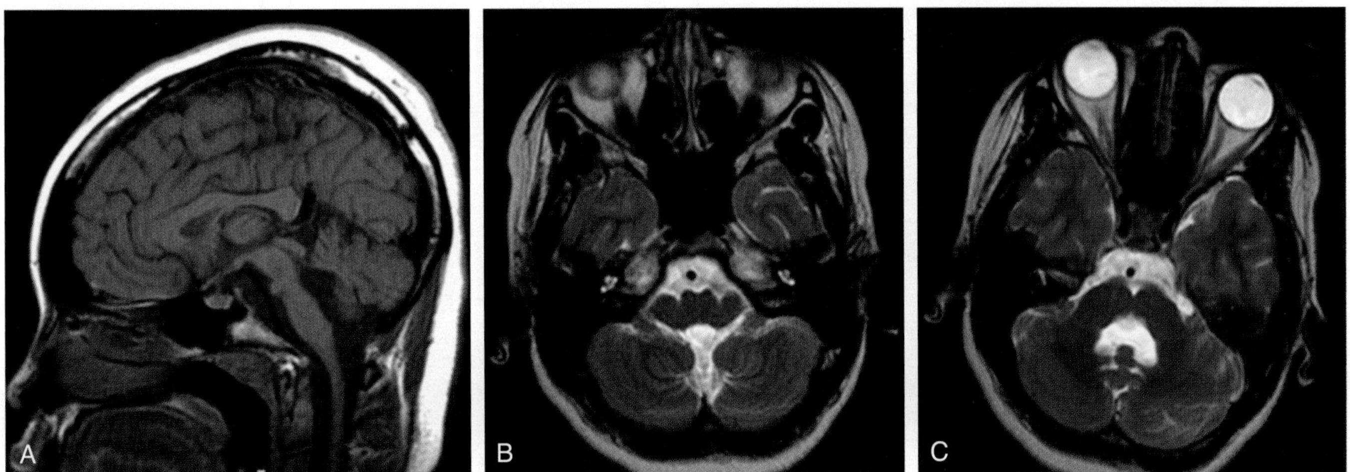

Fig. 2.119 Horizontal Gaze Palsy and Progressive Scoliosis. (A) Sagittal T1W and (B and C) axial T2W MRI of the brain in a child with horizontal gaze palsy and progressive scoliosis with butterfly appearance of the lower brainstem and hypoplastic pons with midline clefting.

Key Points

Background

- Rare autosomal recessive disorder caused by mutations of the *ROBO3* gene that encodes a receptor for axonal guidance.
- Clinically these children present with a congenital absence of horizontal eye movements secondary to a congenital absence of the abducens nucleus, preservation of vertical gaze and convergence, and progressive spinal scoliosis in childhood.

Imaging

- On axial imaging a characteristic butterfly appearance of the lower brainstem is noted secondary to the combination of a lack of the gracile and cuneate nuclei prominence, while the inferior olivary nuclei are prominent with respect to the medullary pyramids. The pons is hypoplastic with a dorsal midline cleft and absence of the bulging contour of the facial colliculi.
- Diffusion tensor imaging and color-coded fractional anisotropy maps typically show absence of the decussation of the corticospinal tracts, pontine sensory tracts, and superior cerebellar peduncles.

REFERENCE

1. Bosemani T, Orman G, Boltshauser E, Tekes A, Huisman TA, Poretti A. Congenital abnormalities of the posterior fossa. *Radiographics*. 2015;35(1):200–220.

RHOMBENCEPHALOSYNAPSIS

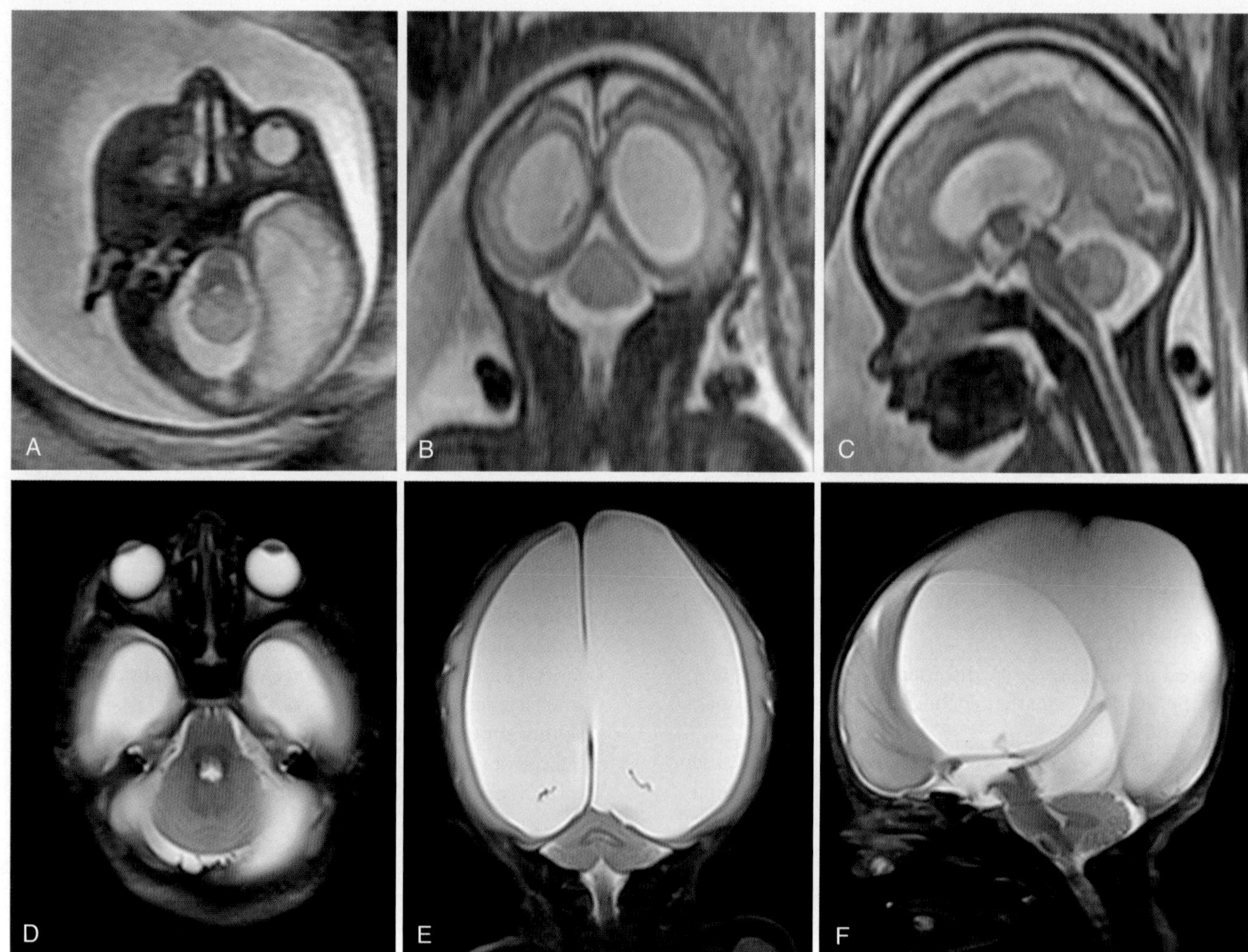

Fig. 2.120 Rhombencephalosynapsis. (A to C) Axial, coronal, and sagittal T2W fetal MRI demonstrate fusion of the cerebellar hemispheres, including dentate nuclei, complete absence of the vermis, aqueductal stenosis, and supratentorial ventriculomegaly. (D to F) Postnatal axial, coronal, and sagittal T2W MRI confirm the findings.

Key Points

Background

- Rhombencephalosynapsis is a rare congenital cerebellar malformation characterized by a complete or near-complete lack of the vermis with fusion of both cerebellar hemispheres. The dentate nuclei are fused in the midline as well as the middle cerebellar peduncles.
- Rhombencephalosynapsis is a constant feature in Gomez-Lopez-Hernandez syndrome (rhombencephalosynapsis, developmental delay, scalp alopecia, and trigeminal anesthesia).
- Severe and early morbidity and mortality.

Imaging

- On coronal and axial imaging, the cerebellar foliae and fissures extend uninterrupted across the midline.
- On sagittal imaging, the normal vermian anatomy is lacking and the gray matter of the fused dentate nuclei is recognized on a midsagittal slice.
- The fourth ventricle is typically small, mimicking a keyhole on axial imaging; a moderate to severe supratentorial ventriculomegaly is present in most cases, usually secondary to a narrowed cerebral aqueduct.
- The overall size of the cerebellum is often smaller than normal; the posterior fossa is normal in size in most cases.
- Additional supratentorial anomalies have been reported and include corpus callosum malformations, absence or rupture of the leaves of the septum pellucidum, and fusion of the thalami.

REFERENCE

1. Bosemani T, Orman G, Boltshauser E, Tekes A, Huisman TA, Poretti A. Congenital abnormalities of the posterior fossa. *Radiographics*. 2015;35(1):200–220.

CEREBELLAR CLEFT

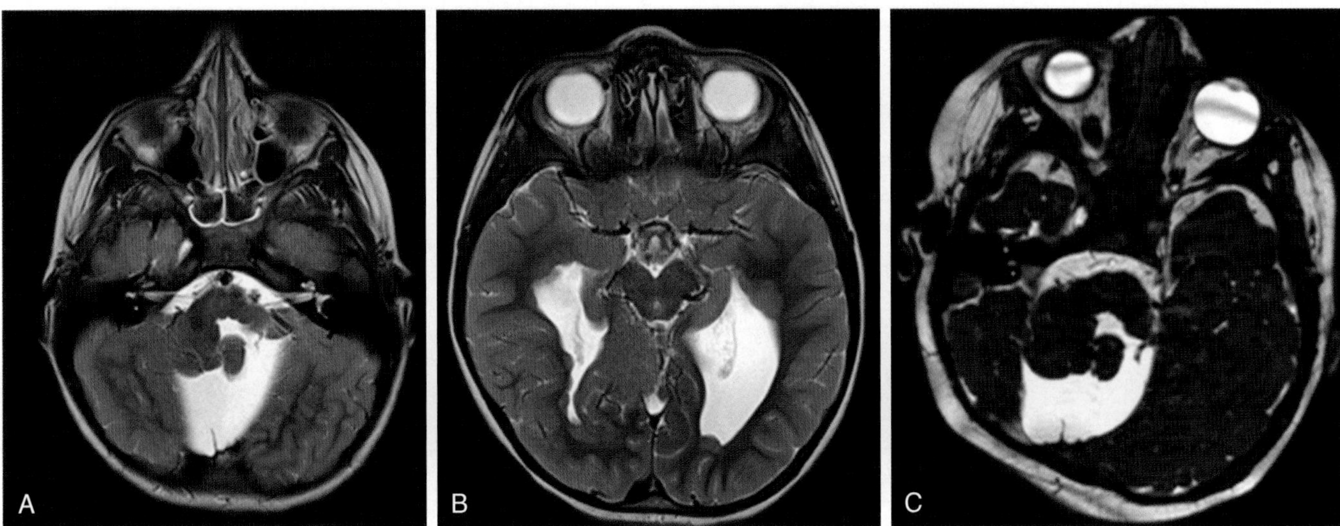

Fig. 2.121 Cerebellar Cleft. (A to C) Axial T2W MRI of the brain in a child with an extensive open-lip left cerebellar cleft with significant disorganization of the adjacent vermis and left cerebellar hemisphere. In addition, extensive supratentorial subependymal gray matter heterotopia is noted along the widened occipital horns of the lateral ventricles.

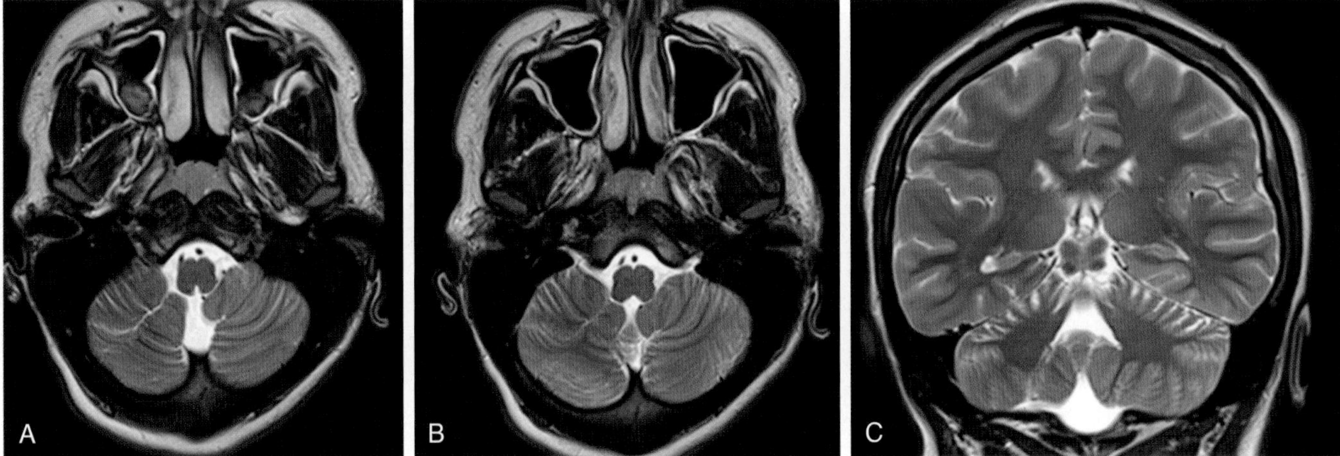

Fig. 2.122 Cerebellar Cleft. (A to C) Axial and coronal T2W MRI of the brain in child with a closed-lip right cerebellar cleft, extending from the subarachnoid space toward the lateral recess of the fourth ventricle.

Key Points

- Currently a cerebellar cleft is considered to be secondary to an early prenatal cerebellar insult (e.g., fetal cerebellar hemorrhage) and consequently belongs in the category of disruptions or destructions rather than being categorized as a true malformation.
- Cerebellar clefts may extend from the surface of the cerebellar hemisphere toward the fourth ventricle, similar to a supratentorial schizencephaly.
- The cleft is typically lined by disorganized, possibly nodular-appearing gray matter; the normal pattern of cerebellar foliae and fissures and white matter arborization is usually disrupted. The affected cerebellar hemisphere and ipsilateral cerebellar peduncles are often hypoplastic. The ipsilateral dentate nucleus may be malformed.
- The vermis is usually spared.
- Supratentorial migrational abnormalities are frequently seen.
- Arachnoid adhesions with resultant arachnoid cysts and an enlarged posterior fossa may coexist.

REFERENCES

1. Bosemani T, Orman G, Boltshauser E, Tekes A, Huisman TA, Poretti A. Congenital abnormalities of the posterior fossa. *Radiographics*. 2015;35(1):200–220.
2. Hayashi M, Poretti A, Gorra M, Farzin A, Graham EM, Huisman TA, Northington FJ. Prenatal cerebellar hemorrhage: fetal and postnatal neuroimaging findings and postnatal outcome. *Childs Nerv Syst*. 2015 May;31(5):705–712.

ECTOPIC CEREBELLAR TISSUE

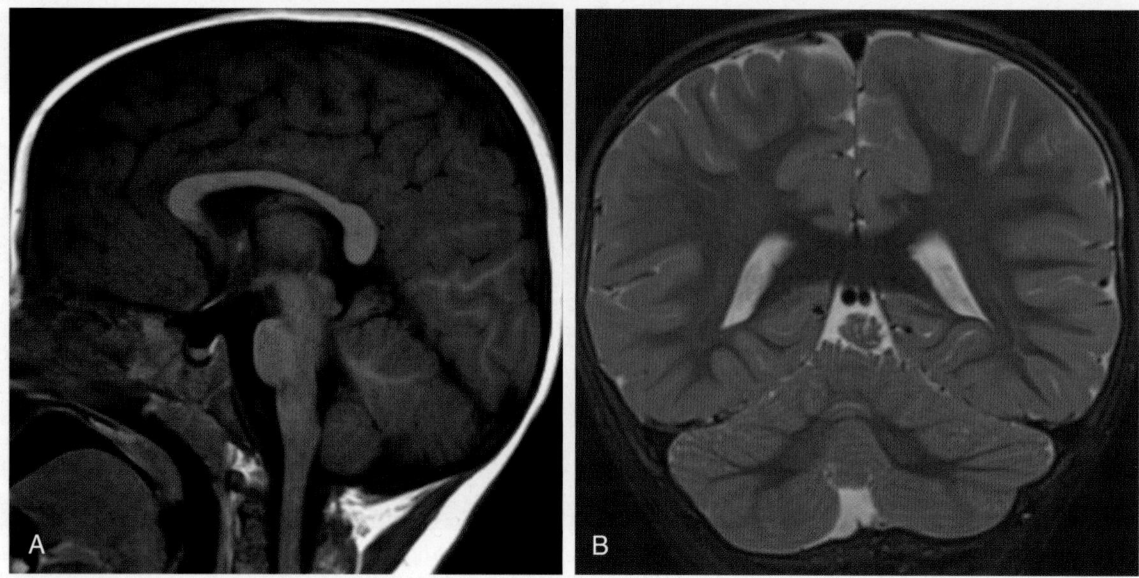

Fig. 2.123 Ectopic Cerebellar Tissue. (A) Sagittal T1W and (B) coronal T2W images demonstrate a pedunculated ectopic cerebellar tissue superior to the cerebellum connected by a thin stalk to the superior cerebellar peduncle.

Key Points

- Rare malformation of the cerebellum
- Most are incidentally detected and no intervention is necessary.
- Most appear as pedunculated cerebellar tissue connected by a stalk to the brainstem or cerebellum.

REFERENCE

1. Orman G, Kralik SF, Battini R, Buchignani B, Desai NK, Goetti R, Meoded A, Mitter C, Wallacher-Scholz B, Boltshauser E, Huisman TAGM. Neuroimaging Features of Ectopic Cerebellar Tissue: A Case Series Study of a Rare Entity. *AJNR Am J Neuroradiol.* 2021 Jun;42(6):1167–1173.

PITUITARY AND SELLA MALFORMATIONS

The pituitary gland is made up of the anterior and posterior pituitary gland and is connected to the hypothalamus by the infundibulum, also known as the pituitary stalk. The anterior pituitary, also known as the adenohypophysis, arises from ectoderm through a process by which the Rathke pouch arising from the ectoderm forms at 3 weeks' gestation, separates at 32 days' gestation, and ~10–12 days later contacts the diencephalon. The anterior wall of the pouch forms the adenohypophysis and the posterior wall forms the pars intermedia. The craniopharyngeal canal is a canal extending from the floor of the sella through the skull base and should disappear by birth. The posterior pituitary, also known as the neurohypophysis, is an extension of the diencephalon. The anterior pituitary also includes the pars intermedia, located in the middle of the pituitary gland, and the pars tuberalis, which is on the exterior of the pituitary infundibulum. The anterior pituitary hormones include ACTH, TSH, LH, FSH, prolactin, growth hormone, and melanocyte stimulating hormone, whereas the posterior pituitary contains vasopressin and oxytocin.

From birth to approximately 6 weeks of age, the pituitary gland is convex at its superior margin and has a diffuse T1 hyperintense appearance. The posterior pituitary T1 bright spot should be easily identified by 2 months of age. The pituitary gland should measure >3 mm in craniocaudal height before puberty. During puberty the pituitary height is typically 6 to 10 mm.

Several malformations can occur in the region of the sella and may be detected incidentally or due to clinical signs and symptoms, such as growth hormone deficiency and precocious puberty. Rathke cleft cysts are remnants of the Rathke pouch, which normally regresses by the 12th week of gestation. Hypothalamic hamartomas are malformations due to gray matter heterotopia in the tuber cinereum. More information on Rathke cleft cysts and hypothalamic hamartomas is found in Chapter 7, Brain Tumors and Treatment Complications. Absence or hypoplasia of the pituitary gland can be isolated or in conjunction with syndromes including Kallman syndrome, CHARGE syndrome, and Coffin-Siris syndrome and malformations including anencephaly, holoprosencephaly, septo-optic dysplasia, and callosal agenesis. This chapter will discuss malformations of the sella, including persistent craniopharyngeal canal, ectopic posterior pituitary gland, and pituitary duplication.

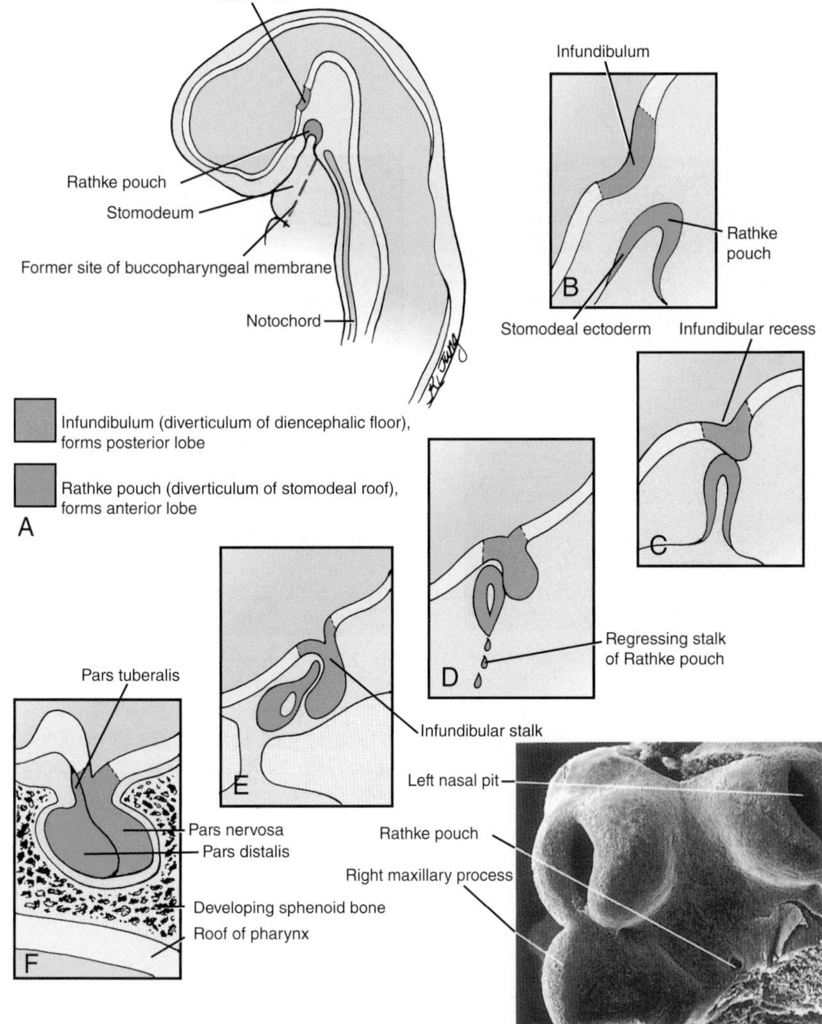

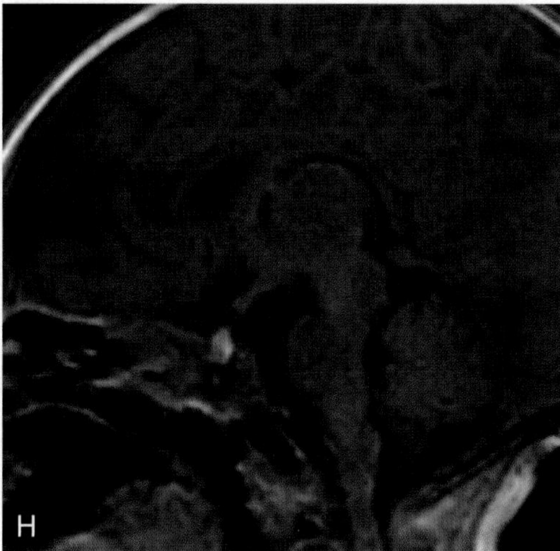

Fig. 2.124 (A–G) Embryologic origin of the pituitary gland with progression of embryologic changes shown in B to F. (H) Normal pituitary gland in a neonate demonstrating convex superior margin and diffuse T1 hyperintense signal. (A From Schoenwolf GC, Bleyl SB, Brauer PR, Francis-West PH. *Larsen's Human Embryology.* 5th ed. Elsevier; 2015.)

ECTOPIC NEUROHYPOPHYSIS

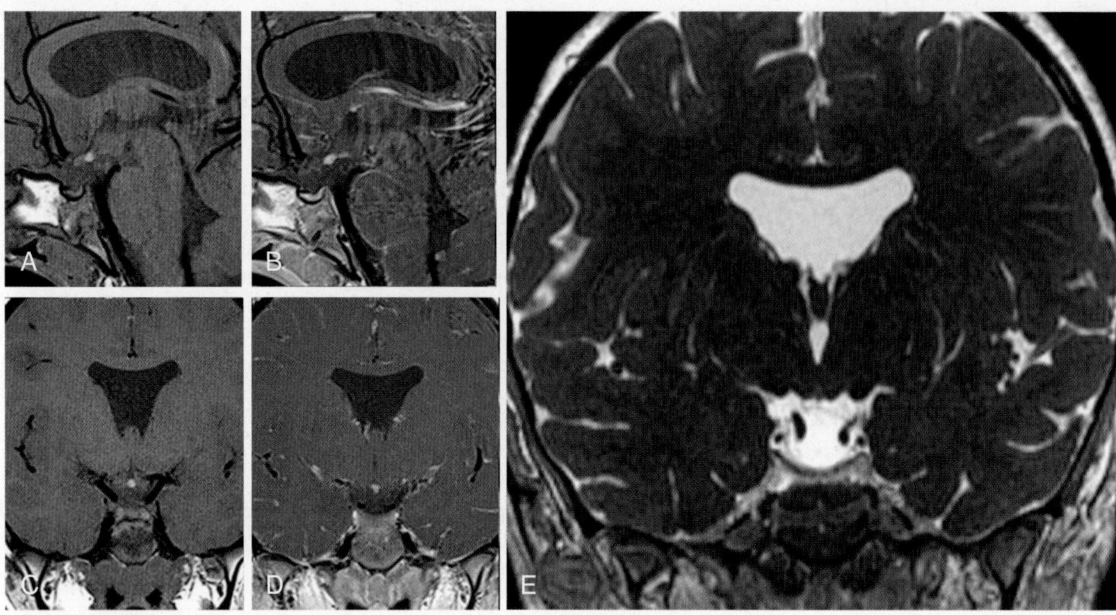

Fig. 2.125 Ectopic Pituitary. (A to D) Sagittal and coronal T1W and T1W+C. (E) Coronal T2W MRI of the sellar region in a child with an ectopic neurohypophysis with a retrochiasmatic T1 hyperintense "dot" along the floor of the third ventricle, in addition to stigmata of septo-optic dysplasia with boxlike configuration of the lateral ventricles and lack of the leaves of the septum pellucidum.

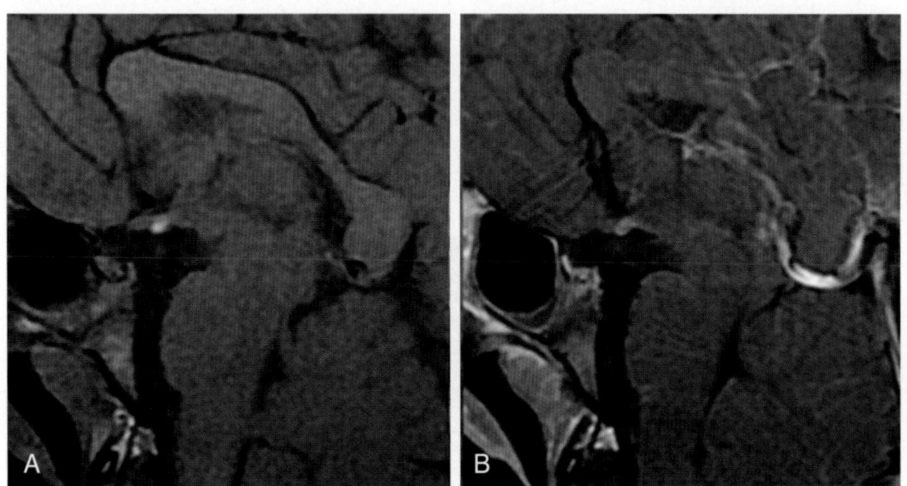

Fig. 2.126 Ectopic Pituitary. (A) Sagittal T1W (B) sagittal T1W+C imaging of the sella region show a precontrast T1 hyperintense neurohypophysis just posterior to the optic chiasm along the floor of the third ventricle compatible with ectopic neurohypophysis. Within the sella region a small contrast enhancing adenohypophysis is noted.

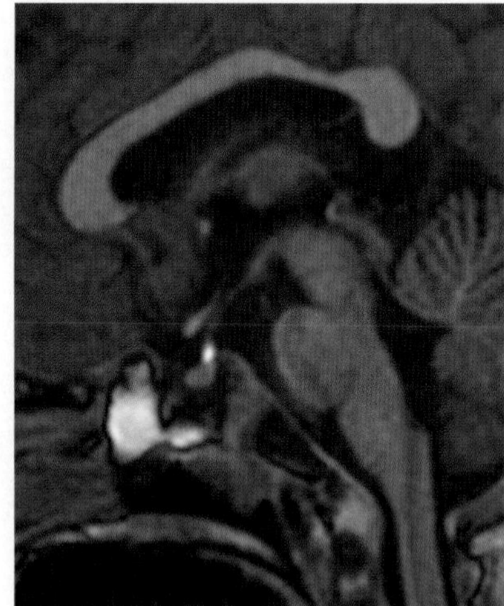

Fig. 2.127 Ectopic Pituitary. Midline sagittal T1W MRI of the sellar region shows a focal T1 hyperintense "dot" within the distal pituitary stalk just superior to the adeno hypophysis compatible with a low ectopic neurohypophysis.

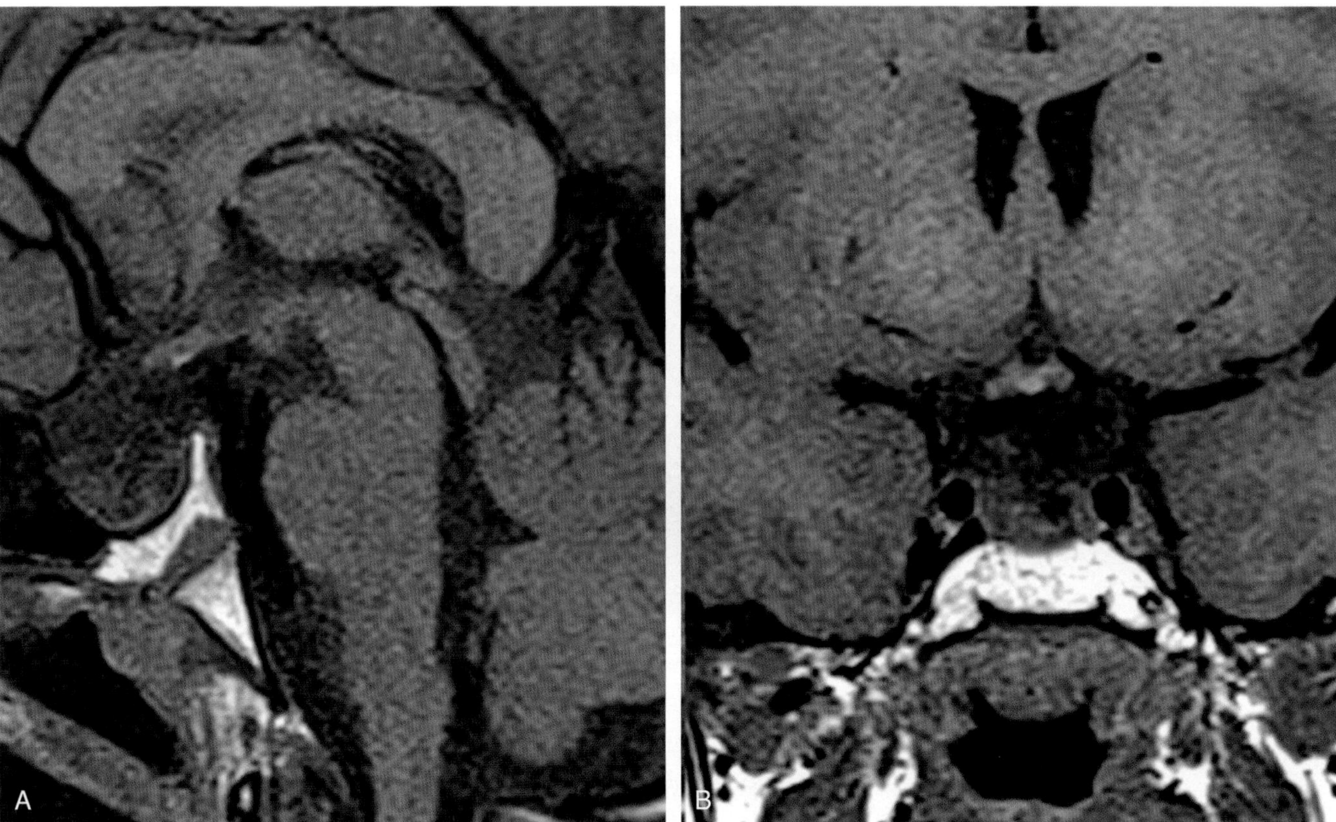

Fig. 2.128 Ectopic Pituitary. (A and B) Sagittal and coronal T1W MRI of the sellar region show an ectopic neurohypophysis along the floor of the third ventricle respectively just posterior to the optic chiasm after surgical resection of a craniopharyngioma. The sella is widened due to the craniopharyngioma. The ectopic location of the neurohypophysis is likely secondary.

Key Points

- Ectopic neurohypophysis refers to an ectopic location of the neurohypophysis distant from its usual location within the sella turcica dorsally to the adenohypophysis.
- An ectopic posterior pituitary gland is often associated with hypoplasia of the anterior pituitary and absent or hypoplastic pituitary infundibulum.
- The neurohypophysis is usually easily detected on precontrast T1-weighted midsagittal MR imaging by its bright T1 signal. The T1-hyperintensity is believed to result from the proteinaceous carrier proteins that transport the antidiuretic hormone (ADH) and oxytocin from the hypothalamic paraventricular and supraoptic nucleus to the neurohypophysis along the pituitary stalk.
- The bright spot of the ectopically located neurohypophysis can be seen anywhere along the hypothalamic-pituitary axis from the medium eminence of the hypothalamus up to the junction between pituitary stalk and adenohypophysis.
- Rarely a neo-appearance of the bright signal is seen after neurosurgical resection of a intrasellar lesion in which the pituitary stalk was injured or transected. In these cases, the bright spot is seen superior to the level of transection.
- In cases of ectopic neurohypophysis, the adenohypophysis may be of normal size despite functional deficiency. Alternatively, the adenohypophysis can be smaller than usual.
- An ectopic neurohypophysis can also be seen in more global malformations, for example, in septo-optic dysplasia with or without corpus callosum anomalies.
- Clinical symptoms are related to the pituitary hormone deficiencies (such as short stature from growth hormone deficiency) and associated brain anomalies.

PITUITARY DUPLICATION

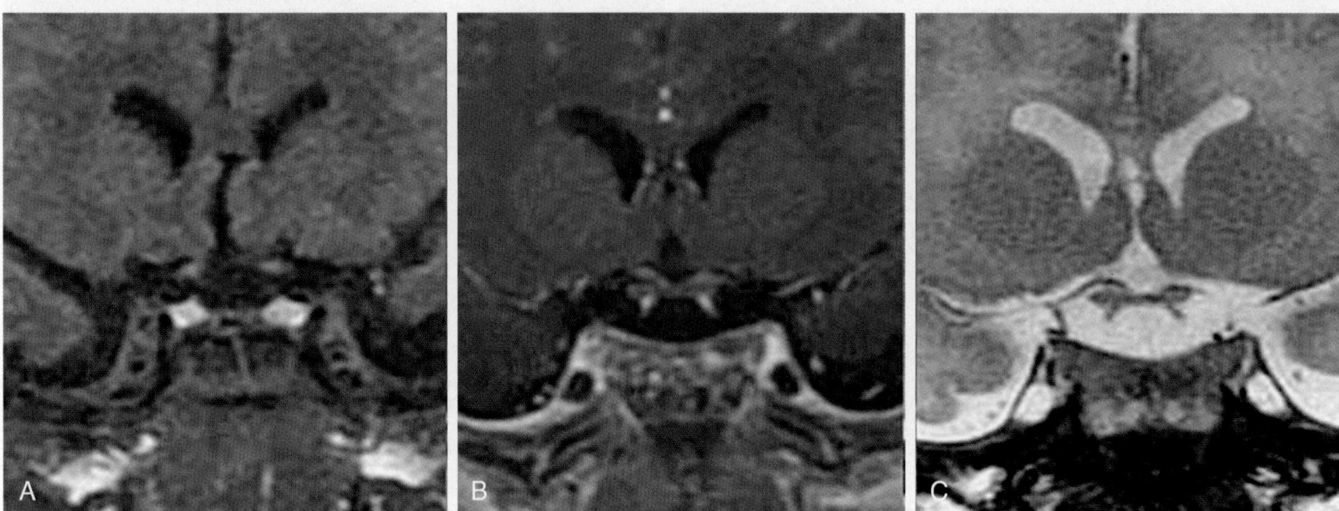

Fig. 2.129 Pituitary Duplication. (A) Coronal T1W, (B) coronal T1W+C and (C) coronal T2W MRI of the sellar region in a child with a duplication of the pituitary gland show a widened sella region with duplication of the T1 hyperintense signal of the neurohypophysis and a duplication of the pituitary stalk in combination with a widening of the optic chiasm.

Key Points

- Pituitary duplication is a rare congenital malformation characterized by a complete duplication of the anterior and posterior lobe of the pituitary gland and pituitary stalk/infundibulum.
- Etiology is suspected to be due to splitting of the notochord.
- Coronal MRI is diagnostic, demonstrating the duplicated infundibulum and pituitary glands and the broad sella.
- Associated findings that have been reported include duplication of the hypothalamus (which may be seen as thickening of the floor of the third ventricle), tuber cinereum hamartoma, anomalies of the circle of Willis with a fenestrated basilar artery, anomalies of the olfactory tracts and bulbs, absent anterior commissure, persistent craniopharyngeal canal, nasopharyngeal teratoma, cleft palate, and hypertelorism.
- Prognosis is poor.

REFERENCE

1. Huisman TA, Fischer U, Boltshauser E, Straube T, Gysin C. Pituitary duplication and nasopharyngeal teratoma in a newborn: CT, MRI, US and correlative histopathological findings. *Neuroradiology*. 2005 Jul;47(7):558–561.

PERSISTENT CRANIOPHARYNGEAL CANAL

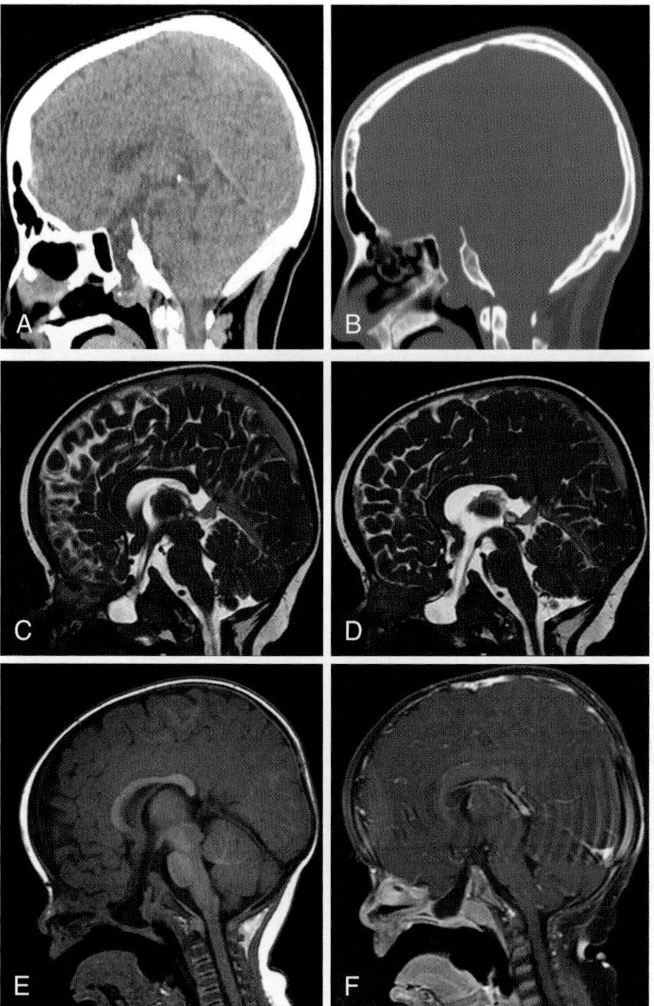

Fig. 2.130 Persistent Craniopharyngeal Canal. (A and B) Sagittal CT images in soft tissue and bone of a child with a persistent craniopharyngeal canal. A fluid-filled osseous defect is present through the sphenoid body and an associated partially calcified soft tissue mass lesion within the nasopharynx. (C and D) Sagittal T2W, (E) sagittal T1W, and (F) T1W+C MRI shows child with a persistent craniopharyngeal canal. An osseous defect is noted in the region of the sella, a CSF-filled space is extending through the defect into the upper nasopharynx, and part of the pituitary gland and floor of the third ventricle herniate through the defect.

Key Points

Background

- Persistent craniopharyngeal canal (CPC) or persistent hypophyseal canal refers to a defect in the midline sphenoid body from the sella turcica to the nasopharynx.
- Embryologic origin is presumed to be due to failure of closure of the Rathke pouch.
- CSF leak and intracranial hypotension may be observed. The pituitary gland can be displaced into the nasopharynx.

Imaging

- Midsagittal imaging is diagnostic demonstrating the bone defect extending from the sella to the nasopharynx; additional malformations including corpus callosum anomalies and midfacial findings like hypertelorism can coexist.
- Three types of CPCs are encountered on imaging:
  1. Small incidental canals
  2. Medium-size canals with ectopic pituitary tissue
  3. Large canals with cephaloceles, tumors, or both

REFERENCES

1. Huisman TA, Poretti A. Chapter 7. Disorders of brain development. In: Magnetic Resonance Imaging of the Brain and Spine, 5th ed. Edited by Scott Atlas, MD. Wolters Kluwer, Lippincott Williams & Wilkins.
2. Tijssen M, Poretti A, Huisman TA. Chiari type 1 malformation, corpus callosum agenesis and patent craniopharyngeal canal in an 11-year-old boy. *The Neuroradiol Journal*. 2016;29(5):307–309.
3. Abele TA, Salzman KL, Harnsberger HR, Glastonbury CM. Craniopharyngeal canal and its spectrum of pathology. *AJNR Am J Neuroradiol*. 2014 Apr;35(4):772–777.

CYSTS AND FLUID SPACES

Intracranial cysts and fluid-filled spaces are commonly encountered on brain imaging, and many are incidental with no intervention is required. Some cysts, such as colloid cysts and Rathke cleft cysts, are discussed in Chapter 7 due to their mass-like properties and because they are often considered in the differential diagnosis of a tumor. Perivascular spaces, cavum septum pellucidum (CSP), cavum vergae, and cavum velum interpositum are additional frequently encountered fluid spaces that are primarily benign anatomic variants. Perivascular spaces are detected in nearly all brain MRIs and are generally insignificant, except in the setting of a potential genetic disorder such as mucopolysaccharidoses or can be seen in increased size and number in the setting of radiotherapy injury to the white matter. The CSP is a midline fluid space whose formation is closely related to the formation of the corpus callosum and is an important structure to identify on fetal imaging. The CSP is present in the majority of neonates and decreases in incidence postnatally. A persistent CSP is considered by most to be an anatomic variant, although an increased incidence is reported in pediatric schizophrenia and developmental delay.

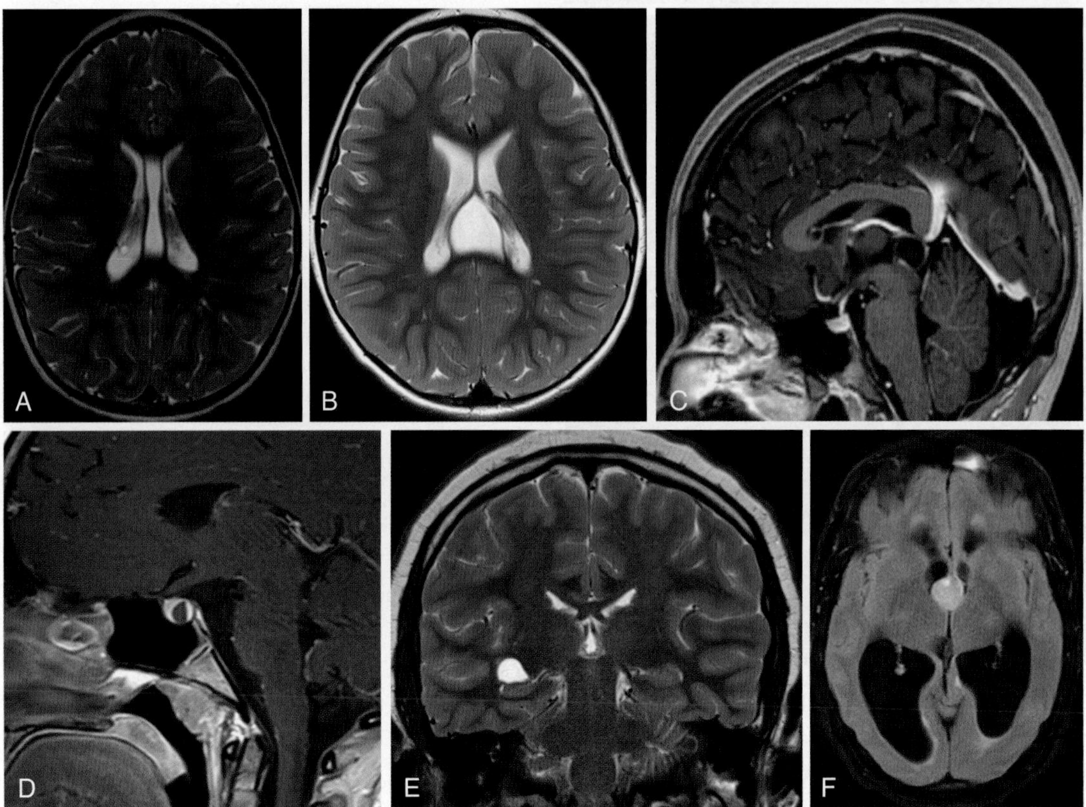

Fig. 2.131 Common Intracranial Cysts and Fluid Spaces. (A) Axial T2W image of a cavum septum pellucidum. (B) Axial T2W image of a cavum velum interpositum. (C) Sagittal T1W+C image of a pineal cyst. (D) Sagittal T1W+C image of a Rathke cleft cyst. (E) Coronal T2W images of a right-sided choroidal fissure cyst. (F) Axial FLAIR image of a colloid cyst.

ARACHNOID CYST

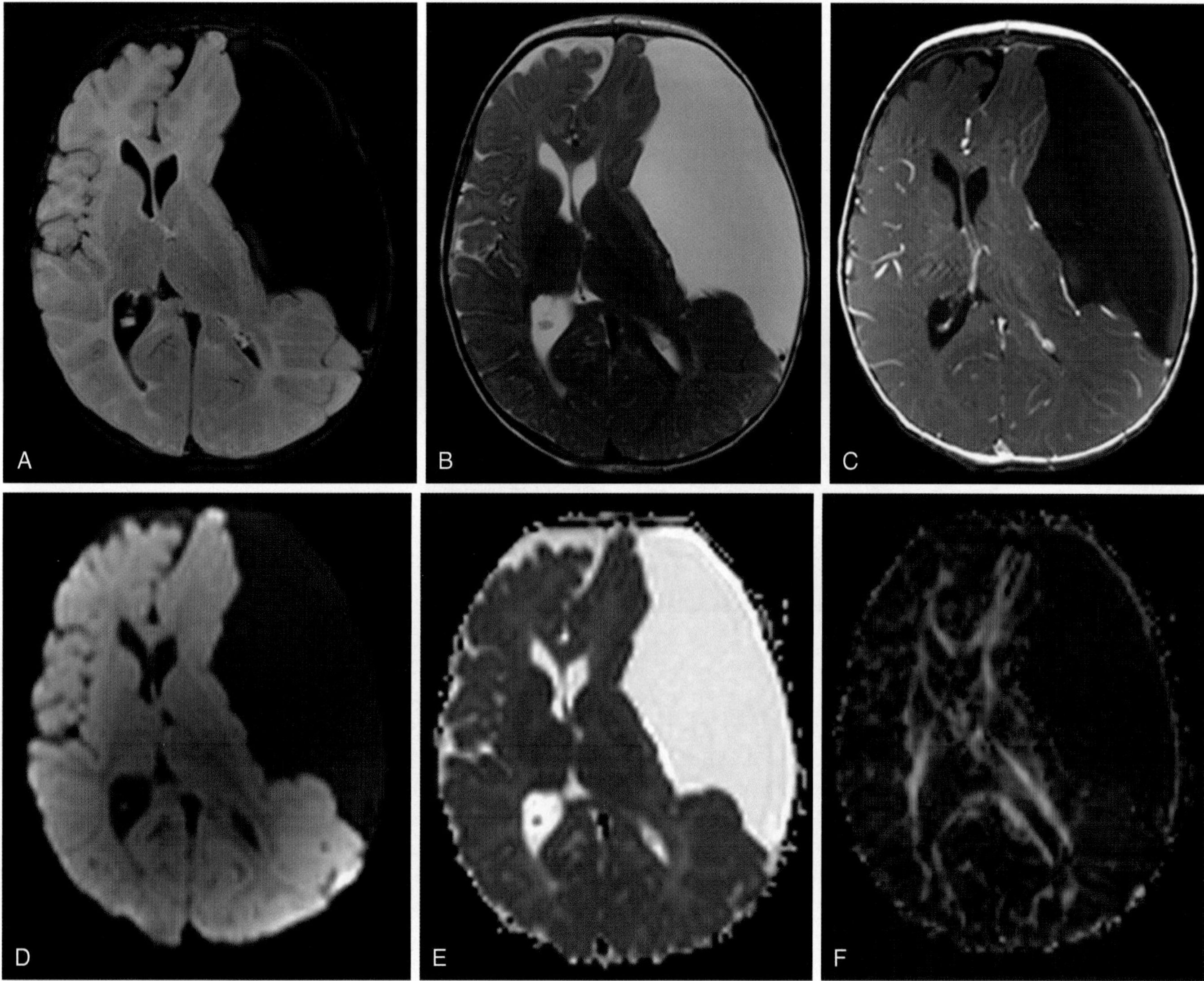

Fig. 2.132 Arachnoid Cyst. (A) Axial FLAIR, (B) T2W, (C) T1W+C, (D) DWI (E) apparent diffusion coefficient and (F) fractional anisotropy maps of a child with a large left-sided Sylvian fissure arachnoid cyst. Significant mass effect on the left cerebral hemisphere with midline shift toward the right, no intraparenchymal signal abnormality. The signal intensity within the arachnoid cyst follows the signal intensity of the cerebrospinal fluid within the lateral ventricles on all sequences.

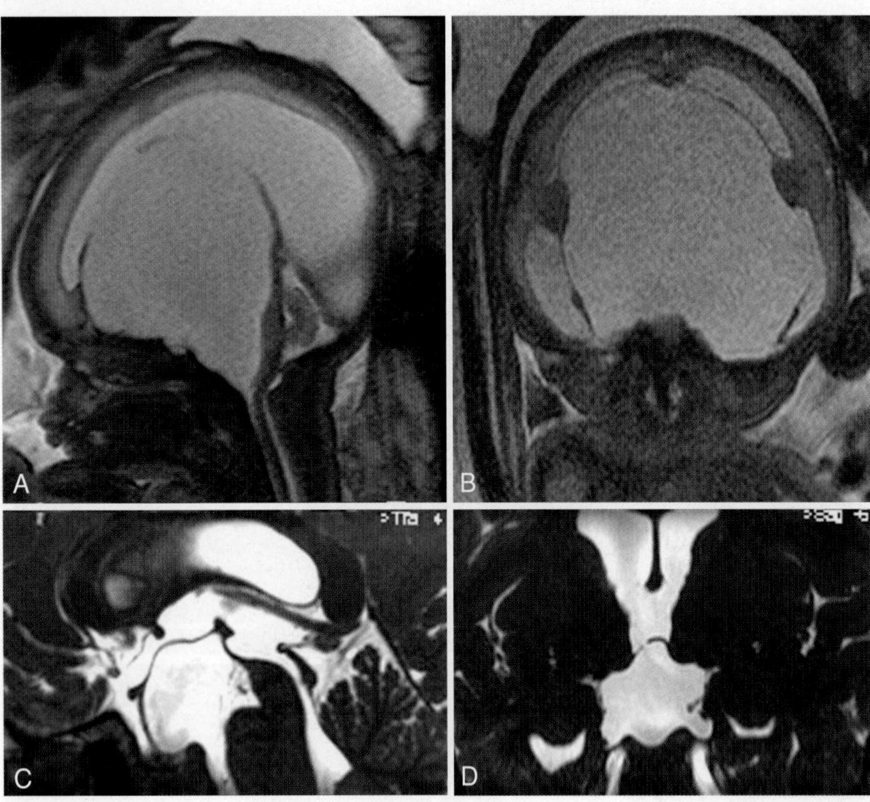

Fig. 2.133 Arachnoid Cyst. (A and B) Sagittal and coronal T2W fetal MRI demonstrates a large suprasellar well-circumscribed cerebrospinal fluid isointense arachnoid cyst. Massive mass effect on the adjacent brainstem, thalami and basal ganglia, and high-grade elevation of the floor of the third ventricle with resultant supratentorial obstructive ventriculomegaly. (C and D) Postnatal sagittal and coronal 3D T2W images after fenestration show the collapse of the suprasellar arachnoid cyst with markedly improved mass effect on the adjacent structures.

Key Points

Background

- Focal fluid collection lined by arachnoidea that does not communicate with the ventricular system or subarachnoid space.
- Arachnoid cysts may be congenital and are intra-arachnoid, meaning the cyst is lined by arachnoidal cells adjacent to the "normal" arachnoidea.
- Arachnoidal cysts may also be seen secondary to a traumatic brain injury or neurosurgical procedures or form as a response to meningitis.
- Depending on the location and mass effect, arachnoid cysts may present with varying neurologic symptoms or hydrocephalus.
- In many cases a conservative "watch-and-follow approach" is sufficient, if neurologic symptoms including hydrocephalus develop endoscopic fenestration, or cystoperitoneal shunting may be indicated.

Imaging

- The lesion is hypoechoic on ultrasound, hypodense on CT, and T2-hyperintense, T1-hypointense on MRI. On diffusion-weighted imaging, the fluid collection follows fluid characteristics with DWI-hypointensity and high ADC values.
- Arachnoid cysts may exert mass effect on the adjacent brain tissue, and the chronicity of the cyst may result in a thinning and/or scalloping of the overlying skull.
- Arachnoid cysts may be solitary or consist of multiple small separate or communicating cysts.
- The lack of a communication with the ventricular system or subarachnoid space or intralesional hemorrhages may result in an increased protein content within the lesion. The lesion consequently may appear mild FLAIR hyperintensity compared to CSF within the ventricular system.
- The arachnoid lining the cyst does not show relevant contrast enhancement.
- Arachnoid cysts may be located anywhere within the cranial vault and may also extend from the supratentorial space into the posterior fossa or from the posterior fossa into the upper cervical spinal canal. Most common locations are the posterior fossa and anterior to the temporal lobes.
- If contrast agents are injected into the subarachnoid space the lack of a communication the ventricles is easily confirmed. Contrast is seen within the ventricles, basal cisterns, and subarachnoid space, but no contrast is seen within the arachnoid cyst.
- Arachnoidal cysts may enlarge over time, especially if an intralesional hemorrhage occurs, for example, after a minor head trauma.
- Congenital arachnoidal cysts may be identified on prenatal ultrasound, or fetal MRI.
- DDx: Arachnoid cysts must be differentiated from epidermoid cysts that may show similar T1- and T2-weighted MRI signal intensities compared to CSF. Diffusion-weighted imaging allows differentiation based upon the differential diffusion characteristics.

REFERENCE

1. Huisman TA, Poretti A. Chapter 7. Disorders of brain development. In: Magnetic Resonance Imaging of the Brain and Spine, 5th ed. Edited by Scott Atlas, MD. Wolters Kluwer, Lippincott Williams & Wilkins.

EPIDERMOID CYST

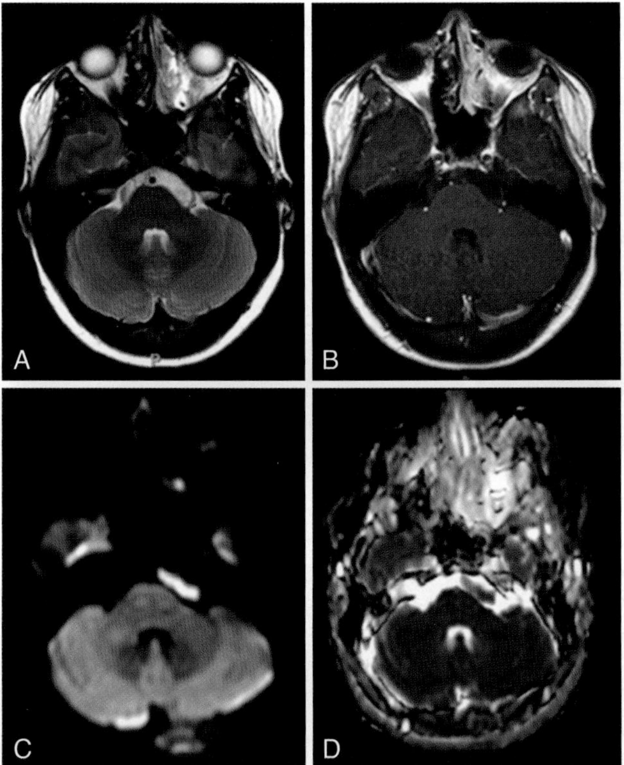

Fig. 2.134 Epidermoid Cyst. (A) Axial T2W, (B) T1W+C, (C) DWI MRI, and (D) ADC map of a child with an epidermoid cyst within the left parapontine cistern. Mild mass effect on the posterior and laterally displaced cisternal segment of the trigeminal nerve. The epidermoid appears T2 and T1 isointense with the cerebrospinal fluid and could be overlooked. The cyst is, however, very conspicuous on the diffusion-weighted imaging by the DWI hyperintensity secondary to the reduced diffusion within the epidermoid, which is confirmed by the low ADC values.

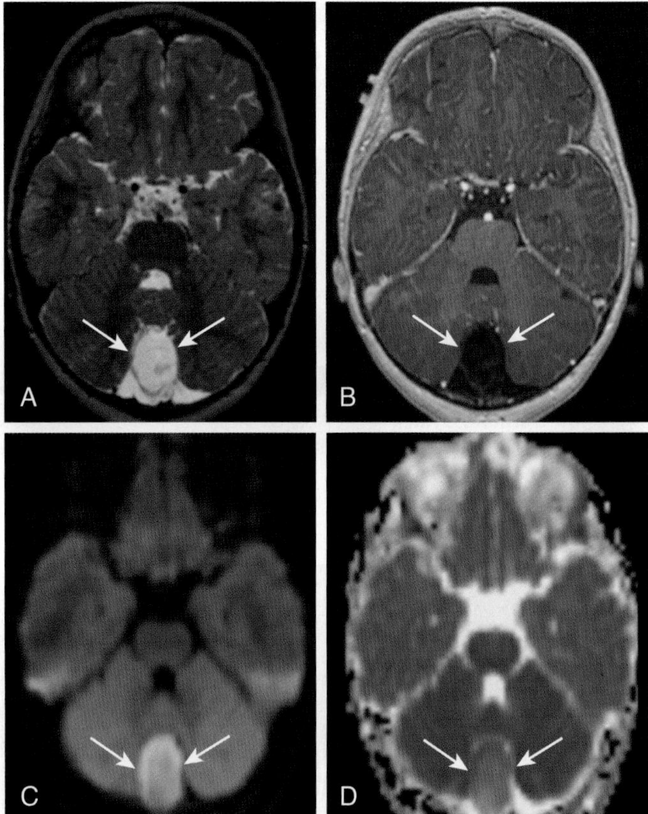

Fig. 2.135 Epidermoid Cyst. (A) Axial T2W, (B) axial T1W+C, (C) DWI, and (D) ADC map of a child with an epidermoid cyst posterior to the cerebellum in the midline. The signal characteristics on T1W and T2W imaging could be mistaken for an arachnoid cyst, however, the DWI and ADC images show reduced diffusion indicative of an epidermoid cyst.

Key Points

Background

- Epidermoid cysts are rare mass-like lesions consisting of squamous epithelium (epidermis) ectopically located within the cranial vault or spinal canal.
- Congenital epidermoid cysts are believed to result from an anomalous inclusion of cutaneous ectodermal during neural tube development.
- Acquired epidermoid cysts result from an iatrogenic inclusion of squamous epithelium in the neuroaxis after, for example, a neurosurgical procedure, open head or spine injury, or after a traumatic lumbar puncture.
- The ongoing epithelial desquamation and keratin accumulation explains the slow growth of the lesion over time.
- Epidermoid cysts may become clinically symptomatic due to progressing mass effect on adjacent neurologic structures like, for example, cranial nerves with resultant cranial nerve palsy.

Imaging

- Epidermoid cysts are most frequently located within the subarachnoid space, in particular within the basal cisterns or along sutures of the face and calvarium, most commonly the superolateral orbit.
- Epidermoid cysts mimic the density and signal intensity of cerebrospinal fluid on CT and T2W MRI, respectively, and can consequently be missed on conventional imaging.
- On diffusion-weighted imaging, the restricted diffusion characterized by DWI-hyperintensity and matching low ADC values significantly improve lesion conspicuity and differentiation from CSF or arachnoid cysts. In cases of "unexplained" focal displacement of the brainstem or cranial nerves, one should always exclude an epidermoid cyst by diffusion-weighted imaging.
- A coexisting dermal sinus tract should be excluded as this communication between the brain and skin can lead to intracranial infection including abscess formation and meningitis.

REFERENCE

1. Agarwal N, Tekes A, Poretti A, Meoded A, Huisman TAGM. Pitfalls in diffusion weighted and diffusion tensor imaging of the pediatric brain. *Neuropediatrics*. 2017 Oct;48(5):340–349.

DERMOID CYST

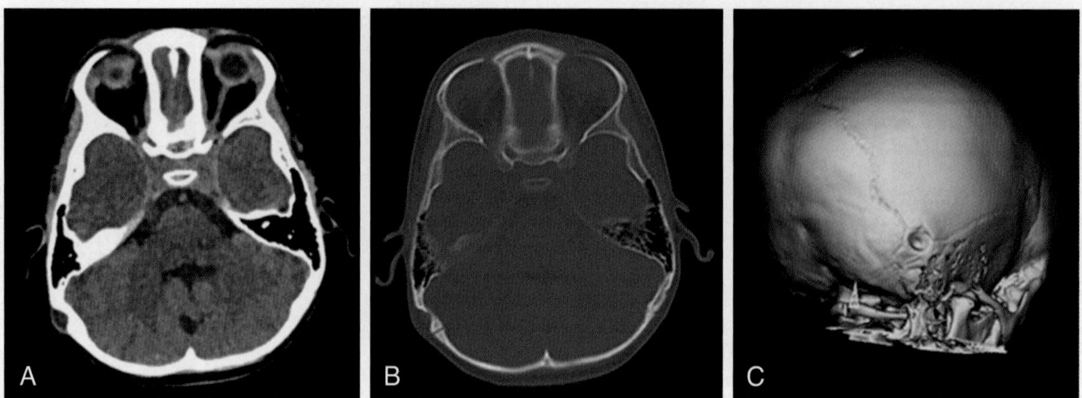

Fig. 2.136 Dermoid Cyst. (A to C) Axial CT including volumetric 3D reconstruction of a child with a dermoid cyst along the right lambdoid suture which appears predominantly hypodense with thinning and scalloping of the adjacent skull.

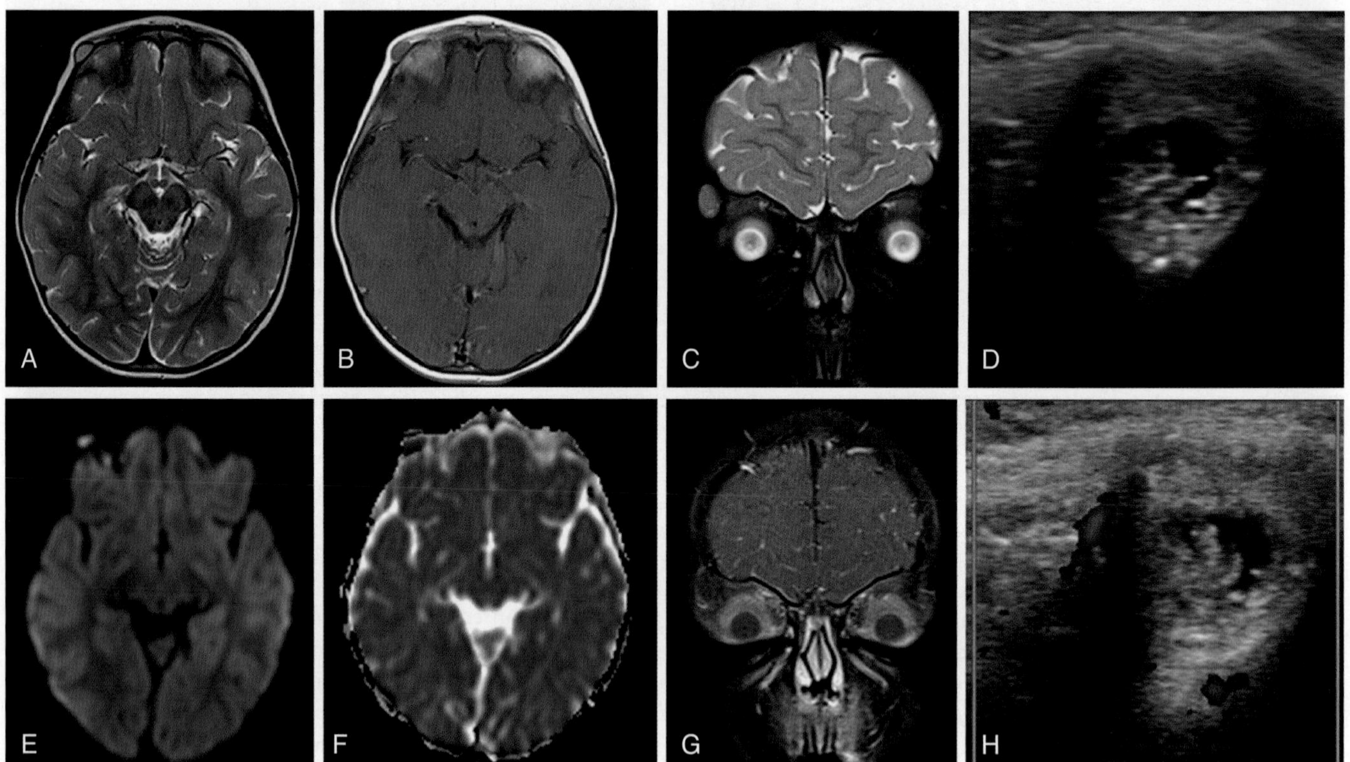

Fig. 2.137 Dermoid Cyst. (A and C) Axial and coronal T2W, (B and G) axial and coronal T1W+C, and (E and F) DWI and ADC map and (D and H) ultrasound study of a child with a dermoid cyst along the superior lateral contour of the right orbit that shows. Typical mild T2 hyperintensity with reduced diffusion and subtle peripheral contrast enhancement. On ultrasound the lesion appears heterogeneous with areas of hyperechogenicity without significant intralesional vascularity.

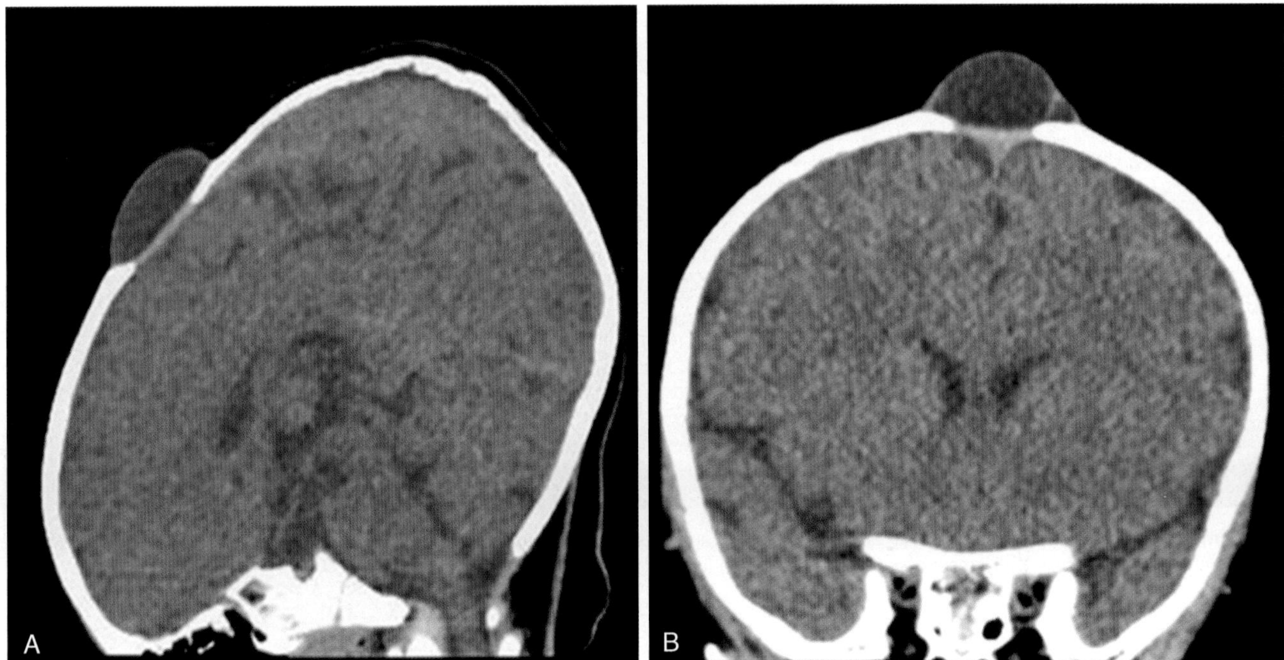

Fig. 2.138 Dermoid Cyst. (A and B) Sagittal and coronal CT of the skull in a child with a dermoid cyst overlaying the anterior fontanelle. The dermoid cyst appears homogeneously hypodense.

Key Points

Background

- Dermoid cysts are similar to epidermoid cysts with the exception that they include dermal appendages like hair follicles, sebaceous and sweat glands, and occasionally dental enamel in addition to the squamous epithelium.
- Within the cyst the mixture of sebaceous secretion and desquamated epithelial cells result in variable neuroimaging features depending on the relative proportion of the various components.

Imaging

- Dermoid cysts classically contain fat and consequently are hypodense to CSF on CT and T1 hyperintense on MRI. Fat-suppressed sequences will confirm the fat inclusions. Dermoid cysts often demonstrate restricted diffusion. Dermoids are often midline, while epidermoids are lateral/off midline. Because imaging features can overlap between dermoid and epidermoid cysts, the authors generally provide a diagnosis of "dermoid/epidermoid cyst" that has to be ultimately determined by pathology.
- Peripheral contrast enhancement may be seen but is thin and mild unless superinfected, in which case there should be surrounding edema.
- Dermoid cysts may exert a mass effect on neuronal structures similar to epidermoids.
- Intracranial dermoids are typically round/oval, less frequently lobulated, and may spontaneously rupture if large, inducing a chemical meningitis.
- Epidermoid and dermoid cysts may also be seen included within the scalp or calvarium.
- Scalp lesions are typically found along sutures, while intraosseous or calvarial lesions may be seen anywhere within the skull. The inner and/or external table may be thinned, resembling a lytic lesion. The skull may be focally remodeled due to the chronic pressure.
- Scalp lesions are often seen along the lateral orbits or along the fontanelles. On ultrasound examination they are hypoperfused with a heterogeneous echogenicity within the center of the lesion.

REFERENCE

1. Agarwal N, Tekes A, Poretti A, Meoded A, Huisman TAGM. Pitfalls in diffusion weighted and diffusion tensor imaging of the pediatric brain. *Neuropediatrics*. 2017 Oct;48(5):340–349.

SUMMARY OF TRISOMIES

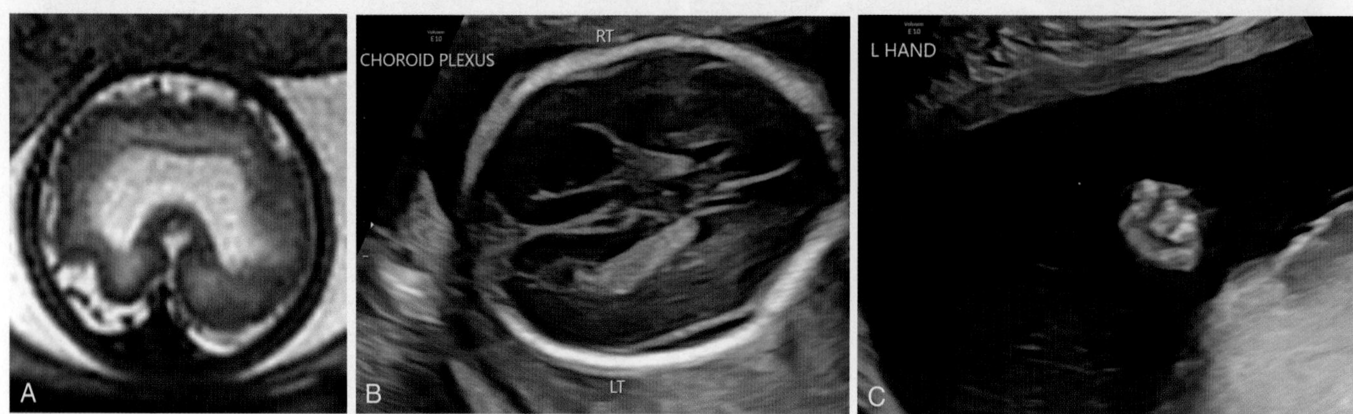

Common imaging findings in trisomies. (A) Axial T2W fetal MRI image of alobar holoprosencephaly. (B) Transverse ultrasound image of the head demonstrating a choroid plexus cyst. (C) Ultrasound image of a clenched fist.

Key Points

Most common trisomies are trisomy 13, 18, and 21. Clues to presence of a trisomy is the presence of multiple fetal anomalies involving multiple structures and organ systems, including the following:

- Brain (malformations, ventriculomegaly, large choroid plexus cysts)
- Orbits (micro-ophthalmia, hypo/hypertelorism)
- Ears (external auditory canal anomalies)
- Face (cleft lip and palate, midface hypoplasia, absent nasal bones)
- Heart (cardiac anomaly)
- GI/GU anomaly
- Limbs (clenched fist, rocker bottom foot)
- Other: In utero growth restriction and nuchal thickening

TRISOMY 13

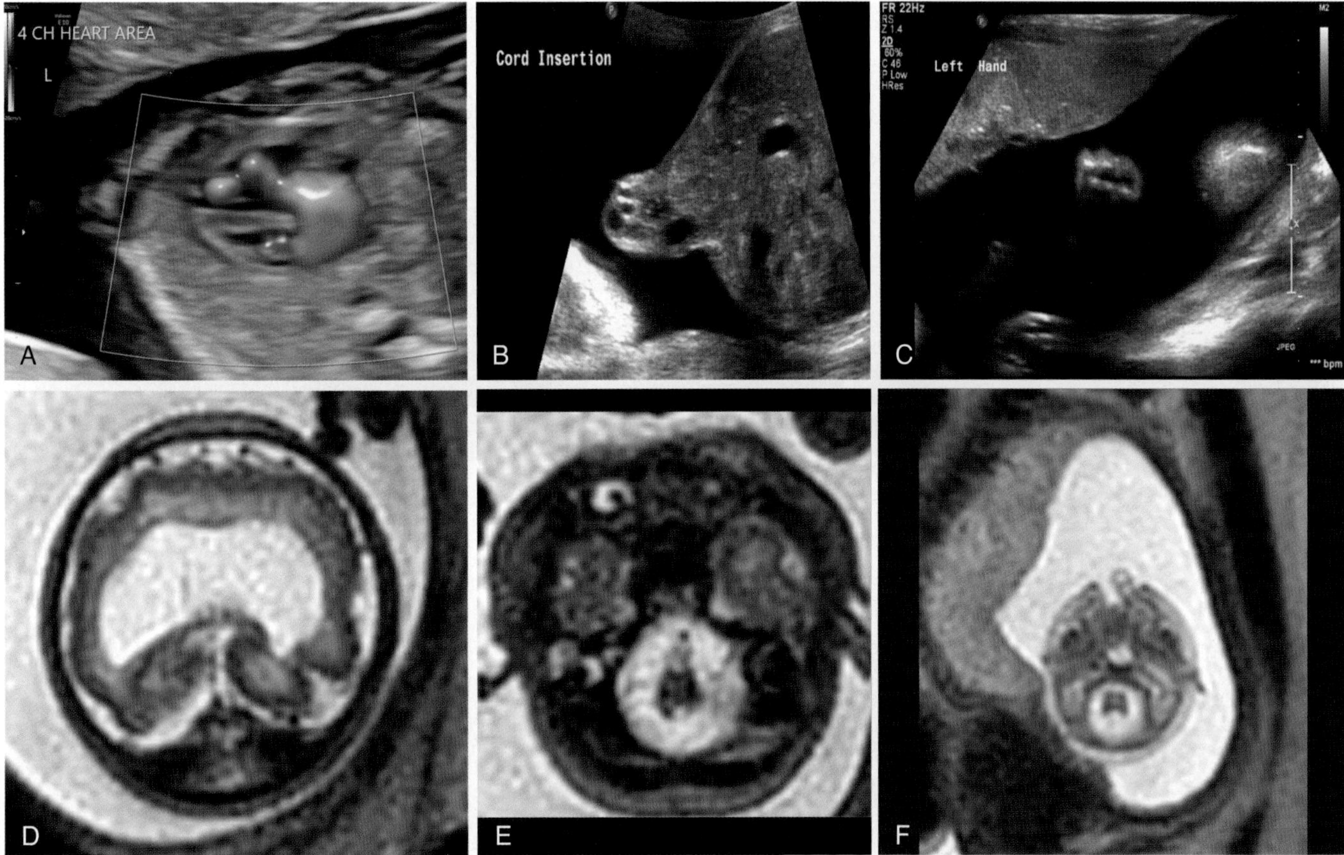

Fig. 2.139 Trisomy 13. Multiple patients with trisomy 13. (A to C) Fetal ultrasound images demonstrate hypoplastic left heart seen as small size of the left ventricle, omphalocele seen on ultrasound image of the abdomen, and clenched fist of the hand. (D to F) Coronal and axial T2W fetal images demonstrate holoprosencephaly, micro-ophthalmia, and cleft lip and palate.

Key Points

Background

- Trisomy 13 also known as Patau syndrome. Caused by nondisjunction (75%) or translocation (25%)
- Third most common autosomal trisomy in newborns: 0.5–1/10,000 live births
- Clues to syndromes include craniosynostosis, encephalocele, large choroid plexus cysts, delayed sulcation, midface hypoplasia, absent nasal bone, hypo/hypertelorism, micrognathia, macroglossia, EAC anomalies, and nuchal thickening

Imaging

- Cardiac defects (50%–80%): VSD, hypoplastic left heart
- CNS anomalies (70%): Holoprosencephaly spectrum, microcephaly, ventriculomegaly, mega cisterna magna
- Craniofacial anomalies: Cleft lip/palate, micro-ophthalmia, micrognathia, hypo/hypertelorism
- GI/GU: Echogenic or polycystic kidneys, omphalocele, bladder exstrophy, echogenic bowel
- Other: IUGR, polydactyly, rocker bottom feet, clenched fist with overlapping digits, increased nuchal thickness

REFERENCE

1. Lhman CD, Nyberg DA, Winter TC, et al. Trisomy 13 syndrome: prenatal US findings in a review of 33 case. *Radiology*. 1995;194:217–222.

TRISOMY 18

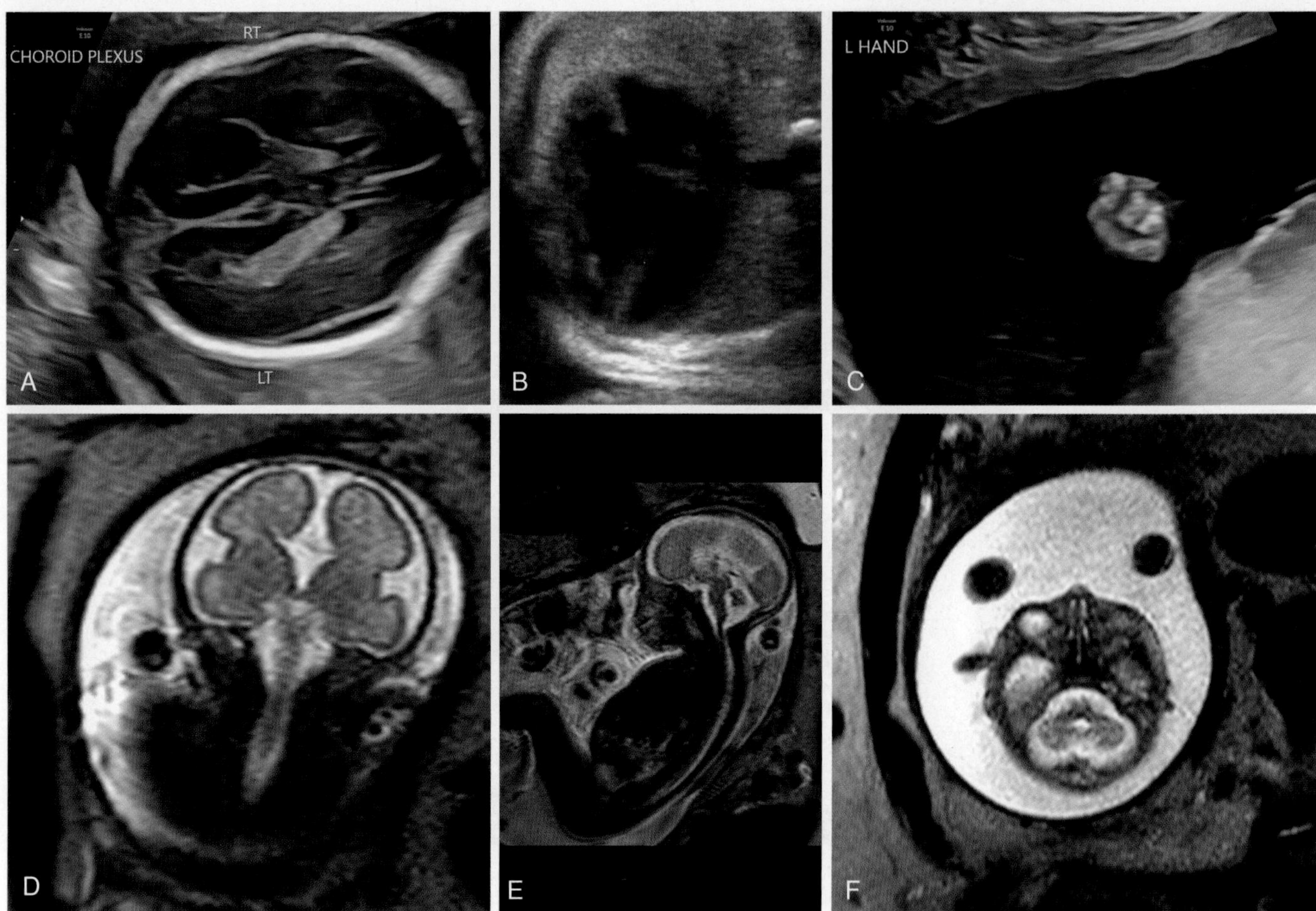

Fig. 2.140 Trisomy 18. Multiple patients with trisomy 18. (A to C) Fetal ultrasound images demonstrating a choroid plexus cyst, VSD, and clenched fist. (D) Multiplanar T2W fetal MR images demonstrate callosal agenesis, hypoplasia of the vermis and pons, and external auditory canal atresia.

Key Points

Background

- Trisomy 18 also known as Edwards syndrome. Second most common trisomy in newborns. Incidence 0.6–2.5/10,000
- More than 90% are due to maternal nondisjunction of chromosome 18
- 50% of neonates survive past the first week of birth. Only 3% to 10% of infants survive past the first year of life.

Imaging

- Multiple systems are affected, including the following:
  - Cardiac: Echogenic intracardiac focus, VSD, ASD
  - GI/GU anomalies: Echogenic bowel, pyelectasis
  - CNS: Choroid plexus cyst, strawberry-shaped skull, ventriculomegaly, Dandy-Walker, agenesis of the corpus callosum, mega cisterna magna
  - Craniofacial: Low-set ears, microcephaly, micrognathia, cleft lip/palate
  - Other: Clenched fist with overlapping digits, rocker bottom foot, clubfeet, syndactyly, short limbs, cystic hygroma IUGR, fetal hydrops

REFERENCE

1. Hsiao CC, Tsao LY, Chen HN, et al. Changing clinical presentations and survival pattern in trisomy 19. *Pediatr Neonatol.* 2009;50:147–151.

TRISOMY 21

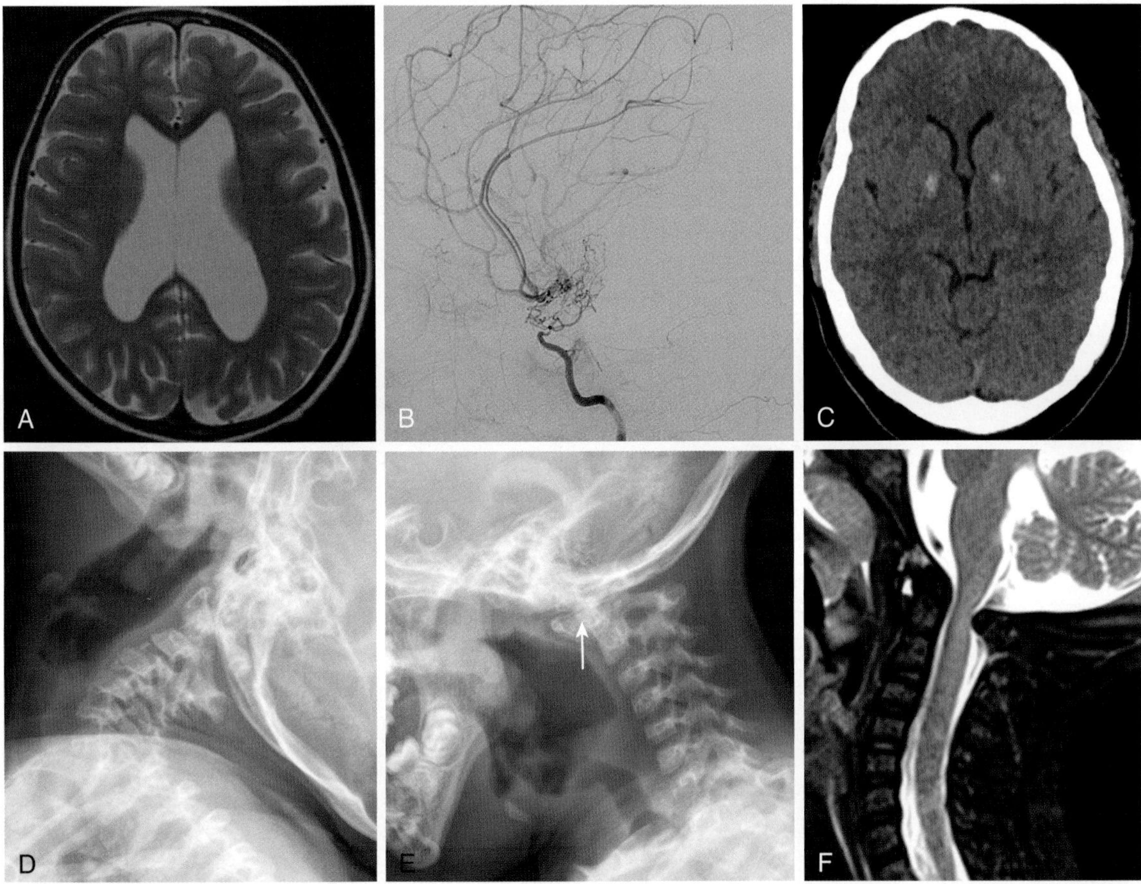

Fig. 2.141 Trisomy 21. Multiple patients with trisomy 21. (A) Axial T2W images demonstrating cerebral volume loss with ventriculomegaly. (B) Lateral catheter angiogram image from a right ICA injection demonstrates moyamoya vasculopathy. (C) Axial CT image demonstrates basal ganglia calcification. (D and E) Lateral radiographs in extension and flexion demonstrate atlantoaxial instability with anterior atlantodental interval measuring 3 mm in extension and 5.5 mm in flexion. (F) Sagittal STIR image of the same patient demonstrates anterior position of the posterior arch of C1, causing posterior cord compression and myelomalacia.

Key Points

Background

- Most common autosomal trisomy in newborns. Incidence 1:319–1000.
- Most commonly from maternal nondisjunction (95%). Strong association with increasing maternal age.
- Characterized by intellectual disability and typical facial appearance. Facial features include flattened face, almond-shaped eyes, macroglossia, downsloping palpebral fissures, and short neck with redundant skin folds.
- Average IQ ranges from 50 to 70. Alzheimer disease occurs in trisomy 21, affecting nearly all those older than 40 years of age.

Imaging

- Multiple systems are affected, including the following:
    - Cardiac (40% of patients): AV canal (45%), VSD (35%), tetralogy of Fallot, echogenic intracardiac focus
    - Brain: Cerebral and cerebellar brain volume, progressive brain atrophy including the hippocampus (Alzheimer), basal ganglia calcification, malformed corpus callosum, moyamoya syndrome, delayed myelination
    - Craniofacial: Microcephaly, brachycephaly, platybasia, macroglossia, inner ear anomalies
    - Spine: Craniocervical junction instability, upper cervical ossification anomalies
    - GI/GU: Echogenic bowel, duodenal atresia (30%), liver calcification, Hirschsprung disease,
    - Other: Increased nuchal fold, polydactyly, clinodactyly, sandal gap foot, clubfoot

REFERENCE

1. Radhakrishnan R, Towbin AJ. Imaging findings in Down syndrome. *Pediatr Radiol*. 2014 May;44(5):506–521.

3 Hypoxic Ischemic Injury and Cerebrovascular Disorders

HYPOXIC ISCHEMIC INJURY

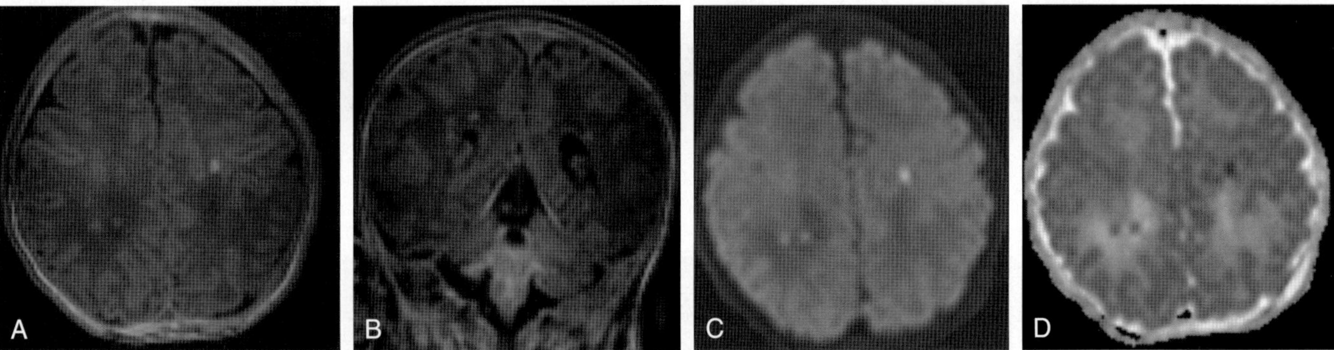

Fig. 3.1 Hypoxic Ischemic Injury. (A and B) Axial and coronal T1W images and (C and D) axial DWI and ADC images demonstrate a few small foci of intrinsic T1 shortening and diffusion restriction in the bilateral periventricular white matter and centrum semiovale indicative of mild hypoxic ischemic injury.

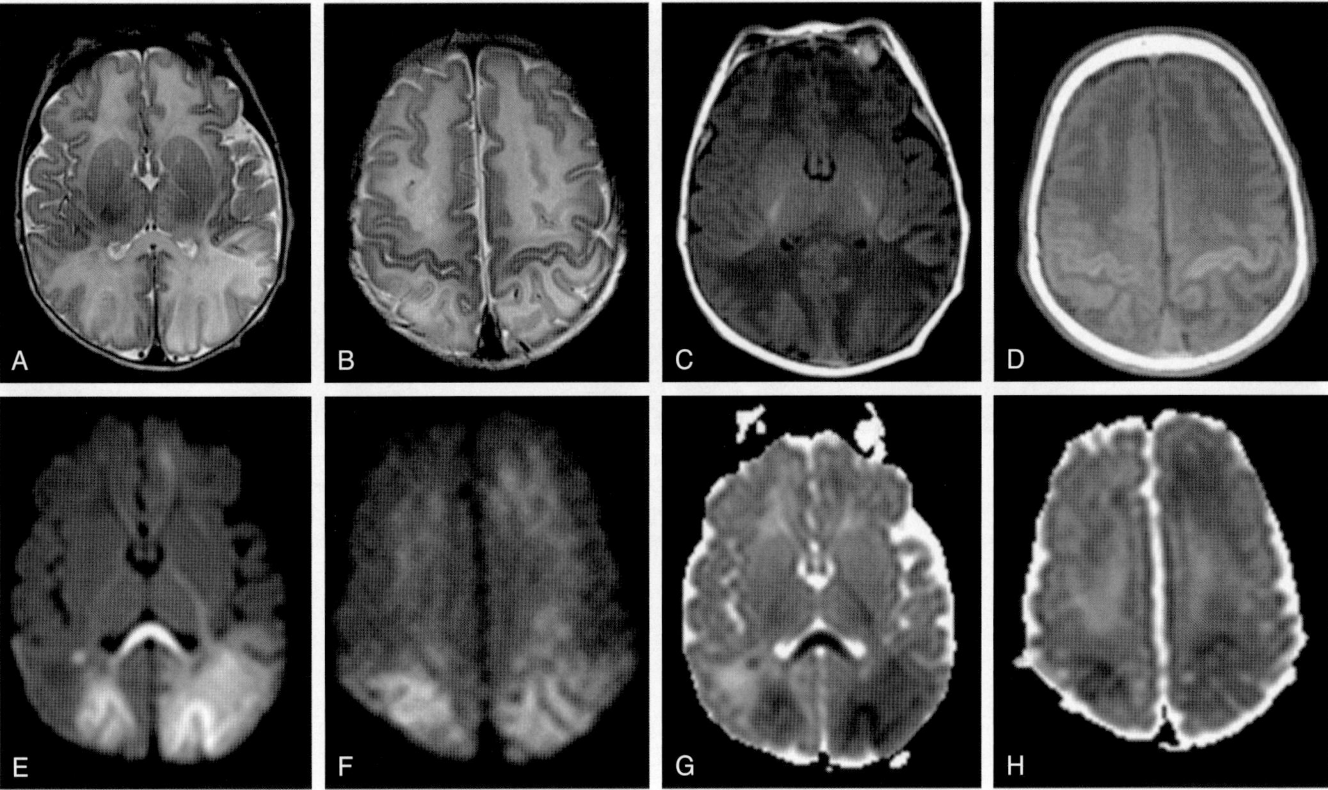

Fig. 3.2 Moderate Hypoxic Ischemic Injury. (A and B) Axial T2W and (C and D) axial T1W images demonstrate subtle T2 hyperintense, T1 hypointense signal in the posterior cerebral hemispheres with areas of cortical thinning. (E and F) axial DWI and (G and H) axial ADC images demonstrate more conspicuous diffusion restriction in a symmetric predominant watershed distribution indicative of moderate acute hypoxic ischemic injury in a term neonate.

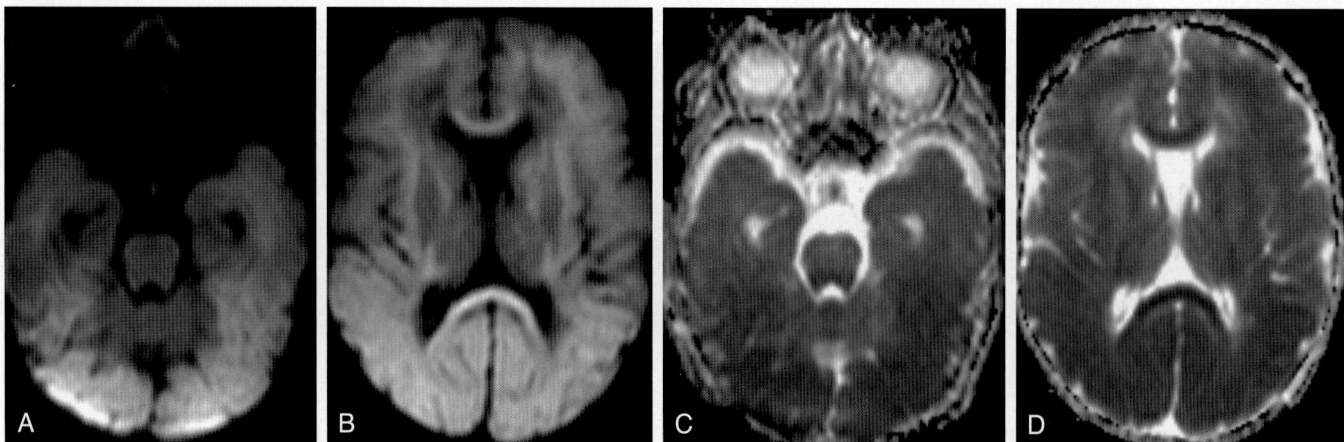

Fig. 3.3 Severe Hypoxic Ischemic Injury. (A and B) Axial DWI, and (C and D) axial ADC images demonstrate diffusion restriction indicative of cytotoxic edema affecting the bilateral cerebral cortex and internal capsules consistent with severe acute hypoxic ischemic injury in a term neonate. The cerebellum frequently provides an internal reference for normal DWI/ADC intensity which is helpful to avoid misdiagnosis that can occur from the diffuse symmetric pattern of injury.

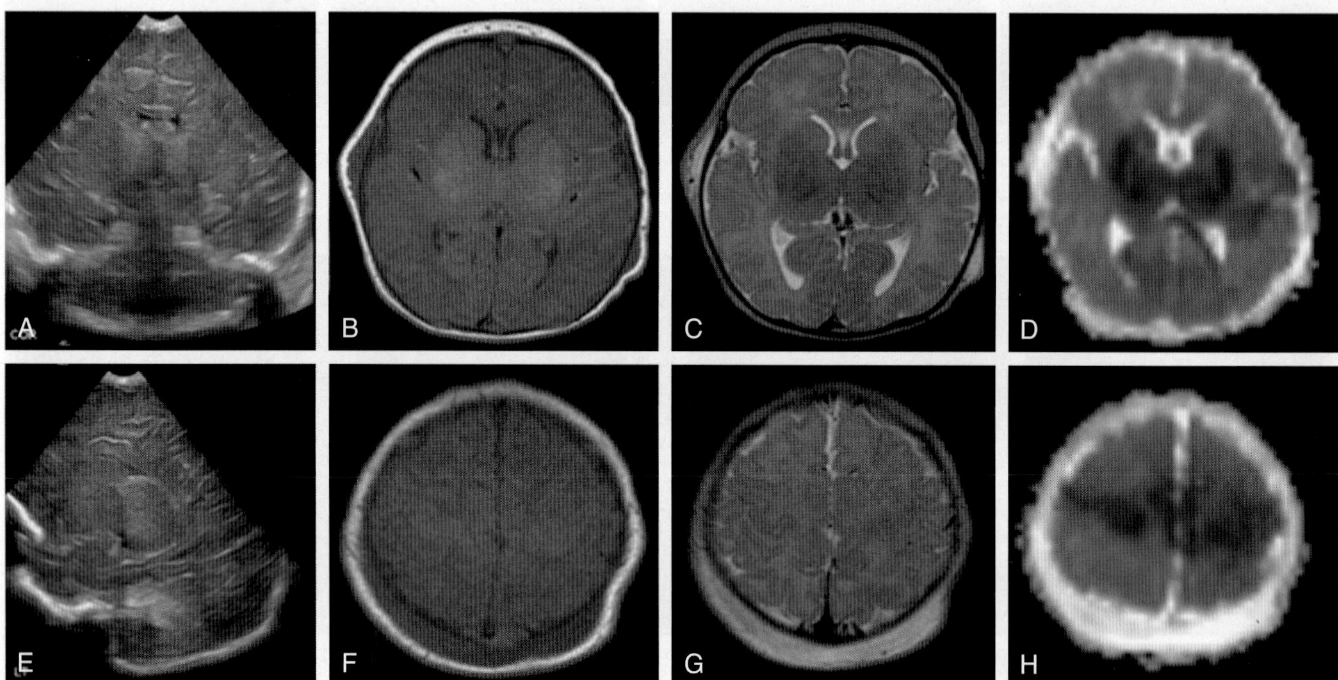

Fig. 3.4 Hypoxic Ischemic Injury. (A and E) Coronal and sagittal head ultrasound images demonstrate subtle hyperechogenicity of the basal ganglia. (B and F) Axial and coronal T1W, (C and G) axial T2W, and (D and H) axial ADC images demonstrate symmetric central gray matter injury characterized by matching T1 hyperintensity, mild T2 hyperintensity, and low ADC values (cytotoxic edema) on the apparent diffusion coefficient maps. Additional cytotoxic edema is seen in the perirolandic cortex. The pattern of ischemic injury is consistent with a severe acute hypoxic ischemic injury in a term neonate.

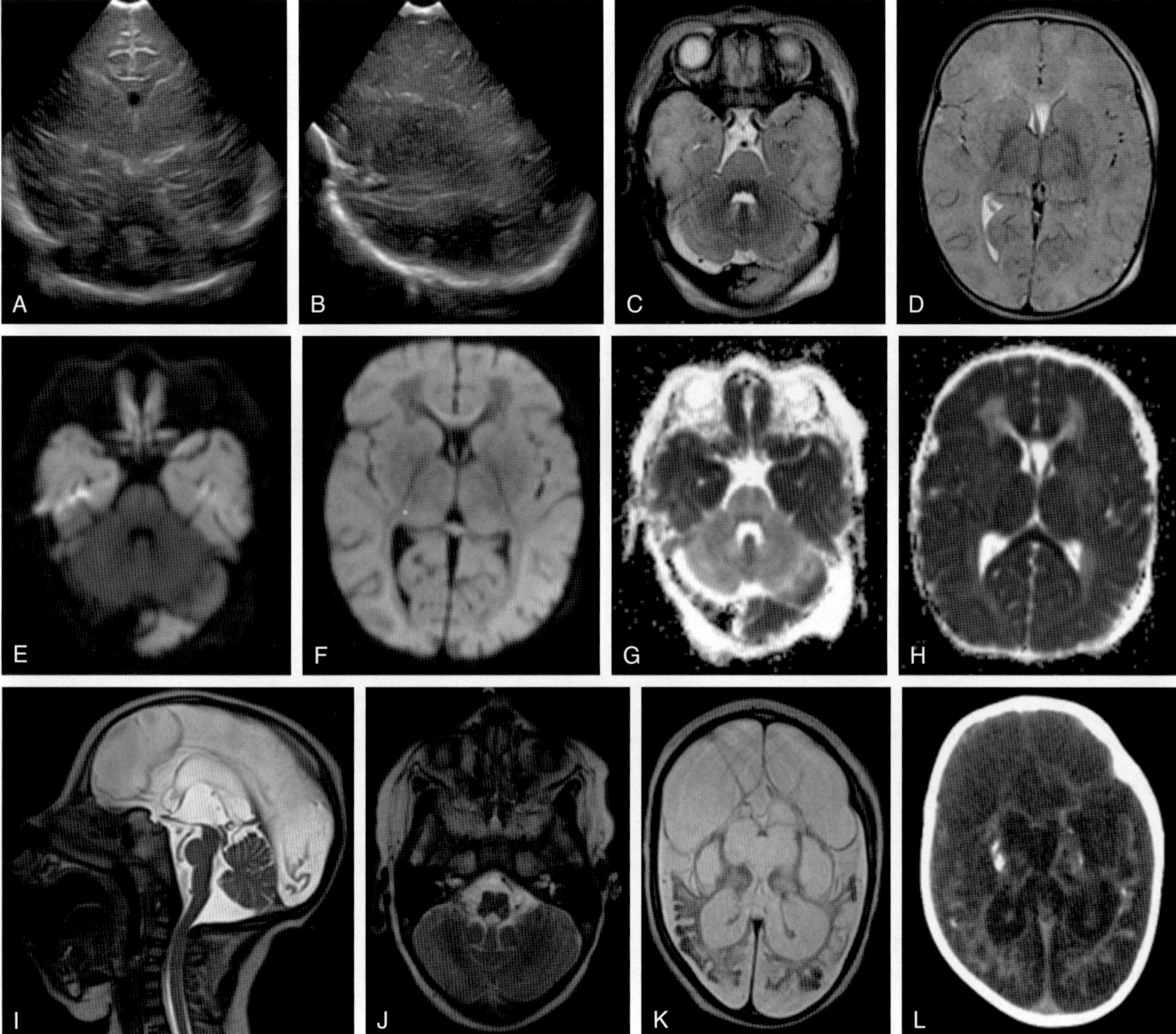

Fig. 3.5 Hypoxic Ischemic Injury. Near total hypoxic ischemic injury to the supratentorial central/cortical gray matter as well as hemispheric white matter in a term neonate. (A and B) Coronal and sagittal head ultrasound demonstrate abnormal hyperechogenic parenchyma with slit-like ventricles. (C and D) Axial T2W, (E and F) axial DWI, and (G and H) axial ADC images demonstrate the supratentorial brain is diffusely T2 hyperintense with extensive cytotoxic edema (DWI hyperintense, low ADC values). The cerebellum and parts of the majority of the brainstem appear spared. DWI-hyperintense Wallerian degeneration is especially well noted along the course of the descending corticospinal tracts in the pons. (I-K) Sagittal and axial T2W images from a follow-up MRI show chronic, near-complete cystic encephalomalacia of the supratentorial brain with preserved cerebellum and brainstem. (L) Follow-up head CT shows dystrophic calcifications within the residual tissue of the thalami and parts of the cortical ribbon.

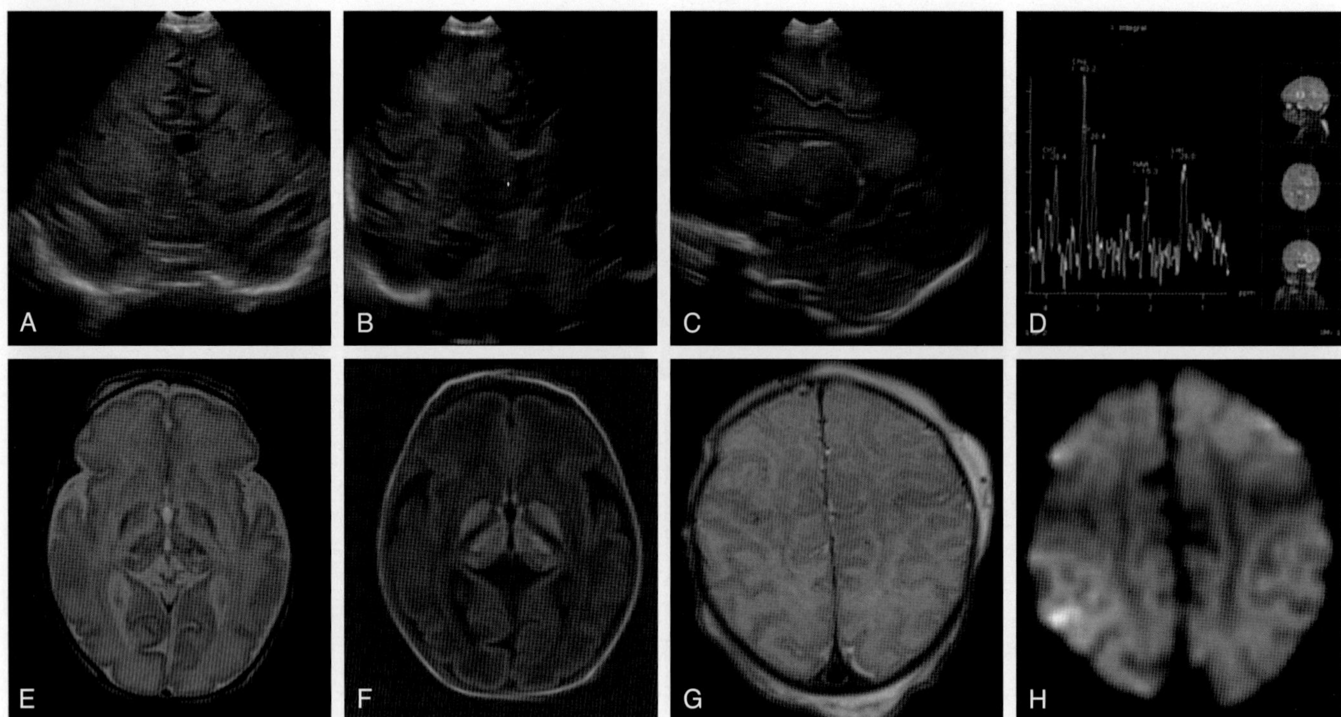

Fig. 3.6 Hypoxic Ischemic Injury. (A-C) Coronal and sagittal transfontanellar head ultrasound show diffuse hyperechogenicity of the injured white matter, increased corticomedullary differentiation, and slit-like ventricles. (D) 1H MR Spectroscopy sampled of the left basal ganglia identifies increased lactate at 1.3 ppm, reduced NAA, and increased choline. (E) Axial T2W and (F) axial T1W images show abnormal T2 hyperintense and T1 hypointense signal relative to the adjacent gray matter in the posterior limb of the internal capsule known as the "lack of the PLIC signal," which is considered to be a predictor of poor outcome. (G) Axial T2W and (H) axial DWI images near the veretx show abnormal parenchymal T2 hyperintensity and diffuse increased signal on diffusion-weighted imaging related to cytotoxic edema. The findings are consistent with near total hypoxic ischemic injury to the supratentorial central/cortical gray matter as well as hemispheric white matter in a term neonate.

Key Points

Background

- Hypoxic ischemic injury (HII) typically refers to a combination of a hypoxic and hypoperfusion injury to the fetal or neonatal brain.
- Clinical manifestations of HII include low Apgar scores (0–3 at 5 minutes and ≤ 5 at 10 minutes), umbilical cord pH < 7.1, poor cry, weak suck, seizures, diminished movement, absent neonatal reflexes, and hypotonia.
- Depending on the maturity of the brain, duration and/or degree of hypoxic-ischemic injury, and coexisting fetal/neonatal or maternal risk factors (e.g., congenital heart disease, neonatal sepsis, chorioamnionitis, placental abruption, surfactant deficiency disease), various patterns of injury may be observed.

Imaging

- In a full-term neonate, mild HII affects the deep white matter (typically periatrial white matter), moderate HII affects the watershed cerebral cortex and subcortical white matter, and severe HII affects the basal ganglia, thalami, and sensorimotor cortex. The combinations of severity and duration of the hypoxia and hypoperfusion has also been reported to follow the following patterns:
  - Mild/moderate, and gradual: cerebral white matter injury
  - Moderate, prolonged and/or intermittent: severe cerebral hemisphere +/- deep gray nuclei
  - Severe, and brief: deep gray nuclei +/- brainstem
  - Severe, and prolonged: cerebral hemirspheres, deep gray matter nuclei, and brainstem
- In a premature infant, mild to moderate HII affects the periventricular white matter leading to periventricular leukomalacia and germinal matrix hemorrhage, and severe HII affects the thalami.
- Transfontanellar ultrasound imaging may show hyperechogenicity of the hemispheric white matter relative to the cortical gray matter with resultant increased corticomedullary differentiation, slit-like ventricles, and lowered resistive index (RI) values sampled within a branch of the circle of Willis 24 to 48 hours after injury. Micro- or macrocystic leukoencephalopathy may be seen starting 8 to 10 days after the initial injury.
- MRI typically shows the distribution of injury in better detail. Diffusion-weighted imaging (DWI) shows reduced diffusion (low ADC) within the first 8 to 10 days after injury followed by pseudonormalization of diffusion (ADC isointensity) followed by progressive increased diffusion (increased ADC) after a brief period of pseudonormalization. DWI is most sensitive for the

extent of injury at 3 to 5 days from the HII. Therapeutic hypothermia may delay the temporal evolution of the diffusion characteristics (pseudonormalization occurring approximately at day 10 with cooling versus day 6–8 without cooling).

- Conventional T1W and T2W MRI may underestimate injury within the first 24 to 48 hours of injury and appear normal in this time frame. Afterwards depending on the type of insult, the hemispheric white matter may be T2 hyperintense, T1 hypointense. Focal T1-hyperintensity may be seen within the cortical or central gray matter, in particular affecting the ventrolateral thalami and posterior putamina as well as perirolandic cortex.
- Relative T2-hyperintensity and T1-hypointensity of the posterior limb of the internal capsule (PLIC-signal) are considered to be linked to a poor prognosis.
- Acute ^{1}H MRS typically reveals increased levels of lactate, while subacute and chronic 1H MRS may show reduced N-Acetyl aspartate (NAA), increased choline (Cho), and decreased Creatine (Cr). A lactate/NAA ratio of >0.3 in the acute phase was associated with poor outcome.
- ASL perfusion has shown increased cerebral blood flow in the deep gray matter at 4 to 7 days after HII and associated with adverse clinical outcome.
- In the chronic phase, various combinations of a micro- or macrocystic hemispheric leukoencephalopathy may be seen accompanied by hemispheric white matter volume loss, size-reduced central gray matter, cortical gray matter thinning, ex vacuo enlargement of the cerebrospinal fluid (CSF) spaces, microcephaly, and global hypomyelination.
- Differential diagnosis includes inborn errors of metabolism, infection/sepsis, and congenital heart disease.

REFERENCES

1. Volpe JJ. Neonatal encephalopathy: an inadequate term for hypoxic-ischemic encephalopathy. *Ann Neurol*. 2012;72:156–166.
2. Salas J, Tekes A, Hwang M, Northington FJ, Huisman TAGM. Head Ultrasound in neonatal hypoxic-ischemic injury and its mimickers for clinicians: A review of the patterns of injury and the evolution of findings over time. *Neonatology*. 2018;114(3): 185–197.

GLOBAL HYPOXIC-ISCHEMIC STROKE AFTER DROWNING OR CARDIAC ARREST

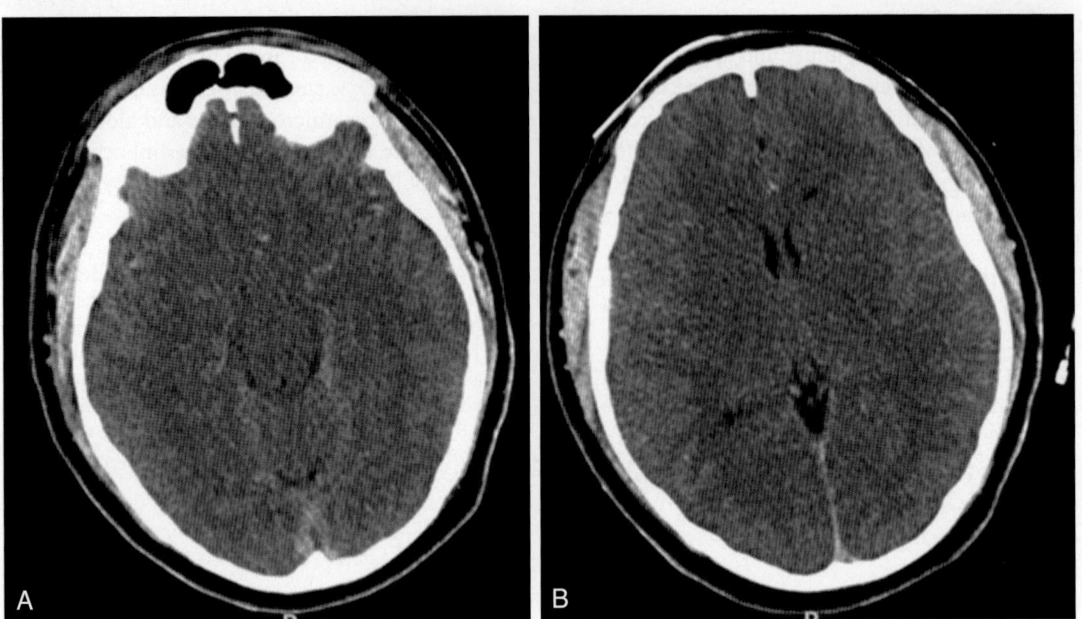

Fig. 3.7 Hypoxic Ischemic Injury. (A and B) Axial head CT performed <12 hours after near-drowning accident with cardiopulmonary arrest reveals faint hypodensity of the central gray matter and brainstem, mild global brain swelling, effaced basal cisterns, relative hyperdensity of the arterial circle of Willis, and venous circle of Trolard (deep veins of the basal cisterns).

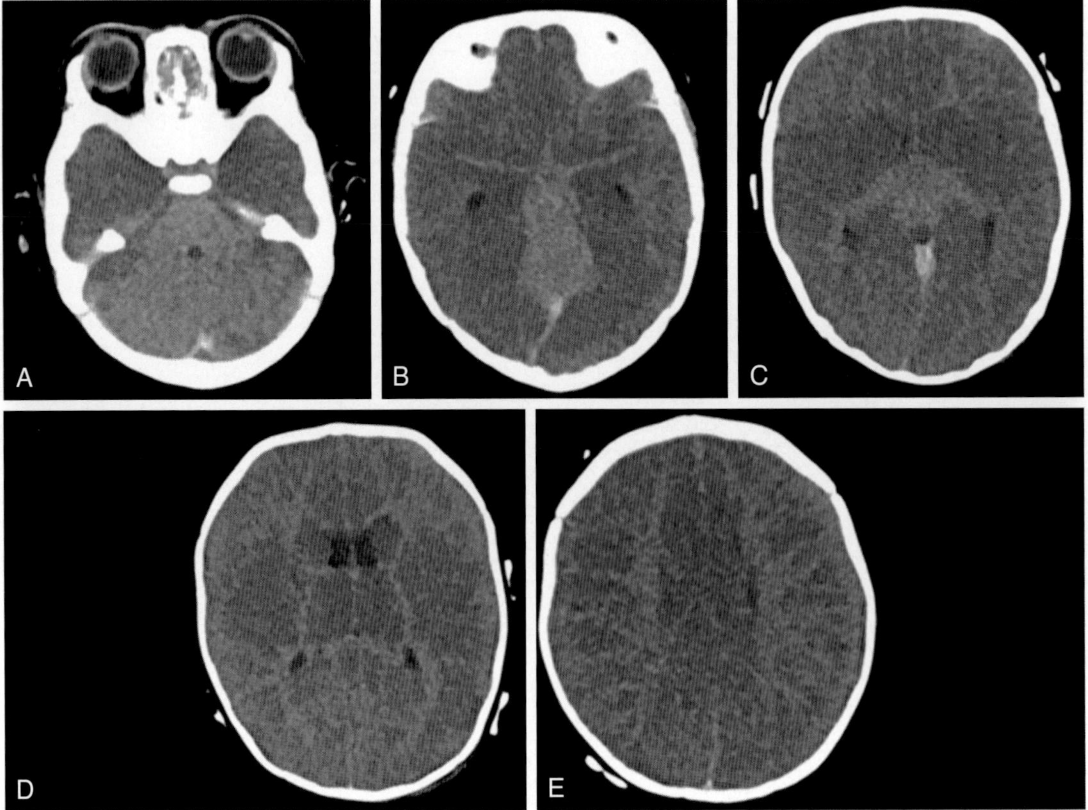

Fig. 3.8 Hypoxic Ischemic Injury. (A-E) Axial head CT images in the subacute phase after prolonged cardiopulmonary arrest show global hypodensity of the supratentorial gray and white matter, relative hyperdensity of the vessels in the basal cisterns, and preserved normal density of the cerebellum and brainstem known as a "white cerebellum."

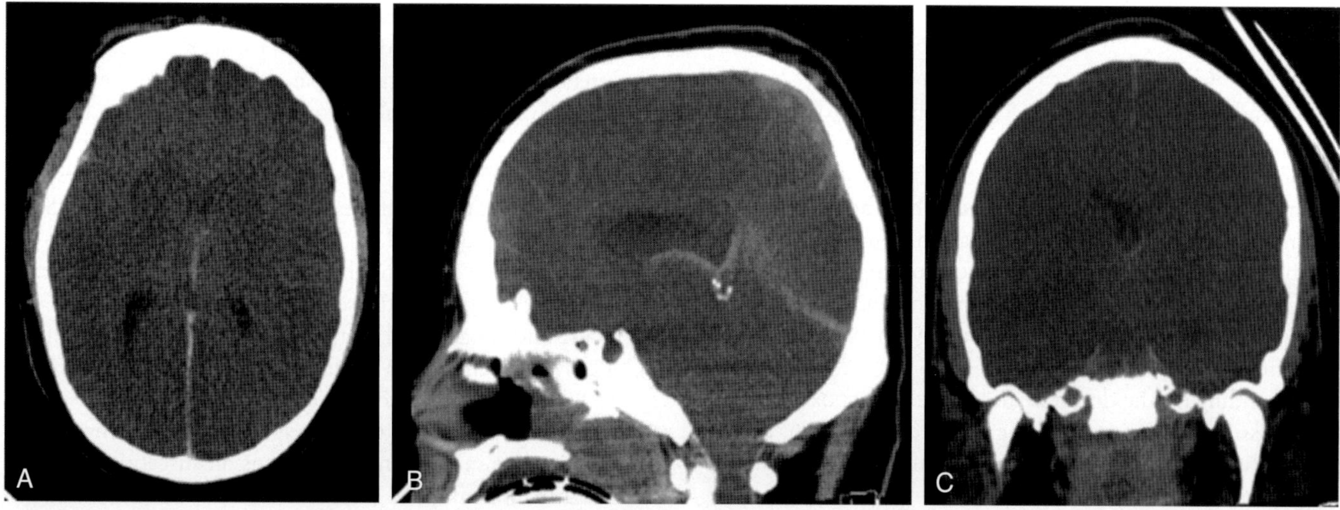

Fig. 3.9 Hypoxic Ischemic Injury. (A-C) Axial, sagittal and coronal reformat head CT images in the subacute phase after severe prolonged cardiopulmonary arrest shows global supra- and infratentorial hypodense brain swelling, complete effacement of all cisterns, and downward herniation of the supratentorial brain through the tentorium cerebelli, and the cerebellum through the foramen magnum. The supratentorial ventricular system is mildly widened secondary to an obstructed cerebrospinal fluid outflow as a result of the downward herniation.

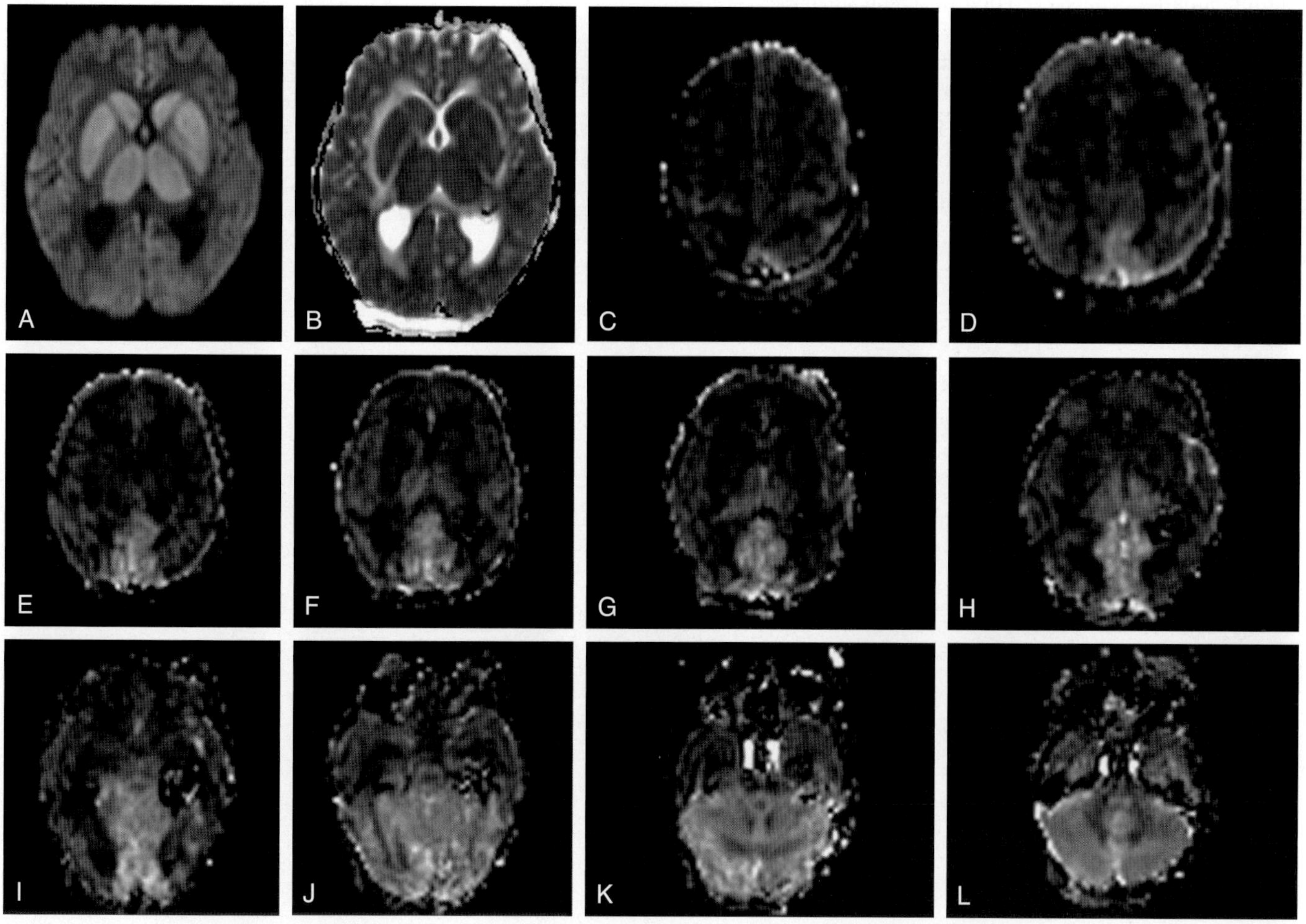

Fig. 3.10 Hypoxic Ischemic Injury. (A) Axial DWI, and (B) axial ADC images demonstrate severe restricted diffusion indicating cytotoxic edema with DWI-hyperintense and low ADC values of the central gray matter and cerebral cortex after cardiopulmonary arrest. (C-L) Multiple ASL CBF images show reduced CBF to the majority of the cerebral hemispheres and preserved CBF to the cerebellum and brainstem.

Key Points

Background

- Beyond the perinatal time period, global hypoxic or anoxic injury may result from a variety of reasons, including a cardiopulmonary arrest, prolonged seizures, strangulation, child abuse, near drowning, severe asthma attack, and smoke or carbon monoxide inhalation.
- Hypoxia refers to a critically reduced or impaired delivery of oxygen to the central nervous system; anoxia is an extreme form of hypoxia with virtually no oxygen delivered to the brain at all.
- Depending on the duration and degree of hypoxia as well as possible coexisting pathologies, different patterns and distributions of injuries may be seen affecting white and gray matter.

Imaging

- CT may be negative within the first 12 to 24 hours after hypoxic injury; MRI and in particular diffusion-weighted imaging may show hypoxic injury within 3 to 6 hours.
- Earliest signs of injury on CT include a global brain swelling with loss of the normal gray-white matter differentiation, effaced cerebral sulci, and small or compressed ventricles. On follow-up, progressive white and gray matter hypodensity will develop with reappearance of the sulci and ventricles. In the chronic phase, progressive volume loss, possibly with cystic transformation of the injured brain tissue, ensues.
- Due to protective rearrangement of the brain perfusion and differing vulnerability of the brain tissue, the brainstem and cerebellum may be partially spared, resulting in the so-called "white cerebellum" sign, also known as reversal sign or dense cerebellum sign on CT due to the contrast of the injured edema low density supratentorial brain with respect to the normal density if the brainstem and cerebellum. Slow flow within the arterial circle of Willis and venous circle of Trolard may result in relative hyperdensity of the vessels compared to the hypodense brain tissue.
- Acute and subacute MRI and DWI typically reveal diffuse T2-hyperintense brain swelling, DWI-hyperintense/ ADC-hypointense cytotoxic edema of the injured tissue, hypoperfusion on perfusion-weighted imaging, engorged hypointense intraparenchymal veins on susceptibility-weighted imaging and increased lactate and decreased N-acetyl aspartate on ^{1}H MRS of the injured tissue. On follow-up, cystic encephalomalacia with volume loss is present.
- Tonsillar and uncal herniation may result from the global supratentorial brain swelling with resultant effacement of the basal cisterns.
- With carbon monoxide poisoning there is injury to the central gray matter, in particular the globus pallidi.

REFERENCE

1. Orru E, Huisman TAGM, Prevalence Izbudak I. Patterns and Clinical Relevance of Hypoxic Ischemic Injuries in Children Exposed to Abusive Head Trauma. *J Neuroimaging*. 2018 Aug 19 [Epub ahead of print].

ACUTE STROKE

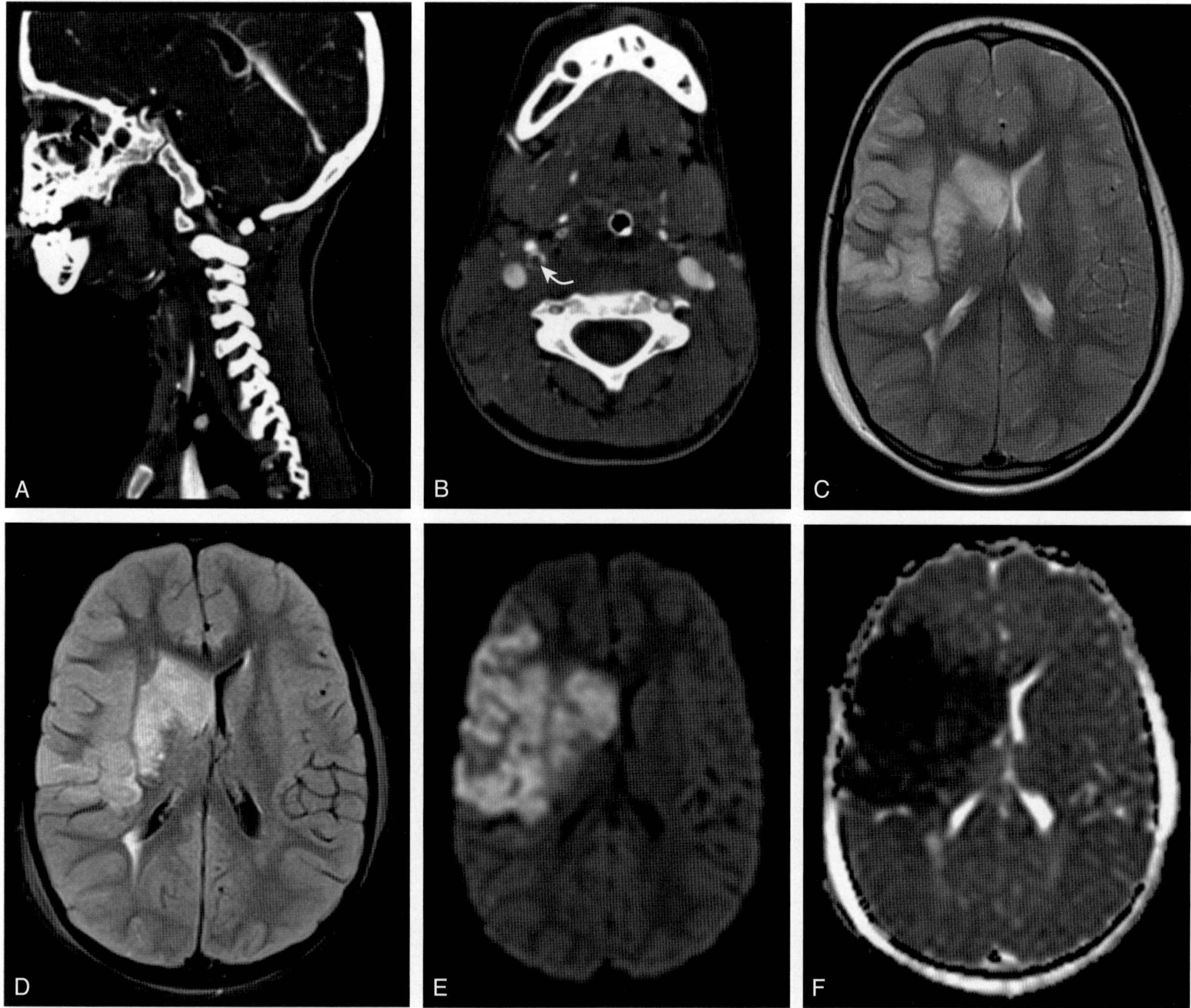

Fig. 3.11 Acute thromboembolic stroke. (A and B) Sagittal reformat and axial CTA images demonstrate a filling defect in the right internal carotid artery extending from the neck into the right middle cerebral artery. Soft tissue air is present from penetrating neck trauma. (C) Axial T2W, (D) axial FLAIR, (E) axial DWI, (F) axial ADC images show an acute right middle cerebral artery infarct with T2/FLAIR/DWI hyperintensity involving parts of the basal ganglia and adjacent frontal and insular cortex. Diffusion restriction/cytotoxic edema is confirmed by the low ADC values.

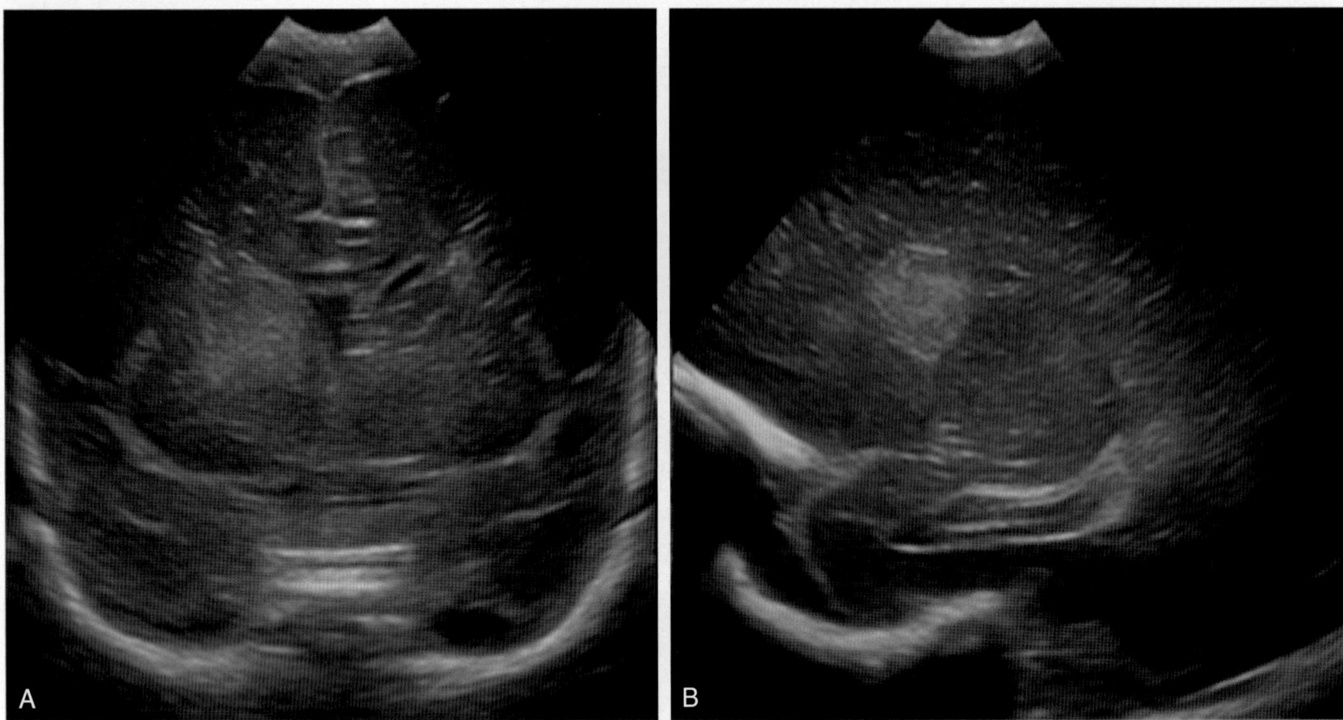

Fig. 3.12 Acute Stroke. (A and B) Coronal and sagittal head ultrasound images demonstrate hyperechogenic, well-circumscribed focal acute stroke involving the right anterior basal ganglia after cardiac surgery.

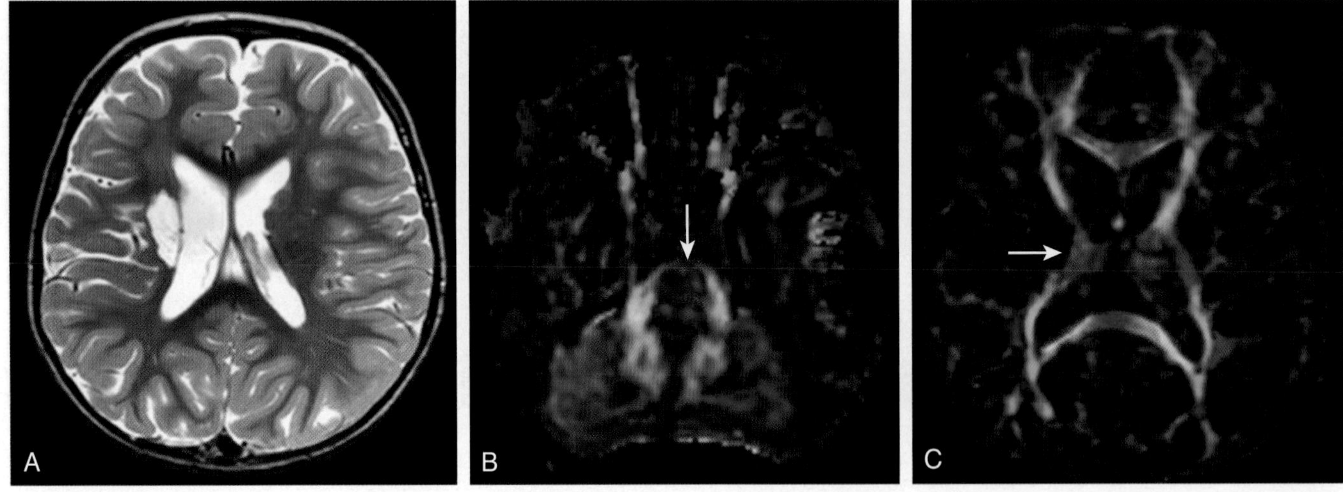

Fig. 3.13 Chronic Stroke. (A) Axial T2W image demonstrates a T2-hyperintense cerebrospinal fluid–filled chronic defect within the body of the right caudate nucleus and adjacent white matter along the course of the corticospinal tract. (B and C) Color coded directional fractional anisotropy maps show volume loss of the blue descending corticospinal tract at the right anterior pons and right internal capsule secondary to the chronic ischemic injury at the level of the corona radiata.

Key Points

Background

- Acute ischemic stroke in children is considered a rare event more common in newborns than older children, occuring in 1/3500 live births compared to 1-2/100,000 during childhood; however, with increasing public and clinical awareness and the wider availability of high-end, sensitive and specific imaging, acute pediatric strokes are increasingly recognized.
- Arterial strokes may be encountered in any age group, including the immediate postnatal and occasionally even fetal period.
- Children may present with a range of symptoms, including minor or major focal neurologic deficits, irritability, and seizures.

- Causes of pediatric arterial ischemic stroke by category include vasculopathy (ex. sickle cell disease, moyamoya, radiotherapy-related vasculopathy, collagen vascular disorders, dissection, focal cerebral arteriopathy, primary and secondary vasculitis, and others), coagulation disorders, congenital and acquired cardiac disease, infection, and genetic disorders.
- Acute stroke in the neonatal period may be of thromboembolic nature, including classic thrombi as complication of a chorioamnionitis, placental infarctions or rarely from amniotic fluid thrombi. In addition, congenital vascular anomalies, including a vein of Galen aneurysmal malformation or a dural arteriovenous malformation or fistula, also increase the incidence of acute strokes, possibly aggravated by steal phenomena.
- Treatment for acute ischemic stroke in children depends on the etiology. Acute thrombotic vascular occlusion can be treated with tissue plasminogen activator if onset is less than 4.5 hours. Prognosis depends on location of the stroke and age at time of injury. Younger patients have less clinical deficits compared to older children with similar infarct size and location. The mortality rate after childhood stroke is ~2-5%.

Imaging

- Focal neonatal strokes appear hyperechogenic on transfontanellar ultrasound on acute imaging with developing hypoechogenicity on progressive evolution and eventual anechoic cystic transformation in the chronic phase.
- CT may be negative within the first 12 to 24 hours, but is useful for excluding acute hemorrhage. In the acute phase, signs of acute ischemic stroke on CT can include hyperdense thrombus, loss of cortical gray-white differentiation including loss of the insular ribbon, hypodense deep gray nuclei, gyral swelling, and wedge shaped parenchymal hypodensity. In the subacute phase ~1-3 weeks after injury, the hypodensity persists but there is decreased swelling. In the chronic phase, there is parnchymal hypodensity and volume loss.
- On MRI, diffusion restriction (DWI hyperintense-ADC hypointense) pattern can be seen within 3-6 hours and persists from ~10-14 days. After 10-14 days the ADC signal will become isointense which is known as pseudonormalization and a few days later the ADC signal will become hyperintense. T2/FLAIR is often normal in the first 6-12 hours of an acute ischemic stroke, after which there is development of T2/FLAIR hyperintensity. Initially, there is no contrast enhancement of the infarct, but at ~3 days there is blood brain barrier breakdown related infarct enhancement which can then persist for 6-12 weeks. Vascular imaging with CTA, or MRA can identify vascular occlusion, stenosis or dissection which can help indicate etiologies such as embolic cause, vasculopathy, or dissection.
- On follow-up imaging the ischemic area will be resorbed and evolve into a cerebrospinal fluid–filled tissue defect. Depending on the location, Wallerian degeneration or distant volume loss may be seen along the course of affected white matter tracts, most commonly the corticospinal tract seen as small size of the cerebral peduncle, ventral pons and medulla.
- If multiple small ischemic lesions are noted, particular etiologies to consider include an embolic source, infection and coagulopathy.
- Hemorrhagic transformation of an ischemic stroke is rarely seen in the pediatric patient population.

REFERENCES

1. Meoded A, Poretti A, Tekes A, Huisman TA. Role of susceptibility weighted imaging in predicting stroke evolution. *Neurographics*. 2013;4(1):159–163.
2. Orman G, Rossi A, Meoded A, Huisman TA. Children with acute neurological emergency. In: Hodler J et al, ed.; 2020. *Diseases if the brain, head and neck, spine 2020-2023, IDKD Springer Series*. 14:179–190.

FOCAL CEREBRAL ARTERIOPATHY OF CHILDHOOD (FCA)

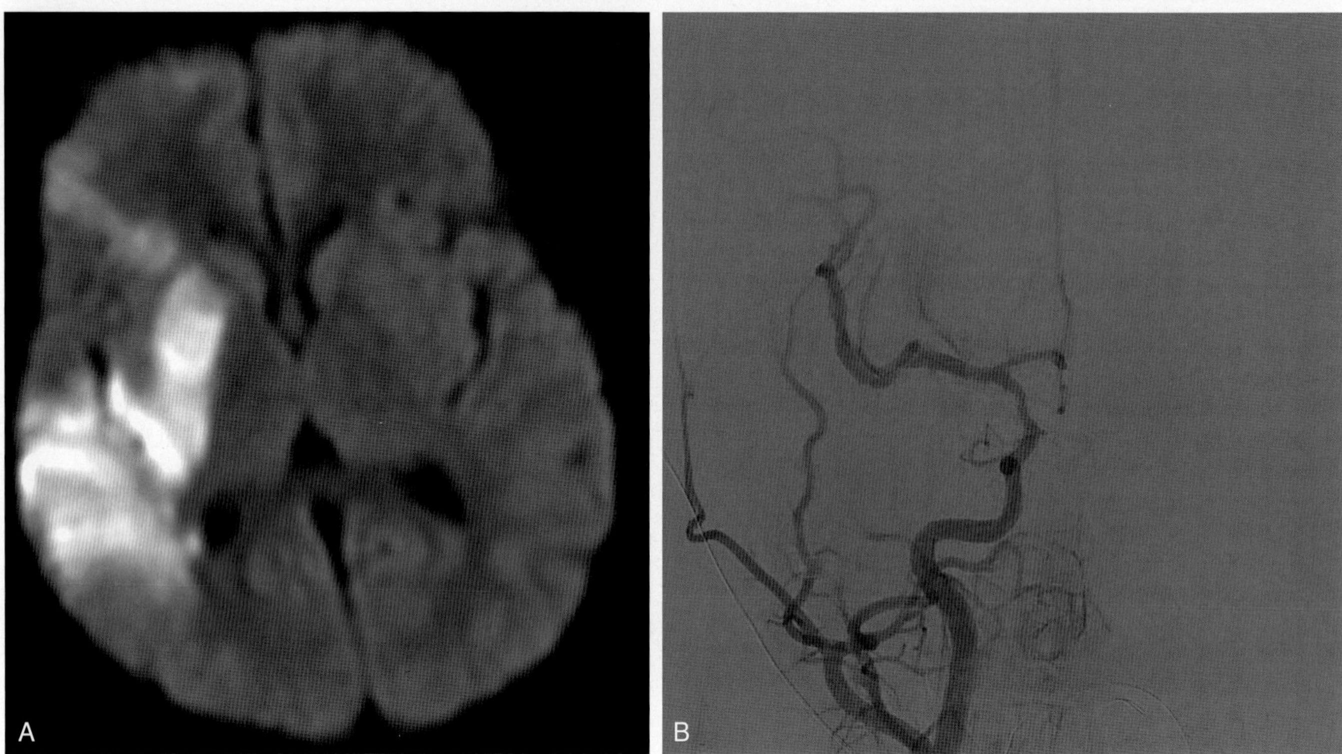

Fig. 3.14 Focal Cerebral Arteriopathy. (A) Axial DWI image demonstrates an acute infarct in the right middle cerebral artery territory. (B) Coronal digital subtraction angiography image demonstrates a moderate stenosis of the right supraclinoid internal carotid artery.

Key Points

Background

- Initially described as an arterial stenotic disease that did not correlate with moyamoya, sickle cell arteriopathy, dissection, vasculitis, post varicella arterioapthy or other known pathologies.
- FCA is monophasic with a stereotypical history of early progression within days to weeks, and nonprogression at 6 months with improvement or resolution in a subset of patients.
- More recent literature by a group of authors seeks to classify this poorly understood entity into three groups based on arterial stenosis/ irregularity to include banding/ occlusion (not attributable to thromboembolism) by definition involving the intracranial ICA and its proximal branches with M1 segment most common. This includes:
  - FCA-inflammation type: includes post varicella arteriopathy, and transient cerebral arteriopathy. FCA may predominately be a function of inflammation that is infectious or postinfectious.
  - FCA-dissection type: sequelae of trauma.
  - FCA-undetermined.

Imaging

- Acute unilateral infarct at presentation predominately involves the lentiform nucleus, caudate nucleus + distal MCA territory is classical. Recurrent strokes may occur in up to 30%. Note that multi-territorial infarcts in a cardiac patient strongly suggest cardioembolic stroke rather than FCA.
- Most patients present with >50% stenosis in the involved segments; vessel occlusion may occur. Vessel wall enhancement may be present.
- Differentiation from primary and secondary CNS vasculitis may be difficult.

REFERENCES

1. Conte G, Righini A, Griffiths PD, et al. Brain-injured survivors of monochorionic twin pregnancies complicated by single intrauterine death: MR findings in a multicenter study. *Radiology.* 2018;288:582–590.
2. Huisman TA, Lewi L, Zimmermann R, Willi UV, et al. Magnetic resonance imaging of the feto-placentar unit after fetoscopic laser coagulation for twin-to-twin transfusion syndrome. *Acta Radiol.* 2005 May;46:328–330.

VASCULAR DISSECTION AND ACUTE STROKE

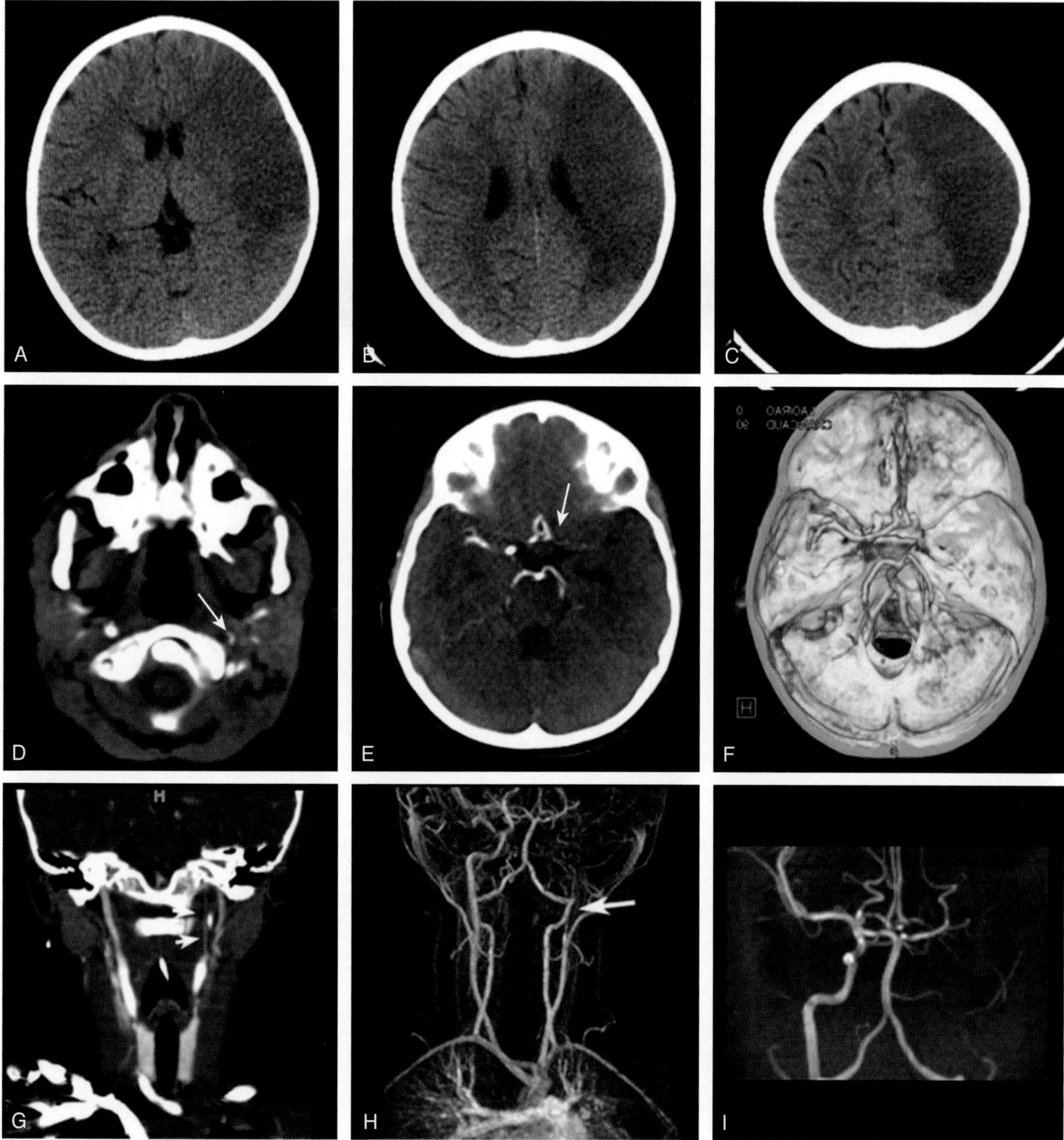

Fig. 3.15 Vascular Dissection. (A-C) Axial head CT images demonstrate a large wedge-shaped area of hypodensity involving the left middle cerebral artery territory. (D-G) Axial, volume rendered, and coronal reformat CT angiography images and (H and I) coronal MR Angiography MIP images show complete lack of opacification of the left internal carotid artery extending from the neck to the level of the distal bifurcation as well as lack of opacification of the left middle cerebral artery.

Key Points

Background

- Vascular dissections are rare in children but may occur after minor trauma to the neck vasculature or may be spontaneous in children with preexistent connective tissue disorders including, Ehlers-Danlos or Loeys-Dietz syndrome.
- Traumatic vascular dissections are more frequently encountered if the pediatric neck is exposed to a sudden acceleration-deceleration or rotatory angulation force. The immature protective reflexes and musculoskeletal stability of the neck relative to the head make young children especially vulnerable for these sudden acceleration-deceleration events.
- Traumatic dissections are often seen at the skull base but may extend into the cranial vault up to the level of the distal internal carotid artery.
- The internal carotid artery is more frequently affected than the vertebral artery.

Imaging

- CTA, and MRA studies are highly diagnostic and show a classic tapering of the injured vessel with a narrowed/compressed true lumen. A T1-hyperintense thrombus within the false, subintimal lumen is best seen on fat-saturated T1-weighted images acquired perpendicular to the longitudinal axis of the affected artery.
- Ultrasound imaging and duplex/doppler sonography may be helpful to evaluate the neck vasculature; however, care should be given to not injure the vessel by the ultrasound probe or possibly dislodge a thrombus.
- Focal strokes typically result from propagation of the thrombus. In addition, a "showering" of peripheral emboli may result in multiple small central or peripheral ischemic lesions.
- The stroke-related parenchymal imaging findings are similar to the previously described acute stroke imaging findings.

REFERENCES

1. Meoded A, Poretti A, Tekes A, Huisman TA. Role of susceptibility weighted imaging in predicting stroke evolution. *Neurographics*. 2013;4(1):159–163.
2. Orman G, Rossi A, Meoded A, Huisman TA. Children with acute neurological emergency. In: Hodler J et al, ed.; 2020. *Diseases if the brain, head and neck, spine 2020-2023, IDKD Springer Series*. 14:179–190.

TWIN-TWIN TRANSFUSION SYNDROME

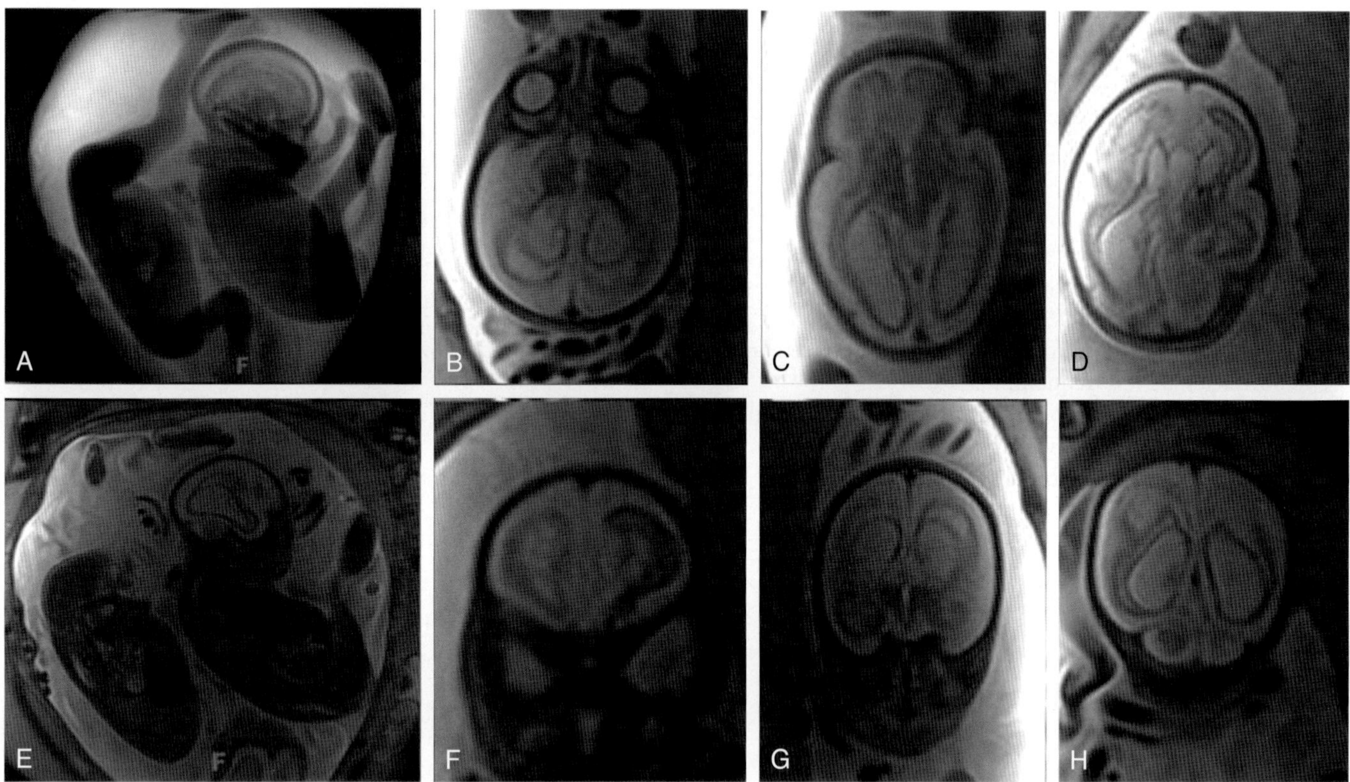

Fig. 3.16 Twin-Twin Transfusion Syndrome. (A-H) Multiplanar T2W fetal MRI images of a twin pregnancy show one fetus with significant supratentorial cystic encephalomalacia, volume loss and widening of the ventricles, and subarachnoid spaces secondary to a twin-twin transfusion syndrome.

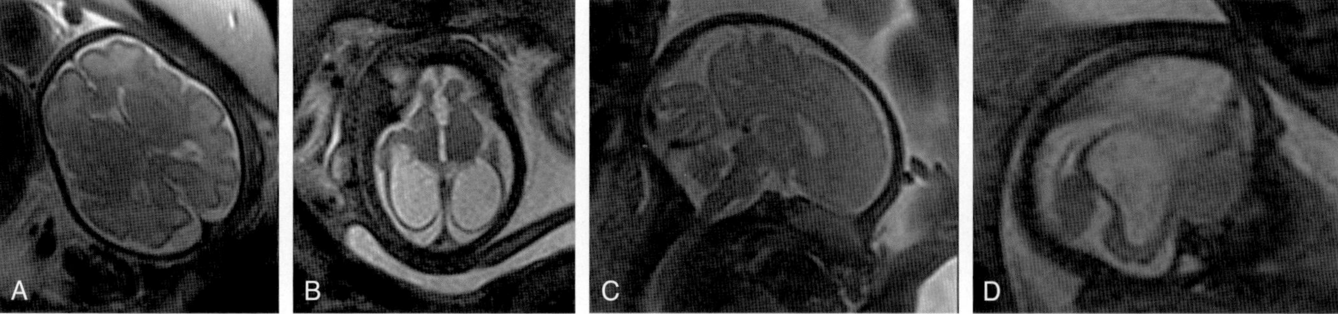

Fig. 3.17 Twin-Twin Transfusion Syndrome. (A-D) Axial and sagittal T2W fetal MRI images shows significant difference in size and integrity of the brains in twin-twin transfusion syndrome. The recipient twin (A, C) brain is normal while the donor twin (B, D) shows severe encephalomalacia.

Key Points

Background

- Twin-twin transfusion syndrome (TTTS) is a rare prenatal complication of a monochorionic-diamniotic twin pregnancy in which anomalous connections between placental blood vessels allow for a hemodynamic imbalance between both twins.
- TTTS occurs in 10%–15% of monochorionic twin pregnancies.
- In TTTS the imbalance results in the shunting of blood from one fetus to the other. The donor fetus typically has a decreased blood volume with resultant low urine output, small urinary bladder, and small amount of amniotic fluid (oligohydramnios), while the recipient fetus has to deal with an increased blood volume, with resultant increased urine output, large urinary bladder, large amount of amniotic fluid (polyhydramnios), and possibly heart failure with hydrops.

- Neurologic complications include focal or global ischemic injury to the brain, cerebral atrophy, ventriculomegaly, and intracerebral hemorrhages. The exact etiology of the cerebral injury remains unclear and is likely multifactorial in origin. Hypoxic-ischemic injury due to cerebral hypoperfusion may be observed in the donor fetus, while hyperviscosity and polycythemia may be causative of cerebral injury in the recipient twin. Arterial strokes typically occur in the recipient.

Imaging

- Fetal MRI may show watershed ischemia, focal strokes, progressive global hemispheric white matter volume loss, ventriculomegaly, possible microcephaly, and overall reduced size of the fetus for gestational age. Intracerebral hemorrhages are less frequent.
- If one fetus dies, thromboembolism over the anomalous placental connections may progressively injure the surviving twin with possible devastating outcome.
- Treatment options include fetoscopic laser coagulation of the anomalous placental connections, allowing for more balanced hemodynamics. Postintervention intracerebral hemorrhages have been reported in the recipient, possibly due to hemorrhagic embolic strokes originating from the placenta.

REFERENCES

1. Oesch G, Perez FA, Wainwright MS, Shaw DWW, Amlie-Lefond C. Focal Cerebral Arteriopathy of Childhood: Clinical and Imaging Correlates. *Stroke*. 2021 Jul;52(7):2258–2265.
2. Wintermark M, Hills NK, DeVeber GA, Barkovich AJ, Bernard TJ, Friedman NR, Mackay MT, Kirton A, Zhu G, Leiva-Salinas C, Hou Q, Fullerton HJVIPS Investigators. Clinical and Imaging Characteristics of Arteriopathy Subtypes in Children with Arterial Ischemic Stroke: Results of the VIPS Study. *AJNR Am J Neuroradiol*. 2017 Nov;38(11):2172–2179.

GERMINAL MATRIX HEMORRHAGE

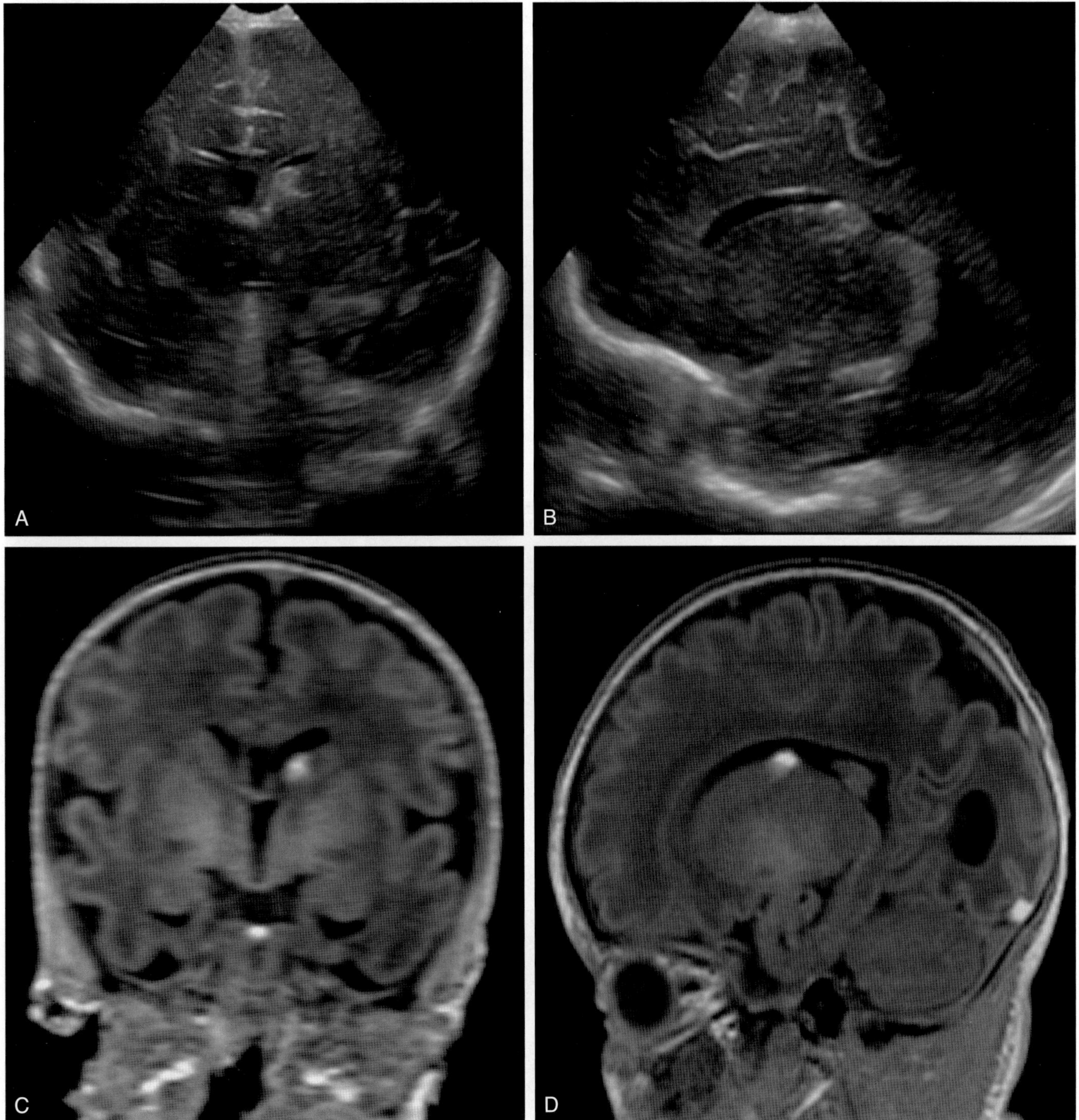

Fig. 3.18 Germinal Matrix Hemorrhage - Grade 1. (A, B) Coronal and sagittal transfontanellar head ultrasound and (C, D) coronal and sagittal T1W images demonstrate focal hyperechogenic and T1-hyperintense hemorrhage in the left caudothalamic sulcus compatible with a grade 1 germinal matrix hemorrhage.

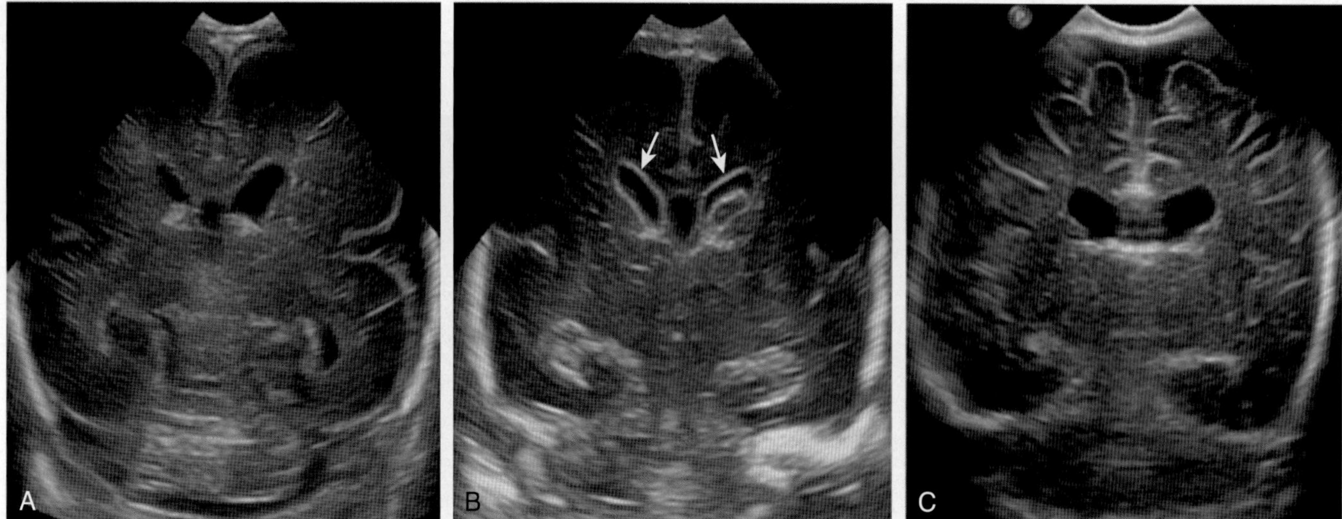

Fig. 3.19 Germinal Matrix Hemorrhage - Grade 2. (A–C) Serial coronal transfontanellar ultrasound images of the brain showing (A) a normal-appearing caudothalamic sulcus on the first image, (B) a focal centrally hypoechogenic hemorrhage in the left caudothalamic sulcus on follow-up, which resolves completely on the third follow-up image (C). The intermittent hyperechogenic lining of the ventricles on the second study (B) indicates intraventricular extension of the hemorrhage with resultant chemical ependymal inflammation. On the follow-up imaging (C) the hemorrhage has completely resolved as well as the hyperechogenic lining. Findings are compatible with a grade 2 germinal matrix hemorrhage given the lack of a ventriculomegaly.

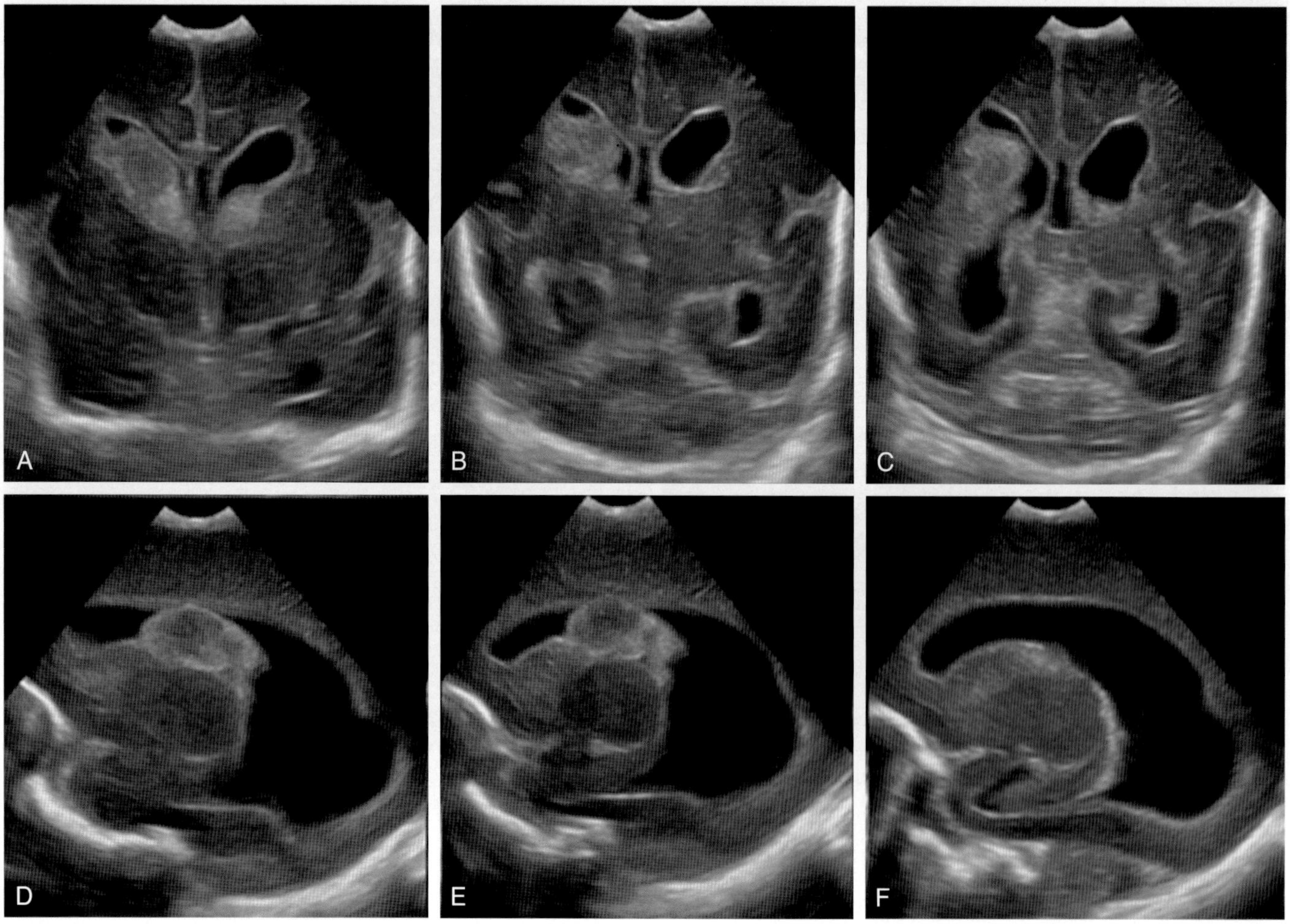

Fig. 3.20 Germinal Matrix Hemorrhage - Grade 3. (A–F) Coronal and sagittal head ultrasound images demonstrate bilateral (right greater than left) hyperechogenic germinal matrix hemorrhages with accompanying ventriculomegaly. The ependymal lining is hyperechogenic due to the intraventricular blood products. The findings are compatible with a grade 3 germinal matrix hemorrhage.

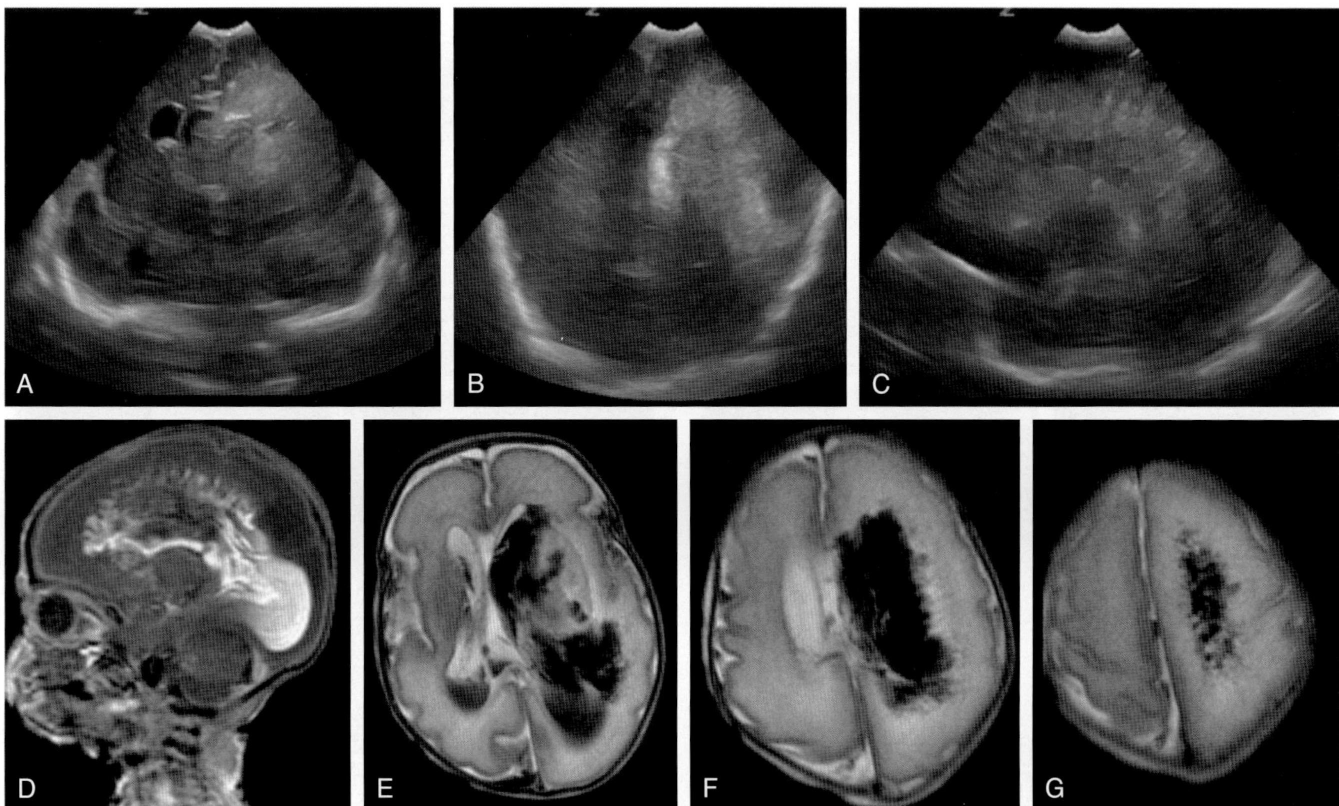

Fig. 3.21 Germinal Matrix Hemorrhage - Grade 4. (A–C) Coronal and sagittal head ultrasound images demonstrate wedge shaped region of abnormal hyperechogenicity in the left periventricular white matter and bilateral (left>right) caudothalamic groove germinal matrix hemorrhage. On the matching (D) sagittal T1W and (E–G) axial T2W images the germinal matrix hemorrhage appears T1 hyperintense and T2 hypointense. In addition, engorged/thrombosed T1-hyperintense/T2-hypointense periventricular veins are noted in the swollen left cerebral white matter due to a periventricular venous hemorrhagic infarct secondary to the germinal matrix hemorrhage.

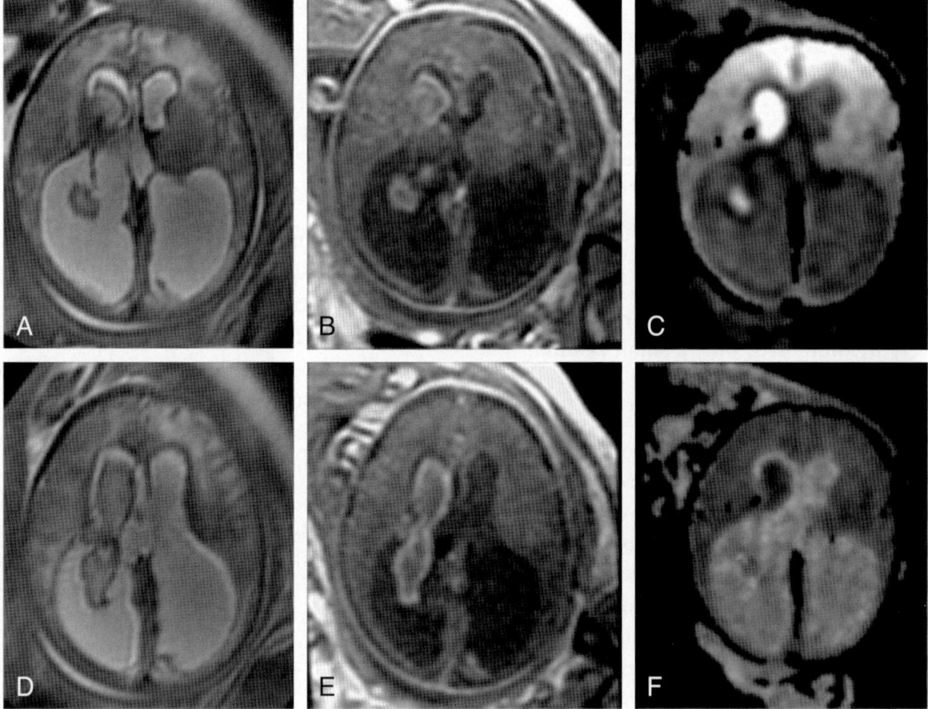

Fig. 3.22 Germinal Matrix Hemorrhage. (A, D) Axial T2W, (B, E) axial T1W, and (C, F) axial DWI and ADC fetal MRI images of a right-sided germinal matrix hemorrhage. The hemorrhage appears T2 mixed hypointense and hyperintense, and T1 hyperintense. The hemorrhage covers the intraventricular choroid plexus. Additional hemorrhages are noted in the occipital horns of the moderately widened ventricles. The hemorrhage shows restricted diffusion with DWI-hyperintensity and low ADC values.

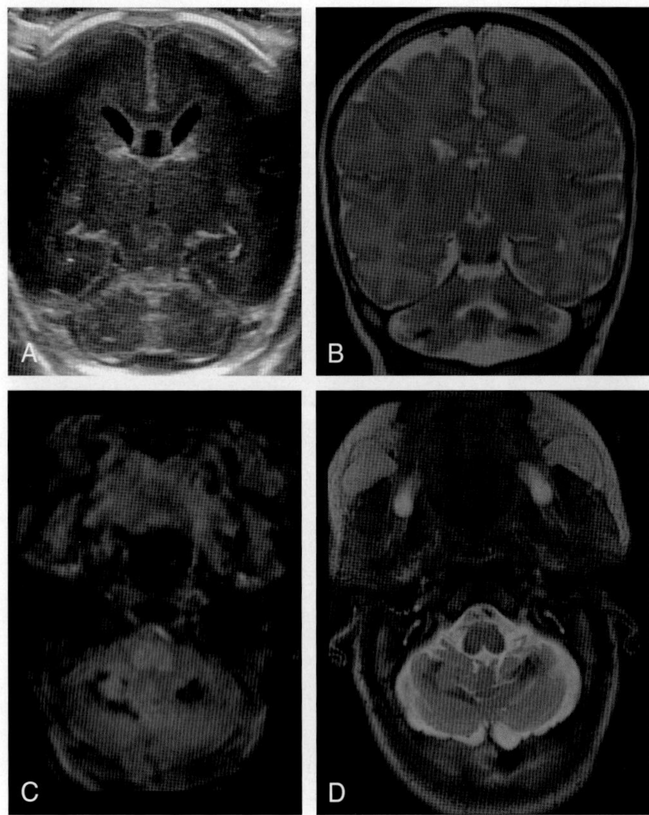

Fig. 3.23 Germinal Matrix Hemorrhage. (A) Coronal head ultrasound in a 23-week premature infant was normal. However, (B) coronal T2W, (C) axial GRE, and (D) axial T2W MRI images performed at 6 months old (full-term equivalent when adjusted for prematurity) demonstrate bilateral hypointense cerebellar germinal matrix hemorrhages and associated cerebellar volume loss.

Fig. 3.24 Germinal Matrix Hemorrhage. (A) Coronal and (B) transmastoid head ultrasound images in a 24-week premature infant demonstrate abnormal hyperechogenic region in the right cerebellar hemisphere. (C) Coronal T2W and (D) axial SWI follow-up MRI at 3 years old demonstrate asymmetric severe right cerebellar hemisphere volume loss and small amount of old blood products caused by the cerebellar germinal matrix hemorrhage.

Key Points

Background

- The germinal matrix is a transient, highly metabolically active, highly perfused cell layer along the ventricles from which the precursors of the cortical neurons and hemispheric glial cells originate and subsequently radially migrate peripherally in a programmed pattern.
- The germinal matrix is most active during early gestation and will progressively involute with only a small residual component at the caudothalamic groove by 32–34 weeks of gestation.
- The high vascularity makes the germinal matrix vulnerable for hemorrhages, especially if concomitant risk factors like congenital heart disease, sepsis, low birth weight, prolonged labor, or coagulation disorders are present.
- The hemorrhage can be confined to the germinal matrix or depending on the size rupture into the ventricular system. In addition, complicating periventricular venous infarction with or without hemorrhagic conversion may occur.
- Intraventricular blood products may result in obstructive supratentorial hydrocephalus due to adhesions, in particular at the level of the sylvian aqueduct.
- Based upon the progressive involution of the germinal matrix, these hemorrhages typically occur in premature children and more frequently in the area of the caudothalamic groove.

Imaging

- Germinal matrix hemorrhages can be classified as grades 1–3, and periventricular (hemorrhagic) venous infarction (formerly known as grade 4).
  - Grade 1: Hemorrhage confined to the germinal matrix
  - Grade 2: Hemorrhage in the germinal matrix with extension into normal-size ventricles
  - Grade 3: Hemorrhage in the germinal matrix with extension into enlarged ventricles
  - Periventricular (hemorrhagic) venous infarction is characterized by a focal hemorrhage in the germinal matrix along the course of the veins that drain the periventricular white matter. The impaired venous drainage results in venous stasis, which may evolve into a venous ischemia possibly complicated by an additional hemorrhagic conversion. On follow-up, the ischemic lesion may evolve to a porencephalic cyst incorporated into the adjacent lateral ventricle.

- Differential diagnosis includes hemorrhage within the choroid plexus, which may also extend into the ventricular system.
- Posterior fossa germinal matrix hemorrhage is less common than supratentorial germinal matrix hemorrhages.
- Transfontanellar ultrasound is the imaging method of choice. Acute hemorrhages appear hyperechogenic and will progressively involute on follow-up examination. The center may become hypoechogenic. A hyperechogenic lining of the ventricles indicates intraventricular blood products, resulting in a chemical inflammation. A periventricular hemorrhagic venous ischemia appears in the acute phase as a fan-shaped hyperechogenicity extending from the germinal matrix into the adjacent white matter. The immediate subcortical white matter is typically spared as well as the overlying cortical ribbon because this part of the brain drains into an unaffected, functional superficial venous system.
- If hydrocephalus develops, hyperechogenic blood products may be noted in the region of the sylvian aqueduct just superior to a normal-size fourth ventricle.
- CT and MRI studies are rarely indicated in the acute phase; follow-up MRI may allow for better depiction of the infarcted periventricular white matter and remaining intraventricular blood products (SWI-hypointense hemosiderin staining).

REFERENCES

1. Poretti A, Huisman TA, eds. *Neonatal head and spine ultrasonography*: Springer, International Publishing Switzerland; 2016.
2. Orman G, Benson JE, Kweldam CF, Bosemani T, et al. Neonatal head ultrasonography today: a powerful imaging tool!. *J Neuroimaging*. 2015, Jan-Feb;25(1):31–55.

PERIVENTRICULAR LEUKOMALACIA

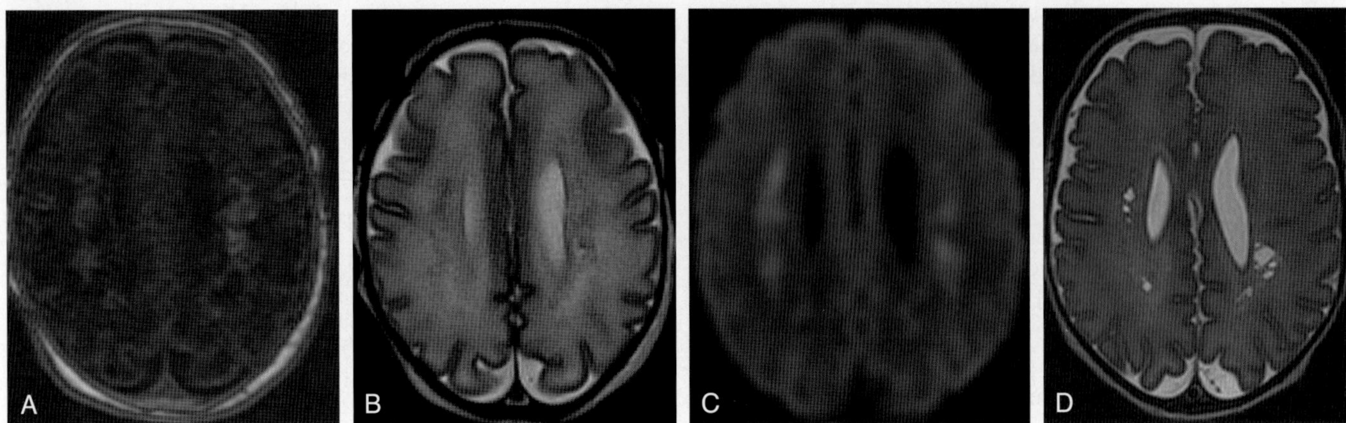

Fig. 3.25 Periventricular Leukomalacia (PVL). 34-week premature infant with PVL seen on (A) axial T1W, (B) axial T2W, and (C) axial DWI images as multiple focal/confluent areas of T1 hyperintensity, T2 iso/hypointensity with reduced diffusion in the deep white matter. (D) Follow-up axial 3D T2W MRI 2 weeks later demonstrated cystic PVL in the white matter.

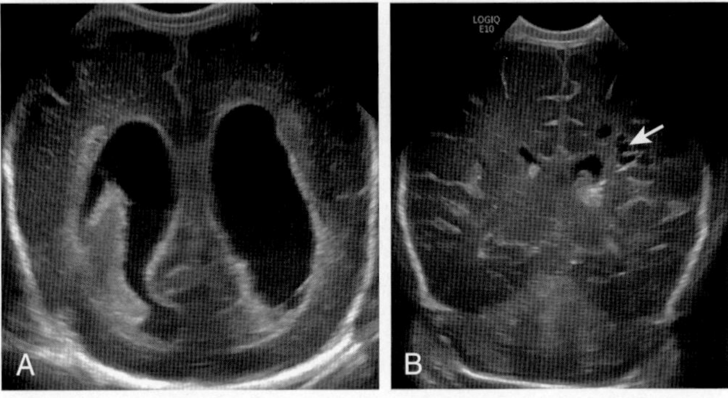

Fig. 3.26 Periventricular Leukomalacia (PVL). Coronal ultrasound appearance of noncystic PVL (A) and cystic PVL (B) in two different premature neonates.

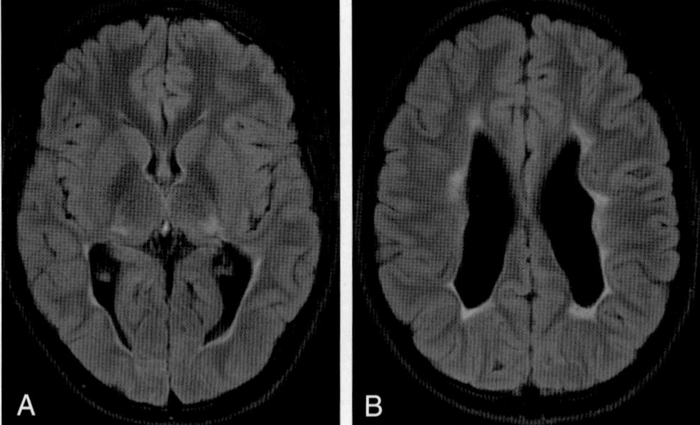

Fig. 3.27 Periventricular Leukomalacia. (A and B) Axial FLAIR images demonstrate chronic bilateral PVL seen as mild confluent FLAIR hyperintensity in the periventricular white matter, central white matter volume loss, ex vacuo dilatation of the lateral ventricles, angulated ventricular margins, mild thalamic volume loss with posterior thalamic FLAIR hyperintensity, and FLAIR hyperintensity in the PLIC bilaterally.

Key Points

Background

- Periventricular leukomalacia (PVL) is periventricular white matter injury in premature neonates that can be caused by hypoxic-ischemic injury, infections, metabolic disorders, and congenital heart disease. The periventricular white matter location has been presumed to be due to the watershed arterial region in premature infants; however, other factors may be important, including location of immature oligodendrocytes, which are susceptible to ischemic injury.
- The severity of white matter injury correlates with clinical motor and cognitive outcomes.
- The periatrial white matter is the most common location of PVL detected on imaging.

Imaging

- On ultrasound, PVL is suspected when the periventricular echogenicity is similar or greater than the choroid plexus. Cystic PVL appears as anechoic rounded areas adjacent to the ventricles.
- MRI is more sensitive and specific for the diagnosis of PVL than ultrasound. Acute and subacute noncystic PVL typically demonstrates focal areas of T1W hyperintense, T2W hypointense signal in the periatrial white matter. Cystic PVL demonstrates focal T2 hyperintensity. Chronic stages of PVL appear as focal or confluent periventricular T2/FLAIR hyperintensities, and depending on the degree of white matter volume loss, are associated with thinning of the corpus callous, ex vacuo dilatation of the lateral ventricles, angulated ventricular margins, thalamic volume loss, and posterior limb internal capsule T2/FLAIR hyperintensity.

REFERENCE

1. Poretti A, Huisman TA, eds. *Neonatal head and spine ultrasonography*: Springer, International Publishing Switzerland; 2016.

ECMO COMPLICATIONS

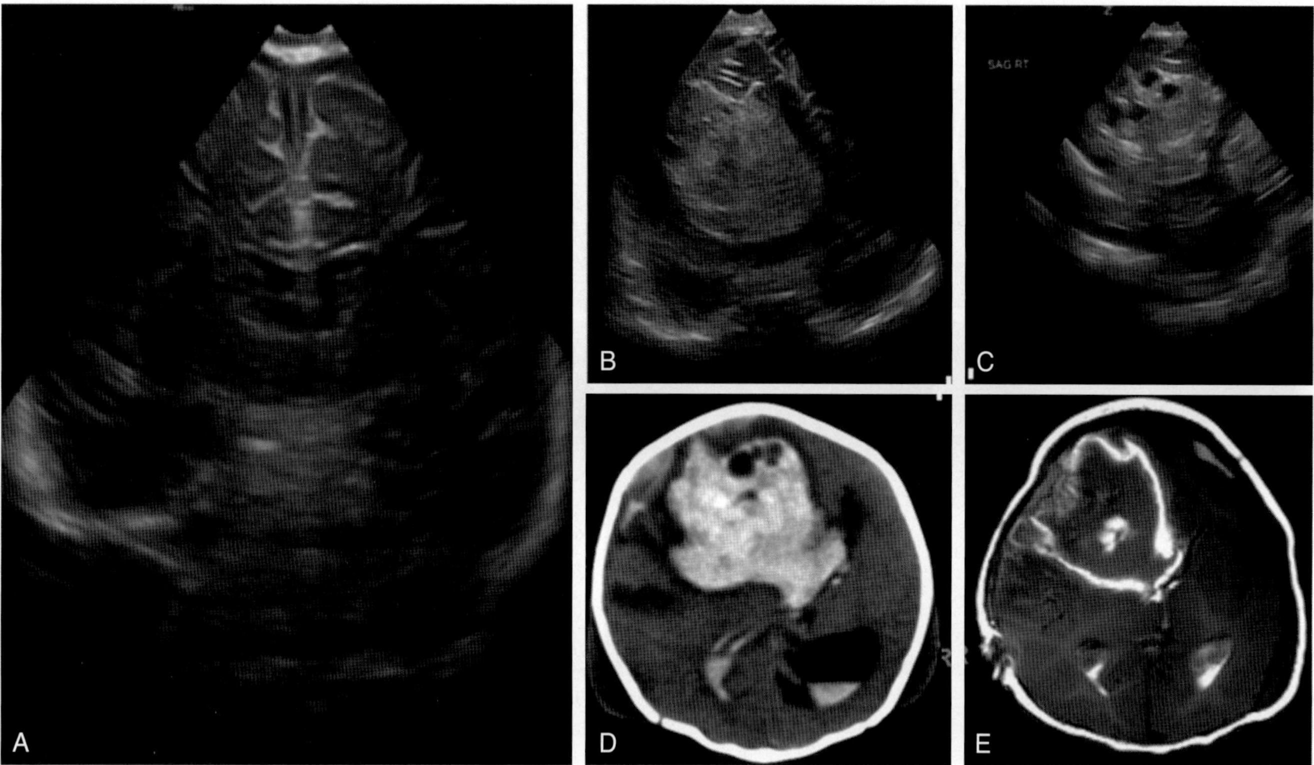

Fig. 3.28 ECMO Complications. (A) Initial coronal transfontanellar head ultrasound appears normal in a neonate on ECMO support. After a sudden drop in the hematocrit the (C and D) follow-up coronal and sagittal ultrasound images show focal predominantly hyperechogenic intraparenchymal hemorrhage in the right cerebral hemisphere with significant midline shift. (D) Axial head CT and (E) axial T1W MRI images confirm the large intracerebral hemorrhage, mass effect, midline shift and intraventricular hemorrhage from extension of the parenchymal hemorrhage.

Key Points

Background

- Extracorporeal membrane oxygenation (ECMO) is progressively being used in critically sick pediatric patients including neonates.
- The indications for ECMO include life-threatening cardiopulmonary failure, congenital heart disease, congenital diaphragmatic hernia, meconium aspiration syndrome, pulmonary hypertension, respiratory distress syndrome, systemic organ failure, and sepsis.
- Common neurologic complications include intracerebral hemorrhage and acute stroke.

Imaging

- Daily transfontanellar head ultrasound (HUS) examination may be used in neonates to identify hemorrhage and stroke early.
- On HUS an acute focal hemorrhage typically appears as a mass-like hyperechogenic area. The size of the bleeding can be substantial and result in compression and displacement of adjacent brain structures, including ventricles. A midline shift and possible downward herniation may occur. Most hemorrhages occur in the supratentorial brain.
- Studies have suggested that the resistive index values measured within branches of the anterior circle of Willis may show an increased variability in the 24 to 48 hours prior to a hemorrhage.
- Focal strokes follow the imaging characteristics of classic strokes; in the acute phase a mild to moderate hyperechogenicity is seen within arterial territories. Mild mass effect may be noted. The cortical ribbon, cerebral white matter, or central gray matter may be affected.
- CT and MRI may identify the extent of the hemorrhage and/or stroke in better detail but are typically less available or contraindicated because of the ECMO system.

REFERENCE

1. Zamora CA, Oshmyansky A, Bembea M, Berkowitz I, et al. Resistive index variability in anterior cerebral artery measurements during daily transcranial duplex sonography: a predictor of cerebrovascular complications in infants on ECMO? *J Ultrasound Med.* 2016;35:2459–2465.

DURAL SINUS OR VEIN THROMBOSIS

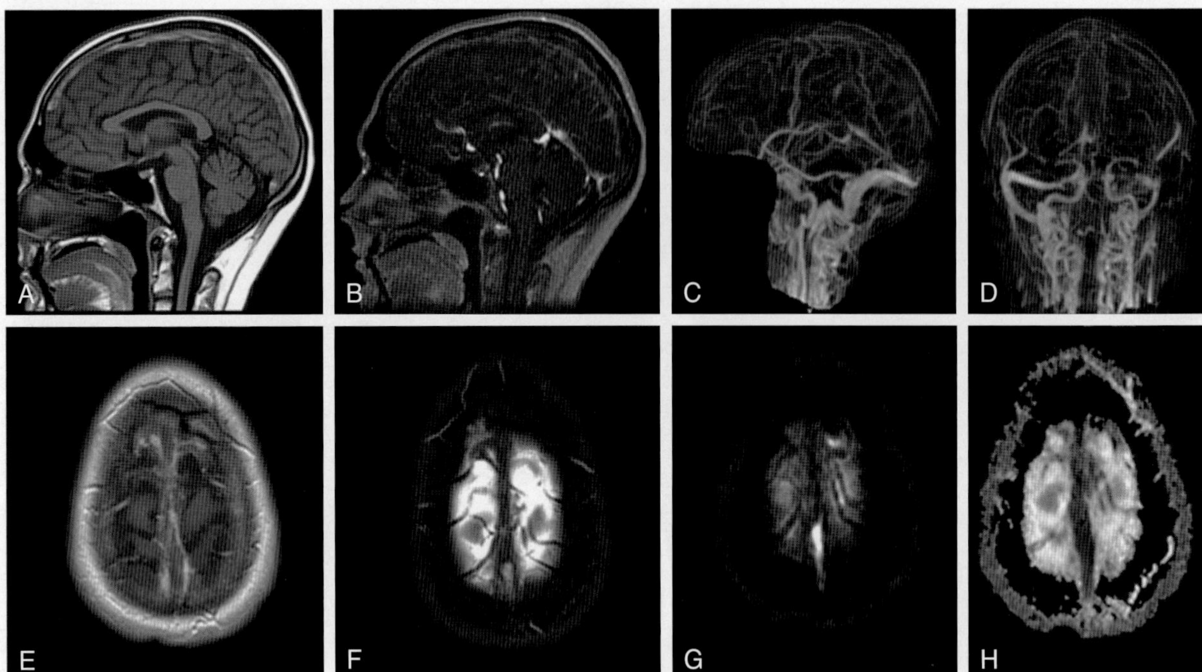

Fig. 3.29 Dural Sinus Thrombosis. (A) Sagittal T1W, (B-D) sagittal and coronal MR venogram , (E) axial T1W+C, (F) axial T2W, (G) axial DWI, and (H) axial ADC images demonstrates abnormal T1-hyperintensity, loss of the normal T2 flow void, restricted diffusion and lack of of flow related signal on MR Venogram indicative of dural sinus thrombosis in the superior sagittal sinus extending into the region of the torcular Herophili.

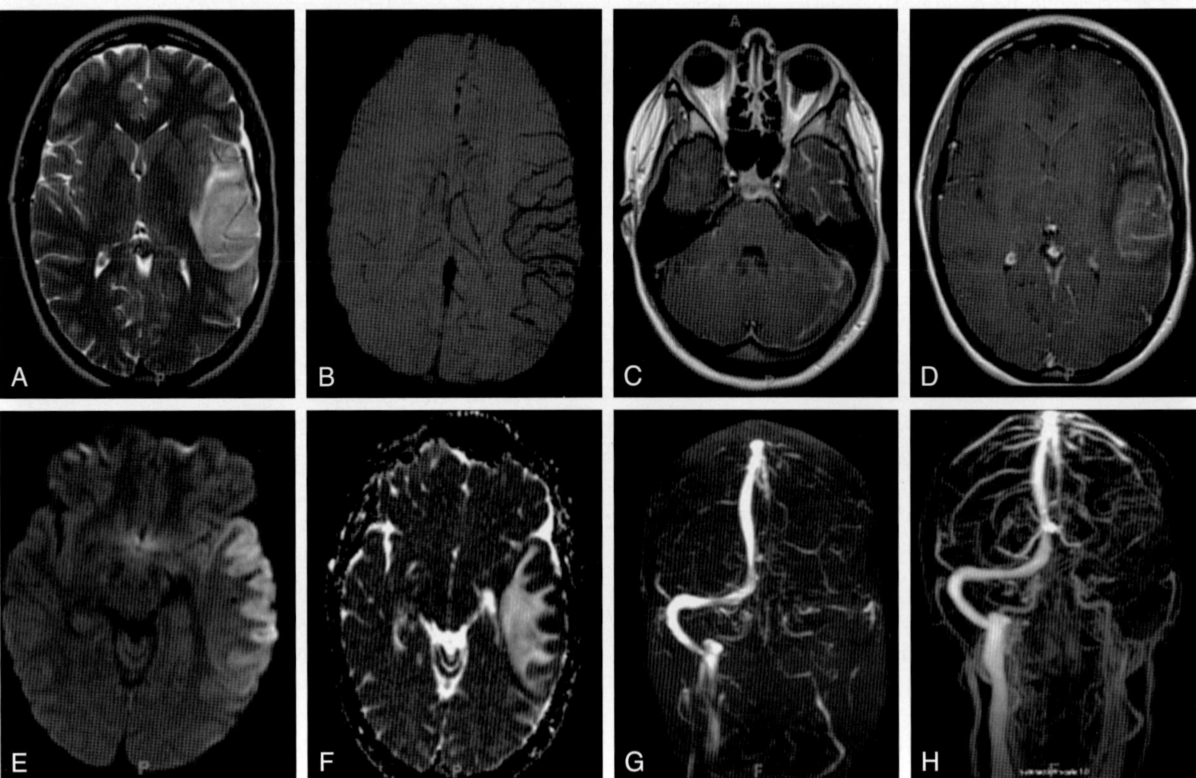

Fig. 3.30 Dural Sinus Thrombosis. (A) Axial T2W image demonstrates an abnormal region of T2-hyperintensity consistent with edema in the cortex and subcortical white matter of the left temporal lobe. (B) Axial SWI demonstrates abnormal prominent hypointense sulcal veins overlying the edematous temporal lobe. (C and D) Axial T1W+C images show a filling defect within the left transverse and sigmoid sinus and mild parenchymal contrast enhancement in the region of abnormal T2 hyperintensity. (E) Axial DWI, and (F) axial ADC images demonstrate predominantly facilitated diffusion (DWI hyperintensity and elevated ADC values) compatible with vasogenic edema. (G and H) Coronal time-of-flight MR venography MIP and dynamic contrast enhanced MIP images show a lack of flow related enhancement is seen in the left transverse and sigmoid sinus and internal jugular vein due to thrombus.

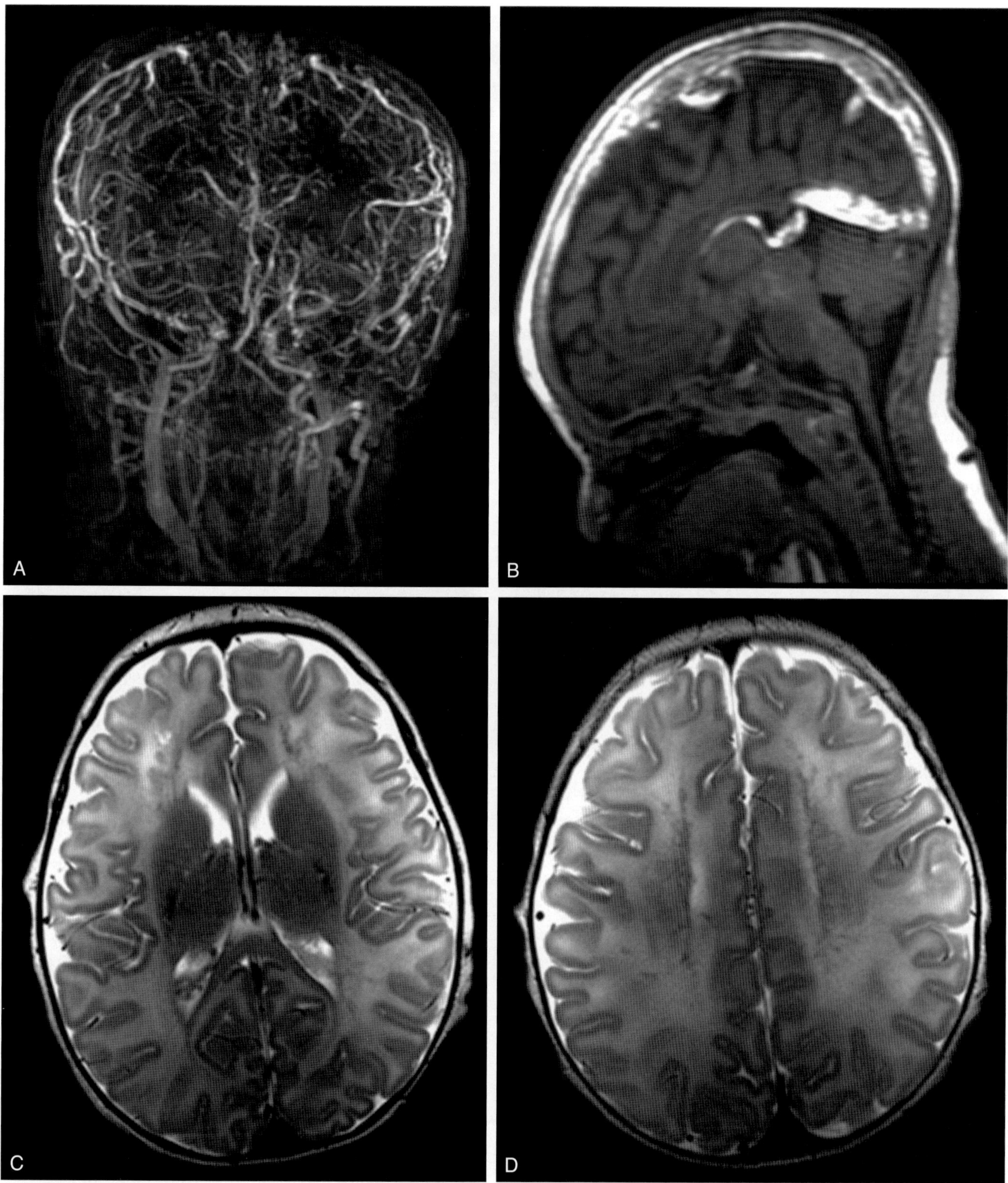

Fig. 3.31 Dural Sinus Thrombosis. (A) Coronal MR Venogram MIP image shows no flow-related enhancement in the superior sagittal sinus and straight sinus. (B) Sagittal T1W image shows abnormal T1-hyperintense thrombus involving the entire superior sagittal sinus, straight sinus, vein of Galen, and internal cerebral veins. (C and D) Axial T2W images demonstrate abnormal T2 hypointense prominence of intramedullary veins in the hemispheric white matter as well as diffuse white matter edema due to venous stasis.

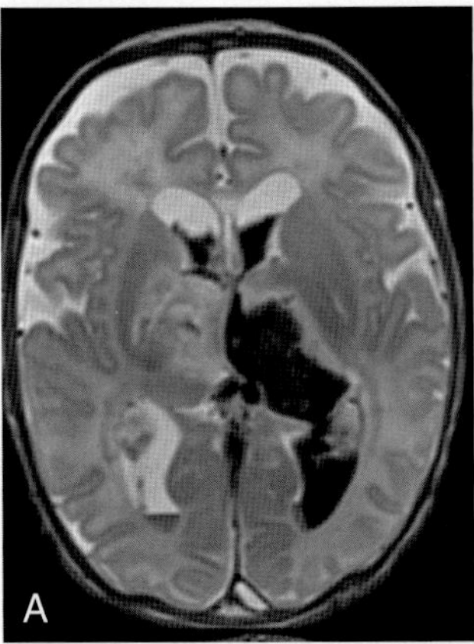

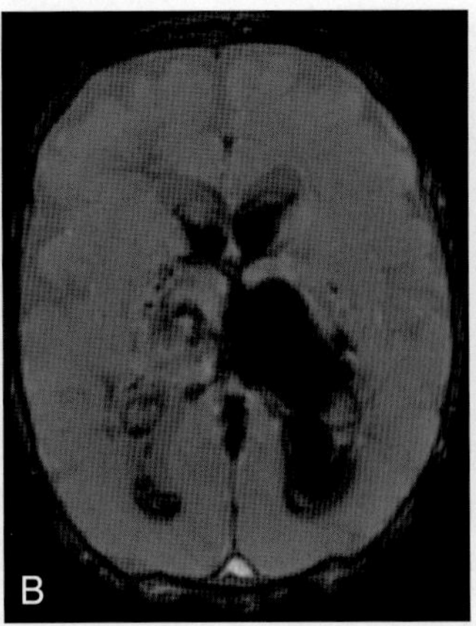

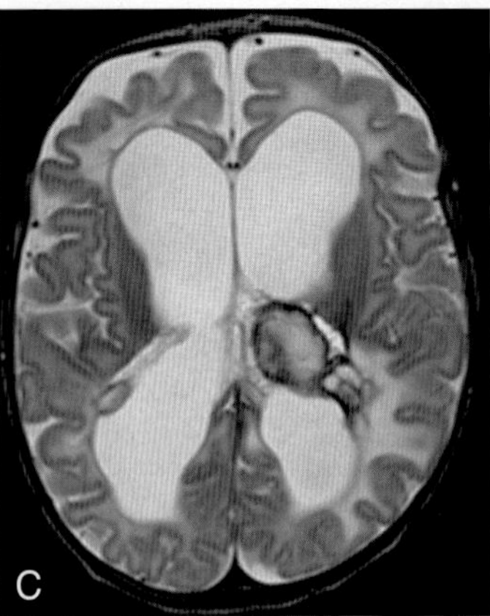

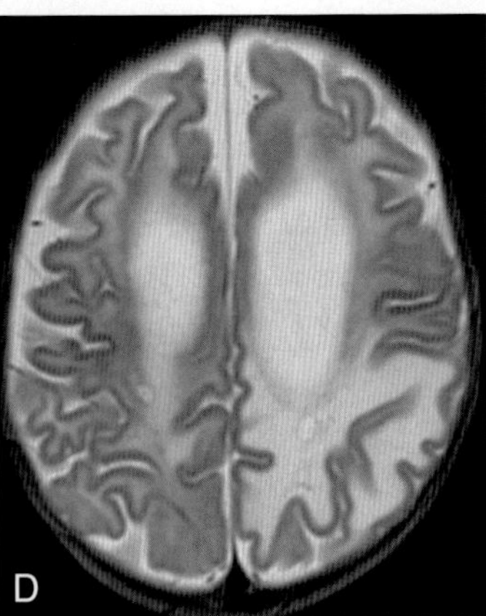

Fig. 3.32 Dural Sinus Thrombosis. Deep venous thrombosis with deep gray matter hemorrhagic infarctions. (A) Axial T2W image and (B) axial SWI image demonstrate abnormal areas of T2 hypointense signal and susceptibility due to hemorrhage in bilateral thalami and basal ganglia with associated abnormal surrounding T2 hyperintensity due to edema. There is associated intraventricular hemorrhage from parenchymal extension of hemorrhage. SWI image also shows engorged hypointense veins in the periventricular white matter and both thalami due to the obstructed deep venous drainage. (C and D) Axial T2W images on follow-up MRI show diffuse hemispheric white matter volume loss, ex vacuo enlargement of the ventricles, mild residual white matter edema, and residual intraventricular blood products.

Key Points

Background

- Dural sinus thrombosis is a venous thrombosis of the major venous drainage pathways of the brain and may involve parts or the multiple segments of the superficial venous system (superior sagittal sinus, transverse sinuses, sigmoid sinuses) as well as the deep venous system (internal cerebral veins, vein of Galen, straight sinus). Thrombosis propagation may be antegrade into the jugular veins, superior ophthalmic veins, pterygoid plexus, or retrograde from the head and neck region as part of an inflammatory process in, for example, Lemierre syndrome.
- Focal thrombosis may also involve smaller, segmental veins, including the cortical veins in, for example, meningoencephalitis or after trauma or may affect the cavernous sinuses and intercavernous sinuses as a complication of a paranasal sinusitis.
- Symptoms depend on the involved segments and the presence and functionality of noninvolved venous collaterals.
- Dural venous thrombosis may result from infection and sepsis, hypercoagulability, trauma, tumor-related compression or infiltration, or dehydration or may be considered iatrogenic/spontaneous. In addition, venous thrombosis has an increased incidence in premature neonates.
- Symptoms vary significantly and can include intermittent headache, seizures, and more severe symptoms such as focal neurologic deficits, signs of raised intracranial pressure, or as severe as coma.

Imaging

- On CT, acute intraluminal thrombus may appear mildly hyperdense; on contrast-enhanced CT/CTV typically a filling defect is seen. The shape of the filling defect follows the configuration and imaging plane of the involved vein and may resemble an empty delta or an empty tube. The differential diagnosis of these defects includes a prominent arachnoid granulation.
- On MRI acute thrombus is typically T1 hyperintense, may be DWI hyperintense with restricted diffusion on ADC maps, and exhibits a lack of flow-related signal void. On susceptibility-weighted imaging (SWI), the thrombus is typically hypointense, and prominent hypointense veins may be seen within the adjacent brain parenchyma. The signal intensity of the thrombus on T2-weighted imaging can vary but is typically mildly hyperintense. Similar to contrast-enhanced CT a central filling defect may be seen within the dural sinus with preserved enhancement of the dural/venous walls. On MRV there is a lack of flow-related enhancement, but the intrinsic T1-hyperintense signal of the blood clot can mimic flow on time-of-flight MRV.
- In neonates a transfontanellar color-coded Doppler study can be helpful by directly identifying the thrombus in combination with a lack of a normal venous flow.
- Intraparenchymal complications of the thrombosis include vassogenic edema, which may eventually evolve into cytotoxic edema and intraparenchymal or intraventricular hemorrhage. In the early phases of venous ischemia, parenchymal edema will be predominantly vasogenic edema rather than cytotoxic edema.
- A superficial venous thrombosis typically results in venous ischemia involving the adjacent cortical ribbon and immediate subcortical white matter in a nonarterial territory distribution.
- A deep venous thrombosis affecting the straight sinus or vein of Galen may result in ischemic injury to both thalami and basal ganglia.

REFERENCES

1. Holzmann D, Huisman TA, Linder TE. Lateral dural sinus thrombosis in childhood. *Laryngoscope*. 1999;109(4):645–651.
2. Wagner MW, Bosemani T, Oshmyansky A, Kubik-Huch RA, et al. Neuroimaging findings in pediatric cerebral sinovenous thrombosis. *Childs Nerv Syst*. 2015 May;31(5):705–712.

POSTERIOR REVERSIBLE ENCEPHALOPATHY SYNDROME (PRES)

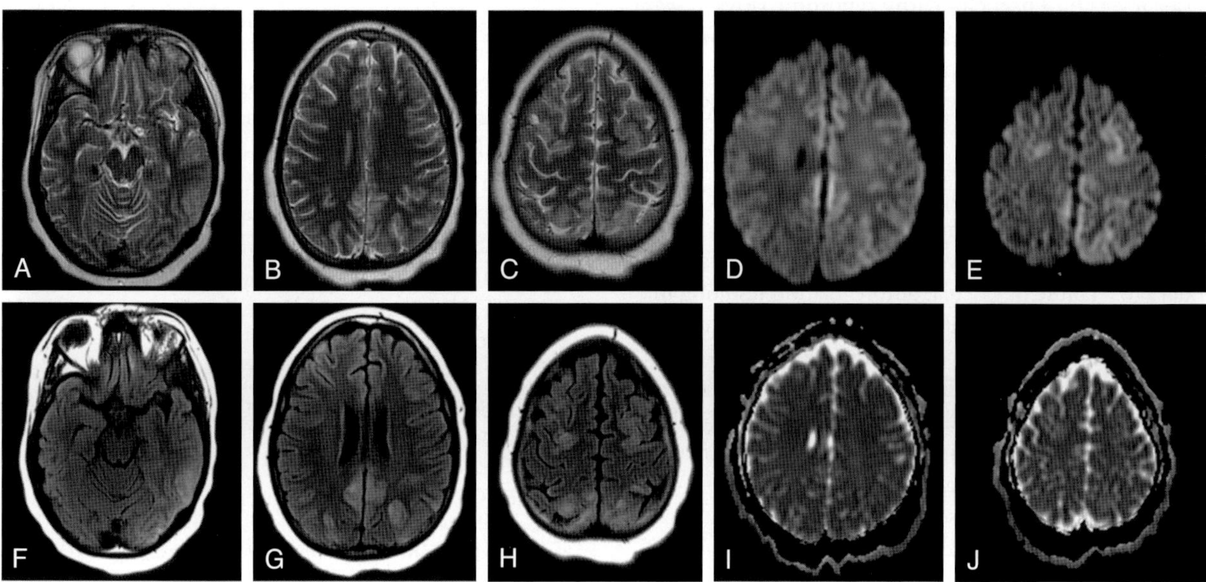

Fig. 3.33 Posterior Reversible Encephalopathy Syndrome (PRES). (A-C) Axial T2W, (D and E) axial DWI, (F-H) axial FLAIR, and (I and J) axial ADC images demonstrate bilateral (left greater than right) symmetric multifocal T2/FLAIR/DWI hyperintense cortex and partial subcortical white matter involvement in a predominantly posterior distribution. On the ADC maps most of the areas are characterized by facilitated diffusion compatible with vasogenic edema.

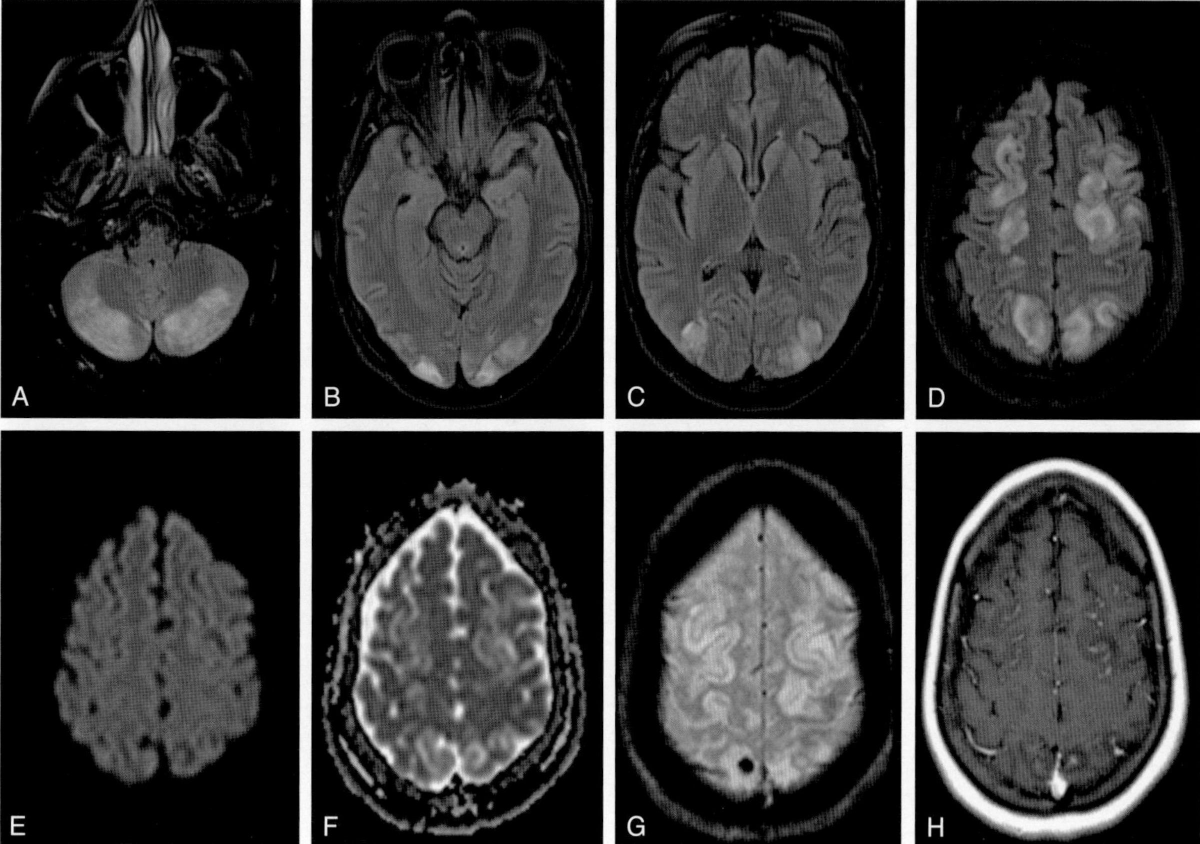

Fig. 3.34 Posterior Reversible Encephalopathy Syndrome (PRES). (A to D) Axial FLAIR, (E) axial DWI, (F) axial ADC, (G) axial GRE, and (H) axial T1W+C images demonstrate multifocal FLAIR/DWI-hyperintense cortical gray matter lesions with posterior distribution affecting both the supratentorial brain as well as cerebellum. On the ADC maps the lesions show increased diffusion (vasogenic edema). On T1W+C there is mild enhancement of engorged sulcal veins adjacent to the swollen/affected cortical ribbon.

Key Points

Background

- Posterior reversible encephalopathy syndrome (PRES) was first described in 1996 as an acute, reversible syndrome characterized by variable combinations of headache, altered mental function, seizures, confusion, drowsiness, and loss of vision.
- PRES typically occurs in patients with renal insufficiency, hypertension or immunosuppression, or as part of a pre-eclampsia-eclampsia syndrome.
- The exact etiology is still not yet fully established but is likely secondary to a failure of vascular autoregulation resulting in a disruption of the blood-brain barrier with extravasation of blood and macromolecules and consequent cortical and subcortical interstitial edema in response to acutely elevated blood pressure. There is a predilection of the vertebrobasilar system secondary to the paucity of a sympathetic innervation compared to the anterior intracranial circulation.
- If systemic blood pressure rises acutely, insufficient protective, sympathetically controlled arteriolar vasoconstriction results in the edema.
- If the vasogenic edema persists, cytotoxic edema may develop.

Imaging

- The clinical presentation is nonspecific; neuroimaging is consequently essential for diagnosis.
- On CT and MRI, the posterior cerebral cortex and subcortical white matter are bilaterally affected; the paramedian posterior superior frontal lobes are also often involved. Brainstem, basal ganglia, and thalami are typically spared.
- There is no or very minimal contrast enhancement; on diffusion-weighted imaging vasogenic edema is seen with facilitated diffusion on the ADC maps. T2 shine-through may mimic restricted diffusion on the isotropic DWI images. Hemorrhage and/or ischemia can occur in 10-20% of patients with PRES.
- With rapid and adequate treatment, the vasogenic edema will resolve with often near-complete resolution of the imaging findings.

REFERENCE

1. Kontzialis M, Huisman TA. Toxic-metabolic neurologic disorders in children: a neuroimaging review. *J. Neuroimaging*. 2018 Jul 31 [Epub ahead of print].

VEIN OF GALEN ANEURSYMAL MALFORMATION

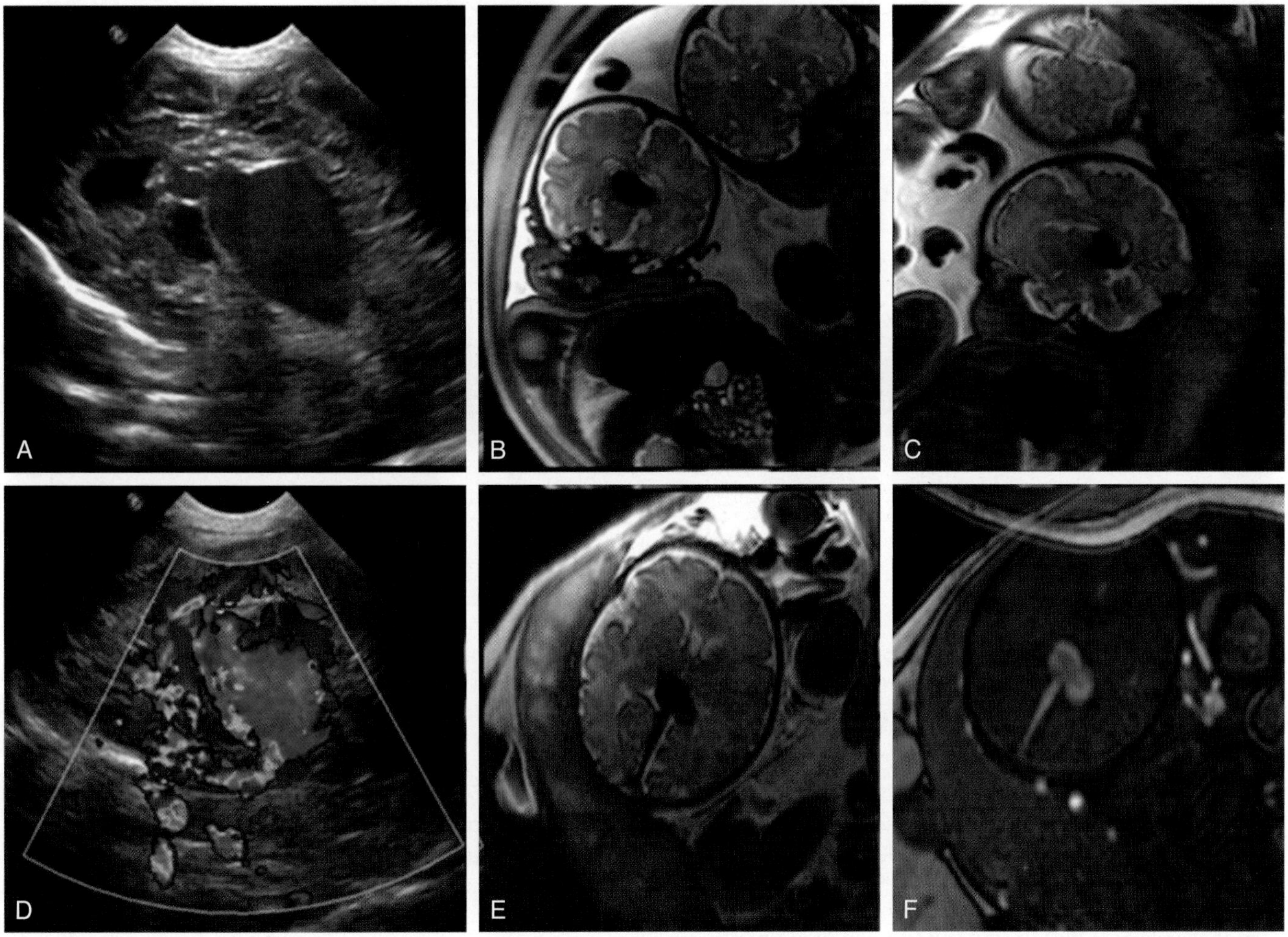

Fig. 3.35 Vein of Galen Malformation. (A and D) Sagittal head ultrasound and color-coded Doppler sonography show a large aneurysmal dilatation of the vein of Galen with turbulent flow. Multiple dilated feeding arteries are seen originating from the anterior and posterior circulation. (B, C, E) Coronal, sagittal and axial T2W fetal MRI images and (F) axial fetal MRA show the vein of Galen aneurysmal malformation is T2 hypointense with intense flow-related signal enhancement on MRA. The brain parenchyma shows no edema, hemorrhage or encephalomalacia. Additional note is made of a twin gestation pregnancy.

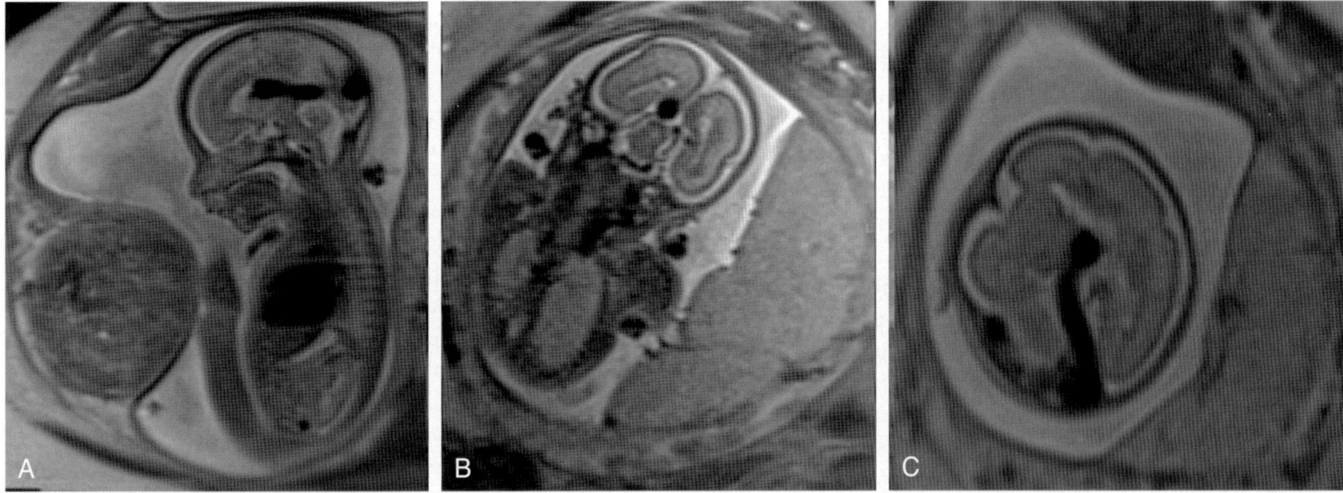

Fig. 3.36 Vein of Galen Malformation. (A-C) Sagittal, coronal and axial T2W fetal MRI shows a marked dilatation of the internal cerebral veins, vein of Galen, and straight sinus compatible with a vein of Galen aneurysmal malformation. The brain parenchyma is unremarkable. Incidental note is made of a uterine myoma.

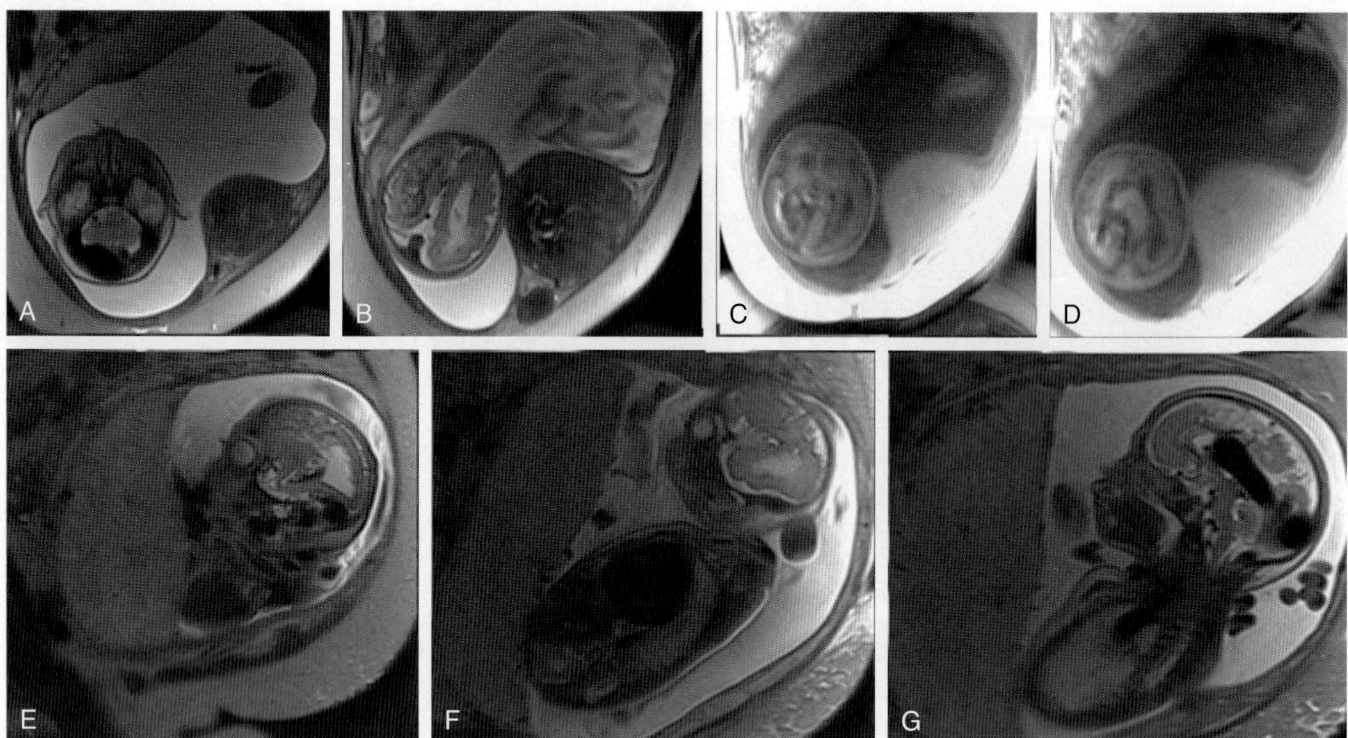

Fig. 3.37 Vein of Galen Malformation. Follow-up fetal MRI for the same patient shown in Fig. 3.35 later in pregnancy with (A, B) axial T2W, (C, D) axial T1W, and (E–G) sagittal T2W images shows progressive white matter volume loss, ex vacuo widening of the ventricles, and intraparenchymal T1-hyperintense dystrophic calcifications known as "melting brain." In addition, polyhydramnios, cardiomegaly, and umbilical cord vessel dilatation have developed.

Key Points

Background

- A vein of Galen aneurysmal malformation is a rare arteriovenous malformation in which one or more arteries of the circle of Willis directly connect and drain into the deep venous system with resultant "aneurysmal" dilatation of the vein of Galen.
- This congenital malformation develops between the sixth and eleventh week of gestation and is believed to result from a fistulous connection between a persisting median prosencephalic vein of Markowski, an embryonic precursor of the vein of Galen, and primitive arachnoideal and choroideal arteries.
- A dilated vein of Galen may be seen in multiple types of malformations, but only one of them is a true vein of Galen aneurysmal malformation (VGAM). In a true VGAM, the vein of Galen is not yet formed. Intermittent deep vein thrombosis with anomalous recanalization and/or venous stenosis may also result in a dilatation of the vein of Galen.
- The arteriovenous shunting may result in progressive ischemic injury to the developing brain due to chronic venous hypertension and parenchymal venous stasis as well as arterial steal phenomena. The progressive injury is also known as "melting brain." In addition, hydrocephalus may develop secondary to an impaired cerebrospinal fluid resorption at the arachnoid granulation due to the elevated "arterialized" venous pressure as well as a direct compression of the sylvian aqueduct by the dilated vein of Galen. Finally, the systemic sequelae of the intracranial arteriovenous shunting may result in progressive heart failure, affecting cerebral perfusion and venous drainage.

Imaging

- A VGAM is typically first identified on routine prenatal ultrasound screening either by directly identifying the dilated vein or by the systemic hemodynamic consequences, including polyhydramnios, cardiomegaly, fetal ascites, pleural effusion, or even fetal hydrops. If the anomaly is not recognized prenatally, children who are born typically present with congestive heart failure, respiratory distress, cyanosis, macrocephaly, prominent scalp veins, and a distinct bruit of the scalp.
- On fetal and postnatal ultrasound, the dilated vein of Galen appears anechoic with turbulent flow on doppler ultrasound. A low resistive index value is sampled within arterial feeders secondary to the shunting. Ventriculomegaly can easily be depicted by enlarged ventricles; the complication of a melting brain is characterized by global white matter volume loss and intra- and subcortical color-coded Doppler sonography calcifications due to the chronic venous stasis.
- Fetal and postnatal MRI imaging findings match the ultrasound findings with a T1/T2-hypointense aneurysmal dilatation of the vein of Galen, ventriculomegaly and chronic hemispheric white and gray matter injury, and

volume loss. The calcifications may be T1 hyperintense, T2 hypointense. On fetal MRI, the umbilical cord is often hydropic; the umbilical vessels are typically dilated; the heart is enlarged; T2-hyperintense fetal pericardial and pleural effusion, ascites, or hydrops may develop.

- Postnatal angiography and possible multiphased embolization remain standard of imaging and care to evaluate and treat these congenital malformations.
- Overall prognosis depends on the hemodynamic significance of the arteriovenous shunting and subsequent impact on the central nervous system and cardiovascular system. If untreated, morbidity and mortality are high. Ideally, treatment is delayed until ~5 months of age when the vascular system is mature. The Bicetre score which includes assessment of cardiac, cerebral, respiratory, hepatic and renal function is used to guide need for intervention. A score <8 suggests near fatal prognosis, a score between 8-12 suggests benefit from emergent embolization, and a score >12 suggests medical management. Lastly, there is positive correlation between increasing medial-lateral diameter of the straight or falcine sinus on fetal or neonatal MRI and likelihood of being in the neonatal at risk cohort.

REFERENCES

1. Alvarez H, Garcia-Monaco R, Rodesch G, Sachet M, et al. Vein of Galen aneursymal malformations. *Neuroimaging Clin N Am*. 2007;17(2):189–206.
2. Hergan F, Huisman TA."Melting brain" as complication of a vein of Galen aneurysmal malformation diagnosed by fetal MRI. *Clinical Obstetrics, Gynecology and Reproductive Medicine*. Printed online.
3. Orman G, Benson JE, Kweldam CF, Bosemani T, et al. Neonatal head ultrasonography today: a powerful imaging tool! *J Neuroimaging*. 2015 Jan-Feb;25(1):31–55.

CAVERNOUS ANGIOMA

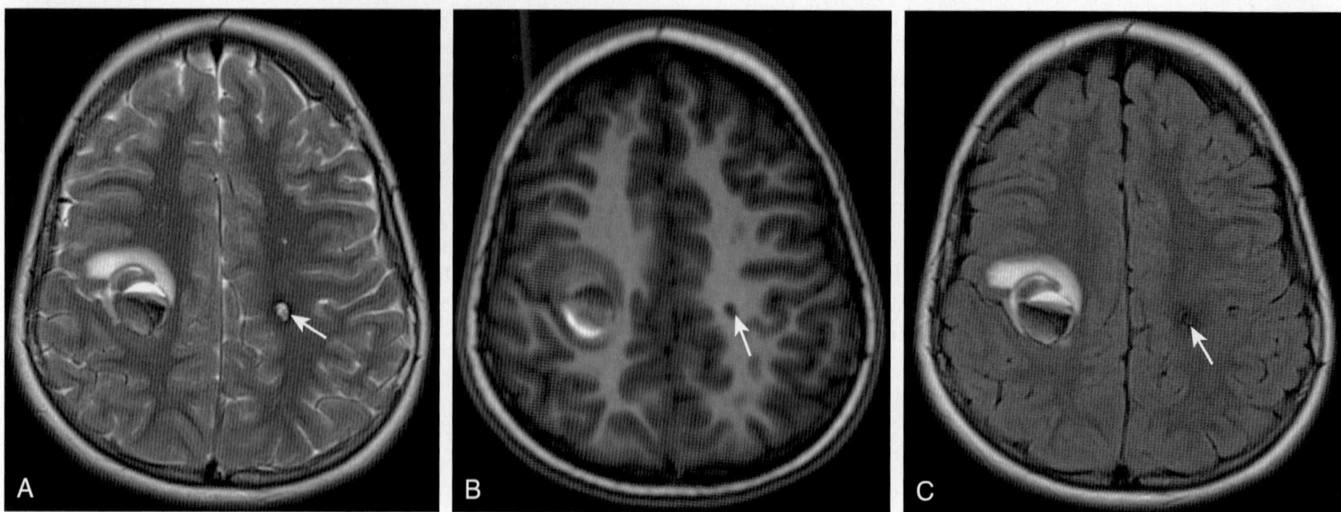

Fig. 3.38 Cavernous Angioma. (A) Axial T2W, (B) axial T1W, and (C) axial FLAIR images demonstrate a rounded intraparenchymal lesion in the right centrum semiovale with T2/T1/FLAIR heterogeneous hyperintense and hypointense signal, layering of internal hemorrhage and mild edema within the right perirolandic subcortical white matter. An additional smaller cavernoma is seen on the left centrum semiovale with classic T2-hypointense hemosiderin staining along the periphery (*arrow*).

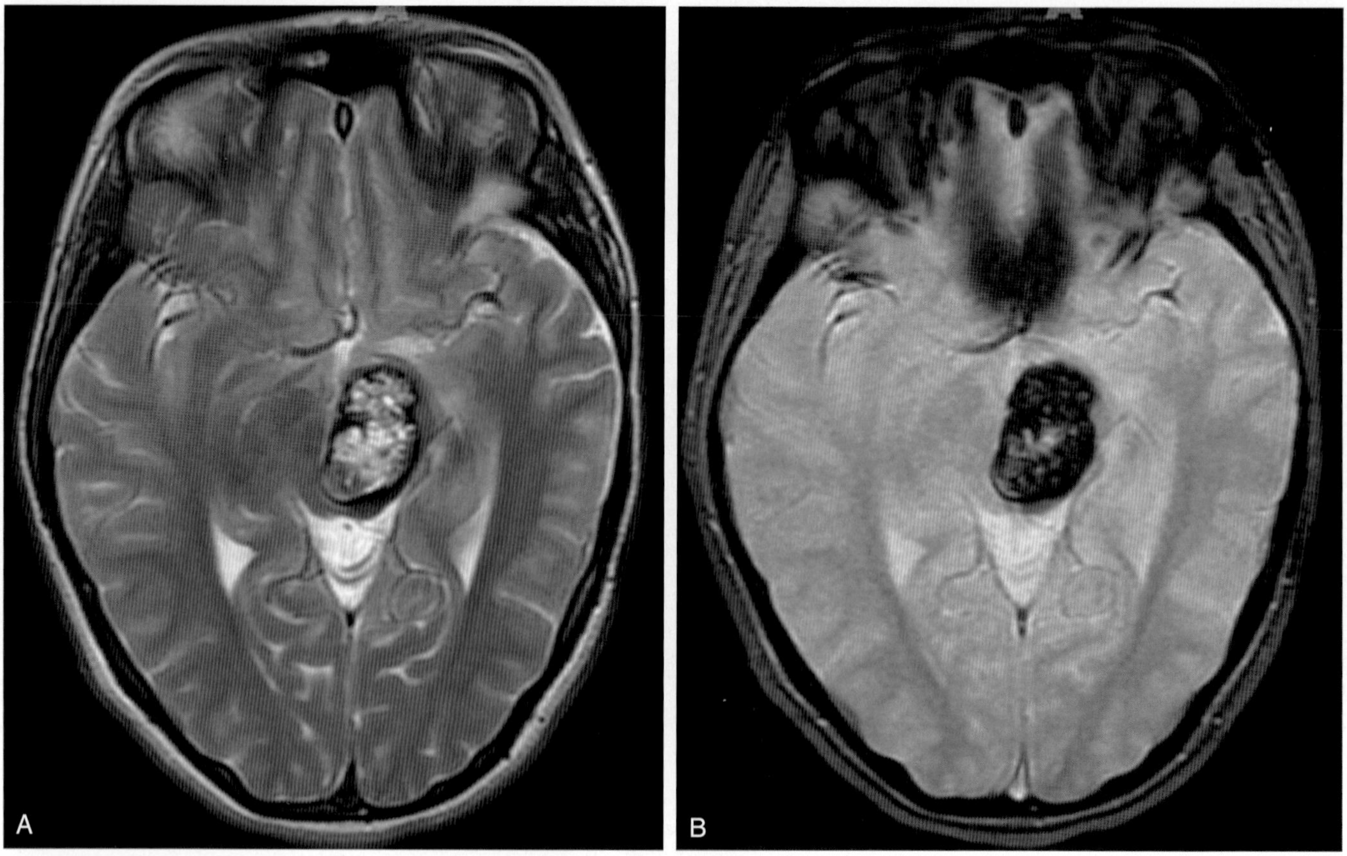

Fig. 3.39 Cavernous Angioma. (A) Axial T2W image demonstrate a large popcorn-like T2-heterogeneous hyper/hypointense cavernoma with peripheral T2-hypointense hemosiderin staining in the left cerebral peduncle. (B) Axial GRE image shows marked hypointense blooming artifact typical of a cavernous angiuoma.

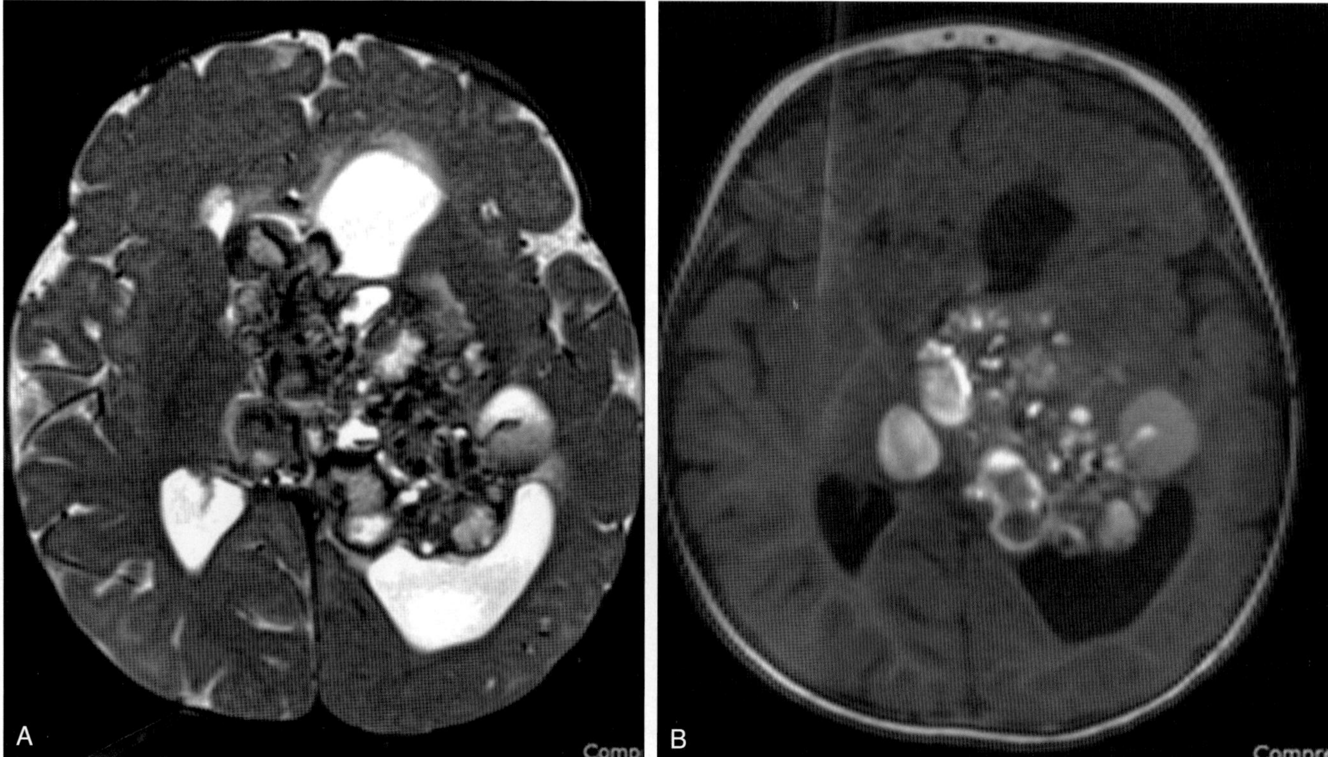

Fig. 3.40 Giant Cavernous Angioma. (A) Axial T2W and (B) axial T1W images demonstrate a giant multilobulated T2- and T1-heterogeneous midline cavernoma, which appears to protrude into the ventricles. Apparent mass effect on the region of the foramen of Monro bilaterally with resultant obstructive, left dominant ventriculomegaly. Mild periventricular interstitial edema is noted along the left lateral ventricle. Multiple compartments of the cavernoma are T1 hyperintense due to methemoglobin. Chronic hemorrhages and calcifications appear T2 hypointense. The case illustrates how a rare giant cavernous angioma could mimic an intracranial tumor and could pose a challenge to radiologists who are not familiar with this possibility.

Key Points

Background

- Cavernous angiomas or cavernomas are venous vascular malformations characterized by low-pressure, slow-flowing sinusoidal enlarged venous compartments. The lesions are primarily located within hemispheric white matter but may also be seen within the brainstem. Cavernomas are expansile rather than infiltrative, and consequently no white or gray matter is included in the lesion.
- Recurrent intralesional venous hemorrhages and thrombosis result in lesion enlargement.
- Cavernous angiomas should be differentiated from cavernous hemangiomas, which are true (benign) neoplasms that grow by mitosis.

Imaging

- On CT, an unruptured cavernoma is mildly hyperdense which can mimic acute hemorrhage, and may have visible calcifications. The density of intralesional hemorrhages follow the classical temporal evolution of intracranial blood products. On delayed contrast-enhanced imaging the cavernoma may enhance.
- On MRI, the cavernoma is typically described as a "mulberry"- or "popcorn"-like focal lesion with mixed T1 and T2 hyper- and hypointense signal characteristic. T2-hypointense hemosiderin staining of adjacent white matter is often noted secondary to microhemorrhages. Fluid-sedimentation levels may be seen in areas with more acute hemorrhaging. Similar to CT, the lesions may show variable degrees of contrast enhancement on delayed imaging. On susceptibility-weighted imaging, prominent blooming of the chronic blood products make the lesion highly conspicuous; however, the blooming may result in an overestimation of the overall size of the lesion. Surrounding edema indicates recent hemorrhage from the cavernoma.
- If the cavernoma is close to overlying cortical gray matter, the hemosiderin staining may extend into the cortical ribbon and is believed to act highly epileptogenic.
- Due to the slow flow, cavernomas are typically barely visible on non–contrast-enhanced magnetic resonance angiography (MRA) or magnetic resonance venography (MRV). Similarly, cavernomas are usually angiographically occult.
- Neighboring developmental venous anomalies should be actively searched for as the mass effect of the cavernoma may impact normal venous drainage of the white matter, resulting in a hemodynamically relevant alternative drainage over preexistent intramedullary or collector veins, mimicking a primary developmental venous anomaly.

REFERENCE

1. Huisman TA, Singhi S, Pinto P. Non-invasive imaging of intracranial pediatric vascular lesions. *Childs Nerv Syst.* 2010 Oct;26(10):1275–1295.

DEVELOPMENTAL VENOUS ANOMALY

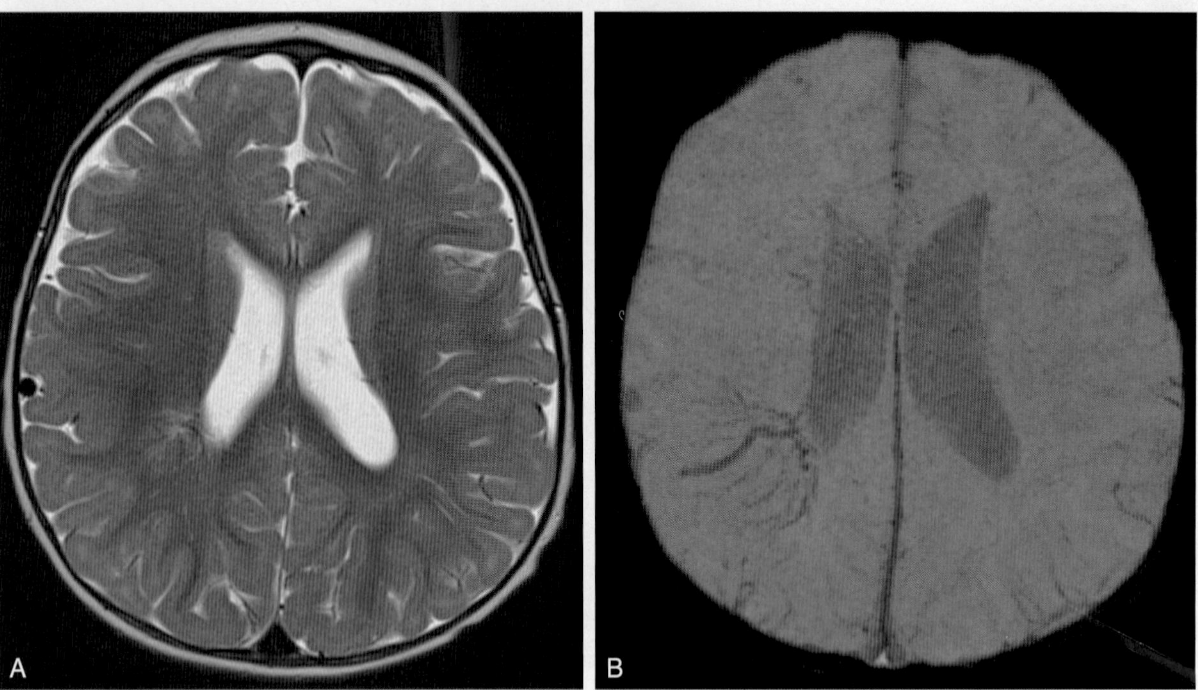

Fig. 3.41 Developmental Venous Anomaly. A right parietal developmental venous anomaly is faintly visible on (A) axial T2W image, but well seen on (B) axial SWI as multiple hypointense intramedullary veins (caput medusa) converging to a wide collector vein, which subsequently drains into the superficial venous system. Mild T2 hyperintensity is seen along the "head" of the developmental venous anomaly.

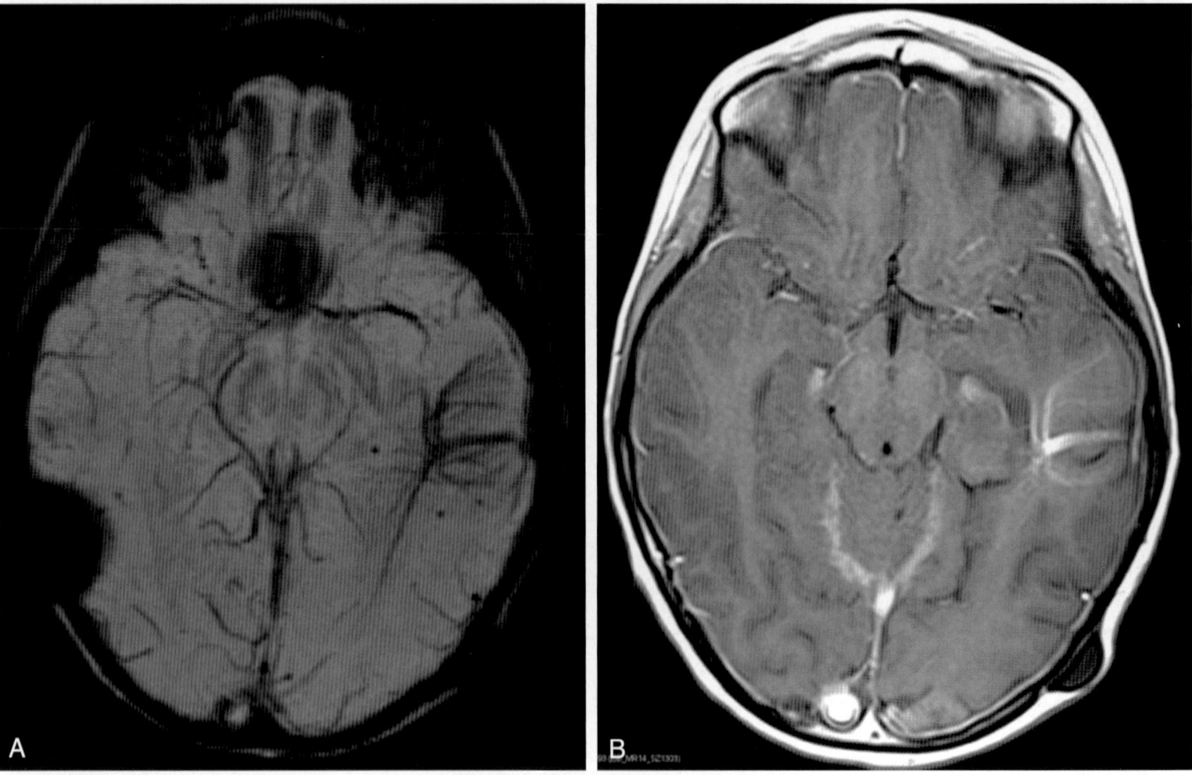

Fig. 3.42 Developmental Venous Anomaly. Left temporal developmental venous anomaly seen on (A) axial SWI with multiple hypointense intramedullary veins draining via a large collector vein into the superficial venous system. On (B) T1W+C image the majority of the developmental venous anomaly enhances because of the slow flow.

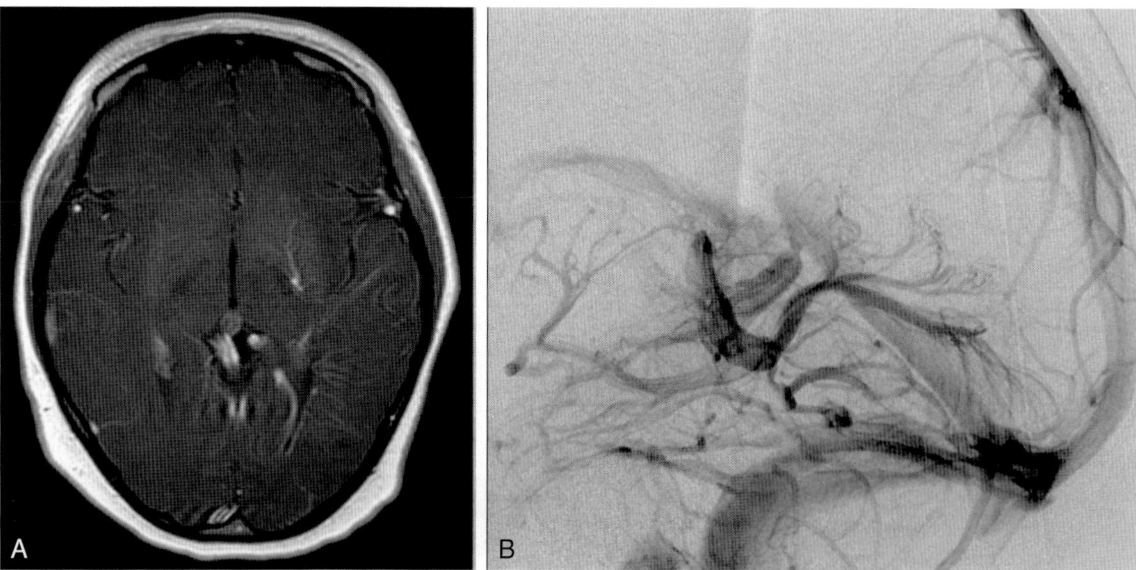

Fig. 3.43 Developmental Venous Anomaly. A large occipital developmental venous anomaly is partially visualized on (A) axial T1W+C image. (B) Sagittal venous phase of a digital subtraction catheter angiography shows the full extent of the DVA with drainage into the deep venous system.

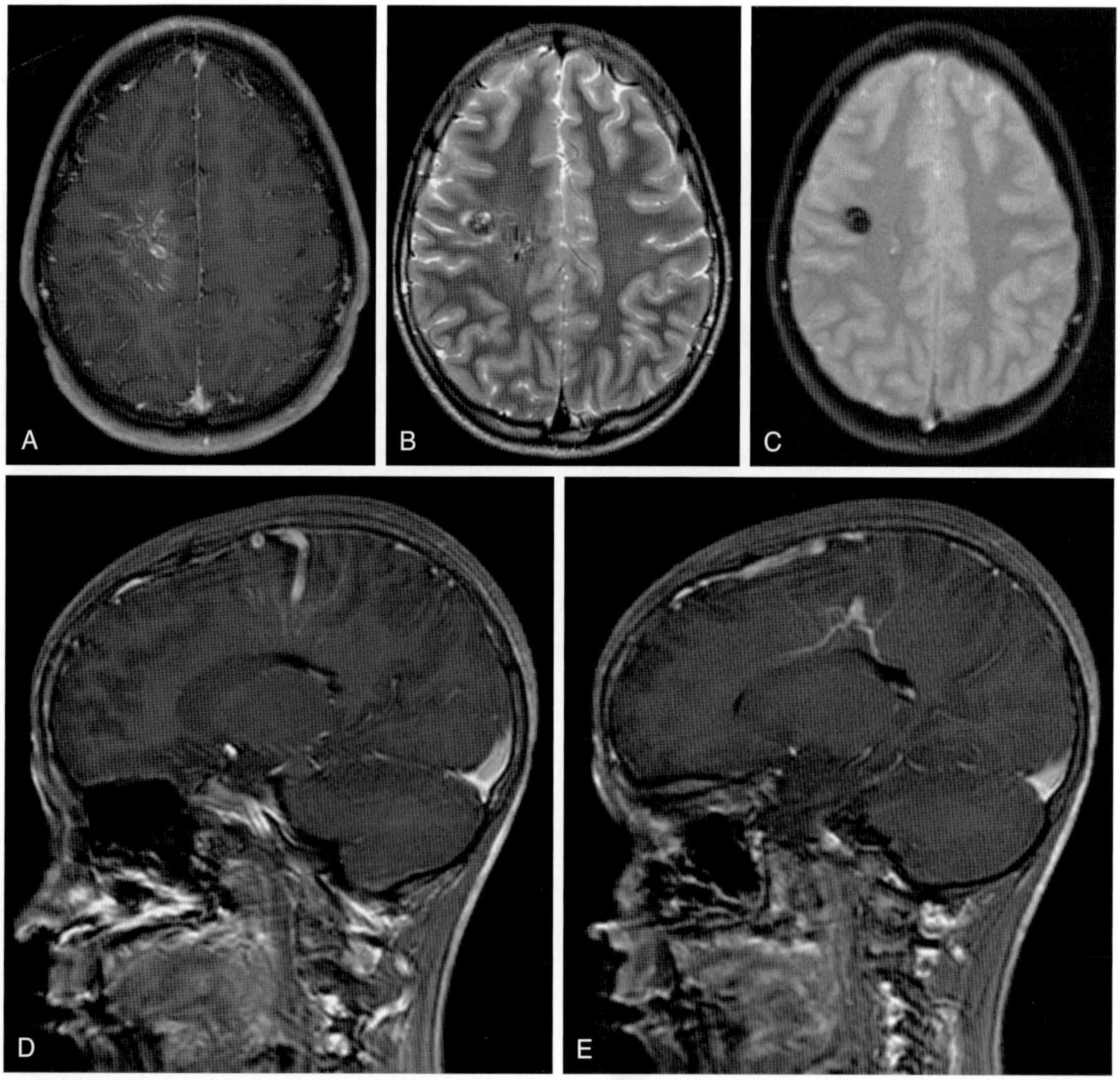

Fig. 3.44 Developmental Venous Anomaly. (A, D, and E) Axial and sagittal T1W+C images show a contrast-enhancing developmental venous anomaly in the right perirolandic region draining into the superior sagittal sinus in combination with a small T2-heterogeneous hypointense, markedly T2*-hypointense adjacent cavernoma seen on (B) axial T2W and (C) axial GRE images.

Key Points

Background

- Developmental venous anomalies (DVAs) represent functional and vital pathways of venous drainage of the white and gray matter of the supra- and infratentorial brain.
- They are characterized by multiple intramedullary veins converging toward a larger collector vein that drains into either the superficial or deep venous system.
- The multiple smaller veins that drain toward this collector vein resemble a "caput medusa."
- Developmental venous anomalies were erroneously believed to represent venous angiomas or venous malformations increasing the risk for intracerebral hemorrhages. Today it is well recognized that these DVAs are benign anomalies of the venous system that drain normal brain tissue and should not be resected. Hemorrhaging is primarily secondary to hemorrhages within adjacent cavernomas or secondary to a thrombosis of the DVA with resultant hemorrhaging venous stroke.
- It is the task of each neuroradiologist to alert neurosurgeons about the exact location and venous territory of the DVA to prevent accidental resection, which would impair the functional venous drainage increasing the likability of postsurgical venous strokes.
- Primary DVAs are believed to be a variation of nature or compensatory because of an incomplete development of the deep or superficial venous system requiring alternative venous drainage.
- DVAs may be seen in various vascular pathologies as a kind of secondary finding: for example, in Sturge-Weber syndrome or with intracranial arteriovenous malformations.
- Based upon the venous nature of the DVAs, intralesional pressure is low and blood flow is slow.

Imaging

- On CT, DVAs are not visible or are barely visible prior to intravenous contrast injection but may be seen on delayed contrast-enhanced series as a linear or curvilinear mildly prominent enhancing vessel with a classical caput medusa of small vessels converging to the collector vein.
- On MRI the DVA is best seen on delayed contrast-enhanced T1-weighted imaging; however, recent studies have shown that susceptibility-weighted imaging may show the lesion based upon the SWI hypointensity of the slow-flowing deoxygenated venous blood with high accuracy and sensitivity.
- Most importantly, contrast-enhanced imaging should be studied to exclude associated lesions, in particular cavernomas.
- Occasionally, mild T2/FLAIR hyperintense gliosis or edema is noted surrounding the DVA.
- DVAs are easily missed on the arterial phase of catheter angiography but are typically well seen on the delayed, venous phase.

REFERENCES

1. Young A, Poretti A, Bosemani T, Goel R, Huisman TAGM. Sensitivity of susceptibility weighted imaging in detecting developmental venous anomalies and associated cavernomas and microhemorrhages in children. *Neuroradiol.* 2017 Aug;59(8):797–802.
2. Huisman TA, Singhi S, Pinto P. Non-invasive imaging of intracranial pediatric vascular lesions. *Childs Nerv Syst.* 2010 Oct;26(10):1275–1295.

FAMILIAL AND POSTRADIATION CAVERNOUS MALFORMATIONS

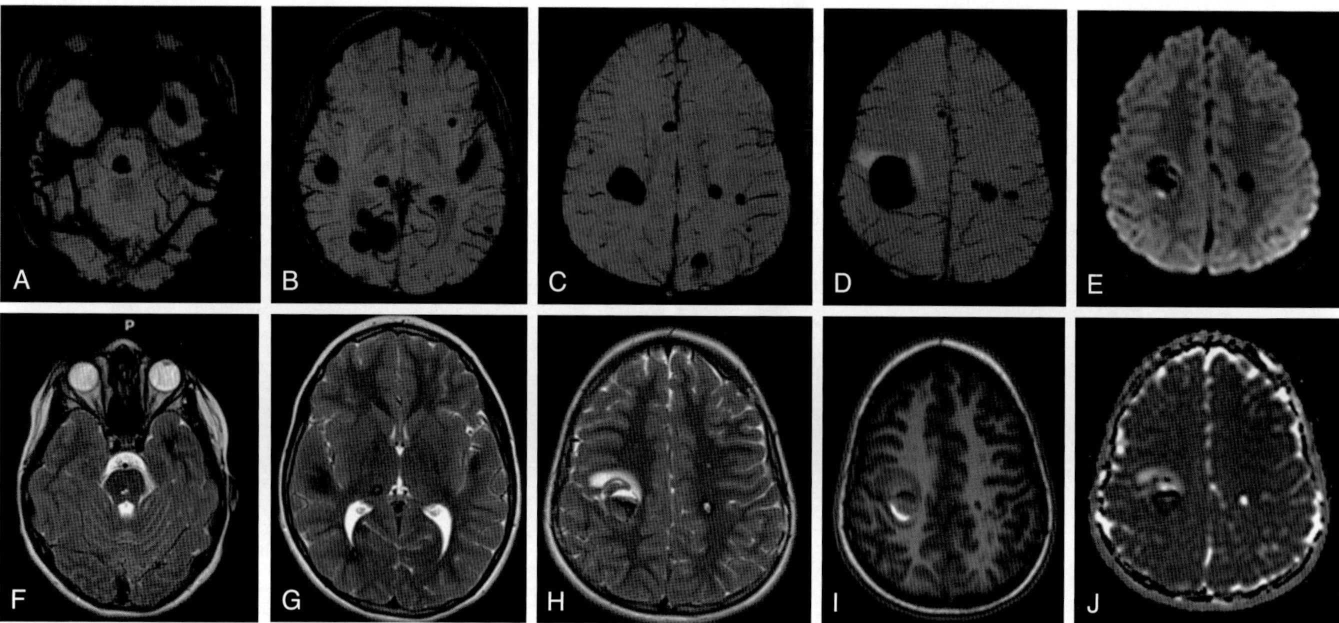

Fig. 3.45 Familial Cavernomas. (A-D) Axial SWI, (E) axial DWI, (F-H) axial T2W, (I) axial T1W, and (J) axial ADC images demonstrate multiple SWI-hypointense, T2 and T1-heterogeneous hyper-/hypointense cavernomas sprinkled throughout the supratentorial white matter bilaterally as well as brainstem. Blood sedimentation leveling is seen in the largest cavernoma in the right perirolandic region surrounded by mild vasogenic edema (high ADC values) typically seen after a recent intralesional hemorrhage. The blood products also result in significant susceptibility related signal loss on diffusion-weighted imaging.

Key Points

Background

- Multiple cavernomas, symptomatic or incidentally noted, should raise the possibility of a genetic disorder known as "familial multiple cavernous malformation syndrome."
- If more than five cavernomas are identified on neuroimaging in one patient or if one cavernoma is identified but at least one related family member has one or more cavernomas, the diagnosis should be called.
- Mutations in several genes have been identified to be linked to this syndrome (*KRIT1, CCM2, PDCD10*).

Imaging

- Imaging features are identical to the isolated cavernoma findings.
- However, multiple cavernomas may also be seen after cranial radiotherapy. Careful review of the clinical history is indicated; cavernomas may be detected within weeks, months, or even years after radiotherapy.

REFERENCE

1. Young A, Poretti A, Bosemani T, Goel R, Huisman TAGM. Sensitivity of susceptibility weighted imaging in detecting developmental venous anomalies and associated cavernomas and microhemorrhages in children. *Neuroradiol.* 2017 Aug;59(8):797–802.

ARTERIOVENOUS MALFORMATIONS (AVMS)

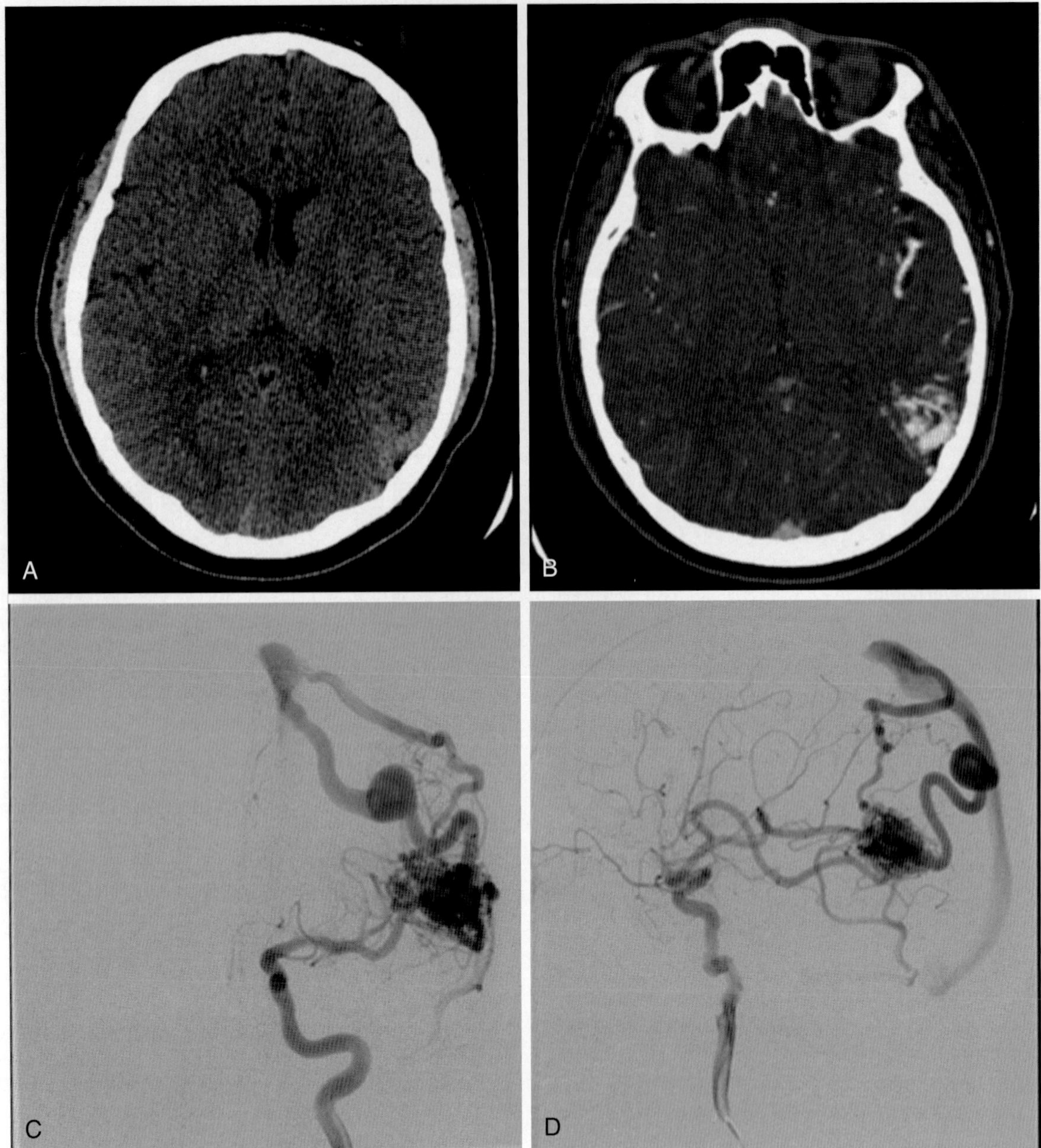

Fig. 3.46 Arteriovenous Malformation. (A) Axial head CT demonstrates subtle hyperdensity in the left temporal-occipital junction. (B) Axial CTA image shows the area corresponds to a tangle of vessels consistent with an arteriovenous malformation with dilated feeding branches of the left middle cerebral artery are seen within the left sylvian fissure. (C and D) AP and lateral digital subtraction catheter angiography shows the arteriovenous malformation nidus with dilated feeding arteries originating from the middle cerebral artery and venous drainage over varicose and elongated veins into the superficial venous system. This case illustrates how a keen radiologist's detection of the subtle finding on the noncontrast CT led to detection of an extremely significant finding of an arteriovenous malformation.

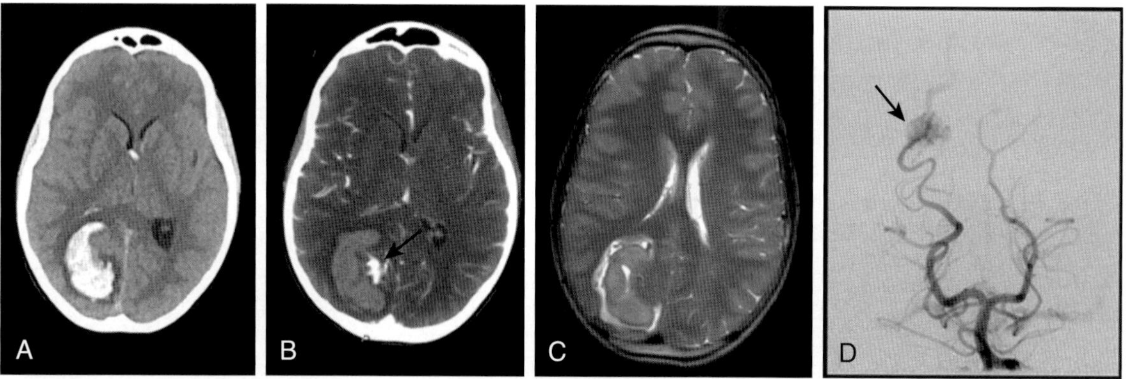

Fig. 3.47 Arteriovenous Malformation. (A) Axial head CT shows acute right occipital lobe intraparenchymal hemorrhage. (B) Axial CTA shows an abnormal enhancing nidus of vessels along the medial contour of the hemorrhage consistent with an arteriovenous malformation. (C) Axial T2W image shows isointense/mildly hyperintense hemorrhage surrounded by mild vasogenic edema. (D) AP digital subtraction catheter angiography shows the small arteriovenous malformation nidus fed by branches of the right posterior cerebral artery.

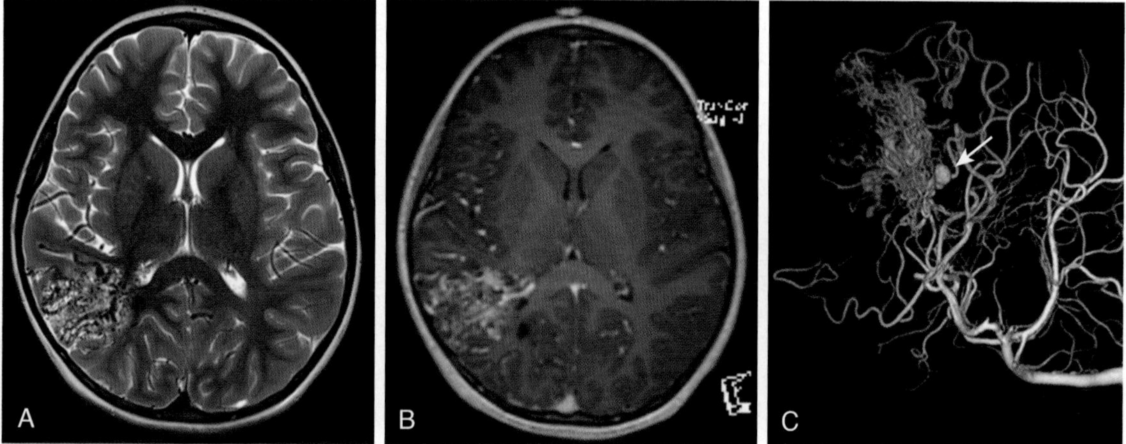

Fig. 3.48 Arteriovenous Malformation. (A) Axial T2W, (B) axial T1W+C, and (C) volume rendered angiography image demonstrate a diffuse right temporal-occipital arteriovenous malformation with multiple T2-hypointense flow voids, partially contrast-enhancing vessels and a flow-related aneurysm well seen on the angiography (*arrow*).

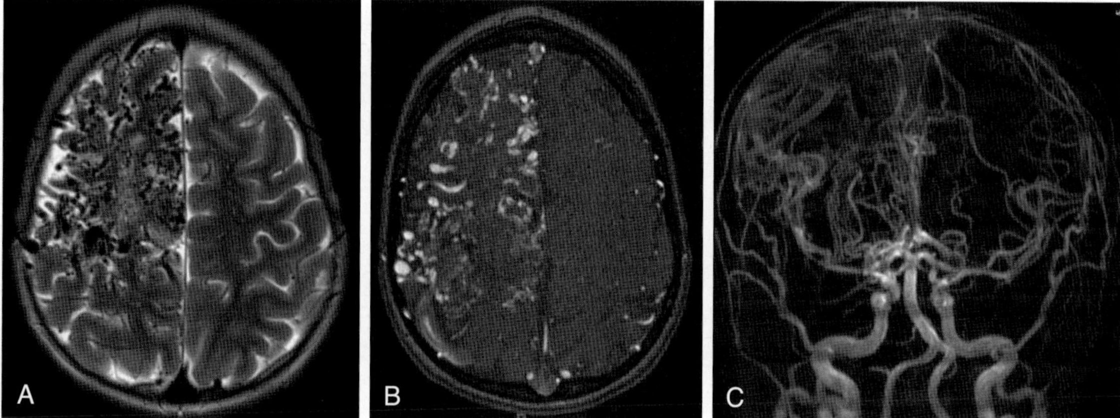

Fig. 3.49 Arteriovenous Malformation. (A) Axial T2W, (B and C) axial source images and coronal MIP time-of-flight MRA image demonstrate diffuse infiltrative hemispheric arteriovenous malformation involving the right frontal and parietal lobe. Mild T2-hyperintense gliosis is also present within the right frontal white matter.

Key Points

Background

- Arteriovenous malformations (AVMs) are anomalous connections between arteries and veins without an intervening capillary network. Depending on the primary location of the AVM, feeding arteries may originate from the anterior or posterior circle of Willis; veins may drain into the deep or superficial venous system. The feeding arteries and/or draining veins are typically enlarged depending on the hemodynamic significance of the arteriovenous shunting.
- If a single arteriovenous connection exists, the malformation is typically known as an arteriovenous fistula (AVF). If multiple vessels are involved, a nidus may be seen, which refers to a complex tangle of numerous arteriovenous shunts.
- The feeding arteries may bear flow-related aneurysms that can be causative of hemorrhages; the draining veins may be elongated and varicose and are at risk for rupturing.
- The arteriovenous shunting may result in ischemic injury to adjacent brain tissue secondary to steal phenomena.
- Depending on the location, AVMs may be subdivided in deep-seated (thalamic/central gray matter), transmantle, superficial (gyral or sulcal), intraparenchymal, or diffuse/mixed variants.
- AVMs may present acutely with hemorrhage; however, slowly progressive ischemic injury or seizures are also reported. In rare cases, the AV-shunting may result in congestive heart failure.

Imaging

- An AVM should be ruled out in children with an acute, unexplained intracranial hemorrhage. Contrast-enhanced CT/CTA typically shows the AVM, including nidus, feeding arteries, and draining veins. Flow-related aneurysms, possibly hidden within the nidus, should actively be ruled out. In the acute phase, a hematoma may compress or obscure the AVM nidus, therefore, follow-up imaging after hematoma retraction should be considered.
- MRI and MRA/MRV are relevant for a more sensitive and specific evaluation of tissue at risk for ischemic injury. Perilesional edema and gliosis may be seen in better detail. MRI, MRA/MRV allow for a detailed evaluation of the vascular architecture of the malformation with T1/T2-hypointensity of the feeding arteries secondary to the flow void; the nidus may be intermediate in signal intensity while mixed signal void may be seen in the draining veins. Furthermore, pulsation artifacts may be seen along the phase encoding gradient. Finally, on susceptibility-weighted imaging the draining vein may show an increased signal intensity compared to veins that are not related to the AVM because of the shunt-related high percentage of oxygenated blood within the draining veins. The AVM may show mixed T1-hyperintense signal on the contrast-enhanced sequences. Dynamic contrast-enhanced MRA/MRV allows for a hemodynamic evaluation of the AVM. Similar to CT, an acute hematoma may compress or obscure the AVM nidus.
- Digital subtraction angiography remains the imaging method of choice for a complete diagnostic workup of the AVM and is the baseline study for endovascular AVM embolizations.
- The Spetzler-Martin grading scale estimates the risk of open surgery for AVMs and consists of the AVM size (1 point: < 3 cm; 2 points: 3-6 cm; 3 points: > 6 cm), venous drainage (0 points: superficial; 1 point: deep), and eloquence of the location in the brain (0 points: no; 1 point: yes). The greater the total number of points is associated with worse outcome.

REFERENCE

1. Huisman TA, Singhi S, Pinto P. Non-invasive imaging of intracranial pediatric vascular lesions. *Childs Nerv Syst*. 2010 Oct;26(10):1275–1295.

DURAL SINUS MALFORMATION

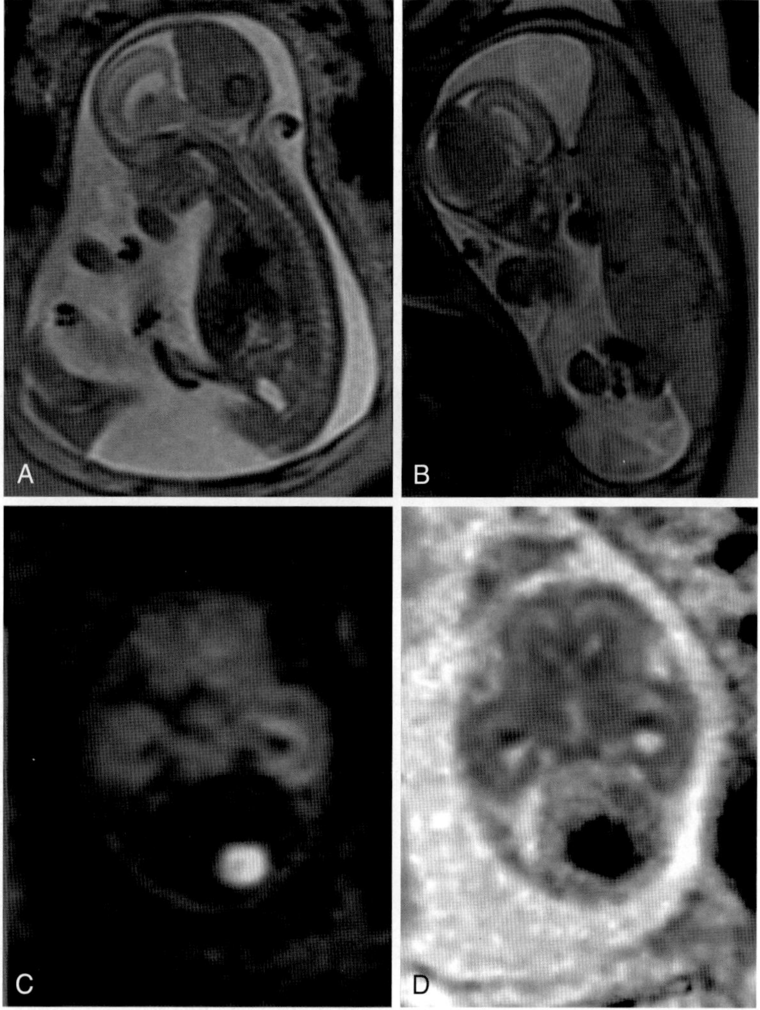

Fig. 3.50 Dural Sinus Malformation. (A and B) Sagittal and coronal T2W fetal MRI images demonstrate an abnormal T2 isointense/mild hypointense extra-axial collection consistent with a dural sinus malformation centered in the torcular Herophili characterized by a significant enlargement of the torcular Herophili with moderate mass effect on the tectal plate and occipital lobes with resultant mild obstructive supratentorial ventriculomegaly. The blood flow within the torcular Herophili results in a flow-related signal loss on T2-weighted imaging. Within the torcular Herophili on sagittal T2W image a rounded T2-hypointense blood clot was present which on (C and D) axial DWI and ADC images has reduced diffusion indicating thrombus. Postnatal imaging confirmed an associated arteriovenous fistula was supplying the malformation.

Key Points

Background

- Dural sinus malformations are rare malformations typically involving the posterior third of the superior sagittal sinus, torcula, and one or both transverse sinuses.

Imaging

- Dural sinus malformations can have an associated arteriovenous fistula; however, the fistula itself is rarely identified on fetal MRI.
- The torcular Herophili is typical dilated with mass effect on the adjacent brain structures.
- Blood flow within the torcular Herophili is usually slow, resulting in an intermediate T1/T2 signal intensity.
- In many cases, the slow flow may result in partial thrombosis of the torcular Herophili. Thrombosis may progress over gestation, resulting in a spontaneous involution/resolution of the AVF.
- The thrombus is often DWI hyperintense with matching low ADC values.
- Intracranial hemorrhage or ischemic lesions due to steal phenomena are rarely seen.
- Hydrocephalus due to mass effect occasionally develops.

REFERENCE

1. Ebert MD, Esenkaya A, Huisman TA, Bienstock J, et al. Multimodality, anatomical and diffusion weighted fetal imaging of a spontaneously thrombosing congenital dural sinus malformation. *Neuropediatrics*. 2012 Oct;43(5):279–282.

CONGENITAL DURAL AV FISTULA

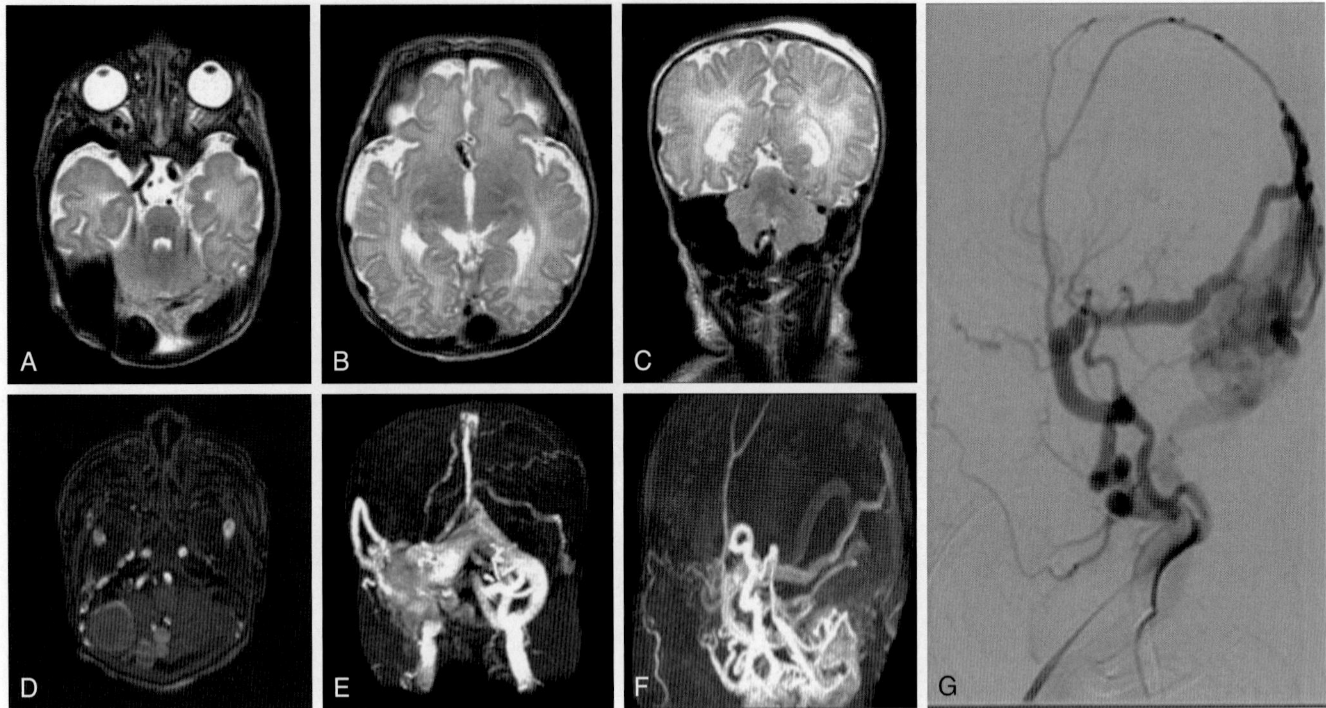

Fig. 3.51 Congenital Dural AV Fistula. (A-C) Axial and coronal T2W images demonstrate abnormal dilated T2-hypointense right transverse sinus, mild dilatation of the torcular Herophili, and left transverse sinus. (D-F) Multiplanar time-of-flight MRA and MRV images and (G) digital subtraction angiography image demonstrate the abnormality is caused by a dural arteriovenous fistula with arterial feeding vessels communicating with the posterior venous system.

Key Points

Background

- Dural arteriovenous (AV) fistula (AVF) may be seen along any dural venous sinus within the cranial vault.

Imaging

- Similar to the more frequent torcular Herophili AVF, the affected dural sinus appears enlarged with possible mass effect on adjacent brain tissue.
- In cases of a moderate- to high-flow AV shunting, the dural sinus may appear T1 and T2 hypointense secondary to the flow-related signal void.
- Superselective digital subtraction angiography is typically required to identify the exact site of the AV connection.
- Spontaneous hemorrhages and/or ischemic steal phenomena are rarely seen.
- Retrograde back pressure may result in widening of the intraparenchymal veins, in rare cases accompanied by white matter edema. Furthermore, the draining jugular veins can enlarge with widening of the jugular foramen.

REFERENCE

1. Ebert MD, Esenkaya A, Huisman TA, Bienstock J, et al. Multi-modality, anatomical and diffusion weighted fetal imaging of a spontaneously thrombosing congenital dural sinus malformation. *Neuropediatrics*. 2012 Oct;43(5):279–282.

INTRACRANIAL ANEURYSM

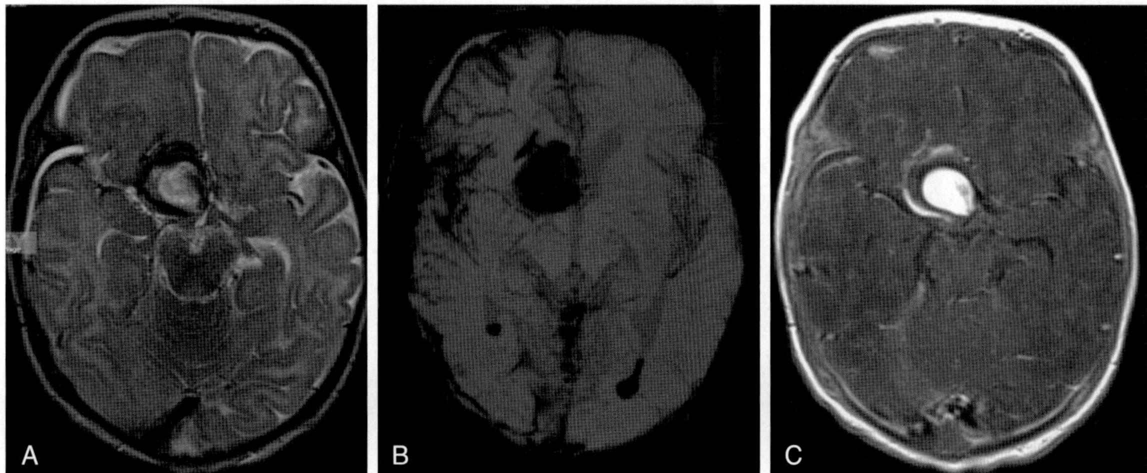

Fig. 3.52 Aneurysm. (A) Axial T2W image demonstrates a rounded mass with central T2-hyperintensity and peripheral T2-hypointensity characteristic of a partially thrombosed aneurysm from the anterior communicating artery. (B) Axial SWI shows the aneurysm is uniformly hypointense indicative of thrombus. In addition, extensive hypointense blood products are present in the subarachnoid space along the right cerebral hemisphere and small amount of hypointense blood products are seen in the occipital horns of the lateral ventricles. (C) Axial T1W+C image demonstrates the central thrombus appears T1 hyperintense indicative of methemoglobin (noncontrast T1W image not shown) and there is mild peripheral contrast enhancement indicating residual perfusion of the aneurysm.

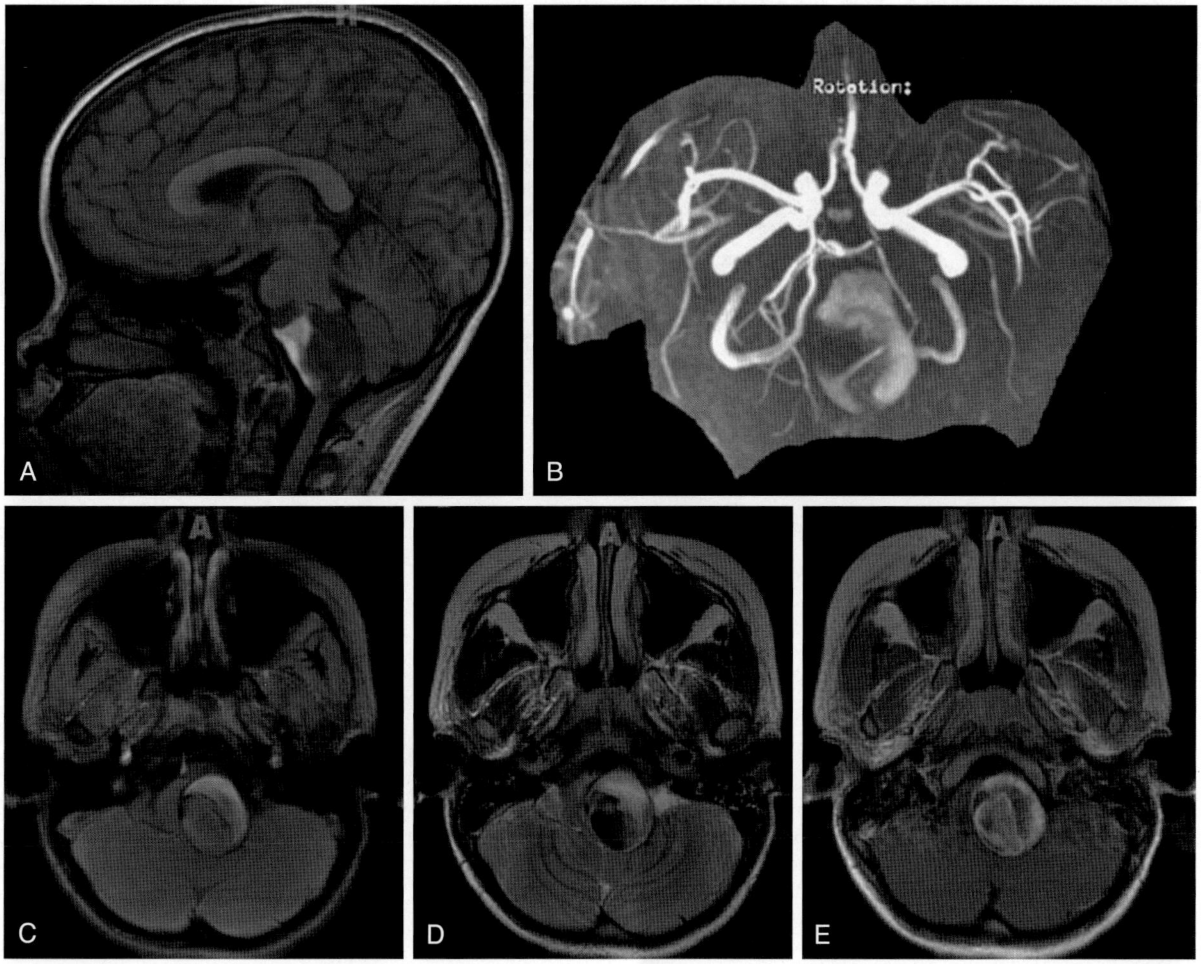

Fig. 3.53 Giant Aneurysm. (A) Sagittal T1W, (B) axial time-of-flight MRA MIP, (C) axial GRE, (D) axial T2W, and (E) axial T1W+C images demonstrate a large, partially thrombosed, T1W/T2W-heterogeneous hyper/hypointense left vertebral artery aneurysm, which exerts significant mass effect on the lower brainstem. T1W+C MRI and 3D time-of-flight MRA confirms partial perfusion of the aneurysm.

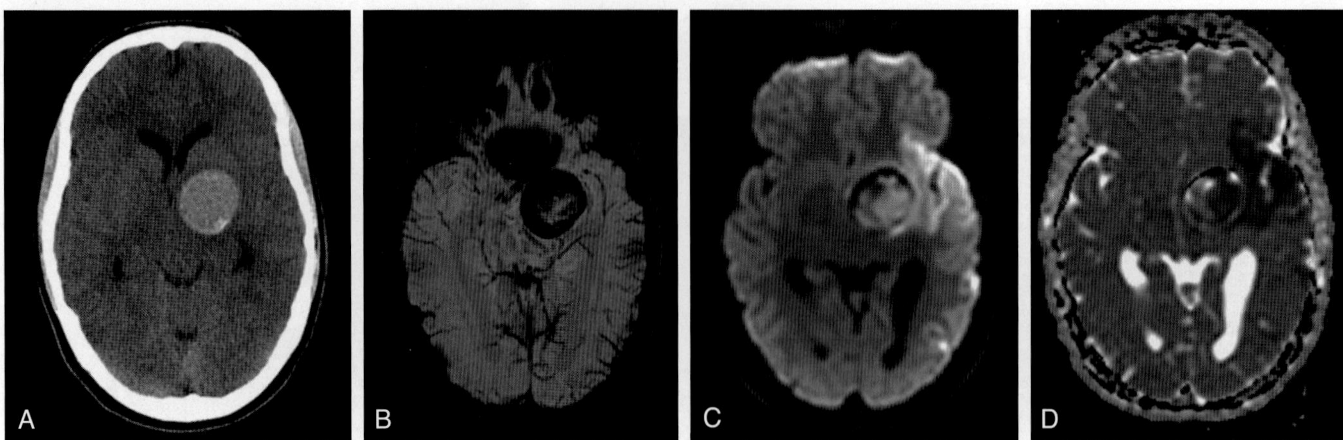

Fig. 3.54 Aneurysm. (A) Axial head CT demonstrates a round, well-circumscribed, hyperdense, thrombosed proximal left middle cerebral artery aneurysm is seen exerting mass effect on the adjacent basal ganglia. (B) Axial SWI image shows the aneurysm is hypointense compatible with thrombosis. (C and D) DWI and ADC images show a wedge shaped region of reduced diffusion indicative of an acute segmental left middle cerebral artery infarct.

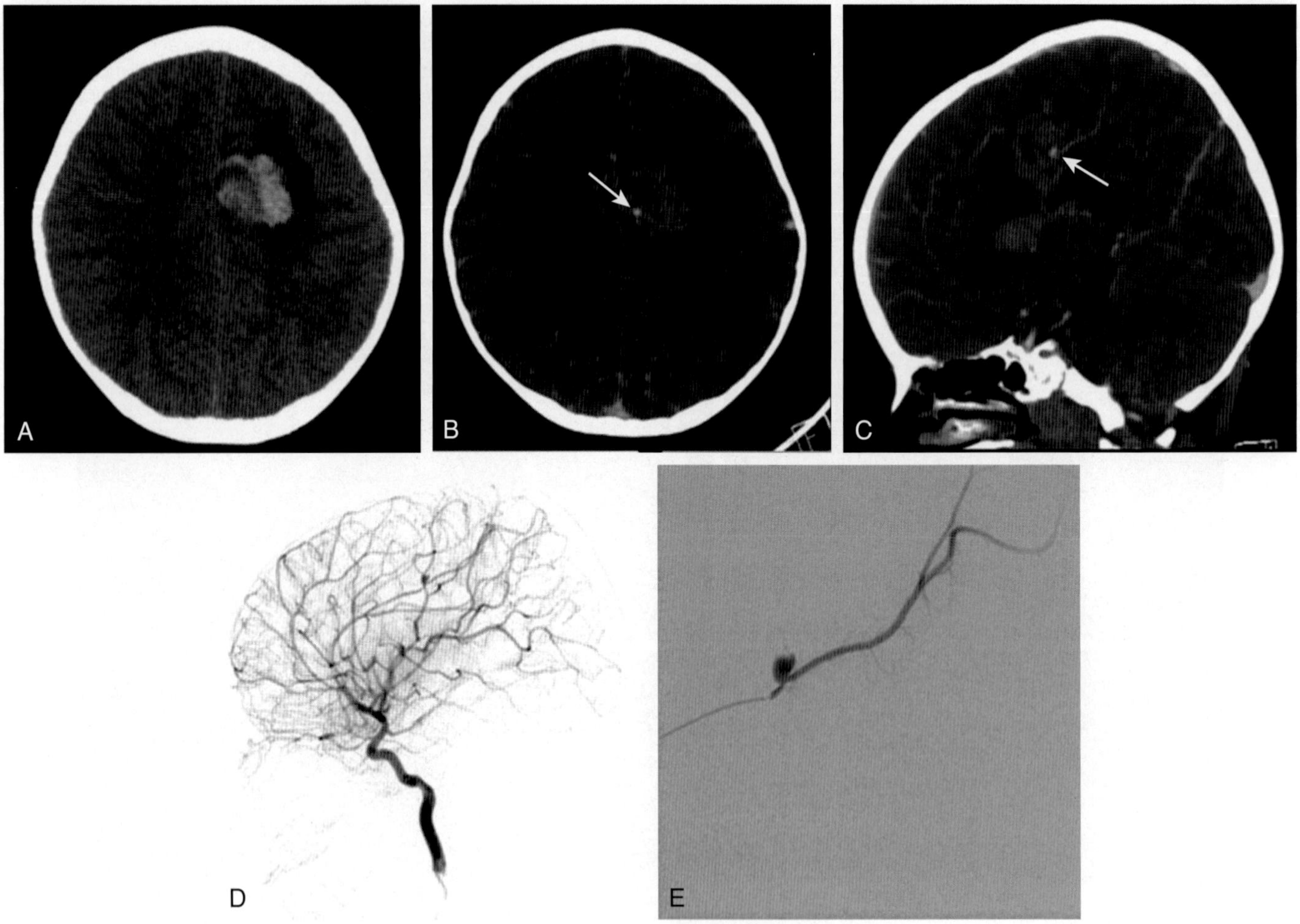

Fig. 3.55 Ruptured mycotic aneurysm. (A) Axial head CT demonstrates acute hyperdense hemorrhage in the left frontal lobe surrounded by small region of hypodensity indicative of vasogenic or cytotoxic edema. (B and C) Axial and sagittal reformat CTA images show a small, well-circumscribed focal enhancement along the medial/posterior contour of the hemorrhage, which was subsequently confirmed as a distal anterior cerebral artery aneurysm on the (D and E) digital subtraction angiography images.

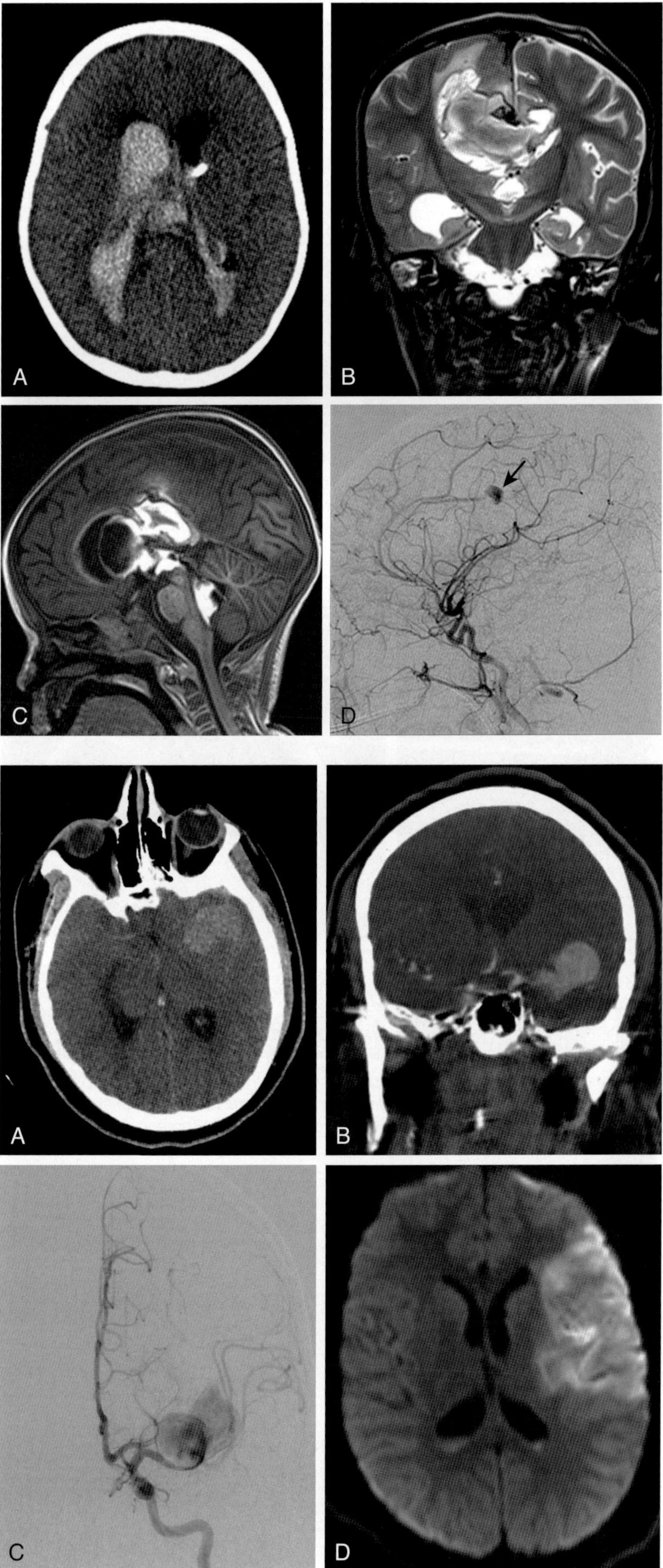

Fig. 3.56 Ruptured mycotic aneurysm. (A) Axial head CT demonstrates hyperdense blood within the body and splenium of the corpus callosum as well as within both lateral ventricles. (B) Coronal T2W, and (C) sagittal T1W images demonstrate the hematoma in the corpus callosum has mixed T2 and T1 hypointense, isointense, and hyperintense signal. Blood is also noted in the third ventricle, Sylvian aqueduct, and fourth ventricle. On coronal T2W image, a focal round hypointense flow void is noted matching the mycotic pericallosal aneurysm, which is best seen on the (D) lateral digital subtraction angiography.

Fig. 3.57 Dissecting pseudoaneurysm. A 16-year-old with headache and vomiting. (A) Axial CT demonstrates lobular acute hemorrhage in the left sylvian fissure. (B) Coronal reformat CTA demonstrates contrast filling a pseudoaneurysm from the left middle cerebral artery aneurysm and indistinct contours of the left middle cerebral artery. (C) Digital subtraction angiography coronal view from left internal carotid artery injection demonstrates the pseudoaneurysm from the left middle cerebral artery. (D) Axial DWI image demonstrates a large left middle cerebral artery infarct as a result of the dissecting pseudoaneurysm.

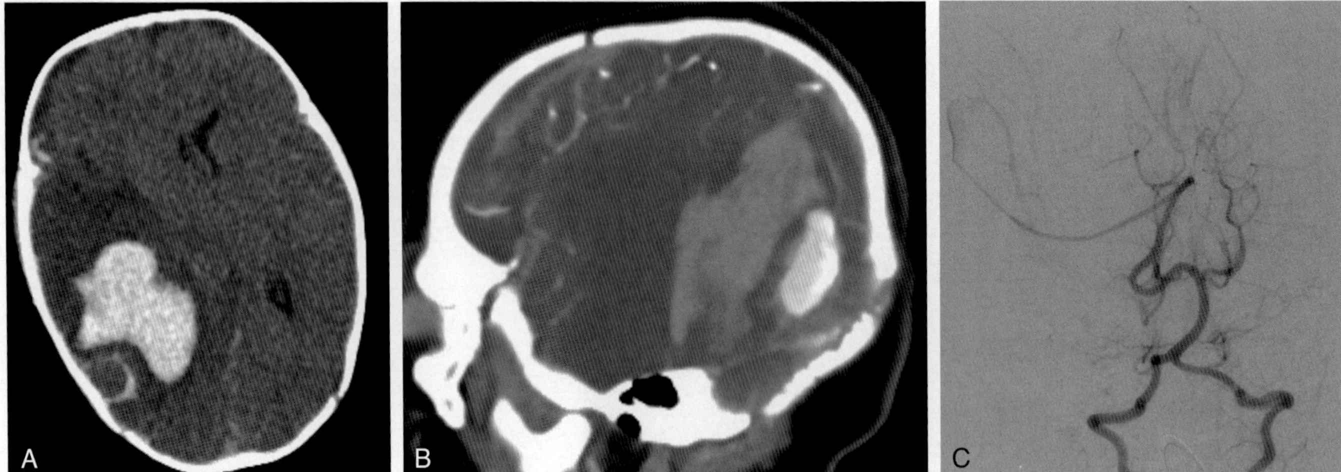

Fig. 3.58 Pseudoaneurysm. A 3-month old with asymmetric pupuils, and bulging fontanelle. (A) Axial CT demonstrates acute hemorrhage in the right temporal and parietal lobes with surrounding low density. A circular structure is surrounded by hemorrhage. (B) Sagittal reformat CTA image demonstrates the contrast filling a tubular structure concerning for an aneurysm posterior to the acute hemorrhage. (C) Coronal digital subtraction angiography injection of the posterior circulation demonstrates slow filling of a distal right posterior cerebral artery pseudoaneurysm from a right posterior cerebral artery branch. Coil embolization was performed however the hemorrhage led to a large region of encephalomalacia in the right cerebral hemisphere (*not shown*).

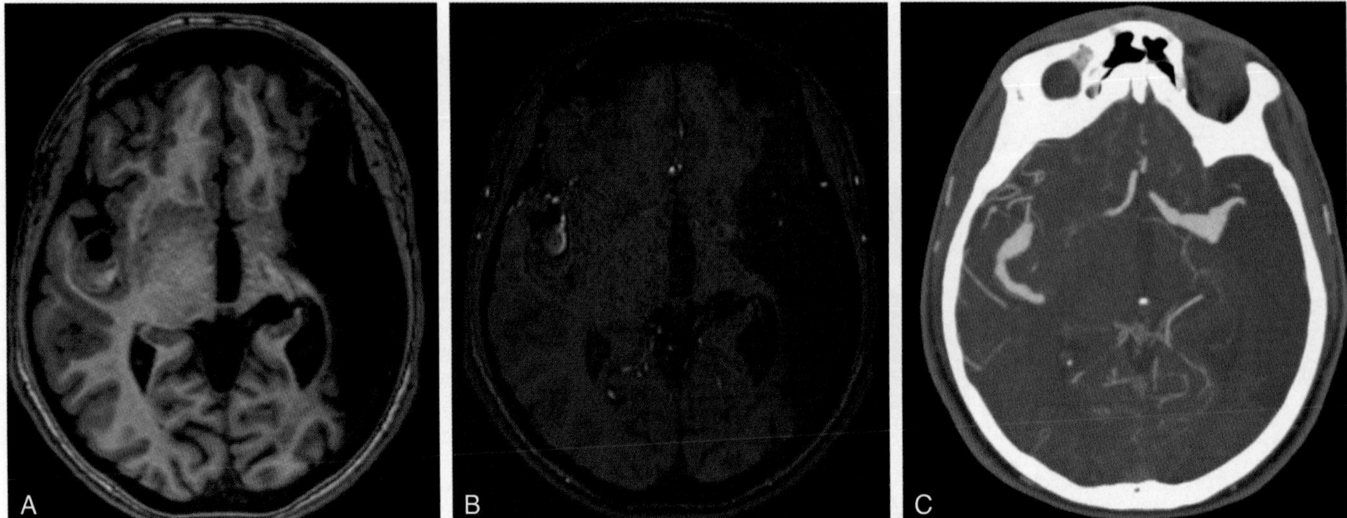

Fig. 3.59 Multiple fusiform aneurysm. 16-year-old with history of an atrial myxoma resected and stroke. A) Axial T1W demonstrates an old left middle cerebral artery territory infarct as well as a rounded lesion in the right sylvian fissure with central hypointensity and peripheral mixed isointensity and hyperintensity. (B) Axial MRA image demonstrates the right sylvian fissure lesion is a partially thrombosed aneurysm. (C) Axial CTA MIP image demonstrates the irregular right sylvian fissure partially thrombosed aneurysm as well as an additional fusiform and saccular aneurysm of the left middle cerebral artery. This represents a rare case of multiple intracranial aneurysms and stoke associated with an atrial myxoma.

Key Points

Background

- Intracranial aneurysms are rare in children and often linked to traumatic head injury or preexistent conditions including connective tissue disorders (Loeys Dietz syndrome, Ehlers-Danlos), infections (e.g. vasculitis or mycotic aneurysms), sickle cell disease, neurocutaneous disorders (Tuberous sclerosis complex, Rendu-Osler-Weber syndrome), moyamoya disease and arteriovenous malformations.
- Compared to the adult population, children have more frequent giant aneurysms (20-50% vs 2%), posterior circulation aneurysms (25% vs 8%), pseudoaneurysms (19% vs 1%), and distal aneurysms. Furthermore, the risk for an intracranial hemorrhage is significantly higher.
- Pediatric aneurysms can clinically present with an intracerebral or subarachnoid hemorrhage with or without ischemic strokes, however because of an increased incidence of giant aneurysms, local mass effect may also be the leading symptom as well as seizures.
- Mycotic or infectious aneurysm refer to acquired aneurysms secondary to an infectious process after bacteremia (streptococcus or Staphylococcus aureus), sepsis or as complication of e.g. endocarditis affecting the intracranial vasculature. Fungal infection is less frequently reported.
- Infectious agents are believed to "embolize" into the vasa vasorum of the intracranial vessels with resultant local infection/arteritis complicated by necrosis of the intima, media and adventitia and pseudo-aneurysm formation.

Imaging

- In case of a spontaneous intracerebral hemorrhage or subarachnoid hemorrhage, an aneurysm should always be included in the differential diagnosis and be excluded preferably by contrast enhanced CTA. The aneurysm may be compressed by the hematoma, so a careful comparison of pre- and post-contrast imaging may help to identify the aneurysm.
- MRI and MRA also allow for identification of the aneurysm with high sensitivity and specificity. MRI has the benefit of diffusion weighted imaging which allows for early detection of concomitant or complicating ischemic injury due to vasospasm or peripheral embolism originating from a partially thrombosed aneurysm.
- Imaging features are often characterized by partial thrombosis and resultant mixed densities and heterogeneous signal intensities on CT respectively MRI.
- Giant aneurysms are more frequently partially thrombosed with an "onion peel" or "onion skin" sign secondary to an intraluminal multi-layered thrombosis. Depending on the age of thrombosis, the aneurysm presents with mixed T1/T2-hypo-and hyperintensity. On susceptibility weighted imaging the aneurysm is typically SWI-hypointense. On contrast enhanced imaging, the patent compartment of the aneurysm may show a vigorous enhancement. On Time-of-Flight MRA, thrombus with intrinsic T1-hyprintense signal from methemoglobin may mimic a perfused aneurysm. Alternatively, a neighboring hematoma may compress or obscure the aneurysm.
- Peripherally located aneurysms are more frequently of infectious etiology but can also occur without infection. Mycotic aneurysms are usually of small cross sectional diameter and may be multiple. Peripheral aneurysms can lead to more distal lobar hemorrhage which leads to a confusing imaging presentation.
- Dissecting pseudoaneurysms are characterized by organizing hematoma and fibrosis outside the true lumen. The artery supplying the pseudoaneurysm may be poorly defined indicating a pseudoaneurysm. Angiography shows a globular aneurysm without a neck, delayed filling and stagnation.
- Skull base internal carotid artery aneurysm are more frequently "false" aneurysms secondary to traumatic acceleration-deceleration forces after a high speed motor vehicle accident resulting in a dissection due to the relative immobility of the internal carotid artery at the skull base relative to the cervical segments.
- Although rare, atrial myxomas have a predilection for resulting in multiple fusiform aneurysms in addition to cerebral embolism.

REFERENCES

1. Sorteberg A, Dahlberg D. Intracranial Non-traumatic aneurysms in children and adolescents. *Curr Pediatr Rev.* 2013;9(40):343–352.
2. Khan A, Wagas M, Nizamani WM, Bari ME. Ruptured mycotic aneurysms: report and outcomes of two surgically managed patients. *Surg Neurol Int.* 2017;8:144.

PRIMARY ANGIITIS OF THE CENTRAL NERVOUS SYSTEM (PACNS)

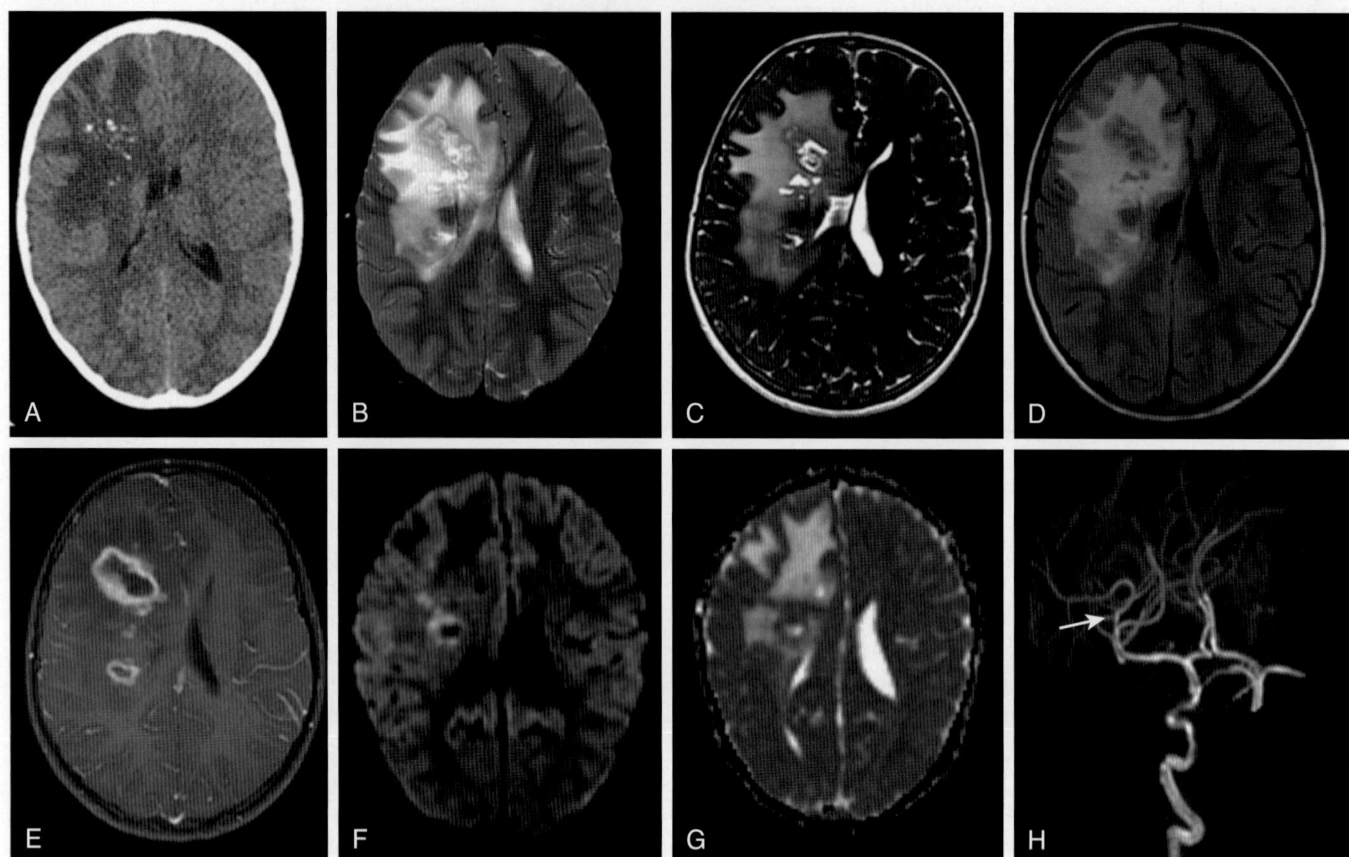

Fig. 3.60 Primary Angiitis of the Central Nervous System (PACNS). (A) Axial head CT demonstrates hypodensity in the right frontal white matter sparing the adjacent cortical ribbon consistent with vasogenic edema. Small hyperdense punctuate calcifications are also present in the right frontal white matter. (B and C) Axial T2W, and (D) axial FLAIR images demonstrate a confluent region of T2/FLAIR hyperintense white matter edema with areas of central necrosis. (E) Axial T1W+C image demonstrates several peripherally enhancing necrotic areas. (F and G) Axial DWI and ADC images demonstrate the broad region of vasogenic edema with relative reduced diffusion at the enhancing areas. (H) Coronal time-of-flight MRA MIP image demonstrates mild contour irregularity affecting the distal middle cerebral artery branches consistent with a primary angiitis of the central nervous system.

Key Points

Background

- Primary angiitis of the central nervous system (PACNS) is believed to be an autoimmune disease affecting the intracranial vasculature, without concomitant systemic involvement.
- PACNS is subdivided in two subtypes: large or medium-size versus small vessel disease. The large/medium-size type typically presents with acute symptoms, whereas the small type appears slowly progressive.
- Clinical symptoms vary and include focal strokes, especially in the large/medium-size vasculitis, whereas seizures, behavioral disorders/psychosis, and headache are more frequently seen in the small-size type.

Imaging

- CT and MRI show areas of perivascular inflammation with ischemia and demyelination. On diffusion-weighted imaging, vasogenic edema of the white matter may be extensive, surrounding areas of restricted diffusion secondary to stroke and necrosis. Peripheral contrast enhancement is seen in the acute phase. Vessel irregularity and vessel wall enhancement is noted on contrast-enhanced black blood MRI.

REFERENCE

1. Benseler SM, Silverman E, Aviv RI, Schneider R, et al. Primary central nervous system vasculitis in children. *Arthritis Rheum.* 2006;54:1291–1297.

SECONDARY CENTRAL NERVOUS SYSTEM VASCULITIS

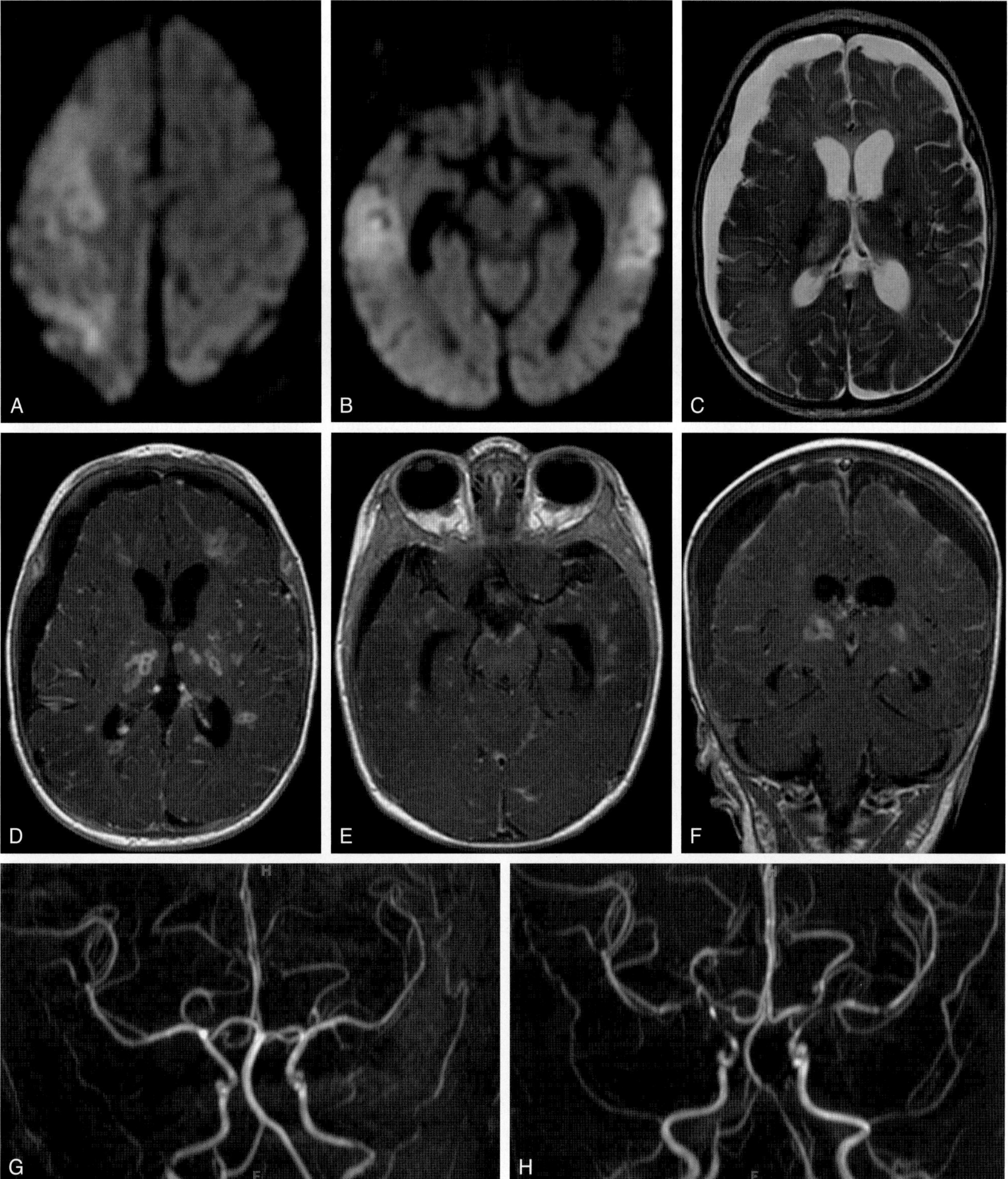

Fig. 3.61 Secondary CNS Vasculitis. A 3-month-old with history of abuse presents with new onset upper respiratory infection symptoms and fever. Patient then developed seizures, altered mental status and drooling and was diagnosed with Streptococcus pneumonia meningitis. (A and B) Axial DWI images demonstrate acute infarcts in the bilateral cerebral hemispheres with MCA and watershed distributions. (C) Axial T2W image demonstrates bilateral subdural collections and multifocal T2 signal abnormality in the bilateral central grey matter and white matter. (D-F) Axial T1W+C images demonstrate multiple regions of confluent and peripheral enhancement are present in the central grey matter and hemispheric white matter with areas of leptomeningeal enhancement. (G) MRA coronal MIP image at baseline prior to the current infection is normal. (H) MRA coronal MIP image at the same time as this MRI brain demonstrates segmental high grade stenosis of the anterior circulation including the supraclinoid ICAs, M1 and A1 segments.

Key Points

Background

- Inflammatory process involving intracranial vasculature secondary to underlying systemic disease or agent. Vascular and perivascular inflammation may occur.
- Causes of secondary CNS vasculitis may be classified as follows:
    - Infection (most common)- infection of the vessel wall with secondary inflammation
    - Bacteria- S. pneumonia, M. tuberculosis among others
    - Viral- EBV among others
    - Fungal- Aspergillus, Candida among others
    - Rheumatologic disease
    - Lupus, Behcet, granulomatosis with polyangiitis, polyarteritis nodosa
    - Other
    - Drug induced
- Clinical symptoms may include new onset of neurologic or psychiatric deficit symptoms vary and include focal strokes, especially in the large/medium sized vasculitis while seizures, behavioral disorders/psychosis and headache are more frequently seen in the small-size type.
- Treatment typically involves treatment of the offending etiology; treatment may include immunosuppression.

Imaging

- Vascular imaging demonstrates vessel wall irregularity, stenosis and possibly vessel wall enhancement. Predisposition for certain arterial segments may occur. For example, post varicella angiopathy has predilection for the supraclinoid ICA, proximal MCA and proximal ACA. Other etiologies such as lupus vasculitis may involve any segment of the arterial tree. Small vessel vasculitis may be angiographically occult.
- Brain parenchyma imaging may be normal. Acute, subacute and/or chronic stroke may be present. Regions of vasogenic edema/ inflammation which may be focal, multifocal and confluent. Areas of contrast enhancement may be present. Imaging findings of CNS infection may be seen.

REFERENCES

1. Gowdie P, Twilt M, Benseler SM. Primary and secondary central nervous system vasculitis. *J Child Neurol.* 2012;27(11):1448–1459.
2. Moharir M, Shroff M, Benseler SM. Childhood central nervous system vasculitis. *Neuroimaging Clin N Am.* 2013;23(2):293–308.

MOYAMOYA VASCULOPATHY

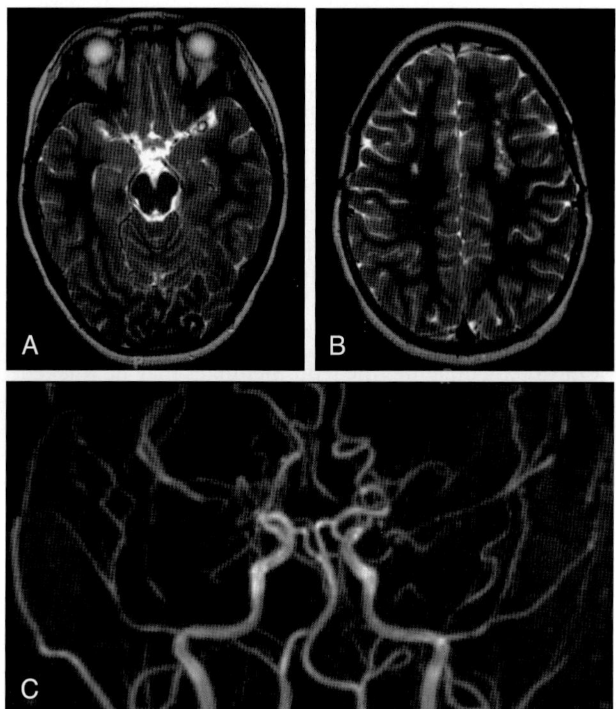

Fig. 3.62 Moyamoya. (A and B) Axial T2W images demonstrate near-complete absence of flow-related T2-hypointense signal void along the expected course of the middle cerebral arteries as well as small caliber distal internal carotid arteries. In addition, small T2-hyperintense chronic ischemic lesions are noted in the frontal hemispheric white matter. (C) Coronal time-of-flight MRA MIP image confirms high-grade stenosis of the distal internal carotid arteries and lack of flow-related enhancement within the M1/M2 segments of the middle cerebral arteries secondary to moyamoya disease.

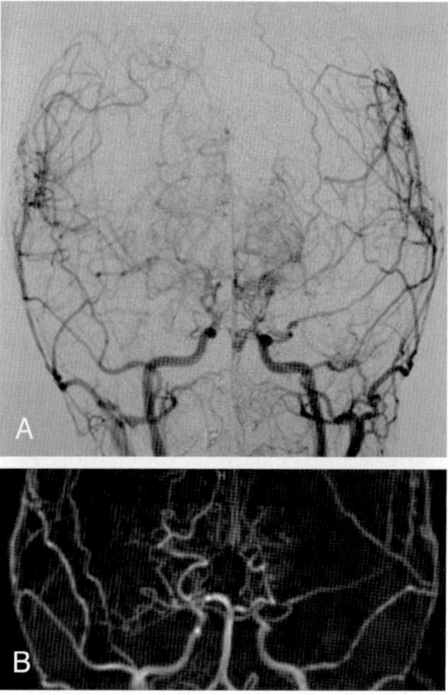

Fig. 3.63 Moyamoya. (A and B) Matching coronal digital subtraction angiography and time-of-flight MRA in a child with confirmed moyamoya disease. The distal internal carotid arteries are diminutive, the middle cerebral arteries nearly occluded, and collateral circulation is provided over branches of the external carotid arteries/middle meningeal arteries after pial synangiosis. A cloud-like enhancement is seen along the lenticulostriate arteries known as the characteristic "puff of smoke" in moyamoya disease.

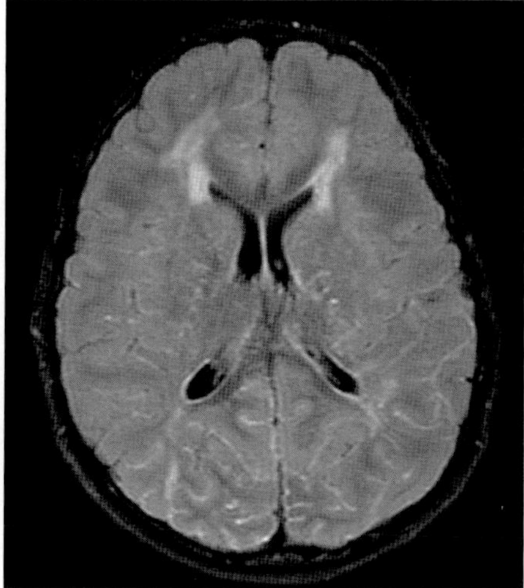

Fig. 3.64 Moyamoya. Classic predominantly parietooccipital FLAIR-hyperintensity of the hemispheric sulci known as "ivy-sign" in child with moyamoya disease which are due to collateral vessels. Chronic FLAIR-hyperintense ischemic lesions are seen within the watershed regions of both cerebral hemispheres.

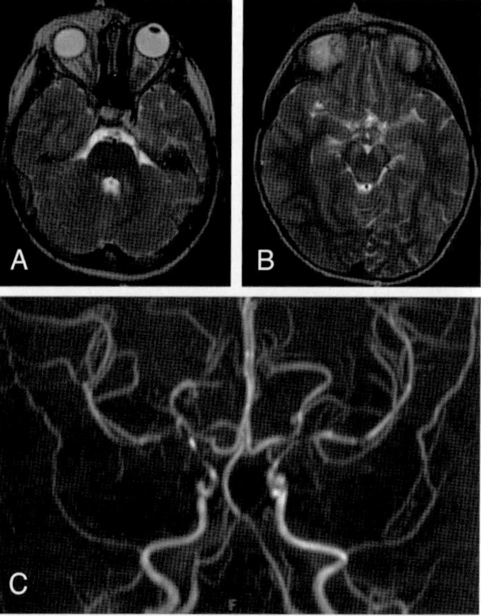

Fig. 3.65 Moyamoya syndrome in a child with confirmed neurofibromatosis type 1. (A and B) Axial T2W images and (C) coronal TOF MRA MIP images demonstrate the typical lack of flow-voids along the course of the middle cerebral arteries, high-grade stenosis of the distal internal carotid arteries, mildly prominent lenticulostriate arteries are seen next to a left-sided optic nerve glioma and a plexiform neurofibroma filling out the right orbit. Furthermore, areas of myelin vacuolization are seen within the cerebral peduncles and cerebellum.

Key Points

Background

- Moyamoya disease is a rare, idiopathic disease characterized by slowly progressive stenosis and occlusion of the distal internal carotid arteries. The proximal M1 and A1 segments can also be affected. The posterior circulation is typically spared.
- Moyamoya disease refers to the primary, idiopathic disease, which has a higher incidence in Asian countries.
- Moyamoya syndrome refers to the constellations of distal internal carotid artery occlusion with extensive collateral network. It may also be seen as a sequelae of cranial radiation therapy or may be associated with neurofibromatosis type 1, tuberous sclerosis complex, Down syndrome, sickle cell disease, and as result of various infectious diseases, for example, tuberculosis.
- The slowly progressive course typically allows for development of an extensive collateral network of perforating lenticulostriate and thalamostriate arteries.
- The marginal perfusion of the supratentorial brain puts the brain at risk for acute and chronic ischemic lesions, typically in watershed distribution. However, territorial infarctions may also be observed.

Imaging

- CT/CTA, MRI/MRA show the tapering and occlusion of the distal internal carotid arteries and adjacent proximal A1 and M1 segments of the anterior and middle cerebral arteries.
- The multiple mildly dilated perforating arteries that supply the central gray matter are typically seen as multiple contrast-enhancing punctuate vessels on CTA, or as T1/T2 hypointense vessels on MRI. On MRA, the conglomerate of perforating arteries appears like a tangle of small vessels that present as a cloud of contrast enhancement on digital subtraction angiography, hence its Japanese name: moyamoya, which refers to "puff of smoke."
- On FLAIR imaging, the leptomeninges may be thickened secondary to the extensive collateral circulation, which limits the normal suppression of the "sulcal signal." The FLAIR hyperintense signal is referred to as "ivy sign."

REFERENCE

1. Li J, Jin M, Sun X, Li J, et al. Imaging of moyamoya disease and moyamoya syndrome: Current status. *J Comput Assist Tomogr*. 2019;43(2):257–263.

SICKLE CELL DISEASE

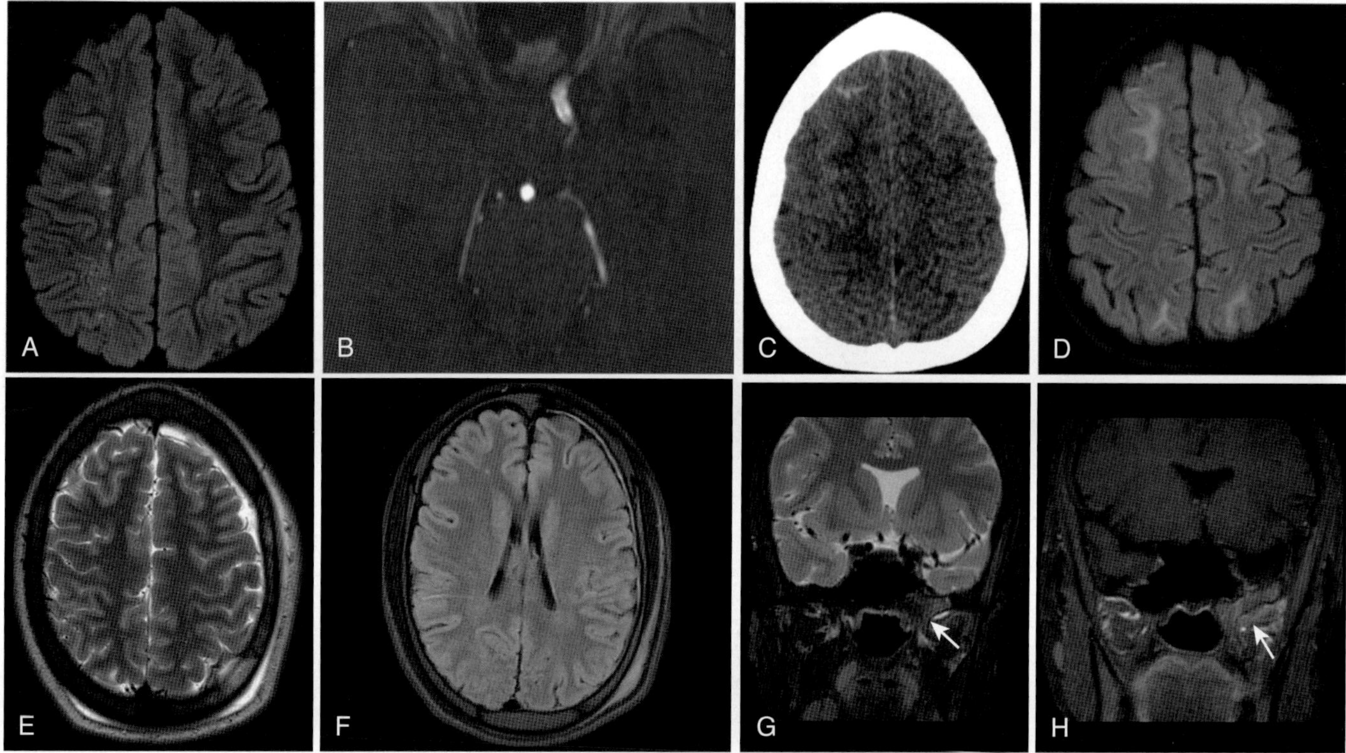

Fig. 3.66 Multiple Patients With Sickle Cell Disease. (A and B) Axial FLAIR and time-of-flight MRA in a 5-year-old with sickle cell anemia found to have multiple deep white matter foci of gliosis and occluded supraclinoid ICAs due to moyamoya vasculopathy. (C) A 7-year-old with sickle cell anemia who presented with altered mental status and seizure found to have small area of acute subarachnoid hemorrhage in the right frontal lobe on head CT (C) and subsequent (D) axial FLAIR MRI image demonstrated relatively symmetric bilateral juxtacortical FLAIR hyperintensity in the frontal and parietal white matter consistent with PRES. (E, F) Axial T2W and FLAIR images in a 17-year-old with sickle cell anemia who presented with headache demonstrates abnormal T2 hyperintensity in the left parietal bone consistent with a bone infarct with adjacent small epidural hemorrhage, subdural effusion, subperiosteal and subgaleal fluid. (G, H) Coronal T2W fat saturation and coronal T1W+C fat saturation images in an 18-year-old with sickle cell disease presenting with facial pain and swelling demonstrate a bone infarct in the left side of the central skull base with presumed inflammation of cranial nerve V2 and V3 contributing to the clinical symptoms.

Key Points

Background

- Sickle cell disease refers to a group of inherited disorders with the hemoglobin S (HbS) point mutation in the beta globin gene, either in both genes referred to as HbSS disease (sickle cell anemia), or in conjunction with another beta globulin mutation including HbSC disease, HbSB+ (beta) and HbSB0 (beta-zero) thalassemia, HbSD, HbSE, and HbSO. Sickle cell trait patients have one sickle cell gene (S) and one normal gene (A).
- Patients with sickle cell disease have chronic anemia and experience vaso-occlusive phenomena, leading to pain, acute chest syndrome, stroke, bone infarction, myocardial infarction, renal insufficiency, and venous thromboembolism and are more prone to infections including osteomyelitis.

Imaging

- CNS manifestations in sickle cell disease include transient ischemic attacks, seizures, ischemic and hemorrhagic infarcts, moyamoya syndrome, posterior reversible encephalopathy syndrome, and sinus thrombosis. Ischemic infarcts are more common in children, whereas hemorrhagic infarcts are more common in adults. Silent infarcts can occur in ~10% of patients and most often involve the deep cerebral white matter.
- Bone infarcts can involve the calvarium and skull base and uncommonly can have associated epidural hemorrhage.

REFERENCE

1. Li J, Jin M, Sun X, Li J, et al. Imaging of moyamoya disease and moyamoya syndrome: Current status. *J Comput Assist Tomogr.* 2019;43(2):257–263.

HEREDITARY HEMORRHAGIC TELANGIECTASIA

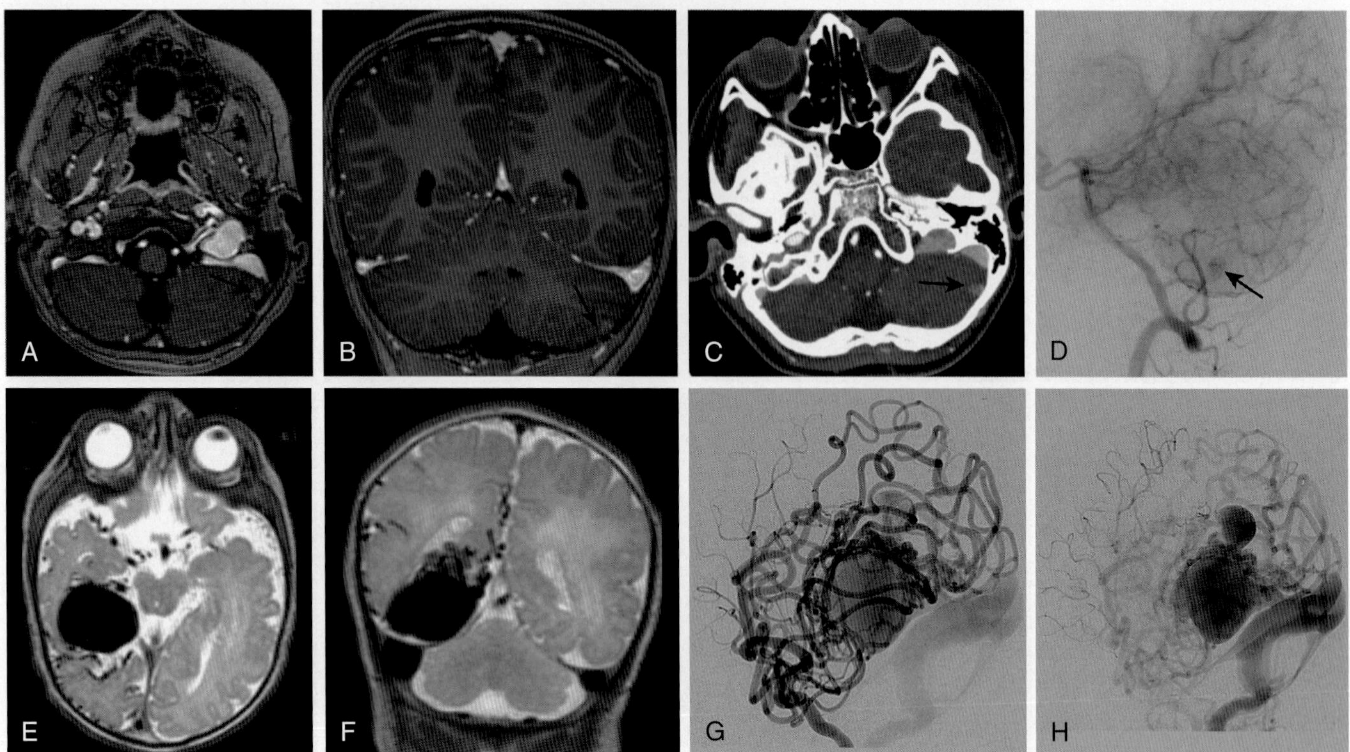

Fig. 3.67 Hereditary Hemorrhagic Telangiectasia (HHT). (A to D) A 7-year-old with HHT found to have a 7-mm vague area of enhancement in the lateral left cerebellar hemisphere on axial and coronal T1W+C (A, B) and enhancement on the CT angiography (C), which was confirmed as a micro-AVM on catheter angiography (D). (E to H) A 1-day-old with HHT found to have a pial arteriovenous fistula with enlarged vessels along the right temporal and occipital lobes, a large posterior temporal venous varix, and enlarged right transverse and sigmoid sinuses on the axial and coronal T2W imaging (E, F) and catheter angiogram (G, H).

Key Points

Background

- Hereditary hemorrhagic telangiectasia (HHT), also known as Osler-Weber-Rendu, is a rare autosomal dominant genetic disorder affecting the vascular system of multiple organ systems with telangiectasias and AVMs.
- 80%–90% of HHT is due to mutations in the *ENG* gene (HHT1) or *ACRL1* gene (HHT2), which affect the transforming growth factor (TGF)-β type III and TGF-β type I receptors, respectively.
- Clinical diagnosis can be made by three of the four Curacao criteria: (1) recurrent spontaneous epistaxis; (2) multiple mucocutaneous telangiectasias involving the lips, oral cavity, face, and fingers; (3) visceral AVMs; (4) first-degree relative with HHT.
- Clinical manifestations include epistaxis, GI bleeding, dyspnea, hemoptysis, and stroke.

Imaging

- CNS manifestations include vascular malformations (pial arteriovenous fistulae, AVMs with a nidus, and micro-AVMs, also known as capillary vascular malformations), as well as stroke and abscesses due to right-to-left pulmonary or intracardiac shunting.
- Pial arteriovenous fistulae in HHT have high shunting, leading to enlarged feeding arteries, feeding artery aneurysm, multiple draining veins, venous ectasia, and a pseudophlebolithic pattern.
- Nidus AVMs in HHT patients typically have a Spetzler-Martin grade of ≤2. Most are 1 to 2 cm and do not have arterial stenosis, aneurysms, multiple draining veins, or venous ectasia.
- Micro-AVMs in HHT patients have an abnormal dilated capillary bed and imaging appearance of a blush of abnormal vessels without dilated arteries or veins. These measure ~5 mm in diameter and are usually superficially located.

REFERENCE

1. Brinjikji W, Iyer VN, Sorenson T, Lanzino G. Cerebrovascular manifestations of hereditary hemorrhagic telangiectasia. *Stroke* 105; 46:3329-3337.

LOEYS-DIETZ SYNDROME

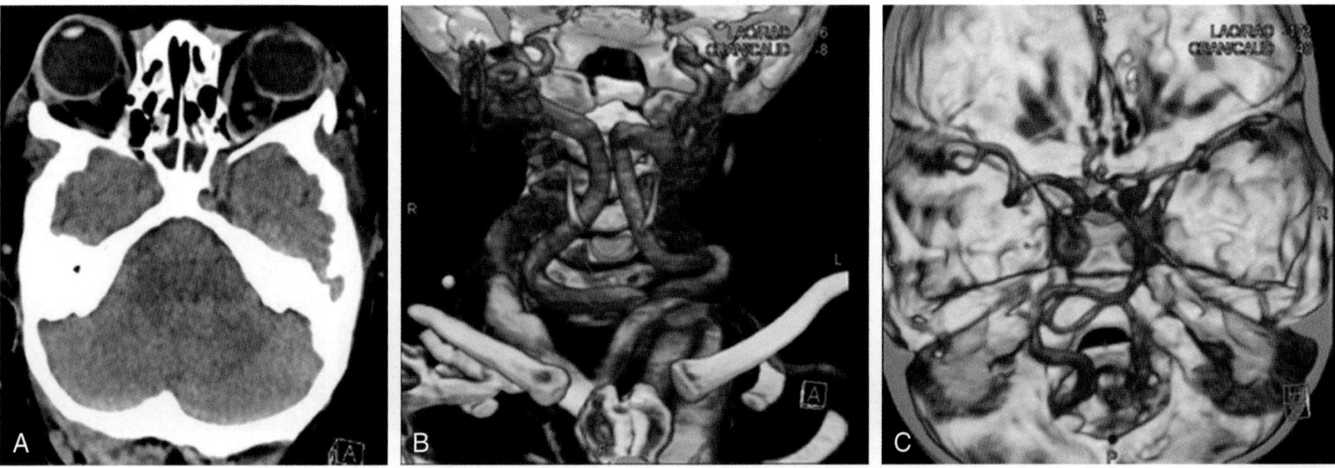

Fig. 3.68 Loeys-Dietz Syndrome. Three children with confirmed Loeys-Dietz syndrome demonstrating key imaging features. (A) Axial head CT demonstrates significant hypertelorism. (B and C) Volume rendered CTA of the head and neck demonstrate severely elongated and tortuous internal carotid arteries, and a focal fusiform aneurysm of the distal left internal carotid artery.

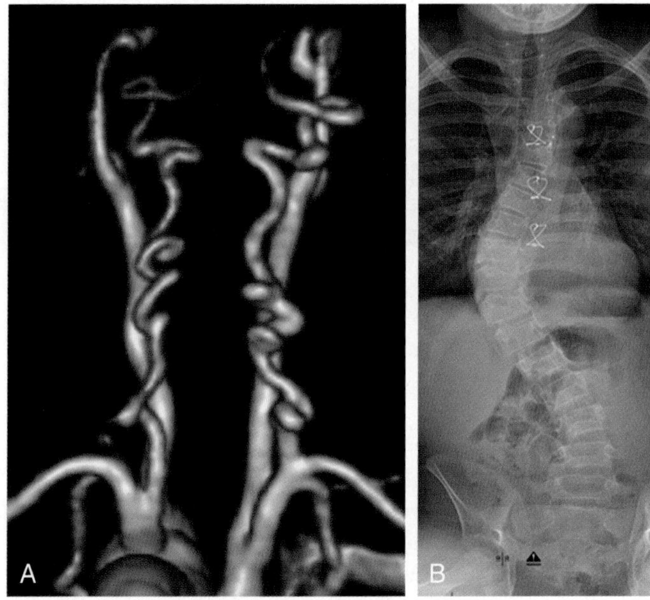

Fig. 3.69 Loeys-Dietz Syndrome. (A) Coronal volume rendered CTA of the neck demonstrates extensive elongation and tortuosity of both vertebral arteries and mild tortuosity of the distal internal carotid arteries in a child with confirmed Loeys-Dietz syndrome. (B) AP radiograph of the spine reveals a moderate S-shaped scoliosis of the thoracic and lumbar spinal column and stigmata of prior cardiac surgery, Amplatz device placement and mild elongation of the thoracic aorta in a second child with LoeysDietz syndrome.

Key Points

Background

- Loeys-Dietz syndrome (LDS) is an autosomal dominant inherited congenital connective tissue disorder described by Dr. Bart Loeys from Leuven, Belgium, and Dr. Hal Dietz from Johns Hopkins, Baltimore, in 2005.
- LDS may affect multiple systems, including the cardiovascular, musculoskeletal, and gastrointestinal system.

Imaging

- Head and neck findings include moderate to severe arterial tortuosity and widening of the supraaortic vessels that may extend into the circle of Willis. Focal aneurysms may develop. Furthermore, hypertelorism and a bifid or broad uvula may be seen; occasionally craniosynostosis, cleft palate, and club feet are present.
- Systemic, extra-CNS findings appear similar to other connective tissue disorders (Ehlers-Danlos and Marfan syndrome) with excessive joint laxity, craniocervical instability, scoliosis, aortic root enlargement, congenital heart disease, and retinal detachment as lead symptoms.
- CT/CTA, MR/MRA of the head and neck are indicated to evaluate the degree of vessel tortuosity and to exclude accompanying aneurysms or spontaneous dissections. For the complete diagnostic workup, the chest, abdomen, and pelvis should also be evaluated.
- Routine surveillance imaging is recommended at least every 2 years.
- Functional views of the craniocervical junction are advised to assess for instability.

REFERENCE

1. Rodrigues VJ, Elsayed S, Loeys BL, Dietz HC, et al. Neuroradiological manifestations of Loeys-Dietz syndrome type 1. *AJNR Am J Neuroradiol.* 2009;30(8):1614–1619.

COL4A1/2 DISORDERS

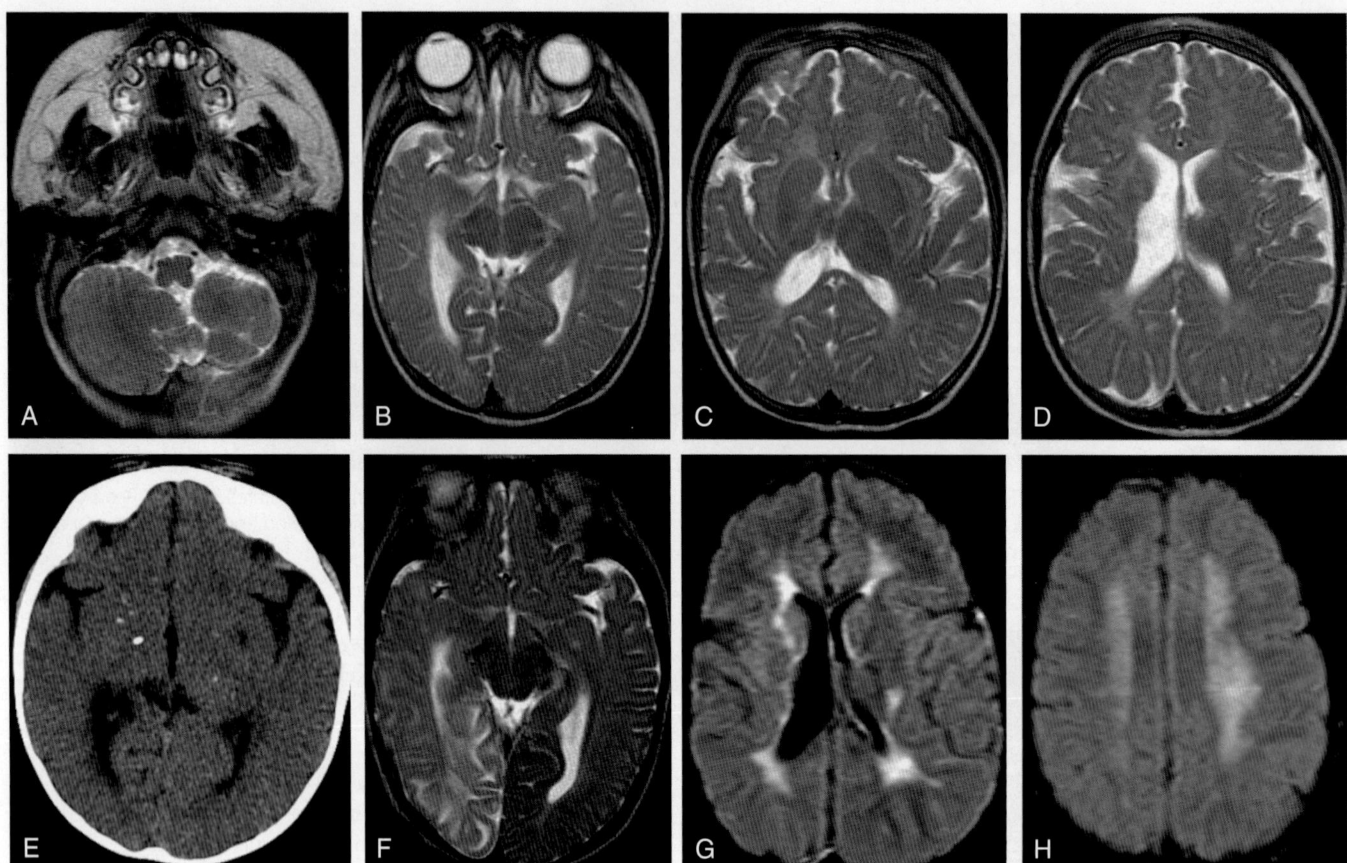

Fig. 3.70 COL4A1 Disorder. (A to D) Axial T2W images in a 5-month-old with COL4A1 disorder demonstrating hypoplasia and dysplasia of the left cerebellar hemisphere, bilateral cataracts, volume loss of the right thalamus, and porencephaly along the right lateral ventricle. (E) Axial head CT demonstrates small calcifications in the deep gray matter. (F) Axial T2W image at 6 months of age demonstrates a new T2 hyperintense region in the right occipital lobe. (G and H) Axial FLAIR images at 2 years of age demonstrate confluent periventricular leukomalacia and old lacunar infarct in the posterior left putamen.

Key Points

Background

- COL4A1/2 disorders refer to autosomal dominant mutations involving collagen type IV alpha 1 (COL4A1) and 2 (COL4A2). These encode extracellular proteins present in nearly all basement membranes.
- Genetic mutations result in multisystem disorders with abnormal blood vessels in the brain, ocular dysgenesis, myopathy, and renal disorders.
- Clinical manifestations include epilepsy, migraine, intellectual and behavioral difficulties, congenital cataracts, and increased serum creation kinase.

Imaging

- Imaging findings include porencephaly, cortical malformations (schizencephaly, polymicrogyria, focal cortical dysplasia, and nodular heterotopia), periventricular leukomalacia, small vessel infarcts, and microhemorrhages in the centrum semiovale, deep gray matter, and/or brainstem.

REFERENCE

1. Zagaglia S, Selch S, Nisevic JR, Mei D, et al. Neurologic phenotypes associated with COL4A1/2 mutations. *Neurology*. 2018 Nov 27;91(22):e2078–e2088.

ACTA2 VASCULOPATHY

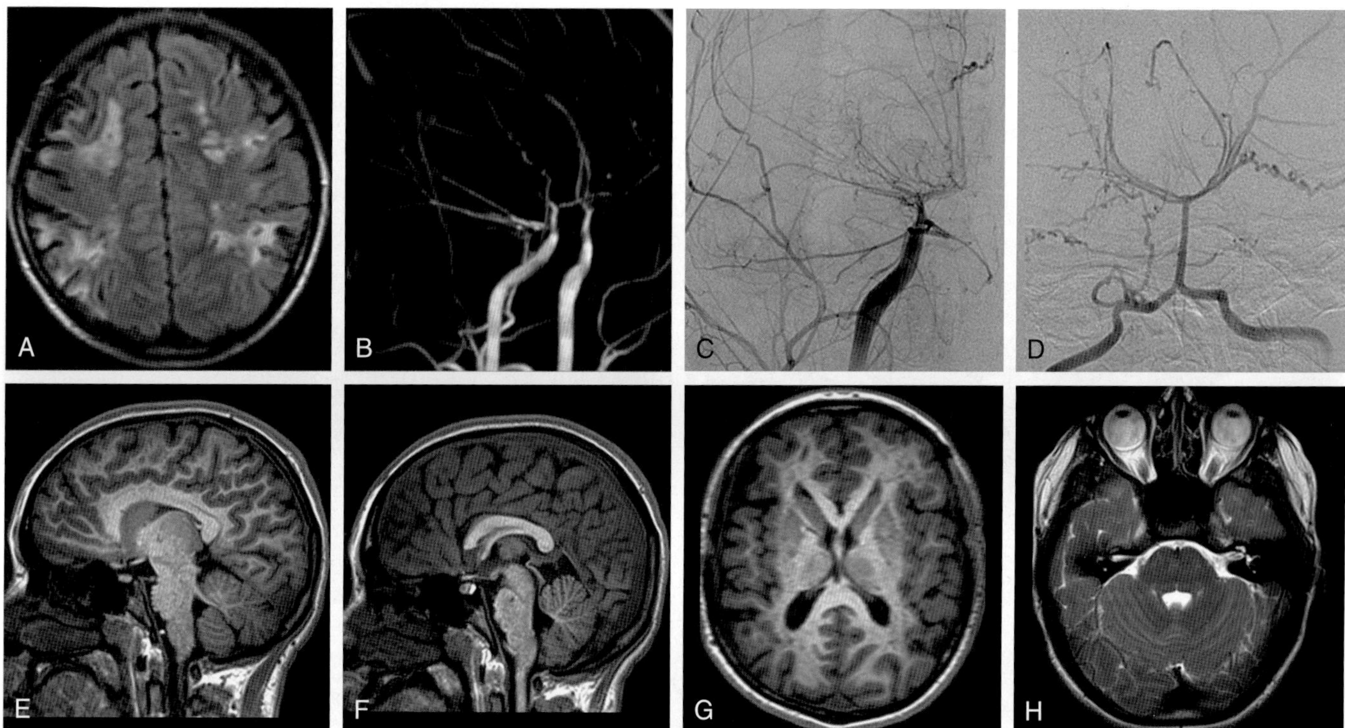

Fig. 3.71 ACTA2 Vasculopathy. (A) Axial FLAIR image demonstrates multifocal FLAIR hyperintense chronic ischemic lesions in watershed distribution within the white matter of both cerebral hemispheres secondary to a high-grade stenosis of the distal internal carotid arteries seen on (B) 3D TOF MRA MIP image and (C) sagittal digital subtraction catheter angiography as well as straightening of the petrous and cavernous segments characteristic for ACTA2 vasculopathy. (D) Coronal catheter angiography of the posterior circulation demonstrates tortuous collateral vessel formation. (E and F) Sagittal T1W, (G) axial T1W, and (H) axial T2W images demonstrate brain findings in ACTA2 including pontine indentations, flattened ventral pons, radial frontal gyri, absent anterior cingulate gyri, and bending of the anterior corpus callosum.

Key Points

Background

- ACTA2 vasculopathy is a distinct cerebral arteriopathy caused by missense mutations in the gene that codes for the smooth muscle actin. The resultant smooth muscle dysfunction results in the ACTA2 cerebral arteriopathy, which resembles a moyamoya disease.
- Because the mutation results in a systemic smooth muscle dysfunction, multiple smooth muscle organs may be affected. Consequently, this syndrome is also referred to as "multisystem smooth muscle dysfunction syndrome" (MSMDS).

Imaging

- On CTA/MRA, there is a fusiform dilatation of the proximal internal carotid arteries, straightening of the petrous and cavernous segments, and severe stenosis of the distal segments.
- The arteriopathy increases the risk for ischemic strokes in children, mimicking the distribution of strokes that may be seen in moyamoya disease (watershed distribution and hemispheric white matter).
- If a patient is suspected of a moyamoya disease and has additional symptoms of dysfunction of smooth muscle organs, ACTA2 genotyping should be initiated.
- Additional brain MRI findings seen with ACTA2 vasculopathy include hypoplasia and bending of the anterior corpus callosum, absence of the anterior cingulate gyrus, radial frontal gyral pattern, flattening of the anterior pons, pons indentations, and transverse narrowing of the cerebral peduncles.

REFERENCES

1. Cuoco JA, Busch CM, Klein BJ, Benko MJ, et al. ACTA2 cerebral arteriopathy: Not just a puff of smoke. *Cerebrovasc Dis.* 2018;46:159–169.
2. D'Arco F, Alves CA, Raybaud C, et al. Expanding the Distinctive Neuroimaging Phenotype of ACTA2 Mutations. *AJNR Am J Neuroradiol.* 2018;39(11):2126–2131.

TAKAYASU ARTERITIS

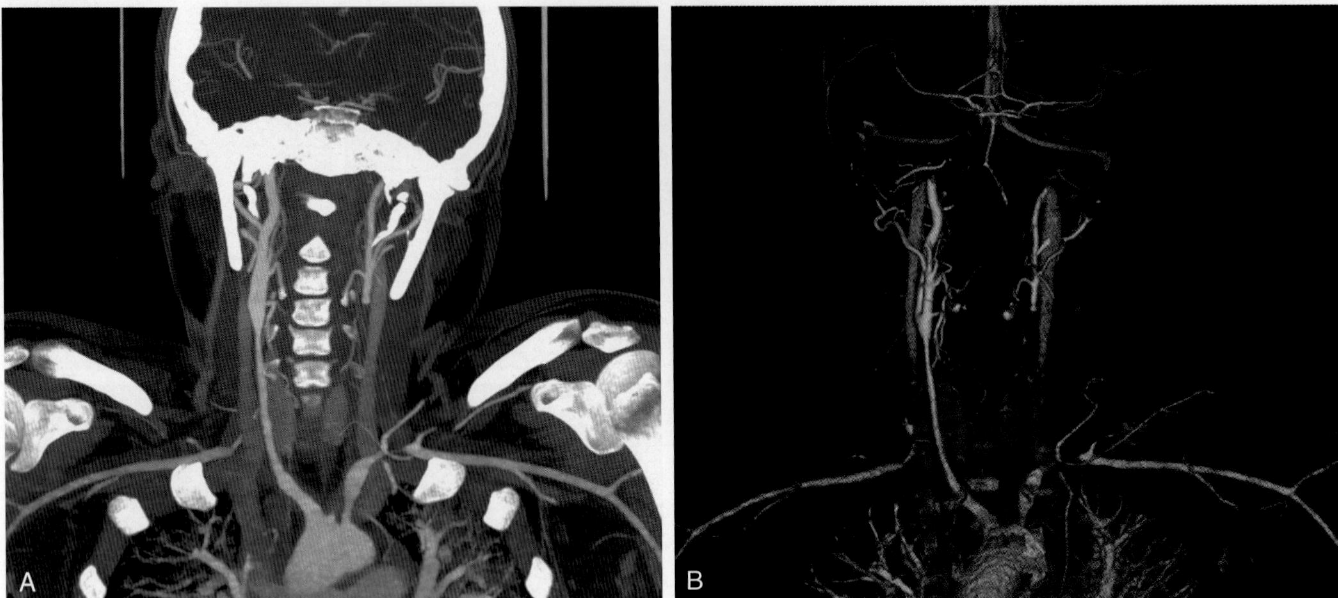

Fig. 3.72 Takayasu Arteritis. A 12-year-old female with known history of Takayasu arteritis. (A) CTA MPR and (B) CTA MIP of the neck demonstrates extensive steno-occlusive disease of the arterial neck vasculature. Findings include occlusion of the proximal right subclavian artery, mild to moderate stenosis of the right common carotid artery with luminal irregularity, occlusion of the left common carotid artery, small caliber of the left ICA and left ECA and high grade stenosis of the proximal and mid left subclavian artery.

Key Points

Background

- Worldwide idiopathic disease with increased incidence in parts of Asia, Africa and South America.
- Majority of cases are diagnosed in the second and third decade of life although the disease may occur in younger children. Female predominance is notable.
- Takayasu arteritis is a rare disorder typified by idiopathic chronic granulomatous medium and large vessel vasculitis that results in transmural fibrous arterial wall thickening. Patients develop arterial stenosis, occlusion, thrombosis with the possibility of organ damage/ ischemic changes. Elastic fiber degradation may result in aneurysm formation.
- The condition may be autoimmune with genetic predisposition.
- Patients may present with a variety of constitutional symptoms including fever, night sweats, fatigue, unintended weight loss and fever. Vascular presentations include stroke, other neurologic or ophthalmic symptoms, hypertension, pulselessness, vascular claudication, and bruit. Additional presentations include cardiomyopathy and renal failure.
- Diagnosis is made angiographically. Elevated inflammatory markers and clinical signs/ symptoms support the diagnosis.

Imaging

- Extracranial arterial neck vasculature: Often long segment bilateral steno-occlusive disease with vessel wall thickening. Common carotid artery narrowing is most common. Internal and external carotid arteries, subclavian and vertebral arteries may be involved.
- Intracranial arterial vasculature: Segmental stenosis and/ or occlusion especially proximally in both the anterior and posterior circulation.
- Brain: Large and small infarcts; parenchymal microhemorrhages.

REFERENCES

1. Millan P, Gavcovich TB, Abitbol C. Childhood-onset Takayasu arteritis. *Curr Opin Pediatr.* 2022;34(2):223–228.
2. Bond KM, Nasr D, Lehman V, Lanzino G, Cloft HJ, Brinjikji W. Intracranial and extracranial neurovascular manifestations of Takayasu arteritis. *AJNR Am J Neuroradiol.* 2017;38(4):766–772.

4 Inherited and Acquired Metabolic Disorders

INTRODUCTION

Background

Inherited metabolic disorders are challenging to diagnose because they have variable clinical severity and age at presentation, are uncommonly encountered, and can have a range of imaging appearances. The variability in clinical manifestation and imaging appearance relates to the underlying genetic mutation and degree of protein function remaining. Some metabolic disorders can have infantile, juvenile, and adult forms. Many of the metabolic disorders can be determined through laboratory studies and genetic evaluation; however, a radiologist may be the first person to trigger this investigation through recognition of imaging findings that suggest a metabolic or genetic etiology. This chapter discusses some of the clinical features most common to each disorder to provide a clinical context for the imaging findings. Last, this chapter discusses toxic disorders that affect children, which are important to recognize because some of these disorders may be reversible if the toxin is removed.

Imaging

Magnetic resonance imaging (MRI) is the primary modality for evaluating metabolic and genetic disorders because MRI provides the greatest assessment of the brain parenchyma through the contrasts in tissue as well as with MR spectroscopy.

As mentioned previously, the variability in genetic mutation and remaining protein function leads to potentially different appearances for the same disorder, which can lead to difficulty in reaching the specific diagnosis. In these situations, excluding or indicating a potential metabolic or genetic disorder has value as it can either prevent or lead to a series of laboratory and genetic testing.

This section illustrates some of the many metabolic disorders in children. Although imperfect, this chapter is organized using an imaging pattern approach to provide manageable differential diagnoses. This provides a starting point for forming a knowledge base of metabolic disorders and emphasizes important structures that should be assessed systematically. This approach combined with clinical information, particularly age of presentation and specific clinical features highlighted in this section, can help lead to an appropriate differential diagnosis or specific diagnosis.

REFERENCE

1. Van der Knaap MS, and Valk J. *Magnetic Resonance of Myelination and Myelin Disorders*. 3rd edition. Berlin: Springer; 2005.

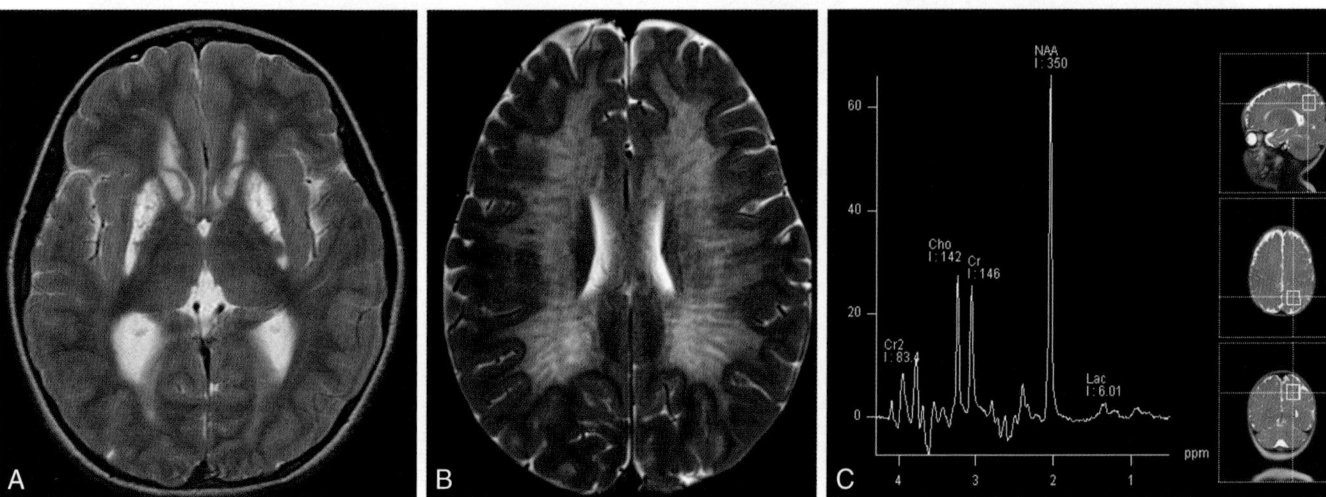

Fig. 4.1 Examples of Metabolic Disorders. Pattern recognition is an important component of recognizing a potential metabolic disorder and a reasonable differential diagnosis. Some common patterns seen with metabolic disorders include deep gray matter involvement such as with mitochondrial disorders (A), confluent white matter abnormality such as with metachromatic leukodystrophy (B), and spectroscopy abnormalities such as with Canavan disease, which has a large NAA peak (C).

METABOLIC DISORDERS: NEONATAL ONSET

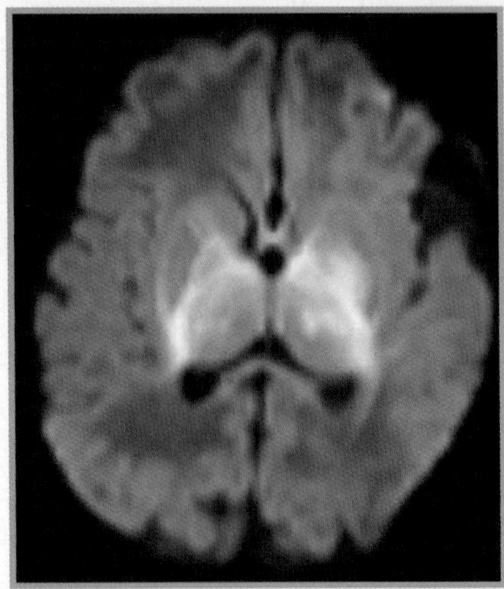

Maple Syrup Urine Disease

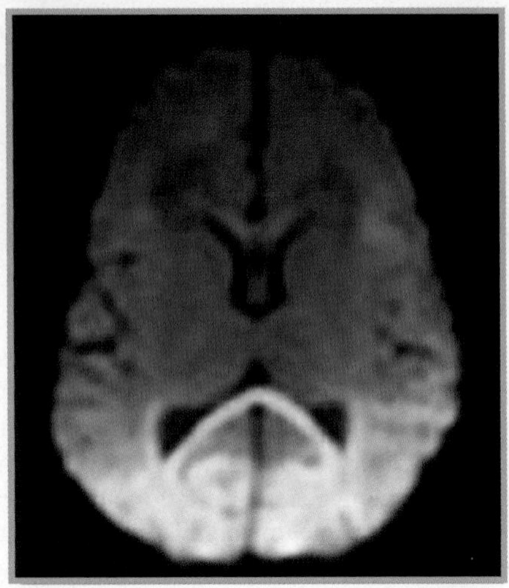

Hypoglycemia

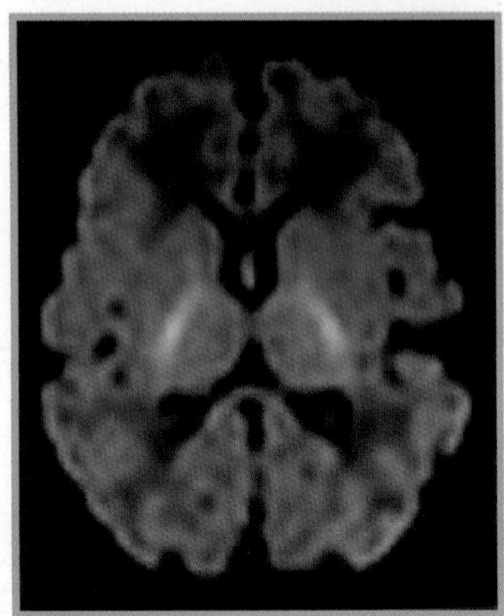

Nonketotic Hyperglycemia

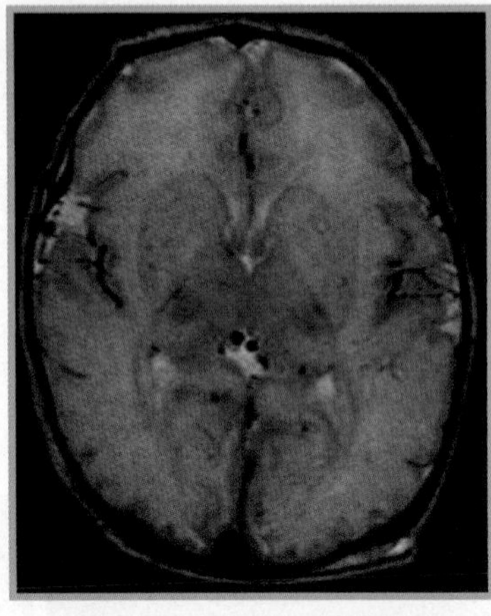

Sulfite Oxidase & Molybdenum Cofactor

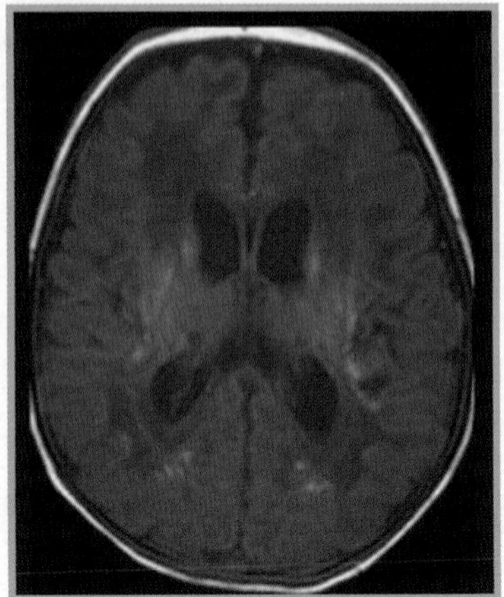

Urea Cycle Disorders

MAPLE SYRUP URINE DISEASE

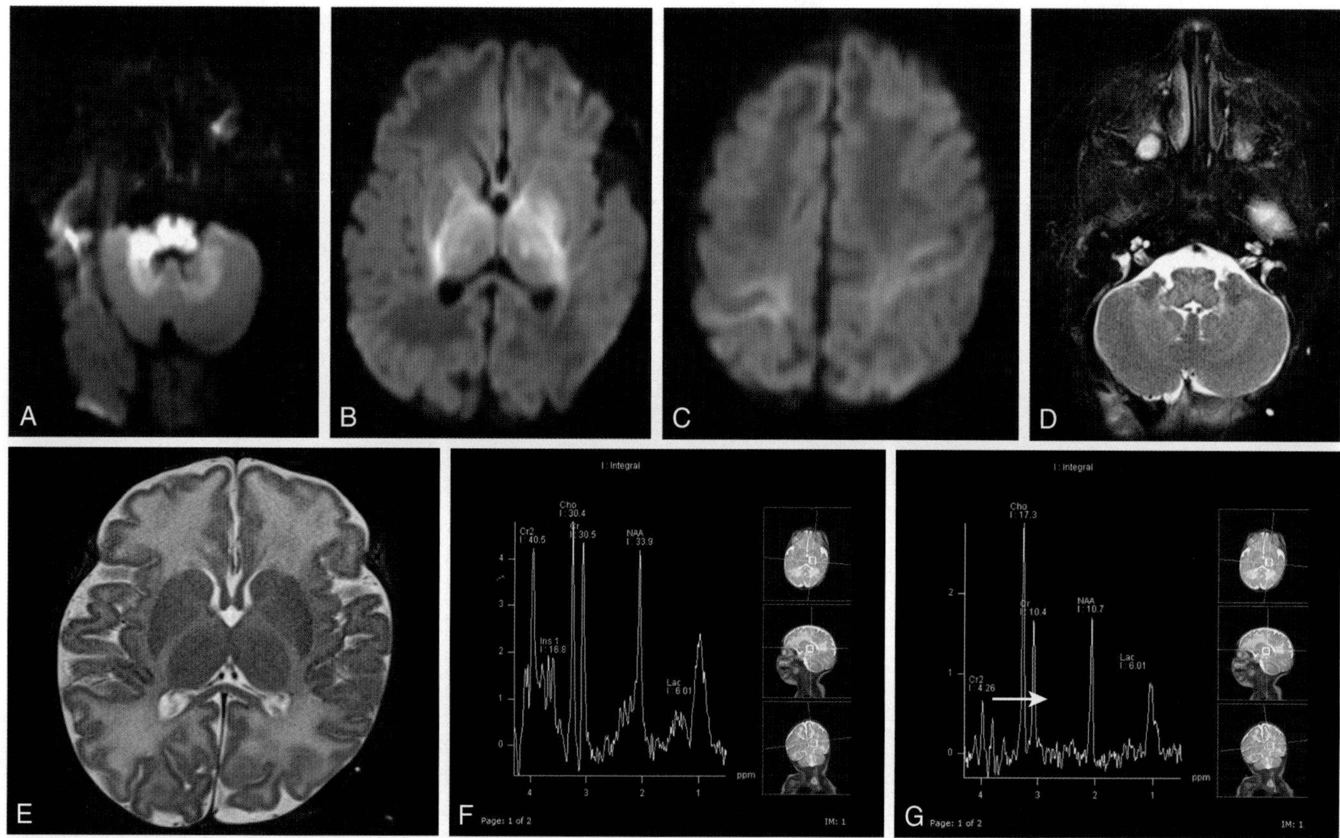

Fig. 4.2 Maple Syrup Urine Disease. 50-day-old with seizures. (A to C) Axial DWI images demonstrate hyperintensity in the perirolandic cortex, internal capsules, thalami, medulla, and deep cerebellar white matter. (D and E) Axial T2W images demonstrate abnormal loss of the T2W hypointense signal in the posterior limb of the internal capsule and abnormal T2W hyperintensity in the medulla. (F and G) Single voxel MR spectroscopy with short and long echo times demonstrates abnormal peak at 0.9 ppm on both short and long echoes, indicative of elevated branched-chain amino acids. A lipid peak would not persist on the long echo MRS.

Key Points

Background

- Autosomal recessive deficiency of branched-chain alpha-keto acid dehydrogenase
- Leads to accumulation of branch chain amino acids, which result in extracellular intramyelin edema and demyelination

Clinical

- Classical form is the most common and presents in the first week of life; disease-free interval of 4 to 7 days followed by lethargy, feeding difficulty, apnea; rapid progression to cerebral edema, coma, and death within 1 month if untreated
- Elevated branched-chain amino acids in the urine, blood, and CSF
- Prognosis is good if detected early and dietary control is maintained

Imaging

- Diffusion restriction along corticospinal tracts and myelinated white matter; T2W-hyperintense signal in areas of normal myelination
- MRS: broad peak at 0.9 ppm on short and long echo, which is caused by branched-chain amino acids

REFERENCES

1. Van der Knaap MS, and Valk J. *Magnetic Resonance of Myelination and Myelin Disorders*. 3rd edition. Berlin: Springer; 2005.
2. Barkovich AJ, Raybaud C. *Pediatric Neuroradiology*. 6th edition. Philadelphia: Wolters-Kluwer; 2019.

NEONATAL HYPOGLYCEMIA

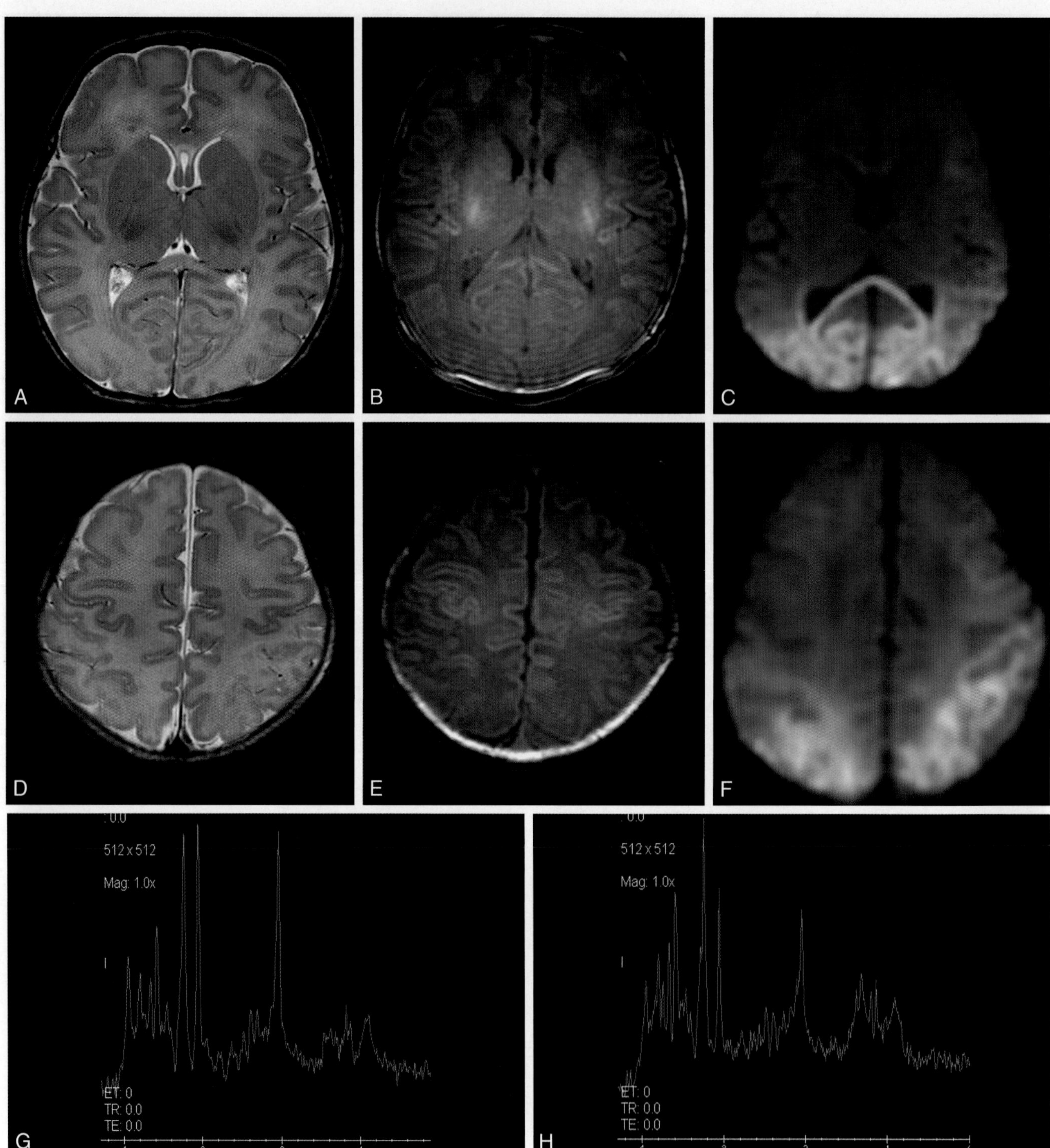

Fig. 4.3 Neonatal Hypoglycemia. (A and D) Axial T2W, (B and E) axial T1W, and (C and F) axial DWI images demonstrate T2W hyperintensity, T1W hypointensity, and diffusion restriction (low ADC not shown) in the parietal and occipital lobe cortex and white matter indicative of a posterior pattern of cytotoxic edema. (G and H) Short TE MRS demonstrating mild elevation of lactate, mild decrease in NAA and choline due to acute parenchymal injury.

NEONATAL HYPOGLYCEMIA

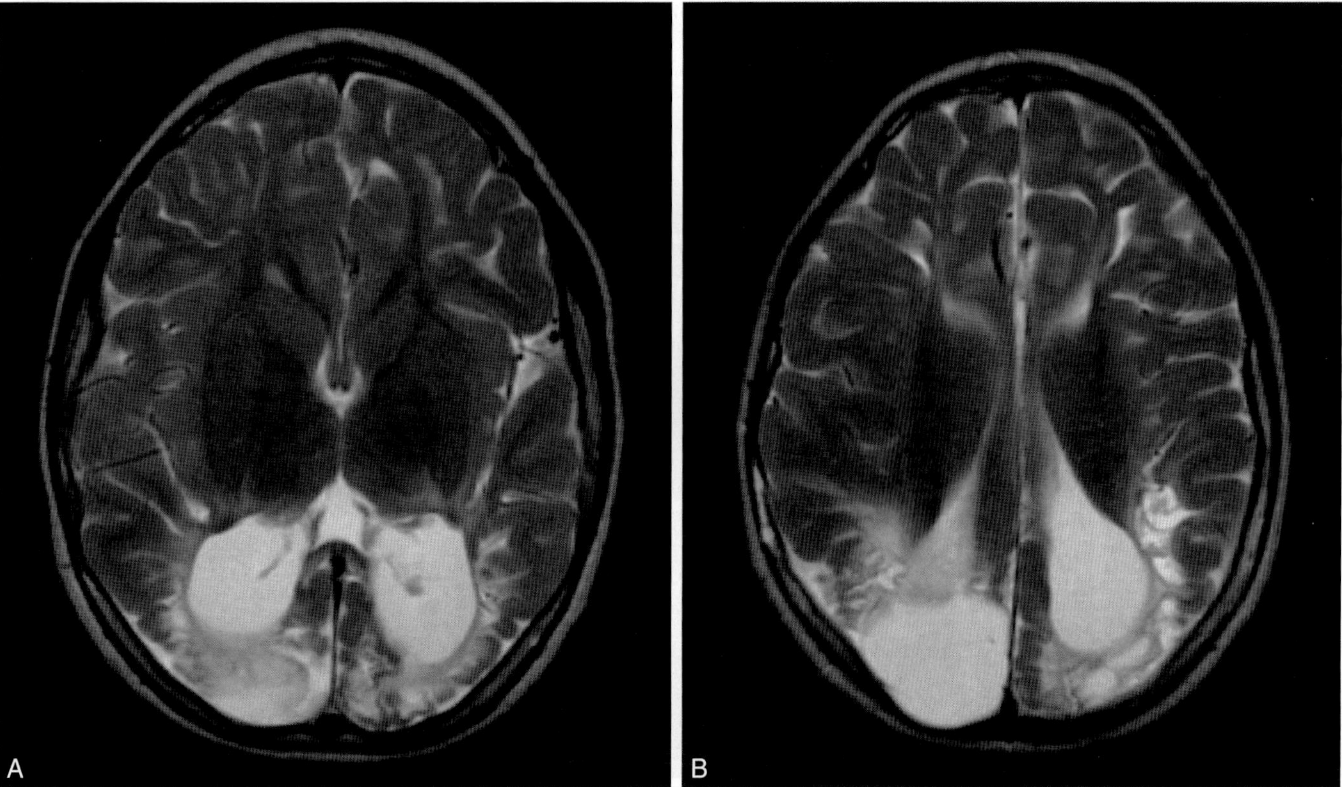

Fig. 4.4 Neonatal Hypoglycemia. (A and B) Axial T2W images demonstrate symmetric volume loss of the posterior parietal and occipital lobes indicative of sequela of injury from neonatal hypoglycemia.

Key Points

Background

- Etiologies include hyperinsulinism, endocrine deficiency, and metabolic disorders.
- Hypoglycemia → decreased pyruvate and lactate → tissue alkalosis → selective neuronal necrosis of the cerebral cortex (typically parietal and occipital lobes), hippocampus, caudate, and potentially the spinal cord. The reason for the predilection of injury to the parietooccipital areas remains unknown.
- Hypoglycemia has a greater effect on the superficial cortical layers, while hypoxic ischemic injury has a greater effect on the middle cortical layers. Axon sparing and dendritic swelling is seen with hypoglycemic injury.

Clinical

- Sequela range from no impairment to epilepsy, visual impairment, mental retardation, and death

Imaging

- Acute phase will demonstrate diffusion restriction and T2W hyperintensity in the occipital lobes and posterior parietal cortex. Chronic phase will demonstrate volume loss and T2/FLAIR hyperintensity in the occipital lobes and posterior parietal lobes indicative of encephalomalacia and gliosis.
- MRS: ↓ NAA and ↑ lactate in acute and subacute phases

REFERENCE

1. Van der Knaap MS, and Valk J. *Magnetic Resonance of Myelination and Myelin Disorders*. 3rd edition. Berlin: Springer; 2005.

NONKETOTIC HYPERGLYCINEMIA

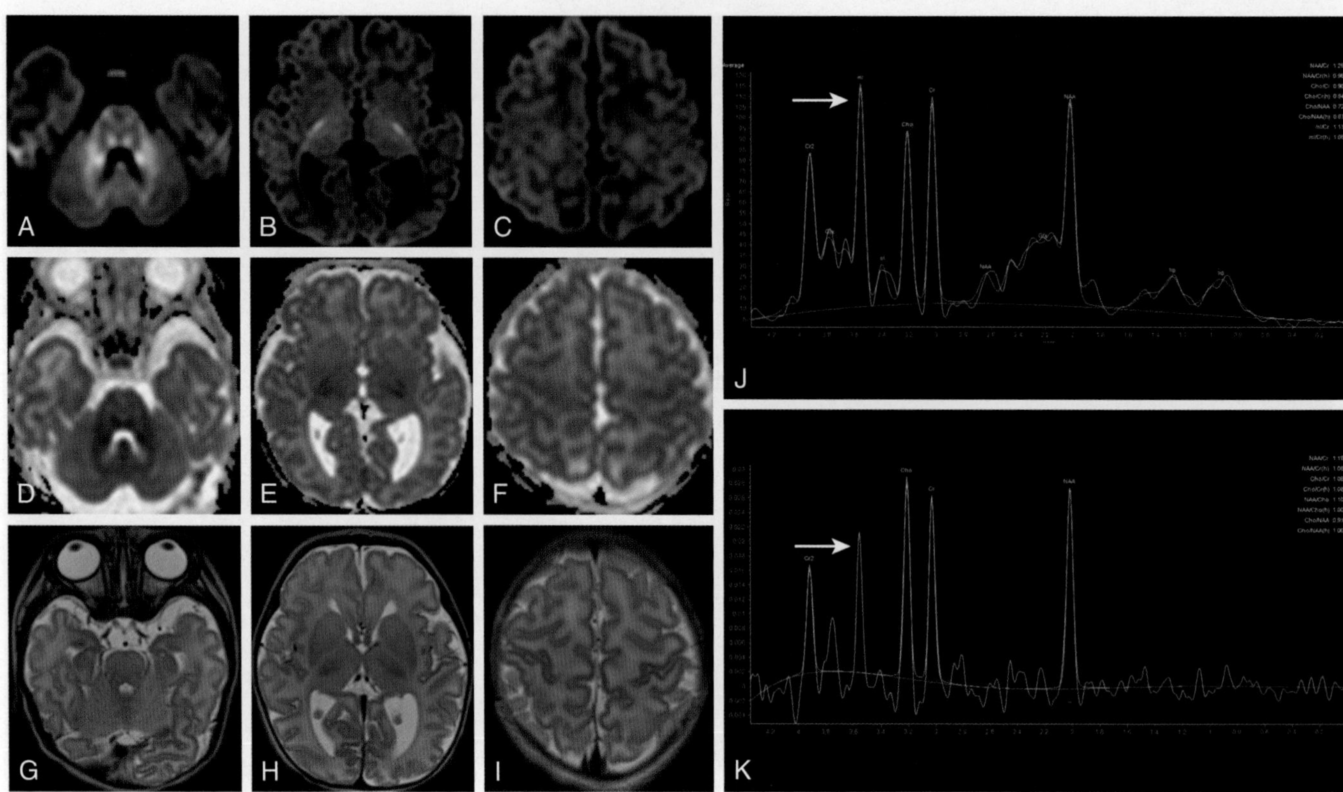

Fig. 4.5 **Nonketotic Hyperglycinemia**. 6-day-old with weakness and lethargy. (A to I) Multiple sections of the brain with rows of axial DWI, ADC, and T2W images demonstrate diffusion restriction in a nonvascular distribution involving the middle cerebellar peduncles, pons, posterior limbs of the internal capsules, and the subcortical white matter of the perirolandic cortex. (J and K) Short and long echo MRS demonstrating a large peak at 3.56 ppm, which persists on long echo, indicating abnormal glycine peak.

Key Points

Background

- Autosomal recessive disorder of the glycine cleavage system (a mitochondrial multi-enzyme complex) leading to glycine accumulation
- Pathologically demonstrates development of vacuoles in the myelin
- Glycine potentiates the excitotoxic action of glutamate in the brain.

Clinical

- Presents within first 4 days of life; signs and symptoms include seizures, hypotonia, apnea, dystonia, and developmental delay.
- Diagnosis made by elevated CSF: Plasma glycine > 0.08 (normal < 0.04)

Imaging

- Neonates present with T2W hyperintensity and *reduced diffusion in the dorsal pons, midbrain, and posterior limb internal capsules.* Older infants demonstrate delayed myelination and volume loss.
- MRS: *Glycine peak at 3.56 ppm is key to diagnosis.* Must perform intermediate or long echo because glycine persists on short and intermediate/long echo while myo-inositol does not persist on intermediate/long echo

REFERENCES

1. Van der Knaap MS, and Valk J. *Magnetic Resonance of Myelination and Myelin Disorders*. 3rd edition. Berlin: Springer; 2005.
2. Huisman TAGM, Thiel T, Steinmann B, et al. Proton magnetic resonance spectroscopy of the brain of a neonate with nonketotic hyperglycinemia: in vivo-in vitro (ex vivo) correlation. *Eur Radiol.* 2002 Apr;12(4):858–861.

ISOLATED SULFITE OXIDASE DEFICIENCY

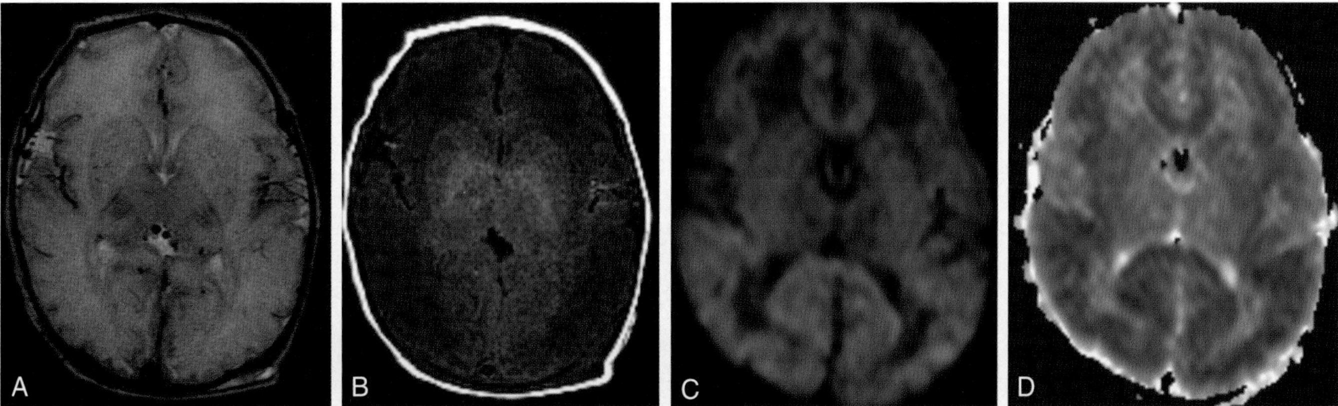

Fig. 4.6 Isolated Sulfite Oxidase Deficiency. A 4-day-old with seizures. (A) Axial T2W, (B) axial T1W, (C) axial DWI, (D) axial ADC images demonstrate diffuse edema seen as cortical, deep gray matter, and white matter T2W hyperintensity, poor visualization of cortical gray matter-white matter interface, and mild DWI hyperintensity and diffusely low ADC in the cortex.

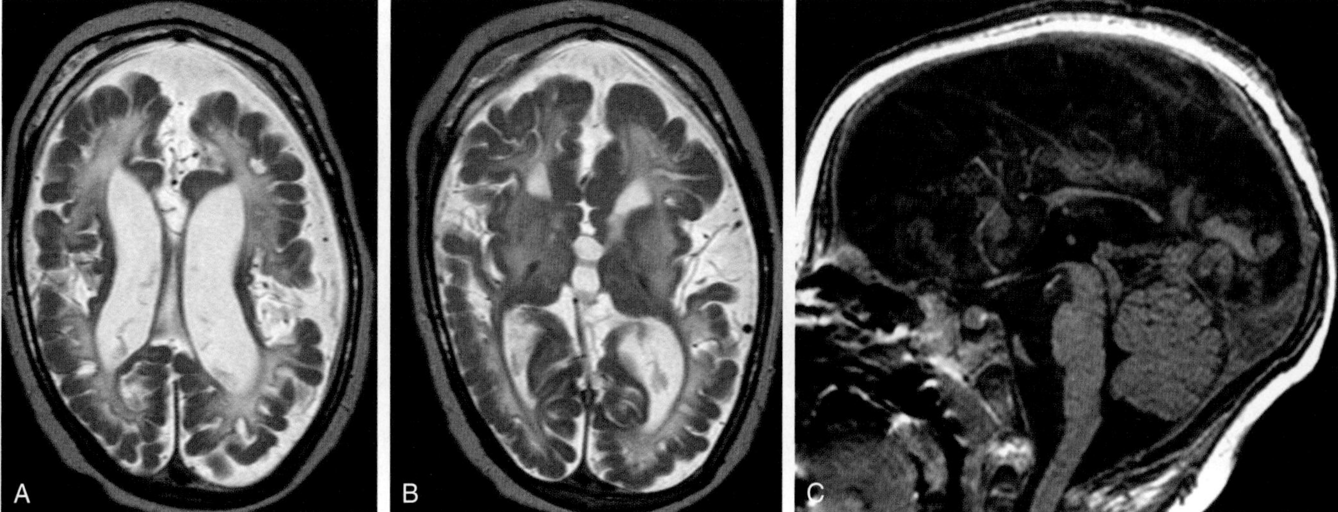

Fig. 4.7 Isolated Sulfite Oxidase Deficiency. 10-month-old with seizures and myoclonic jerks. (A and B) Axial T2W, and (C) sagittal T1W images demonstrate sequela of cytotoxic edema from sulfite oxidase deficiency seen as severe cerebral volume loss and thinning of the corpus callosum.

Key Points

Background

- Autosomal recessive mutation in the SUOX gene which makes the enzyme sulfite oxidase. Loss of oxidation of sulfite to sulfate preventing the breakdown of sulfur-containing amino acids. It is uncertain whether pathogenesis is due to a toxic metabolite or deficient product

Clinical

- Variable clinical manifestation from neonatal onset with encephalopathy, seizure, and early death to late infantile onset with dystonia, hypotonia, and developmental delay
- Elevated urinary excretion of sulfite, thiosulfate, and taurine
- No effective treatment to date. Limitation of sulfur amino acids and cysteamine may help absorb excess sulfite

Imaging

- Acute presentation in the neonate period with *diffusion restriction* and T2W hyperintense signal in the cerebral cortex *mimicking HIE*
- Chronic phase demonstrates *diffuse atrophy and cystic degeneration* of the cerebral hemispheres, cerebellar and deep gray matter atrophy
- MRS: ↓ NAA and ↑ lactate in acute and subacute phases

REFERENCES

1. Van der Knaap MS, and Valk J. *Magnetic Resonance of Myelination and Myelin Disorders*. 3rd edition. Berlin: Springer; 2005.
2. Barkovich AJ, Raybaud C. *Pediatric Neuroradiology*. 6th edition. Philadelphia: Wolters-Kluwer; 2019.
3. Poretti A, Blaser SL, Lequin MH, et al. Neonatal neuroimaging findings in inborn errors of metabolism. *J Magn Reson Imaging*. 2013 Feb;37(2):294–312.

MOLYBDENUM COFACTOR

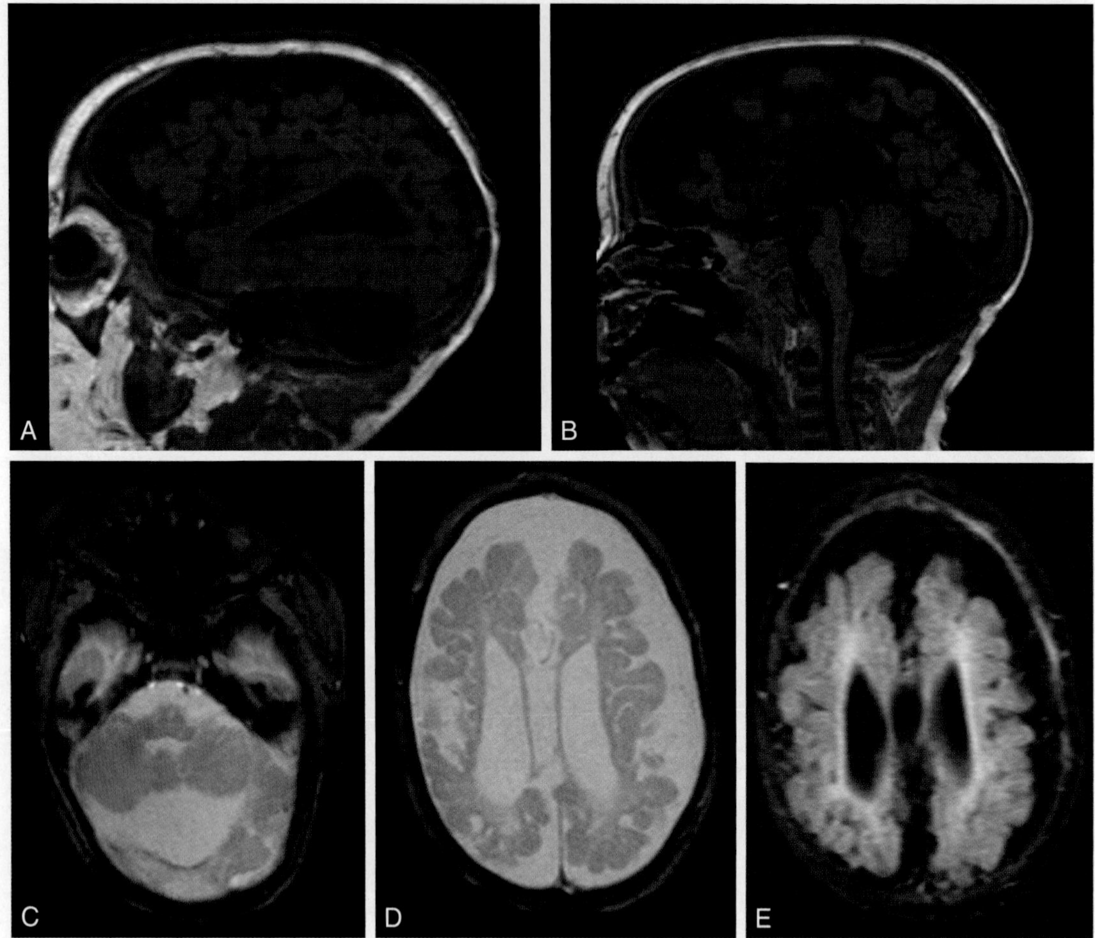

Fig. 4.8 Molybdenum Cofactor. 9-month-old. (A and B) Sagittal T1W, (C and D) axial T2W, and (E) axial FLAIR images demonstrate sequela of cytotoxic edema seen as severe cerebral volume loss, thinning of the corpus callosum, cerebellar and brainstem atrophy, periventricular gliosis, ex vacuo enlargement of the ventricles, and secondary prominence of the subarachnoid spaces.

Key Points

Background

- Autosomal recessive. The cofactor is formed by molybdopterin and molybdenum
- Results in simultaneous loss of all cofactor-dependent enzymes, including sulfite oxidase, xanthine dehydrogenase, and aldehyde oxidase
- Uncertain whether pathogenesis is due to a toxic metabolite or deficient product

Clinical

- Neonatal presentation with seizure, axial hypotonia, limb hypertonia, and feeding difficulty. Most patients die at an early age.

Imaging

- Similar imaging pattern to sulfite oxidase that resembles severe hypoxic ischemic injury
- MRS: ↓ NAA and ↑ lactate in acute and subacute phases

REFERENCES

1. Van der Knaap MS, and Valk J. *Magnetic Resonance of Myelination and Myelin Disorders*. 3rd edition. Berlin: Springer; 2005.
2. Barkovich AJ, Raybaud C. *Pediatric Neuroradiology*. 6th edition. Philadelphia: Wolters-Kluwer; 2019.

UREA CYCLE DISORDERS

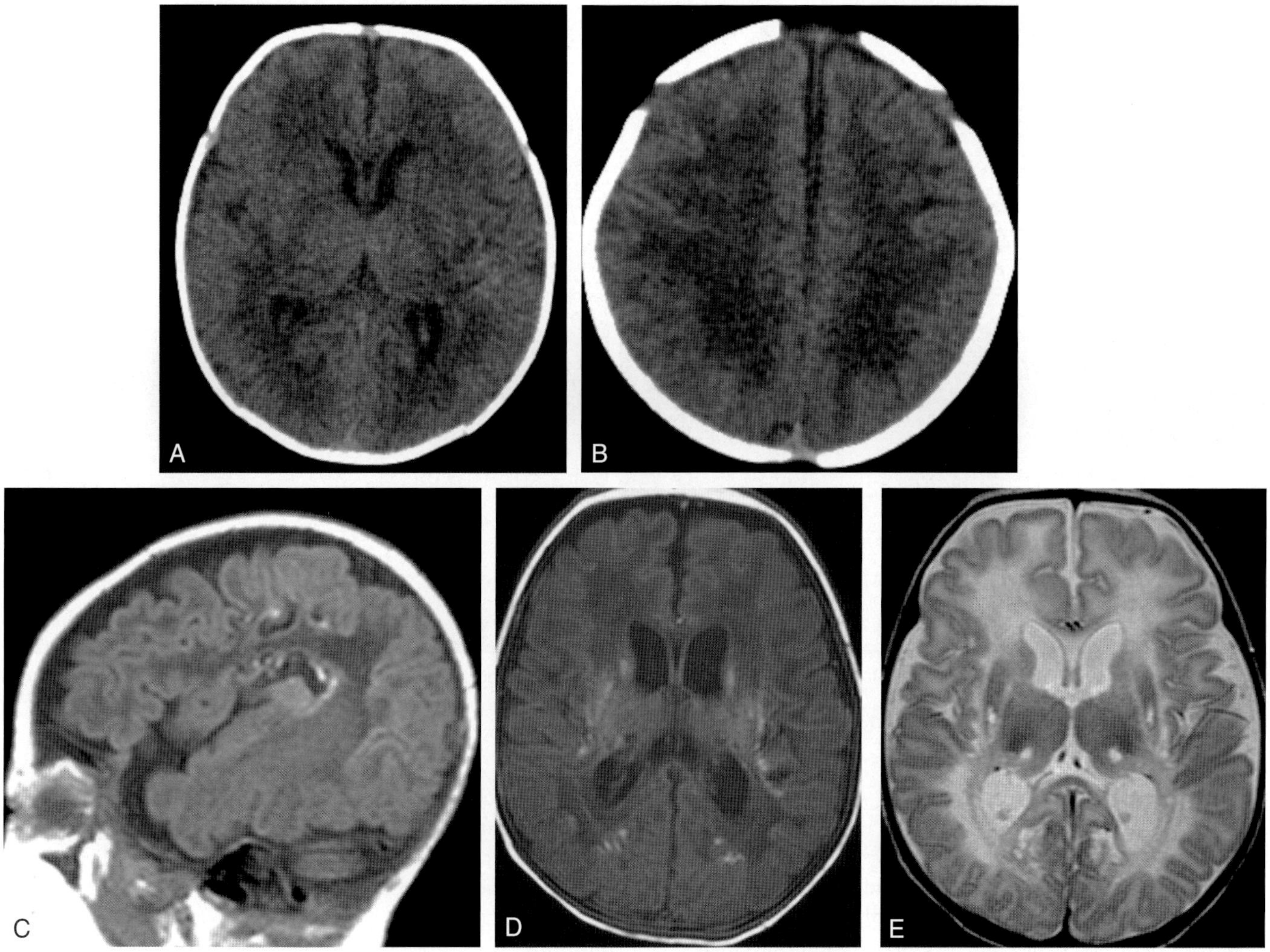

Fig. 4.9 Urea Cycle Disorder. 1-month-old with encephalopathy, and hyperammonemia (>1000 μmol/L) due to carbamyl phosphate deficiency. (A and B) Axial CT images demonstrate white matter, posterior thalamic, and posterior insular cortex hypodensity. Follow-up MRI (C and D) sagittal and axial T1W and (E) axial T2W images demonstrate volume loss and cortical T1W hyperintensity in the posterior insula and perisylvian frontal, temporal, and parietal cortex and diffuse white matter T2W hyperintensity; and volume loss of the basal ganglia and thalami.

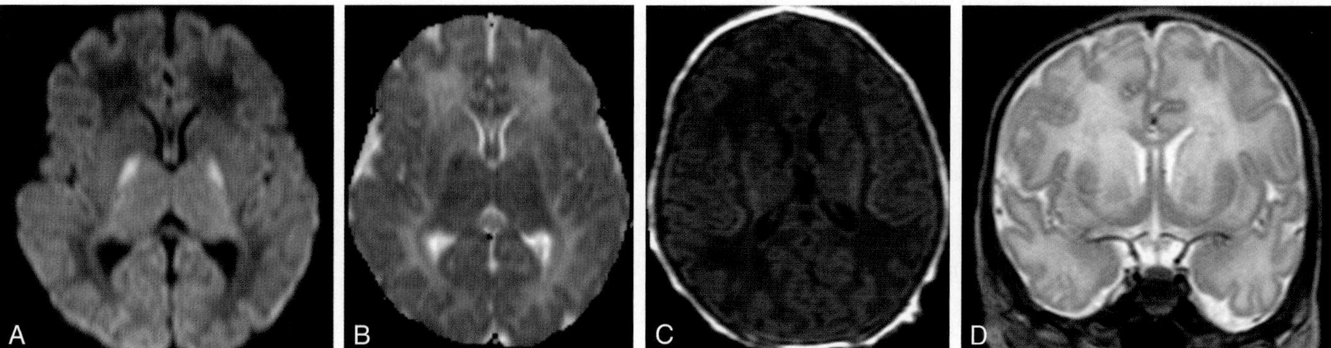

Fig. 4.10 Urea Cycle Disorder. 14-day-old with seizure, lethargy, poor feeding, and hyperammonemia (367 μmol/L) due to citrullinemia. (A and B) Axial DWI and ADC, (C) axial T1W, and (D) coronal T2W images demonstrate diffusion restriction in the globus pallidi and genu of the internal capsules, posterior insular cortex T1W hyperintensity, and T2W hyperintensity in the basal ganglia in addition to diffuse white matter T2W hyperintensity.

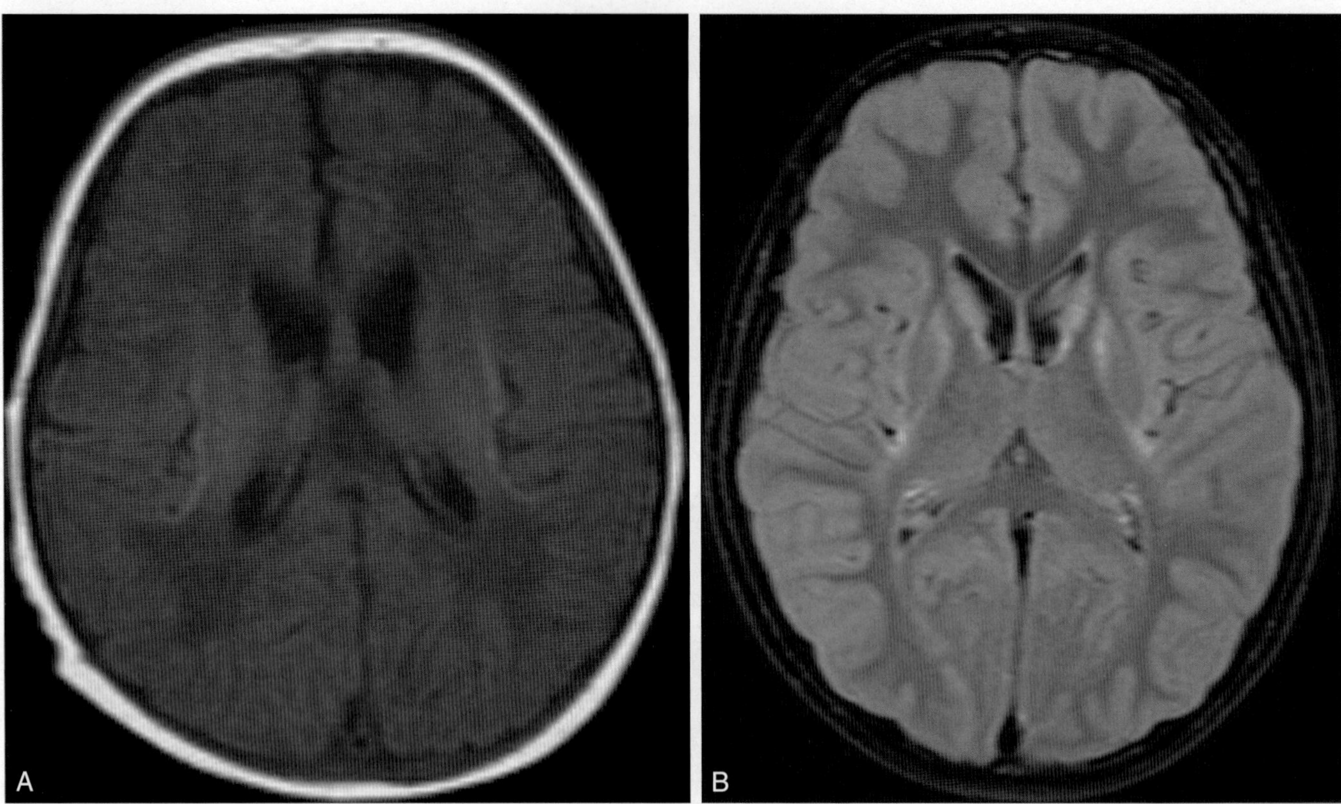

Fig. 4.11 Urea Cycle Disorder: Sequela. (A) Axial T1W and (B) axial FLAIR images demonstrate insular cortex T1W and FLAIR hyperintensity with volume loss in the basal ganglia.

Key Points

Background

- Five common urea cycle defects include: carbamoyl phosphate synthetase deficiency (CPSD), ornithine transcarbamylase deficiency (OTCD), argininosuccinate synthetase deficiency (ASSD/citrullinemia), argininosuccinate lyase deficiency (ASLD), arginase deficiency
- Autosomal recessive, except OTCD, which is X-linked recessive
- Histopathology: Elevated ammonia leads to astrocyte swelling and accumulation of glutamine

Clinical

- Clinical features are similar with exception of ASLD, which has a slow, progressive course; hyperammonemia is present except in arginase deficiency; most present in the neonatal period with lethargy, hypotonia, seizure, coma, and rapid progression to death or severe neurologic sequela. Late-onset disease is chronic and episodic in response to infection, high protein intake, trauma, surgery, or valproate.
- Treatment includes limiting protein intake as well as dialysis and lactulose medication.

Imaging

- Neonates often demonstrate diffuse edema in the cerebral hemispheres and basal ganglia, and *T1W shortening in the insula* and perirolandic regions.
- Older infants and children may demonstrate asymmetric infarct-like patterns of cortical and subcortical involvement.
- Chronic stage demonstrates atrophy and gliosis.
- MRS: Acute phase may demonstrate ↑ lactate and glutamate/glutamine.

REFERENCES

1. Van der Knaap MS, and Valk J. *Magnetic Resonance of Myelination and Myelin Disorders*. 3rd edition. Berlin: Springer; 2005.
2. Barkovich AJ, Raybaud C. *Pediatric Neuroradiology*. 6th edition. Philadelphia: Wolters-Kluwer; 2019.

METABOLIC DISORDERS WITH REGIONAL WHITE MATTER PATTERNS

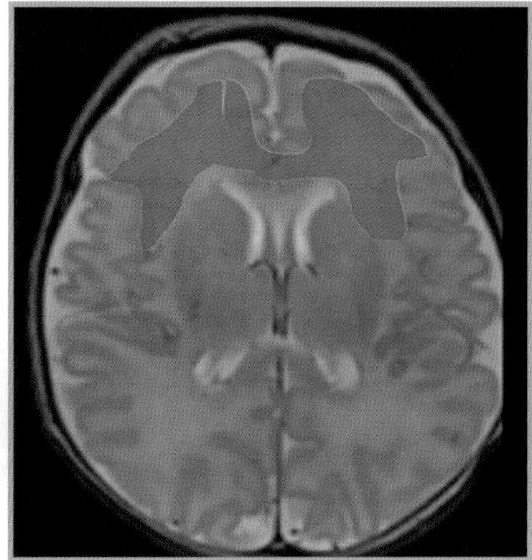

Anterior
Alexander's disease

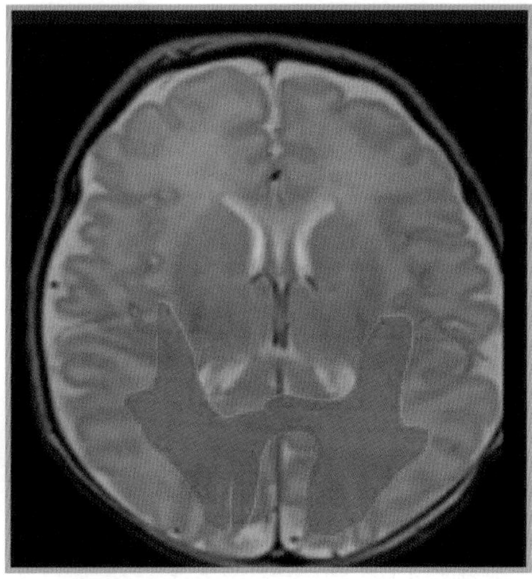

Posterior
X-linked Adrenoleukodystrophy

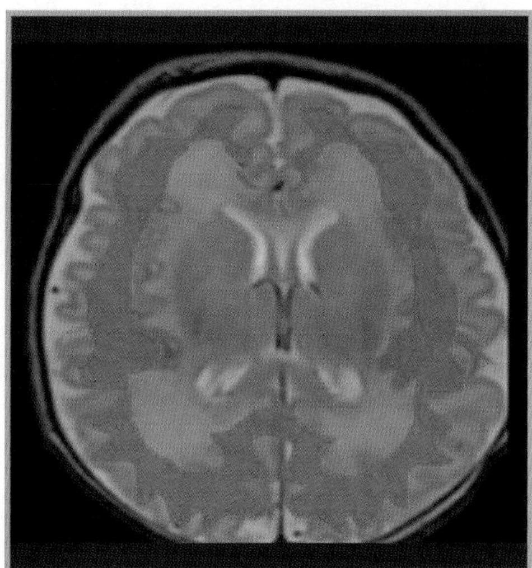

Peripheral
Canavan
L-2-hydroxyglutaric aciduria

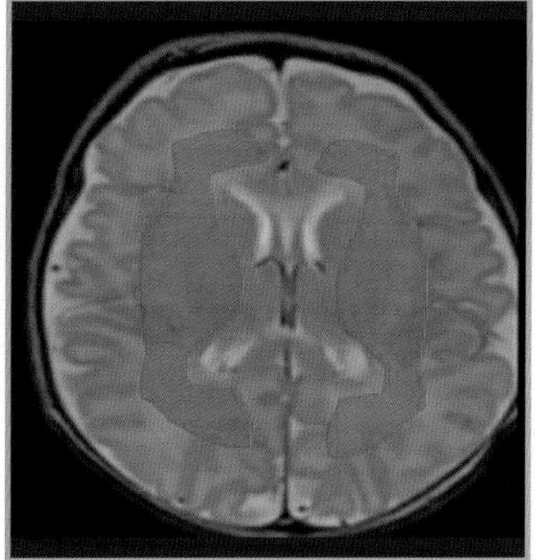

Deep White Matter
Krabbe disease
Metachromatic leukodystrophy
Vanishing white matter
Lowe syndrome
Mucopolysacharridoses

ALEXANDER DISEASE

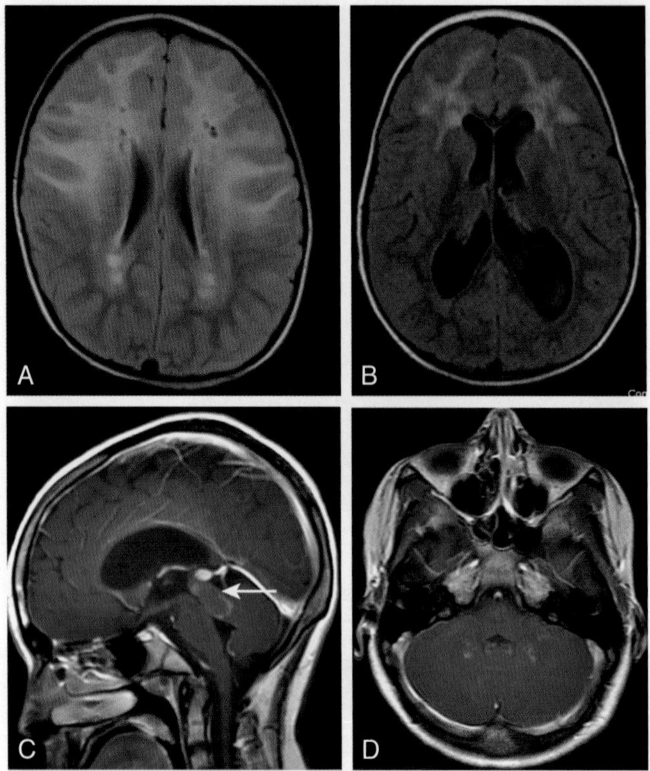

Fig. 4.12 Alexander Disease in a 12-Year-Old With Seizure. (A and B) Axial FLAIR and (C and D) sagittal and axial T1W+C images demonstrate anterior pattern of white matter FLAIR hyperintensity, expansion of the tectal plate, and small foci of parenchymal enhancement in the cerebellum. The expansion of the tectal plate is due to deposition of Rosenthal fibers and could be erroneously mistaken for a tectal glioma.

Fig. 4.13 Alexander Disease in an 8-Month-Old With Macrocephaly, Developmental Delay, and Seizures. (A) Axial CT demonstrates confluent white matter hypodensity with areas of deep white matter increased density. (B) Axial T2W, (C) axial DWI, and (D) sagittal T1W+C images demonstrate a diffuse white matter T2W hyperintensity with abnormal enhancement of the periventricular white matter, which demonstrated mild relative diffusion restriction (ADC hypointensity not shown).

Key Points

Background

- Most cases are caused by a sporadic de novo mutation.
- Deficiency of glial fibrillary acidic protein (GFAP) leads to astrocyte dysfunction white matter destruction, and accumulation of Rosenthal fibers (subependymal, subpial, and perivascular locations).
- Laboratory assessment is not helpful. Biopsy demonstrates Rosenthal fibers.

Clinical

- Infantile onset (ranging from birth to early childhood) is the most common (typically presents at 6 months) and presents with macrocephaly, seizures, spasticity, and feeding difficulty.
- Juvenile onset (4–14 years of age) often presents with bulbar and pseudobulbar symptoms.
- Adult onset (second to seventh decade) has variable clinical features; no specific treatment.

Imaging

- *Confluent anterior white matter T2 FLAIR* hyperintense signal and can also involve periventricular white matter, fornix, basal ganglia (BG), thalami, dentate, and brainstem
- *Parenchymal enhancement* can occur from *Rosenthal deposition* (presumably from impaired blood-brain barrier due to dysfunction of astrocyte foot processes caused by Rosenthal fiber accumulation), can result in expansion of the tectal plate and narrowing of the cerebral aqueduct, mimicking a tectal glioma
- Diffusion restriction not typically seen
- MRS: Nonspecific ↓ NAA, ↑ lactate

REFERENCE

1. Van der Knaap MS, and Valk J. *Magnetic Resonance of Myelination and Myelin Disorders*. 3rd edition. Berlin: Springer; 2005.
2. van der Knaap MS, Naidu S, Breiter SN, et al. Alexander disease: diagnosis with MR imaging. *AJNR Am J Neuroradiol*. 2001 Mar;22(3):541–552.

X-LINKED ADRENOLEUKODYSTROPHY

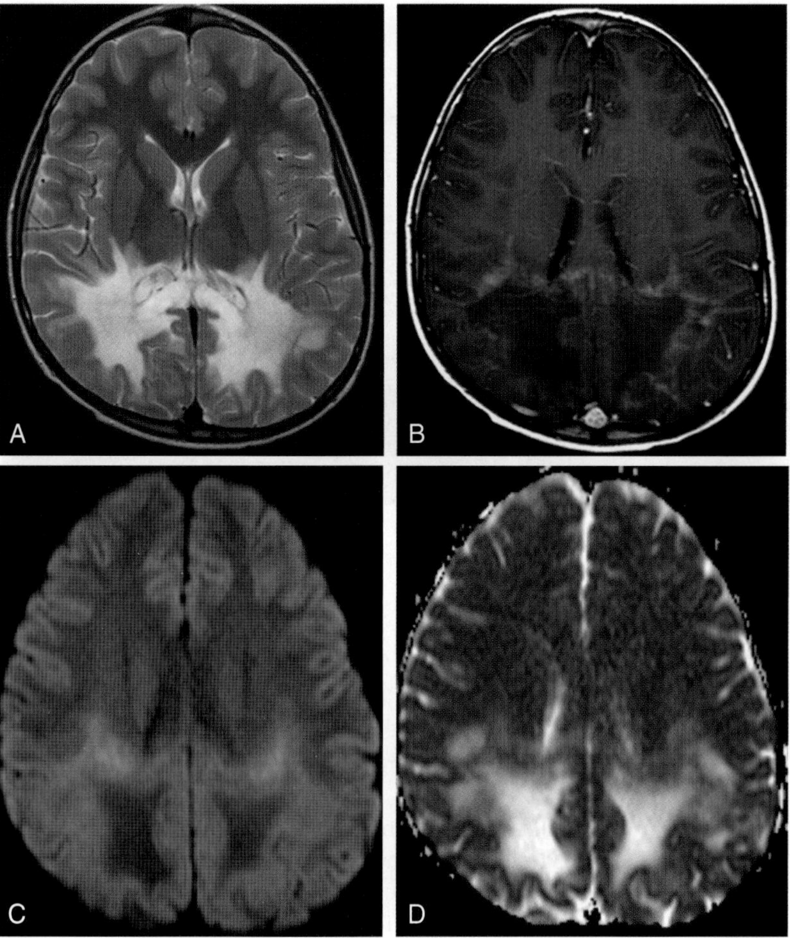

Fig. 4.14 X-linked Adrenoleukodystrophy. (A) Axial T2W, (B) axial T1W+C, (C) axial DWI, and (D) axial ADC map images demonstrate posterior pattern of white matter T2W hyperintensity in the splenium, peritrigonal white matter, and parieto-occipital white matter with peripheral "leading edge" enhancement, and reduced diffusion at the anterior margin.

Key Points

Background

- X-linked recessive disorder of adrenoleukodystrophy (ALDP), a peroxisome membrane protein, involved in peroxisome metabolism leading to impaired beta-oxidation of very long chain fatty acids (VLCFA); VLCFA accumulation in myelin → demyelination → microglial response
- Pathology demonstrates a leading edge of demyelination with axonal sparing, middle zone of active inflammation, and central area of necrosis
- Loes scoring system used to assess disease severity and guide decision on bone marrow transplantation

Clinical

- Presentation usually age 4 to 8 years; early neurologic manifestations include vision loss, gait abnormality, and auditory symptoms, which progress to spastic quadriplegia, epilepsy, dementia, and vegetative state or death within 1 to 5 years; adolescent and adult presentation can also occur
- Diagnosed by detecting elevated plasma VLCFA; treated with replacement of adrenal hormones, and dietary restriction of saturated VLCFA combined with Lorenzo's oil (a 4:1 mixture of glyceryl trioleate and glyceryl trierucate), and bone marrow transplantation
- Outcome of bone marrow transplantation depends on degree of cerebral involvement at time of transplantation

Imaging

- Demyelination of splenium and posterior peritrigonal white matter, with sparing of the subcortical U fibers
- Progresses to involve corticospinal tracts, fornices, commissures, visual and auditory pathways
- Pathognomonic "leading edge" enhancement and reduced diffusion at active edge of demyelination
- MRS: Nonspecific; depends on region evaluated; affected areas show ↑ Cho; ↓ NAA, ↑ lactate; late stage shows ↓ metabolites except ↑ myoI

REFERENCES

1. Loes DJ, Fatemi A, Melham ER, et al. Analysis of MRI patterns aids prediction of progression in X-linked adrenoleukodystrophy. *Neurology*. 2003;61:369–374.
2. Van der Knaap MS, and Valk J. *Magnetic Resonance of Myelination and Myelin Disorders*. 3rd edition. Berlin: Springer; 2005.

CANAVAN DISEASE

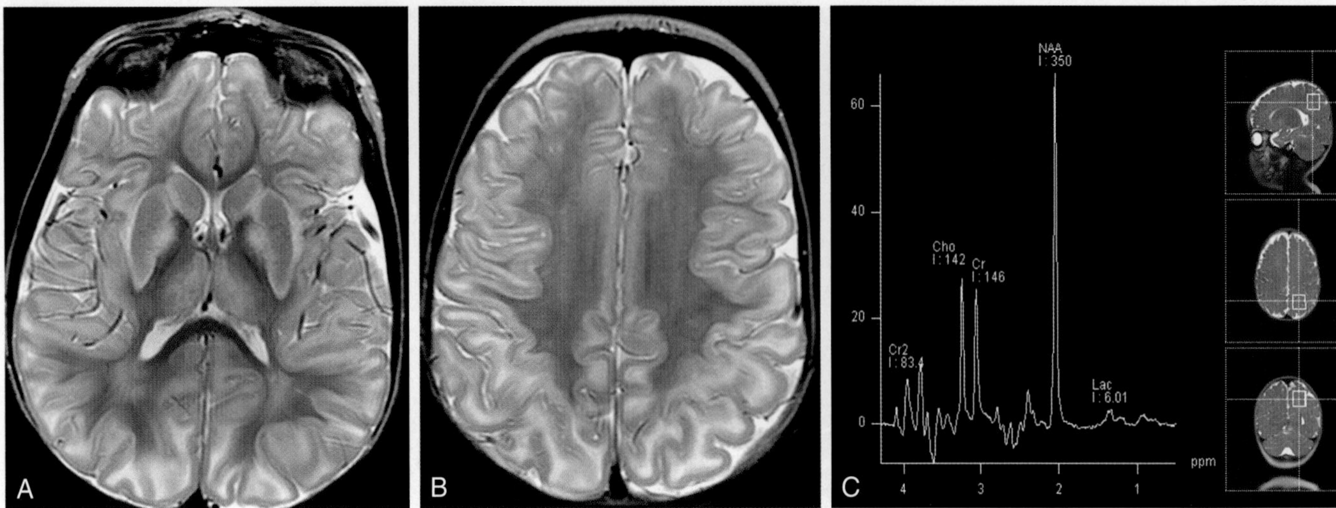

Fig. 4.15 Canavan Disease. (A and B) Axial T2W images demonstrate a pattern of peripheral white matter T2W hyperintensity as well as hyperintensity in the thalami and basal ganglia. (C) MRS long echo spectroscopy demonstrates significantly elevated NAA peak (>2× the choline and creatine peaks).

Key Points

Background

- Autosomal recessive mutation in aspartoacylase gene. Deficiency of aspartoacylase → elevated NAA brain. Pathogenesis of elevated NAA is unknown but includes acting as an osmolyte and leading to water accumulation in the brain, altered neurotransmission, synthesis of myelin lipids, and/or molecular water pump in myelinated neurons.
- Elevated NAA in the urine and plasma is diagnostic.
- Pathology demonstrates intramyelinic vacuole formation.

Clinical

- Infant presentation (age 6 months) is most common; macrocephaly, hypotonia, blindness, and seizures; rapidly progressive; leads to a vegetative state and often death before age 4.
- No therapy presently exists for Canavan disease.

Imaging

- T2/FLAIR hyperintensity in the *subcortical WM before deep WM*
- T2/FLAIR hyperintensity in the globus pallidi (typically sparing caudate and putamen) and thalami
- Diffusion restriction can be seen in acute phase and may represent intramyelinic edema
- MRS: Characteristic *large NAA peak* is a key finding

REFERENCES

1. Van der Knaap MS, and Valk J. *Magnetic Resonance of Myelination and Myelin Disorders*. 3rd edition. Berlin: Springer; 2005.
2. Barkovich AJ, Raybaud C. *Pediatric Neuroradiology*. 6th edition. Philadelphia: Wolters-Kluwer; 2019.

L-2-HYDROXYGLUTARIC ACIDURIA

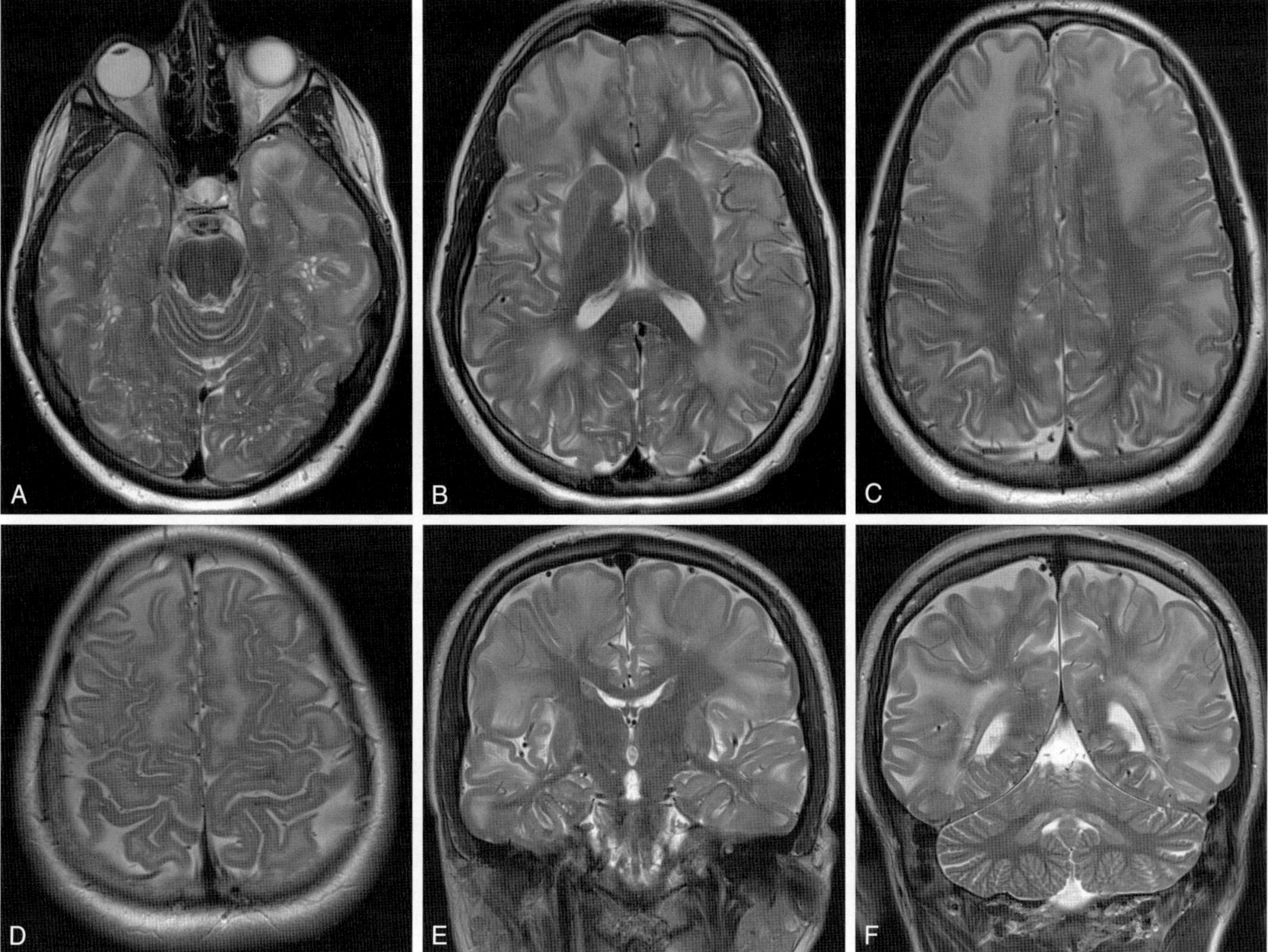

Fig. 4.16 L-2-Hydroxyglutaric Aciduria. A 17-year-old with ataxia. Initial presentation at age 3 with developmental delay and macrocephaly. (A to F) Axial and coronal T2W images demonstrate a peripheral pattern of white matter T2W hyperintensity in the subcortical white matter and sparing the central white matter. Abnormal T2W hyperintensity is also present in the globus pallidi and dentate nuclei. Increased numbers of perivascular spaces are seen in the temporal and occipital lobes as well.

Key Points

Background

- Autosomal recessive mutation in gene for L-2-hydroxyglutarate dehydrogenase, which is a mitochondrial protein.
- Pathology demonstrates spongiform degeneration of the cerebral and cerebellar white matter with gliosis and vacuole formation.

Clinical

- Usually presents in the second year of life with macrocephaly, developmental delay, abnormal gait, and febrile seizures. Slowly progressive ataxia, tremor, and other neurologic signs and symptoms, including extrapyramidal signs.
- Diagnosis made by detection of elevated urine L-2-hydroxyglutaric acid.

Imaging

- T2/FLAIR hyperintensity in the U fibers and subcortical WM before deep WM
- T2/FLAIR hyperintensity in the globus pallidi
- MRS: Nonspecific; normal or mild reduction in NAA

REFERENCES

1. Van der Knaap MS, and Valk J. *Magnetic Resonance of Myelination and Myelin Disorders*. 3rd edition. Berlin: Springer; 2005.
2. Barkovich AJ, Raybaud C. *Pediatric Neuroradiology*. 6th edition. Philadelphia: Wolters-Kluwer; 2019.

METACHROMATIC LEUKODYSTROPHY

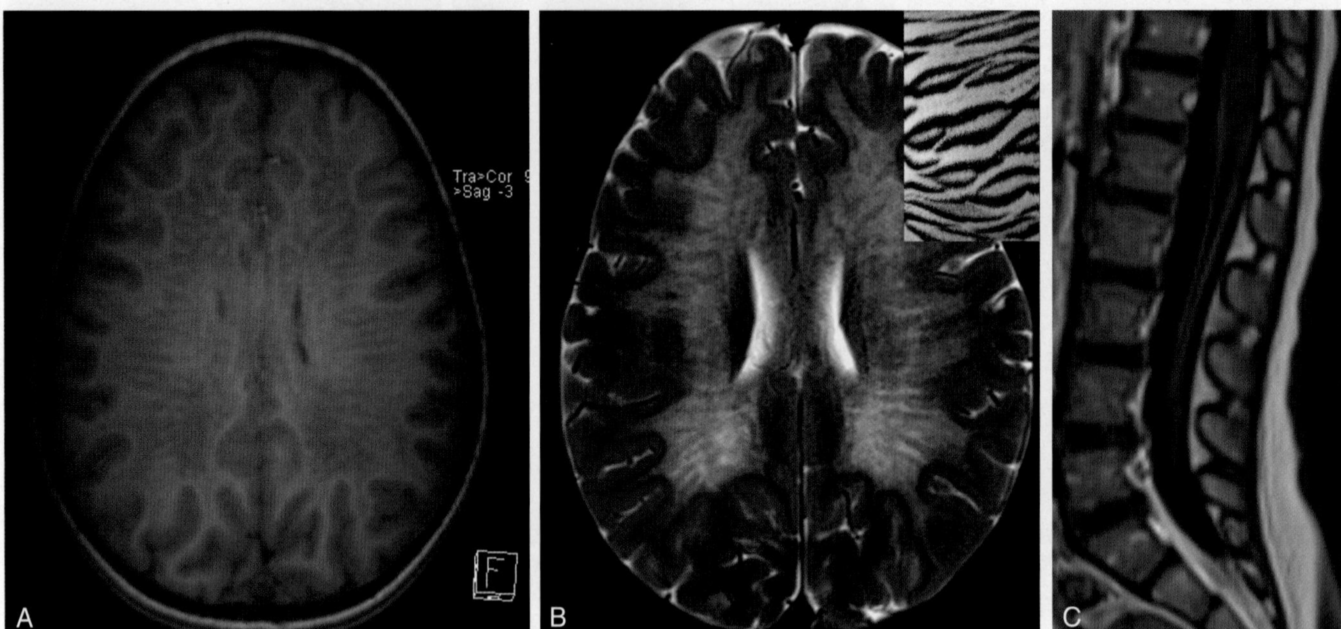

Fig. 4.17 Metachromatic Leukodystrophy. 20-month-old with ataxia, no lower extremity reflexes. (A) Axial T1W, and (B) axial T2W images demonstrate a pattern of central white matter T2W hyperintensity with linear areas of sparing, resulting in a "tigroid" pattern. (C) Sagittal T1W+C of the lumbar spine demonstrates enhancing cauda equina. (C, Tiger stripe. Copyright © iStock.com/anankkml.)

Key Points

Background

- Autosomal recessive; lysosomal disorder; decreased arylsulfatase A or cofactor prevents hydrolysis of sulfatides
- Name comes from the deposition of metachromatic staining material (sulfatides) in the white matter
- Increased urinary sulfatides is used for diagnosis
- Pathology of the brain demonstrates demyelination of affected areas, astrocyte proliferation, gliosis, and absence of inflammation. Peripheral nerves can demonstrate segmental demyelination

Clinical

- Late infantile: Most common (40%) with onset around age 2 and steady progression over 4 years, difficulty walking, hypotonia, progressive polyneuropathy, cerebellar ataxia, nystagmus, and flaccid paresis, leading to spasticity, blindness, and death after 5 years from onset
- Juvenile: Onset age 5 to 7 with steady progressive decline in school, language, coordination, and emotional and behavioral disturbances, leading to epilepsy in 50%, quadriplegia, dementia, and death 5 to 10 years from onset
- Adult: Onset between age 16 and 30 years; begins with emotional, behavioral, and psychiatric symptoms progressing to spastic paresis, extrapyramidal symptoms, and then to vegetative state with course lasting 15 years

Imaging

- Symmetric deep white matter T2W hyperintensity; subcortical WM later in disease
- Stripes of unaffected WM result in "tigroid" or "leopard skin" pattern
- Cauda equina can demonstrate enhancement
- MRS: Nonspecific; ↑ myoI, ↓ NAA
- Differential Diagnosis: Tigroid pattern can also be seen with Krabbe disease, Pelizaeus-Merzbacher, and Cockayne syndrome

REFERENCE

1. Van der Knaap MS, and Valk J. *Magnetic Resonance of Myelination and Myelin Disorders*. 3rd edition. Berlin: Springer; 2005.

KRABBE DISEASE

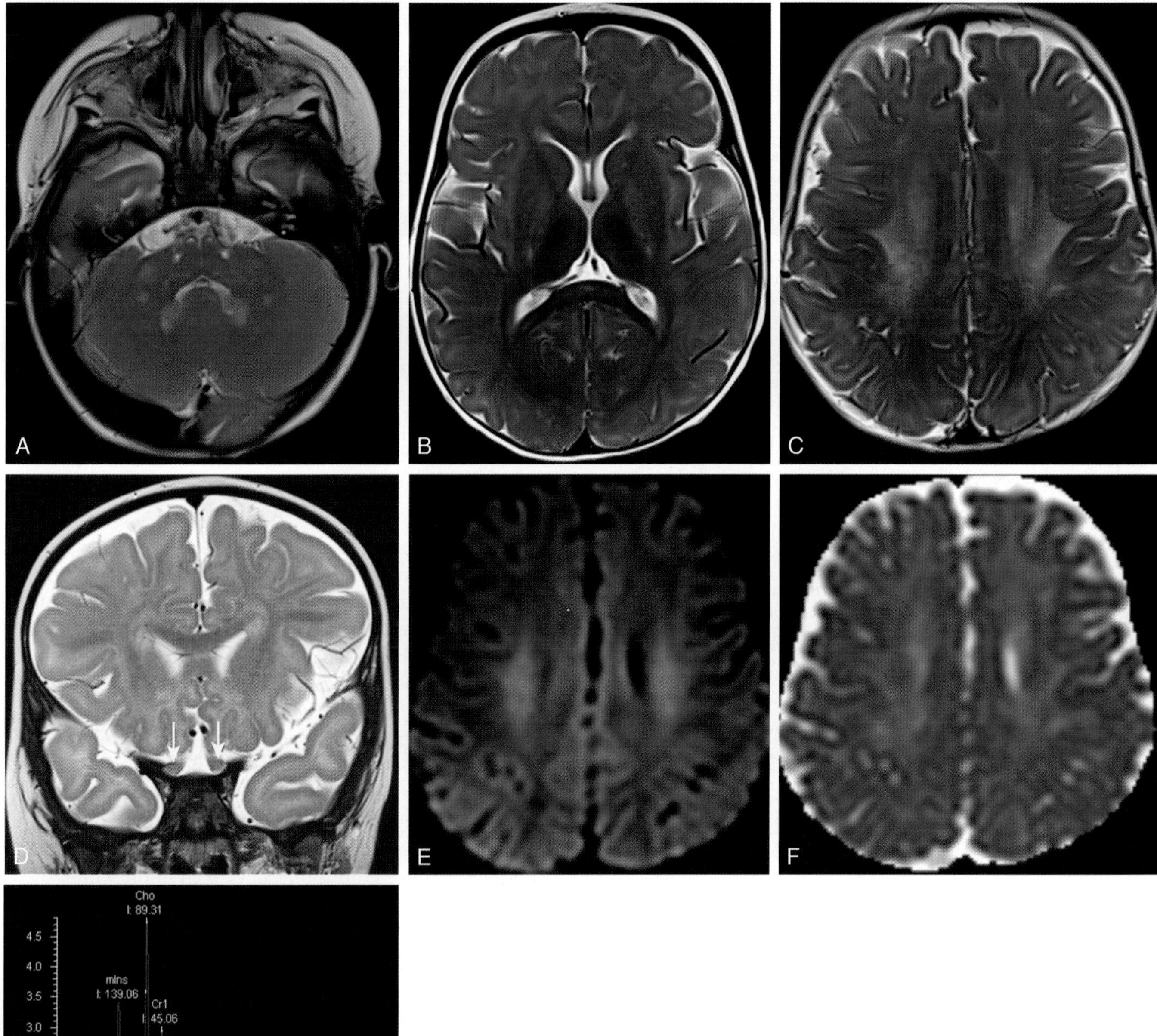

Fig. 4.18 Krabbe Disease. 8-month-old with stiff arms and legs, central hypotonia, decreased voluntary movements, and irritability. (A to D) Axial and coronal T2W images demonstrate a pattern of confluent T2W hyperintensity in the centrum semiovale, patchy areas in the splenium, foci the middle cerebellar peduncles, medial cerebellar white matter, and thickened optic nerves. (E) Axial DWI and (F) axial ADC map demonstrate areas of relative reduced diffusion in the central deep white matter. (G) MRS short echo obtained from the central white matter demonstrates elevated choline and myo-inositol, reduced NAA, and presence of a lactate peak (1.3 ppm) and a lipid peak (0.9 ppm).

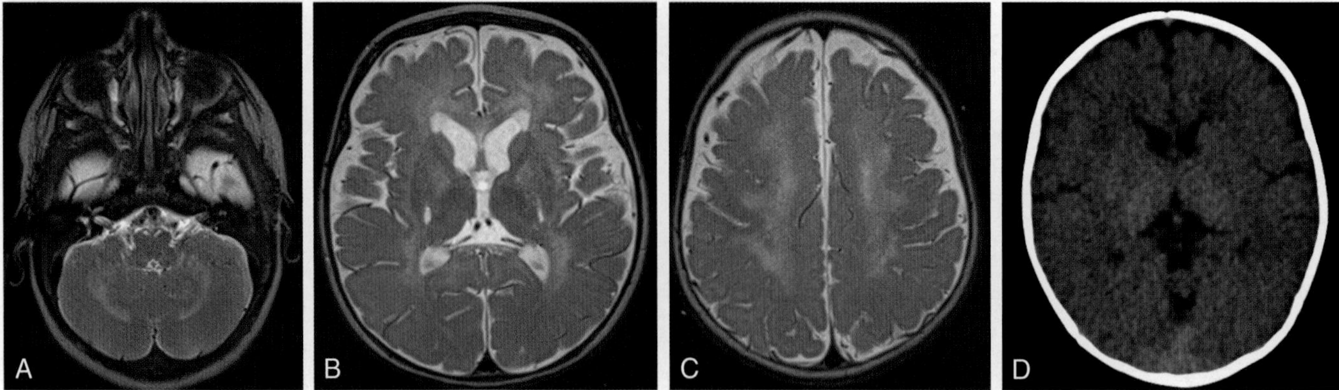

Fig. 4.19 Krabbe Disease. (A to C) Axial T2W images demonstrate a pattern of confluent central white matter T2W hyperintensity, foci of hyperintensity putamen and caudate, atrophy of the thalami. (D) Axial CT image demonstrates mild hyperdense thalami.

Key Points

Background

- Also known as globoid cell leukodystrophy; autosomal recessive; deficiency of lysosomal enzyme galactocerebrosidase → accumulation of cerebroside leading to transformation of phagocytic cells into globoid cells and accumulation of galactosyl sphingosine (psychosine), which leads to apoptosis in oligodendrocytes and loss of myelination. Cerebroside is almost exclusively found in oligodendrocytes, Schwann cells, and myelin. Process of myelination corresponds to rises in galactocerebrosidase activity in normal brains.
- Pathology demonstrates diffuse demyelination, diffuse fibrillary gliosis, and accumulation of globoid cells; peripheral nervous system demonstrates demyelination and variable axonal degeneration

Clinical

- Variable time of onset and progression.
- Early infantile/classic form is most common with normal first few months of life followed by symptom onset at 1 to 6 months in three stages; stage 1 demonstrating hyperirritability, noise and light sensitivity, excessive startle response, febrile episodes without infection, hypertonia; stage 2 occurring within 2 to 4 months from onset, demonstrating rapid and severe motor and mental deterioration, opisthotonus, hypertonic limb flexion, frequent fevers and sweats, lung infections, myoclonic jerks, seizures, vision failure, and optic atrophy; stage 3 vegetative state with decerebrate posture, blindness, and absent voluntary movements; death occurs between 5 months to 3 years of age
- Less common are neonatal onset, late-infantile, juvenile, and adolescent onset.
- Stem cell transplantation is performed in late-onset forms.
- Early onset form demonstrates high CSF protein with normal cell count.

Imaging

- Stage 1 (early stages) may demonstrate *CT hyperdensity in the thalami*, and T2/FLAIR hyperintensity in the corona radiata, and less commonly posterior limb of the internal capsule (PLIC), and basal ganglia.
- Stage 2 demonstrates abnormal *deep white matter T2/ FLAIR hyperintensity* in the periventricular white matter, corpus callosum, and *cerebellar* white matter. There is typical sparing of the subcortical U fibers. A "tigroid" pattern similar to metachromatic leukodystrophy can be seen in the deep white matter. Brainstem and cerebellar abnormalities often precede the supratentorial white matter findings. Reduced diffusion can be seen in the white matter in early stages of the disease.
- Stage 3 demonstrates diffuse atrophy; *optic nerve enlargement* due to high number of globoid cells.
- Adults may exhibit changes limited to the corticospinal tracts; subtle enhancement can occasionally be detected at the interface of normal and abnormal white matter.
- MRS: Nonspecific; ↑ Cho and myoI, ↓ NAA, and abnormal lactate

REFERENCES

1. Van der Knaap MS, and Valk J. *Magnetic Resonance of Myelination and Myelin Disorders*. 3rd edition. Berlin: Springer; 2005.
2. Barkovich AJ, Raybaud C. *Pediatric Neuroradiology*. 6th edition. Philadelphia: Wolters-Kluwer; 2019.

VANISHING WHITE MATTER DISEASE

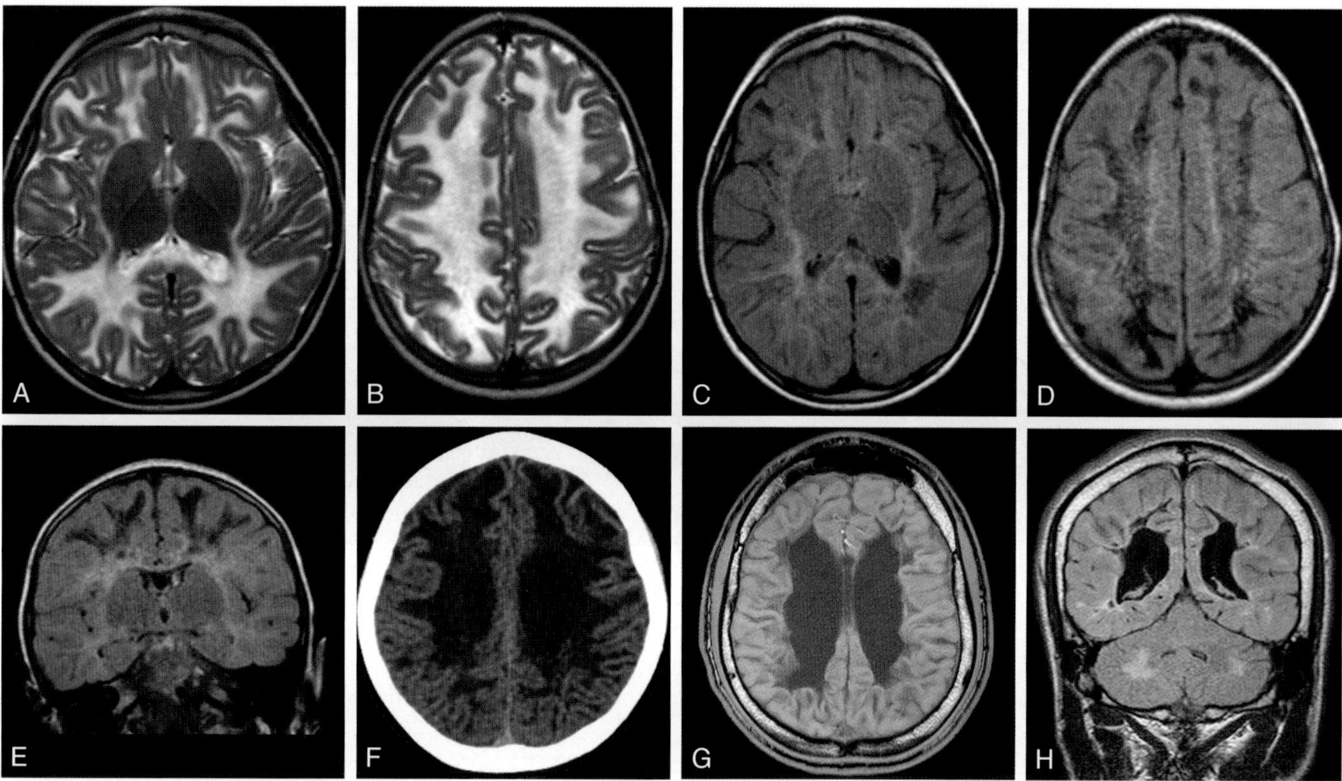

Fig. 4.20 Vanishing White Matter Disease. (A to F) A 4-year-old with progressive neurologic decline. (A and B) Axial T2W, and (C to E) axial and coronal FLAIR images demonstrates a pattern of confluent central and peripheral white matter T2W hyperintensity, with areas of FLAIR hypointensity indicating significant liquefaction, and sparing of the deep gray matter. (F) Axial CT image demonstrates the CT appearance of very low density diffusely in the cerebral white matter. (G and H) Axial and coronal FLAIR images in a 17-year-old with vanishing white matter disease demonstrating late-stage severe supratentorial white matter volume loss and cerebellar white matter confluent FLAIR hyperintensity. The calvarium is also diffusely thickened due to the volume loss.

Key Points

Background

- Also known as childhood ataxia with central nervous system hypomyelination
- Autosomal recessive; defective eukaryotic translation initiation factor eIF2B
- Histopathology demonstrates gelatinous, cystic and cavitary cerebral white matter with myelin pallor, vacuoles, cyst formation, and rarely active demyelination; no significant inflammation

Clinical

- Age of onset typically 2 to 6 years; chronic progressive neurologic deterioration with ataxia, less prominent spasticity, and mild mental decline; superimposed episodes of rapid decline following head trauma or febrile infection with loss of motor function and hypotonia. Epilepsy is frequently seen but uncommonly the predominant feature. Severe clinical variant such as in Cree leukoencephalopathy has onset between 3 and 9 months and death by 2 years of age.
- CSF glycine may be elevated, presumably due to excitatory injury.
- Treatment is supportive and avoidance of stress conditions.

Imaging

- Confluent T2/FLAIR hyperintensity of the cerebral white matter greatest in the frontal and parietal lobes, which progresses to *low FLAIR signal due to high water content* then to *disappearance of the white matter* without internal collapse of the cortex.
- Areas of spared white matter include temporal lobes, anterior limbs of the internal capsules, anterior commissure, and cerebellum. Central tegmental tracts often demonstrate abnormal T2W hyperintensity.
- MRS: White matter metabolites progressively decrease; cortex maintains a more normal pattern.

REFERENCE

1. Van der Knaap MS, and Valk J. *Magnetic Resonance of Myelination and Myelin Disorders*. 3rd edition. Berlin: Springer; 2005.

MEGALENCEPHALY WITH SUBCORTICAL CYSTS

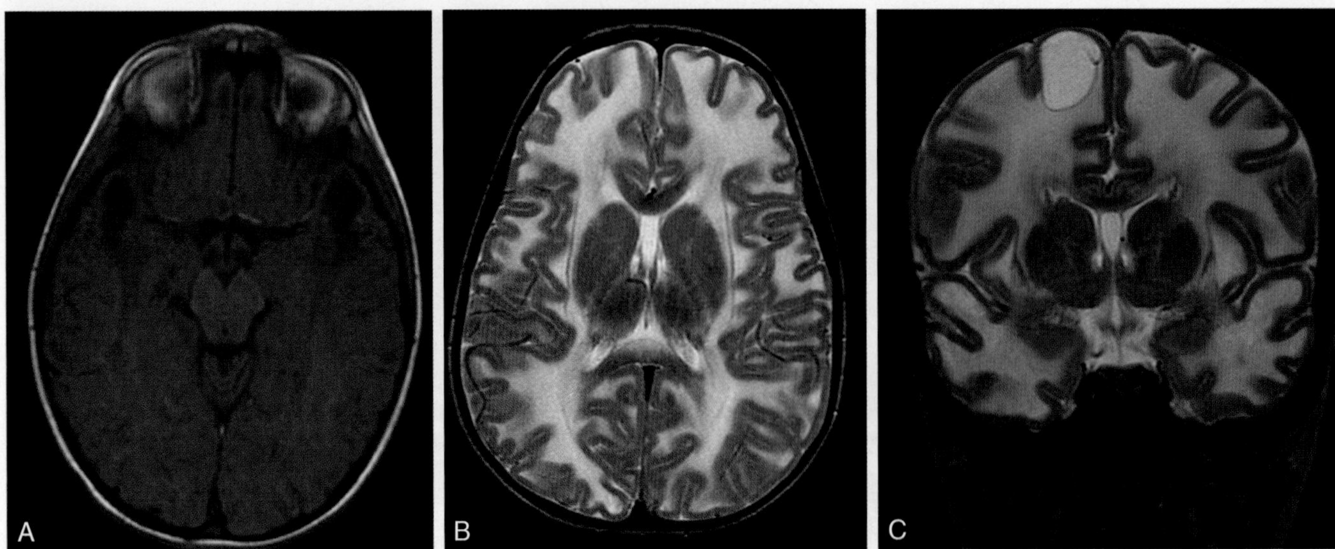

Fig. 4.21 Megalencephaly with subcortical cysts. (A) Axial T1W, and (B, C) axial and coronal T2W images demonstrates a pattern of confluent central and peripheral white matter T2W hyperintensity with anterior temporal and superior frontal cyst formation.

Key Points

Background

- Also known as van der Knaap disease; autosomal recessive
- Abnormal *MLC1* gene, which encodes a membrane protein express in astrocyte end feet in the perivascular, subependymal, and subpial regions. The protein function remains unknown.
- No laboratory abnormalities. Diagnosis by MRI and genetic testing
- Pathology demonstrates intramyelin vacuole formation and fibrillary astrogliosis

Clinical

- *Macrocephaly* in the first year of life, which later parallels normal curve. Delayed and unstable walking is an early sign followed by slow deterioration of motor function, epilepsy, decreasing school performance, dysarthria, developmental delay presenting at age 2 with gradual progression with ataxia and dysarthria between ages 8 and 12.
- No treatment currently exists.

Imaging

- Absent myelin in subcortical white matter (WM) and less involvement of deep WM, callosum, cerebellar WM and occipital lobes
- *Subcortical cysts* typically in the anterior temporal, frontal, and parietal lobes
- MRS: Nonspecific; ↓ NAA, ↑ myoI
- Differential Diagnosis: Anterior temporal subcortical cyst can also occur with utero CMV infection although head size should be small or normal rather than macrocephalic

REFERENCES

1. Van der Knaap MS, and Valk J. *Magnetic Resonance of Myelination and Myelin Disorders*. 3rd edition. Berlin: Springer; 2005.
2. Barkovich AJ, Raybaud C. *Pediatric Neuroradiology*. 6th edition. Philadelphia: Wolters-Kluwer; 2019.

MUCOPOLYSACCHARIDOSES

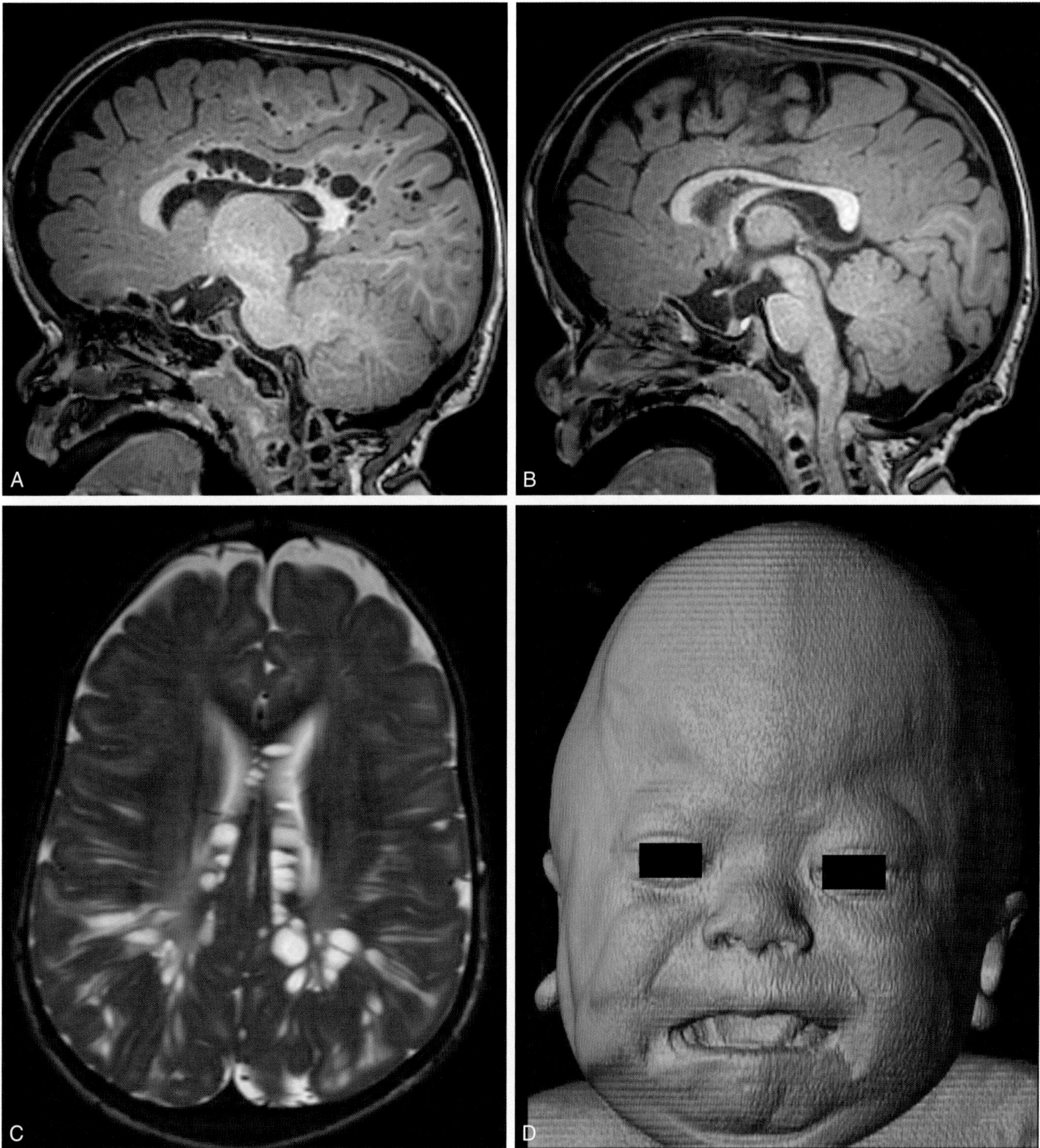

Fig. 4.22 Mucopolysaccharidoses. 18-month-old with macrocephaly and abnormal head shape. (A and B) Sagittal T1W and (C) axial T2W images demonstrate enlarged perivascular spaces in the cerebral white matter, including the corpus callosum, J-shaped sella, shortened clivus, foramen magnum stenosis, and frontal bossing. (D) 3D volumetric CT image demonstrating facial appearance of mucopolysaccharidosis. Genetic testing confirmed type 1H (Hurler) subtype.

Key Points

Background

- A group of lysosomal storage disorders with enzyme deficiencies resulting in failure to degrade mucopolysaccharides (MPS, also known as glycosaminoglycans/GAGs)
- Accumulation of GAGs around vessels and leptomeninges may result in the perivascular spaces and/or impaired resorption of CSF in the arachnoid granulations
- Autosomal recessive except MPS-2 (Hunter syndrome), which is X-linked

Classification

- Seven distinct types that are further divided into subtypes according to enzyme deficiency and clinical severity. MPS-5 was reclassified as MPS-1S and MPS-8 was retracted
- MPS-1: 1H (Hurler) subtype is the most severe with cognitive and multisystemic involvement; 1H/S (Hunter/Scheie) subtype has intermediate severity; 1S (Scheie) subtype is the least affected and no cognitive decline; all due to alpha-L-iduronidase deficiency
- MPS-2: Hunter syndrome due to iduronate-2-sulfatase deficiency; mild and severe subtypes depending on neurologic impairment
- MPS-3: Sanfilippo syndrome A–D (subtypes) due to multiple enzymes deficiency
- MPS-4: Morquio syndrome A and B (subtypes) due to N-acetylgalactosamine-6-sulfatase and galactose 6-sulfatase deficiency
- MPS-6: Maroteaux-Lamy syndrome due to N-acetylgalactosamine-4-sulfatase deficiency
- MPS-7: Sly syndrome due to beta-glucoronidase deficiency
- MPS-9: Natowicz syndrome due to hyaluronidase deficiency; most rare of the MPS

Clinical

- Urinary GAG testing done for screening and enzyme assay for confirmation.
- MPS 1–3 and 7 have cognitive impairment in the first year of life.
- MPS 4 and 6 usually do not have cognitive impairment but more frequent spinal stenosis.
- Multiple organ systems are involved, leading to hepatosplenomegaly, mental retardation, and skeletal anomalies (also known as dysostosis multiplex; MPS 1, 2, 4, 6, 7).
- Some MPS can be treated with intravenous enzyme replacement or stem cell transplantation.

Imaging

Brain Findings

- *Enlarged perivascular spaces* particularly in the corpus callosum and seen in MPS 1–3, and 6; not shown to correlate with cognitive decline
- Hydrocephalus (MPS 1–3); presumably from impaired arachnoid granulations and/or foramen magnum stenosis, and/or volume loss
- White matter gliosis (1st year of life in MPS 1–3, 7 and 2nd decade for MPS-4 or 6)
- Skull and skull base: *Foramen magnum stenosis, J-shaped sella*, hyperostosis along the metopic suture, sagittal craniosynostosis, and enlarged emissary veins
- Other: Enlarged optic nerve sheaths, closed cephaloceles (MPS-2), arachnoid cysts, and enlarged cisterna magna (MPS-2)

Spine Findings

- *Craniocervical junction abnormalities*: Odontoid hypoplasia, ligament laxity, atlantoaxial instability, ligament thickening, and anterior position of the C1 posterior arch lead to cervical canal stenosis and myelopathy/myelomalacia
- *Vertebral body wedge shape, anterior beaking, or bullet-shape appearance*
- *Thoracolumbar kyphosis* (gibbous deformity)

REFERENCES

1. Nicolas-Jiwan M, Al Sayed M. Mucopolysaccharidoses: overview of neuroimaging manifestations. *Pediatr Radiol.* 2018;48:1503–1520.
2. Reichert R, Goncalves Campos L, Vairo F, et al. Neuroimaging findings in patients with mucopolysaccharidosis: What you really need to know. *Radiographics.* 2016 Sept-Oct;36(5):1448–1462.

METABOLIC DISORDERS WITH DIFFUSE HYPOMYELINATION

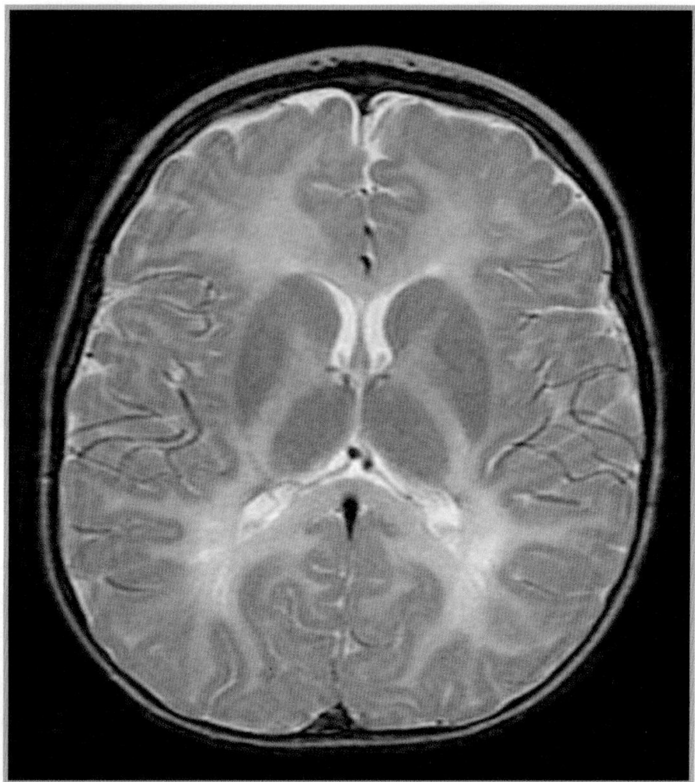

- **Pelizaeus-Merzbacher**
- **Pelizaeus-Merzbacher-like disease**
- **4H syndrome**
- **Salla disease**
- **Hypomyelination with atrophy of the basal ganglia and cerebellum (HABC)**
- **Hypomyelinatin with congenital cataracts**
- **18q deletion**
- **GM1 and GM2 gangliosidosis**
- **Trichothiodystrophy**

PELIZAEUS-MERZBACHER

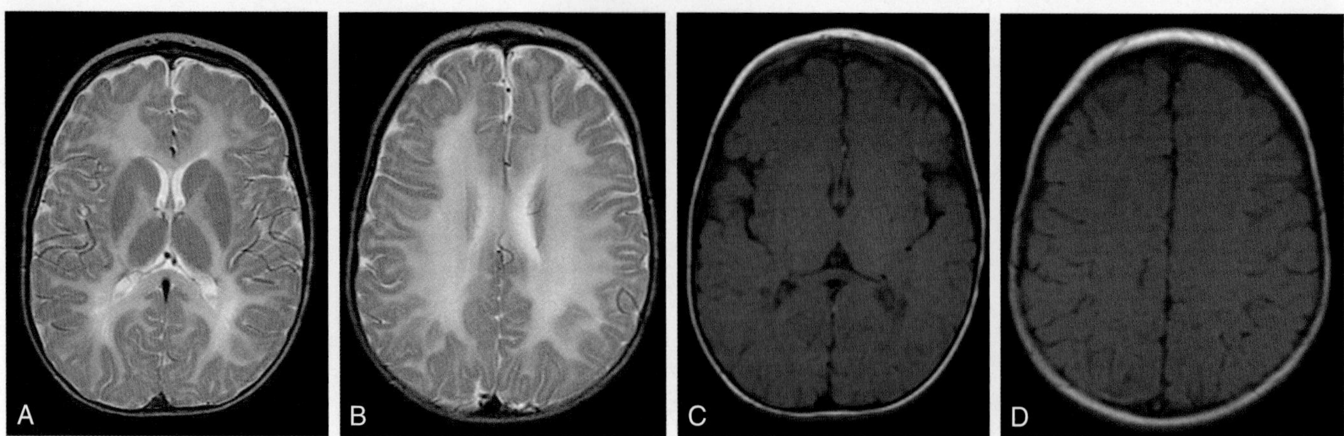

Fig. 4.23 Pelizaeus-Merzbacher. 21-month-old. (A and B) Axial T2W and (C and D) axial T1W images demonstrate abnormal diffuse T2W hyperintense, T1W hypointense white matter indicative of absence of myelination.

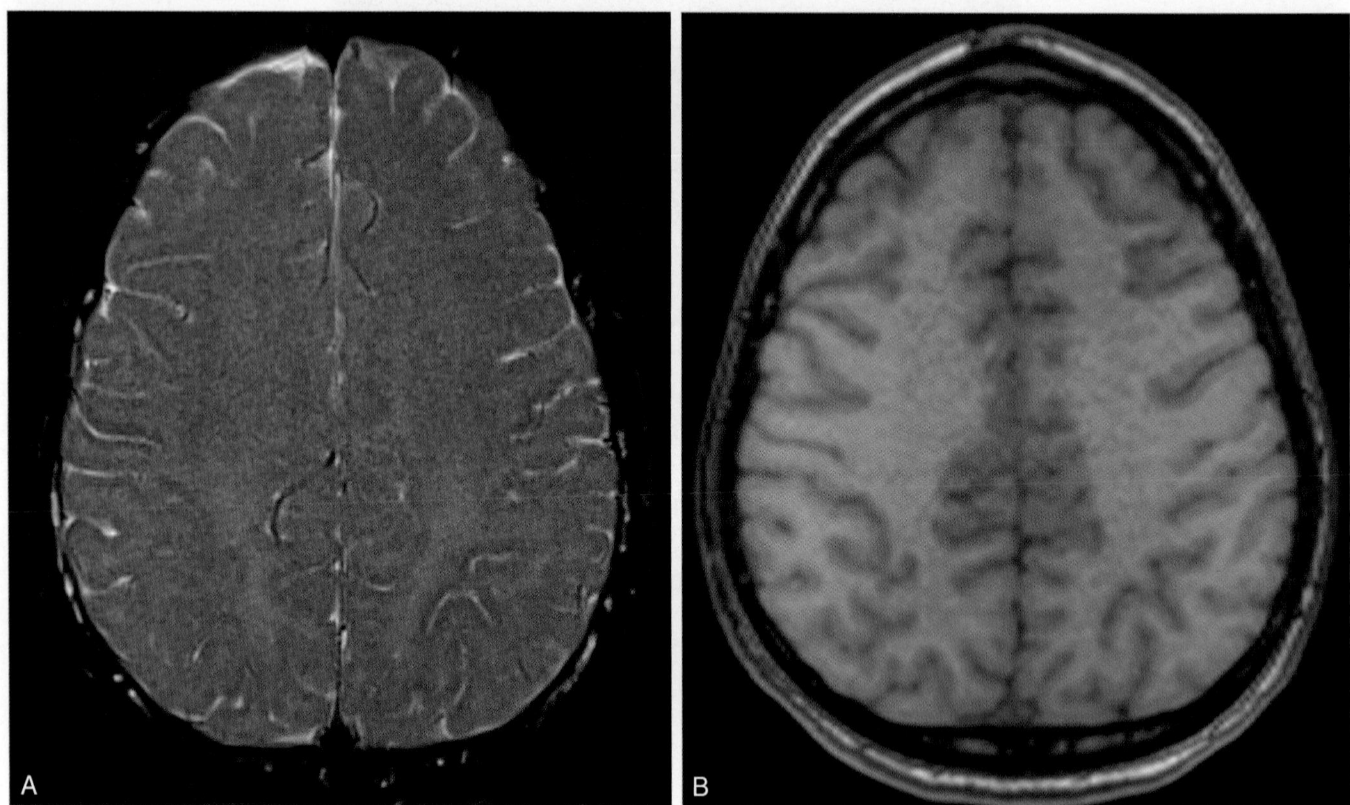

Fig. 4.24 Pelizaeus-Merzbacher: Mild Form. 4-year-old. (A) Axial T2W and (B) axial T1W images demonstrate abnormal intermixed areas of T2W hyperintense signal in the central and peripheral white matter while T1W signal pattern indicates areas of myelination are present.

Key Points

Background

- X-linked recessive disorder of the *PLP1* gene, which encodes the myelin-specific proteolipid protein 1, which normally constitutes 40% to 50% of CNS myelin protein. Diagnosis made by genetic testing.
- Clinical severity is related to the nature of the genetic mutation. Gene deletions or null mutations lead to more benign course, gene duplication to an intermediate course, and missense mutations to a severe course (due to accumulation of mutated protein in the endoplasmic reticulum that triggers apoptosis in oligodendrocytes).

Clinical

- Connatal form: Almost exclusively seen in boys; diffuse lack of myelin; hypotonia, absent neonatal reflexes, feeding difficulty, rapid progression, microcephaly, and death in the first decade
- Classical form has onset in the first year of life; less severe myelin deficiency with islands of normal myelin surrounding blood vessels that can give a tigroid pattern; abnormal eye movement, seizures, developmental delay, and slow progression with death in early to mid-adulthood
- Transitional form has onset between neonatal and early infantile time with less rapid course, and abnormalities intermediate with respect to the connatal and classical forms
- Rate of progression is the most useful in determining the different types

Imaging

- Degree of myelination correlates with disease severity.
- Connatal form demonstrates *diffuse absence of myelination* with absent T1W hyperintense signal in the white matter.
- Classical form may demonstrate myelination in the cerebellum, brainstem, PLIC, thalami, and basal ganglia and even more mild forms can demonstrate patchy a tigroid pattern of myelination in the deep white matter.

Differential Diagnosis Hypomyelination Disorders

- Pelizaeus-Merzbacher–like disorder: diffuse hypomyelination including the brainstem
- 18q deletion: Dysmorphic features
- Cockayne syndrome: Calcifications, cataracts, hearing loss
- HABC: Atrophy of basal ganglia and cerebellum
- Hypomyelination with congenital cataracts: cataracts
- 4H syndrome: Thin callosum, cerebellar atrophy, dental abnormalities, and delayed puberty
- Salla disease: Thin callosum, coarse facial features, and hepatosplenomegaly
- Trichothiodystrophy: Thin brittle hair, ichthyosis, and photosensitivity

REFERENCES

1. Van der Knaap MS, Valk J. *Magnetic Resonance of Myelination and Myelin Disorders*. 3rd edition. Berlin: Springer; 2005.
2. Pouwels PJW, Vanderver A, Bernard G, et al. Hypomyelinating leukodystrophies: Translational research progress and prospects. *Ann Neurol.* 2014;76:5–19.
3. Barkovich AJ, Raybaud C. *Pediatric Neuroradiology*. 6th edition. Philadelphia: Wolters-Kluwer; 2019.

HYPOMYELINATION, HYPODONTIA, AND HYPOGONADOTROPIC HYPOGONADISM (4H SYNDROME)

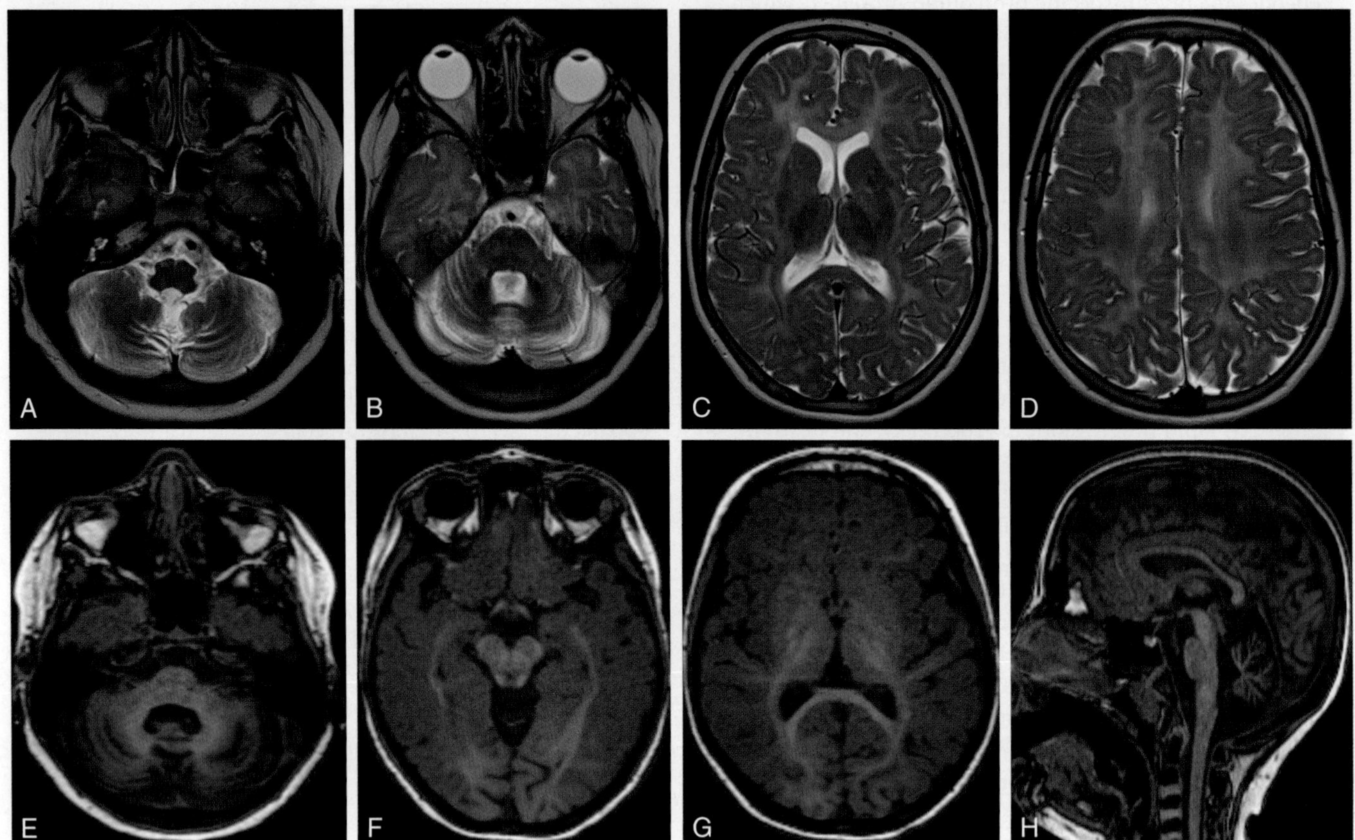

Fig. 4.25 4H Syndrome. (A to D) Axial T2W and (E to H) axial and sagittal T1W images demonstrate abnormal diffuse T2W hyperintense, T1W hypointense white matter but sparing optic radiations, and thin corpus callosum.

Key Points

Background

- Autosomal recessive; mutations in *POL3RA*, *POL3RB*, and *POLR1C* genes (POL3-related leukodystrophy)

Clinical

- Characterized by *hypomyelination, hypodontia,* and *hypogonadotropic hypogonadism*
- Varying degrees of developmental delay; spastic ataxia; *missing or delayed tooth eruption*; *absent, arrested or delayed puberty*; *low LH and FSH*; no response to stimulation with GnRH; progressive cerebellar dysfunction and cognitive impairment; ocular abnormalities.
- No specific treatment exists.

Imaging

- *CNS hypomyelination* with preserved myelination in the optic radiations, cerebellar atrophy, and thinning of the corpus callosum

REFERENCE

1. Thomas A, Thomas AK. POLR3-related Leukodystrophy. *J Clin Imaging Sci*. 2019 Oct 24;9:45.

SALLA DISEASE

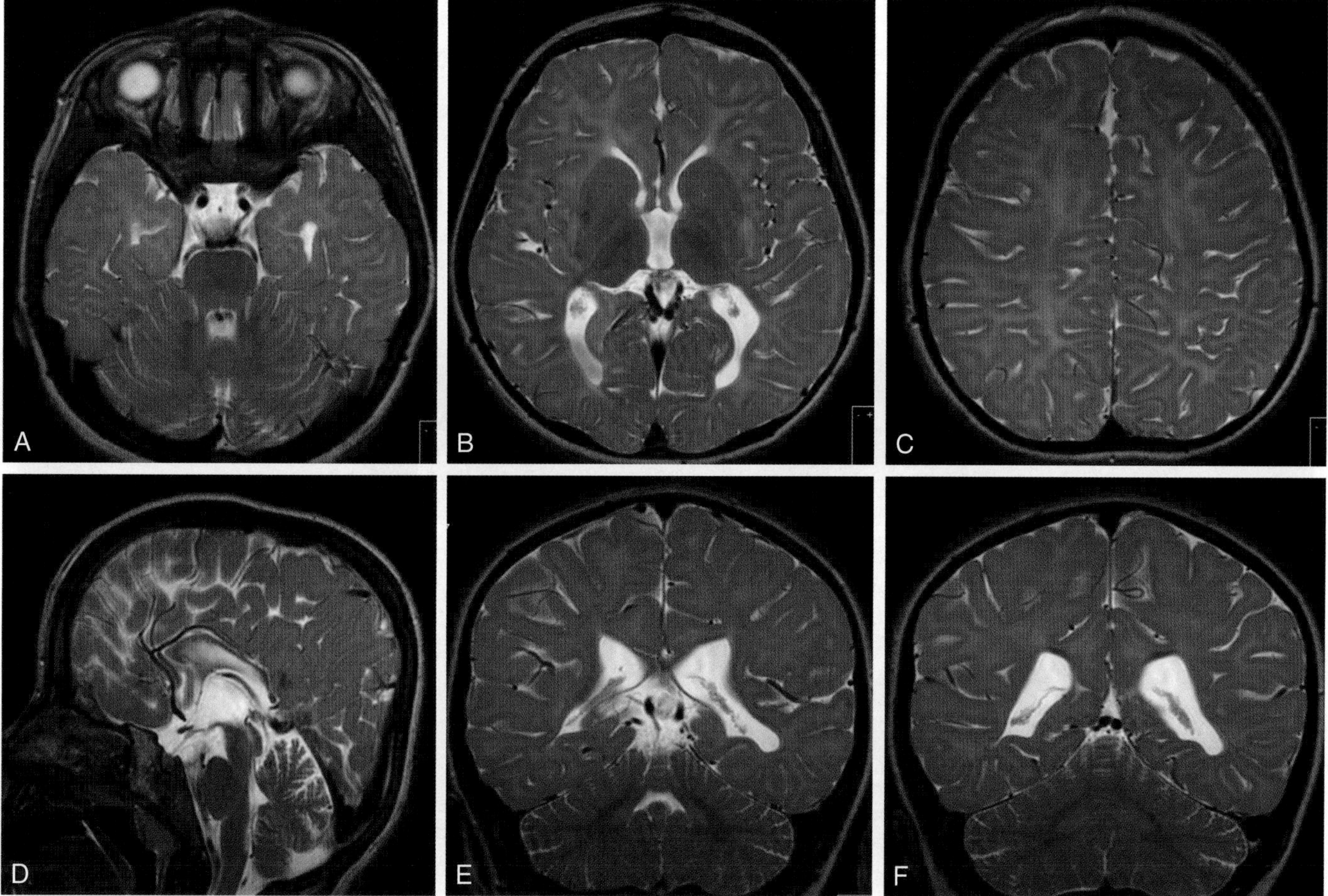

Fig. 4.26 Salla Disease. 2-year-old with developmental delay and ataxia. (A to F) Axial and coronal T2W images demonstrate abnormal diffuse T2W hyperintense white matter indicative of absence of myelination, periatrial white matter volume loss, and thin corpus callosum.

Key Points

Background

- Autosomal recessive lysosomal storage disorder caused by defective protein sialin, a lysosomal free sialic acid transporter that functions to remove sialic acid from lysosomes
- Increased urinary sialic acid used for diagnosis
- Histopathology demonstrates large amount of lipofuscin in the neuronal cell body in the cerebral and cerebellar cortex, thalami, basal ganglia, brainstem nuclei, and spinal cord, severe loss of myelin, and axonal loss

Clinical

- Onset at 6 to 9 months with hypotonia, nystagmus, ataxia then speech and motor delay, spasticity, and later coarse facial features. Many patients have a static clinical course and live into adulthood.
- Treatment is supportive.

Imaging

- Hypomyelination, reduced white matter volume, and thin corpus callosum
- Imaging severity correlates with clinical severity
- MRS: Can show a large peak at 2.02 ppm as sialic acid co-resonates with NAA

REFERENCES

1. Van der Knaap MS, and Valk J. *Magnetic Resonance of Myelination and Myelin Disorders*. 3rd edition. Berlin: Springer; 2005.
2. Barkovich AJ, Raybaud C. *Pediatric Neuroradiology*. 6th edition. Philadelphia: Wolters-Kluwer; 2019.

HYPOMYELINATION WITH ATROPHY OF BASAL GANGLIA AND CEREBELLUM (H-ABC)

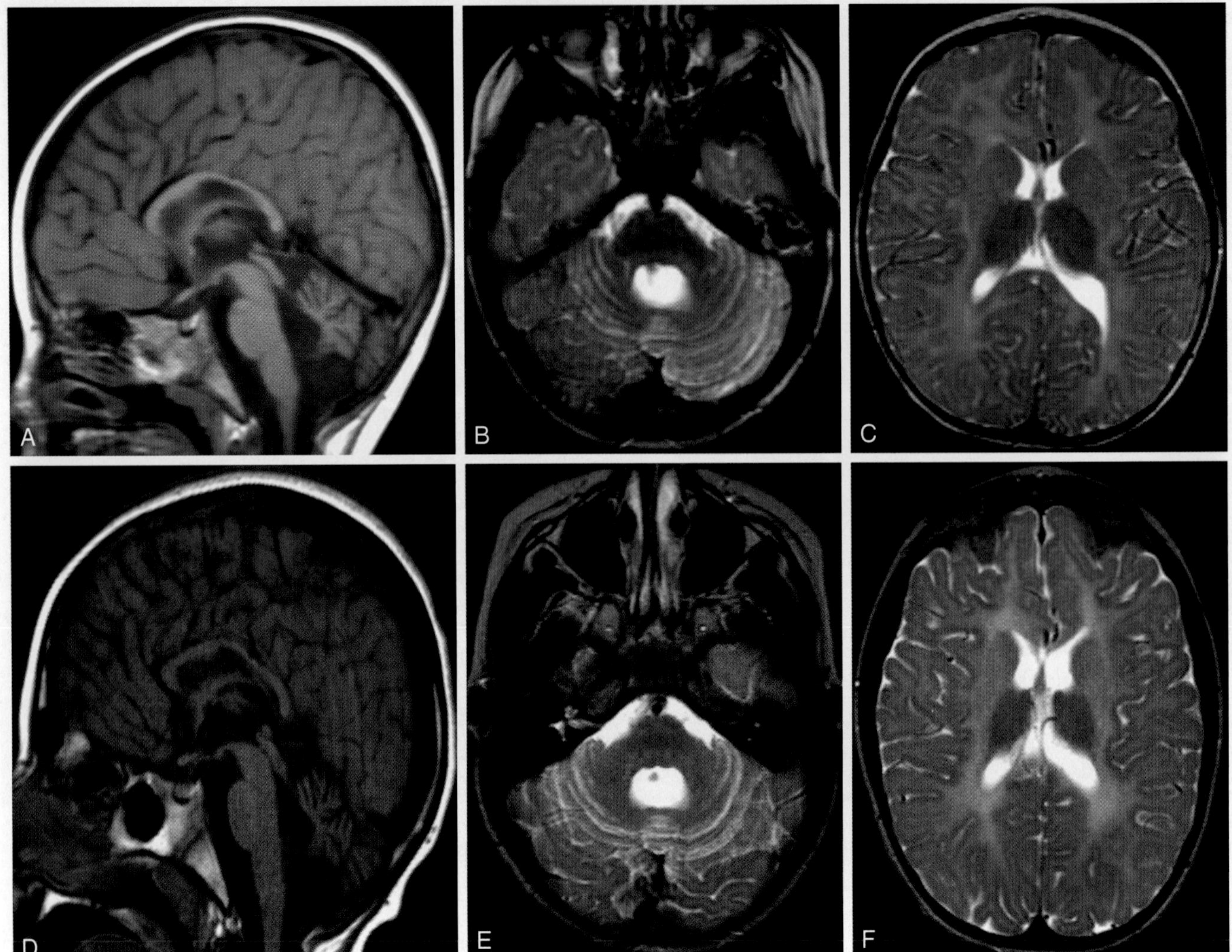

Fig. 4.27 H-ABC. (A to C) Sagittal T1W, and axial T2W images at 2 years 8 months demonstrate atrophy of basal ganglia and cerebellum and diffuse T2W hyperintense white matter indicative of hypomyelination with progression of volume loss and persistence of hypomyelination on follow-up MRI at 8 years 2 months of age seen on sagittal T1W and axial T2W images at similar levels of the brain (D to F).

Key Points

Background

- Mutations in TUBB4A which encodes tubulin B-4A has been found in patients with H-ABC. Mutations are autosomal dominant but most cases are new mutations in the patient affected.

Clinical

- Variable disease severity with onset in infancy or early childhood
- Severe cases demonstrate infantile onset with poor vision function, pale optic discs, and absent motor development progressing to spasticity and extrapyramidal movement disorders.
- Milder cases present in early childhood with slower manifestation of neurologic dysfunction.
- Laboratory studies are unremarkable.
- Treatment is supportive.

Imaging

- Diffuse white matter *hypomyelination*, *progressive atrophy of basal ganglia and cerebellum* without evidence of gliosis (suggests apoptosis mechanism)
- Degree of atrophy correlates with clinical severity
- MRS: Normal NAA and Cho, ↑ myoI and Cr

REFERENCE

1. Van der Knaap MS, and Valk J. *Magnetic Resonance of Myelination and Myelin Disorders*. 3rd edition. Berlin: Springer; 2005.

GM2 GANGLIOSIDOSIS

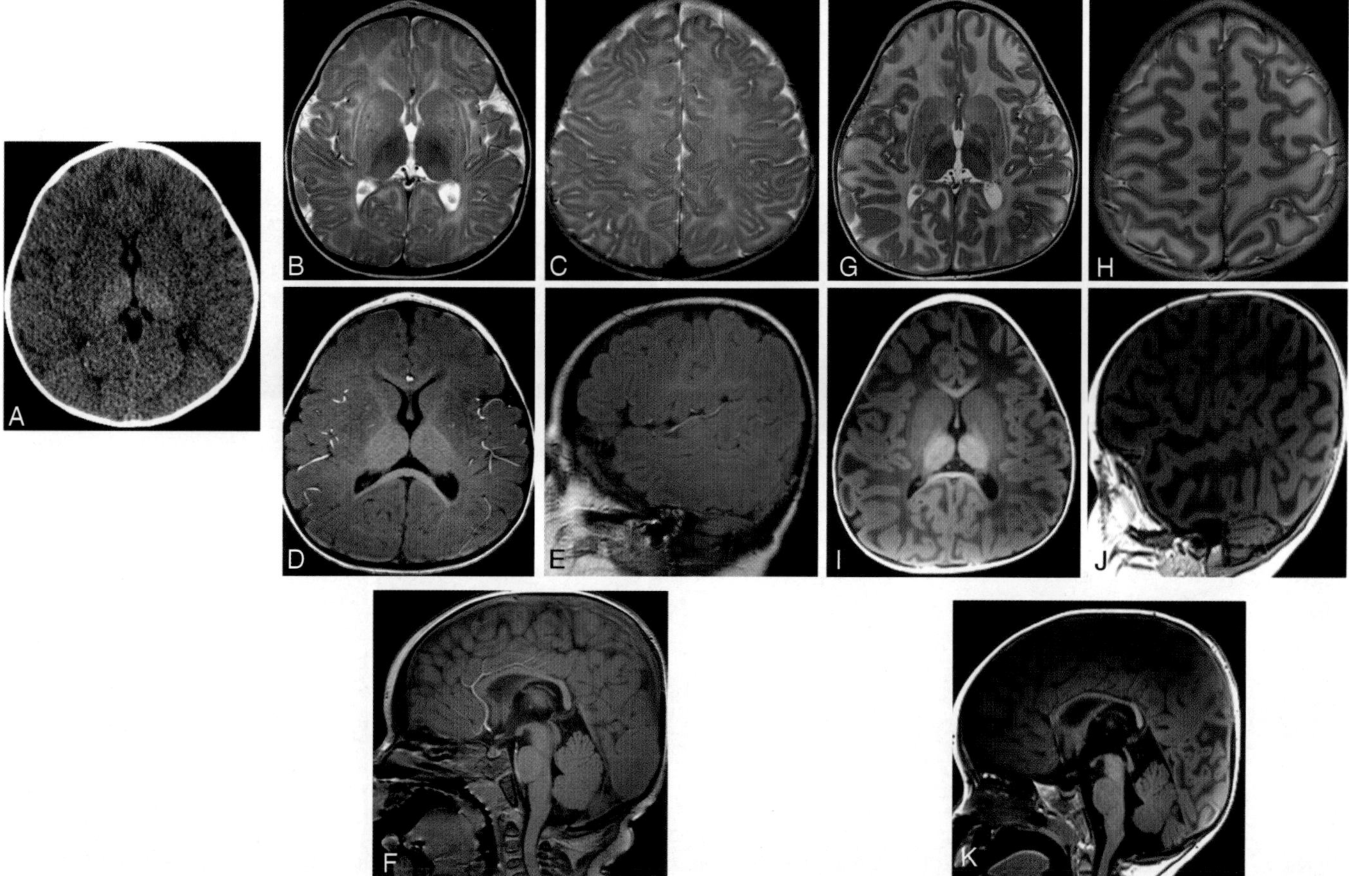

Fig. 4.28 GM2 Gangliosidosis (Sandhoff Disease). 14-month-old with developmental delay. (A) Axial CT image demonstrates mild hyperdensity in the thalami. (B and C) Axial T2W and (D to F) axial and sagittal T1W images demonstrate abnormal T1W hypointense, T2W hyperintense white matter indicative of hypomyelination, mild T1W hyperintense, T2W hypointense thalami, and heterogeneous T2W hyperintensity in the basal ganglia. Corpus callosum is myelinated but thin. Follow-up MRI at 19 months old: (G and H) axial T2W, and (I to K) axial and sagittal T1W images demonstrate progressive T2W hyperintense white matter with more expansion from edema, more conspicuous T1W hyperintense thalami, thinning of the corpus callosum, and development of mild volume loss of brainstem and cerebellum.

Key Points

Background

- GM2 gangliosidosis is an autosomal recessive lysosomal disorder due to deficiency of hexosaminidase. Three types: type B (Tay-Sachs), type O (Sandhoff disease), and type AB. Tay-Sachs is common in Ashkenazi Jews (1 in 30).
- Pathology: Accumulation of GM2 ganglioside, a glycosphingolipid, causes cortical neuronal swelling and eventual neuronal loss, and myelin deficiency.

Clinical

- Tay-Sachs disease infants are normal until 6 months of age when they develop an exaggerated startle response and progressive psychomotor decline, progressive vision loss, optic atrophy, *cherry-red spot on the maculae (90%),* progressive weakness, which in the first year of life results in previous abilities, such as sitting up or standing, to decline to lying in bed and, in the second year, to paralysis and rigidity.
- Sandhoff disease and subtype AB are similar to Tay-Sachs, except Sandhoff also has hepatosplenomegaly.
- Infantile (most common), juvenile, and adult forms exist and depend on degree enzyme activity that is present.

Imaging

- Imaging patterns on GM1 (not discussed here) and 2 gangliosidosis are similar.

CT:

- Diffuse white matter hypodensity and *mild thalamic hyperdensity*

MRI:

- *Hypomyelination* of the cerebral white matter with progressive edema resulting in *macrocephaly* in year 2 of life; corpus callosum remains myelinated but undergoes progressive thinning
- *Thalami appear T1W hyperintense/T2W hypointense*
- T2W hyperintense basal ganglia
- Progressive brainstem and cerebellar volume loss in later stages
- MRS: ↑ myoI and Cho, ↓ NAA

REFERENCES

1. Van der Knaap MS, and Valk J. *Magnetic Resonance of Myelination and Myelin Disorders*. 3rd edition. Berlin: Springer; 2005.
2. Barkovich AJ, Raybaud C. *Pediatric Neuroradiology*. 6th edition. Philadelphia: Wolters-Kluwer; 2019.

AICARDI-GOUTIÈRES SYNDROME

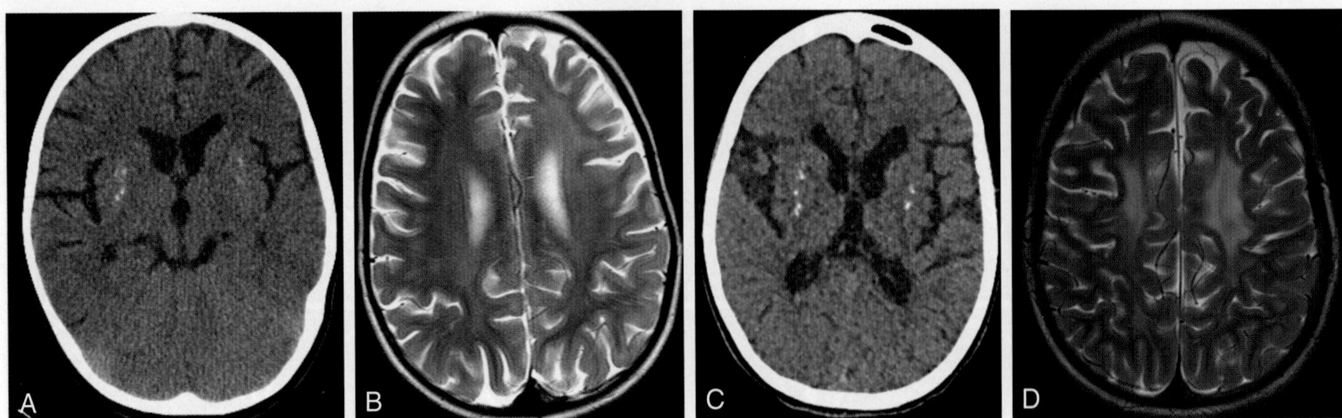

Fig. 4.29 Aicardi-Goutières. 2-year-old with loss of developmental milestones. (A) Axial CT image demonstrates small foci of calcification in the putamen bilaterally. (B) Axial T2W image demonstrates mild central white matter T2W hyperintensity indicative of hypomyelination. Follow-up MRI at 8 years old: (C) Axial CT image demonstrates stable small foci of calcification in the putamen bilaterally but progression of central white matter volume loss. (D) Axial T2W demonstrates progression of central white matter T2W hyperintensity.

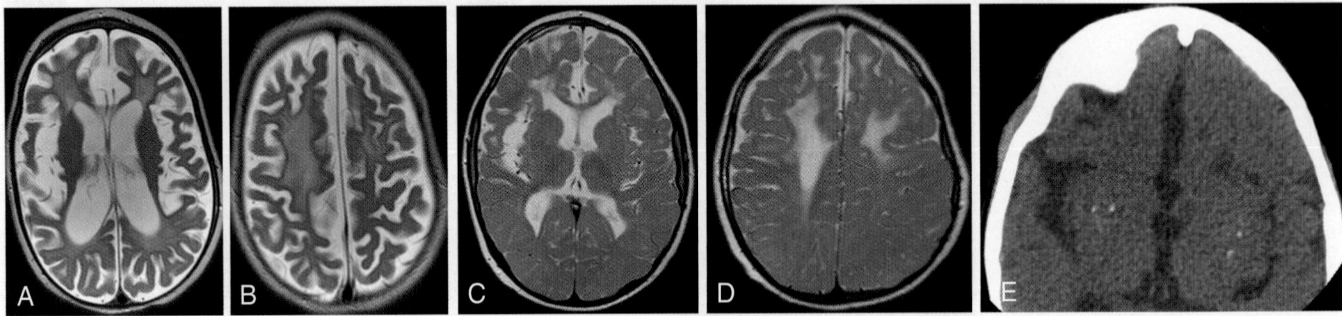

Fig. 4.30 Aicardi-Goutières. (A and B) Axial T2W image at 15 months old demonstrates severe cerebral volume loss with central white matter hypomyelination. (C and D) Axial T2W images at 6 years of age demonstrate striking improvement in cerebral volume but areas of severe subinsular white matter volume loss and periventricular gliosis. (E) Punctate calcifications were present on CT imaging in the basal ganglia.

Key Points

Background

- Autosomal recessive in majority of patients. Several genes have been found which are involved in breakdown of molecules of DNA and RNA and for immune system proteins. It is hypothesized that an abnormal immune response leads to inflammatory damage to the brain, skin and other organs.
- Histopathology demonstrates vascular and perivascular calcification greatest in the basal ganglia, thalami, and dentate nuclei, patchy areas of myelin deficiency (without signs of active myelin breakdown), astrocytosis, occasional cavitation of the white matter, and wedge-shaped microinfarctions in the cerebral and cerebellar cortex

Clinical

- Neonatal presentation with feeding difficulty, failure to thrive, irritability, recurrent fever, abnormal tone, and cutaneous lesions. Most patients have a progressive disease course and die within months to a few years.
- A chronic CSF lymphocytosis (10–300 cells/mm^3) and elevated interferon-alfa are consistently present.

Imaging

- *Punctate parenchymal calcifications* (typically in the basal ganglia, thalami, and dentate), which may coalesce to form large concretions
- Abnormal cerebral and cerebellar white matter with varying degrees of T2W hyperintense signal from areas of hypomyelination and gliosis
- Atrophy of the brain
- Occasional anterior temporal white matter subcortical cysts
- Differential Diagnosis: Cockayne syndrome, TORCH infection

REFERENCE

1. Van der Knaap MS, and Valk J. *Magnetic Resonance of Myelination and Myelin Disorders*. 3rd edition. Berlin: Springer; 2005.

COCKAYNE SYNDROME

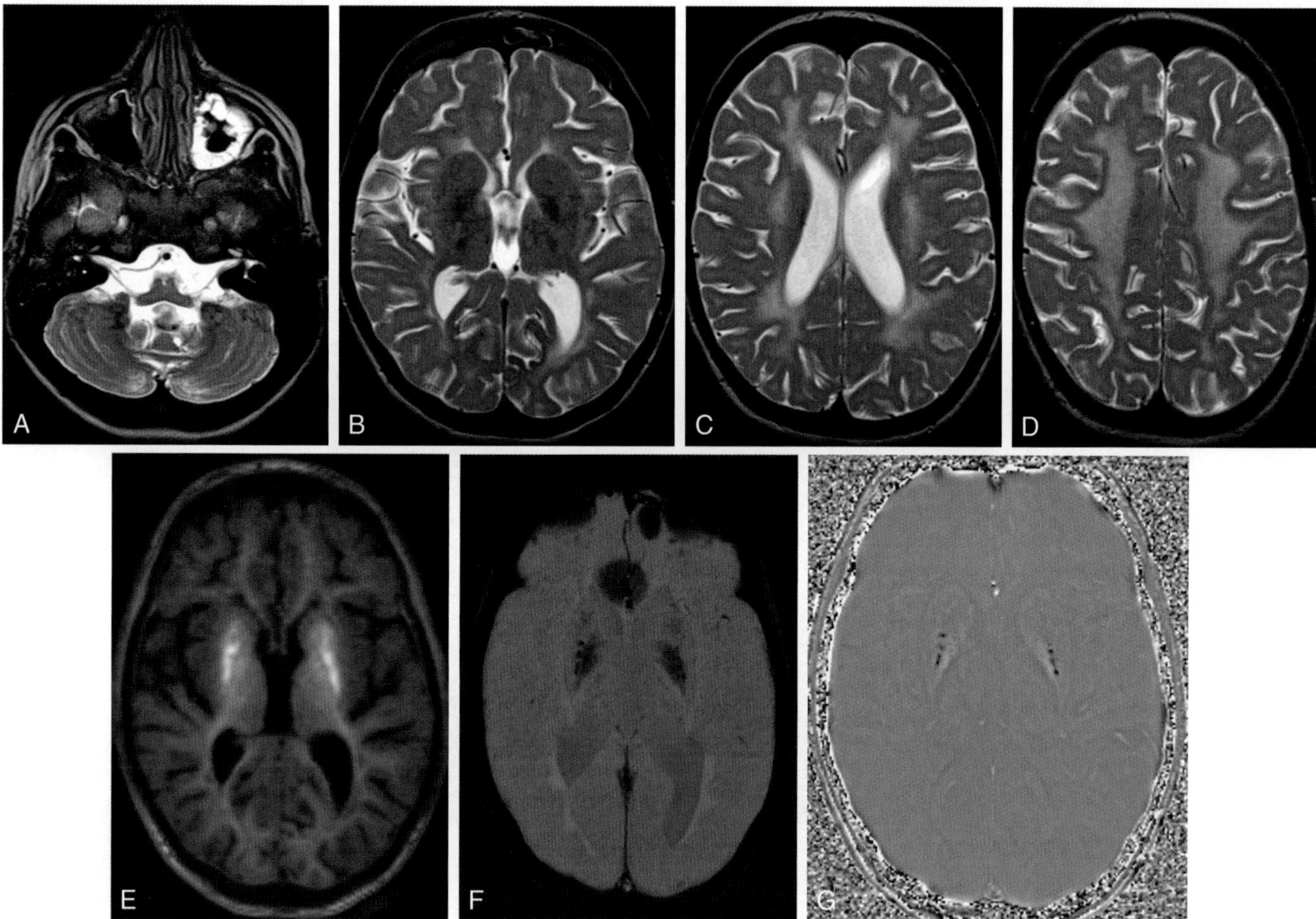

Fig. 4.31 Cockayne Syndrome. (A to D) Axial T2W images demonstrate confluent white matter T2W hyperintensity indicative of hypomyelination and atrophy of the brainstem and cerebellum. A few speckles of normal myelin are present, which can form a "tigroid" appearance. (E) Axial T1W, (F) axial SWI, and (G) axial SWI phase image demonstrate basal ganglia T1W hyperintensity and susceptibility with dark phase signal indicative of calcification.

Key Points

Background

- Autosomal recessive disorder due to mutations in ERCC6 or ERCC8 genes that leads to a defect in DNA repair
- Histopathology of the brain demonstrates thick and fibrotic leptomeninges, hypomyelination, calcium deposition, while peripheral nerve biopsy demonstrates demyelination and remyelination with onion bulb formation

Clinical

- Photosensitivity, cachexia, short stature, severe neurodegenerative disorder; classical (type 1) and severe (type 2) forms
- No effective therapy to date

Imaging

- *Calcification* (often homogeneous in appearance) in the basal ganglia, dentate, cerebral and cerebellar cortex, and white matter
- Atrophy of the brainstem and cerebellum
- *Hypomyelination* and white matter T2W hyperintense signal sometimes with a tigroid pattern due to presence of myelin
- Differential Diagnosis: Aicardi-Goutières (calcification typically more punctate); Metachromatic Leukodystrophy, Pelizaeus-Merzbacher, and Krabbe could have a tigroid pattern of white matter would not have similar calcification pattern

REFERENCE

1. Van der Knaap MS, and Valk J. *Magnetic Resonance of Myelination and Myelin Disorders*. 3rd edition. Berlin: Springer; 2005.

METABOLIC DISORDERS WITH PREDOMINANT BASAL GANGLIA INVOLVEMENT

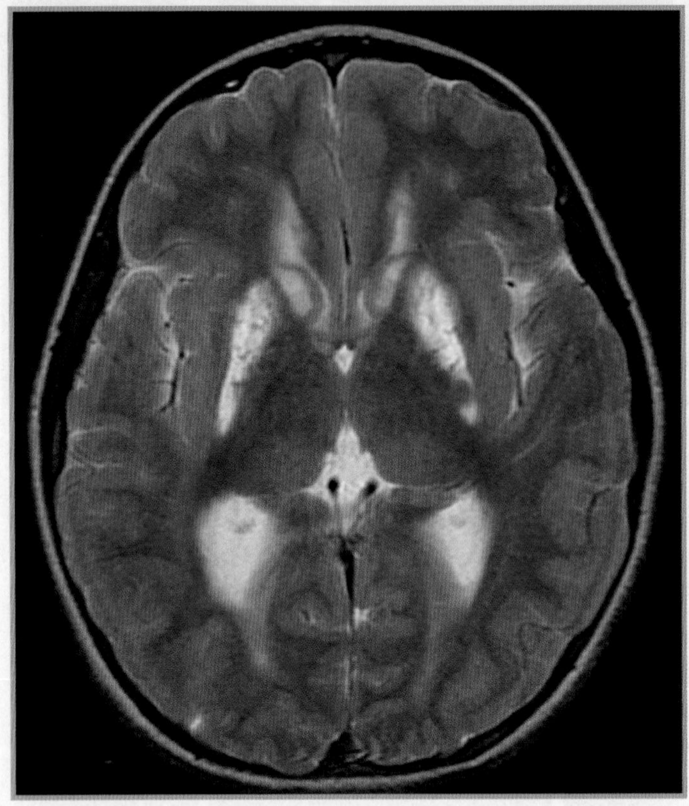

- Mitochondrial disorders
- Organic acidurias: ethylmalonic aciduria, methylmalonic aciduria, propionic aciduria
- Glutaric aciduria type 1 and 2
- Wilson disease
- PKAN

MITOCHONDRIAL DISORDERS: OVERVIEW

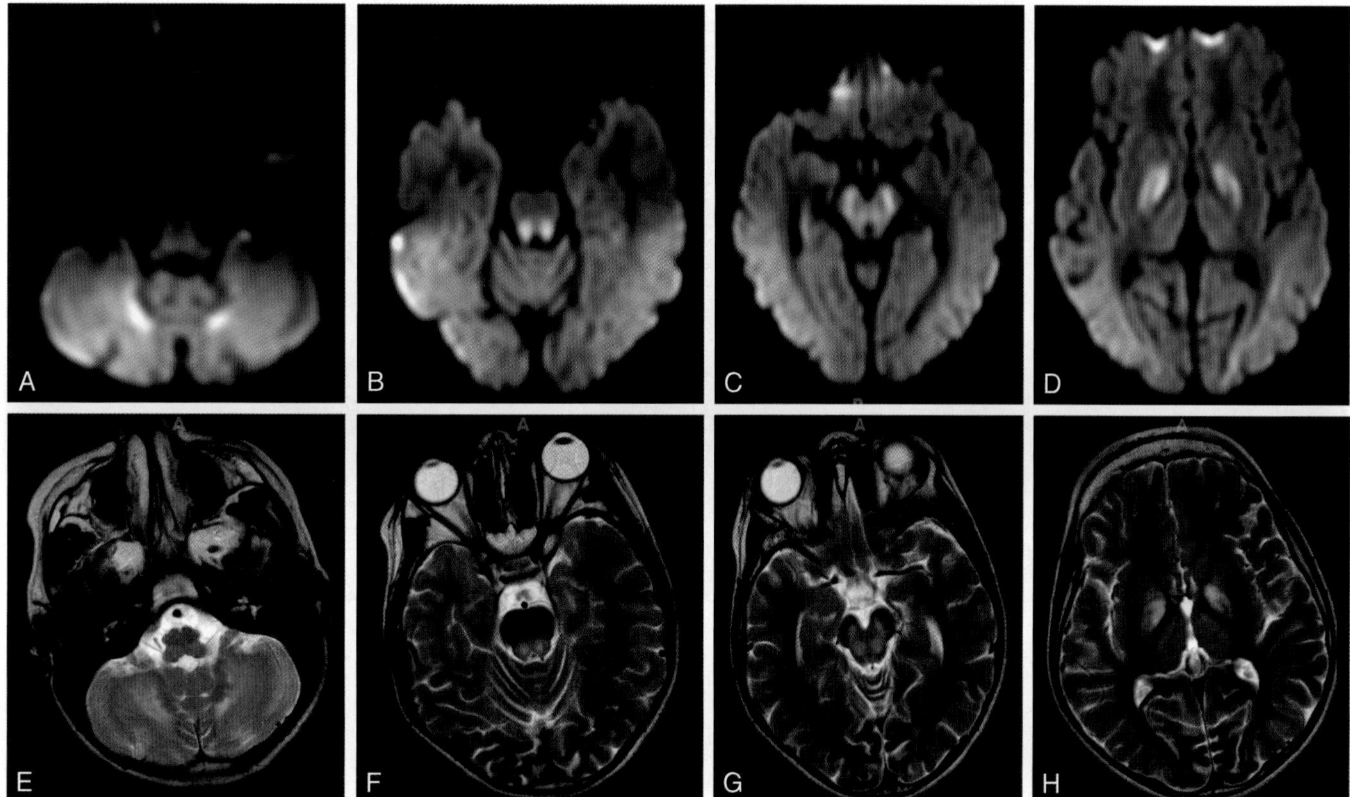

Fig. 4.32 Mitochondrial Disorder. Cytochrome C oxidase deficiency. (A to D) Axial DWI, and (E to H) axial T2W images demonstrate diffusion restriction (ADC not shown) and T2W hyperintensity in the deep cerebellar white matter, dorsal pons, cerebral peduncles, and globus pallidi.

Key Points

Background

- Typically refers to disorders of the respiratory chain

Clinical

- Associated with short stature, sensorineural hearing loss, progressive external ophthalmoplegia, axonal neuropathy, diabetes mellitus, hypertrophic cardiomyopathy, or renal tubular acidosis

Imaging

- A broad spectrum of imaging findings have been reported with mitochondrial disorders, however, a mitochondrial disorder should be suspected in any infant or child who has abnormalities of the deep cerebral gray matter or dorsal brainstem, in particular if white matter disease or cerebellar atrophy is present, as well.
- The finding of significantly *increased lactate* in the brain parenchyma or CSF by MRS also supports the possibility of mitochondrial disease.

MITOCHONDRIAL DISORDERS: MELAS

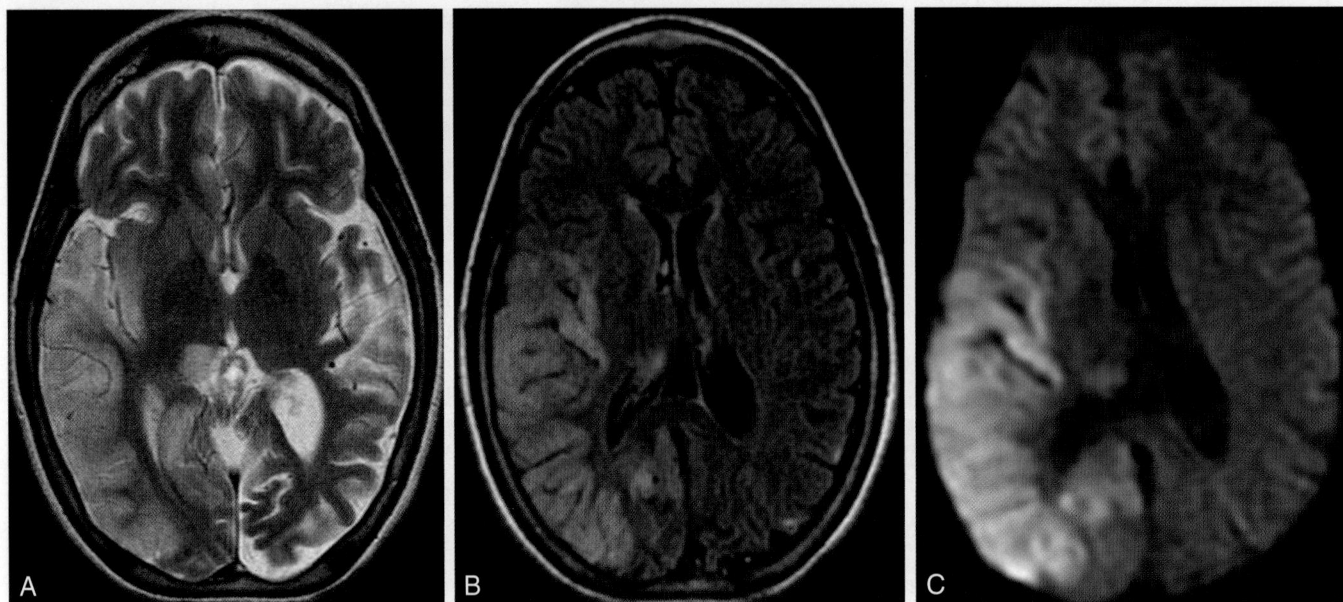

Fig. 4.33 Mitochondrial Disorder: MELAS. (A) Axial T2W, (B) axial FLAIR, and (C) axial DWI images demonstrate diffusion restriction (ADC not shown) and T2W hyperintensity in the right insula, thalamus, temporal and occipital lobes indicative of cytotoxic edema in a nonvascular distribution as well as evidence of cerebral volume loss in the left occipital and temporal lobes from prior cytotoxic edema.

Key Points

Background

- Mitochondrial encephalomyopathy with lactic acidosis and stroke-like episodes (MELAS)
- Number of mitochondrial DNA mutations, most common tRNA *Leu* gene. Likely affect function of cytochrome oxidase function

Imaging

- *Cortical diffusion restriction* in the acute phase or T2W/FLAIR hyperintensity with atrophy in the chronic phase (often parietal and occipital cortex) not conforming to arterial distribution.
- Diffusion restriction and T2/FLAIR hyperintensity can also be present in the basal ganglia, and dorsal brainstem.

MITOCHONDRIAL DISORDERS: SURF1

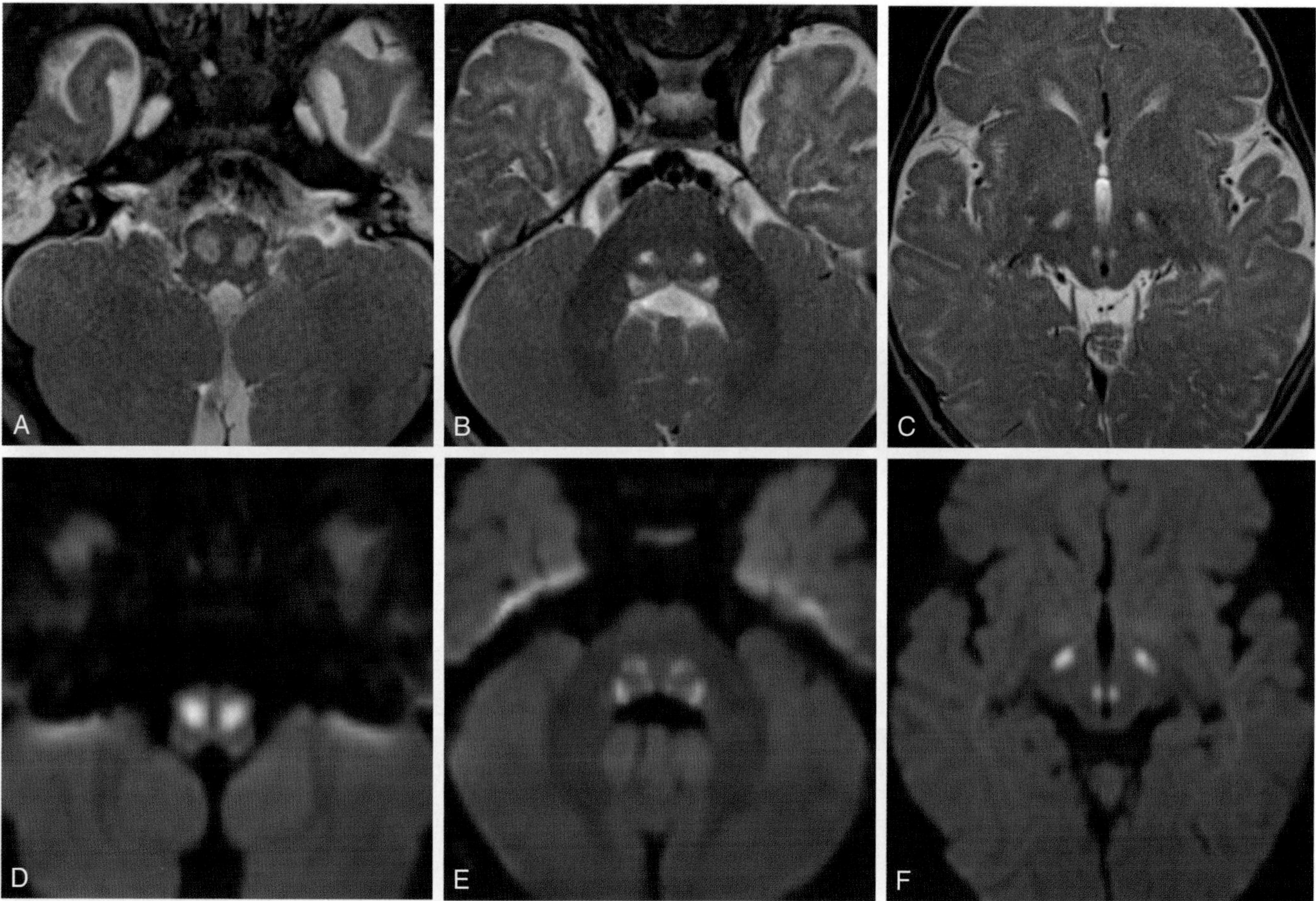

Fig. 4.34 Mitochondrial Disorder: SURF1. (A to C) Axial T2W and (D to F) axial DWI images demonstrate diffusion restriction (ADC not shown) and T2W hyperintensity in the bilateral subthalamic nuclei, cerebral peduncles, periaqueductal gray matter, dorsal pons, and central medulla.

Key Points

Background

- Both autosomal recessive and x-linked inheritance patterns exist.

Clinical

- Leigh syndrome: Symptom complex with characteristic, but variable clinical and pathologic manifestations. Affected infants and children typically present toward the end of the first year of life with hypotonia and psychomotor deterioration. Ataxia, ophthalmoplegia, ptosis, dystonia, and swallowing difficulties almost inevitably ensue.
- Many disorders can result in Leigh syndrome. Most common are pyruvate dehydrogenase, cytochrome oxidase (SURF1), complex 5 deficiency with mitochondrial ATPase gene 6m mutation, complex 1 deficiency, thiamine deficiency, and succinate dehydrogenase deficiency

Imaging

- SURF1: Diffusion restriction and/or T2W hyperintensity in the *subthalamic nuclei*, medulla, inferior cerebellar peduncles, inferior olivary nucleus, central tegmental tract, and periaqueductal gray;
- +/– lactate peak on MRS

MITOCHONDRIAL DISORDERS: PYRUVATE DEHYDROGENASE

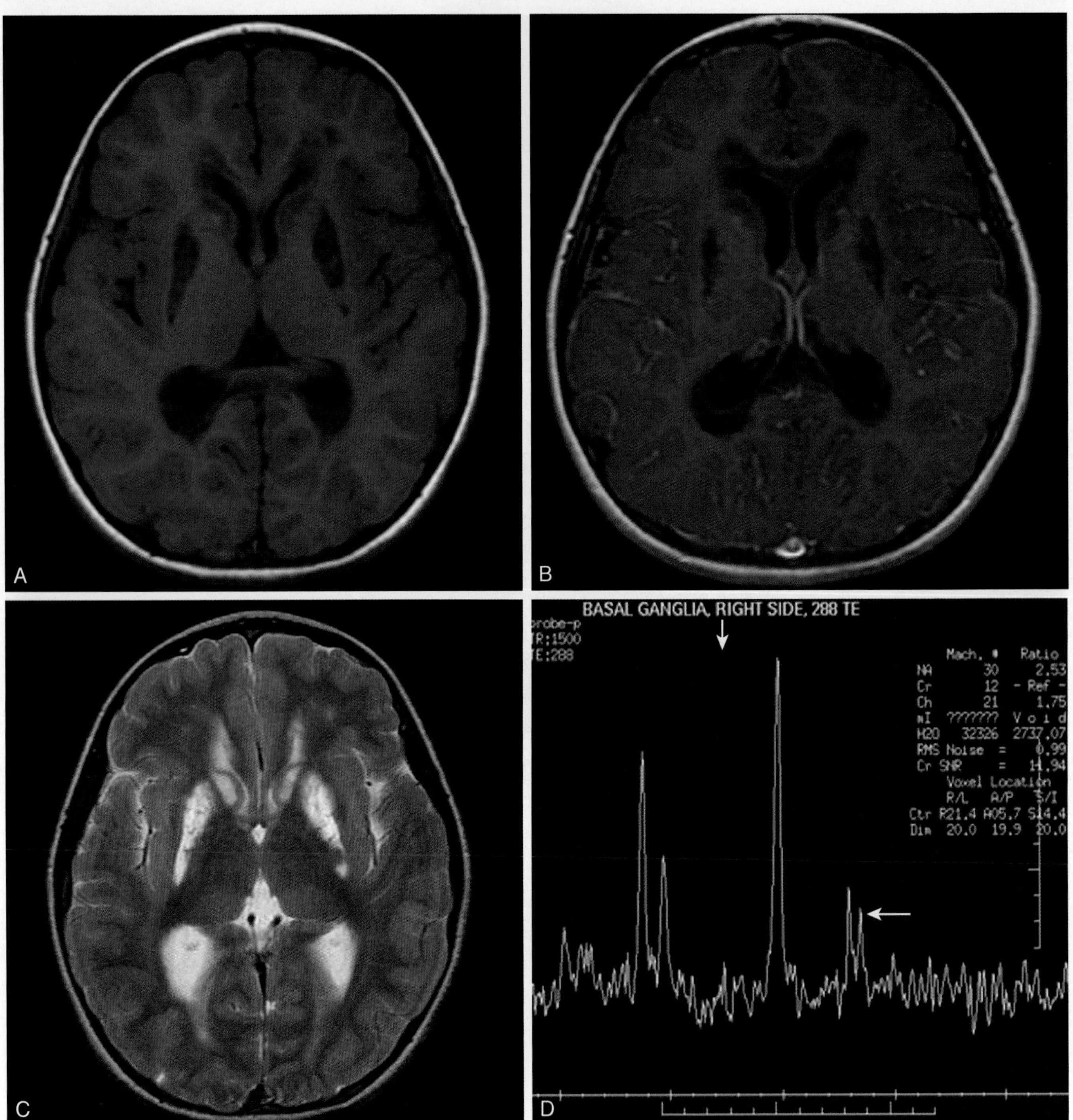

Fig. 4.35 Mitochondrial Disorder: Pyruvate Dehydrogenase. (A and B) Axial T1W and axial T1W+C, (B) axial T2W images demonstrate T1W hypointensity, T2W hyperintensity in the caudate and putamen. (D) MRS with long echo time demonstrates a high lactate peak. Additional findings that can be seen in other patients with pyruvate dehydrogenase include cortical volume loss, delayed myelination, cavitation in white matter, and possible malformations, including callosal dysgenesis.

PROPIONIC ACIDEMIA

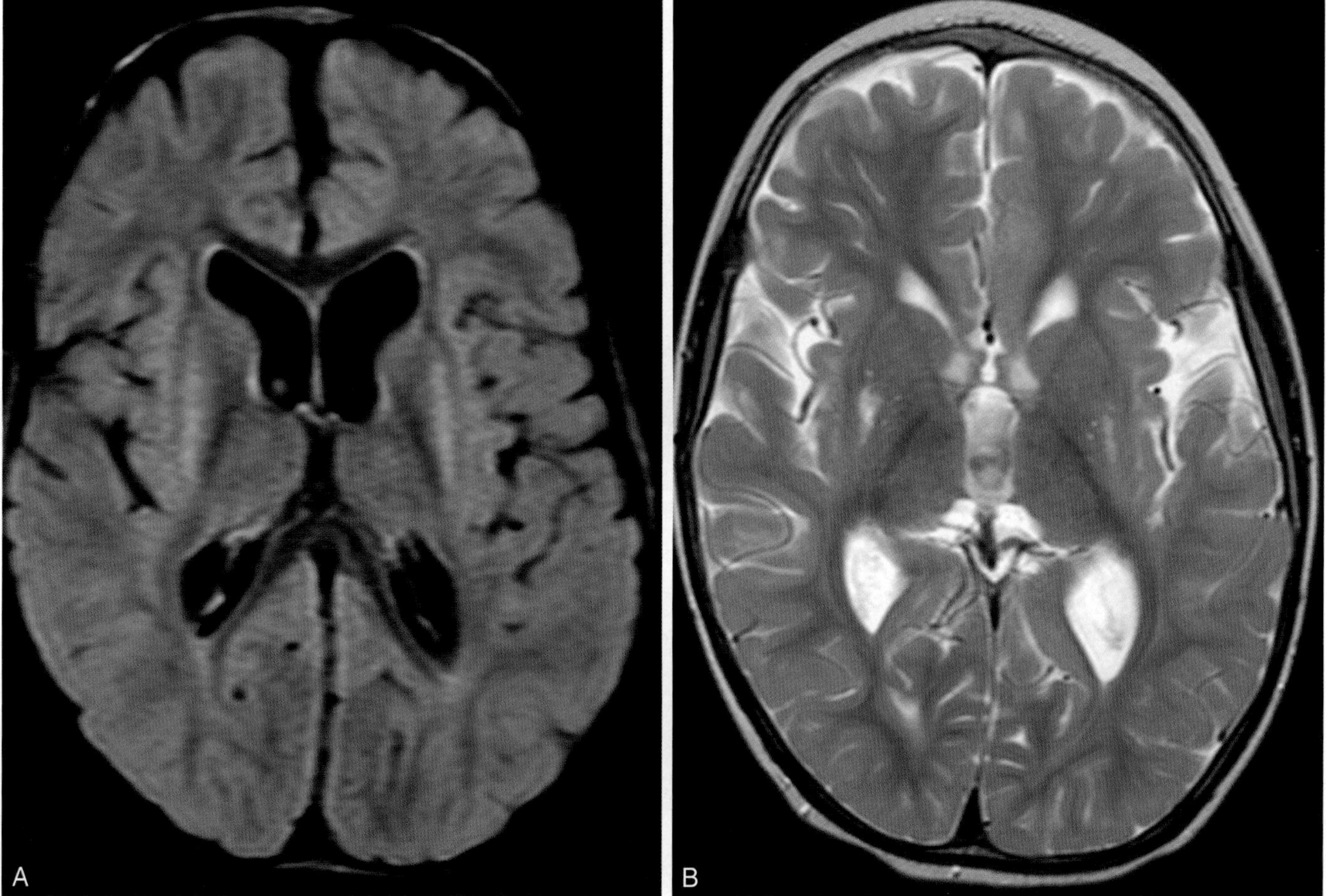

Fig. 4.36 Propionic Aciduria. 3-Year-Old. (A and B) Axial FLAIR and axial T2W images demonstrate T2/FLAIR hyperintensity in the lateral putamen.

Key Points

Background

- Autosomal recessive; deficient activity of the mitochondrial enzyme propionyl-CoA carboxylase
- Pathology demonstrates myelin vacuolization in neonates and atrophy of caudate and putamen in older children

Clinical

- Neonatal presentation most common; progressive encephalopathy, feeding difficulty, lethargy, vomiting, tachypnea, abnormal tone and movement; late-onset form presents after age 1 to adulthood with episodes of encephalopathy
- Acute episodes treated with dialysis, parenteral nutrition, and insulin infusion while long-term dietary protein restriction
- Elevated plasma and urinary propionate

Imaging

- Neonatal presentation can demonstrate restricted diffusion in areas of myelination (brainstem, PLIC, GP, thalami, central corona radiata); hemorrhage possible due to thrombocytopenia
- Older children demonstrate T2W hyperintensity and atrophy in the basal ganglia, dentate, and substantia nigra.
- MRS: ↑ Glutamate/glutamine, ↓ NAA and myoI

REFERENCES

1. Van der Knaap MS, and Valk J. *Magnetic Resonance of Myelination and Myelin Disorders*. 3rd edition. Berlin: Springer; 2005.
2. Barkovich AJ, Raybaud C. *Pediatric Neuroradiology*. 6th edition. Philadelphia: Wolters-Kluwer; 2019.

METHYLMALONIC ACIDEMIA

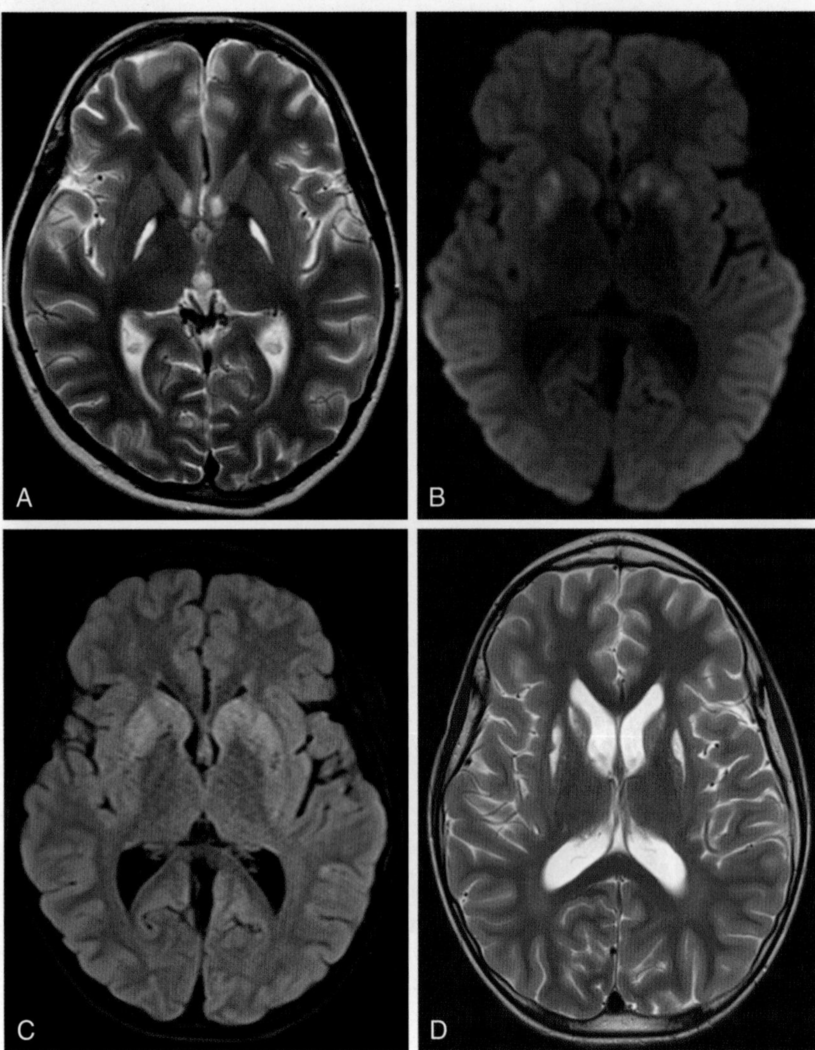

Fig. 4.37 Methylmalonic Aciduria. (A) Axial T2W image in a 16-year-old with methylmalonic acidemia demonstrating classic volume loss and T2W hyperintensity in the globus pallidus. (B to D) Atypical pattern of methylmalonic acidemia in a 6-year-old presenting with altered mental status, stiffness, lethargy. (B) Axial DWI and (C) axial FLAIR images demonstrate T2/FLAIR hyperintensity and diffusion restriction in the caudate head and putamen. Three-month follow-up MRI axial T2W image (D) demonstrates volume loss and cavitation in the caudate and putamen.

Key Points

Background

- Autosomal recessive; methylmalonic acid is created during metabolism of certain amino acids and odd chain fatty acids. Deficient activity of the methylmalonic CoA mutase; elevated plasma and urinary methylmalonic acid.
- Elevated methylmalonic acid is a competitive inhibitor of succinate dehydrogenase, a key enzyme in mitochondrial aerobic oxidation. This may lead to elevation of lactic acid and injury to the basal ganglia.

Clinical

- Neonatal presentation most common; metabolic acidosis, vomiting seizures, lethargy leading to quadriplegia, encephalopathy, hypotonia, extrapyramidal signs, coma, and death.
- Treated with protein restriction, carnitine, and parenteral B12.

Imaging

- T2W hyperintensity and atrophy in the basal ganglia (most commonly the *globus pallidi*)
- Cerebral and cerebellar volume loss, subcortical and periventricular gliosis
- MRS: ↓ NAA ↑ lactate
- Differential Diagnosis: Propionic acidemia, mitochondrial disorders, ethylmalonic acidemia, carbon monoxide poisoning, and methanol poisoning (more commonly putamen)

REFERENCES

1. Michel SJ, Given CA, Robertson WC. Imaging of the brain, including diffusion-weighted imaging in the methylmalonic acidemia. *Pediatr Radiol.* 2004;34:580–582.
2. Radmanesh A, Zaman T, Ghanaati H, et al. Methylmalonic acidemia: brain imaging findings in 52 children and a review of the literature. *Pediatr Radiol.* 2008;38:1054–1061.
3. Baker EH, Sloan JL, Hauser NS, et al. MRI Characteristics of Globus Pallidus Infarcts in isolated methylmalonic acidemia. *AJNR Am J Neuroradiol.* 2015;36(1):194–201.

ETHYLMALONIC ACIDEMIA

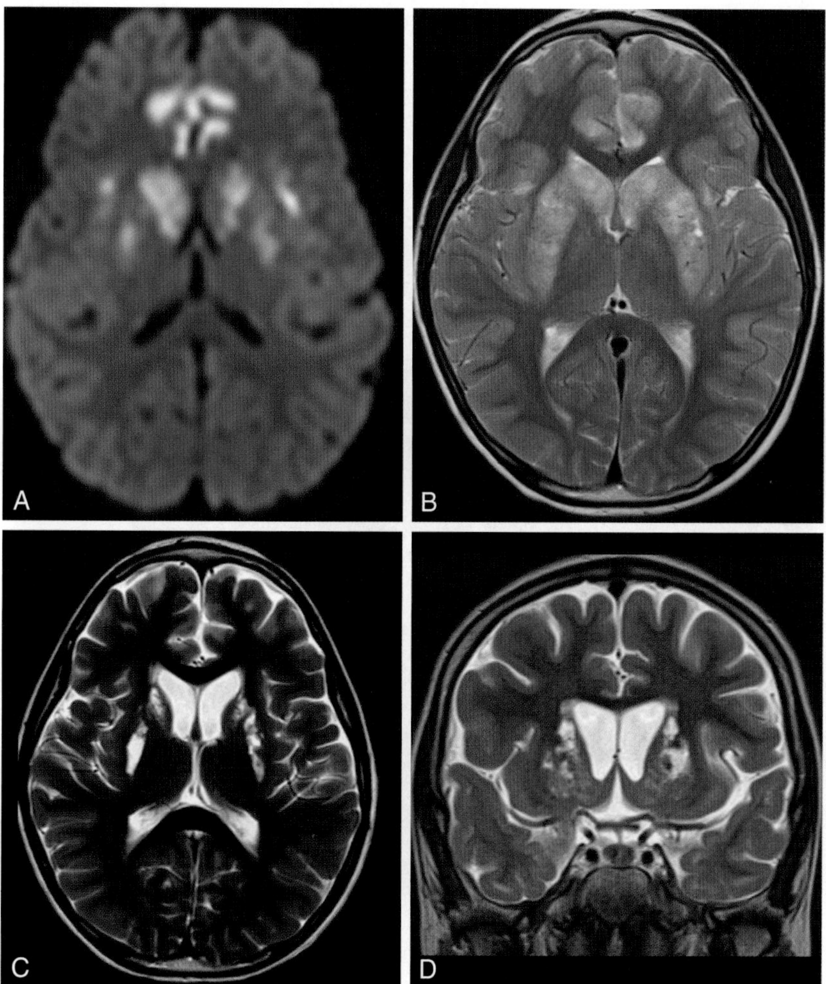

Fig. 4.38 Ethylmalonic Aciduria. (A) Axial DWI and (B) axial T2W images demonstrate T2W hyperintensity and diffusion restriction in the caudate heads, putamen, insula, and anterior cingulate gyri. (C and D) Follow-up axial and coronal T2W images demonstrate greater T2W hyperintensity and increased size of the ventricles in the basal ganglia indicative of neuronal volume loss.

Key Points

Background

- Autosomal recessive mitochondrial disorder; defective *ETHE1* gene → deficiency of mitochondrial sulfur dioxygenase → accumulation of hydrogen sulfide → inhibits function of cytochrome c oxidase and short-chain acyl-CoA dehydrogenase.

Clinical

- Variable clinical manifestations and clinical course; classic features include acrocyanosis, petechiae, chronic diarrhea; neurologic manifestations include developmental regression, spastic diplegia, ataxia, extrapyramidal signs; death in early childhood
- Laboratory findings include elevated C4 and C5 acylcarnitines and C4–C6 acylglycines in the serum and elevated ethylmalonic acid in urine.

Imaging

- Abnormal T2/FLAIR hyperintense signal in the basal ganglia, predominantly the caudate and putamen, and cerebral white matter, which can progress to cavitation and atrophy
- Acute episodes can demonstrate diffusion restriction.

REFERENCE

1. Lim J, Shayota BJ, Lay E, et al. Acute stroke-like presentation and long term evolution of diffusion restriction pattern in ethylmalonic encephalopathy.

WILSON DISEASE

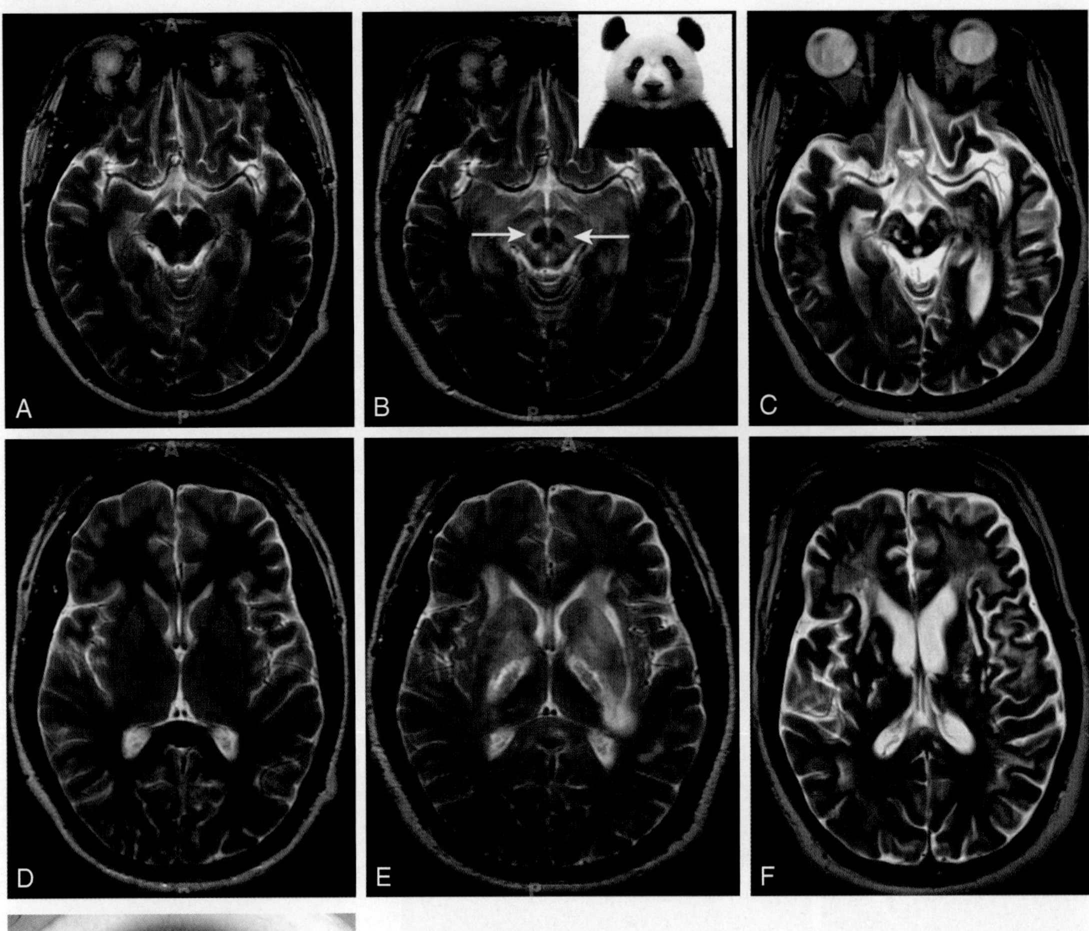

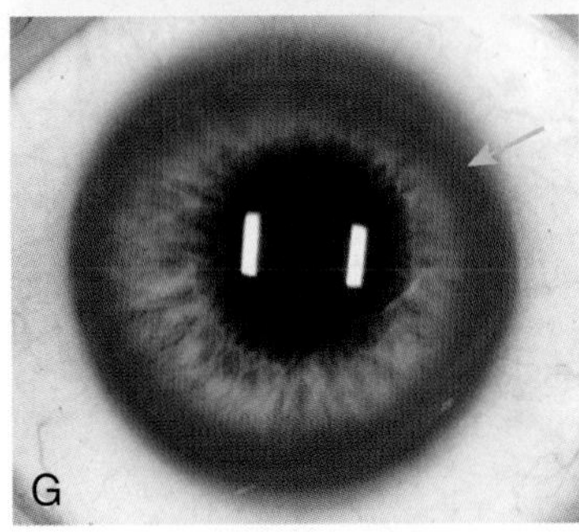

Fig. 4.39 Wilson Disease. (A and D) Initial presentation MRI T2W images are normal. (B and E) Axial T2W follow-up MRI demonstrate confluent T2W hyperintensity due to edema centered in the basal ganglia and extending into the midbrain, internal capsules, subinsular white matter, and medial temporal lobes. The "panda" sign is seen in image B in the midbrain. (C and F) Late follow-up T2W images demonstrate progressive T2W hyperintensity in the frontal white matter and now volume loss in the midbrain, basal ganglia, internal capsules, medial temporal lobes, and subinsular white matter. (G) Clinical image of a Kayser-Fleischer ring. (B, inset image of panda © istock.com/olgalT. G, From Pyeritz RE, Kork BR, Grody WW: Emery and Rimoin's principles and practice of medical genetics and genomics: metabolic disorders, ed 7, London, 2021, Academic Press.)

Key Points

Background

- Autosomal recessive defect in copper metabolism leading to *accumulation of copper* in the liver, and brain

Clinical

- Rings of green pigmentation in the cornea (Kayser-Fleischer rings), extrapyramidal symptoms and signs (tremor, dystonia, chorea), and seizure

Imaging

- Brain MRI can be normal or demonstrate *symmetric bilateral T1W and/or T2W hyperintense signal in the basal ganglia and midbrain* and less commonly the thalami and pons. The "panda" sign refers to the appearance of the red nuclei and substantia nigra in the midbrain are surrounded by edema simulating the face of a panda
- MRS: ↑ myoI:creatine ratio; ↓ metabolites

REFERENCE

1. Kim TJ, Kim IO, Kim WS, et al. MR Imaging of the brain in Wilson Disease of childhood: Findings before and after treatment with clinical correlation. *Am J Neuroradiol.* Jun-Jul 2006;27(6):1373–1378.

GLUTARIC ACIDURIA TYPE 1

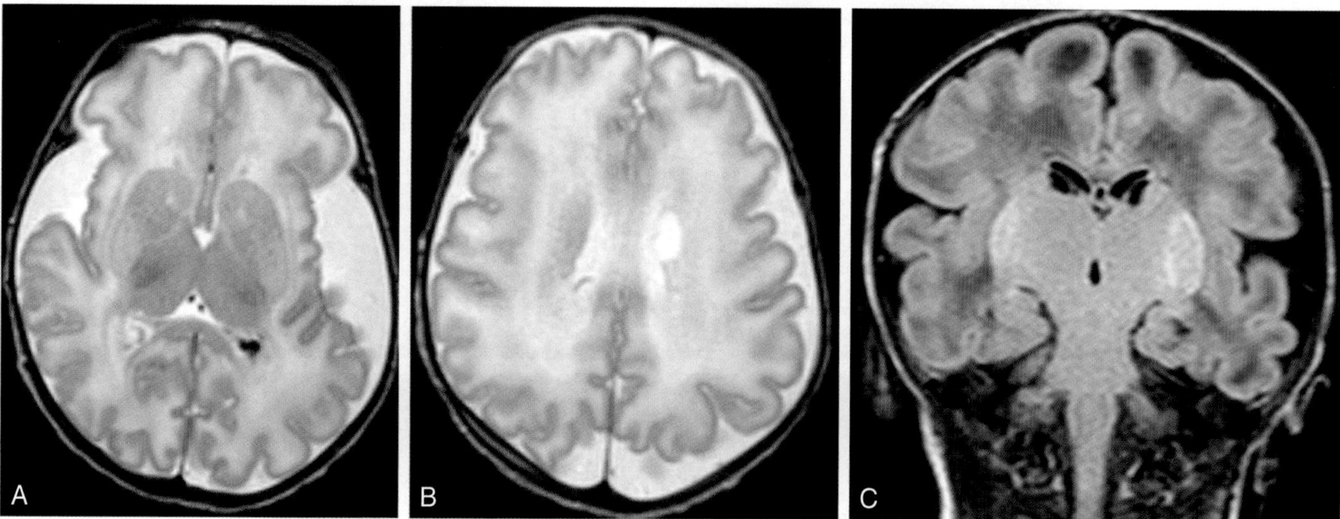

Fig. 4.40 Glutaric Aciduria Type 1. (A and B) Axial T2W, and (C) coronal FLAIR images demonstrate open sylvian fissures, diffuse white matter T2W hyperintensity, and posterior putamen T2W hyperintensity as well as bilateral caudothalamic groove germinolytic cysts.

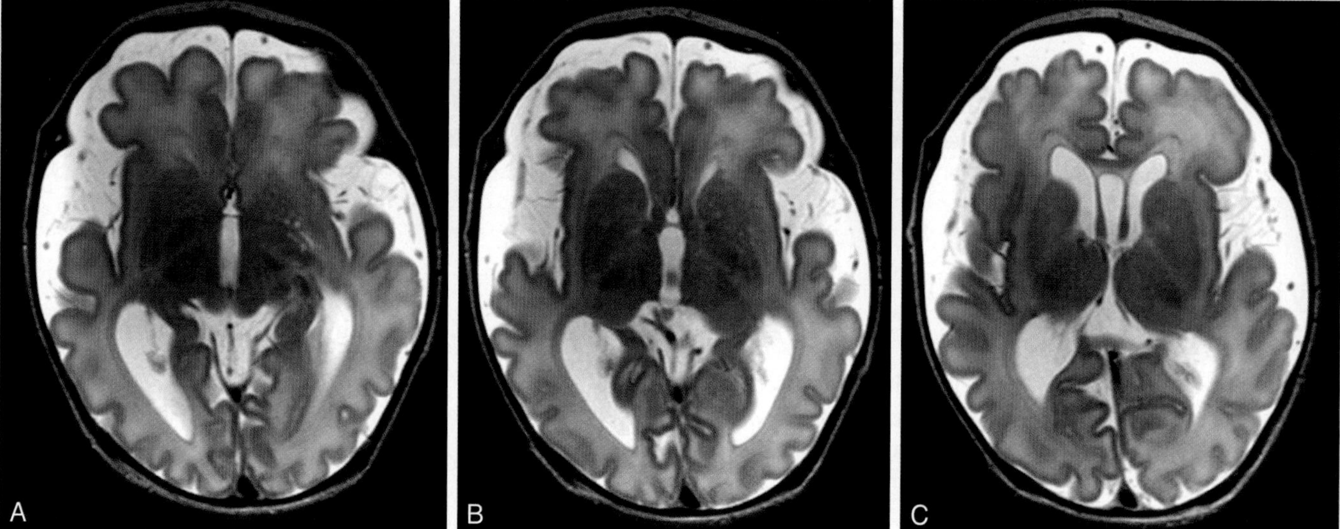

Fig. 4.41 Glutaric Aciduria Type 1. (A to C) Axial T2W images demonstrate open sylvian fissures, cerebral volume loss, and bilateral subdural hygromas.

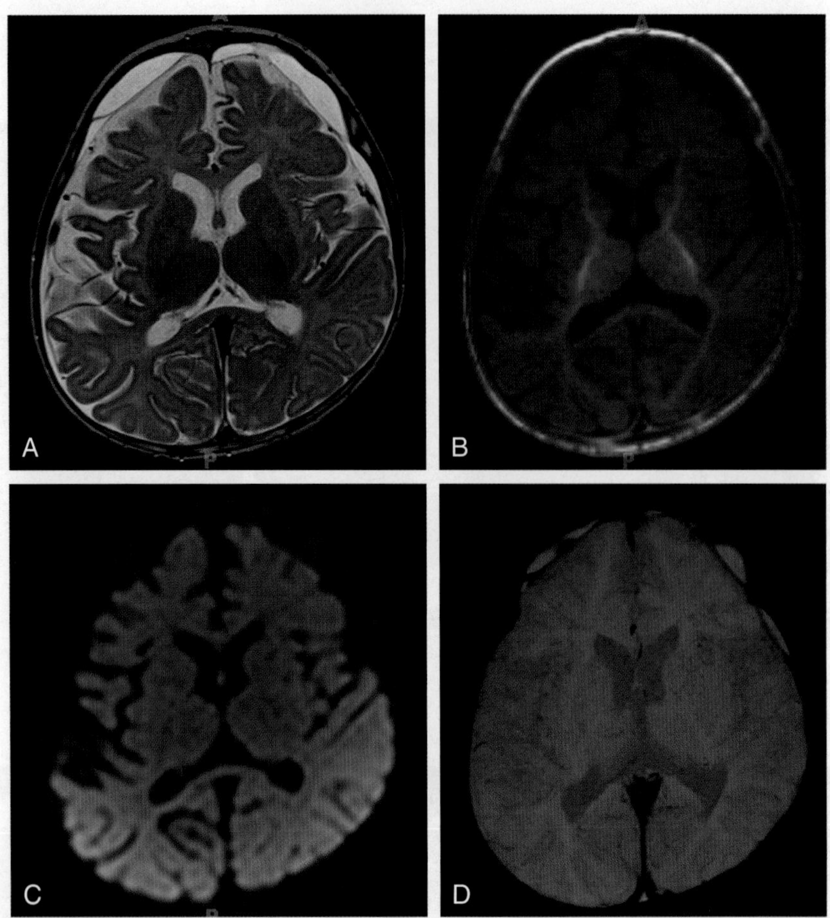

Fig. 4.42 Glutaric Aciduria Type 1. (A) Axial T2W, (B) axial T1W, (C) axial DWI, (D) axial SWI images demonstrate cerebral volume loss, bifrontal subdural hematomas.

Key Points

Background

- Also known as D-2 hydroxyglutaric aciduria; autosomal recessive; deficiency of the mitochondrial enzyme D-2 hydroxyglutarate dehydrogenase; inability to break down amino acids hydroxylysine, lysine, and tryptophan

Clinical

- Mild variant has variable clinical presentation with hypotonia, epilepsy, developmental delay, and *macrocephaly*; severe variant has neonatal or early infantile presentation with epilepsy, hypotonia, poor vision, facial dysmorphism, and absent development
- *May mimic child abuse due to spontaneous subdural fluid collections*
- Elevated urinary D-2 hydroxyglutaric acid
- Treatment is supportive

Imaging

- Delayed myelination and gyration (particularly occipital lobes)
- Expanded CSF spaces, and wide sylvian fissures
- Subdural effusions and/or hematomas
- Germinolytic cysts along caudothalamic groove (seen prior to 6 months of age)
- Basal ganglia and white matter T2W hyperintensities
- Large ventricles
- MRS: Pattern depends on clinical phase; early subacute phase mild ↑ lactate; late subacute ↓ Cho and ↓ NAA chronic phase ↓ NAA

REFERENCE

1. Van der Knaap MS, and Valk J. *Magnetic Resonance of Myelination and Myelin Disorders*. 3rd edition. Berlin: Springer; 2005.

PANTOTHENATE KINASE-ASSOCIATED NEURODEGENERATION (PKAN)

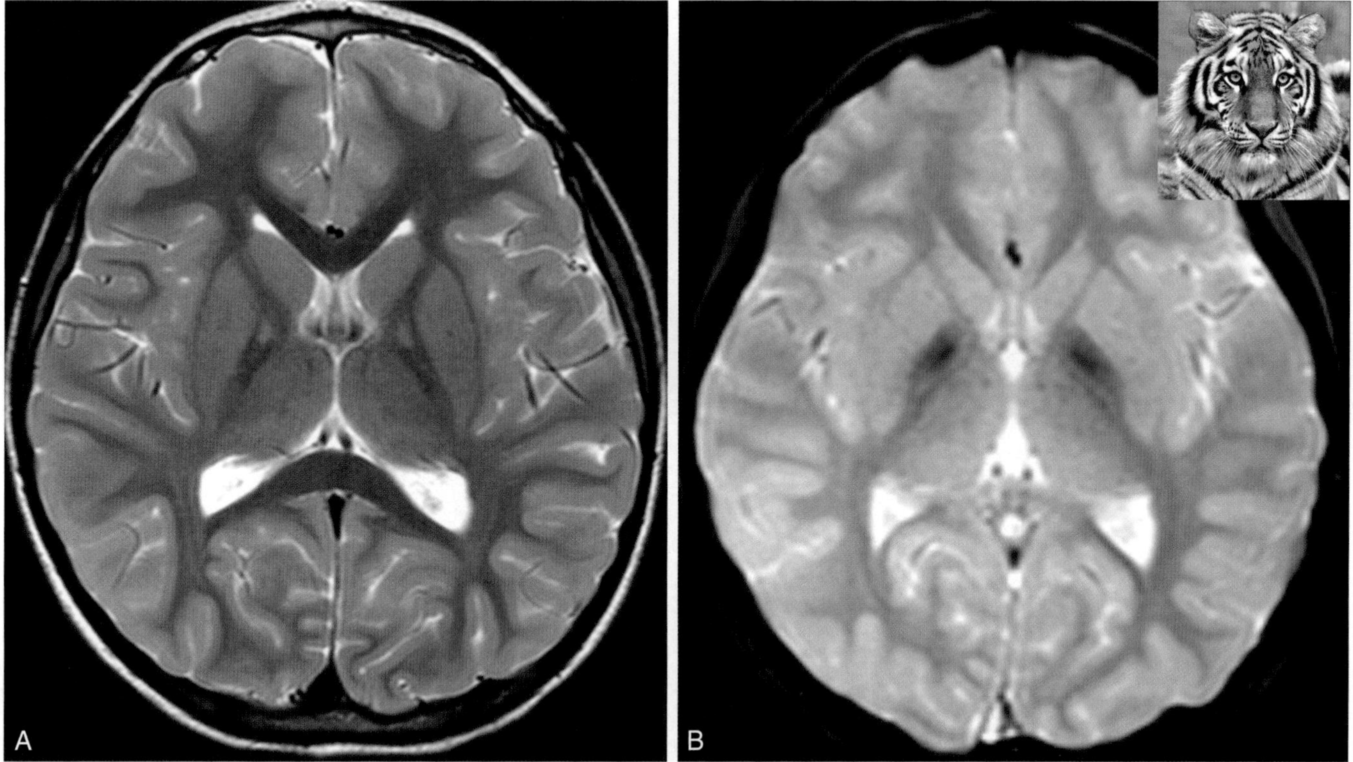

Fig. 4.43 PKAN. 4-year-old with developmental delay, and difficulty walking. (A) Axial T2W and (B) axial GRE images demonstrate T2W hyperintensity in the globus pallidi associated with susceptibility from increased iron deposition also known as the "eye of the tiger" sign. The patient's symptoms slowly progressed to inability to walk, dystonia, and bradykinesia by age 8 years. (B, inset image of tiger © istock.com/Histoirdemy Photography.)

Key Points

Background

- A form of neurodegeneration with brain iron accumulation (NBIA) also known as NBIA type 1, or previously Hallervorden-Spatz.
- PKAN is the most common type of NBIA.
- Autosomal recessive mutation in the *PKAN2* gene. Pantothenate kinase is a regulatory enzyme in the biosynthesis of coenzyme A leading to abnormal metabolism of vitamin B5 resulting in problems with energy and lipid metabolism and iron accumulation.
- Pathology: Iron deposition in the globus pallidi, tissue necrosis, and edema within iron accumulation results in the "eye of the tiger" pattern.

Clinical

- Classic and atypical forms. Treatment is related to symptomatic management.
- Classic form has age of onset before 10 years (mean 3{1/2} years); majority have extrapyramidal symptoms (dysarthria, dystonia, rigidity, choreoathetosis), gait impairment, spasticity, loss of ability to walk 10 to 15 years after onset, and retinopathy (66%). All have *PKAN2* mutations.
- Atypical form has onset after 10 years of age (mean 13 years), less severe and slower progression, uncommon retinopathy, frequent psychiatric symptoms, loss of ability to walk 15 to 40 years after onset of symptoms. Only {1/3} have *PKAN2* mutation.

Imaging

- *PKAN2* mutation patients demonstrate the *"eye of the tiger" pattern* of T2W hypointensity with central T2W hyperintensity, and diffuse increased susceptibility in the globus pallidi.
- "Eye of the tiger" pattern is not seen with other NBIA types.

REFERENCE

1. Hayflick SJ, Westaway SK, Levinson B, et al. Genetic, Clinical, and Radiographic delineation of Hallervorden-Spatz syndrome. *N Engl J Med.* 2003 Jan;348:33–40.

METABOLIC AND GENETIC DISORDERS WITH CEREBELLAR ATROPHY

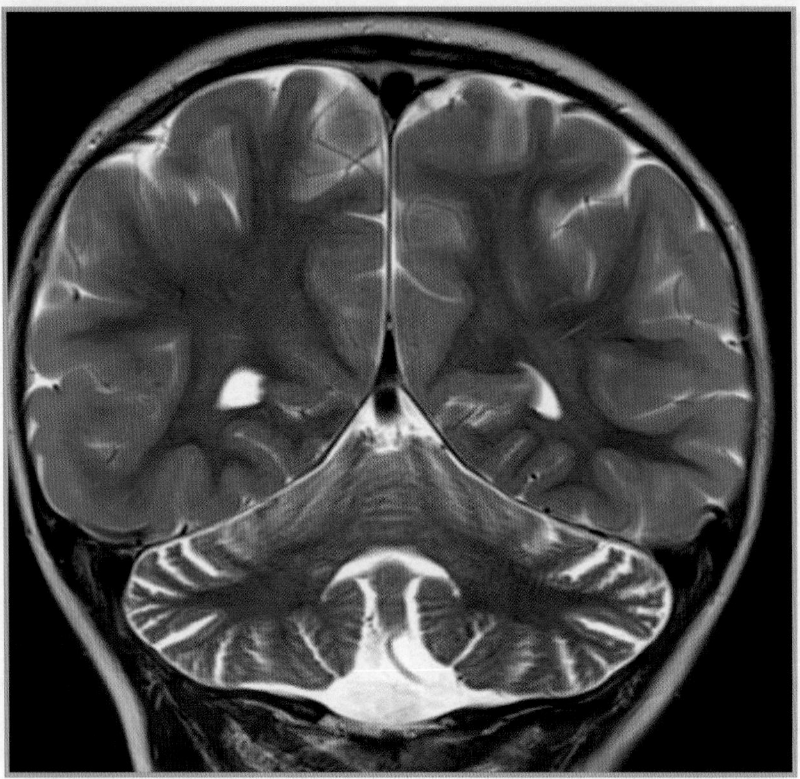

- Neuronal ceroid lipofuscinosis
- Spinocerebellar ataxia
- Congenital glycosylation disorder
- Infantile neuroaxonal dystrophy
- Ataxia telangiectasia
- 4H syndrome
- HABC
- CASK mutation
- VLDLR mutation
- Mitochondrial disorders
- Pontocerebellar hypoplasia

NEURONAL CEROID LIPOFUSCINOSIS

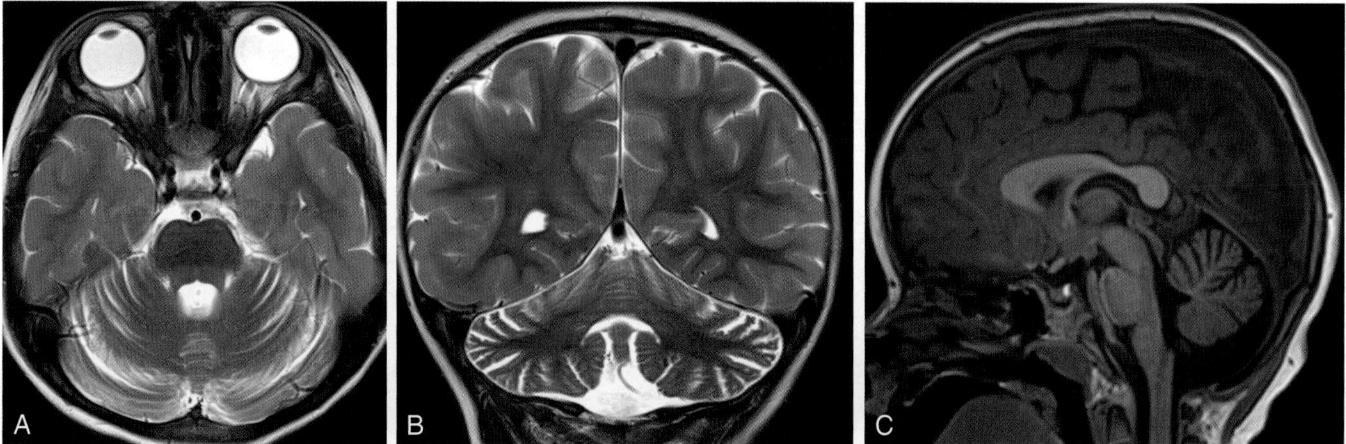

Fig. 4.44 Neuronal Ceroid Lipofuscinosis. 3-year-old with seizure. (A and B) Axial and coronal T2W and (C) sagittal T1W images demonstrate cerebellar volume loss. Genetic testing revealing CLN2-related Batten disease.

Key Points

- Also known as Batten disease

Background

- Ten main types (CLN1–10), which are due to different gene mutations

Clinical

- Clinical presentation depends on the type and age of onset; infants present with microcephaly, epilepsy, and early death; progressive encephalopathy

Imaging

- *Cerebral and cerebellar atrophy* and T2W hyperintensity along the margins of the ventricles
- T2W hypointensity in the thalami and globus pallidi
- MRS:
  - Infantile form demonstrates loss of NAA, severe reduction of Cr and Cho, ↑ myoI and lactate
  - Late infantile form demonstrates reduced NAA, ↑ myoI, Cr, and Cho in the white matter

REFERENCE

1. Barkovich AJ, Raybaud C. *Pediatric Neuroradiology*. 6th edition. Philadelphia: Wolters-Kluwer; 2019.

CONGENITAL GLYCOSYLATION DISORDER

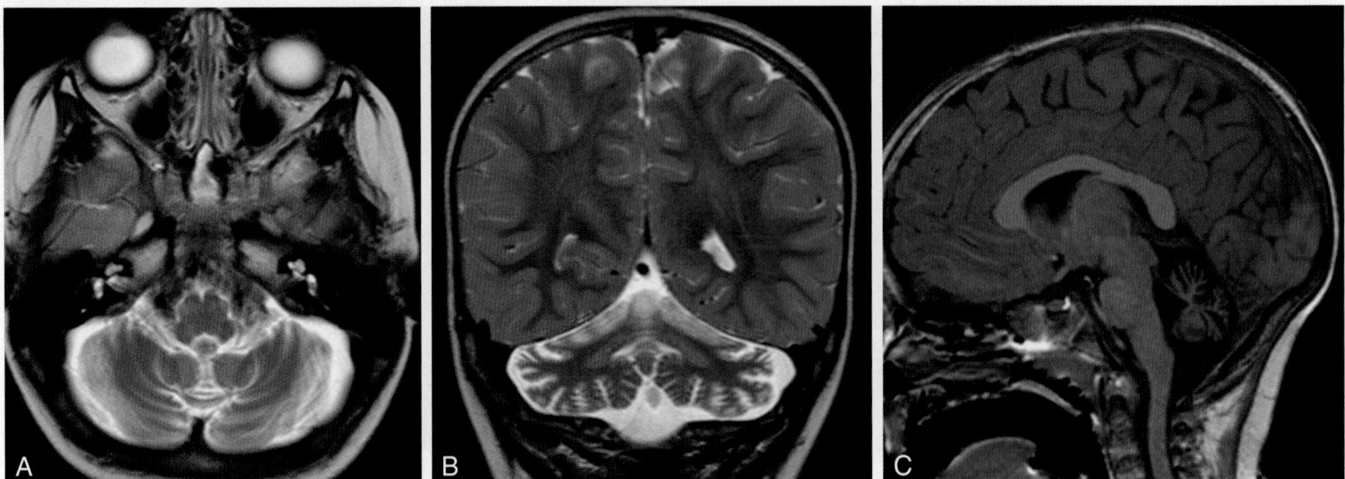

Fig. 4.45 Congenital Glycosylation Disorder. 3-year-old with developmental delay and abnormal movements. (A and B) Axial and coronal T2W and (C) sagittal T1W images demonstrate cerebellar volume loss with T2W hyperintensity in the cerebellar cortex, superior vermis, and dentate nuclei. Genetic testing revealed *PMM2* gene mutations causing CDG 1a.

Key Points

Background

- Autosomal recessive disorders caused by abnormal glycosylation of N-linked oligosaccharides
- Congenital disorder of glycosylation 1a (CDG-1a) is the most common form and caused by mutations in the gene *PMM2*

Clinical

- Variable from severe infantile to mild late onset. Clinical features include hypotonia, developmental delay, strabismus, dysmorphic features, abnormal fat distribution, inverted nipples, and stroke-like episodes.

Imaging

- Cerebellar hypoplasia and progressive pontine and cerebellar atrophy with T2/FLAIR hyperintense cortex and subcortical white matter
- Differential Diagnosis: Neuroaxonal dystrophy, neuronal ceroid lipofuscinosis, and pontocerebellar hypoplasia

REFERENCE

1. Feraco P, Mirabelli-Badenier M, Severino M, et al. The shrunken, bright cerebellum: A characteristic MRI finding of congenital disorders of glycosylation type 1a. *AJNR Am J Neuroradiol.* 2012 Dec;33(11):2062–2067.

INFANTILE NEUROAXONAL DYSTROPHY

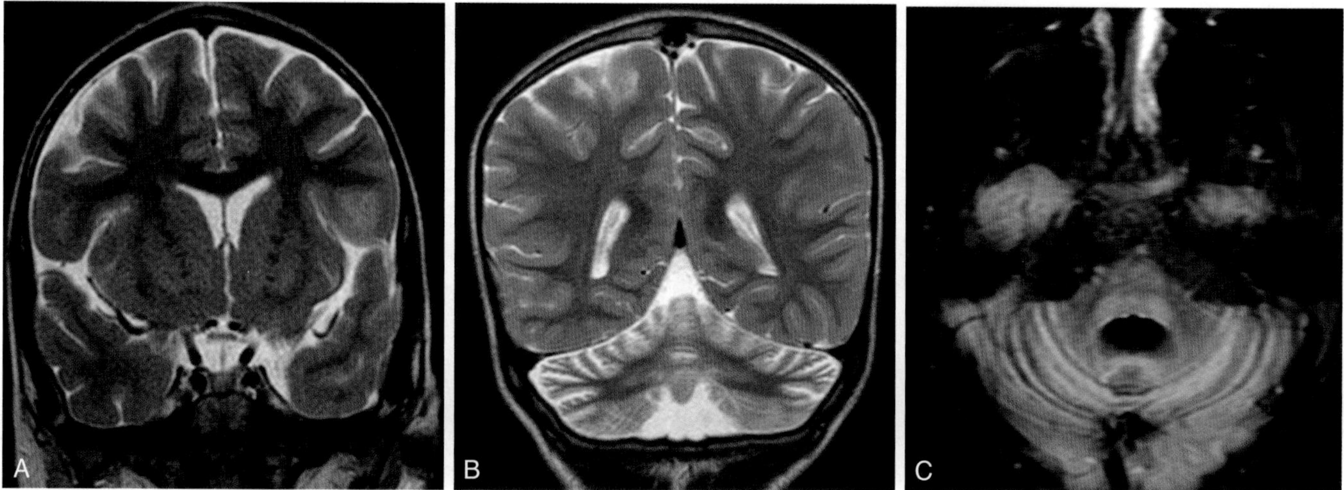

Fig. 4.46 Infantile Neuroaxonal Dystrophy. 4-year-old with cerebellar ataxia and delayed milestones. (A and B) Coronal T2W and (C) axial FLAIR images demonstrate cerebellar volume loss with cortical T2W hyperintensity and atrophy of the optic chiasm. Genetic testing revealed mutation in the *PLA2G6* gene.

Key Points

Background

- Autosomal recessive neurodegenerative disorder that remains incompletely characterized, but most cases are due to mutations in *PLA2G6* gene, which encodes an A2 phospholipase that metabolizes phospholipids
- Pathology demonstrates axonal swelling and spheroid bodies in the central and peripheral nervous system

Clinical

- Onset within first 2 to 3 years of life. Neurodegeneration leads to psychomotor regression, hypotonia, tetraplegia, vision impairment, dementia, and seizures.

Imaging

- Most common finding is symmetric cerebellar atrophy with T2/FLAIR hyperintense signal in the cortex.
- Additional findings can include T2/FLAIR hyperintensities in the PLIC, corticospinal tracts, and frontal periventricular white matter.
- Optic nerves and chiasm can be atrophic.
- Iron deposition in the globus pallidi, causing T2W hypointense signal, also reported.
- DWI can demonstrate restriction in some cases.

REFERENCES

1. Nardocci N, Zorzi G, Farina L, et al. Infantile neuroaxonal dystrophy: Clinical spectrum and diagnostic criteria. *Neurology*. 1999 Apr 22;52(7):1472–1478.
2. Sener RN. Diffusion-weighted and conventional MR imaging findings of neuroaxonal dystrophy. *AJNR Am J Neuroradiol*. 2004 Aug;25(7):1269–1273.

SPINOCEREBELLAR ATAXIA

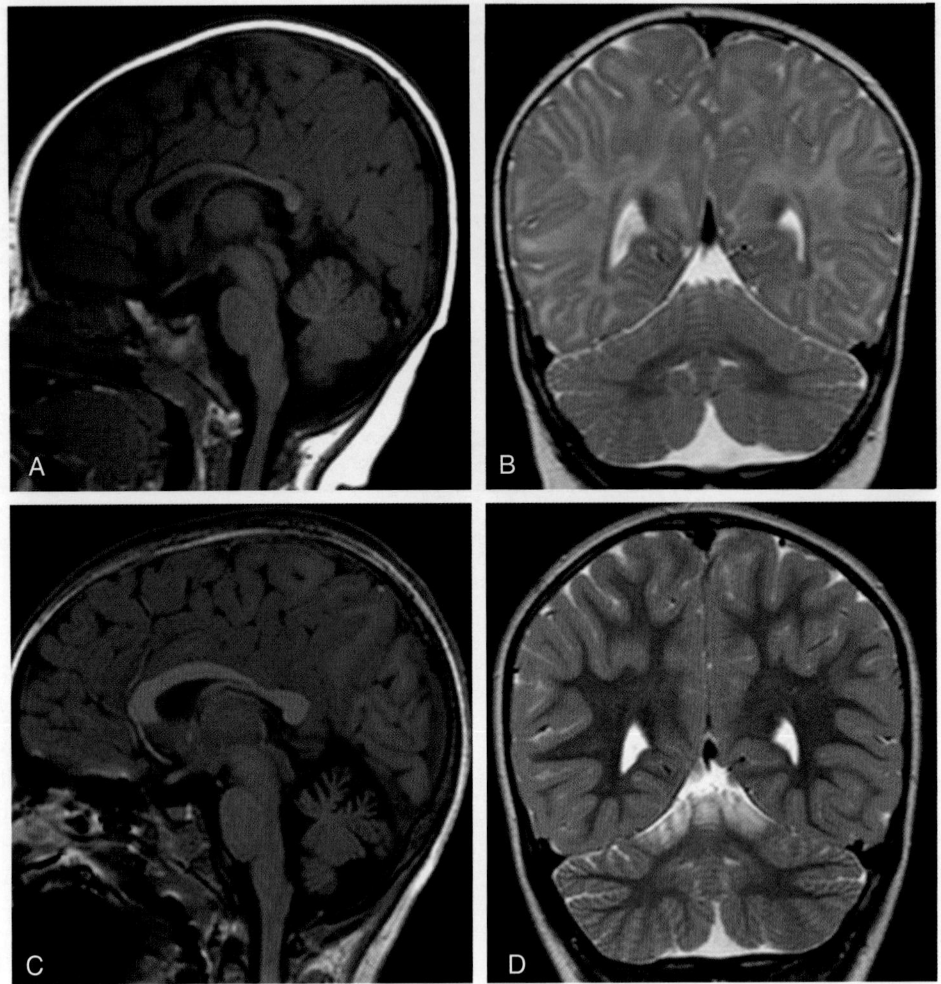

Fig. 4.47 Spinocerebellar Ataxia. (A) Sagittal T1W image and (B) coronal T2W image at 5 months old and (C and D) sagittal T1W and coronal T2W images at 5 years old demonstrate progressive atrophy and cortical T2W hyperintensity of the superomedial cerebellar hemispheres and superior vermis.

Key Points

Background

- Group of autosomal dominant neurodegenerative diseases with cerebellar ataxia caused by different gene mutations (SCA 1–SCA 48).

Clinical

- Symptoms include ataxia, dysarthria, decreased vision, difficulty learning, and processing information.

Imaging

- Most common finding is *cerebellar and spinal atrophy* without or with additional findings including olivopontocerebellar atrophy, spinal cord atrophy, "hot cross bun" sign, and dentate calcification.
- Advanced imaging using diffusion tensor imaging (DTI) and volumetric analysis has demonstrated alterations in the cerebellum, brainstem, striatum, thalamus, and cervical spinal cord.

REFERENCE

1. Meira AT, Arruda WO, Ono SE, et al. Neurological findings in the spinocerebellar ataxias. *Tremor Other Hyperkinet Mov (NY)*. 2019;9:10.

GENETIC SYNDROMES WITH CEREBELLAR HYPOPLASIA

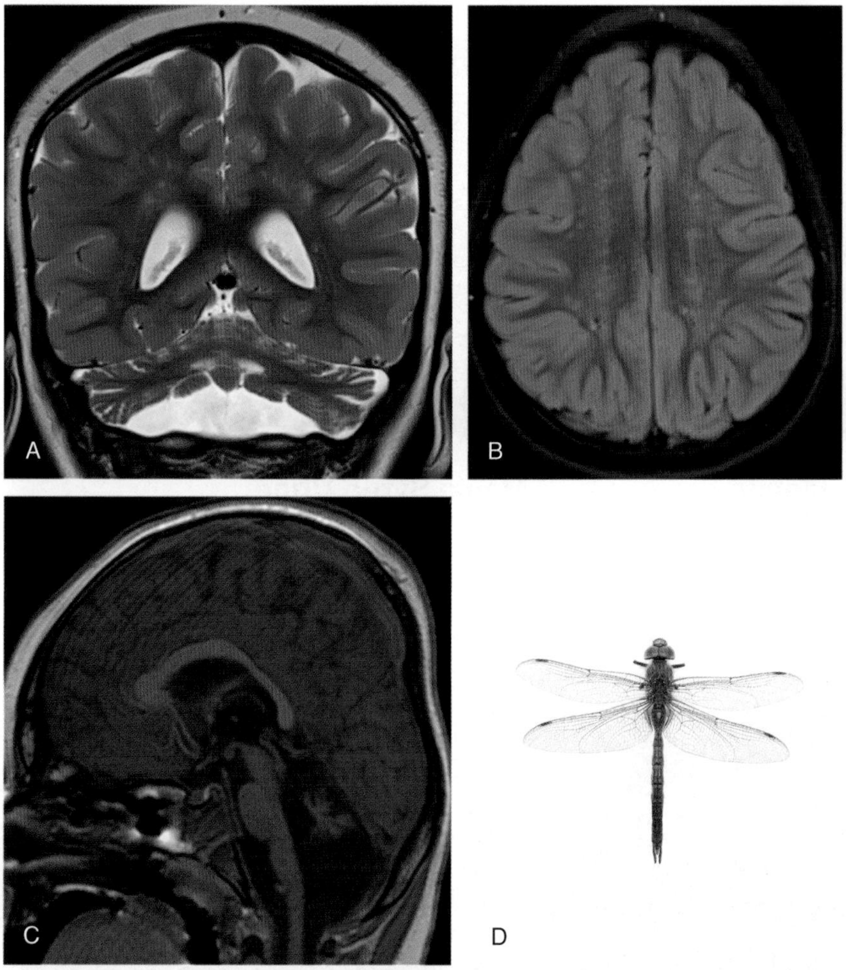

Fig. 4.48 CASK Mutation. X-linked inheritance disorder seen in females due to lethality in males. Clinical features include ataxia, nystagmus, microcephaly, severe cognitive impairment, seizures, retinopathy, sensorineural hearing loss. (A) Coronal T2W and (B) axial FLAIR, and (C) sagittal T1W imaging demonstrate pontocerebellar hypoplasia with "dragonfly appearance," and simplified gyral pattern in the frontal lobes. (D, Copyright © iStock.com/Serg_Velusceac.)

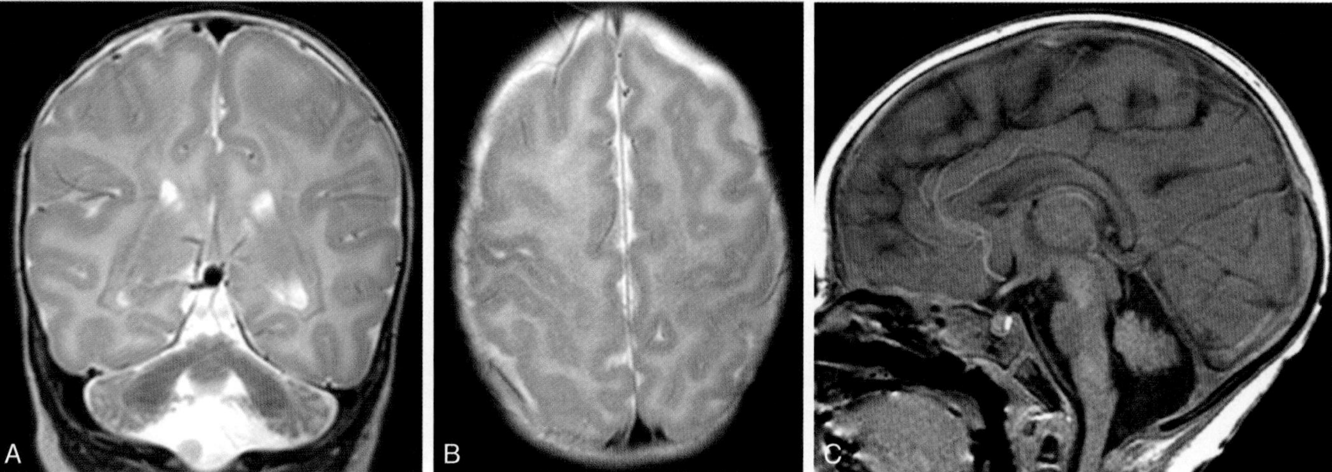

Fig. 4.49 VLDLR Mutation. VLDLR mutation encodes a very-low-density lipoprotein receptor, which is a coreceptor in the reelin pathway. Clinical features include nonprogressive cerebellar ataxia, moderate to profound intellectual disability, strabismus, dysarthria, and seizures. (A) Coronal and axial T2W, and (C) sagittal T1W imaging demonstrate pontocerebellar hypoplasia with frontal pachygyria (more severe pattern seen in RELN mutations).

REFERENCE

1. Poretti A, Bolthauser E, Huisman TAGM. Cerebellar and brainstem malformations. *Neuroimaging Clin N Am*. 2016 Aug;26(3):341–357.

Differential Diagnoses: SPECTROSCOPY PATTERNS OF METABOLIC DISORDERS

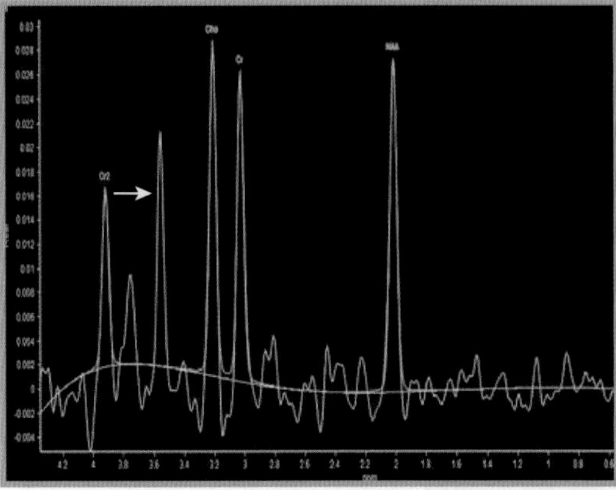

Nonketotic Hyperglycinemia
Abnormal glycine peak at 3.56 on long echo

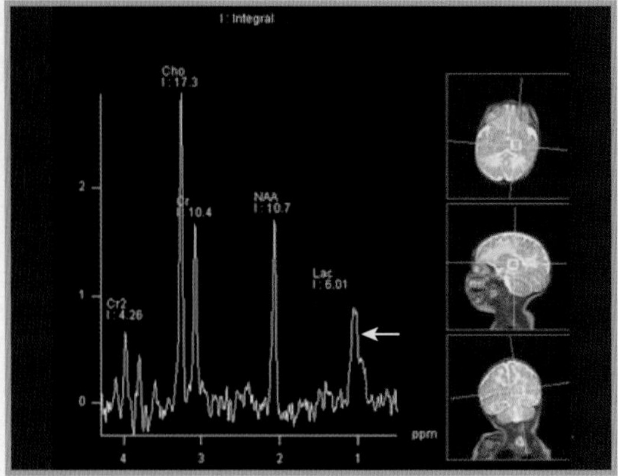

Maple Syrup Urine
Abnormal branch chain amino acid peak at 0.9 ppm on long echo

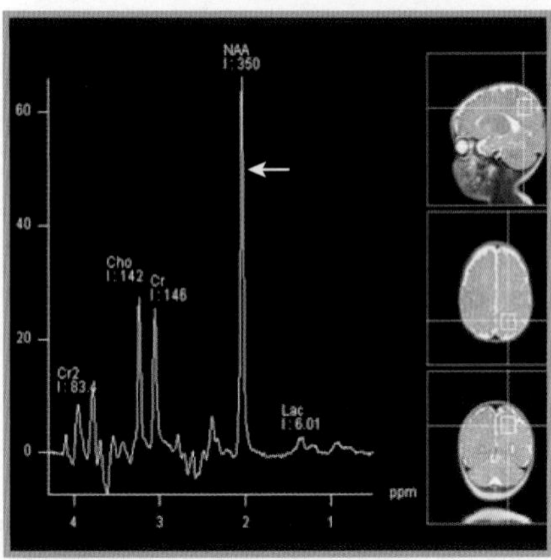

Canavan Disease
Abnormal large NAA peak at 2.0 ppm

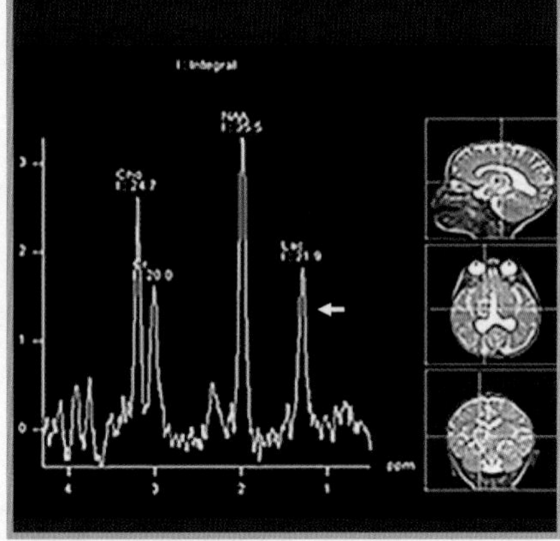

Mitochondrial
Abnormal elevation of lactate peak at 1.3 ppm

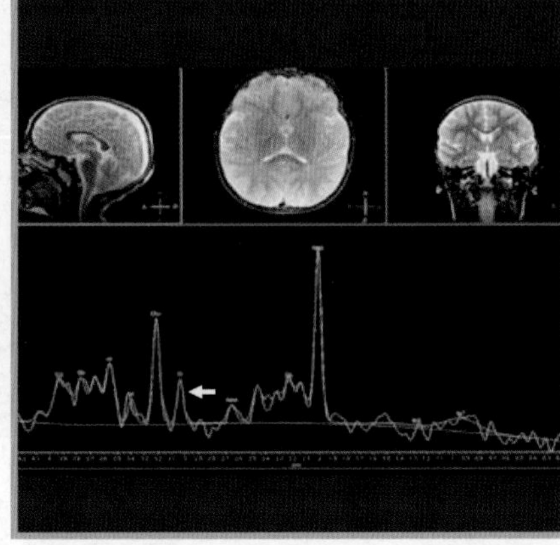

Creatine Deficiency
Abnormal severe reduction in creatine peak at 3.0 ppm

CREATINE DEFICIENCY

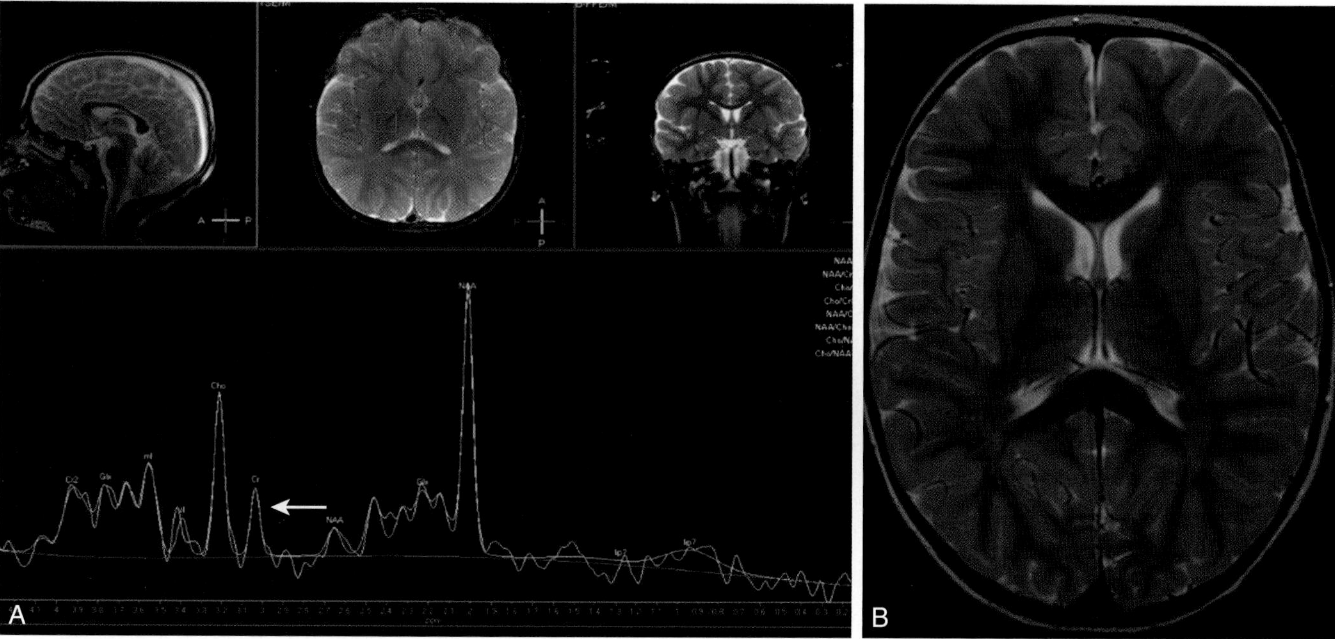

Fig. 4.50 **Creatine Deficiency**. (A) MRS short echo demonstrates severely reduced creatine peak. (B) Axial T2W image demonstrates normal appearance of the brain.

Key Points

Background

- Caused by autosomal recessive defect in the creatine synthesis in guanidinoacetate methyltransferase (GAMT) or arginine:glycine amidinotransferase (AGAT) or X-linked defect in creatine transport protein.
- Creatine is essential for storage and transmission of phosphate bound energy in muscle and brain.

Clinical

- Developmental delay, hypotonia, extrapyramidal disorders, epilepsy; creatine transport protein deficiency can demonstrate severe language delay, hypotonia, seizures, and autism spectrum;
- AGAT and GAMT can be treated with oral creatine supplementation.

Imaging

- GAMT deficiency can demonstrate *T2W hyperintensity and diffusion restriction* in the *globus pallidi and central tegmental tracts,* and T2/FLAIR hyperintensity in the cerebral white matter
- MRI often normal in AGAT deficiency
- MRS: *Absent or severely reduced creatine peak,* which can reappear with supplementation; GAMT disorder can demonstrate a broad guanidinoacetate peak at 3.78 ppm

REFERENCE

1. Barkovich AJ, Raybaud C. *Pediatric Neuroradiology*. 6th edition. Philadelphia: Wolters-Kluwer; 2019.

TOXIC DISORDERS

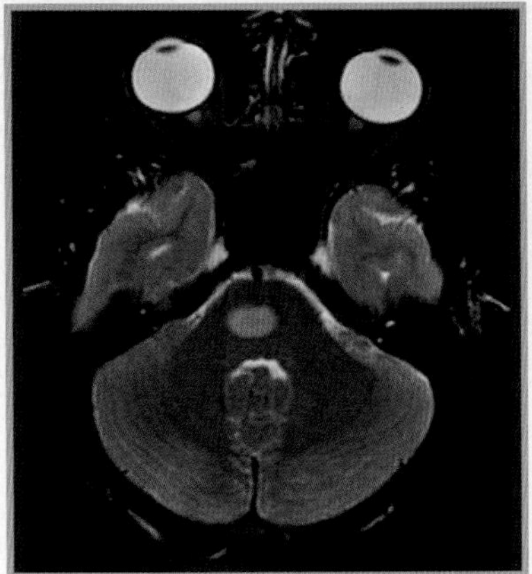

Electrolyte
- Diabetic ketoacidosis
- Hyponatremia
- Hyperbilirubinemia
- Hyperammonemia
- Uremia

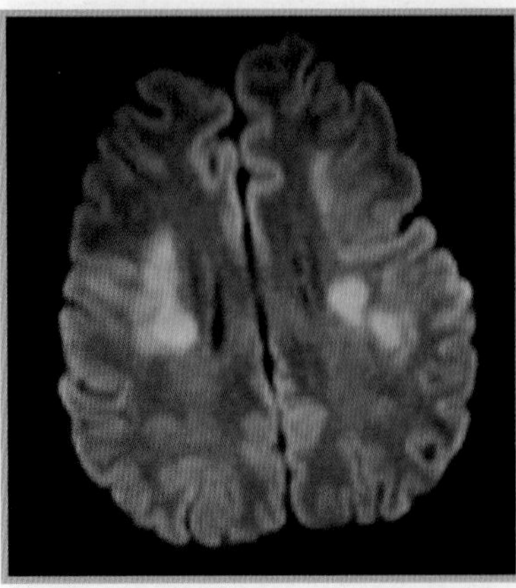

Medication Treatment
- Methotrexate
- Vigabatrin

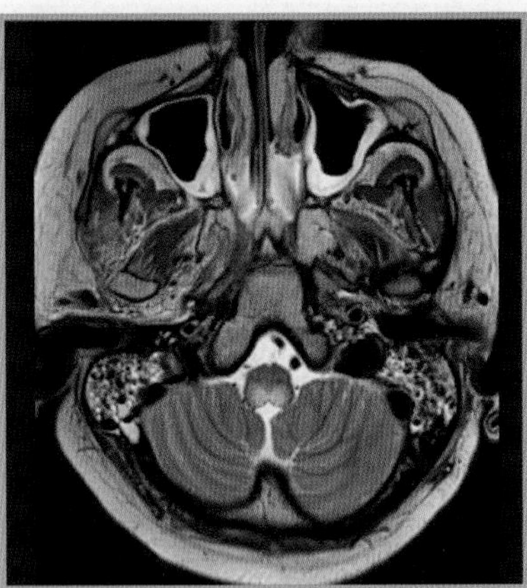

Vitamin Deficiency
- Vitamin B1
- Vitamin B6
- Vitamin B12

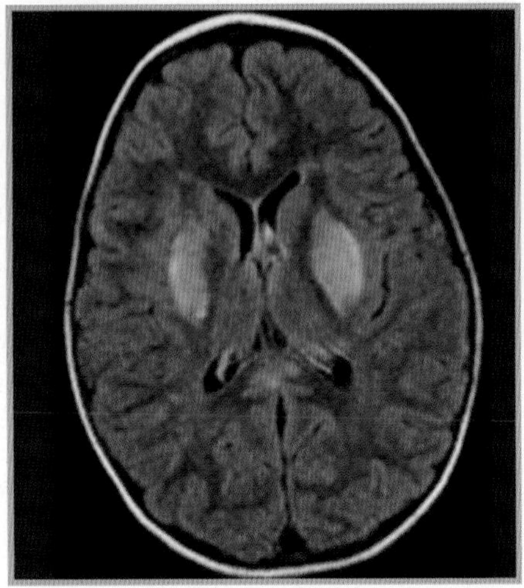

Infection
- Hemolytic uremic syndrome

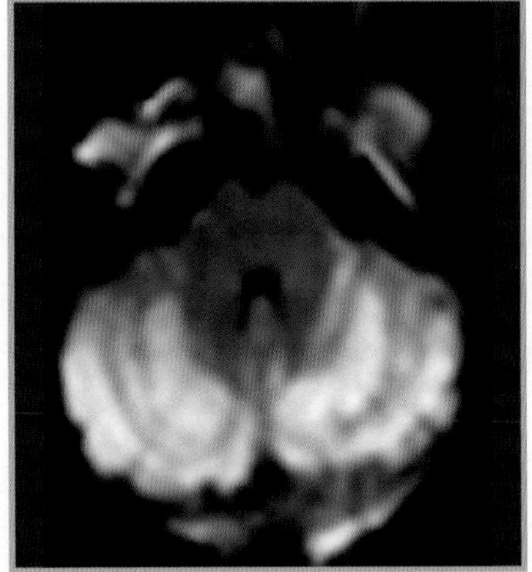

Illicit Drug Abuse
- Multiple drugs including cocaine, heroin, and fentanyl

DIABETIC KETOACIDOSIS

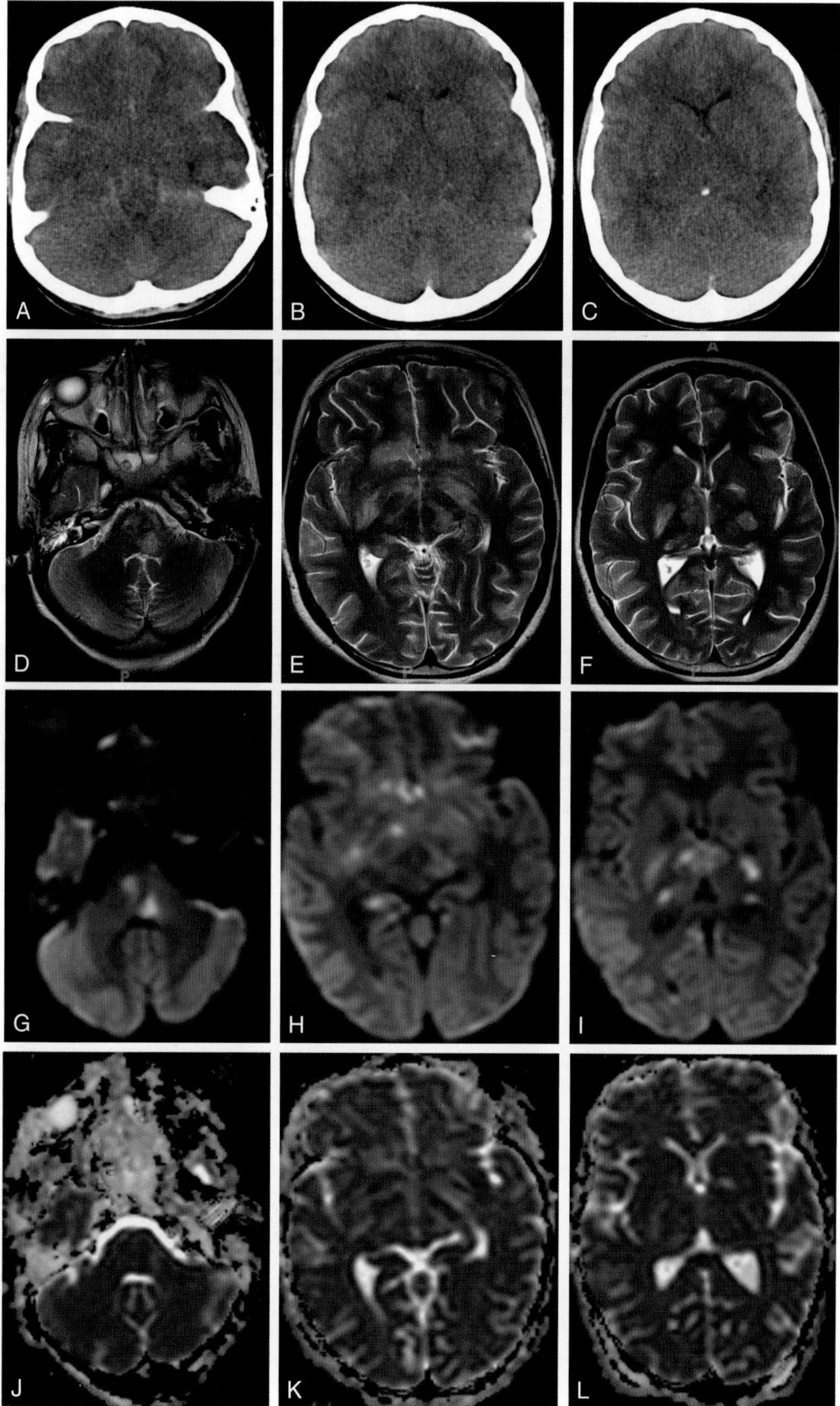

Fig. 4.51 Diabetic Ketoacidosis. 10-year-old with waxing and waning mental status, 2-week history of polydipsia and polyuria, and new diagnosis of type 1 diabetes mellitus. (A to C) Axial CT images demonstrate diffuse cerebral edema with effaced sulci and basal cisterns. (D to F) Axial T2W, (G to I) axial DWI, and (J to L) axial ADC images demonstrate T2W hyperintensity in the pons, midbrain, thalami, internal capsules, basal ganglia, and basal frontal lobes with areas of diffusion restriction indicative of a combination of cytotoxic and vasogenic edema.

DIABETIC KETOACIDOSIS

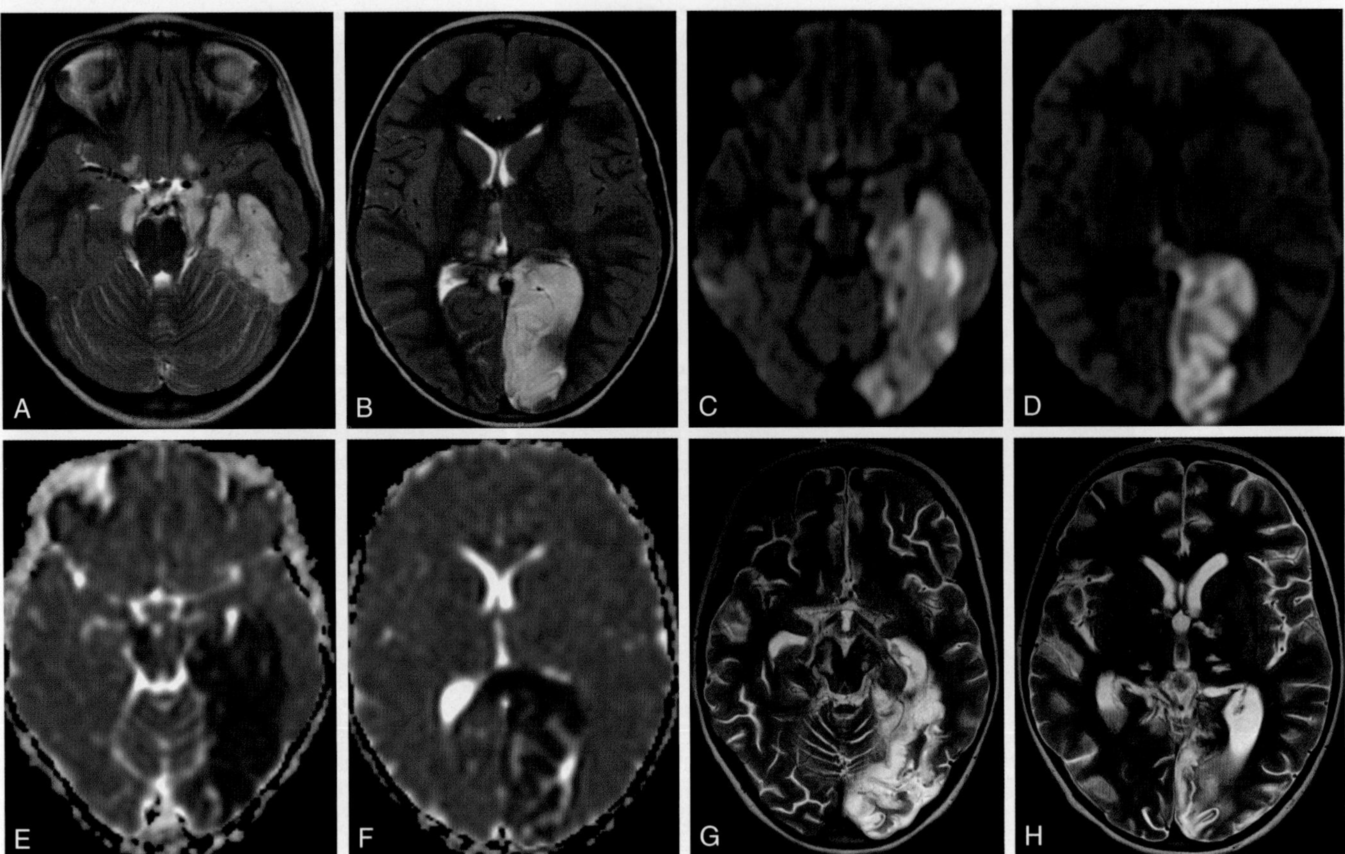

Fig. 4.52 Diabetic Ketoacidosis. (A and B) Axial T2W, (C and D) axial DWI, and (E and F) axial ADC images demonstrate a region of T2W hyperintensity and diffusion restriction in the medial temporal lobes, left occipital lobe, midbrain, splenium of the corpus callosum, and bilateral thalami indicative of posterior circulation large and small vessel infarcts and smaller areas in the posterior orbitofrontal gyri. (G and H) Follow-up axial T2W images demonstrate encephalomalacia in these areas.

Key Points

Background

- Serious complication that occurs in type 1 diabetics due to severe insulin deficiency resulting in hyperglycemia, acidosis and systemic inflammation. Approximately 1% of pediatric DKA is complicated by CNS injury.
- Pathogenesis may be related to osmotic gradients, intracellular accumulation of sodium and water, and vasodilatation and reperfusion.

Clinical

- Cerebral edema manifesting with headache, altered mental status, apnea, bradycardia, posturing and absent pupillary reflexes.
- Stroke like signs and symptoms.

Imaging

- *Cerebral edema* (occurs almost exclusively in pediatric patients) with imaging findings of effaced sulci and cisterns. Although determination of effaced sulci in children can be challenging, the effacement of cerebral sulci at the vertex often best seen on sagittal imaging are a reliable indicator of the presence of diffuse cerebral edema.
- Acute ischemic typically consisting of small vessel infarcts involving the medial basal ganglia, thalami, and brainstem
- Hemorrhagic infarcts without or with sinus thrombosis
- Extrapontine myelinolysis demonstrated as T2/FLAIR hyperintensity in the claustrum, and putamen
- Up to 40% of children with DKA and acute neurologic symptoms may not demonstrate abnormality on head CT.

REFERENCE

1. Barrot A, Huisman TAGM, Poretti A. Neuroimaging findings in acute pediatric diabetic ketoacidosis. *The Neuroradiology journal.* 2016;29(5):317–322.

CENTRAL PONTINE MYELINOLYSIS

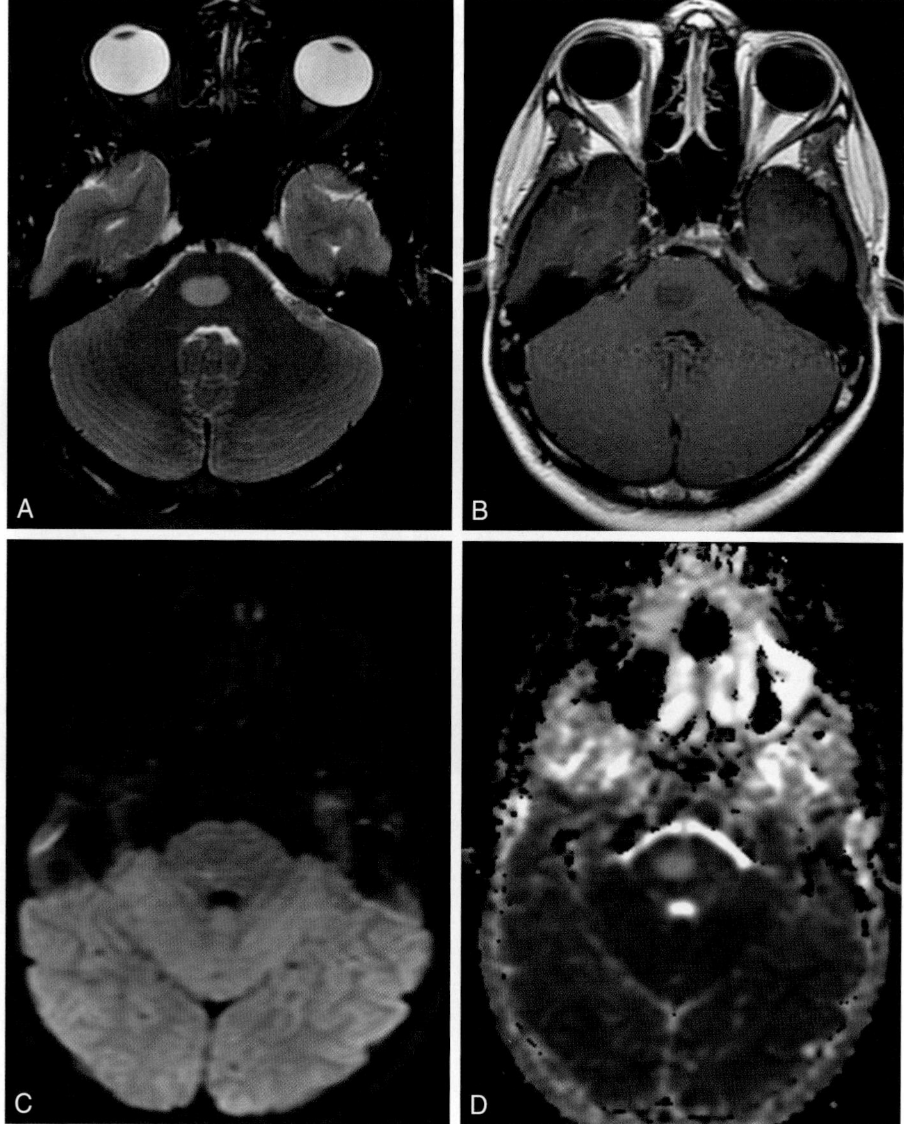

Fig. 4.53 Central Pontine Myelinolysis. (A) Axial T2W, (B) axial T1W+C, (C) axial DWI, and (D) axial ADC images demonstrate nonenhancing non-mass-like T2W hyperintensity without diffusion restriction in the central pons.

Key Points

Background

- Uncommon disorder typically occurring in the setting of rapid correction of sodium levels

Clinical

- Spastic quadriparesis, pseudobulbar palsy, delirium, horizontal gaze palsy, and coma; prognosis has no apparent correlation with clinical and imaging findings

Imaging

- Central pons T2W hyperintense signal, classically trident shaped, that spares the corticospinal tracts
- Diffusion restriction has been reported to occur within 24 hours of symptom onset
- No enhancement
- Extrapontine myelinolysis can involve the basal ganglia, thalami, midbrain, cerebellum, and gray-white matter junctions

REFERENCE

1. Howard SA, Barletta JA, Klufas RA, et al. Osmotic demyelination syndrome. *Radiographics*. 2009 May-Jun;29(3):933–938.

KERNICTERUS

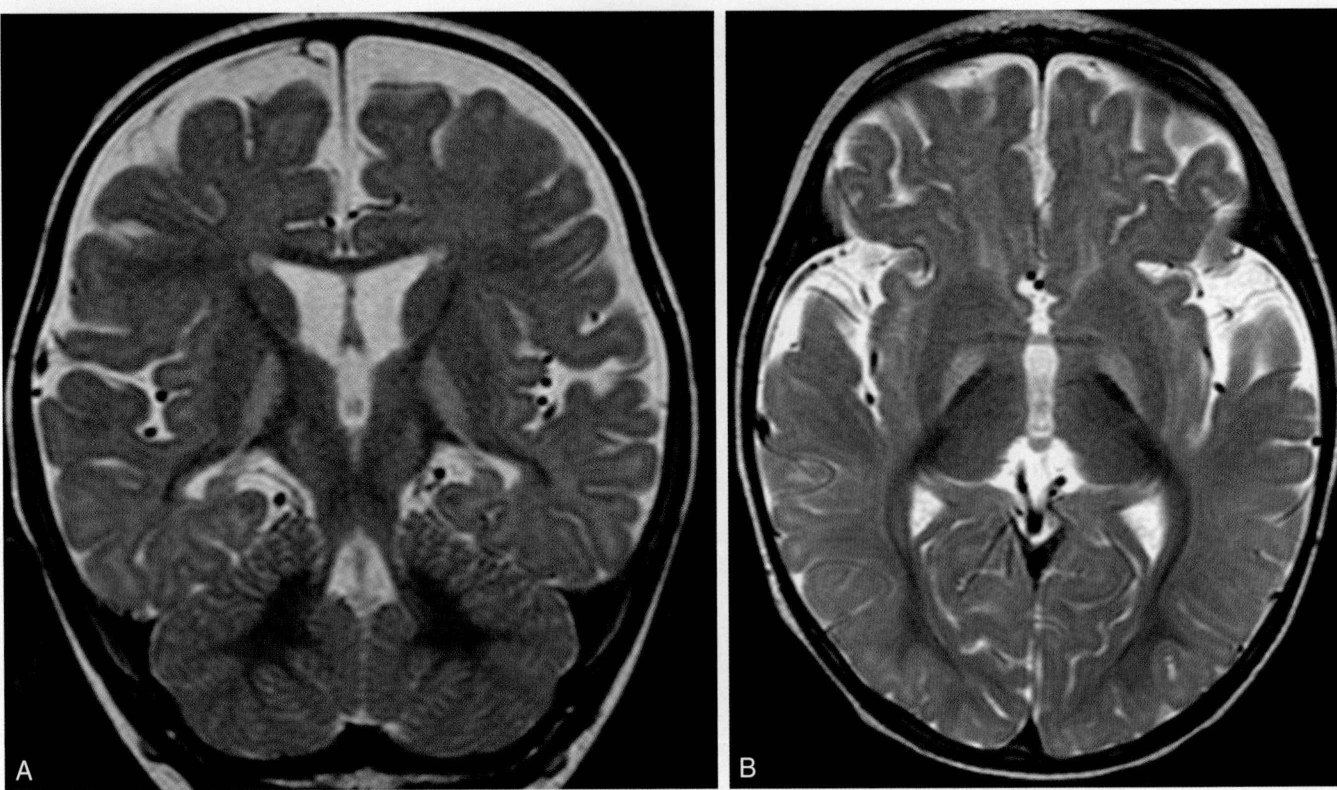

Fig. 4.54 Kernicterus. 10-month-old with dystonia and hyperbilirubinemia at birth. (A) Coronal T2W, and (B) axial T2W images demonstrate symmetric T2W hyperintensity in the bilateral globus pallidi indicative of chronic stage injury.

Key Points

Background

- Cerebral deposition of unconjugated bilirubin seen in the setting of hyperbilirubinemia in newborns. Causes of hyperbilirubinemia include erythroblastosis fetalis or other hemolytic anemias.

Clinical

- Manifestations appear at 2 to 5 days of age
- Occurs in infants with serum bilirubin >20 mg/dL (lower levels in premature infants); jaundice, lethargy, hypotonia, and high-pitched cry.
- 100% of babies with symptoms at 10 months of age will continue to have symptoms later in life. The severity cannot be predicted until 4-5 years old.
- Treated with phototherapy and transfusions when severe

Imaging

- Acute phase T1W hyperintense signal in the globus pallidi and subthalamic nuclei
- Chronic stage more often T2W hyperintense signal in the globus pallidi, subthalamic nuclei, hippocampi, and less commonly thalami, putamen, caudate, cerebellar nuclei, substantia nigra, and cranial nerve nuclei (particularly CN III, IV, VI)

REFERENCE

1. Martich-Kriss V, Kollias SS, Ball WS. MRI findings in kernicterus. *Am J Neuroradiol.* 1995 Apr;16:819–821.

DRUG TOXICITY: METHOTREXATE

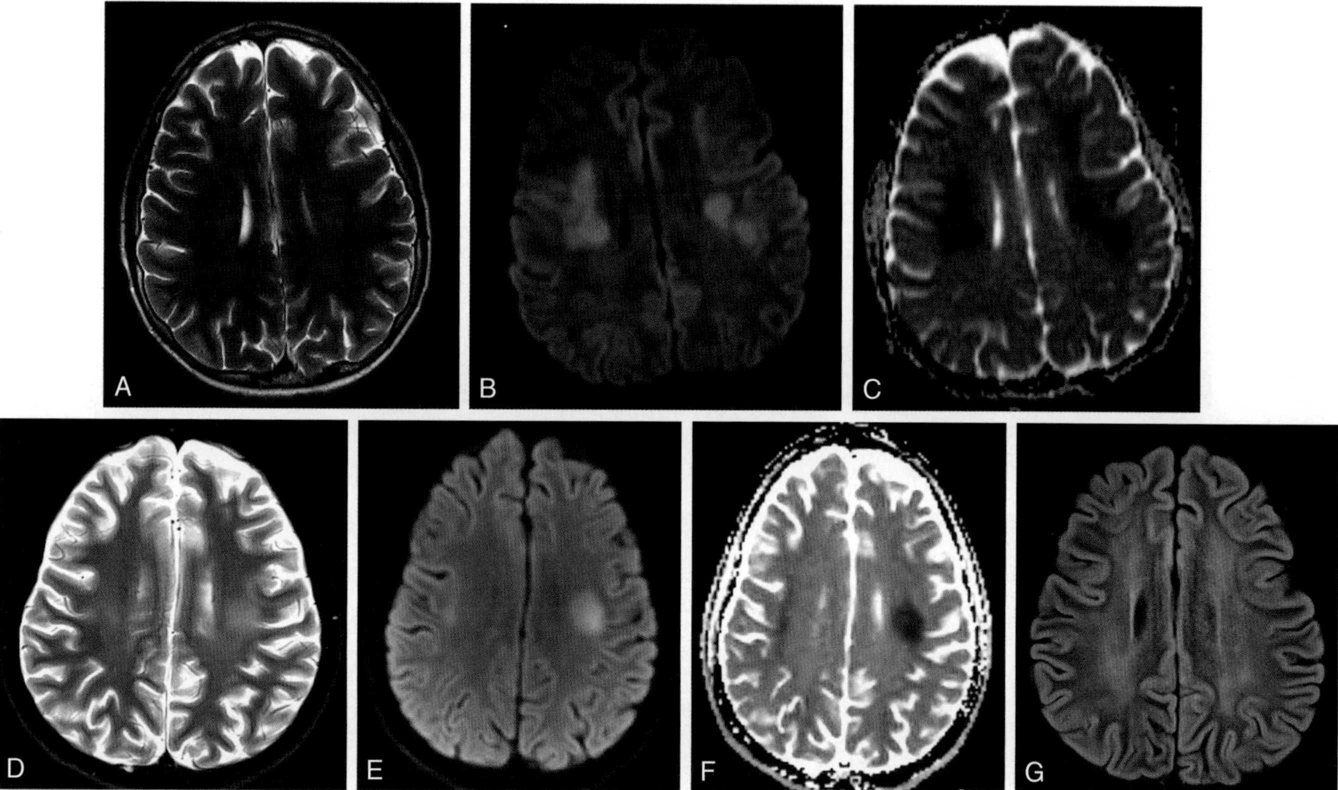

Fig. 4.55 Methotrexate Toxicity. 14-year-old with leukemia and new-onset facial droop. (A) Axial T2W, (B) axial DWI, (C) axial ADC images demonstrate bilateral centrum semiovale diffusion restriction with minimal T2W hyperintensity consistent with acute methotrexate toxicity. (D to F) 11-year-old with leukemia with (D) axial T2W, (E) axial DWI, and (F) axial ADC images demonstrating focal T2W hyperintensity with diffusion restriction in the left centrum semiovale. (G) A 10-year-old with leukemia and confluent white matter FLAIR hyperintensity secondary to chronic methotrexate toxicity.

Key Points

Background

- Methotrexate (MTX) is used in the treatment of acute lymphocytic leukemia. MTX inhibits dihydrofolate reductase, preventing conversion of folic acid to tetrahydrofolic acid and inhibiting cell replication.
- High-dose intravenous and intrathecal MTX are associated with demyelination, white matter necrosis, loss of oligodendroglia, axonal swelling, microcystic encephalomalacia, and atrophy.
- MTX also results in excess homocysteine, which may induce a small vessel vasculopathy.

Clinical

- Incidence of 3% to 10% and depends on dose, frequency, and route of administration
- Stroke-like symptoms (weakness, aphasia, ataxia, sensory deficits), and seizure
- Time from induction to toxicity varies from 2 to 127 weeks; typically occurs 10 to 11 days following intrathecal MTX
- Occurrence of MTX toxicity does not predict likelihood of recurrence with repeat administration

Imaging

- Acute phase: DWI restriction in the centrum semiovale/corona radiata
- Subacute/chronic phase: Patchy or confluent T2/FLAIR hyperintensity. No enhancement
- Unknown why some white matter changes are reversible while others persist or progress

REFERENCE

1. Rollins N, Winick N, Bash R, et al. *AJNR Am J Neuroradiol.* 2004 Nov-Dec;25(10):1688–1695.

DRUG TOXICITY: VIGABATRIN

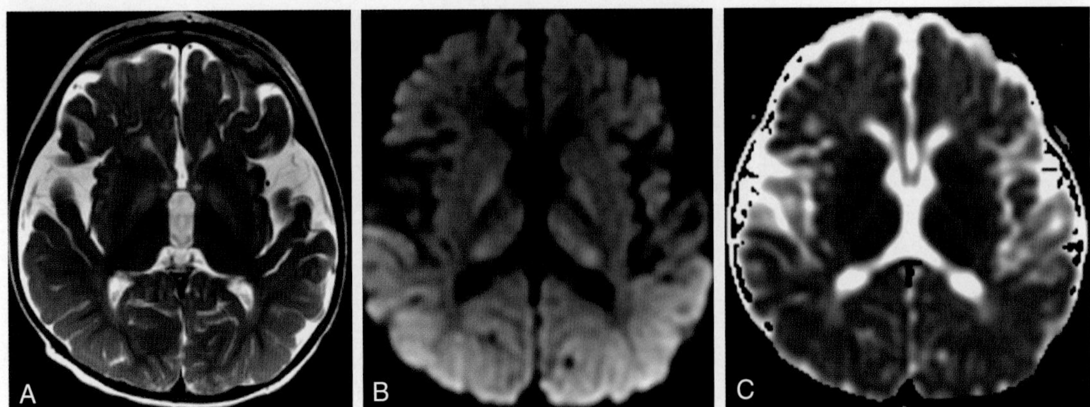

Fig. 4.56 Vigabatrin Toxicity. (A) Axial T2W, (B) axial DWI, and (C) axial ADC images demonstrate symmetric T2W hyperintensity with diffusion restriction in the bilateral globus pallidi and thalami.

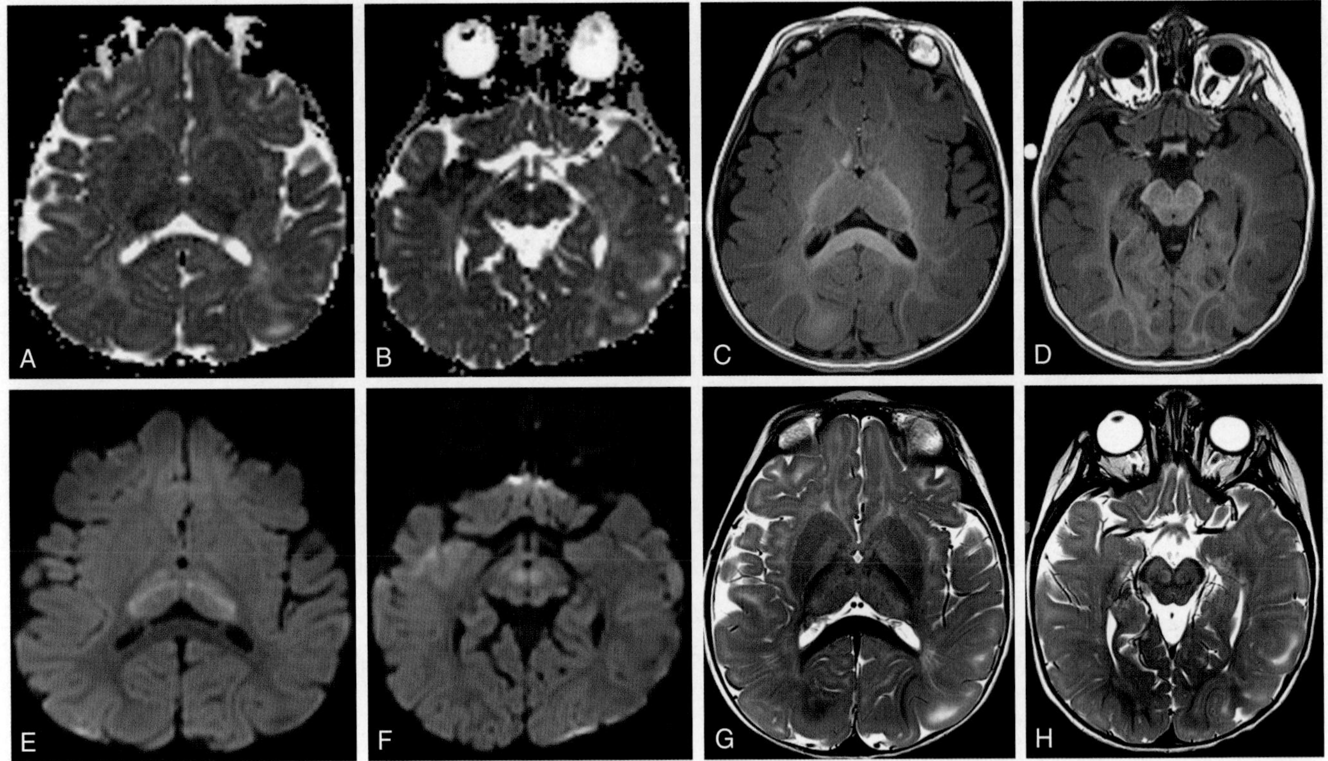

Fig. 4.57 Vigabatrin Toxicity. (A and B) Axial ADC, (C and D) axial T1W, (E and F) axial DWI, and (G and H) axial T2W images demonstrate symmetric T2W hyperintensity with diffusion restriction in the bilateral globus pallidi, thalami, and midbrain.

Key Points

Background

- Vigabatrin is a GABA analog that inhibits GABA transaminase and increases GABA, an inhibitory neurotransmitter

Clinical

- Affects children <2 years; symptoms range from asymptomatic to extrapyramidal symptoms, hypotonia, and bradycardia

Imaging

- Reversible T2W hyperintensity and diffusion restriction involving globus pallidi, thalami, dentate nuclei, brainstem (midbrain), and corpus callosum
- Abnormalities resolve with cessation of vigabatrin

REFERENCE

1. Dracopoulos A, Widjaja E, Raybaud C, et al. Vigabatrin-associated reversible MRI signal changes in patients with infantile spasms. *Epilepsia*. 2010 Jul;51(7):1297–1304.

WERNICKE ENCEPHALOPATHY

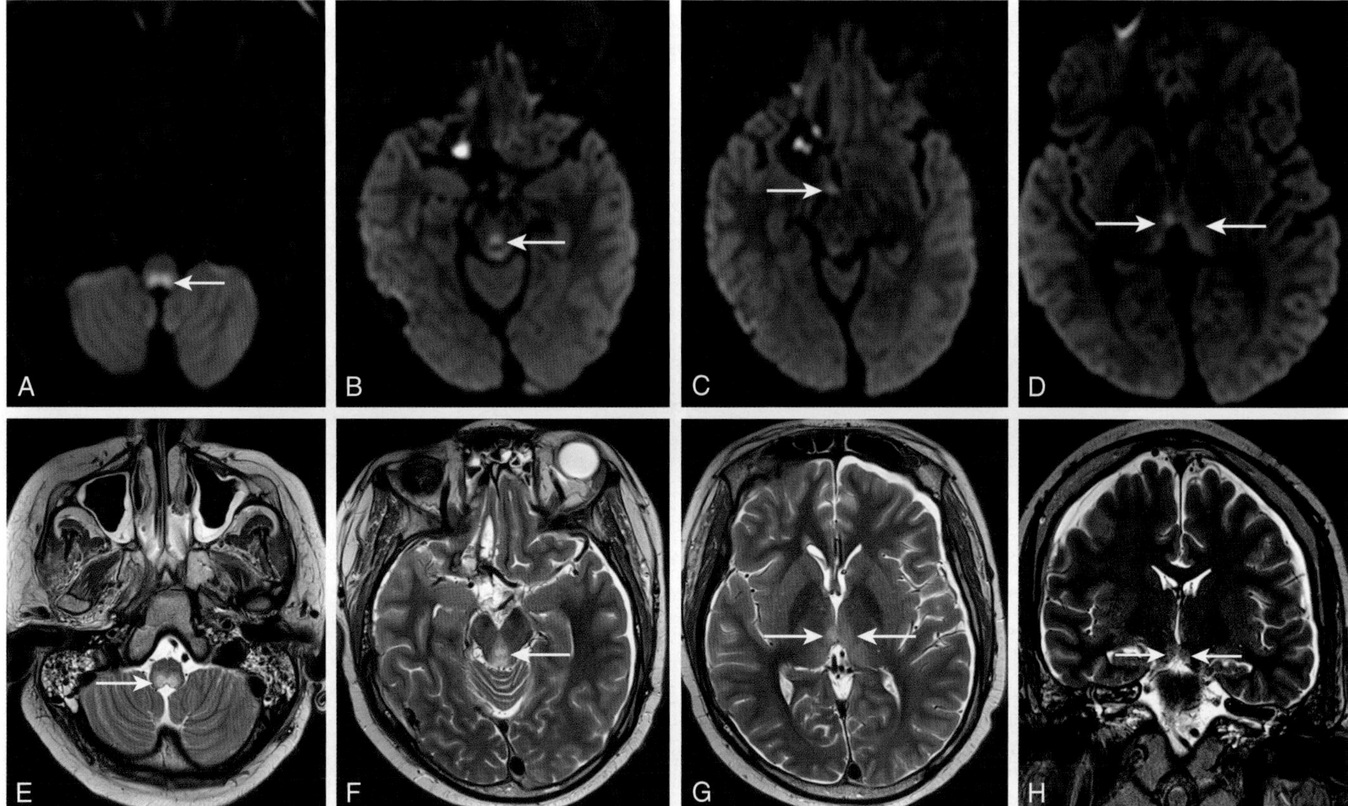

Fig. 4.58 Wernicke Encephalopathy. 15-year-old with past medical history of metastatic retinoblastoma presenting with altered mental status, and unresponsive. (A to D) Axial DWI, (E to H) axial and coronal T2W images demonstrate T2W hyperintensity and diffusion restriction in the medial thalami, mammillary bodies, periaqueductal gray, and dorsal medulla. Focal DWI restriction in the right frontal lobe with volume loss was secondary to previous treatment of intracranial metastasis. Patient was found to be thiamine deficient with serum vitamin B1 measuring 45 nmol/L (normal range 70–180 nmol/L).

Key Points

Background

- Deficiency of thiamine (vitamin B1); can occur with malnutrition and prolonged parenteral nutrition in children

Clinical

- Triad of encephalopathy, ataxia, and ocular dysfunction
- Prognosis depends on time from diagnosis to thiamine supplementation

Imaging

- T2/FLAIR hyperintense signal in the mammillary bodies, medial thalami, tectal plate, and periaqueductal gray matter

REFERENCE

1. Zuccoli G, Siddiqui N, Bailey A, et al. Neuroimaging findings in pediatric Wernicke encephalopathy: a review. *Neuroradiology*. 2010 Jun;52(6):523–529.

HEMOLYTIC UREMIC SYNDROME

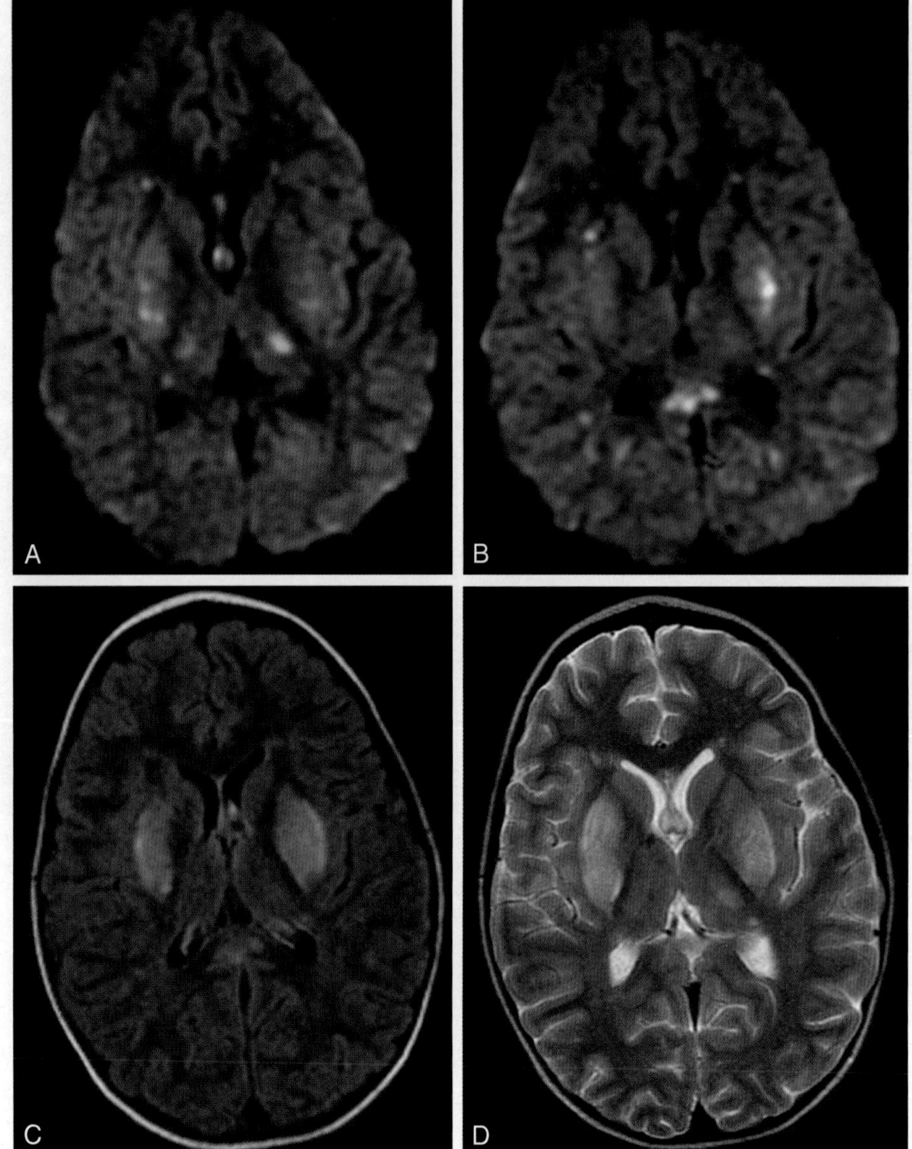

Fig. 4.59 Hemolytic Uremic Syndrome. (A and B) Axial DWI and (C) axial FLAIR and (D) axial T2W images demonstrate small foci of diffusion restriction in the splenium, thalami, and basal ganglia and more confluent T2/FLAIR hyperintensity in the basal ganglia.

Key Points

Background

- Multisystem disorder secondary to capillary thromboses, leading to triad of acute renal failure, hemolytic anemia, and thrombocytopenia.

Clinical

- Most common cause of renal failure in infancy and childhood requiring dialysis. Most common affects children <5 years old.
- Diarrhea-positive HUS is seen in >90% of HUS and is caused by *E. coli* Shiga toxin.
- Long-term mild to severe neurologic impairment occurs in 50% of survivors.

Imaging

- *Symmetric DWI restriction and/or T2/FLAIR hyperintensity in the basal ganglia (usually putamen) and centrum semiovale*

REFERENCE

1. Gitaux C, Krug P, Grevent D, et al. Brain magnetic resonance imaging pattern and outcome in children with haemolytic-uraemic syndrome and neurological impairment treated with eculizumab. *Dev Med Child Neurol.* 2013 Aug;55(8):758–765.

ILLICIT DRUG ABUSE AND DRUG OVERDOSE

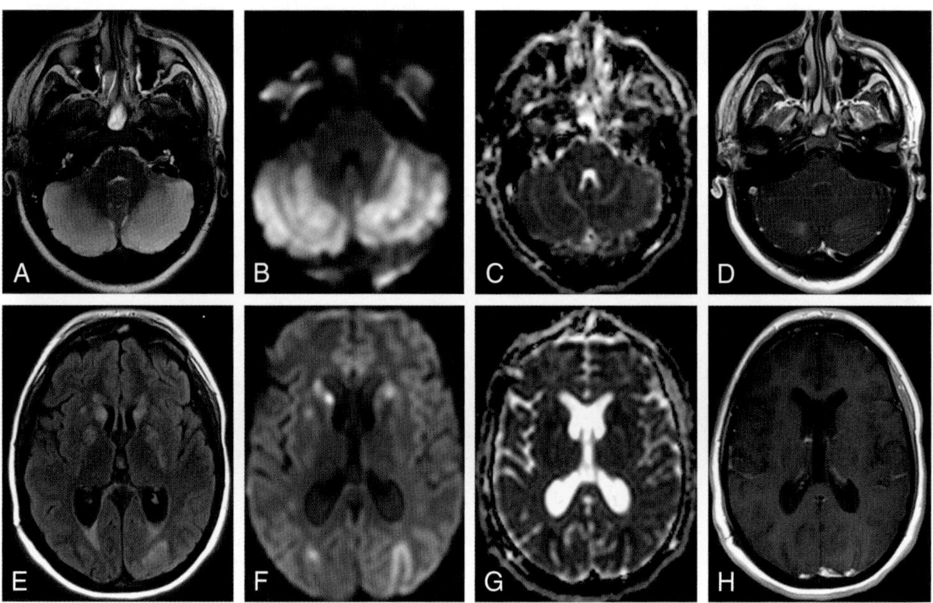

Fig. 4.60 Methadone Toxicity. (A to D, *top row*) Axial T2W, DWI, ADC map and T1W+C, and (E to H, *bottom row*) axial FLAIR, DWI, ADC map, and T1W+C images demonstrate abnormal symmetric nonenhancing T2/FLAIR hyperintensity with diffusion restriction in the cerebellum, caudate, putamen, and posterior occipital lobes indicative of cytotoxic edema from drug toxicity.

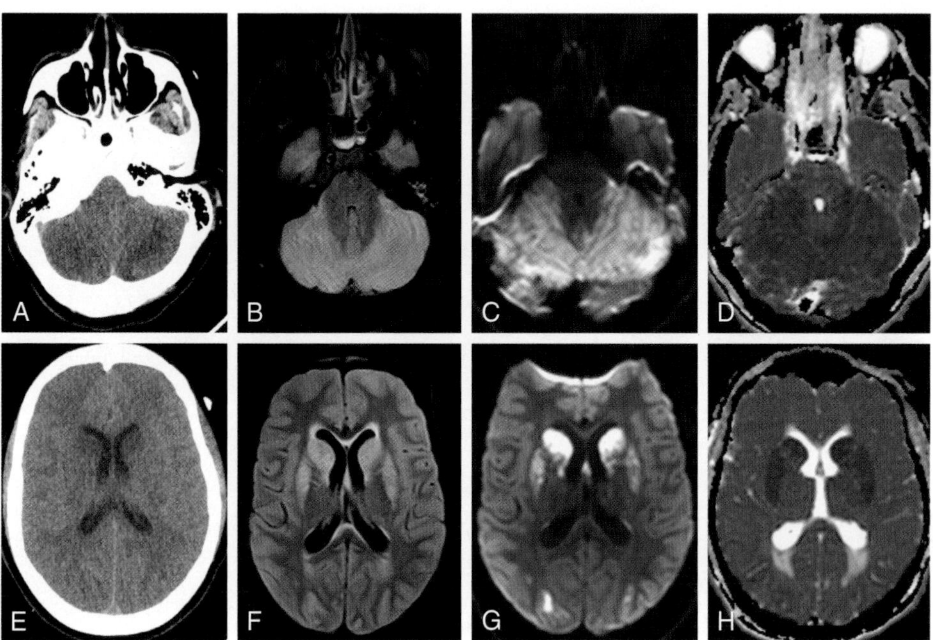

Fig. 4.61 Bupropion Overdose Toxicity. (A and E) Axial CT images demonstrate low density in the bilateral caudate and cerebellar hemispheres. (B and F) Axial FLAIR, (C and G) axial DWI, and (D and H) axial ADC images demonstrate symmetric FLAIR hyperintensity with diffusion restriction in the bilateral basal ganglia, and cerebellar hemispheres.

Key Points

Background

- Although uncommon in pediatric patients, illicit drug abuse and medication overdose can occur.

Imaging

- Patterns of injury include diffuse symmetric subcortical white matter injury, multiple foci of ischemic infarcts in nonarterial territory distributions, and *cerebellar edema and ischemia.*

REFERENCE

1. Shrot S, Poretti A, Tucker EW, et al. Acute brain injury following illicit drug abuse in adolescent and young adult patients: spectrum of neuroimaging findings. *Neuroradiol J.* 2017 Apr;30(2):144–150.

5 Infectious Disorders of the Brain

INTRODUCTION

Background

Central nervous system (CNS) infections can be due to multiple pathogens; however, viral and bacterial infections are the most common (Table 5.1). The CNS injury that results from the infection depends on the timing of infection, pathogen, immune response, and medical treatment.

Viral infections can lead to brain malformations when acquired in utero or lead to meningoencephalitis in infants and children. Congenital infections that occur earlier in pregnancy typically have more severe brain developmental sequelae than those occurring later in pregnancy. Although improvements in laboratory testing have improved detection of viruses, in many viral infections the causative pathogen goes unidentified. Several viral infections are discussed in this chapter, with a focus on those viral infections that cause in utero infections, perinatal infections, and infections later in childhood.

Bacterial infections can lead to meningitis, abscesses, and empyemas and can result in significant injury to the brain. Unfortunately, bacterial meningitis can lead to death in approximately 10% of patients, and survivors remain at high risk for neurologic sequela. Bacterial meningitis is most common in the first year of life, which leads to challenges for clinical diagnosis. Neonates and infants may present with a wide range of nonspecific clinical symptoms of meningitis, including fever, hypothermia, poor feeding, irritability, seizure, and bulging fontanelle. Fortunately, pediatricians are well trained to consider meningitis as the cause of these signs and symptoms and to appropriately perform blood cultures, and lumbar puncture for cerebrospinal fluid (CSF) analysis and culture to diagnose meningitis. Imaging is performed to assess for complications of meningitis, provide supportive evidence of meningitis, and assess for adequacy of treatment. Bacterial meningitis can occur through hematogenous seeding and direct extension from an extracranial source. The bacterial toxins and inflammatory response can subsequently cause complications, including vascular occlusions leading to infarcts, cerebritis, abscess formation, CSF obstruction, and disruption of CSF absorption leading to hydrocephalus.

Atypical infectious pathogens include fungi, tuberculosis, parasites, and amoebic infections. These are much less commonly clinically encountered. They are discussed briefly in this chapter to highlight some features that should alert the radiologist to the potential for an atypical infection.

Imaging

Neuroimaging is often performed to assess safety of lumbar puncture procedure; identify findings supportive of bacterial meningitis when CSF culture is negative; assess for complications of meningitis, including abscess, empyema, infarct, and hydrocephalus; and to reevaluate the status of a known infection.

Ultrasound, CT, and MRI are commonly used neuroimaging techniques for CNS infections. Ultrasound is often used in neonates and infants when the anterior fontanelle remains open. Ultrasound is useful for following ventricular size; however, other imaging findings are often difficult to identify. Noncontrast CT is often used at initial presentation to assess safety of a lumbar puncture and prevent delay in obtaining CSF and starting antibiotics. CT is also commonly performed to assess complications of meningitis including hydrocephalus. Noncontrast CT and contrast-enhanced CT (CECT) are less commonly performed when MRI is available because of the ionizing radiation and reduced accuracy of CT compared to MRI for detection of findings and complications of meningitis. MRI is the modality of choice for definitive evaluation of intracranial infection. This chapter illustrates the common and uncommon causes of CNS infections in children with emphasis on imaging patterns and helpful clinical features, including the age of the patient.

TABLE 5.1 Etiologies of CNS Infections

Developmental Stage	Pathogenic Agents
Congenital (TORCH)	**Viral** Cytomegalovirus (CMV) Toxoplasmosis Herpes simplex virus (HSV) Rubella Syphilis Varicella Human immunodeficiency virus (HIV) Lymphocytic choriomeningitis virus infection Zika virus
Perinatal	**Bacterial** Group B *Streptococcus* (GBS) *Escherichia coli* *Listeria monocytogenes* **Viral** Herpes simplex virus (HSV) Fungal Candidiasis
Infants	**Bacterial** Group B *Streptococcus* *Staphylococcus aureus* *Escherichia coli* *Pseudomonas aeruginosa*
Children/adolescents	**Bacterial** *Haemophilus influenzae* type B *Streptococcus pneumoniae* *Neisseria meningitides* *Mycobacterium tuberculosis*

SUMMARY: CONGENITAL INFECTIONS "TORCHEZ"

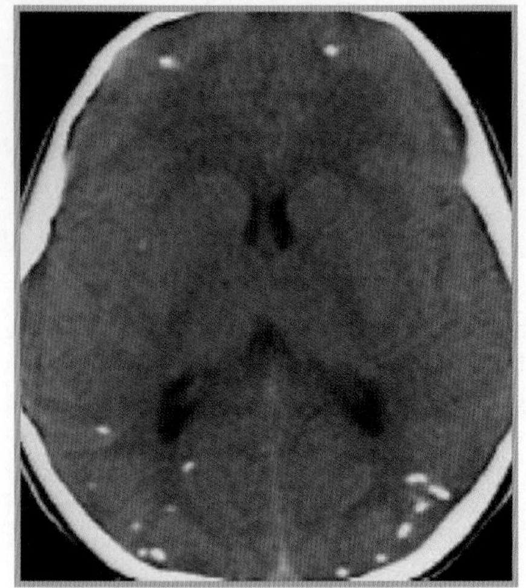

Toxoplasmosis

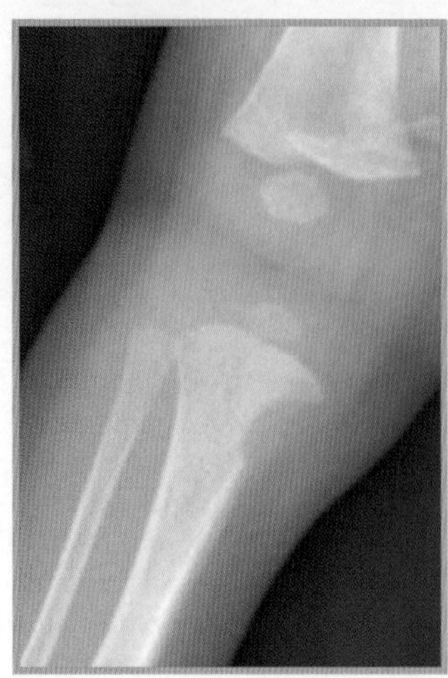

Other (Syphilis, Varicella Zoster Virus, Parvovirus B19)

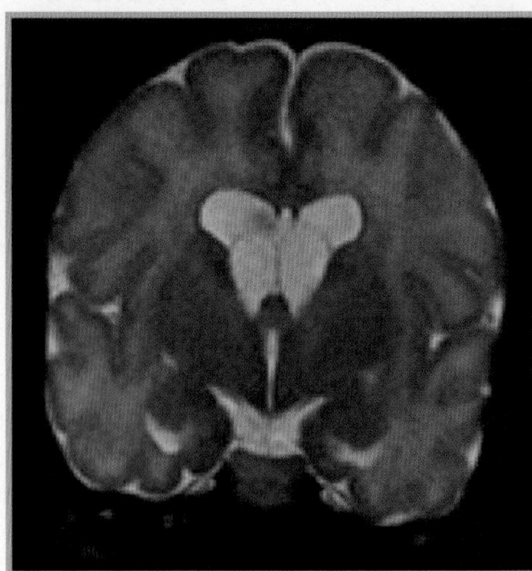

Rubella

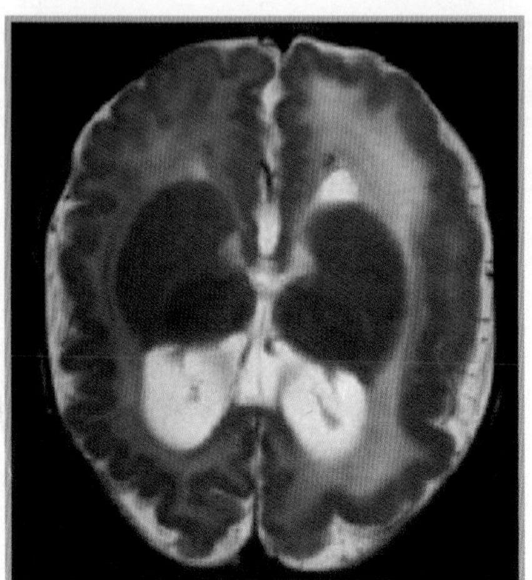

Cytomegalovirus

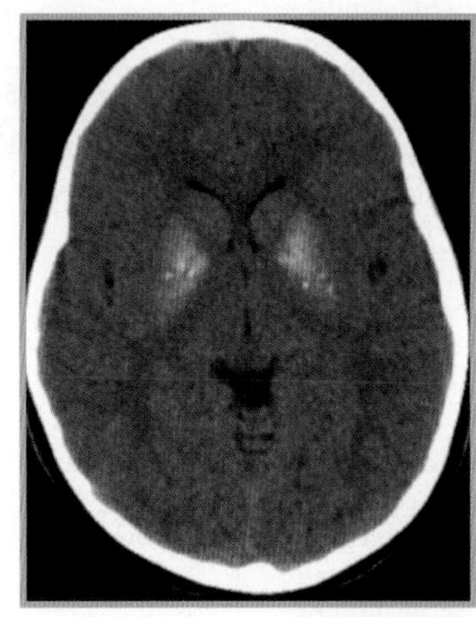

Herpes and Human Immunodeficiency Virus

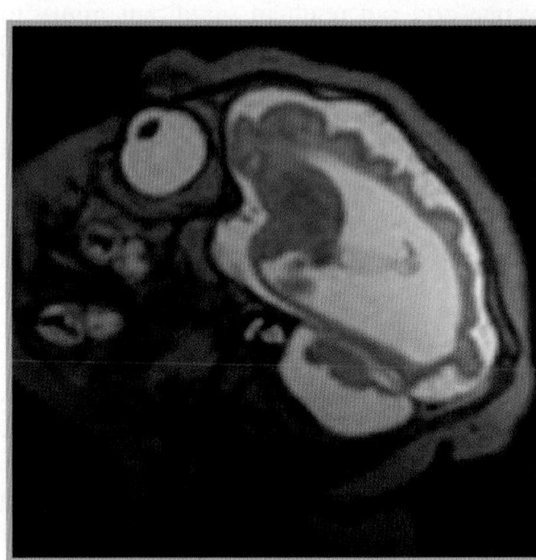

Zika

CONGENITAL CYTOMEGALOVIRUS (CMV) INFECTION

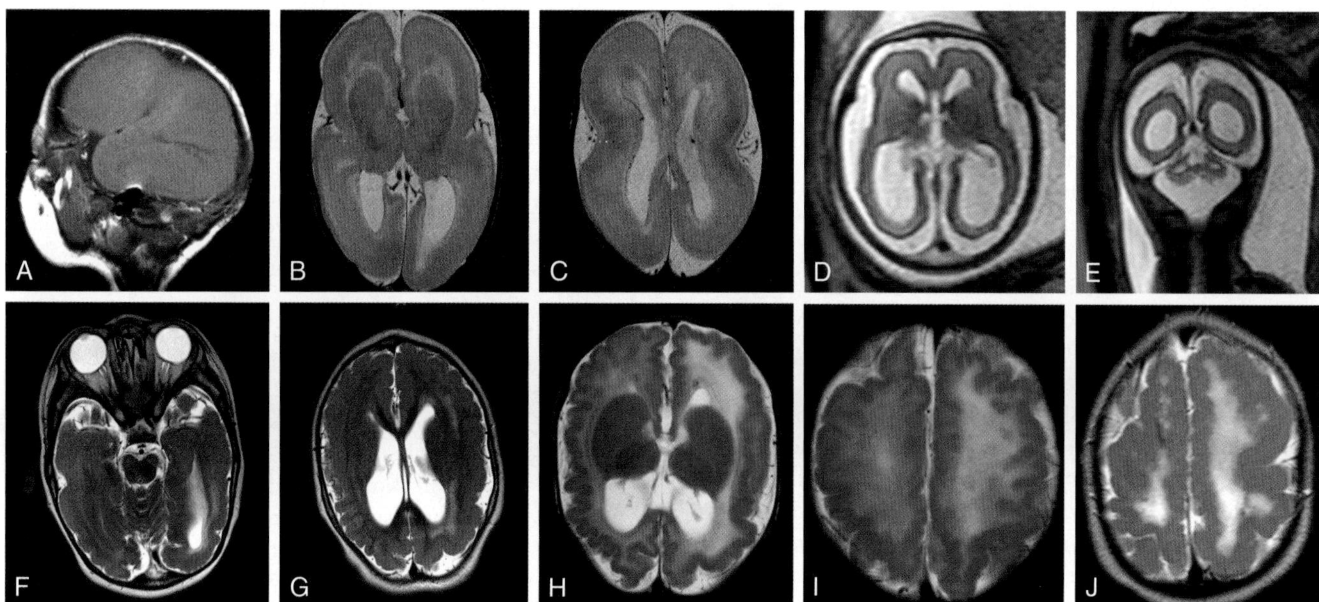

Fig. 5.1 Congenital Cytomegalovirus (CMV): Cortical Malformations. (A to C) Sagittal T1W (A) and (B and C) axial T2W images demonstrate an infant with classical lissencephaly indicative of a first trimester of early second trimester infection and dysmorphic central gray matter. (D and E) Axial and coronal T2W fetal MR images at 29 weeks' gestation demonstrate diffuse polymicrogyria indicative of a second trimester infection in addition to lateral ventriculomegaly from severe loss of white matter, and T2W hyperintense cerebellar destructive lesions. (F to J) Axial T2W images in multiple patients demonstrating diffuse cortical malformations and associated leukodystrophy.

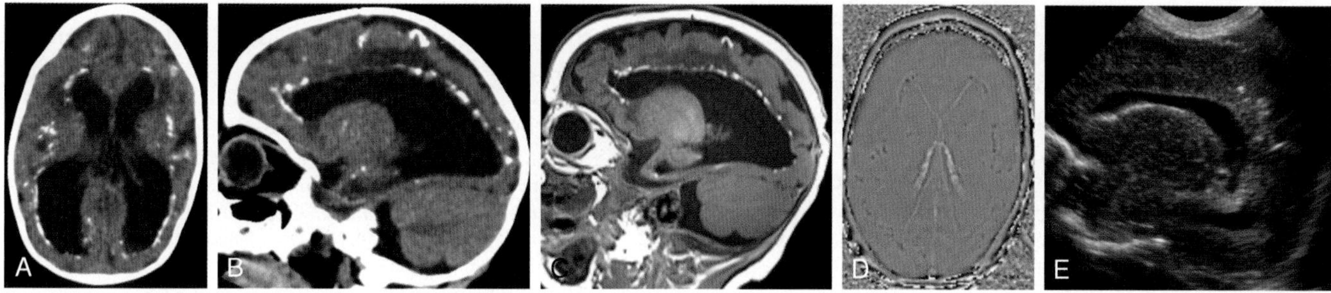

Fig. 5.2 Congenital Cytomegalovirus (CMV): Calcifications. (A to D) A 4-month-old with congenital CMV infection. (A and B) Axial and sagittal reformat CT, (C) sagittal T1W, and (D) axial SWI phase map demonstrate parenchymal calcifications (CT hyperdense foci; T1W hyperintense foci and SWI phase map hypointense foci) with predilection for the periventricular white matter. (E) Sagittal ultrasound in a 6-day-old with congenital CMV demonstrates multiple left posterior periventricular hyperechoic foci due to calcification.

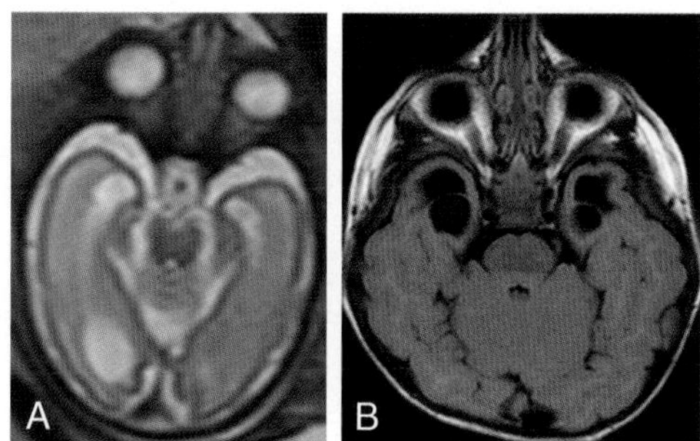

Fig. 5.3 Congenital Cytomegalovirus (CMV): Temporal Cyst. (A) Axial T2W fetal MRI and (B) postnatal axial FLAIR image demonstrate bilateral temporal pole cysts.

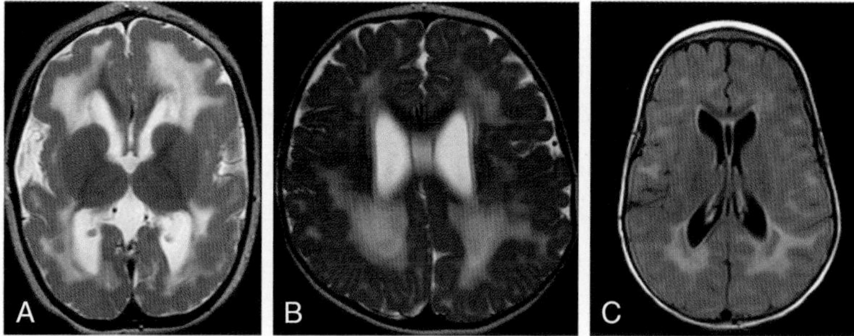

Fig. 5.4 Congenital Cytomegalovirus (CMV): Leukodystrophy. (A to C) Axial T2W and axial FLAIR images in multiple patients demonstrate confluent white matter hyperintensity indicative of leukodystrophy. Polymicrogyria is also present in the first patient (A).

Key Points

Background

- Cytomegalovirus (CMV) is a member of the herpesvirus family and is acquired by direct contact of mucosal surfaces with the virus via infected body fluids and, similar to other herpesviruses, has the potential for latency and reactivation.
- Congenital CMV is the most common congenital viral infection in children and most common cause for nongenetic sensorineural hearing loss.
- Maternal-fetal transmission is primarily due to a primary maternal CMV infection, which has a 32% risk of transmission compared to 1% with recurrent CMV infection. Primary maternal infection results in greater number of symptomatic infants.
- Approximately 10% of congenital CMV infections are symptomatic at birth. Clinical findings include hepatosplenomegaly, petechiae, jaundice, small size for gestational age, microcephaly, sensorineural hearing loss, seizure, and chorioretinitis. Laboratory studies include thrombocytopenia, elevated liver transaminases, and elevated direct and indirect bilirubin.
- Long-term neurologic outcomes include cerebral palsy, developmental delay, intellectual disability, sensorineural hearing loss, seizures, and vision impairment.
- Sensorineural hearing loss is present in 33% to 50% of symptomatic infants, has a delayed onset in 18% to 30%, and is bilateral in 71% of symptomatic and 43% of asymptomatic infants. Progressive hearing loss occurs in 18% to 63% of patients, and hearing loss becomes severe to profound in 78% of affected ears.
- Timing of infection during pregnancy correlates with the severity of disease.
  - Presence of abnormal imaging findings portends abnormal neurodevelopmental outcome.
- Confirmed diagnosis is made by detection of CMV with polymerase chain reaction (PCR) or shell vial culture of newborn saliva, or urine within 3 weeks of birth. Intrauterine infection may be diagnosed with PCR of amniotic fluid.
- Treatment with antiviral medication may improve hearing and developmental outcomes.

Imaging

- Normal fetal MRI and normal fetal neurosonology are good predictors of favorable neurodevelopmental outcome.
  - Third trimester or perinatal infection may result in an anatomically normal appearing brain.
- Fetal MRI is superior to fetal US, especially regarding dysplasia and myelination abnormalities.
- MRI
  - Ventricles: Ventriculomegaly, ventriculitis (rare), intraventricular septations, and hemorrhage
  - Parenchyma
    - *Cortical malformations:* Lissencephaly, polymicrogyria, schizencephaly
      - Early infections around 16 to 18 weeks of gestation result in microlissencephaly.
      - Infections around 18 to 24 weeks of gestation may cause polymicrogyria (most common).
    - *Leukodystrophy*: Periventricular T2W hyperintensity
    - *Temporal polar cysts and germinolytic cysts*
    - *Calcifications* (predominantly periventricular, may also be seen in central gray matter and elsewhere in white matter)
    - Parenchymal volume loss; porencephaly
    - Cerebellar dysplasia/hypoplasia
    - Hemorrhage
- Differential Diagnosis (DDx): Other TORCH infections, and Aicardi syndrome

REFERENCES

1. Capretti MG, Lanari M, Tani G, et al. Role of cerebral ultrasound and magnetic resonance imaging in newborns with congenital cytomegalovirus infection. *Brain Dev.* 2014 Mar;36(3):203–211.
2. Nickerson JP, Richner B, Santy K, et al. Neuroimaging of pediatric intracranial infection–part 2: TORCH, viral, fungal, and parasitic infections. *J Neuroimaging.* 2012 Apr;22(2):e52–e63.
3. Diogo MC, Glatter S, Binder J, et al. The MRI spectrum of congenital cytomegalovirus infection. *Prenat Diagn.* 2020 Jan;40(1):110–124.

CONGENITAL ZIKA VIRUS INFECTION

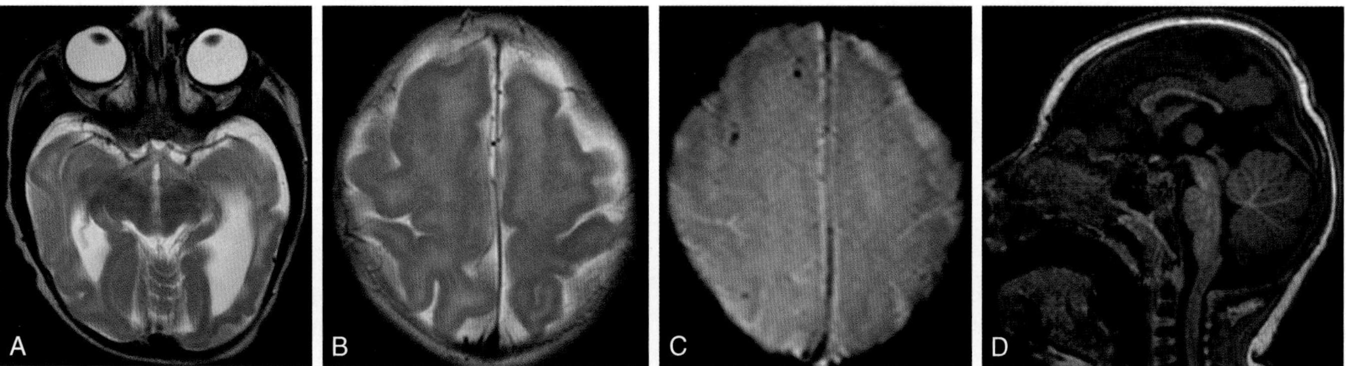

Fig. 5.5 Congenital Zika: 9–month-old with severe microcephaly. (A and B) Axial T2W, (C) axial GRE, and (D) sagittal T1W images demonstrate severe microcephaly, simplified gyral pattern, and peripheral white matter susceptibility foci indicative of calcifications.

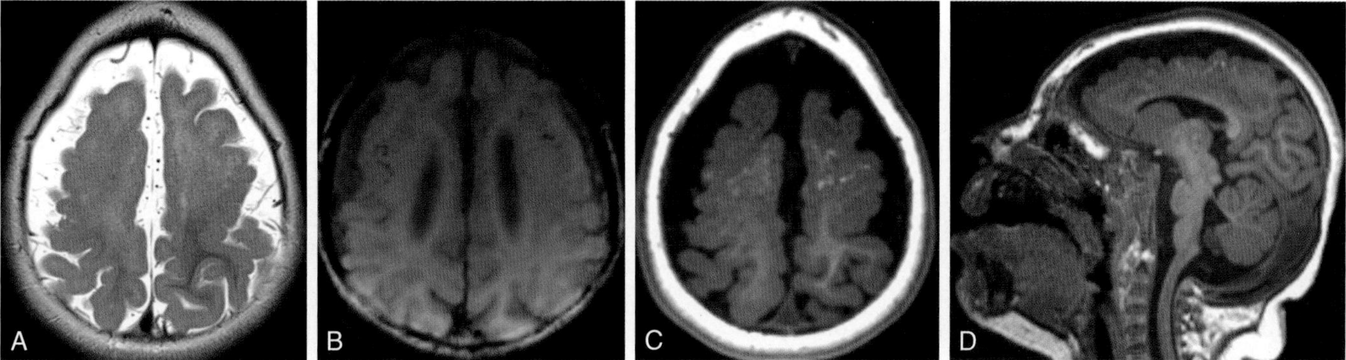

Fig. 5.6 Congenital Zika: 10-month-old with severe microcephaly. (A) Axial T2W, (B) axial SWI, (C and D) axial and sagittal T1W images demonstrate severe microcephaly, frontal lobe cortical malformation, and peripheral white matter foci with susceptibility and T1W hyperintense calcifications.

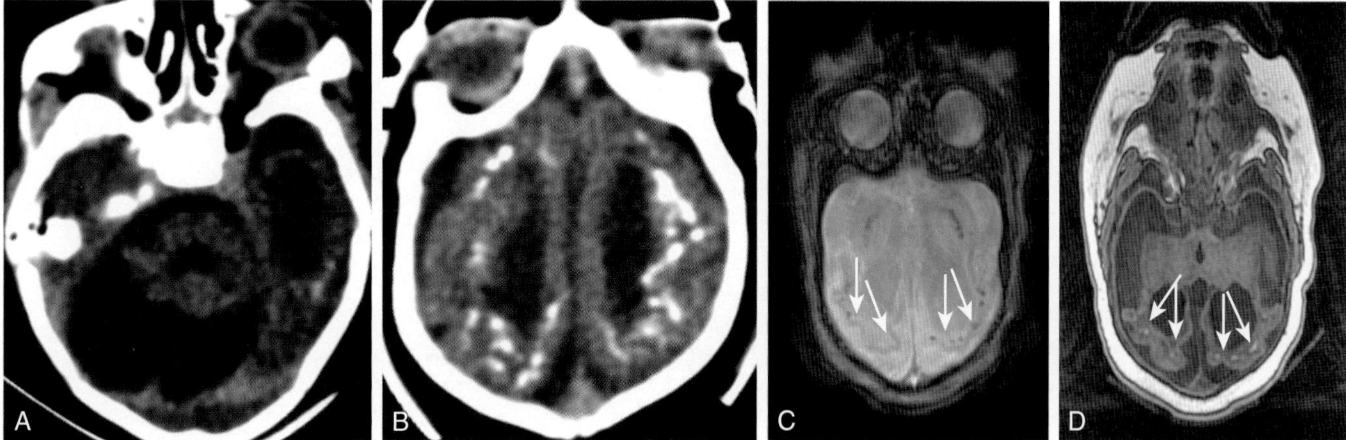

Fig. 5.7 Congenital Zika. (A and B) Axial noncontrast CT, (C) axial SWI, (D) axial T1W images demonstrate microcephaly, cerebellar hypoplasia, and numerous foci of calcification *(arrows)* predominantly at the gray-white junction.

Key Points

Background

- First discovered in 1947 in Zika Forest in Uganda
- Single-strand RNA virus transmitted by female *Aedes aegypti* mosquito
- Endemic in Asia, and Africa
- Historical outbreaks have occurred; large outbreak in the Americas in 2014–2016
- 80% of infections are asymptomatic, 20% are symptomatic
    - Fever, headache, joint/muscle pain, rash, conjunctivitis, and Guillain-Barré (rare)
- Maternal infection may cross the fetal placenta barrier and cause fetal neural infection; fetuses may be normal despite maternal infection
    - Maternal infection may occur via the mosquito transmission or by unprotected sex with an infected partner, even if partner is asymptomatic
- Zika infection in the first trimester has a 1% to 13% risk of microcephaly
- Confirmed diagnosis is made by positive detection of Zika virus in the infant serum, urine, or CSF within first 2 days after birth. A probable diagnosis is made in the setting of negative PCR with positive immunoglobulin M (IgM) antibodies. Diagnosis is excluded if both PCR and IgM are negative.

Imaging

- Brain
    - *Microcephaly*, overlapping sutures with secondary redundancy of scalp tissue
    - Ventricles: Ventriculomegaly, intraventricular septations especially in occipital horns, subependymal cysts
    - Parenchyma
        - Cortical malformation: Lissencephaly/microlissencephaly, pachygyria, polymicrogyria
        - Parenchymal volume loss
        - *Calcifications predominantly and characteristically peripheral* at gray-white junction, may also be seen in central gray matter and elsewhere in white matter (less common in posterior fossa)
        - Corpus callosum: Agenesis/dysgenesis/hypoplasia
        - Cerebellar dysplasia/hypoplasia
        - Brainstem hypoplasia/volume loss
- Other
    - Arthrogryposis
    - Spine: Spinal cord volume loss, decreased number of ventral nerve roots
    - Orbits: Herniation of orbital fat into the cranial vault, intraocular calcifications, coloboma, cataracts, microphthalmia, and lens subluxation

REFERENCES

1. Zare Mehrjardi M, Keshavarz E, Poretti A, et al. Neuroimaging findings of Zika virus infection: a review article. *Jpn J Radiol.* 2016 Dec;34(12):765–770.
2. Henderson AD, Ventura CV, Huisman TAGM, et al. Characterization of Visual Pathway Abnormalities in Infants With Congenital Zika Syndrome Using Computed Tomography and Magnetic Resonance Imaging. *J Neuroophthalmol.* 2020 Oct 27.
3. de Souza AS, de Oliveira-Szjenfeld PS, de Oliveira Melo AS. Imaging findings in congenital Zika virus infection syndrome: an update. *Childs Nerv Syst.* 2018 Jan;34(1):85–93.
4. Soares de Oliveira-Szejnfeld P, Levine D, Melo AS, et al. Congenital Brain Abnormalities and Zika Virus: What the Radiologist Can Expect to See Prenatally and Postnatally. *Radiology.* 2016 Oct;281(1):203–218.
5. Aragao MFVV, Brainer-Lima AM, Holanda AC, et al. Spectrum of Spinal Cord, Spinal Root, and Brain MRI Abnormalities in Congenital Zika Syndrome with and without Arthrogryposis. *AJNR Am J Neuroradiol.* 2017 May;38(5):1045–1053.
6. Johansson MA, Mier-y-Teran-Romero L, Reefhuis J, et al. Zika and the Risk of Microcephaly. *N Engl J Med.* 2016 Jul 7;375(1):1–4.

CONGENITAL TOXOPLASMOSIS

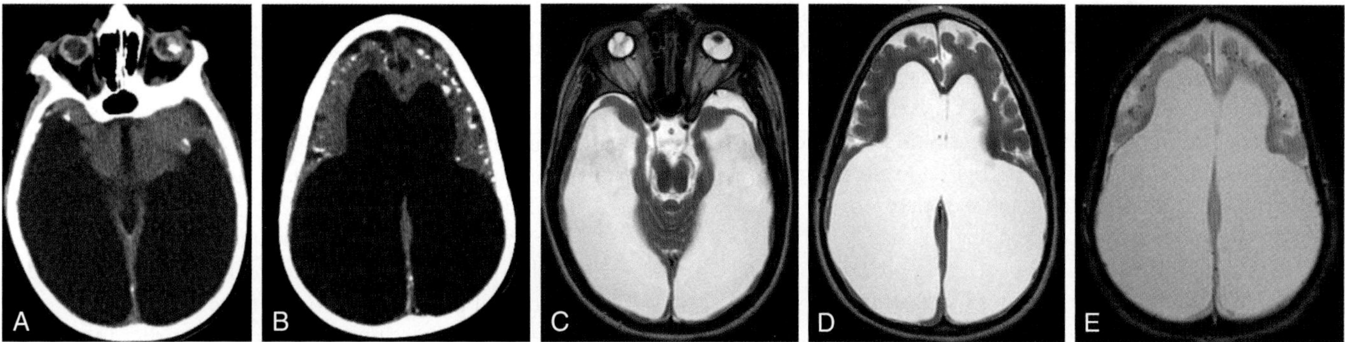

Fig. 5.8 Congenital Toxoplasmosis. (A and B) Axial noncontrast CT, (C and D) axial T2W, and (E) axial GRE images demonstrate severe microphthalmia with calcifications, lateral ventriculomegaly greatest at the atria, severe cerebral volume loss, and multiple parenchymal calcifications.

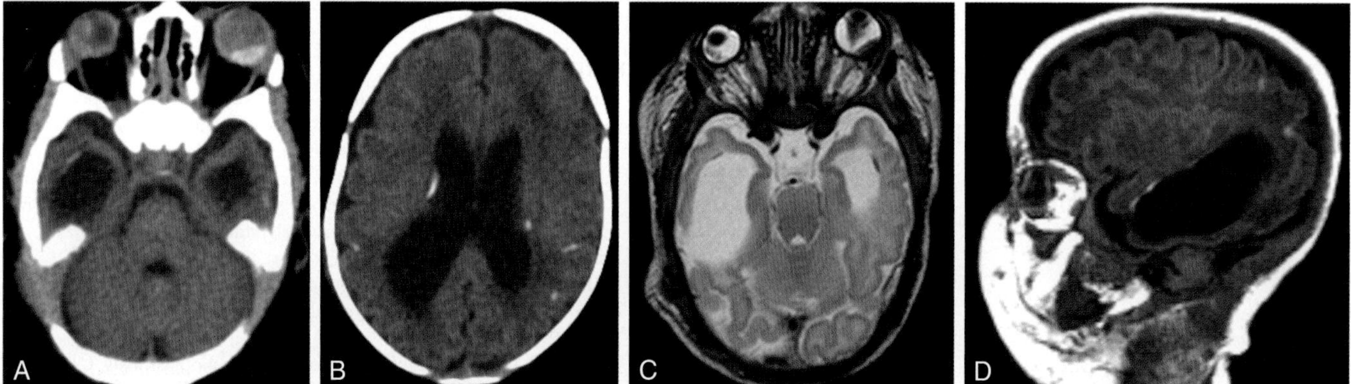

Fig. 5.9 Congenital Toxoplasmosis. (A and B) Axial noncontrast CT, (C) axial T2W, and (D) sagittal T1W images demonstrate multiple foci of scattered calcification within the brain parenchyma, ventriculomegaly, which is less severe in this patient and is greatest in the temporal and atrial regions, microphthalmia (right worse than left) with intraocular hemorrhage.

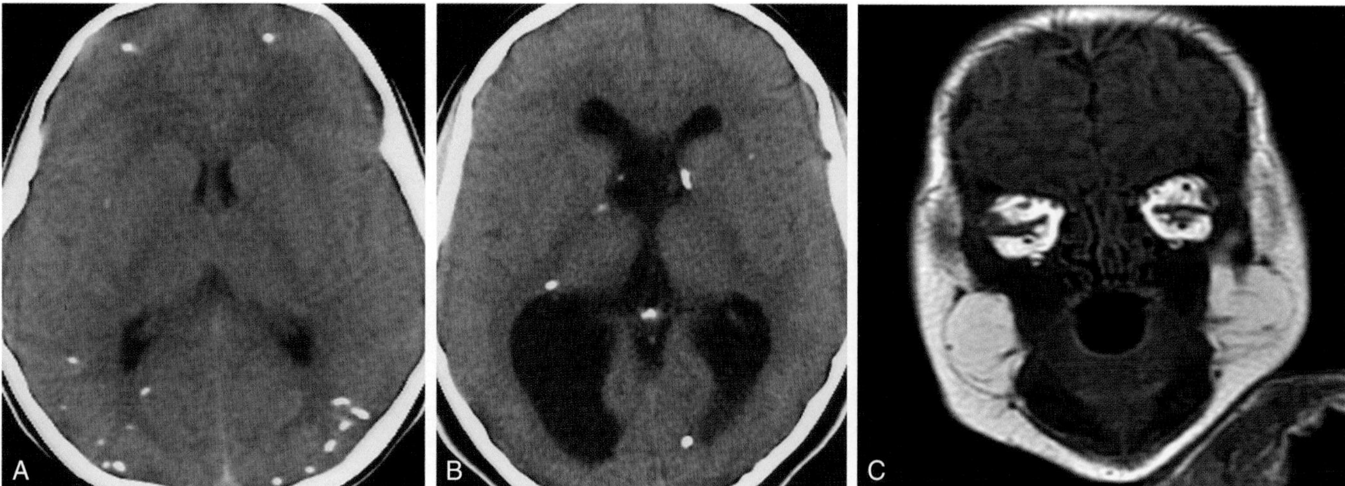

Fig. 5.10 Congenital Toxoplasmosis. (A and B) Axial noncontrast CT and (C) coronal T1W images demonstrate multiple foci of scattered calcification within the brain parenchyma, ventriculomegaly more affecting the right lateral ventricle, and severe ocular injury seen in (C) as collapsed slit-like globes.

Key Points

Background

- *Toxoplasma gondii* is a protozoan parasite with infection occurring through infected domestic cats, ingestion of meats containing viable parasite, or contaminated water or soil.
- Maternal infection may be asymptomatic; infection may cross the fetal placenta barrier and result in adverse neurologic and ophthalmologic sequelae.
  - In utero infection occurs in approximately 1/1000 to 1/10,000 births.
  - Transplacental infection rates increase during progressing pregnancy.
  - Infection later in pregnancy is more common but results in less severe disease.
- If the fetus is infected before 20 weeks of gestation, findings may be severe, including the presence of microcephaly, hydrocephalus, tetraparesis, seizures, cognitive impairment, migrational disorders, microphthalmia, and blindness due to chorioretinitis.
- Confirmed diagnosis is made with positive IgG with positive IgM and/or IgA, positive PCR, increasing IgG titers in the first year or relative to maternal IgG titer, or positive IgG beyond 12 months.

Imaging

- Classic triad:
  - *Chorioretinitis, hydrocephalus,* and *intracranial calcification* occur in a minority of patients; the majority of infected neonates have subclinical infection.
- Ventricles
  - *Ventriculomegaly*, hydrocephalus (rare with infection after second trimester); ventriculitis that causes hydrocephalus. Predilection for dilatation of the atria of the ventricles
- Parenchyma
  - Parenchymal volume loss, parenchymal injury/necrosis
    - Parenchymal injury may be severe and diffuse with early in utero infection
    - Volume loss may be mild, especially in late in utero infection
  - *Calcifications* are scattered throughout the basal ganglia, periventricular white matter, and cortical and subcortical parenchyma without site predilection
    - Larger calcification associated with earlier infection
  - Migrational anomalies are not present
    - Cysts
- Orbits
  - Microphthalmia, chorionic calcifications, and lens deformity

REFERENCES

1. Nickerson JP, Richner B, Santy K, et al. Neuroimaging of pediatric intracranial infection–part 2: TORCH, viral, fungal, and parasitic infections. *J Neuroimaging*. 2012 Apr;22(2):e52–e63.
2. Barkovich AJ, Raybaud C. *Pediatric Neuroimaging*: LWW; 2011:1144.
3. Neuberger I, Garcia J, Meyers ML, Feygin T, Bulas DI, Mirsky DM. Imaging of congenital central nervous system infections. *Pediatr Radiol.* 2018 Apr;48(4):513–523.
4. Malinger G, Werner H, Rodriguez Leonel JC, et al. Prenatal brain imaging in congenital toxoplasmosis. *Prenat Diagn.* 2011 Sep;31(9):881–886.
5. Diebler C, Dusser A, Dulac O. Congenital toxoplasmosis. Clinical and neuroradiological evaluation of the cerebral lesions. *Neuroradiology*. 1985;27(2):125–130.

CONGENITAL RUBELLA

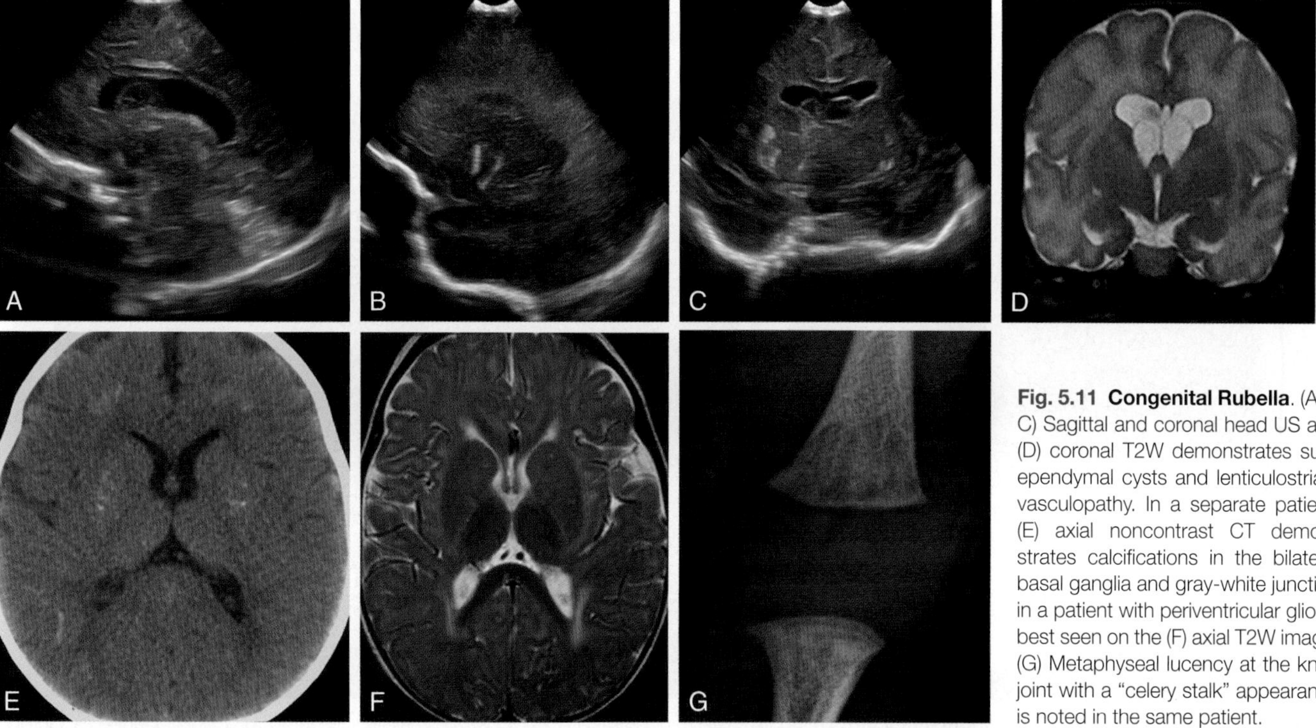

Fig. 5.11 Congenital Rubella. (A to C) Sagittal and coronal head US and (D) coronal T2W demonstrates subependymal cysts and lenticulostriate vasculopathy. In a separate patient, (E) axial noncontrast CT demonstrates calcifications in the bilateral basal ganglia and gray-white junction in a patient with periventricular gliosis best seen on the (F) axial T2W image. (G) Metaphyseal lucency at the knee joint with a "celery stalk" appearance is noted in the same patient.

Key Points

Background

- Caused by a togavirus of the genus *Rubivirus*, which can infect and replicate within the placenta.
- Congenital rubella is rare in countries with rubella immunization.
- Maternal-fetal transmission occurs from maternal viremia and placental transmission and is spread through the fetal vasculature. The greatest risk of maternal-fetal transmission risk occurs during the first 10 weeks of gestation.
- Clinical manifestations depend on timing of maternal infection. Maternal infection prior to 8 weeks typically results in cardiac and eye defects and hearing loss in maternal infections up to 18 weeks. Infections after 18 to 20 weeks are unlikely to cause defects.
- Congenital rubella syndrome classically includes cataracts/glaucoma (25%), congenital heart disease (50% of patients; usually patent ductus arteriosus or peripheral pulmonary artery stenosis), and sensorineural hearing loss (66%) but can also include:
  - Brain injury, microcephaly
  - Neurocognitive, motor abnormality
  - Liver, spleen, lung, hormonal abnormalities
  - Low birth weight
  - Skin rash (blueberry muffin rash) due to extramedullary hematopoiesis
- Diagnosis of congenital rubella syndrome made when one or more clinical signs or symptoms are present and laboratory evidence of congenital rubella infection through detection of rubella IgM antibodies, infant rubella IgG antibody that does not drop at an expected rate of twofold dilution per month, culture isolation of rubella virus, or PCR positive testing for rubella.

Imaging

- Ventricles: Ventriculomegaly, *subependymal cysts*
- Parenchyma
  - Parenchymal volume loss, parenchymal injury/necrosis may be due to vasculitis
    - Parenchymal injury may be severe and diffuse with early in utero infection
    - Volume loss may be mild, especially in late in utero infection
    - White matter T2 signal abnormality from edema, gliosis, necrosis, myelination abnormalities
  - *Calcifications* in basal ganglia, periventricular white matter, cortex
  - *Migrational anomalies are not a feature*
  - Cysts
- Orbits: Chorioretinitis
- Bones: Radiolucent metaphyseal bands known as "celery stalk metaphysis"

REFERENCES

1. Nickerson JP, Richner B, Santy K, et al. Neuroimaging of pediatric intracranial infection–part 2: TORCH, viral, fungal, and parasitic infections. *J Neuroimaging*. 2012 Apr;22(2):e52–e63.
2. Barkovich AJ, Raybaud C. *Pediatric Neuroimaging*: LWW; 2011:1144.
3. Yamashita Y, Matsuishi T, Murakami Y, et al. Neuroimaging findings (ultrasonography, CT, MRI) in 3 infants with congenital rubella syndrome. *Pediatr Radiol*. 1991;21(8):547–549.
4. Neuberger I, Garcia J, Meyers ML, et al. Imaging of congenital central nervous system infections. *Pediatr Radiol*. 2018 Apr;48(4):513–523.

CONGENITAL HUMAN IMMUNODEFICIENCY VIRUS (HIV) INFECTION

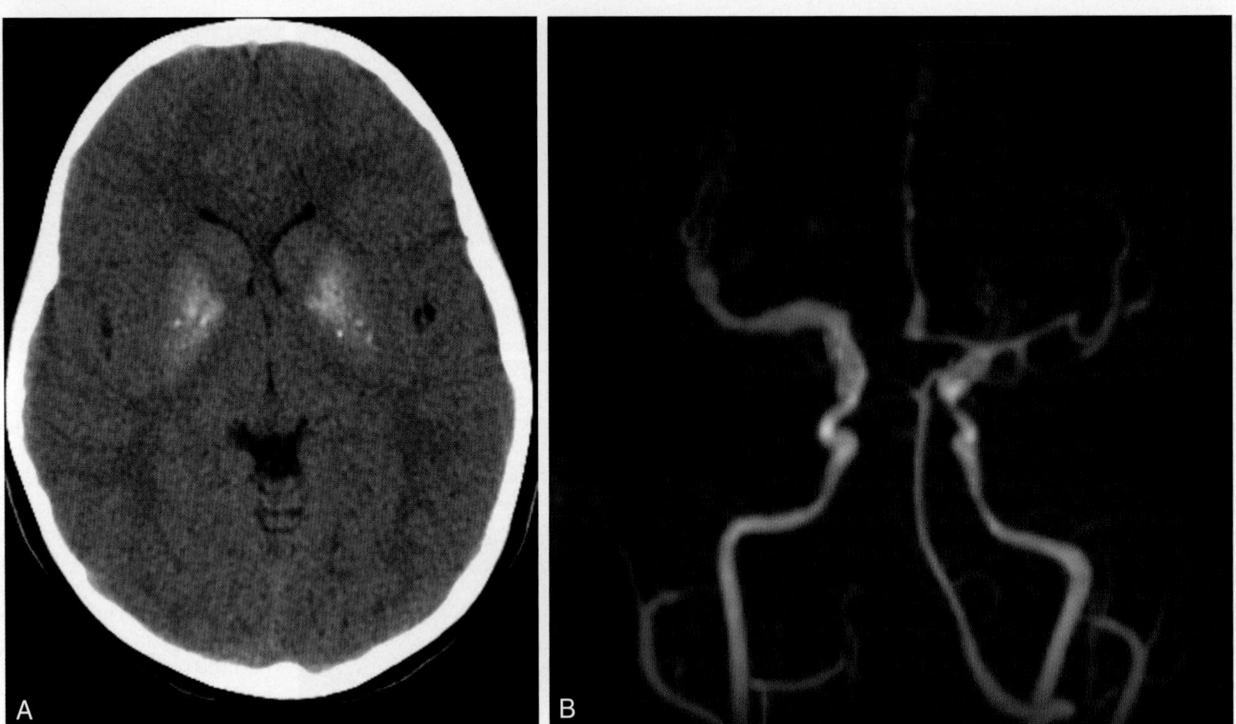

Fig. 5.12 Congenital Human Immunodeficiency Virus (HIV). (A) Axial noncontrast CT demonstrates calcification in bilateral basal ganglia. (B) Coronal MRA volumetric image demonstrating vascular ectasia and irregular fusiform aneurysms of the internal carotid arteries, right middle cerebral artery, and left anterior cerebral artery.

Key Points

Background

- Vertical transmission may occur at any time during gestation, during delivery (majority), and via breastfeeding.
- Congenital HIV has remarkably decreased in the developed world due to screening, mitigation measures including antiretroviral, and avoiding breastfeeding but remains a significant public health issue elsewhere, especially sub-Saharan Africa.
- Manifestations in neonates and children differ significantly from those encountered in the adult population.
  - Neonates are commonly asymptomatic.
  - Infants and children may go on to develop variety of symptoms, including systemic symptoms and neurologic symptoms in up to 50%, including such as encephalopathy, spasticity, motor weakness, seizures, and microcephaly.
  - Opportunistic infections are less common than in adult acquired HIV but CMV, progressive multifocal leukoencephalopathy (PML), varicella zoster virus (VZV), and fungal infection may occur.
  - CNS lymphoma occurs in a minority.

Imaging

- Ventricles: Ventriculomegaly
- Parenchyma
  - *Calcifications of the basal ganglia and subcortical white matter* with congenital HIV; degree of calcification correlates with viral load
  - Volume loss (long term)
- Vascular (long term)
  - Vasculopathy with alternating stenosis and ectasia/aneurysmal dilatation
  - May result in infarction, and/or hemorrhage
- Other (long term): Lymphadenopathy, lymphoepithelial cysts
- Differential Diagnosis of basal ganglia calcification: Aicardi-Goutieres, Cockayne syndrome, sequela of hypoxic ischemic injury, Down syndrome, hyper- or hypoparathyroidism, mitochondrial disorders, toxoplasmosis, and idiopathic

REFERENCES

1. Nickerson JP, Richner B, Santy K, et al. Neuroimaging of pediatric intracranial infection–part 2: TORCH, viral, fungal, and parasitic infections. *J Neuroimaging.* 2012 Apr;22(2):e52–e63.
2. George R, Andronikou S, du Plessis J, et al. Central nervous system manifestations of HIV infection in children. *Pediatr Radiol.* 2009 Jun;39(6):575–585.

PARECHOVIRUS

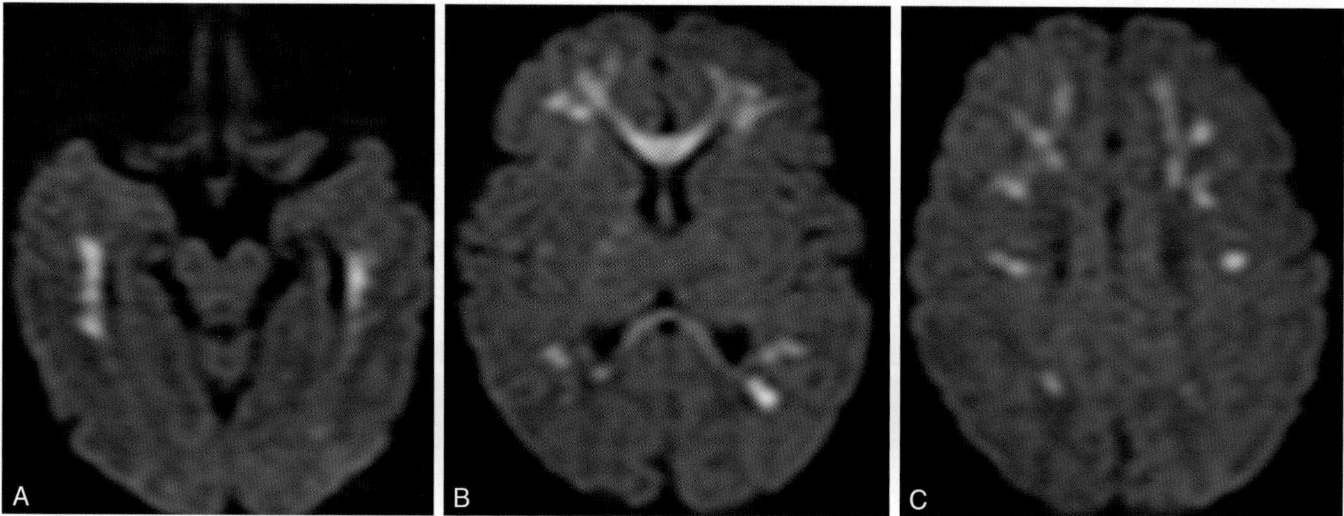

Fig. 5.13 Parechovirus. Seven-day-old with seizure and skin rash on the chest and axilla. (A to C) Axial DWI images demonstrate striated diffusion restriction in the periventricular white matter with more confluent restricted diffusion in the corpus callosum.

Key Points

Background

- Single-strand RNA virus of the Picornaviridae family; HPeV-3 most commonly identified in CNS infections of young infants
- Infection occurs via respiratory or gastrointestinal (fecal-oral) mechanisms with hematogenous spread to the CNS
- Second most common cause of viral meningoencephalitis after enterovirus in infants younger than 2 months
- Presentation
    - Gastroenteritis
    - Respiratory symptoms
    - Severe CNS infection: Fever, rash, irritability, seizures, sepsis-like features
    - Acute flaccid paralysis
- Adverse neurodevelopmental outcome may occur

Imaging

- *Mimics mild-moderate hypoxic ischemic encephalopathy (HIE):* striated, nonenhancing T1W and T2W shortening in the periventricular white matter (frontal predominant) with intense restricted diffusion; corpus callosum is diffusely involved; variable involvement of the thalamus
- May have foci of susceptibility within signal abnormality
- Imaging is not pathognomonic; may be seen with other viruses such as rotavirus, and enterovirus. White matter injury from other causes such as congenital heart disease, prematurity may resemble this pattern
- Permanent parenchymal injury may occur

REFERENCES

1. Amarnath C, Helen Mary T, Periakarupan A, et al. Neonatal parechovirus leucoencephalitis- radiological pattern mimicking hypoxic-ischemic encephalopathy. *Eur J Radiol.* 2016 Feb;85(2):428–434.
2. Sarma A, Hanzlik E, Krishnasarma R, et al. Human Parechovirus Meningoencephalitis: Neuroimaging in the Era of Polymerase Chain Reaction-Based Testing. *AJNR Am J Neuroradiol.* 2019 Aug;40(8):1418–1421.

HERPES ENCEPHALITIS (HSV-1)

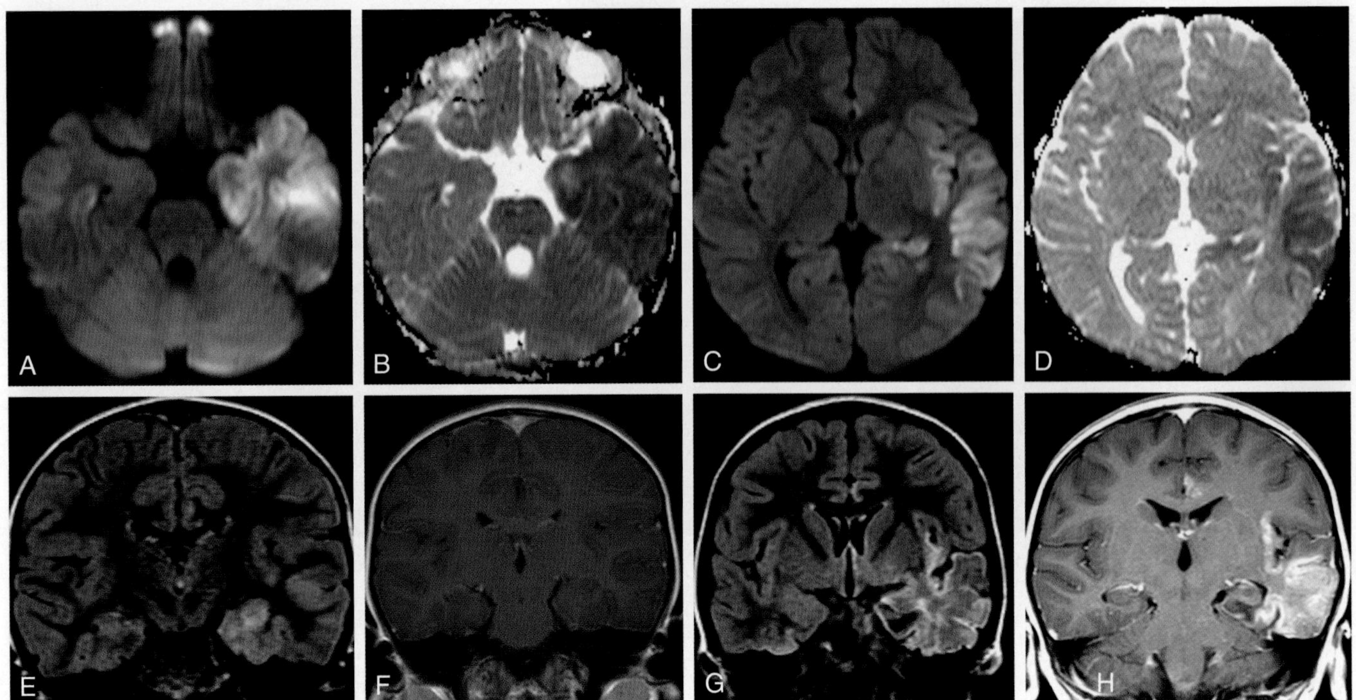

Fig. 5.14 Herpes Encephalitis (HSV-1): 3-year-old with fever and seizure. (A to D) Initial presentation axial DWI and ADC maps demonstrate cortical and subcortical reduced diffusion in the left temporal lobe, insula, and left cingulate gyrus (not shown) and (E) coronal FLAIR demonstrating T2W hyperintensity but (F) coronal T1W+C demonstrating no significant enhancement. Subtle cortical reduced diffusion also involves the right temporal lobe near the ventricle seen on (A) and (B). (G and H) Follow-up MRI 11 days later demonstrates progressive T2W signal abnormality on coronal FLAIR image (G) and avid associated enhancement on coronal T1W+C image (H). Subtle involvement of the right temporal lobe involves the fusiform gyrus seen on the coronal FLAIR image.

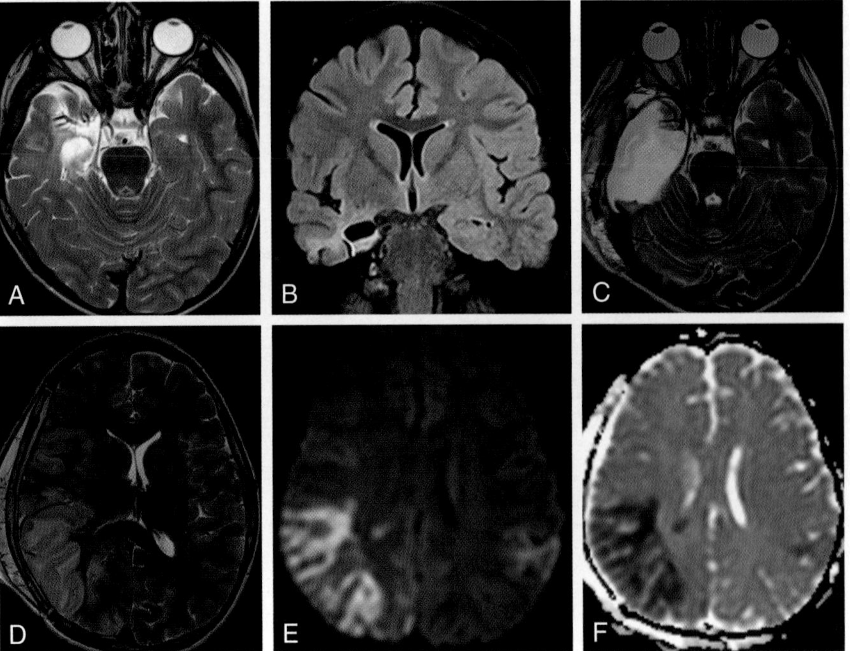

Fig. 5.15 Herpes Encephalitis (HSV-1): 4-year-old with rare HSV-1 reactivation. (A) Axial T2W and (B) coronal FLAIR images demonstrate severe encephalomalacia of the right temporal lobe from prior HSV-1 encephalitis. Because of chronic epilepsy, the patient underwent right temporal lobectomy as seen on axial T2W image (C). Four days after surgery the patient developed fevers and seizure and MRI brain (D) axial T2W, (E) axial DWI, and (F) axial ADC demonstrate a new region of reduced diffusion and T2 hyperintensity in the right parietal lobe, mimicking an arterial infarction and smaller area on the left parietal lobe. CSF and blood HSV-1 PCR were found to be positive, confirming reactivation.

Key Points

Background

- Ubiquitous DNA virus belonging to Herpesviridae family with nearly 80% to 90% seroconversion in general population
- Infection of mucosal surface or nonintact skin, usually orolabial route
    - Primary infection typically asymptomatic
    - Reactivation may be symptomatic or asymptomatic; cold sores most common but rarely may result in meningoencephalitis
- Mechanism of meningoencephalitis
    - Reactivation at the level of the trigeminal ganglion with axonal spread to frontal and temporal lobes
    - Reactivation of latent virus within the brain parenchyma
    - Primary infection of the CNS
    - CNS entry may occur via olfactory or trigeminal nerves
- Most common cause of sporadic fatal viral encephalitis
    - 70% mortality in untreated patients
    - 30% mortality in treated patients
- High incidence of permanent neurologic deficits
- Bimodal age distribution: Childhood and age >50 years with peak in late adulthood
- Patients present with headache, fever, nausea, vomiting, seizures, encephalitis
- Diagnosis made by CSF PCR; CSF is abnormal in more than 95% of patients and includes lymphocytic pleocytosis and increased protein

Imaging

- CT may be normal in the early phase of the disease.
- MRI is the gold standard of imaging.
    - Bilateral asymmetric involvement of the cortical-subcortical *inferior frontal lobes, temporal lobes (medial> lateral), insula, and cingulate gyri.* Patchy bilateral hemispheric involvement may occur, mimicking thromboembolic infarct given the presence of restricted diffusion.
    - DWI imaging is very sensitive demonstrating restricted diffusion; may mimic multifocal thromboembolic infarcts.
    - T2W hyperintensity of involved parenchyma; multifocal susceptibility from hemorrhage.
    - Avid parenchymal and leptomeningeal enhancement well seen on T1W and T2W FLAIR postcontrast imaging.
    - Basal ganglia involvement is rare.
    - Encephalomalacia of affected areas is the end result.

REFERENCES

1. Steiner I, Benninger F. Manifestations of Herpes Virus Infections in the Nervous System. *Neurol Clin.* 2018 Nov;36(4):725–738.
2. Rath TJ, Hughes M, Arabi M, et al. Imaging of cerebritis, encephalitis, and brain abscess. *Neuroimaging Clin N Am.* 2012 Nov;22(4):585–607.

HERPES ENCEPHALITIS (HSV-2)

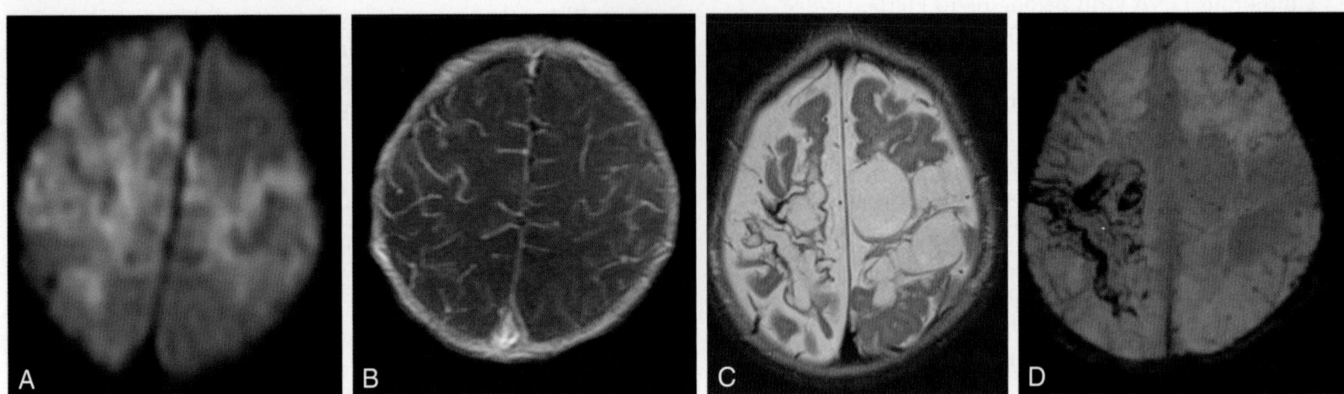

Fig. 5.16 Herpes Encephalitis (HSV-2). (A) Axial DWI image demonstrates confluent regions of reduced diffusion and (B) axial T1W+C image demonstrates diffuse leptomeningeal enhancement. (C) Axial T2W and (D) axial SWI demonstrates eventual development of hemosiderin-laden encephalomalacia.

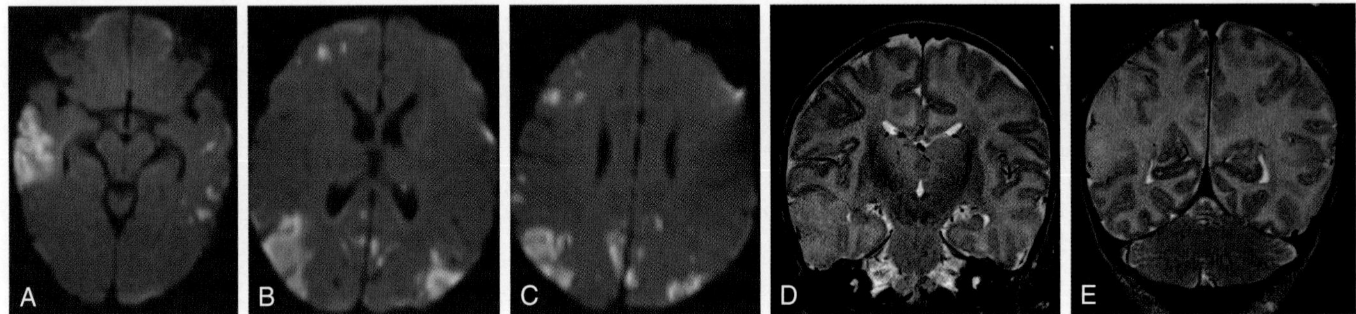

Fig. 5.17 Herpes Encephalitis (HSV-2). (A to C) Axial DWI image demonstrates patchy and confluent regions of restricted diffusion bilaterally. (D to E) Coronal T2W demonstrated corresponding T2W hyperintensity. Findings may mimic thromboembolic infarct. 3D time of flight (TOF) MRA was normal (not shown).

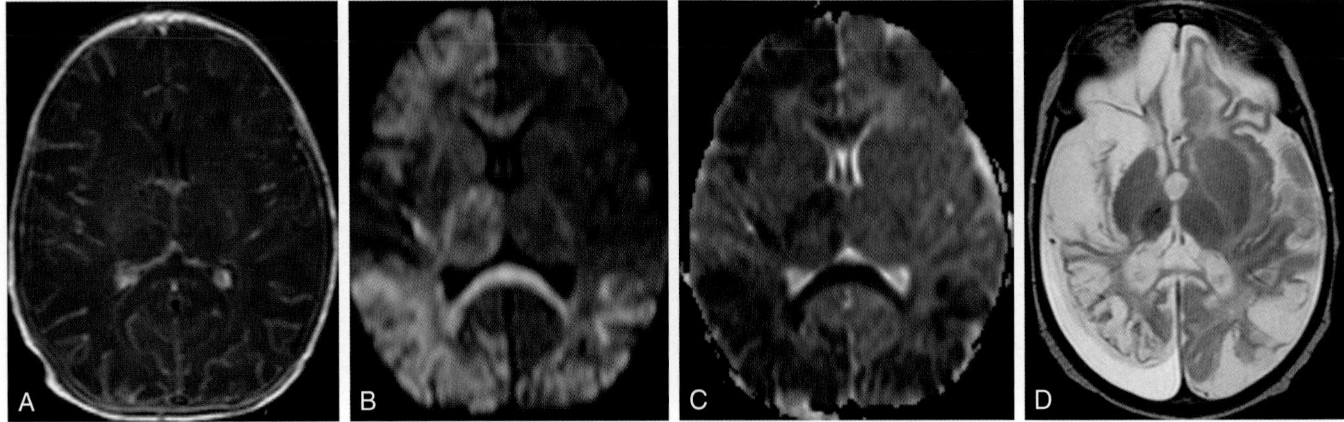

Fig. 5.18 Herpes Encephalitis (HSV-2): 16-day-old with seizures and congestion. (A) Axial T1W+C demonstrates mild diffuse leptomeningeal enhancement. (B) Axial DWI, and (C) axial ADC map demonstrate multifocal extensive areas of diffusion restriction, which may mimic arterial infarcts but in conjunction with the abnormal leptomeningeal enhancement and clinical history should raise concern for HSV-2 encephalitis. (D) Axial T2W image on 1-month follow-up MRI demonstrates the extensive encephalomalacia that can result with an HSV-2 meningoencephalitis.

Key Points

Background

- Accounts for 80% of encephalitis in infants.
- HSV-2 infections in neonates occur in the perinatal/neonatal period and result from exposure to maternal HSV type 2 genital lesions at the time of vaginal birth.
- Infants may present with systemic findings of seizure, lethargy, respiratory distress, vomiting, cyanosis, anorexia, and body temperature alteration.
- CSF PCR gold standard. Up to 25% of neonatal HSV can have negative PCR in the early phase of infection requiring potential repeat CSF testing.

Imaging

- Variable, multifocal, watershed, or diffuse brain involvement without predilection for certain brain regions as seen in HSV-1
  - Cortex, white matter, central gray matter
  - Brainstem and cerebellum may be involved
- Ultrasound and Computed Tomography
  - Nonspecific, includes the presence of both focal edema and diffuse edema
- MRI
  - DWI imaging is very sensitive demonstrating restricted diffusion; *may mimic multifocal thromboembolic infarcts or HIE*
    - T2W hyperintensity of involved parenchyma; multifocal susceptibility may occur
    - Avid leptomeningeal enhancement well seen on T1W and T2 FLAIR postcontrast imaging
    - Encephalomalacia is present long term

REFERENCES

1. Nickerson JP, Richner B, Santy K, et al. Neuroimaging of pediatric intracranial infection–part 2: TORCH, viral, fungal, and parasitic infections. *J Neuroimaging*. 2012 Apr;22(2):e52–e63.
2. Barkovich AJ, Raybaud C. *Pediatric Neuroimaging*: LWW; 2011:1144.

HUMAN HERPESVIRUS 6 (HHV-6)

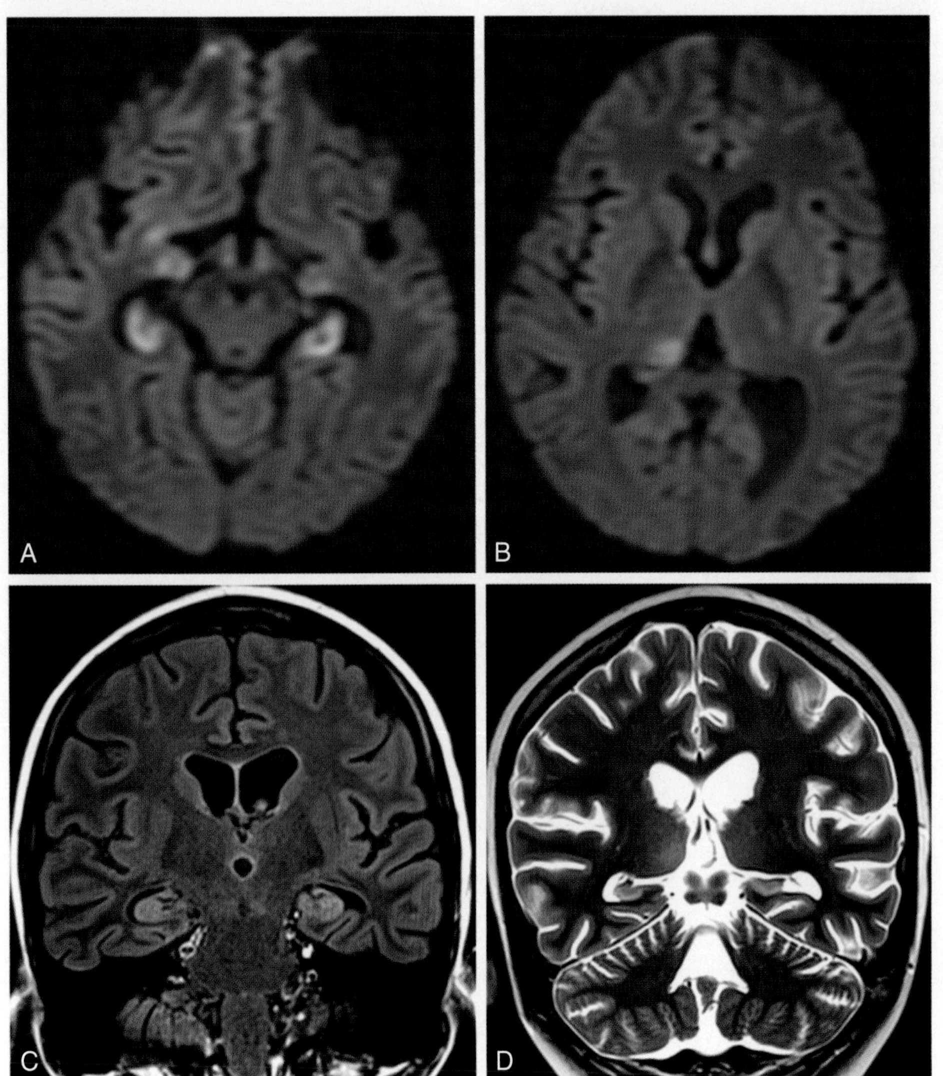

Fig. 5.19 Human Herpesvirus 6 Encephalitis. 12-year-old with Glanzmann thrombasthenia, severe bleeding phenotype, one month after bone marrow transplant presented with new-onset seizure, altered mental status, and fever. (A and B) Axial DWI images demonstrate restricted diffusion of the bilateral hippocampi and right thalamus with corresponding T2W signal abnormality on the (C) coronal FLAIR and (D) coronal T2W images. CSF PCR testing revealed HHV-6.

Key Points

Background

- Pathogen resulting in roseola infantum (sixth disease) and exanthem subitum in children
- Most infections are asymptomatic; 90% of the general population is seropositive by age 2.
- Virus remains latent in brain, white blood cells, salivary glands
- HHV-6 encephalitis can occur in immunocompromised patients, especially in stem cell transplant patients
- Diagnosis by PCR analysis
- Treatment with ganciclovir or foscarnet; without treatment >60% mortality

Imaging

- May be normal in early stage of the disease
- May involve the mesial temporal lobes, limbic system, and central gray matter
- Nonenhancing T2W hyperintensity and less frequently the other areas of the cerebral cortex that may appear similar to HSV-1
- Lack of enhancement
- Differential Diagnosis: Autoimmune encephalitis, status epilepticus, herpes encephalitis

REFERENCES

1. Noguchi T, Yoshiura T, Hiwatashi A, et al. CT and MRI findings of human herpesvirus 6-associated encephalopathy: comparison with findings of herpes simplex virus encephalitis. *AJR Am J Roentgenol.* 2010 Mar;194(3):754–760.
2. Soares BP, Provenzale JM. Imaging of Herpesvirus Infections of the CNS. *AJR Am J Roentgenol.* 2016 Jan;206(1):39–48.

ENTEROVIRUS

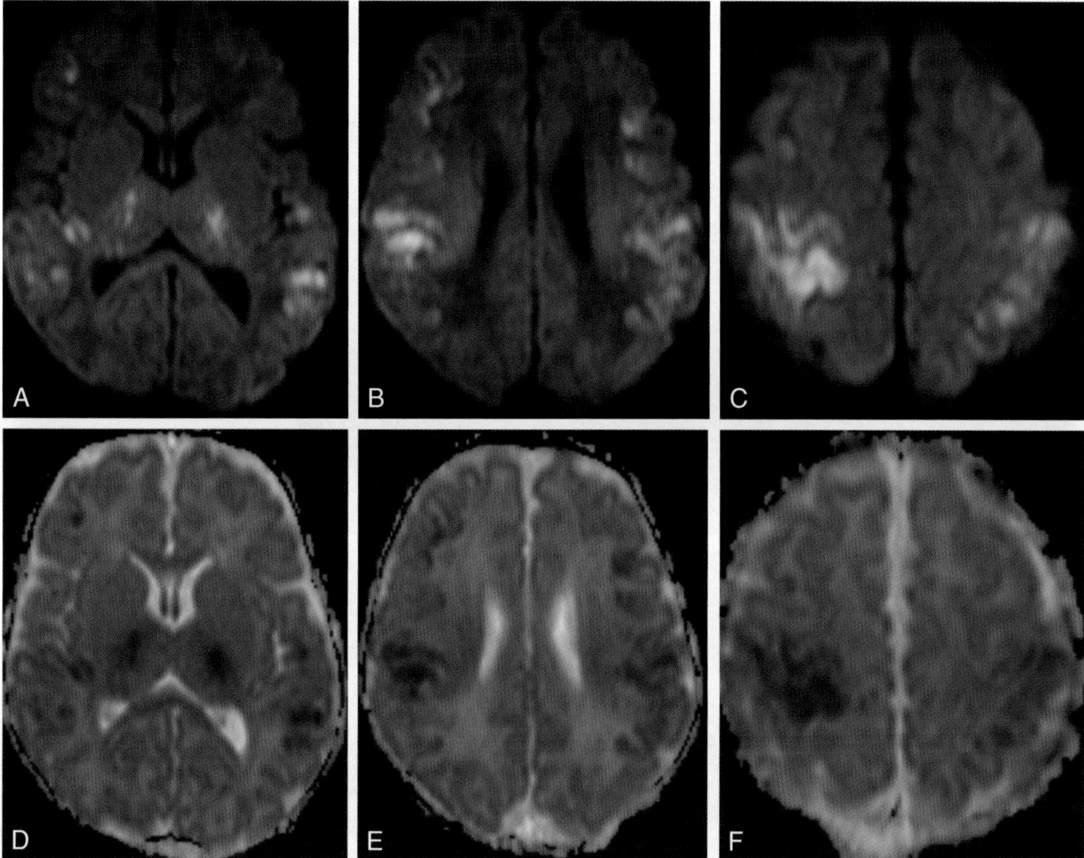

Fig. 5.20 Enterovirus. A 1-month-old with fever, cough, and seizure found to have enterovirus meningitis. (A to C) Axial DWI, and (D to F) axial ADC images demonstrate multifocal reduced diffusion involving the frontal, temporal, and parietal lobes and the thalami. CSF enterovirus PCR was positive.

Key Points

Background

- Human enteroviruses include poliovirus, coxsackie A and B viruses, echoviruses, and enteroviruses but are reclassified as enteroviruses serotypes A to J.
- Transmission is through fecal-oral contact.
- Greater than 90% of infections are asymptomatic or result in a febrile illness. Some serotypes are associated with a rash.
- CNS infections can result in a viral meningitis, encephalitis, or acute paralysis/myelitis. Enterovirus causes >90% of viral meningitis in infants and >50% of viral meningitis in older children and adults. Viral meningitis is most often from the enterovirus B serotype.
- Viral meningitis symptoms in infants include fever and irritability and in children include fever, headache, stiff neck, nausea, and vomiting. The vast majority have complete recovery within 3 to 7 days. About 5% to 10% have an encephalitis pattern with seizures and altered consciousness. Acute paralysis/myelitis is seen with poliovirus and enterovirus D68 and D71 and is discussed in the acute flaccid myelitis section.
- Diagnosis can be made through PCR.

Imaging

- Majority of imaging is normal. Some cases demonstrate mild leptomeningeal enhancement, brainstem T2W hyperintensity, and cerebellitis.
- Enterovirus D68 and D71 have been associated with acute flaccid myelitis, which is discussed in Chapter 18, Infectious, Inflammatory, Demyelinating, and Vascular Disorders.
- Differential Diagnosis: Autoimmune encephalitis, status epilepticus, herpes encephalitis

REFERENCE

1. Shen WC, Chiu HH, Chow KC, et al. MR Imaging findings of enteroviral encephalomyelitis: an outbreak in Taiwan. *AJNR Am J Neuroradiol.* Nov-Dec 1999;20(10):1889–1895.

WEST NILE VIRUS

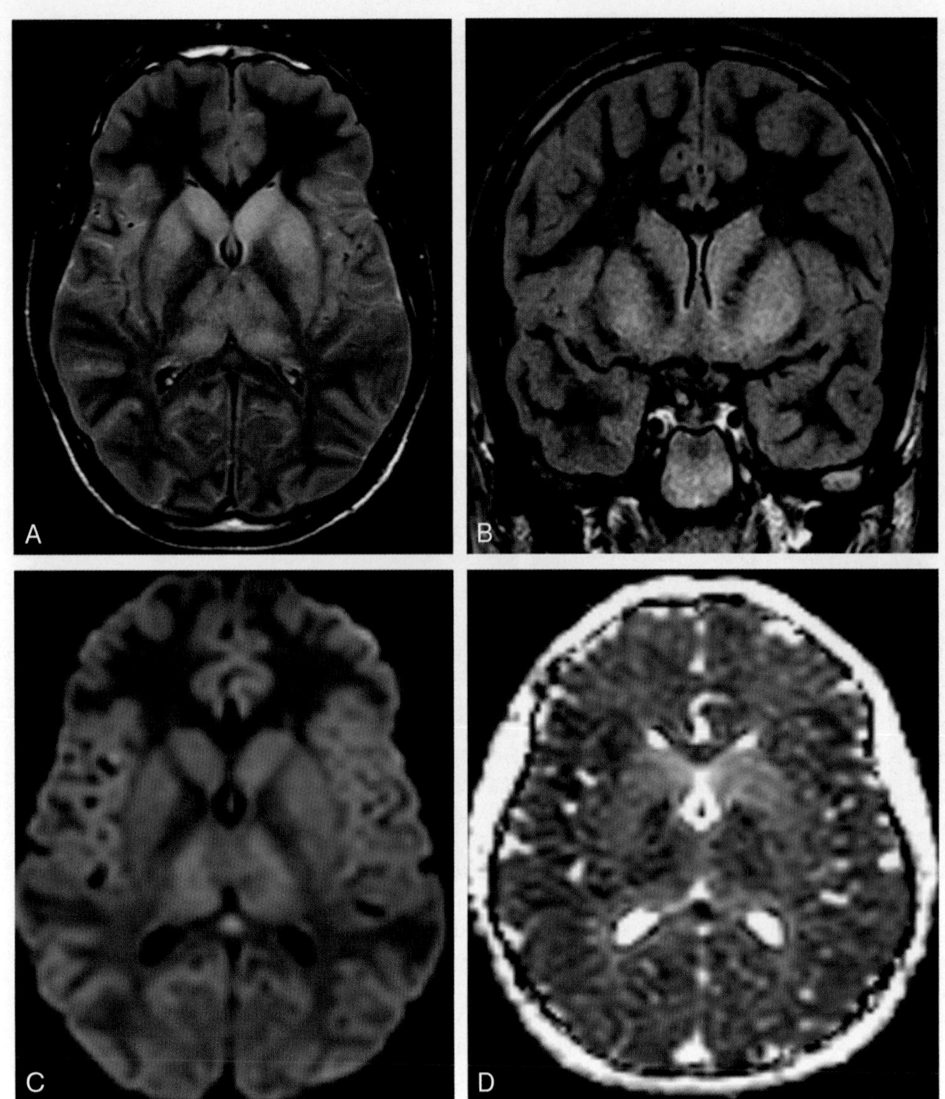

Fig. 5.21 West Nile Virus. An 18-year-old with fever, altered mental status, dystonia, and autonomic storming. (A and B) Axial and coronal FLAIR demonstrate confluent hyperintensity in the central gray matter and subtle cortical hyperintensity. (C) Axial DWI and (D) axial ADC demonstrate elevated diffusion in the basal ganglia and mixed areas of elevated and mildly reduced diffusion in the thalami.

Key Points

Background

- Mosquito-borne flavivirus; most common arbovirus in North America; most common form of transmission
- Transmission has been reported via organ transplantation
- May cause meningitis, encephalitis, or meningoencephalitis
- Present with fever, headache, vomiting, abdominal pain, altered mental status with obtundation, seizures, myoclonus, tremors, and Parkinsonism

Imaging

- Bilateral basal ganglia and thalami (symmetric or asymmetric and patchy)
- Mesial temporal lobe involvement may occur
- Brainstem, cerebellum, and white matter may be involved
- T2W hyperintensity most commonly without restricted diffusion although restricted diffusion may be seen
- Enhancement is uncommon but may be present in leptomeninges and pachymeninges
- Spine
  - T2W hyperintensity with or without enhancement in central gray matter with predilection for anterior horn cells
  - Polyradiculitis with enhancing nerve roots may be seen

REFERENCE

1. Herring R, Desai N, Parnes M, et al. Pediatric West Nile Virus-Associated Neuroinvasive Disease: A Review of the Literature. *Pediatr Neurol.* 2019 Mar;92:16–25.

RABIES VIRUS

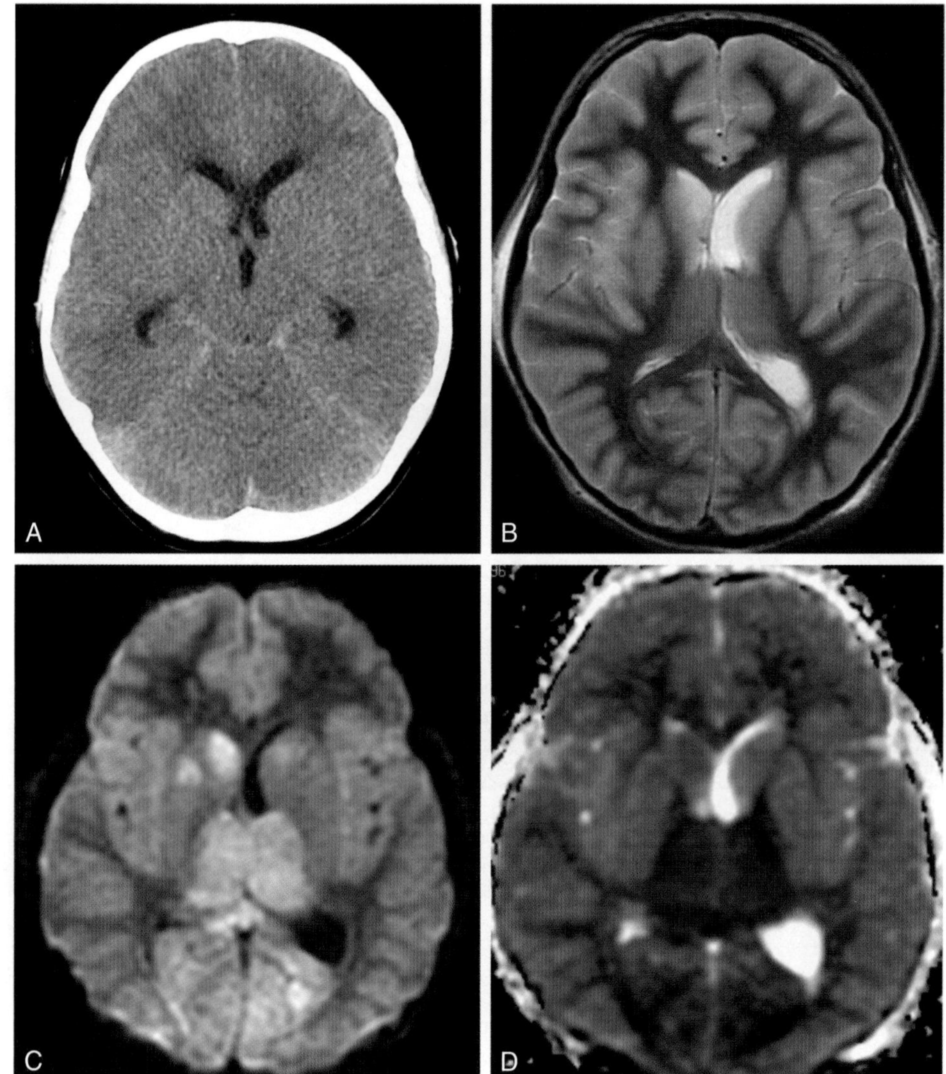

Fig. 5.22 Rabies Virus. (A) Axial noncontrast CT and (B) axial T2W images demonstrate diffuse cerebral edema with cortical T2W hyperintensity, and compressed quadrigeminal cistern. (C) Axial DWI and (D) axial ADC demonstrate restricted diffusion of the thalami, portions of the basal ganglia, and throughout the white matter.

Key Points

Background

- RNA virus of the Rhabdoviridae family
- Transmitted to humans via a bite from an infected animal; nonbite exposure can occur when there is contact with an open wound or mucus membrane; aerosol, and organ transplant transmission have been reported
- Encephalitic and paralytic forms:
  - Encephalitic: Episodes of arousal and hyperexcitability separated by lucid intervals, and autonomic dysfunction
  - Paralytic: Motor weakness starting in the extremity progressing to quadriparesis and facial weakness
  - Virus enters the CNS resulting in gray matter infection with progressive encephalitis

Imaging

- Central gray matter, limbic system, brainstem (especially pons and midbrain), hypothalami, hippocampi, and cortical involvement especially of the frontal and parietal lobes
- Symmetric (often the central gray matter) nonenhancing T2W signal of the involved brain parenchyma typically without enhancement, although enhancement may occur
- Spine
  - Symmetric T2W signal of the central gray matter of the cord
  - Nerve root enhancement

REFERENCES

1. Co SJ, Mackenzie IR, Shewchuk JR. Rabies encephalitis. *Radiographics*. 2015 Jan-Feb;35(1):235–238.
2. Awasthi M, Parmar H, Patankar T, et al. Imaging findings in rabies encephalitis. *AJNR Am J Neuroradiol*. 2001 Apr;22(4):677–680.
3. Jackson AC. *Rabies*. *Neurol Clin*. 2008 Aug;26(3):717–726.
4. Kalita J, Bhoi SK, Bastia JK, et al. Paralytic rabies: MRI findings and review of literature. *Neurol India*. 2014 Nov-Dec;62(6):662–664.

CHIKUNGUNYA ENCEPHALITIS

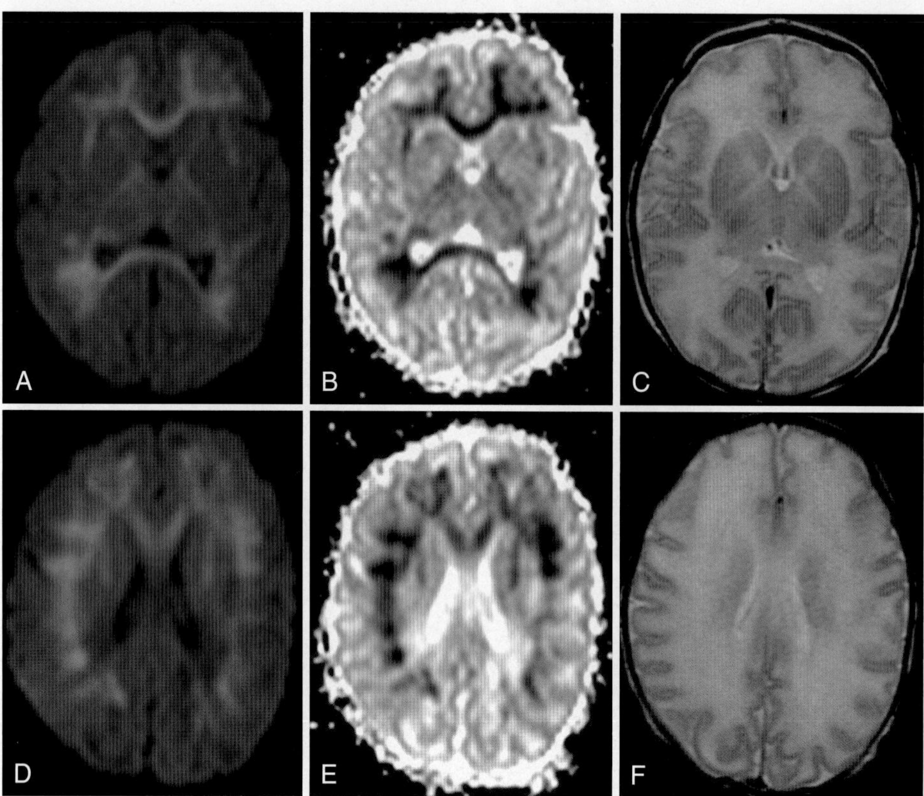

Fig. 5.23 Chikungunya virus. A pregnant mother experienced a high grade fever, joint pain at 36 weeks of gestation and Chikungunya serology was positive for IgG and negative for IgM. Uncomplicated C-section was performed after 5 days later. On the 4th day of life, neonate developed generalized seizure activities with mild fever. RT-PCR for Chikungunya was positive in CSF and blood. MRI brain was then performed. (A and D) Axial DWI and (B and E) axial ADC map images demonstrate restricted diffusion in supratentorial white matter, corpus callosum, thalami and internal capsules. (C, F) Axial T2W images demonstrate increased white matter signal.

Key Points

Background

- Numerous tropical infections may be transmitted by mosquitos to humans including viral infections such as Zika, dengue fever, yellow fever, chikugunya (all of which are Arboviruses) and malaria among others. CNS infection may occur with these entities.
- Chikugunya is an Arbovirus, of the genus Alphavirus transmitted by Aedes aegypti and Aedes albopictus. Outbreaks have occurred in Africa, Asia, and the Americas.
- Infection typically results in fever and joint pain. Additional symptoms include headache, muscle pain, rash, joint edema. Newborns with perinatal infection, elderly patients and patients with comorbidities are at risk for more severe infection. Death may rarely occur.
- Rarely CNS infection may occur including meningitis, encephalitis, meningoencephalitis, encephalomyelitis and optic neuritis. Guillain Barre syndrome has also been reported. CNS infection may result in seizures, behavioral changes, encephalopathy, altered level of consciousness, hypotonia, paresis and coma.
- Symptomatic neonatal infection generally thought to occur by intrapartum infection,

Imaging

- Limited literature on imaging with CNS infection. Imaging is not pathognomonic; imaging may be normal.
- Perinatal/neonatal infection may result in confluent, extensive or multifocal restricted diffusion in the cerebral white matter (perivascular distribution) to include the corpus callosum which may progress to cystic leukomalacia. Foci of hemorrhage may occur.
- Cortical/cerebral edema, focal/ multifocal white matter signal abnormality which may have restricted diffusion and enhancement, limbic encephalitis

REFERENCES

1. Corrêa DG, Freddi TAL, Werner H JM, et al. Brain MR Imaging of Patients with Perinatal Chikungunya Virus Infection. *AJNR Am J Neuroradiol.* 2020 Jan;41(1):174–177.
2. Ortiz-Quezada J, Rodriguez EE, Hesse H, et al. Chikungunya encephalitis, a case series from an endemic country. *J Neurol Sci.* 2021 Jan 15;420:117279.
3. Almeida Bentes A, Kroon EG, Romanelli RMC. Neurological manifestations of pediatric arboviral infections in the Americas. *J Clin Virol.* 2019 Jul;116:49–57.
4. Robin S, Ramful D, Le Seach' F, et al. Neurologic manifestations of pediatric chikungunya infection. *J Child Neurol.* 2008 Sep;23(9):1028–1035.

DENGUE ENCEPHALITIS

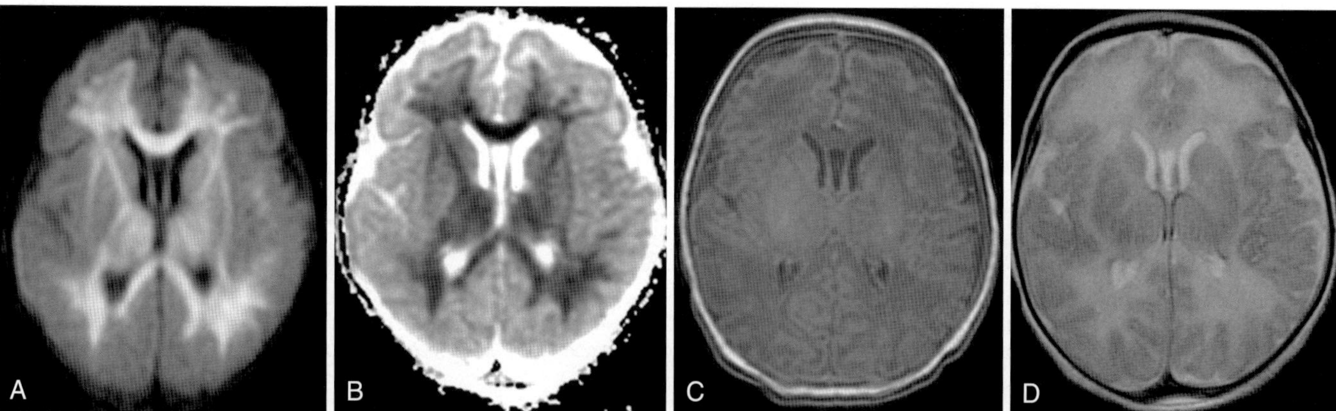

FIG. 5.24 Dengue Fever. Pregnant mother at 37 week gestation experienced high grade fever, rash, increased liver enzymes with positive Dengue serology for both IgG and IgM. Uncomplicated C-section was performed after 3 days of positive serology result. On the 7th day of life, neonate developed mild fever, thrombocytopenia, generalized seizure activities. RT-PCR for Dengue was positive in CSF and blood. RT-PCR for HSV and Chikungunya virus were all negative. MRI Brain was then performed. (A) Axial DWI and (B) axial ADC map demonstrates confluent restricted diffusion in the bilateral supratentorial white matter, thalami, internal capsule and subinsular parenchyma. (C) Axial T1W and (D) axial T2W images do not show definitive abnormality.

Key Points

Background

- Numerous tropical infections may be transmitted by mosquitos to humans including viral infections such as Zika, dengue fever, yellow fever, chikugunya (all of which are Arboviruses) and malaria among others. CNS infection may occur with these entities.
- Arbovirus, genus Alphavirus transmitted by Aedes aegypti and Aedes albopictus. Infection caused by Dengue virus 1-4. Disease is common in the Americas, Asia, Pacific Islands. Per the CDC, up to 400 million people per year are infected with dengue, 100 million are symptomatic and 40,000 die from the infection.
- Infection classified into multiple types including
  - Dengue without warning signs
  - Dengue with warning signs
  - Severe dengue
- Infection typically mild resulting in nausea, vomiting, headache, fatigue, rash and musculoskeletal pain. Infants, pregnant patients and those with history of prior infection are most at risk for severe infection. Multisystem involvement may occur in severe dengue. CNS infection is rare and may result in seizures, behavioral changes, encephalopathy, altered level of consciousness, hypotonia, paresis and coma.
- CNS infection may result in meningitis, encephalitis, meningoencephalitis, parenchymal hemorrhage/ hemorrhagic encephalitis, encephalomyelitis, myelitis, and neuro-opthalmologic manifestations. ADEM has been described with dengue.

Imaging

- Imaging is not pathognomonic; imaging may be normal
- Limited literature on imaging with CNS infection
- Variable encephalitic pattern including involvement of the cortical-subcortical cerebral hemispheres and central grey matter. Confluent/multifocal/ focal white matter signal abnormality. Regions of signal abnormality may have restricted diffusion and enhancement.
- Parenchymal micro- or macrohemorrhage may occur

REFERENCES

1. https://www.cdc.gov/dengue/about/index.html Centers for Disease Control and Prevention, National Center for Emerging and Zoonotic Infectious Diseases (NCEZID), Division of Vector-Borne Diseases (DVBD)
2. Vyas S, Ray N, Maralakunte M, et al. Pattern Recognition Approach to Brain MRI Findings in Patients with Dengue Fever with Neurological Complications. *Neurol India*. 2020 Sep–Oct;68(5):1038–1047.

ACUTE NECROTIZING ENCEPHALOPATHY

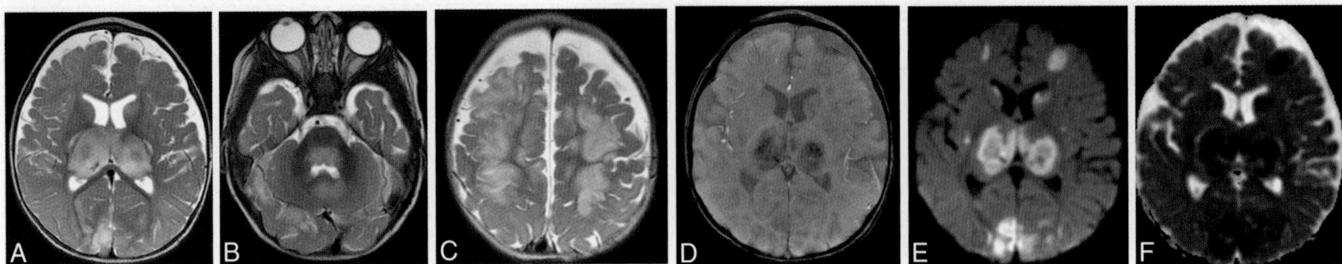

Fig. 5.25 Acute Necrotizing Encephalopathy (ANE). A 7-month-old with fever, seizure, influenza A positive, and elevated liver enzymes. (A to C) axial T2W, (D) axial SWI, (E) axial DWI, and (F) axial ADC images demonstrate T2W hyperintensity with reduced diffusion in the bilateral thalami, dorsal pons, cerebellum, and cortical and juxtacortical areas of the cerebral cortex. Petechial hemorrhages are present in the bilateral thalami as well as dorsal pons and some cortical areas (not shown).

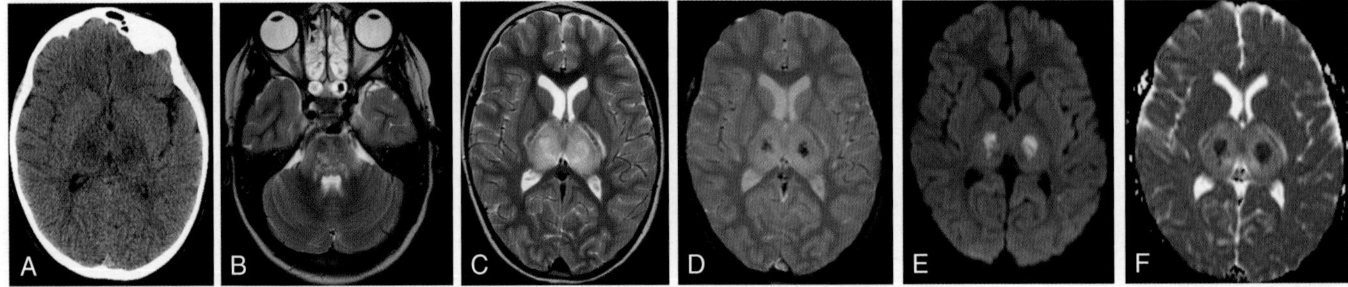

Fig. 5.26 Acute Necrotizing Encephalopathy (ANE). A 7-year-old with encephalopathy, fever, seizure, and recent viral upper respiratory infection. (A) Axial noncontrast CT of the head demonstrates symmetric low density in the thalami. (B and C) Axial T2W, (D) axial GRE, (E) axial DWI, and (F) axial ADC images demonstrate T2W hyperintensity in the bilateral thalami and pons with hemorrhages in the central thalami with reduced diffusion. The patient was found to be positive for Chikungunya virus which is an extremely rare cause of ANE.

Key Points

Background

- Reported in association with coxsackie virus, influenza A virus, *Mycoplasma* infection, herpes simplex virus, Chikungunya virus, and human herpesvirus 6.
- Etiology and pathogenesis of this disease remain unknown but are presumed immune mediated.
- Genetic predisposition has been reported in patients with repeated or familial forms due to missense mutation in *RANBP2* gene.
- Clinical presentation includes rapid onset convulsions, fever, vomiting, and altered consciousness within 12 to 72 hours of a preceding illness. Hepatic dysfunction can be present. ANE has a high morbidity and mortality. Survivors often have spasticity and weakness.
- Pathology demonstrates edema, petechial hemorrhage, necrosis, and absence of inflammatory cells, which differentiates this from ADEM and acute hemorrhagic encephalitis.

Imaging

- Multiple, symmetric lesions showing T2W prolongation in the *bilateral thalami*, frequently with accompanying lesions in the brainstem tegmentum, periventricular white matter, putamen, and cerebellum.
- Hemorrhage and cavitation are classically seen in the thalami.
- May show restricted diffusion.

REFERENCES

1. Mizuguchi M, Abe J, Mikkaichi K, et al. Acute necrotising encephalopathy of childhood: a new syndrome presenting with multifocal, symmetric brain lesions. *J Neurol Neurosurg Psychiatry*. 1995 May;58(5):555–561.
2. Wong AM, Simon EM, Zimmerman RA, et al. Acute necrotizing encephalopathy of childhood: correlation of MR findings and clinical outcome. *AJNR Am J Neuroradiol*. 2006 Oct;27(9):1919–1923.

BACTERIAL MENINGITIS

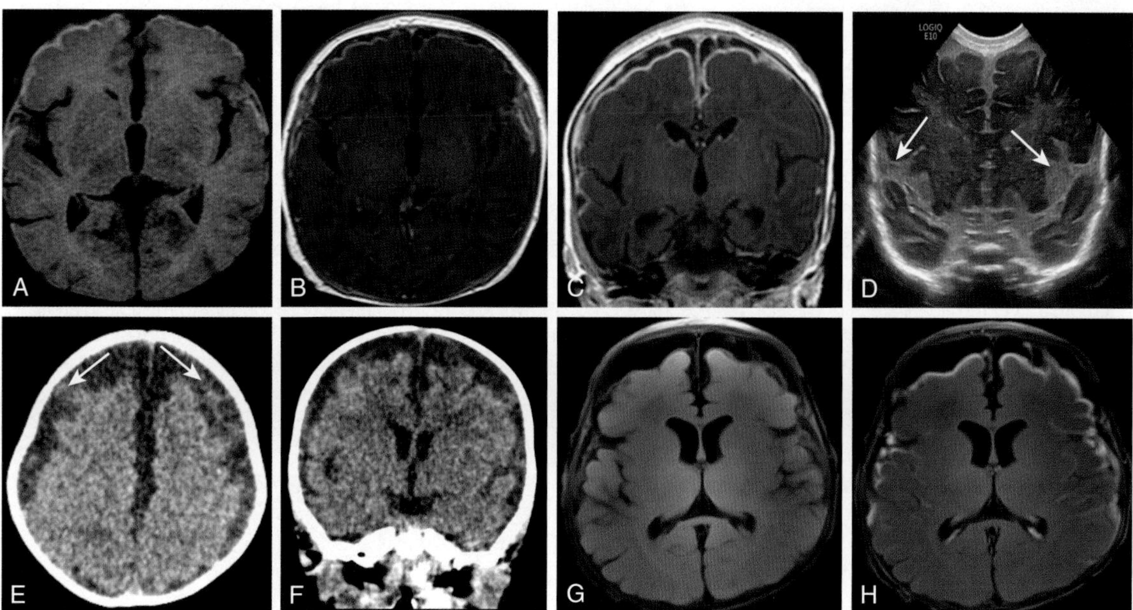

Fig. 5.27 Bacterial Meningitis Finding: Leptomeningitis. (A to C) A 2-month-old with group B streptococcus with abnormal leptomeningeal hyperintensity on axial precontrast FLAIR (A) and typical abnormal enhancement on axial and coronal T1W+C (B, C). (D) A 25-day-old with Group B Streptococcus meningitis and coronal ultrasound image demonstrating hyperechogenic and widened meninges, which is a challenging diagnosis on ultrasound. (E to H) A 3-month-old with GBS meningitis with axial and coronal reformat noncontrast CT head images demonstrating subtle abnormal density to the CSF in the extra-axial spaces in addition to thick web-like densities that should raise suspicion for meningitis. The axial precontrast FLAIR (G) demonstrates isointense material in the subarachnoid spaces, and postcontrast FLAIR (H) demonstrates significant leptomeningeal enhancement. The use of postcontrast FLAIR can be very helpful in demonstrating meningitis, and in some cases better than T1W+C imaging.

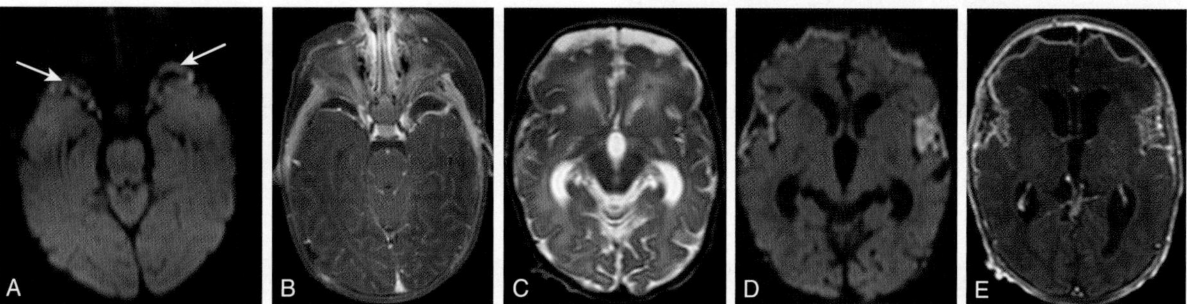

Fig. 5.28 Bacterial Meningitis Finding: Empyema/Purulent Extraaxial Material. (A and B) Two-month-old with Group B Streptococcus meningitis with abnormal reduced diffusion in the subdural spaces anterior to the temporal lobes with peripheral enhancement consistent with subdural empyemas seen on (A) axial DWI and (B) axial T1W+C images. (C to E) Axial T2W, axial DWI, and axial T1W+C images in an infant with *Streptococcus pneumoniae* meningitis with imaging demonstrating widened frontal extraaxial spaces, and purulent material in the subarachnoid spaces best seen in the sylvian fissures in addition to leptomeningeal enhancement.

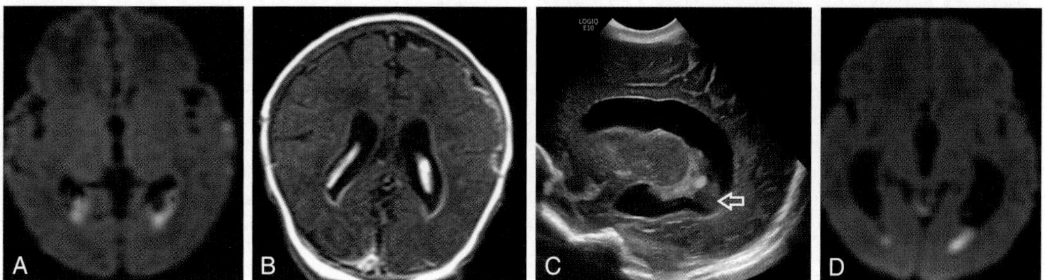

Fig. 5.29 Bacterial Meningitis Finding: Ventriculitis. (A and B) One-month-old with *E. coli* meningitis with (A) axial DWI demonstrating purulent material in the atria of the ventricles and associated ependymal enhancement seen on (B) coronal T1W+C images. (C and D) A 25-day-old with *E. coli* meningitis with sagittal ultrasound (C) demonstrating isoechoic material in the lateral ventricle posterior to the choroid plexus and axial DWI (D) confirming purulent material in the ventricles.

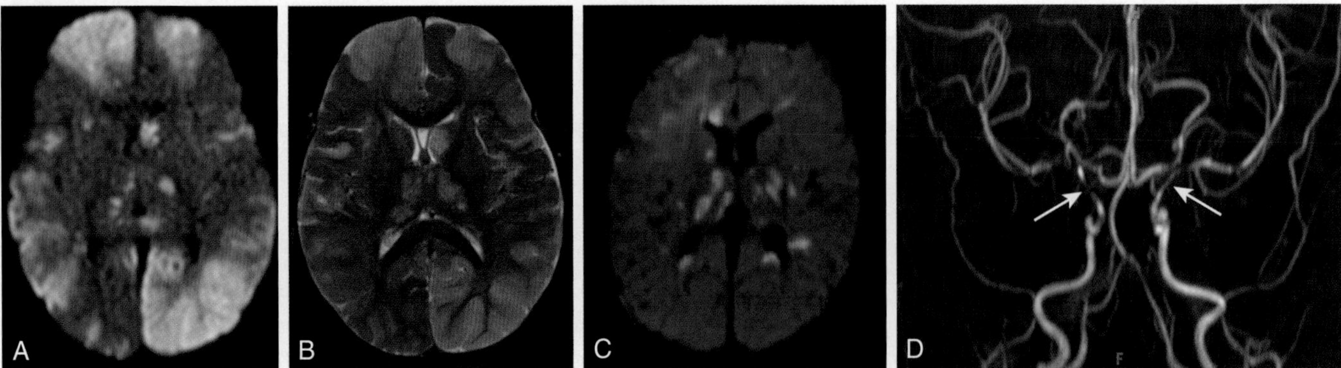

Fig. 5.30 Bacterial Meningitis Finding: Infarcts. (A and B) An 8-month-old with *Streptococcus pneumoniae* meningitis with (A) axial DWI and (B) axial T2W images demonstrating multifocal areas of diffusion restriction (ADC not shown) and T2 hyperintensity secondary to multiple infarcts. (C and D) Axial DWI and coronal volumetric MRA images of an infant with *S. pneumoniae* meningitis demonstrate multifocal infarct with restricted diffusion (ADC not shown) in the central gray matter and periventricular white matter. High-grade stenosis of the anterior circulation secondary to arteritis and/or vasospasm is present on MRA.

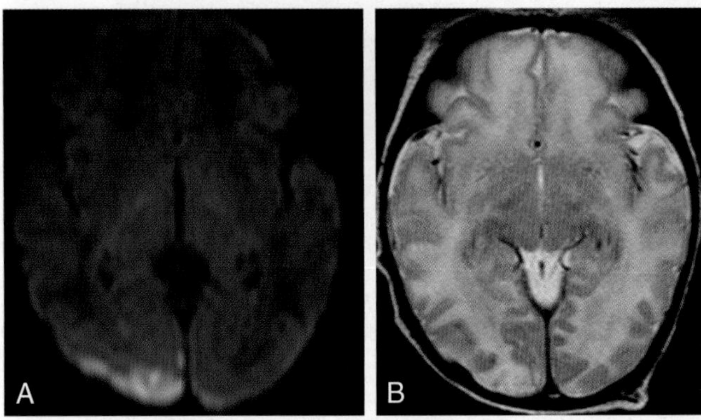

Fig. 5.31 Bacterial Meningitis Finding: Cerebritis. (A and B) A 1-month-old with Group B Streptococcus meningitis areas of cortical diffusion restriction in the occipital lobes (right greater than left) on axial DWI (A) and associated T2W hyperintensity on T2W image (B), which does not conform to an arterial infarct distribution but rather is due to cytotoxic edema from local purulent material.

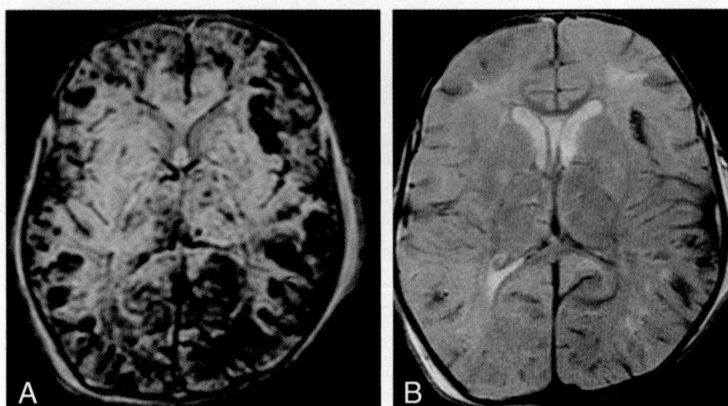

Fig. 5.32 Bacterial Meningitis Finding: Hemorrhage. (A and B) A 19-day-old with Group B Streptococcus meningitis and extensive cortical hemorrhage seen on axial SWI image (A) and associated cortical edema on T2W image (B) with loss of the cortical gray-white matter differentiation.

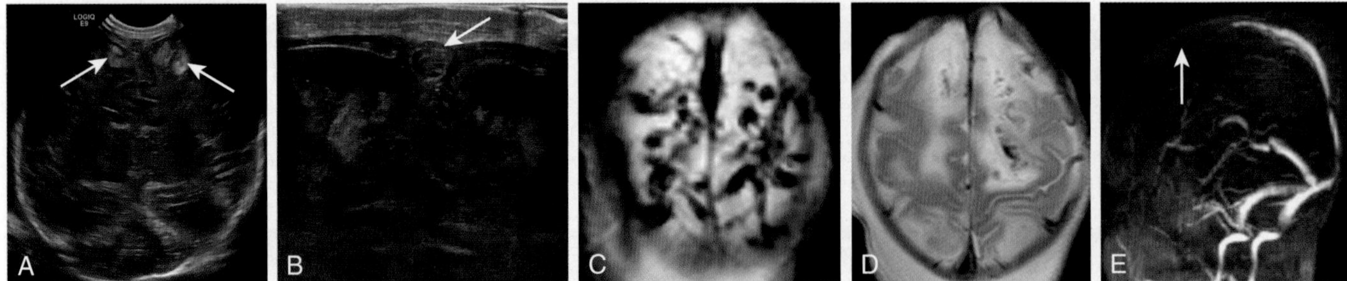

Fig. 5.33 Bacterial Meningitis Finding: Venous Thrombosis. (A to E) A 19-day-old with Group B Streptococcus meningitis. (A) Coronal ultrasound image demonstrates abnormal hyperechogenic areas in the medial frontal lobes (left greater than right) concerning for hemorrhage. (B) Small field of view coronal ultrasound image demonstrates abnormal hyperechoic material in the superior sagittal sinus concerning for thrombus. (C) Axial gradient echo (GRE) demonstrates multiple linear areas of susceptibility due to cortical vein and superior sagittal sinus thrombosis. (D) Axial T2W image demonstrates confluent parenchymal T2W hyperintensity in the superior frontal gyri with loss of cortical visualization indicating venous infarcts as well as small foci of hypointensity due to hemorrhage. (E) Oblique sagittal MR venogram volumetric image demonstrates loss of flow-related signal in the anterior third of the superior sagittal sinus indicative of thrombus.

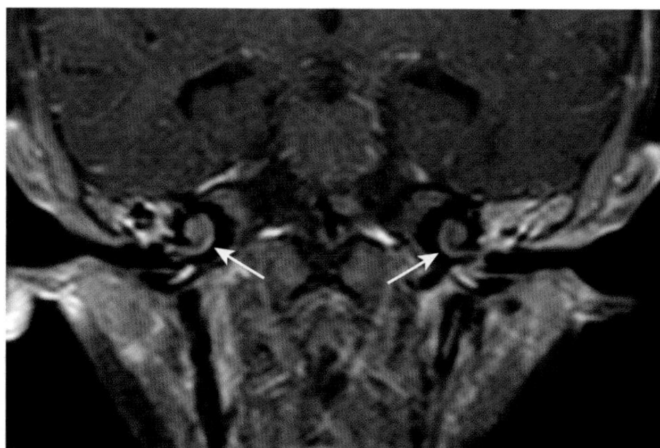

Fig. 5.34 Bacterial Meningitis Findings: Inner Ear Enhancement. An 8-month-old with *S. pneumoniae* meningitis with coronal T1W+C demonstrating abnormal enhancement in the bilateral cochlea. Abnormal enhancement is highly specific but is less sensitive for eventual hearing loss.

TABLE 5.2 Bacterial Meningitis

Age Group	Pathogen
Neonates (<1 month)	Group B *Streptococcus* (GBS) *Escherichia coli* *Listeria monocytogenes* Gram-negative bacilli
Infants (1–3 months)	GBS *E. coli* *L. monocytogenes* Gram-negative bacilli *Streptococcus pneumonia* *Neisseria meningitides* *Haemophilus influenzae*
3 months–3 years	*S. pneumonia* *N. meningitides* *H. influenzae*
3–19 years	*S. pneumonia* *N. meningitides*

Key Points

Background

- Meningitis is the most common form of bacterial infection of the CNS in children.
- The causative organism varies by age group:
  - Neonates: Group B *Streptococcus*, *Escherichia coli*
  - Infants-children: Streptococcus pneumonia, *Haemophilius influenzae* type b, or *Neisseria meningitidis*
  - Postsurgery: *Staphylococcus aureus*, coagulase-negative *Staphylococcus* infection, *Haemophilius influenza* type b, *Streptoccous pneumoniae*, or *Neisseria meningitidis*
- Symptoms include high fever, headache, photophobia, nausea, vomiting, and meningismus. Young children and infants may present with fever, hypothermia, lethargy, seizures, irritability, poor feeding, bulging fontanelle. Young children may not present with meningismus.
- Bacterial meningitis can be diagnosed through a positive CSF culture for bacteria, or a blood culture positive for bacteria with an elevated CSF WBC count (>20 WBC/μL for neonates less than 30 days old, >9 WBC/μL for 30 to 90 days of age, and >6 WBC/μL for older than 90 days).

Imaging

- Ultrasound findings depend on the severity of the infection. Imaging may be normal or may demonstrate hyperechoic widening of the sulci, extraaxial fluid collections, debris in the ventricles, hydrocephalus, infarcts, and hemorrhage.
- Noncontrast-enhanced CT may be normal, or demonstrate hydrocephalus and/or increased attenuation of subarachnoid space due to hypercellularity/increased protein in the CSF.
- Meningeal enhancement: Both leptomeningeal and pachymeningeal enhancement may be seen; pachymeningeal enhancement has been reported to potentially persist for months following complete clinical recovery.
- Incomplete suppression of CSF, especially overlying the cerebral convexities on FLAIR images; subarachnoid space may have restricted diffusion due to purulent debris.
- Ependymitis/ventriculitis with ependymal enhancement and diffusion restricting layering purulent debris within the ventricles.
- Infarcts and cerebritis: Foci of cortical-subcortical or central gray matter T2W hyperintensity with restricted diffusion and possible enhancement indicating parenchymal injury.
- Subdural effusion or empyemas and subarachnoid purulent material.
- Venous sinus thrombosis.
- Enhancement in the inner ear may occur due to membranous labyrinthitis, increasing risk for labyrinthitis ossificans and sensorineural hearing loss.
- Hemorrhage: Parenchymal, subarachnoid, and intraventricular are the most common locations.

REFERENCES

1. Nickerson JP, Richner B, Santy K, et al. Neuroimaging of pediatric intracranial infection–part 1: techniques and bacterial infections. *J Neuroimaging*. 2012 Apr;22(2):e42–e51.
2. Barkovich AJ, Raybaud C. *Pediatric Neuroimaging*: LWW; 2011:1144.
3. Agrawal S, Nadel S. Acute bacterial meningitis in infants and children: epidemiology and management. *Paediatr Drugs*. 2011 Dec 1;13(6):385–400.
4. Kralik SF, Kukreja MK, Paldino MJ, et al. Comparison of CSF and MRI Findings among Neonates and Infants with E coli or Group B Streptococcal Meningitis. *AJNR Am J Neuroradiol*. 2019 Aug;40(8):1413–1417.

ABSCESS

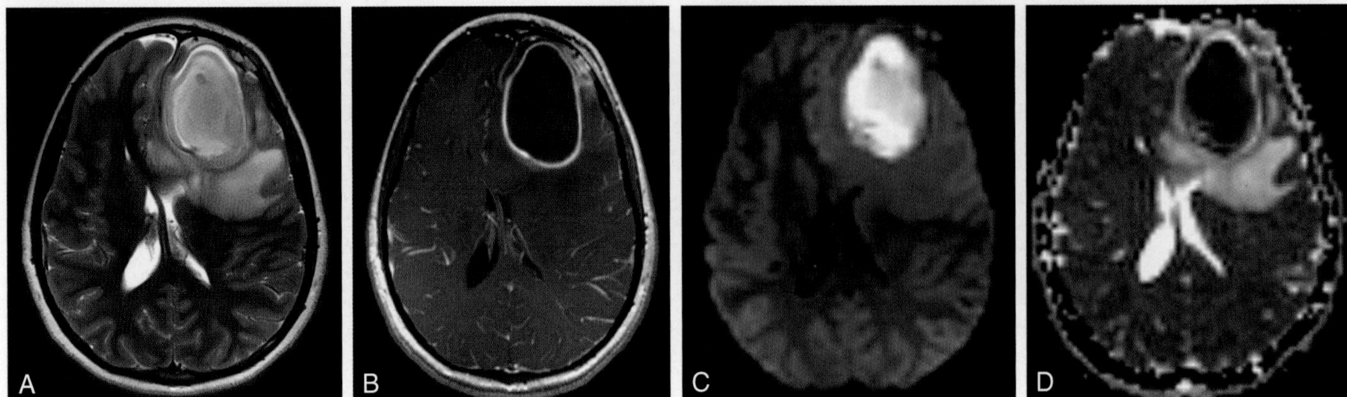

Fig. 5.35 Abscess. (A) Axial T2W demonstrates a large abscess in the left frontal lobe. Note the hypointense wall of the early capsular stage and intense regional edema. (B) Axial T1+C shows avid enhancement of the abscess wall with overlying enhancing cerebritis. (C) Axial DWI and (D) axial ADC demonstrate intense restricted diffusion within the abscess.

Key Points

Background

- Cerebritis and intracerebral abscesses are part of a four-stage spectrum of parenchymal brain infections: early cerebritis, late cerebritis, early capsular, and late capsular phase
- Several primary routes through which bacteria may reach the brain parenchyma:
  - Hematogenous dissemination in association with sepsis
  - Direct inoculation by penetrating trauma or surgery
  - Extension from an adjacent infection (sinusitis, otomastoiditis)
- Symptoms associated with parenchymal brain infection are variable, but include fever, headache, nausea, vomiting, seizures, focal neurologic deficit
- Most common organisms include *Staphylococcus aureus* and *Streptococcus* species. Rarely can be seen with amoebic infections.
- Risk factors for CNS abscess include congenital heart disorders, immunosuppression, and spread from the sinuses or mastoids.

Imaging

- Early cerebritis: Inflammatory edema results in ill-defined low attenuation or T2W signal with no enhancement or ill-defined nodular/ring-like enhancement
- Late cerebritis: Inflammatory edema results in ill-defined low attenuation or T2W signal with thick ring-like or nodular enhancement
- Capsular phases on CT
  - Centrally hypodense with a faint capsule sometimes seen on noncontrast CT; ring-like enhancement surrounded by extensive hypodense vasogenic edema
- Capsular phases on MRI
  - Early capsular: T2W hypointense ring with avid enhancement, central T2W prolongation with restricted diffusion, and extensive surrounding vasogenic edema. Ring is thinner on the deep margin.
  - Late capsular: Abscess cavity is collapsing with thicker wall enhancement than in the early capsular stage transitioning to nodular enhancement, which may be persistent for long periods, decreased or resolved vasogenic edema.

REFERENCE

1. Nickerson JP, Richner B, Santy K, et al. Neuroimaging of pediatric intracranial infection–part 1: techniques and bacterial infections. *J Neuroimaging*. 2012 Apr;22(2):e42–e51.

DIRECT INTRACRANIAL SPREAD OF INFECTION

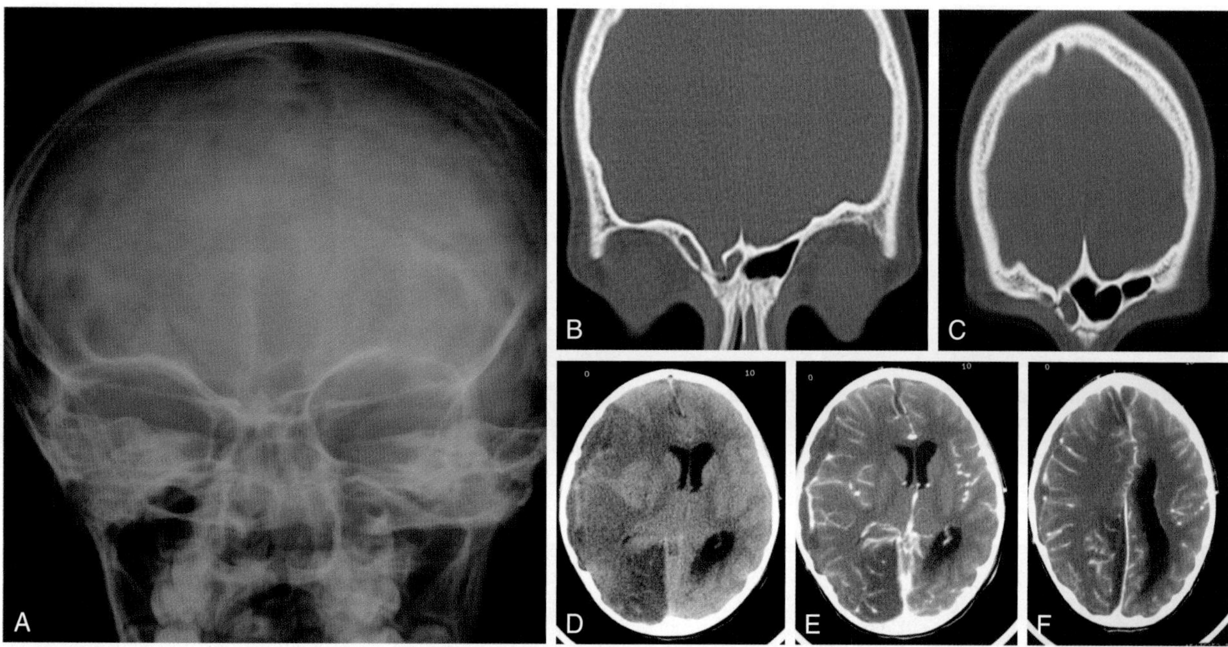

Fig. 5.36 Direct Intracranial Spread of Infection: *Staphylococcus aureus* Empyema due to Skull Fracture. (A) AP skull radiograph demonstrates a right frontal bone fracture traversing the right frontal sinus. (B and C) Noncontrast coronal reformat CT images demonstrating inferiorly displaced fracture through the right frontal sinus. (D) Noncontrast axial head CT and (E and F) axial contrast-enhanced head CT images demonstrate extensive right subdural, interhemispheric, and left frontal subdural empyema. A large region of hypodensity involves the right cerebral hemisphere due to ischemic injury. A component of cerebritis may be present. Left lateral ventricle is trapped due to midline shift.

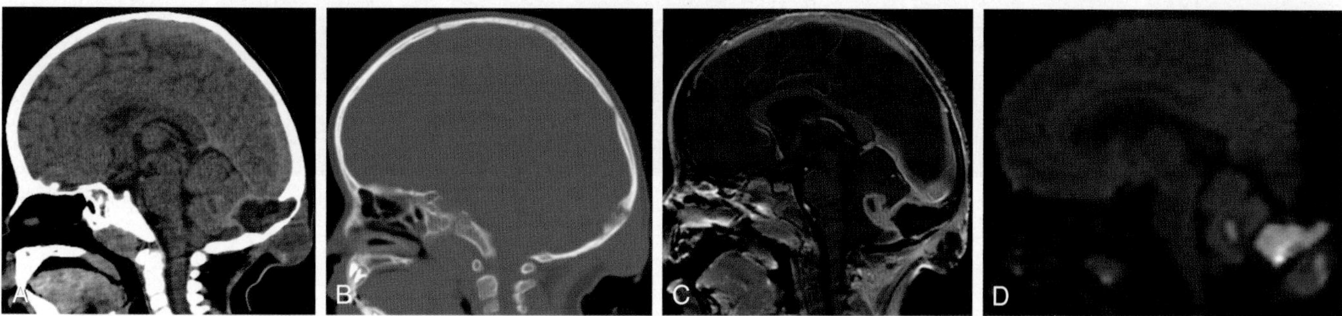

Fig. 5.37 Direct Intracranial Spread of Infection: Dermal Sinus Tract. (A, B) Sagittal reformat CT images demonstrate a posterior scalp mass and low-density intracranial mass in the bone and posterior fossa. A thin, linear lucent channel is seen in the occipital bone communicating both masses. (C) Sagittal T1W+C and (D) sagittal DWI images demonstrate peripheral enhancement and central reduced diffusion of the masses indicative of abscess formation in the scalp and brain as a result of infection entering through the dermal sinus tract.

Key Points

- Direct extension of infection most commonly occurs from primary infection in the sinus, orbits, or temporal bone. These are discussed in more detail in Chapter 15 Infectious and Inflammatory Disorders of the Head and Neck.
- Less common causes include infections due to trauma disrupting the skin of the scalp or extending into the sinuses, or infection entering through a dermal sinus tract.
- Meningitis due to *Staphylococcus aureus* is uncommon, occurring primarily in patients with known preexisting abnormalities of the CNS (including patients who have undergone previous neurosurgery or trauma).

SUBDURAL AND EPIDURAL EMPYEMA

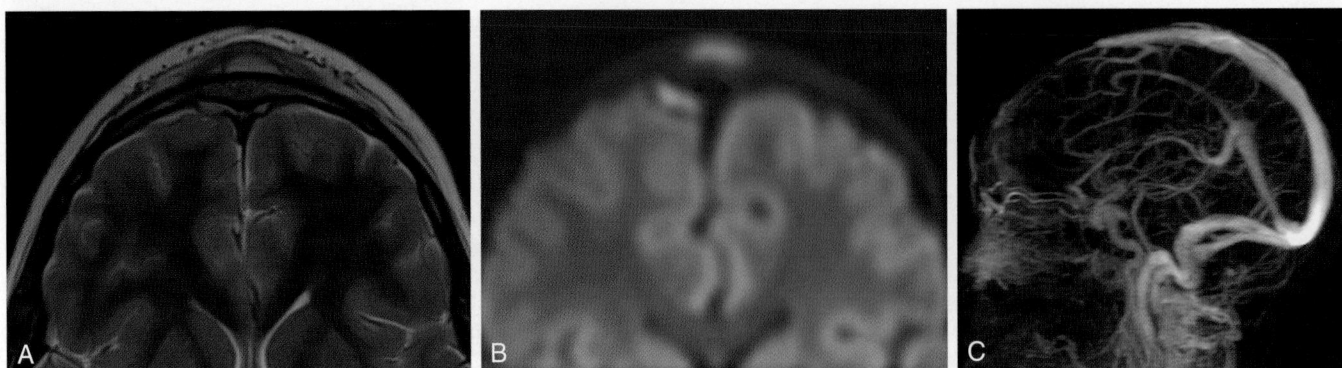

Fig. 5.38 Sinusitis Complications: Pott's Puffy Tumor, Empyema, and Sinus Thrombosis. (A) Axial T2W, (B) axial DWI, and (C) sagittal MR venogram volumetric image demonstrate subgaleal soft tissue thickening with diffusion restricting fluid collection consistent with an abscess (also known as Pott's puffy tumor), right frontal extra axial diffusion restriction (empyema), and thrombosis of the anterior superior sagittal sinus.

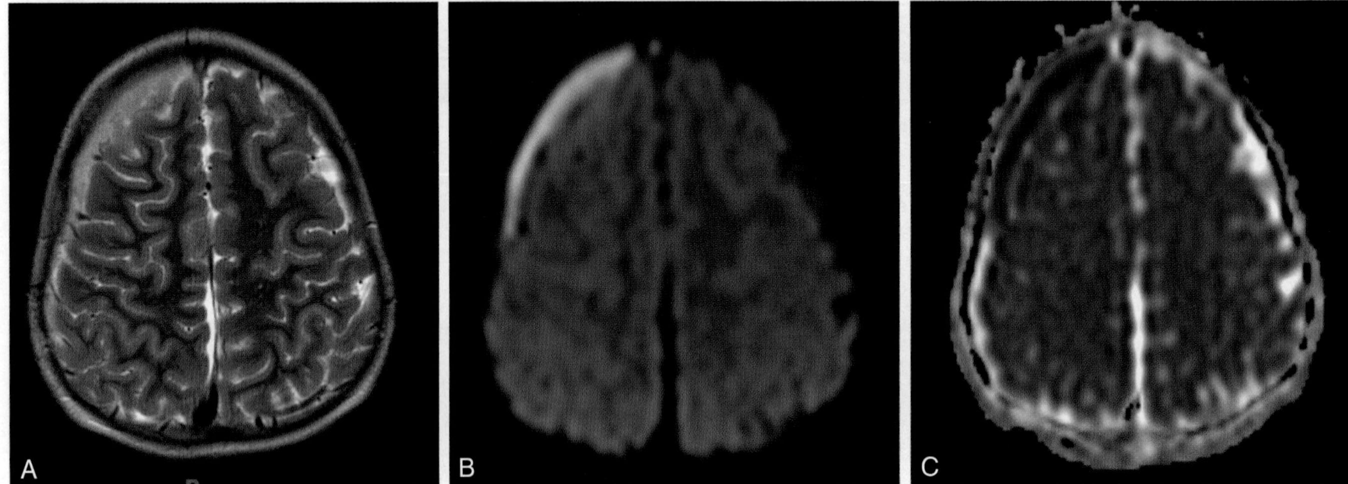

Fig. 5.39 Sinusitis Complications: Subdural Empyema. (A) Axial T2W, (B) axial DWI, and (C) axial ADC image demonstrate a T2W hyperintense diffusion restricting right frontal subdural fluid collection consistent with an empyema.

Key Points

- Subdural and epidural empyemas are most commonly due to extension from paranasal sinusitis. Other potential etiologies are from meningitis and surgical procedures.
- Antibiotics and often surgical intervention are necessary for treatment.
- Subdural empyemas constitute a neurosurgical emergency as the infection can spread widely, spread via emissary veins resulting in infarcts, cerebral edema, sinus thrombosis, and elevated intracranial pressure.
- Epidural empyemas do not always require drainage as the dura can act as a mechanical barrier. An epidural empyema is unlikely to enlarge enough to cause elevated intracranial pressure.
- Subdural empyemas are most often treated with a craniotomy while epidural empyemas can be treated with burr hole drainage.
- Although at times imaging differentiating epidural from subdural empyema can be difficult, a subdural empyema will have acute neurologic symptoms as opposed to epidural empyemas, which can assist in the diagnosis.

REFERENCE

1. Lundy P, Kaufman C, Garcia D, et al. Intracranial subdural empyemas and epidural abscesses in children. *J Neurosurg Pediatr*. 2019 Mar 22;24(1):14–21.

SHUNT INFECTION

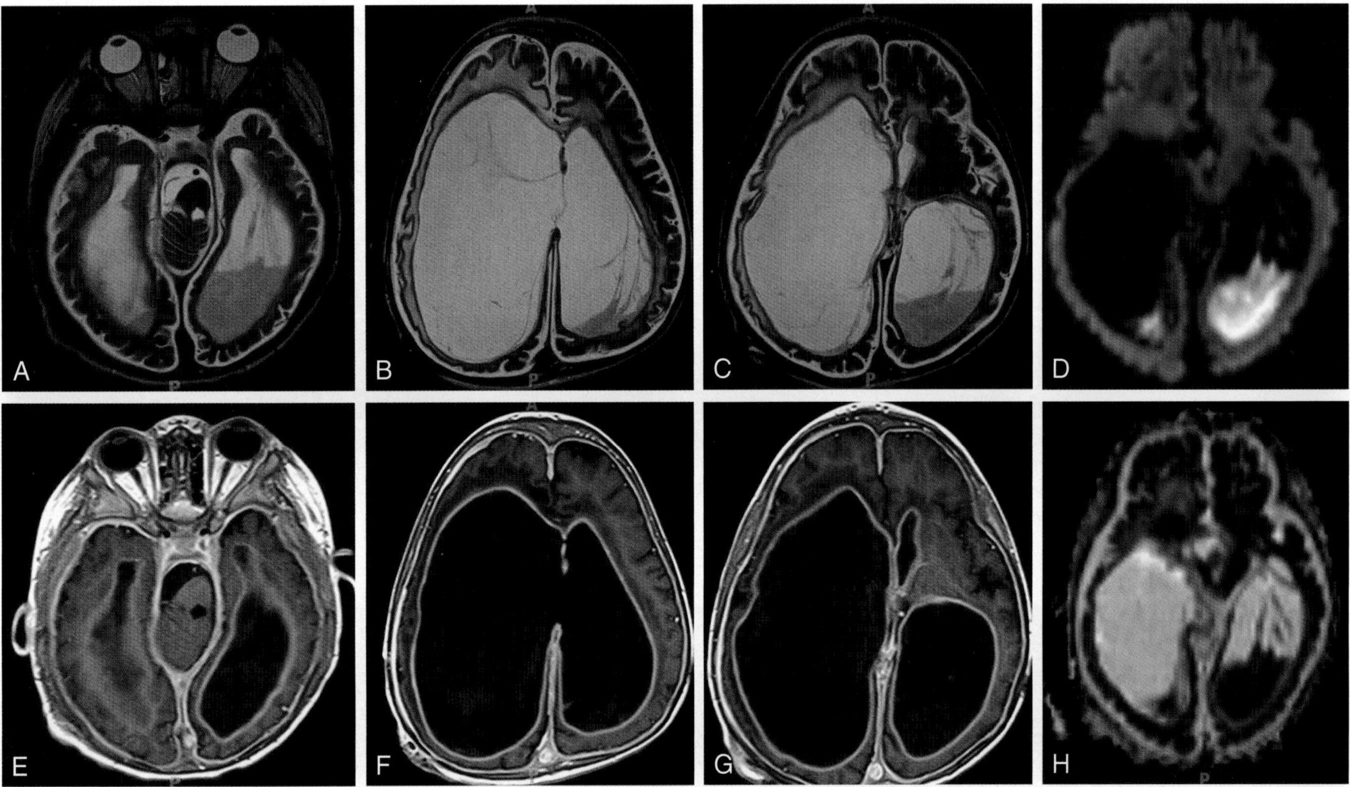

Fig. 5.40 Shunt Infection. (A to C) Axial T2W images in patient with shunt malfunction demonstrating extensive internal septations, purulent layering debris, which demonstrates restricted diffusion on (D) axial DWI and (H) axial ADC. Severe edema is present in the periventricular white matter edema in this patient with severe ventriculomegaly. (E to G) Axial T1W+C images demonstrate avid enhancement of the ependyma due to advanced ependymitis. Diffuse pachymeningeal enhancement is also present.

Key Points

Background

- CSF shunt placement is the most common procedure performed by pediatric neurosurgeons; shunts remain among the most failure-prone life-sustaining medical devices implanted in modern medical practice.
- Majority of infections are caused by skin flora seeded onto the shunt hardware at the time of surgery.
- Shunt infection risk factors include younger patient age, history of prior neurosurgical procedures/shunt revisions, and the presence of the gastrostomy tube.

Imaging

- Hydrocephalus often with periventricular interstitial edema.
- Ventriculitis-ependymal enhancement and diffusion-restricting purulent debris.
- Septations may be present.

REFERENCE

1. Hanak BW, Bonow RH, Harris CA, et al. Cerebrospinal Fluid Shunting Complications in Children. *Pediatr Neurosurg.* 2017;52(6):381–400.

UNCOMMON BACTERIAL INFECTIONS

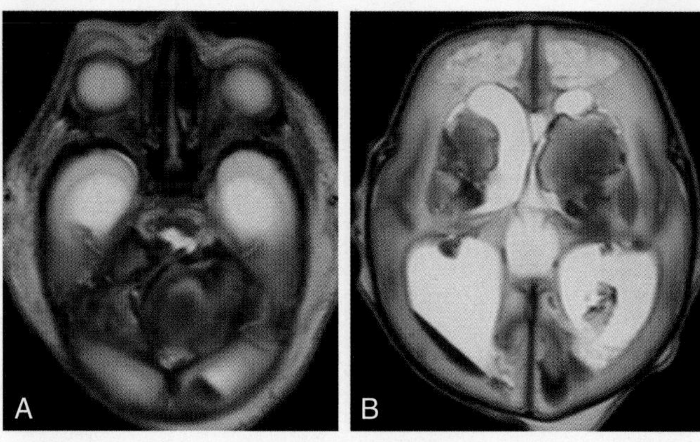

Fig. 5.41 A 1-Month-Old With *Citrobacter freundii*. (A and B) Axial T2W images demonstrate extensive supratentorial and infratentorial hemorrhage with liquefactive necrosis of the bilateral frontal white matter. Note the diffuse hyperintensity of the brain parenchyma and hydrocephalus. Severe scalp edema is present inferiorly.

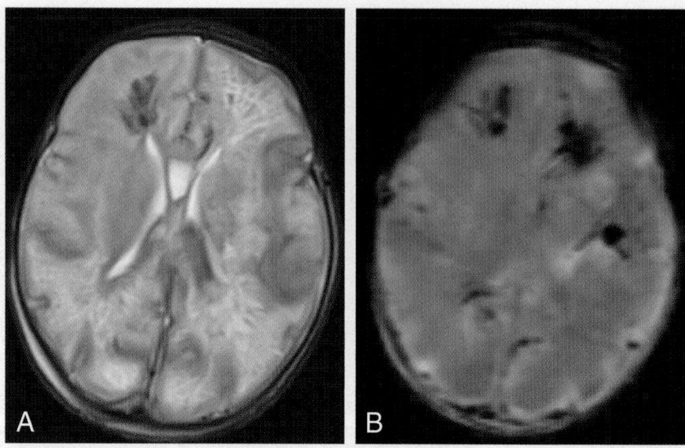

Fig. 5.42 An 8-Day-Old With *Serratia marcescens*. (A) Axial T2W and (B) axial GRE T2* demonstrate multifocal parenchymal hemorrhage and liquefactive T2W hyperintensity of the white matter.

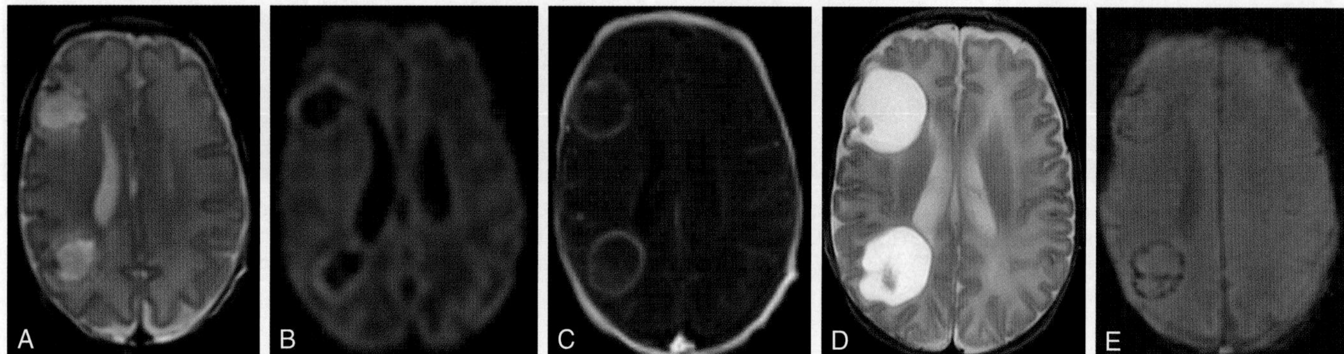

Fig. 5.43 A 7-Week-Old With History of 26-Week Prematurity and *Bacillus cereus* Infection. Initial MRI with (A) Axial T2W, (B) axial DWI, and (C) axial T1W+C demonstrate peripherally enhancing and peripherally diffusion restricting T2W hyperintense rounded masses in the right frontal and parietal lobes. Similar findings were seen in the bilateral temporal lobes (not shown). A 4-week follow-up MRI with (D) axial T2W and (E) axial GRE demonstrate cavitary lesions with peripheral blood products and eccentric nodularity within the cavities.

Key Points

- *Citrobacter*: A gram-negative rod; uncommon aggressive infection occurring in neonates leading to abscesses and hemorrhagic destruction of the brain parenchyma
- *Serratia marcescens*: A gram-negative rod; uncommon neonatal infection leading to liquefactive necrosis and hemorrhage
- *Listeria monocytogenes*: A gram-positive rod; classically a result of contaminated unpasteurized foods; leads to infection of the brainstem and cerebellum
- *Bacillus cereus*: A gram-positive rod found in food; rare CNS infections can occur in neonates and lead to hemorrhagic meningoencephalitis due to the bacterial enterotoxin, phospholipases, proteases, and hemolysin, which cause liquefactive necrosis

REFERENCE

1. Lequin MH, Vermeulen JR, van Elburg RM, et al. Bacillus cereus meningoencephalitis in preterm infants: neuroimaging characteristics. *AJNR Am J Neuroradiol.* 2005 Sep;26(8):2137–2143.

ROCKY MOUNTAIN SPOTTED FEVER

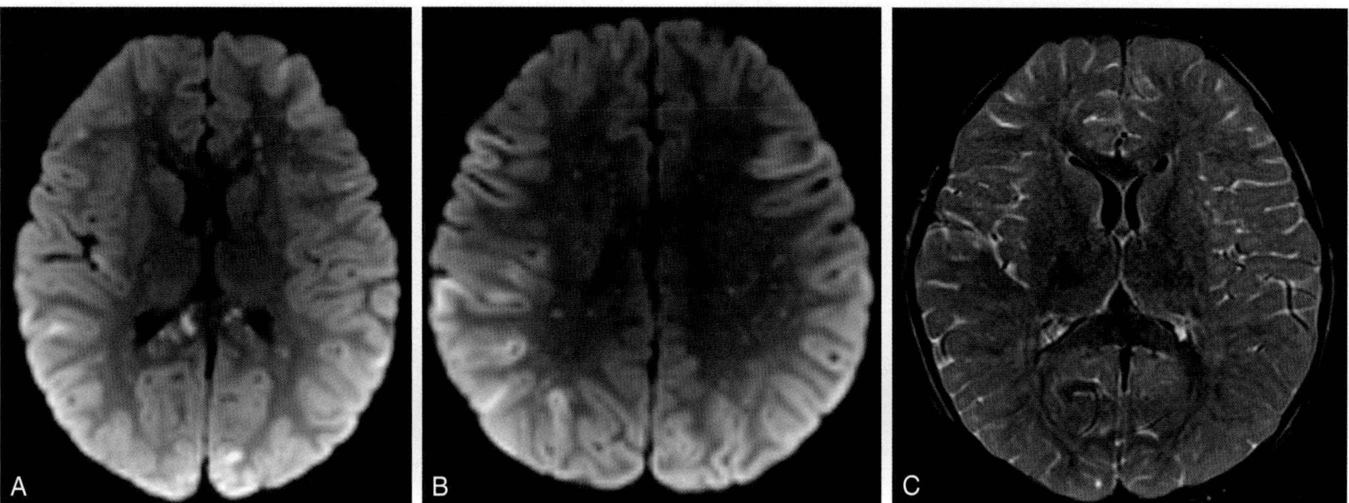

Fig. 5.44 Rocky Mountain Spotted Fever. A 35-month-old with altered mental status. (A and B) Axial DWI demonstrates multifocal cortical, white matter and callosal restricted diffusion with diffuse leptomeningeal enhancement consistent with leptomeningitis on the (C) axial T2 FLAIR+C sequence. The speckled diffusion restriction in the white matter creates the "starry sky" pattern reported with Rocky Mountain Spotted Fever.

Key Points

- Causative agent is *Rickettsia rickettsii*, a gram-negative bacteria, which is transferred to humans by a tick bite
- Presentation with rash, headache, focal neurologic deficits, stroke, seizures, coma; long-term sequelae include permanent neurologic deficits, deafness, and limb amputation
- *Rickettsia rickettsii* injures endothelial and vascular smooth muscle cells, causing damage to the microcirculation of virtually all organs
- CNS involvement: Vasculitis, white matter microinfarctions, and a predominantly mononuclear cell leptomeningitis

Imaging

- Punctate nonenhancing parenchymal DWI restricting T2W hyperintense foci described as "starry sky" pattern
- Leptomeningeal enhancement best seen on FLAIR+C

REFERENCES

1. Akgoz A, Mukundan S, Lee TC. Imaging of rickettsial, spirochetal, and parasitic infections. *Neuroimaging Clin N Am.* 2012 Nov;22(4):633–657.
2. Crapp S, Harrar D, Strother M, et al. Rocky Mountain spotted fever: 'starry sky' appearance with diffusion-weighted imaging in a child. *Pediatr Radiol.* 2012 Apr;42(4):499–502.
3. Bradshaw MJ, Byrge KC, Ivey KS, et al. Meningoencephalitis due to Spotted Fever Rickettsioses, Including Rocky Mountain Spotted Fever. *Clin Infect Dis.* 2020 Jun 24;71(1):188–195.

ATYPICAL INFECTIONS

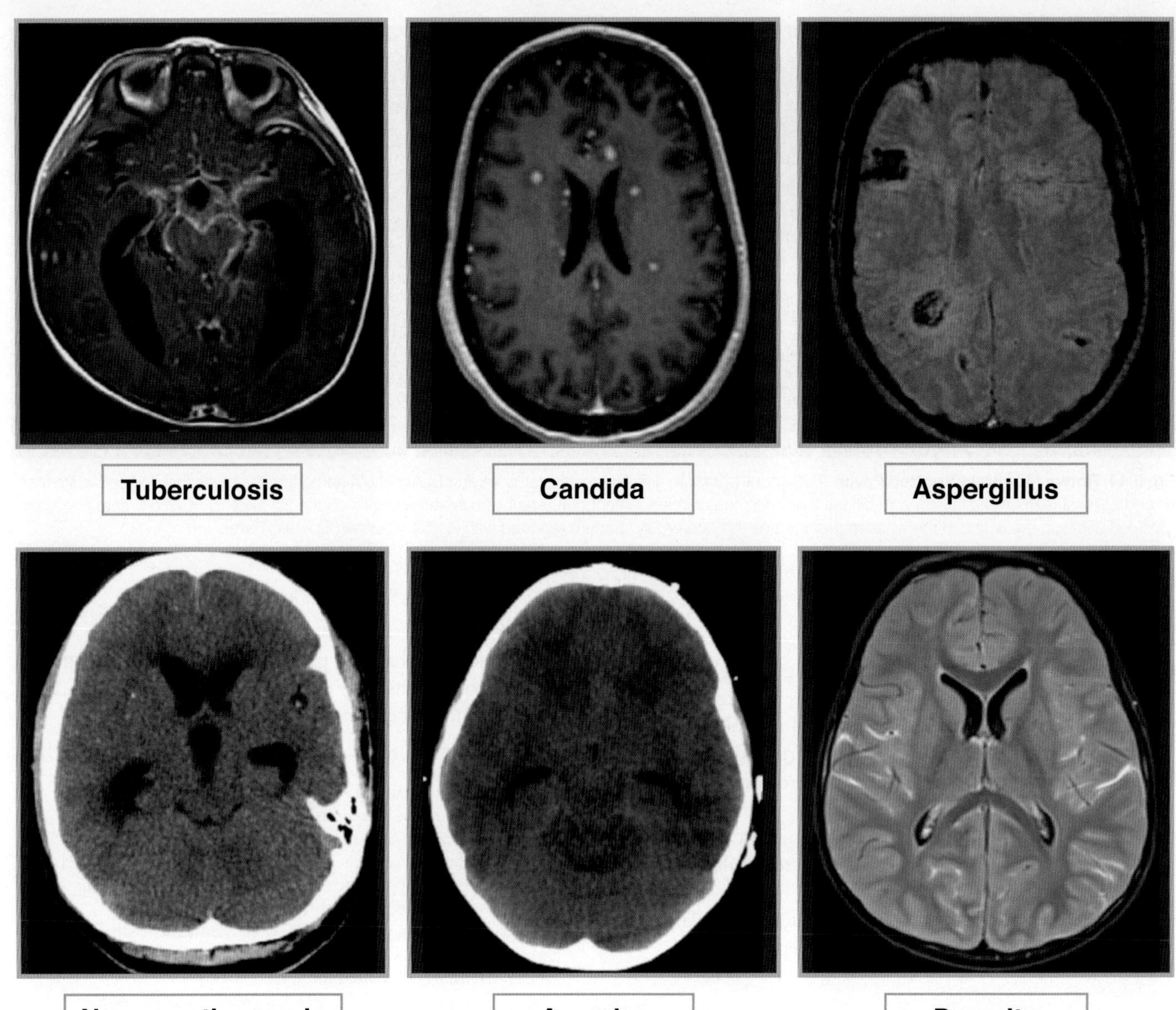

CNS TUBERCULOSIS

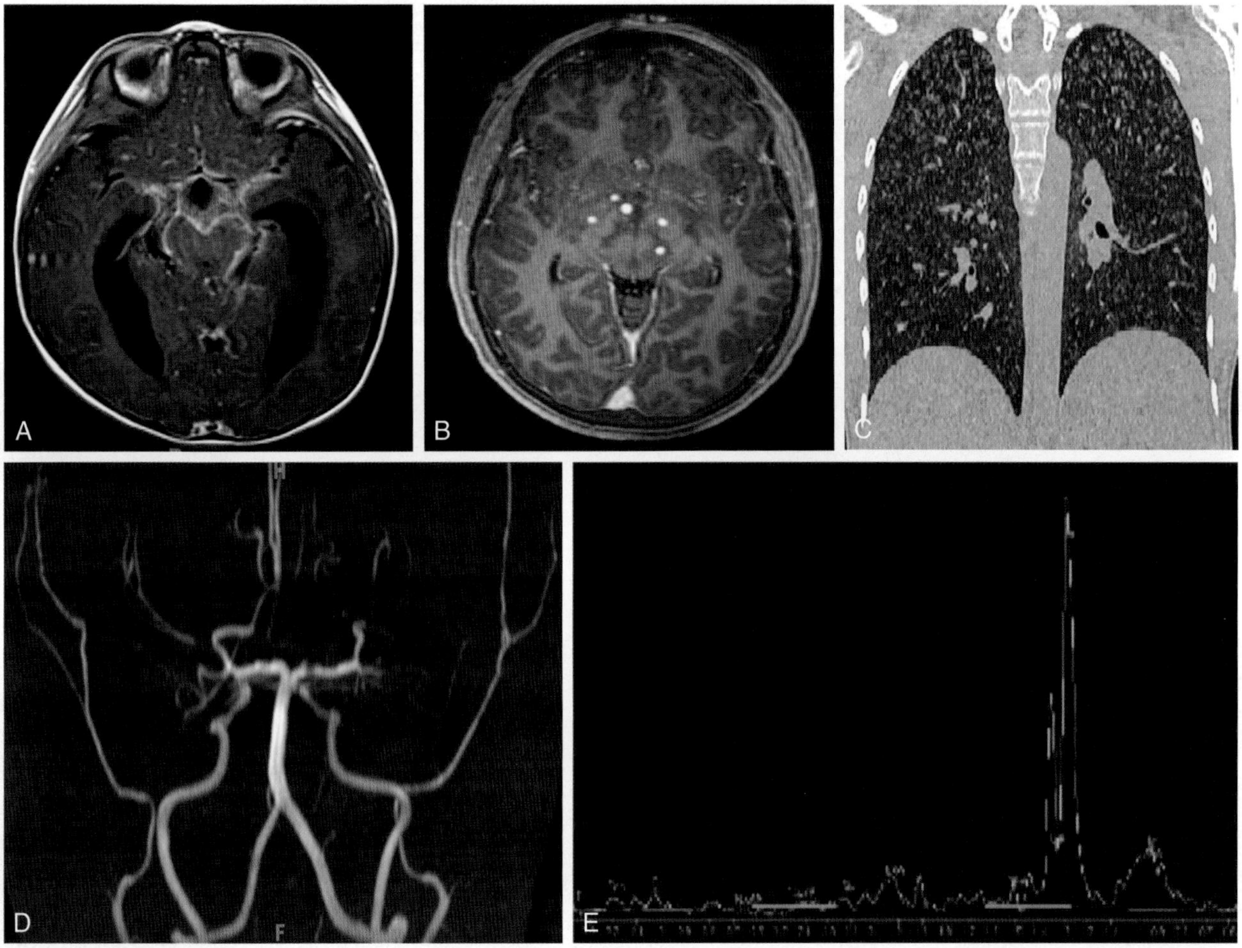

Fig. 5.45 CNS Tuberculosis. (A and B) Axial T1W+C demonstrates advanced basal meningitis and multifocal tuberculomas in the central brain parenchyma. (C) Coronal CT chest demonstrates a military pattern of disease in the bilateral lungs. (D) 3D time of flight (TOF) MRA demonstrates high-grade stenosis of the bilateral anterior circulation and left P1 segment due to arteritis and/ or vasospasm. (E) Elevated lipid peak is present on short TE MRS.

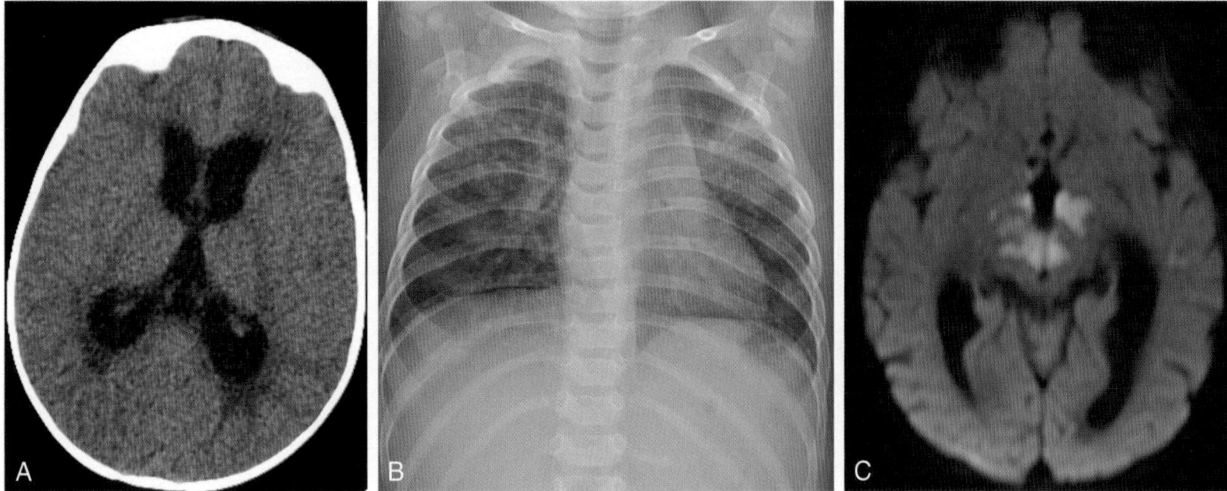

Fig. 5.46 CNS Tuberculosis. An 8-month-old with vomiting and dysconjugate gaze. (A) Axial noncontrast CT demonstrates hydrocephalus. (B) Chest x-ray demonstrates military pattern of lung disease. (C) Axial DWI demonstrates extensive multifocal infarcts of the central brain and brainstem.

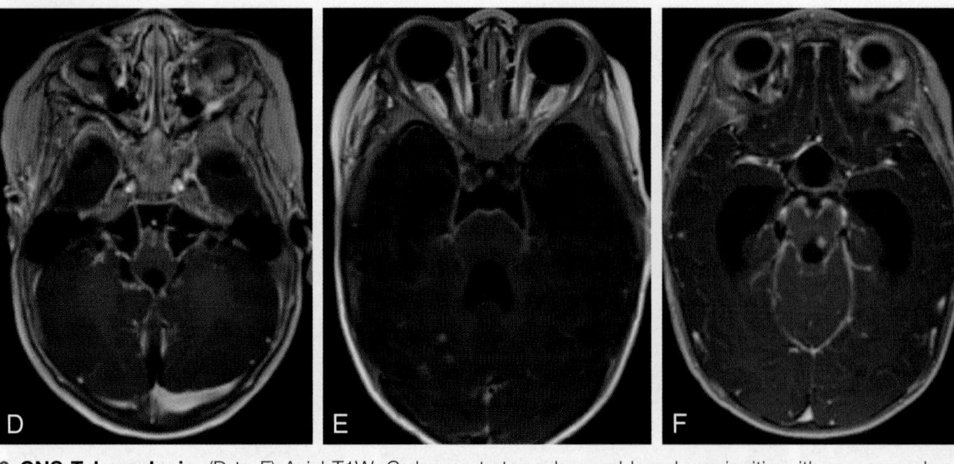

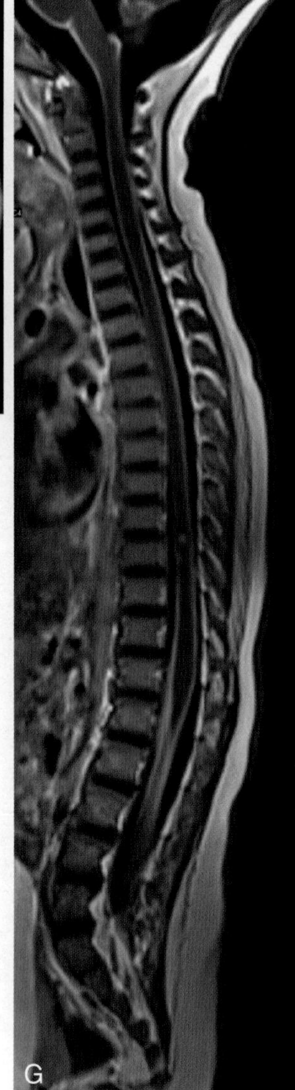

Fig. 5.46 CNS Tuberculosis. (D to F) Axial T1W+C demonstrates advanced basal meningitis with numerous leptomeningeal tuberculomas. (G) Diffuse leptomeningitis, polyradiculitis is present in the spine on the sagittal T1W+C image. Note the tuberculomas in lower thoracic cord.

Key Points

Background

- Acid-fast bacillus
- Most common cause of subacute meningitis and involves the CNS in 0.5% to 2.0% of untreated children
- Symptoms present between 2 and 6 months following primary pulmonary infection, including headaches, seizures, meningismus
- The most common involvement of the CNS by tuberculosis is meningitis, occurring in 95% of cases. Involvement of the brain parenchyma by tuberculosis occurs in approximately 5% of cases, and tuberculous abscesses are seen in less than 1% of patients.

Imaging

- Basal cistern/sylvian fissure predominant meningitis; proteinaceous debris demonstrates lack of suppression on T2 FLAIR with avid enhancement
- Parenchymal or leptomeningeal tuberculomas (round enhancing nodules T2W hypointense, mildly hyperdense on noncontrast CT); long-term tuberculomas may calcify
- Tuberculous abscesses/large tuberculomas are rare
- Stenosing vasculopathy leading to infarcts (often brainstem and deep gray matter nuclei)
- Hydrocephalus
- Concurrent pulmonary tuberculosis common (check chest imaging)
- Spine
  - Infection occurs via dissemination from distant source or by reactivation
  - Enhancing T2W hyperintensity of the involved marrow; disk may be variably involved-normal, expanded with T2W hyperintensity or height loss with destruction; disk sparing is likely an overreported finding
  - Paraspinal, epidural abscess formation may occur; subligamentous spread is characteristic
  - Leptomeningitis, and polyradiculitis

REFERENCES

1. Nickerson JP, Richner B, Santy K, et al. Neuroimaging of pediatric intracranial infection–part 1: techniques and bacterial infections. *J Neuroimaging*. 2012 Apr;22(2):e42–e51.
2. Barkovich AJ, Raybaud C. *Pediatric Neuroimaging*: LWW; 2011:1144.
3. Nguyen I, Urbanczyk K, Mtui E, et al. Intracranial CNS Infections: A Literature Review and Radiology Case Studies. *Semin Ultrasound CT MR*. 2020 Feb;41(1):106–120.
4. Kilborn T, Janse van Rensburg P, Candy S. Pediatric and adult spinal tuberculosis: imaging and pathophysiology. *Neuroimaging Clin N Am*. 2015 May;25(2):209–231.

CANDIDA

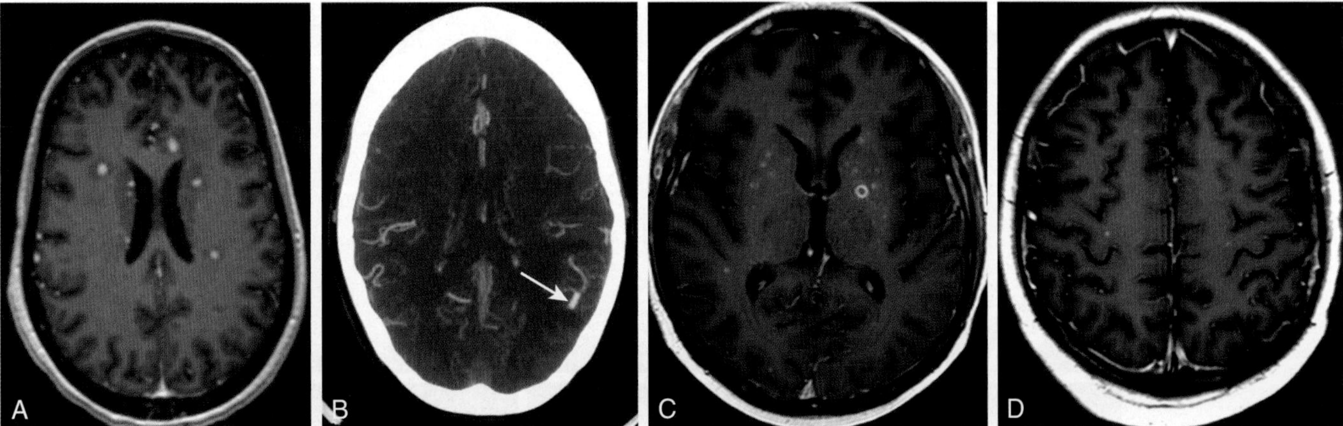

Fig. 5.47 ***Candida.*** (A) Axial T1W+C demonstrates multifocal enhancing nodules in the brain parenchyma. (B) Axial CTA image shows mycotic aneurysm in a left posterior MCA branch vessel. (C and D) A 16-year-old with lymphoma and disseminated *Candida* with multiple small parenchymal-enhancing foci seen on (C and D) axial T1W+C due to CNS candidiasis.

Key Points

Background

- *Candida albicans* is a diploid fungus found in normal flora of skin, oral cavity, intestines, and mucus membranes.
- Infection may occur due to systemic antibiotics, immunosuppression including from diabetes mellitus, prolonged indwelling catheter, and intravenous drug use.
- Vaginally delivered premature infants are at risk of infection due to inoculation during birth (normal vaginal flora overgrowth predisposes to such inoculation).
  - Risk increases with birth defects exposing the CNS (e.g., myelomeningocele).
- Invasion occurs via large vessels but with focal necrosis of microvasculature.

Imaging

- Most common imaging pattern is microabscess formation seen as small homogeneous or peripherally enhancing intraparenchymal foci. Less commonly leptomeningeal and ependymal enhancement can be seen.
- Mycotic aneurysm formation is an uncommon complication and can lead to intracranial hemorrhage.

REFERENCES

1. Nickerson JP, Richner B, Santy K, et al. Neuroimaging of pediatric intracranial infection–part 2: TORCH, viral, fungal, and parasitic infections. *J Neuroimaging*. 2012 Apr;22(2):e52–e63.
2. Barkovich AJ, Raybaud C. *Pediatric Neuroimaging*: LWW; 2011:1144.
3. Palacios E, Rojas R, Rodulfa J, et al. Magnetic resonance imaging in fungal infections of the brain. *Top Magn Reson Imaging*. 2014 Jun;23(3):199–212.

ASPERGILLUS

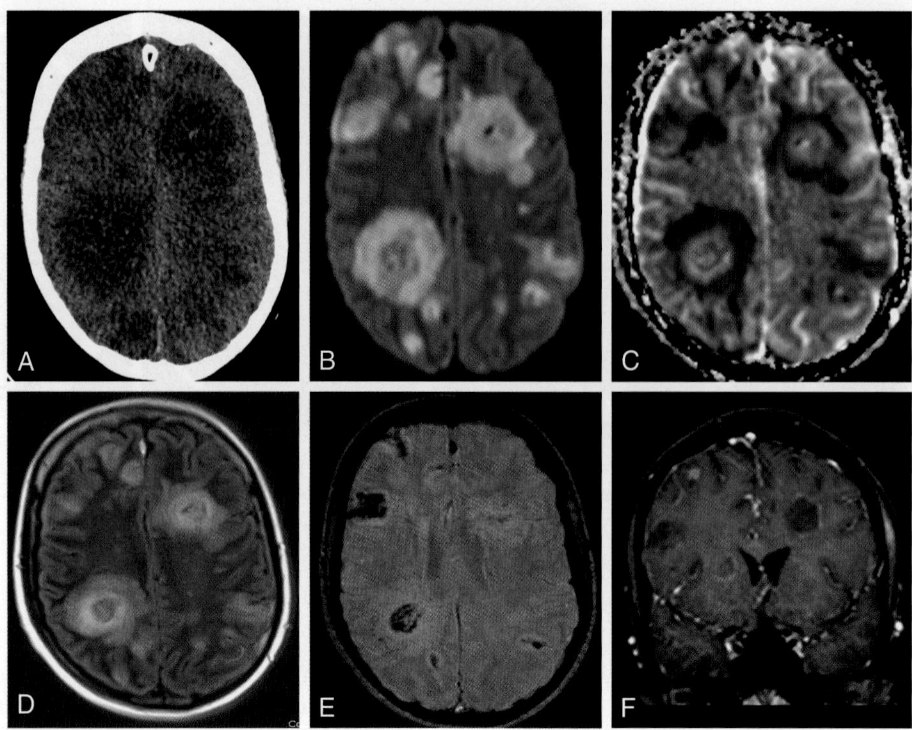

Fig. 5.48 ***Aspergillus.*** (A) Axial noncontrast CT demonstrates multifocal regions of hypodensity. (B) Axial DWI and (C) axial ADC and (D) axial FLAIR images demonstrate intense cytotoxic edema is present surrounding each lesion due to the angioinvasive nature of the organism. (E) Axial SWI image demonstrates significant hemorrhage is associated with each lesion. (F) Coronal T1W+C image demonstrates a relative paucity of enhancement secondary to the angioinvasive nature of the infection thwarting contrast delivery to the region and possibly a limited patient immune response.

Key Points

Background

- Large filamentous fungus, ubiquitous in soil
- Infection occurs in immune suppressed, diabetes; rarely in immunocompetent; infection occurs by inhalation of spores
- Three forms of infections
  - Allergic aspergillosis-sinonasal isolated
  - Aspergilloma-concentrated focus of fungal elements most commonly in lungs
  - Invasive aspergillosis- hematogenous or direct spread from primary site of infection including extension from invasive sinonasal disease
    - Angioinvasion capable as able to produce elastase
    - High mortality

Imaging

- Hematogenous dissemination may result in multifocal lesions throughout the brain
  - Punctate and ring enhancing lesions especially in central gray matter and brainstem
  - Abscess, which may mimic pyogenic abscess
    - Mildly T1W hyperintense, T2W hypointense enhancing ring; enhancement may not occur if host is not responding to lesion
    - Central T2W hypointensity may occur due to hemorrhage/susceptibility from hyphae
  - Cerebritis: T2W hypointensity with susceptibility artifact may similarly be seen as a result of the paramagnetic effect of elements within the hyphae or secondary to associated hemorrhage
- Leptomeningitis
- Vascular
  - Small or large vessel infarcts/ hemorrhagic infarcts due to vascular occlusion
  - Mycotic aneurysm

REFERENCES

1. Nickerson JP, Richner B, Santy K, et al. Neuroimaging of pediatric intracranial infection–part 2: TORCH, viral, fungal, and parasitic infections. *J Neuroimaging*. 2012 Apr;22(2):e52–e63.
2. Barkovich AJ, Raybaud C. *Pediatric Neuroimaging*: LWW; 2011:1144.
3. Palacios E, Rojas R, Rodulfa J, et al. Magnetic resonance imaging in fungal infections of the brain. *Top Magn Reson Imaging*. 2014 Jun;23(3):199–212.

NEUROCYSTICERCOSIS

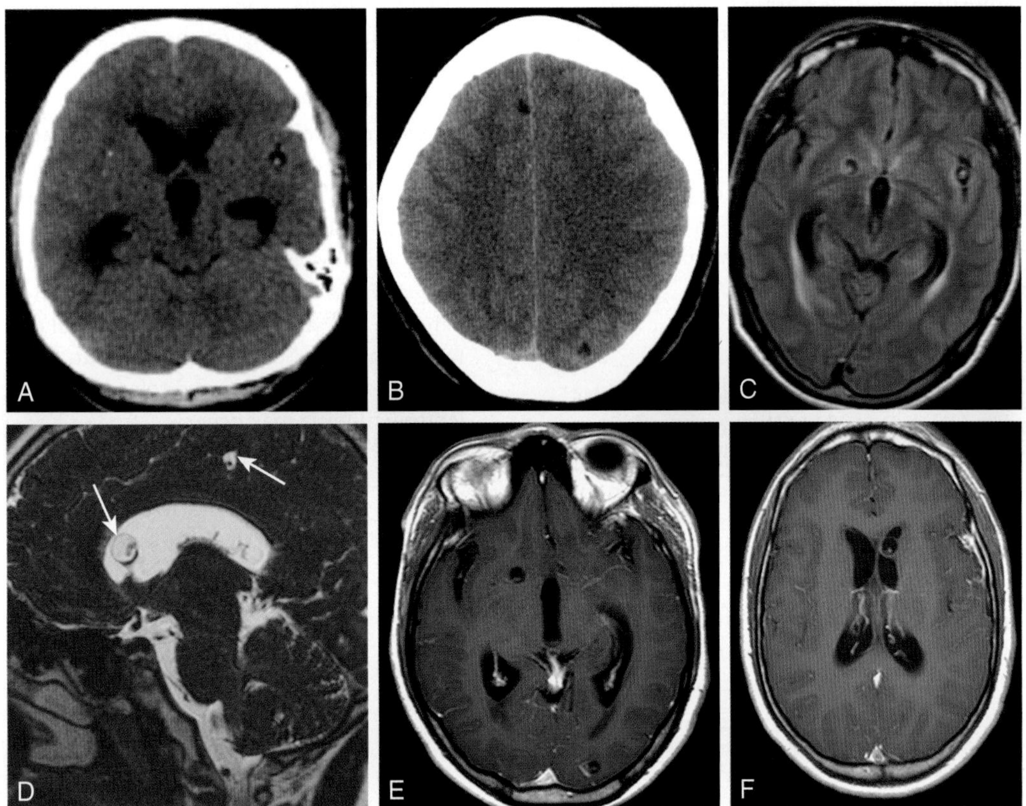

Fig. 5.49 Neurocysticercosis: Multiple Lesions in Multiple Stages. (A and B) Axial noncontrast CT images demonstrate calcifications in the right subinsular white matter without cyst formation, cyst and calcification in the left sylvian fissure, and noncalcified lesions in the right medial frontal and left posterior parietal cortex. Acute hydrocephalus is also present. Granular nodular stage lesion is present along the right caudate nucleus and a subarachnoid vesicular stage lesion is present in the left sylvian fissure. (C) Axial FLAIR image demonstrates lesions in the right frontal lobe and left sylvian fissure as well as periventricular edema. (D) Sagittal 3D T2W image demonstrates the cyst and scolex of lesions in the left lateral ventricle and left cingulate gyrus. (E and F) Axial T1W+C images demonstrate cyst with scolex lesions in the right frontal lobe, left occipital lobe, and left lateral ventricle with varying enhancement related to the stage of infection.

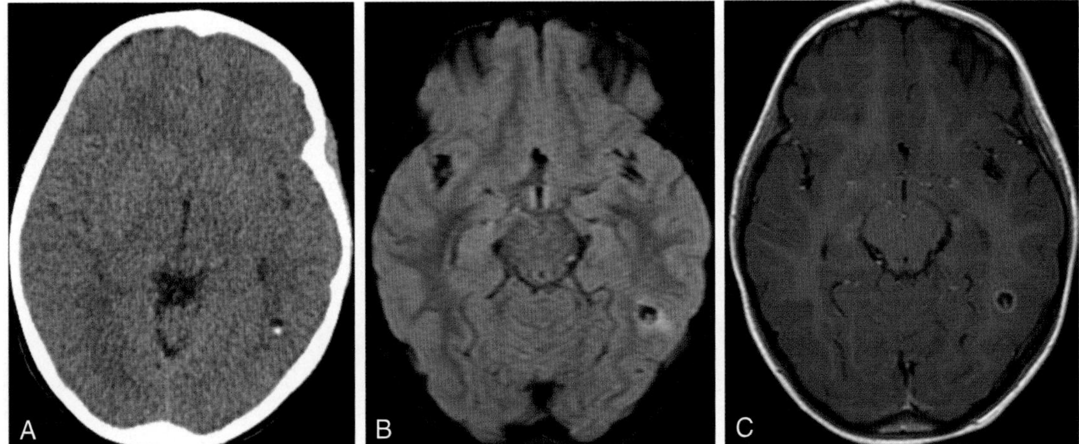

Fig. 5.50 Neurocysticercosis: Solitary Lesion. (A) Axial CT, (B) axial FLAIR, (C) axial T1W+C images demonstrate a cyst with calcification in the left posterior temporal-occipital junction with mild surrounding edema and peripheral enhancement.

Key Points

Background

- Infection and implantation by ingestion of undercooked pork containing the larval form of the cestode *Taenia solium* (pork tapeworm) with human as the definitive host
- One of the most common causes of epilepsy in endemic regions, including Latin America, parts of Asia, Europe, and Africa
- Disseminates in bloodstream and infects the CNS; referred to as neurocysticercosis
- Initial asymptomatic stage followed by seizures and focal neurologic signs

Imaging

- Multiple stages of infection: Vesicular, colloidal vesicular, granular nodular, nodular calcified. The imaging findings vary depending on the life stage of the parasite.
- *Vesicular stage:* Scolex with a cyst that may enlarge up to 1 cm, lack of enhancement or minimal enhancement of the cyst wall, fluid in cyst follows CSF signal intensity/ density, lack of perilesional edema.
- *Colloidal vesicular:* Degeneration occurs after several months, resulting in destruction of the scolex, proteinaceous changes in the cyst (hyperdense on CT, T1W shortening may be seen but without restricted diffusion, occasional fluid-fluid level), ring enhancement, and perilesional edema.
- *Granular nodular:* Degenerating active form in which cyst further contracts and becomes nodular with small ring-enhancing or nodular focus; perilesional edema has decreased but still present.
- *Nodular calcified:* End stage of degeneration; small, calcified nodule without edema or enhancement.
- *Intraventricular:* Often solitary; most common fourth ventricle followed by third ventricle; may migrate; hydrocephalus, and ependymitis may occur.
- *Subarachnoid* form is third mostcommon form after parenchymal and intraventricular; basal cisterns most common. Scolex is often absent. Clustering in subarachnoid space referred to as racemose cysticercosis; leptomeningitis may occur.

REFERENCES

1. Nickerson JP, Richner B, Santy K, et al. Neuroimaging of pediatric intracranial infection–part 2: TORCH, viral, fungal, and parasitic infections. *J Neuroimaging*. 2012 Apr;22(2):e52–e63.
2. Barkovich AJ, Raybaud C. *Pediatric Neuroimaging*: LWW; 2011:1144.
3. Lerner A, Shiroishi MS, Zee CS, et al. Imaging of neurocysticercosis. *Neuroimaging Clin N Am*. 2012 Nov;22(4):659–676.

AMEBIC MENINGOENCEPHALITIS

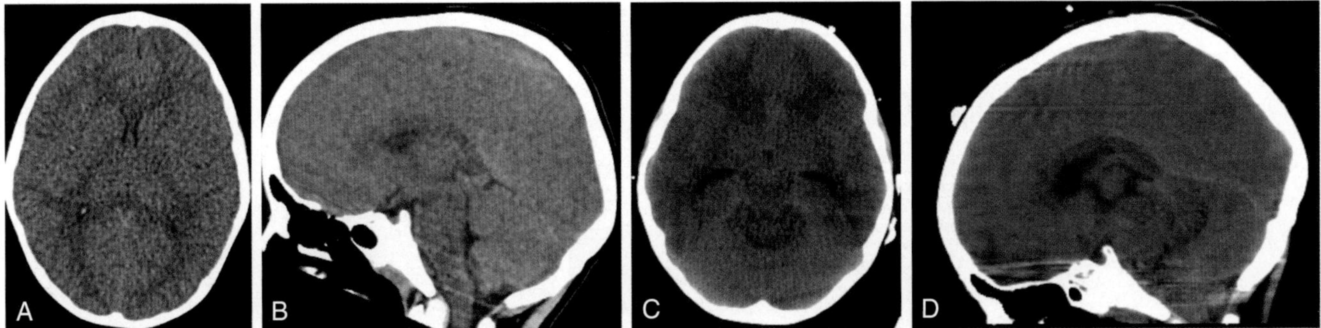

Fig. 5.51 Amebic Meningoencephalitis. 6-year-old with vomiting fever, meningismus diagnosed with *Naegleria fowleri*. Initial (A to D) axial and sagittal noncontrast CT head demonstrates diffuse cerebral edema, which progresses at 24 hours to gross transtentorial herniation on follow-up CT images (C and D).

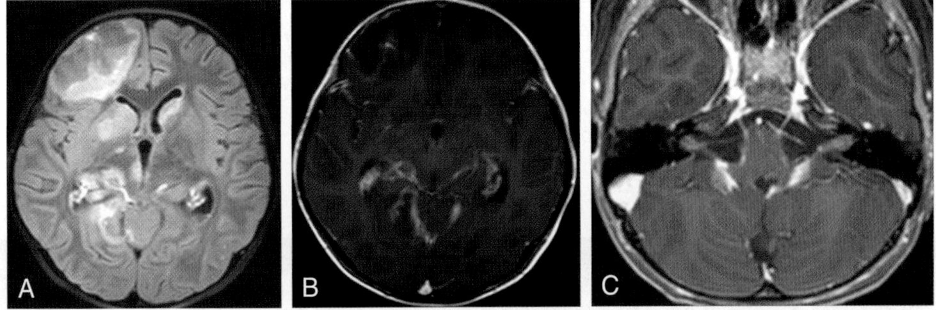

Fig. 5.52 Amebic Meningoencephalitis. 5-year-old with Balamuthia mandrillaris infection. (A) Axial FLAIR and (B and C) axial T1W+C images demonstrate a large necrotic lesion in the right frontal lobe and right mesial temporal lobe that partially enhances. Additional T2/FLAIR hyperintense lesions are present in the basal ganglia and avid leptomeningeal enhancement is seen along cranial nerves VI, VII, and VIII.

Key Points

- Rare infections caused by *Naegleria*, *Acanthamoeba*, and *Balamuthia* species
- Two major subtypes of infection
- Primary amebic meningoencephalitis (acute, caused by *Naegleria fowleri*)
  - Rare rapid progression over 48 to 72 hours with high mortality in children and young adults
  - Entry through the cribriform plate with infection of olfactory mucosa/nerves when in contact with infected, warm fresh water
- Granulomatous amebic meningoencephalitis (subacute to chronic with months of symptoms, caused by *Acanthamoeba*, *Balamuthia mandrillaris* species)
  - *Acanthamoeba:* Rare granulomatous amebic meningoencephalitis, may spread from contact lens solution, skin ulcer, pulmonary, or hematogenous. Affects immunocompromised patients. Duration 2 to 3 months
  - *Balamuthia mandrillaris:* Rare granulomatous amebic meningoencephalitis. Organism is found in soil and fresh water

Imaging

- Primary amebic meningoencephalitis *(Naegleria fowleri)*
  - Leptomeningitis with basal predominance, purulent leptomeningeal exudate, and extensive cerebral edema and hemorrhagic necrosis of the brain, brainstem, upper cord, hydrocephalus, and cerebral edema
- Granulomatous amebic meningoencephalitis
  - Multifocal lesions with heterogeneous or ring-like enhancement and severe edema with predilection for gray-white junction, posterior fossa and thalami, cortical-subcortical cerebritis, and leptomeningeal enhancement. Single focal lesion may also occur. Hemorrhage is common. May mimic septic embolic disease, infection, and neoplasm.

REFERENCE

1. Singh P, Kochhar R, Vashishta RK, et al. Amebic meningoencephalitis: spectrum of imaging findings. *AJNR Am J Neuroradiol.* 2006 Jun-Jul;27(6):1217–1221.

INFECTIOUS EOSINOPHILIC MENINGITIS

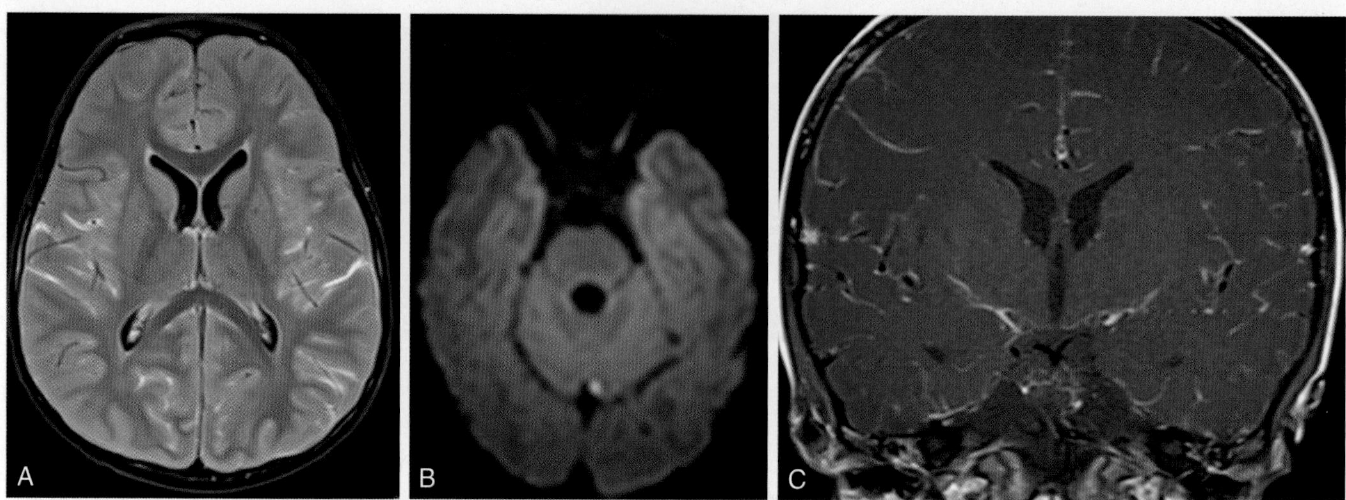

Fig. 5.53 Eosinophilic meningitis: *Angiostrongylus cantonensis*. A 4-year-old child with acute syndrome of inappropriate antidiuretic hormone secretion (SIADH). CSF WBC count 630 with 49% eosinophils. (A) Axial FLAIR+C demonstrates extensive leptomeningitis with (B) axial DWI demonstrating diffusion restricting exudate along the superior vermis. Note the improved identification of the leptomeningeal enhancement on the T2 FLAIR postcontrast sequence compared to the (C) coronal T1W+C where vascular enhancement confounds leptomeningeal enhancement. Additional revealed a history of recently playing with snails. CSF PCR was positive for *Angiostrongylus cantonensis*.

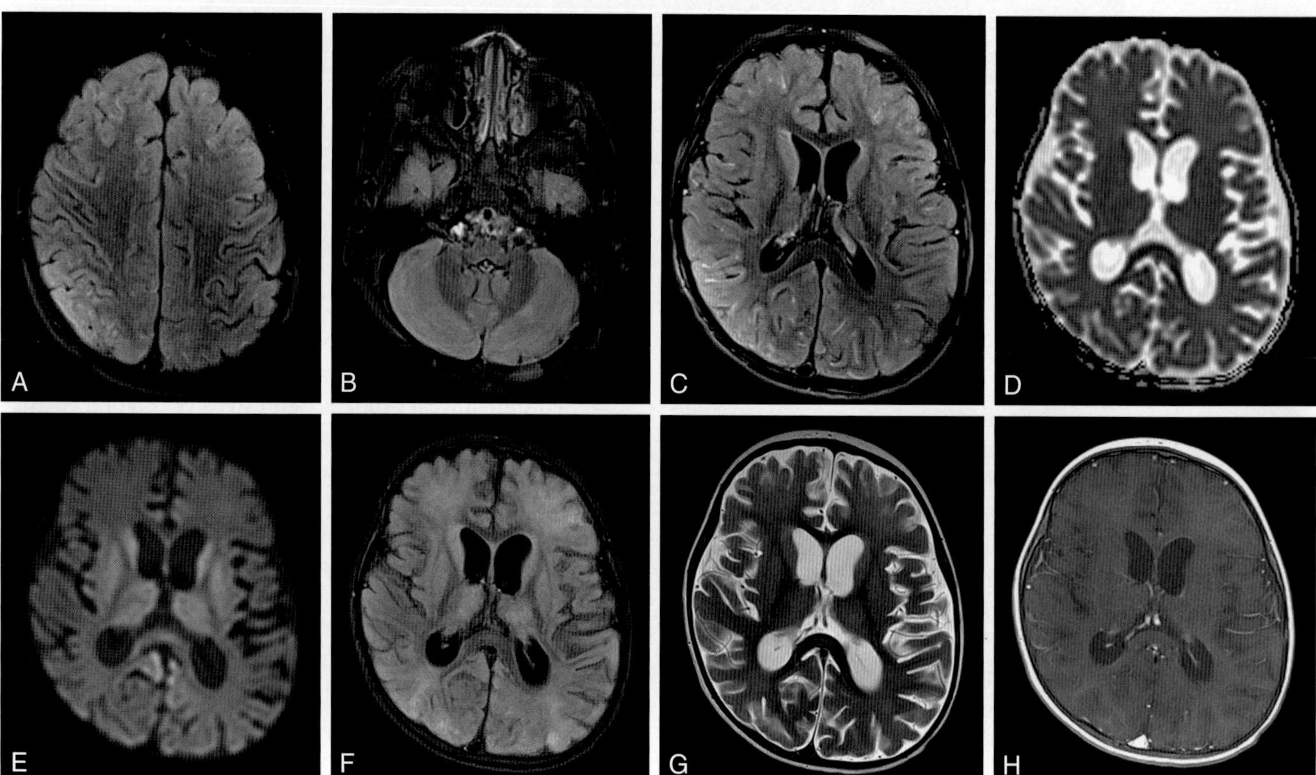

Fig. 5.54 Eosinophilic meningitis: *Baylisascaris procyonis*. A 17-month-old child lives on a rural farm presents with acute onset of fevers, fussiness, progressive axial hypotonia, appendicular hypertonia with elevated serum and CSF eosinophils. Brain MRI at day 1 was normal. (A–C) MRI brain at Day 7. (D–H) MRI brain at day 17. (A–B) Axial T2 FLAIR demonstrates ill-defined regions of cortical T2W signal in the bilateral frontal lobes, right parietal lobe and cerebellar hemispheres. (C) Axial T2 FLAIR C+ demonstrates abnormal leptomeningeal enhancement. (D) Axial ADC and (E) axial DWI demonstrate increased diffusion signal on DWI with equivocal mild decreased ADC signal in the central gray matter. (F) Axial T2W FLAIR and (G) axial T2W images demonstrate broad regions of T2W signal abnormality involving the cortical and central grey matter as well as the cerebral hemispheric white matter with marked volume loss. (H) Axial T1W+C demonstrates resolution of abnormal leptomeningeal enhancement.

Key Points

Background

- Eosinophilic meningitis is defined as at least 10% eosinophils in the total CSF WBC count.
- Most common pathogens are Angiostrongylus cantonensis, Gnathostoma spinigerum, and Baylisascaris procyonis.

Angiostrongylus cantonensis

- Rat lungworm is the most common cause of eosinophilic meningitis in the world. The parasite is endemic in Southeast Asia and Pacific regions and is acquired by eating raw snails, or vegetables containing the larvae. May also occur by accidental oral ingestion from touching snails.
- Symptoms include nausea, weakness, cranial nerve palsies, low grade fever, stiff neck. Young patients may present with upper respiratory symptoms, seizure and altered mental status.

Imaging

- Linear or nodular leptomeningeal enhancement; Small infarcts; Small parenchymal areas of enhancement; Focal T2 hyperitensities in the parenchyma from gliosis

Baylisascaris procyonis

- Raccoons are commonly infected with B. procyonis, an intestinal roundworm. Human infection occurs by ingestion of B. procyonis eggs from raccoon feces or objects contaminated by feces including soil, barns, wood piles used by raccoons. Eggs can survive for years in soil. After ingestion, eggs develop into larvae which may enter CNS and eyes.
- Infection may be asymptomatic, mild, or severe. Infants and those with developmental delay are at greatest risk of severe infection due to the potential of large quantity ingestion. This is similarly true for patients with geophagia/pica.
- Symptoms include nausea, motor weakness and/or rigidity, fever, seizures, ataxia, encephalopathy, coma and visual disturbances including blindness. Profound long term neurologic deficits may occur. Death may occur.
- Diagnosis occurs via ELISA testing of CSF for B. procyonis antibody
- Treatment is albendazole with steroids; early treatment is paramount for best outcome

Imaging

- Imaging is not pathognomonic
- Diffuse T2W hyperintensity of cerebral white matter, especially periventricular white matter, may be progressive. Focal or multifocal T2W signal may occur. T2W signal abnormality may occur in the cortex, central grey matter, brainstem, and cerebellum. Parenchymal and leptomeningeal enhancement may occur. Extensive gliosis and atrophy can be seen as sequela of infection.
- Retinitis/chorioretinitis.

REFERENCES

1. Tsai HC, Tseng YT, Yen CM, et al. Brain magnetic resonance imaging abnormalities in eosinophilic meningitis caused by Angiostrongylus cantonensis infection. *Vector Borne Zoonotic Dis.* 2012 Feb;12(2):161–166.
2. Kanpittaya J, Jitpimolmard S, Tiamkao S, et al. MR findings of eosinophilic meningoencephalitis attributed to Angiostrongylus cantonensis. *AJNR Am J Neuroradiol.* 2000 Jun-Jul;21(6):1090–1094.
3. Rowley HA, Uht RM, Kazacos KR, Sakanari J, Wheaton WV, Barkovich AJ, Bollen AW. Radiologic-pathologic findings in raccoon roundworm (Baylisascaris procyonis) encephalitis. *AJNR Am J Neuroradiol.* 2000 Feb;21(2):415–420.
4. Mehta P, Boyd Z, Cully B. Raccoon roundworm encephalitis. *Pediatr Radiol.* 2010 Nov;40(11):1834–1836.

6 Demyelinating and Inflammatory Disorders

INTRODUCTION

Background

Demyelinating and inflammatory disorders are neuroimmunologic disorders in which there is an exaggerated immune response to the central nervous system (CNS, Fig. 6.1). Neuroimmune disorders have become increasingly recognized as more prevalent than was previously understood, and the understanding of these disorders is rapidly changing and continually evolving. Advances in autoantibodies detection, combined with imaging, clinical signs and symptoms, and cerebrospinal fluid (CSF) findings have led to better understanding and characterization of several of these disorders. Neuroimmune disorders may be triggered by a recent infection or presence of a tumor or may be unknown. Genetic contributions remain to be investigated, but some associations have been found, such as the association between herpes simplex virus (HSV) encephalitis with inborn errors of antiviral interferon immunity, and influenza-mediated acute necrotizing encephalopathy with mutations in heat-shock protein. Most neuroimmune disorders occur in children who are otherwise previously healthy and had normal development. Clinical features include abrupt onset of neurologic signs and symptoms and often a recent history of illness. CSF testing is important for detecting autoantibodies as well as excluding an acute infection. The initial treatment of most neuroimmunologic disorders includes corticosteroids, intravenous immunoglobulin, or plasma exchange, depending on the diagnosis and severity, and has the primary goal of immunosuppression and immunomodulation.

Imaging

The primary imaging modality for detection of demyelinating and inflammatory disorders is MRI, typically of the brain and spine performed without and with contrast. This allows for detection of the full extent of disease, detection of all imaging features, differentiation from disorders that may mimic a demyelination or inflammatory process, and establishment of baseline imaging against which to compare to future imaging. Understanding that there is a wide range of imaging patterns possible with many of these disorders is the first step in the consideration of these neuroimmune disorders in children. Several of these disorders have imaging patterns that can mimic infections or even tumor. Although these disorders involve a wide range of brain, optic nerve, and spine involvement, recognition of patterns of involvement provides clues to the diagnosis. For example, lesions in multiple sclerosis predominate in the white matter and more typically have short-segment spinal cord lesions, whereas neuromyelitis optica (NMO) more often involves the thalamus, hypothalamus, and brainstem and has long segment spinal cord lesions. This chapter discusses the common demyelinating and inflammatory disorders in the brain in children and emphasizes several of the clinical and imaging predilections.

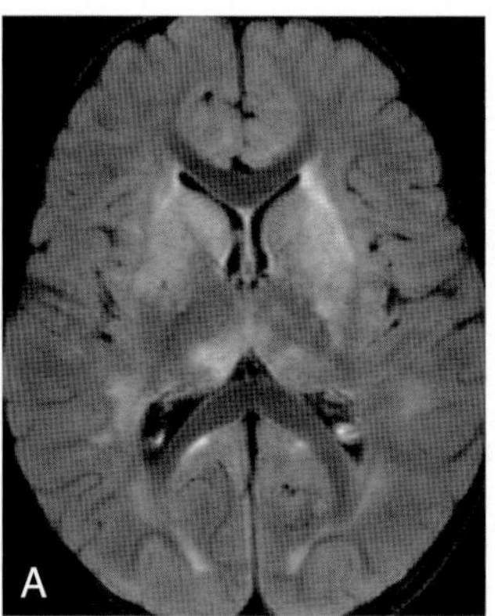

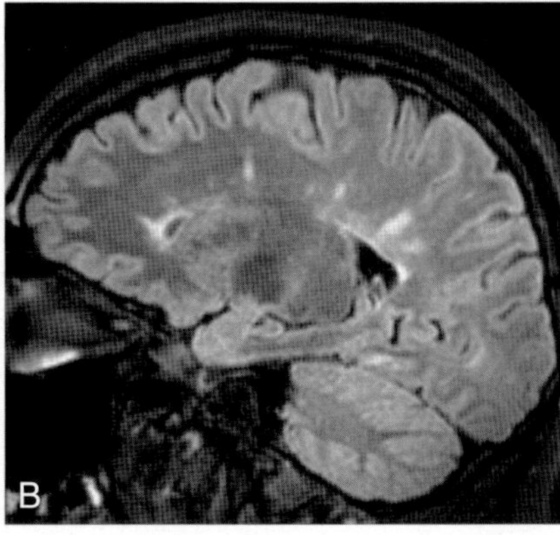

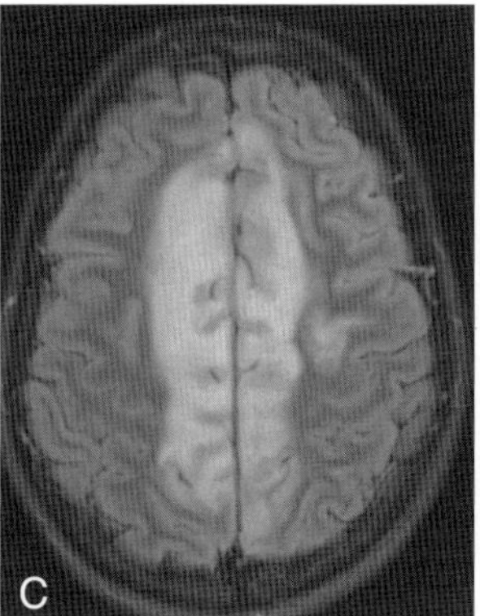

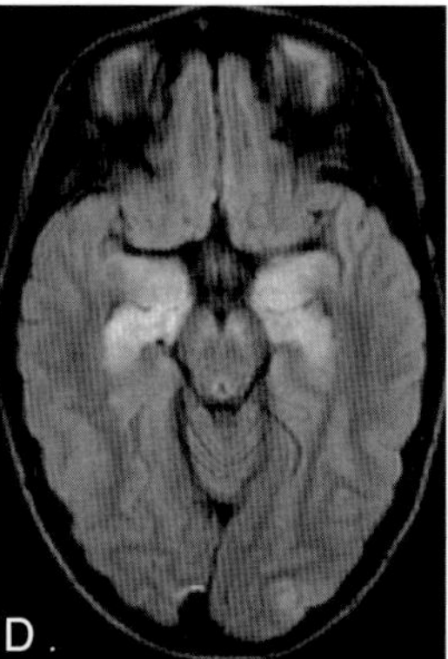

Fig. 6.1 Wide range of imaging findings seen with representative demyelinating and inflammatory disorders of (A) ADEM, (B) multiple sclerosis, (C) anti-MOG demyelination, and (D) autoimmune encephalitis.

ACUTE DISSEMINATED ENCEPHALOMYELITIS (ADEM)

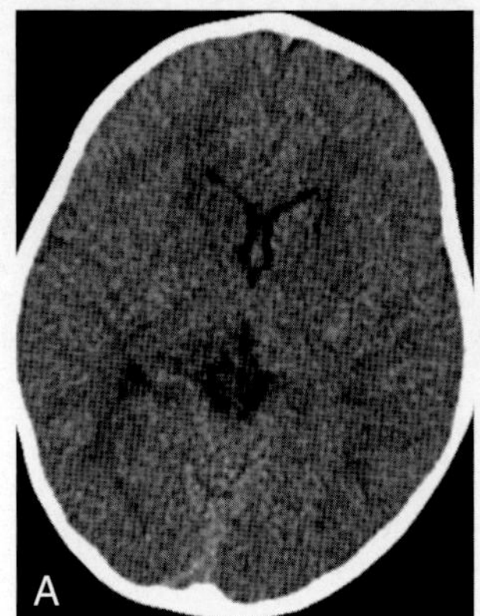

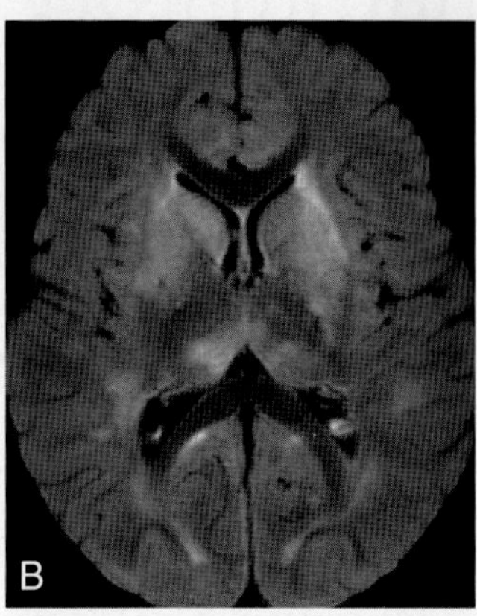

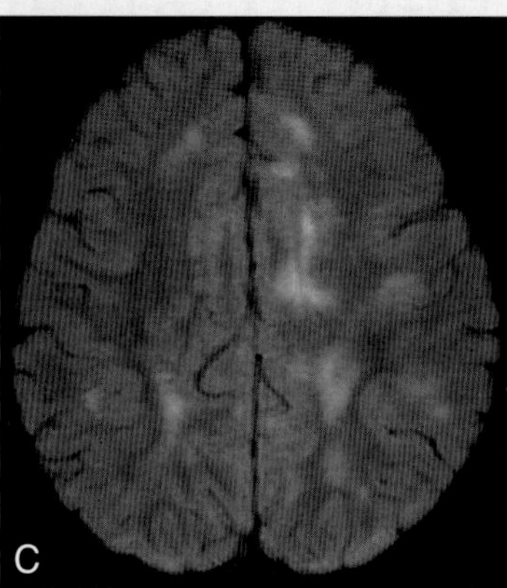

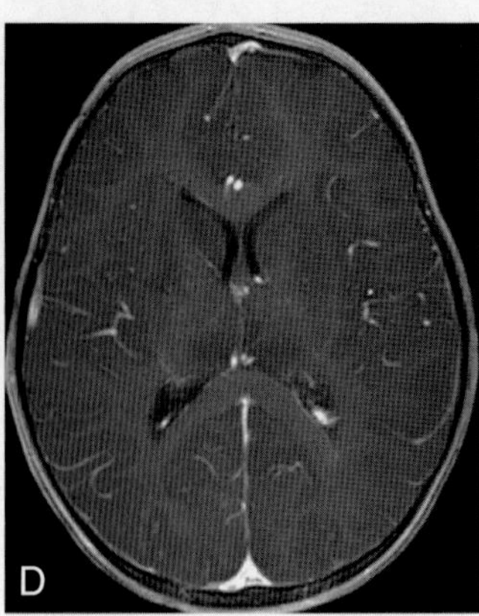

Fig. 6.2 Acute Disseminated Encephalomyelitis (ADEM). A 22-month-old presenting with ataxia and vomiting. CSF analysis demonstrated WBC count 27, normal glucose and protein. (A) Axial noncontrast CT demonstrates patchy hypodensity in the bilateral central gray matter and subcortical white matter similarly seen on the (B and C) axial T2 FLAIR sequence. (D) Axial T1W+C image demonstrates no associated enhancement of the lesions. The patient was diagnosed with ADEM and improved with IV corticosteroids.

Key Points

Background

- Immune-mediated, monophasic inflammatory and demyelinating disorder involving gray and white matter
- Typically (~75%) occurs within 2 to 4 weeks of viral infection or immunization
- Most commonly seen in pediatric patients; may occur in adults
- Less common multiphasic pattern defined as two episodes separated by 3 months, not followed by additional events (<10%). Repeat episodes should raise concern for demyelinating disorders, such as multiple sclerosis (MS), anti–myelin oligodendrocyte glycoprotein (MOG), or NMO.
- Symptoms include encephalopathy that cannot be explained by fever, headache, meningismus, nausea, vomiting, pyramidal signs, cranial nerve palsies, vision loss due to optic neuritis, speech impairment, or hemiparesis
- Anti-MOG antibodies may be transiently positive
- Early use of corticosteroid therapy improves symptoms and prognosis; 10% to 20% have persistent or chronic symptoms

Imaging

- T2W hyperintense ill-defined to well-defined lesions of variable size (often 1–2 cm) involving white matter > gray matter, preferentially juxtacortical white matter; occasionally lesions may show restricted diffusion; variable contrast enhancement
- Rarely symmetric central gray matter involvement may occur
- Spinal cord involvement is often longitudinally extensive, involving gray and white matter; may have dominant central gray matter involvement
- Differential Diagnosis: Encephalitis, vasculitis, posterior reversible encephalopathy syndrome (PRES), other demyelinating disorders (MS, NMO)

REFERENCES

1. Baumann M, Sahin K, Lechner C, et al. Clinical and neuroradiological differences of paediatric acute disseminating encephalomyelitis with and without antibodies to the myelin oligodendrocyte glycoprotein. *J Neurol Neurosurg Psychiatry*. 2015 Mar;86(3):265–272.
2. Marin SE, Callen DJ. The magnetic resonance imaging appearance of monophasic acute disseminated encephalomyelitis: an update post application of the 2007 consensus criteria. *Neuroimaging Clin N Am*. 2013 May;23(2):245–266.
3. Krupp LB, Tardieu M, Amato MP, et al. International Pediatric Multiple Sclerosis Study Group. International Pediatric Multiple Sclerosis Study Group criteria for pediatric multiple sclerosis and immune-mediated central nervous system demyelinating disorders: revisions to the 2007 definitions. *Mult Scler*. 2013 Sep;19(10):1261–1267.

MULTIPHASIC ACUTE DISSEMINATED ENCEPHALOMYELITIS (ADEM)

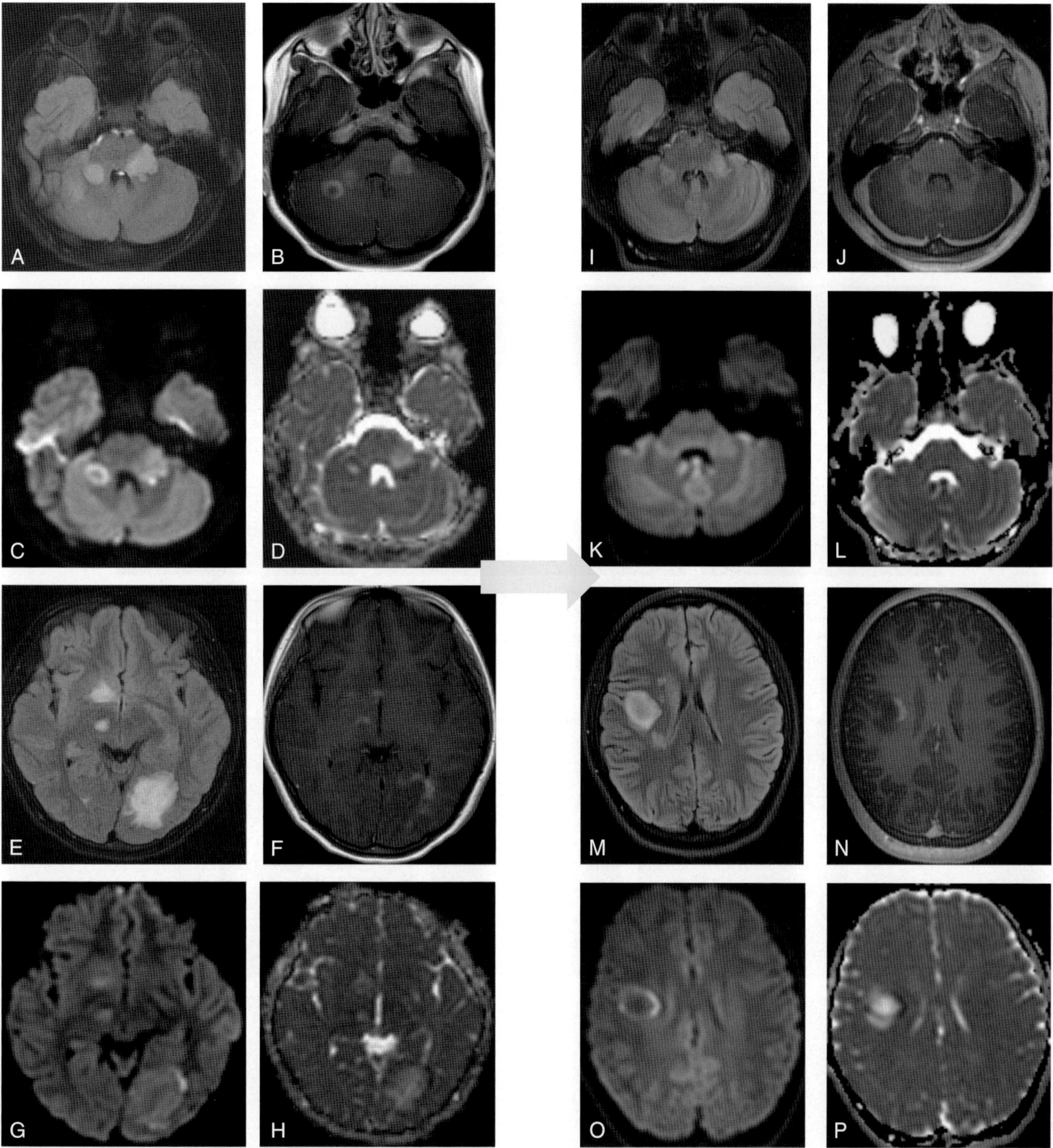

Fig. 6.3 Multiphasic Acute Disseminated Encephalomyelitis (ADEM). A 7-year-old with ataxia. Initial MRI (A to H). (A and E) Axial FLAIR, (B and F) ax T1W+C (C and G) axal DWI, (D and H) axial ADC images demonstrate multifocal lesions in the middle cerebellar peduncles, left posterior pons, right thalamus, right globus pallidus, and left occipital lobe with peripheral areas of reduced diffusion and enhancement. A 4-month follow-up MRI (I to P). (I and M) Axial FLAIR, (J and N) axial T1W+C, (K and O) axial DWI, (L and P) axial ADC images demonstrate decreased T2/FLAIR hyperintensity and resolution of enhancement of the posterior fossa lesions and normalization of diffusion signal but new lesion in the right centrum semiovale with similar incomplete peripheral enhancement and reduced diffusion.

MULTIPLE SCLEROSIS

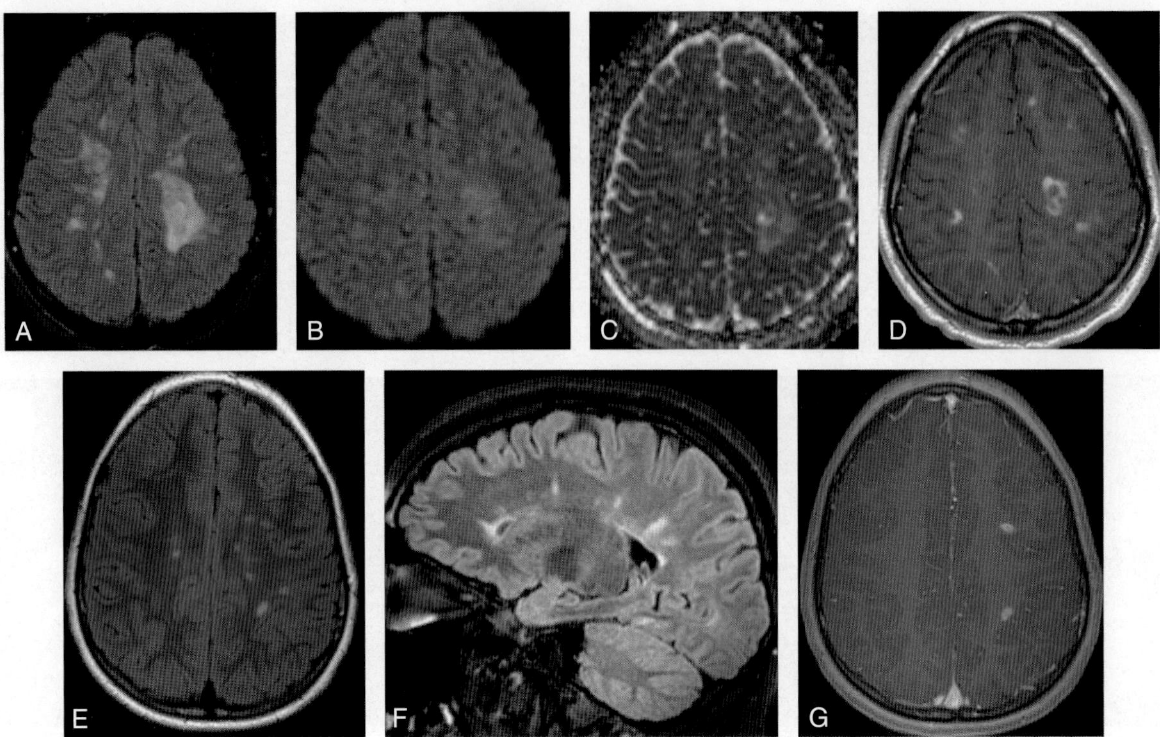

Fig. 6.4 Multiple Sclerosis. An 11-year-old patient. Initial MRI (A to D). (A) Axial T2 FLAIR, (B) axial DWI, (C) axial ADC and (D) axial T1W+C demonstrate focal and confluent T2/FLAIR hyperintense demyelinating lesions with incomplete enhancement without restricted diffusion. Follow-up MRI 5 years later (E to G). (E) Axial FLAIR, (F) sagittal FLAIR, and (G) axial T1W +C images demonstrate characteristic Dawson's fingers along the periventricular white matter and two acute enhancing plaques in the left centrum semiovale. Less T2/FLAIR signal in the centrum semiovale likely represents decreased edema from previous acute demyelinating lesions.

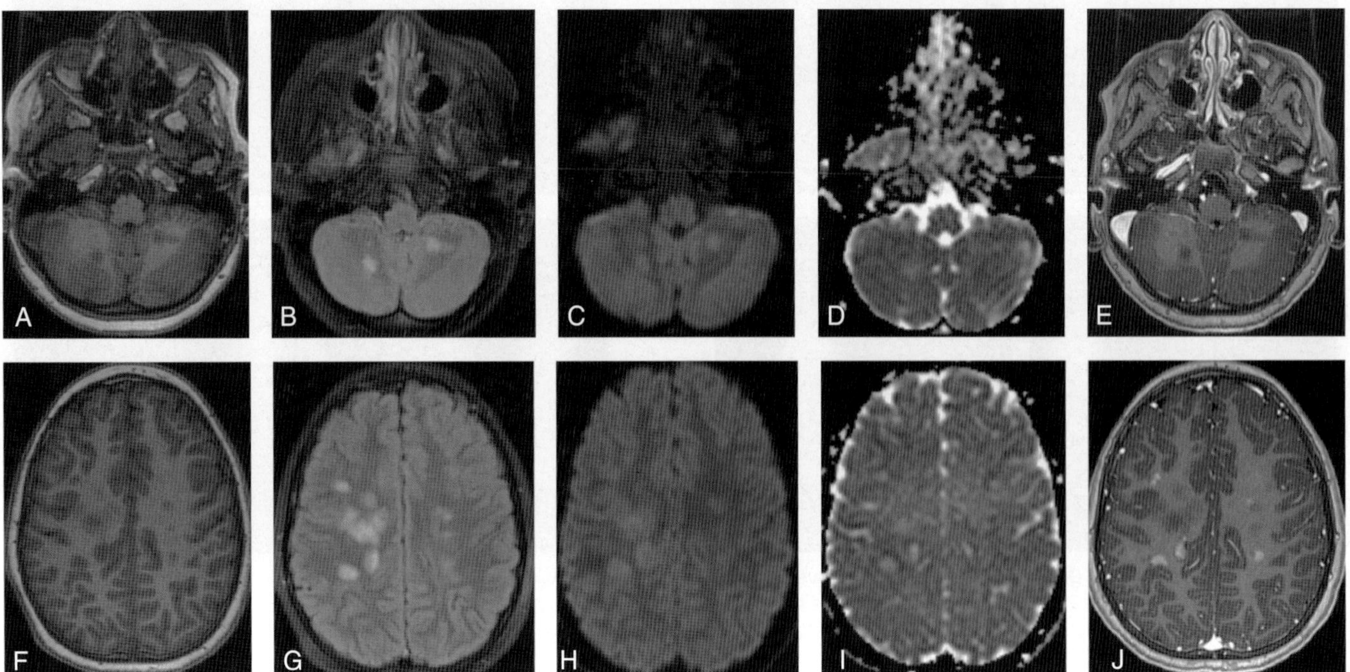

Fig. 6.5 Multiple Sclerosis. A 9-year-old patient with MS. (A and F) Axial T1W, (B and G) axial FLAIR, (C and H) axial DWI, (D and I) axial ADC, (E and J) axial T1W+C images demonstrate multiple focal ovoid T1W hypointense, T2 FLAIR hyperintense supratentorial and infratentorial demyelinating lesions with several lesions demonstrating enhancement. Majority of lesions demonstrate facilitated diffusion and a few demonstrate peripheral reduced diffusion.

Key Points

Background

- Chronic autoimmune condition with genetic predisposition triggered by unknown factors affecting patients typically between the ages of 20 and 40 years
- Highest prevalence in North America and Europe
- 15% primary progressive (PPMS) course, 85% relapsing-remitting (RRMS) course
- CIS (clinically isolated syndrome): First presentation isolated in time and not preceded by prior neurologic event, often presenting with optic neuritis, brainstem syndrome, or transverse myelitis
- Lesions per the McDonald criteria are >3 mm
- Dissemination in space
    - can be demonstrated by one or more T2W-hyperintense lesions that are characteristic of multiple sclerosis in two or more of four areas of the CNS: (1) periventricular, (2) cortical or juxtacortical, and (3) infratentorial brain regions, and (4) the spinal cord
- Dissemination in time
    - can be demonstrated by the simultaneous presence of gadolinium-enhancing and nonenhancing lesions at any time or by a new T2W-hyperintense or gadolinium-enhancing lesion on follow-up MRI, with reference to a baseline scan, irrespective of the timing of the baseline MRI
- Clinical diagnostic criteria for RRMS and PPMS are per the 2017 revisions of the McDonald criteria
- Cognitive dysfunction, including problems with attention, language, memory, and executive functions, occurs in 30% to 50% of pediatric MS and is associated with lesion load
- Pediatric MS versus adult MS:
    - Male:female ratio is closer to 1 in children <10 to 12 years of age
    - Greater ADEM-like onset, more brainstem and cerebellar involvement, and less destructive lesions (less T1 hypointense supratentorial lesions) with pediatric MS
    - Children <12 years have greater numbers of relapses, more severe clinical involvement, worse prognosis, and polysymptomatic onset
    - Oligoclonal bands are detected in 40% to 70% of pediatric MS compared to 90% of adult patients with MS

Imaging

- Brain
    - T2/FLAIR hyperintense ovoid lesions most commonly involving the juxtacortical, subcortical, and periventricular white matter and corpus callosum. Dawson's fingers refers to white matter lesions perpendicular to the ventricles.
    - Posterior fossa lesions often in the cerebellar white matter and middle cerebellar peduncles.
    - Enhancement of lesions is nodular, homogenous, or incomplete ring-like.
    - Tumefactive MS lesions are more common in children than adults.
    - Thalamic and basal ganglia lesions may occur with extensive disease.
- Spine
    - Upper cervical cord and lower thoracic cord most commonly affected; often located in the lateral and posterior columns of the cord; gray matter may be involved; multifocal and short craniocaudal cord involvement
- Differential Diagnoses
    - NMO, ADEM, anti-MOG, Susac, cerebral autosomal dominant arteriopathy with sub-cortical infarcts and leukoencephalopathy (CADASIL), cerebral amyloid angiopathy (CAA), Lyme disease, primary angiitis of the central nervous system (PACNS), chronic lymphocytic inflammation with pontine perivascular enhancement responsive to steroids (CLIPPERS), PML, methotrexate leukoencephalopathy, neurosarcoidosis, and vasculitis

REFERENCES

1. Dekker I, Wattjes MP. Brain and Spinal Cord MR Imaging Features in Multiple Sclerosis and Variants. *Neuroimaging Clin N Am.* 2017 May;27(2):205–227.
2. Thompson AJ, Banwell BL, Barkhof F, et al. Diagnosis of multiple sclerosis: 2017 revisions of the McDonald criteria. *Lancet Neurol.* 2018 Feb;17(2):162–173.
3. Ghassemi R, Narayanan S, Banwell B, et al. Quantitative determination of regional lesion volume and distribution in children and adults with relapsing-remitting multiple sclerosis. *PLoS One.* 2014 Feb 26;9(2):e85741.
4. Ghezzi A, Baronicini D, Zaffaroni M, et al. Pediatric versus adult MS: similar or different. Multiple Sclerosis and Demyelinating Disorders. 2017;2(1).

ANTI-MYELIN OLIGODENDROCYTE GLYCOPROTEIN (MOG) DEMYELINATION

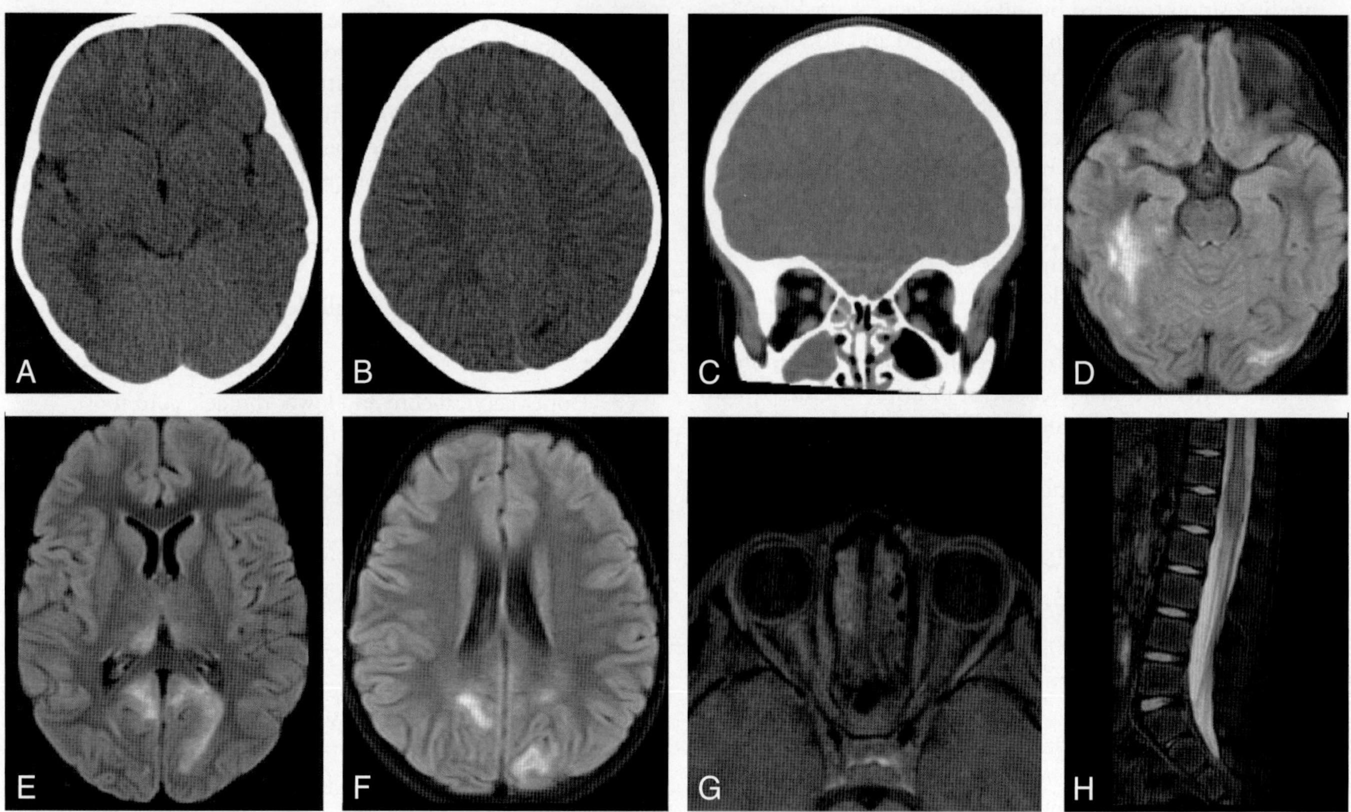

Fig. 6.6 Anti-MOG Demyelination. ADEM pattern with optic neuritis and transverse myelitis. A 5-year-old with acute-onset right eye vision loss, headache, and altered mental status. (A to C) Axial and coronal CT images demonstrate focal confluent hypodensities in the right temporal lobe and left parietal lobe as well as subtle right optic nerve enlargement and perineural inflammation. (D to F) Axial FLAIR images demonstrate multifocal confluent FLAIR hyperintensities in the juxtacortical, subcortical, and periventricular white matter and in the right thalamus. (G) Axial T1W+C fat saturation image of the orbits demonstrates non-mass-like right optic nerve enhancement consistent with optic neuritis. (H) Sagittal STIR image of the spine was performed in the evaluation for demyelination and demonstrates a mildly expansile T2 hyperintense lesion in the conus that involved majority of the transverse spinal cord consistent with myelitis.

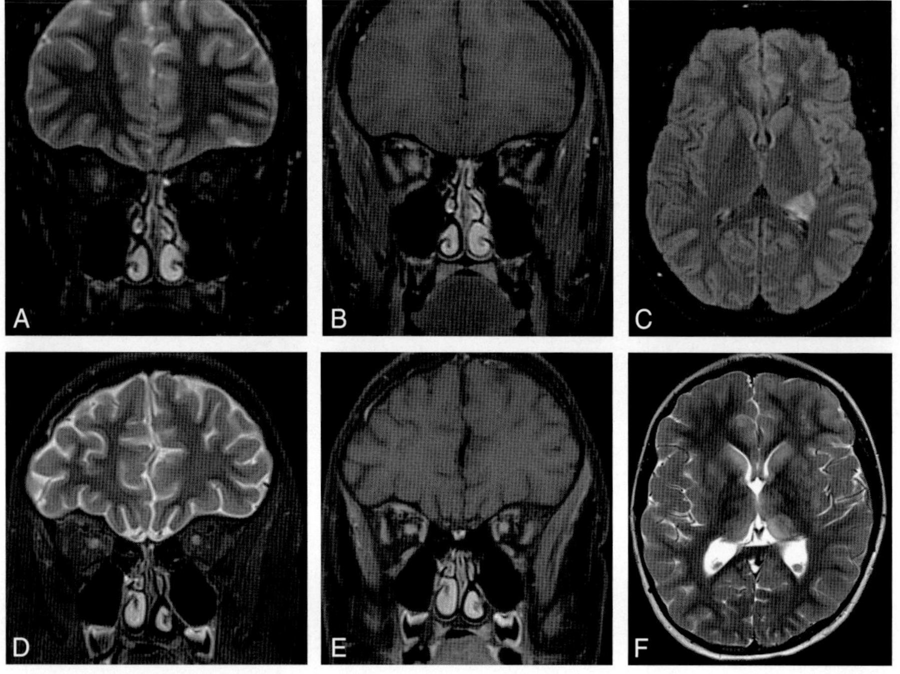

Fig. 6.7 Anti-MOG Demyelination: Optic Neuritis Patterns. (A to C) A 13-year-old acute right eye vision loss found to have anti-MOG antibodies and imaging with (A) coronal STIR, (B) coronal T1W+C fat saturation, and (C) axial FLAIR demonstrating non–mass-like right optic nerve and perineural T2 hyperintensity and enhancement consistent with optic neuritis and perineuritis as well as a parenchymal FLAIR hyperintense lesion in the left posterolateral thalamus. (D to F) A 7-year-old with acute onset bilateral vision loss found on (D) coronal STIR and (E) coronal T1W+C fat saturation to have bilateral non–mass-like T2W hyperintensity and enhancement of the intraorbital optic nerve segments consistent with bilateral optic neuritis. Anti-MOG antibodies were detected in the CSF while aquaporin-4 antibodies were not detected. Three months later the patient returned with new symptoms of altered mental status and was found to have new T2W hyperintensities in the bilateral basal ganglia and thalami seen on (F) axial T2W image.

ANTI-MYELIN OLIGODENDROCYTE GLYCOPROTEIN (MOG) DEMYELINATION

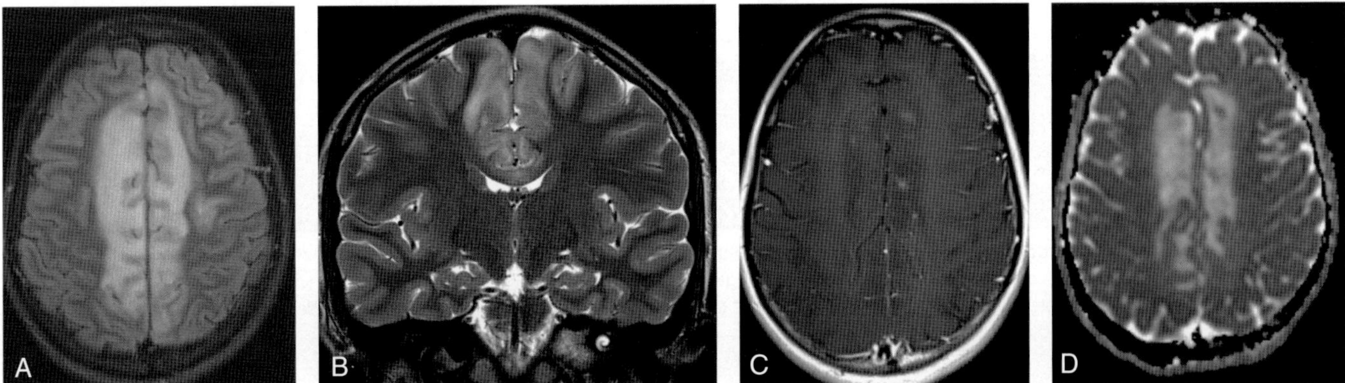

Fig. 6.8 Anti-MOG Demyelination. Encephalitis/tumefactive callosal lesion. A 14-year-old with new onset of seizure. (A) Axial T2 FLAIR, (B) coronal T2W (C) axial T1W+C and (D) axial ADC demonstrate a large confluent partially enhancing region of demyelination in the bilateral parasagittal cerebral hemispheres crossing the corpus callosum. Anti-MOG antibody was found to be positive with titer 1:100.

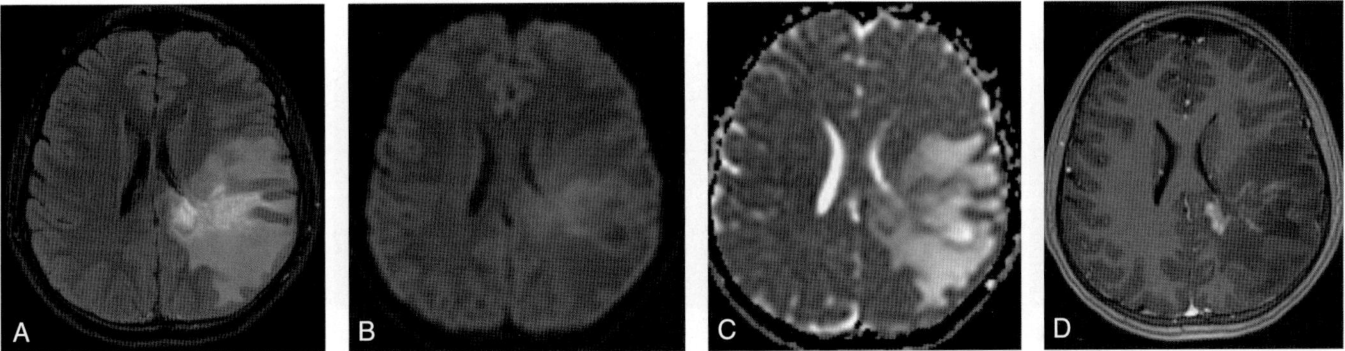

Fig. 6.9 Anti-MOG Demyelination. Encephalitis/FLAMES pattern. A 13-year-old with 1-week history of difficulty walking, right-sided numbness, nystagmus, dizziness, and seizure. (A) Axial FLAIR, (B) axial DWI, (C) axial ADC map, and (D) axial T1W+C images demonstrate a large confluent region of T2 FLAIR hyperintensity in the left frontal and parietal lobe peripheral and deep white matter with internal region with peripheral reduced diffusion and heterogeneous enhancement. Anti-MOG antibody was found to be positive with titer 1:1000.

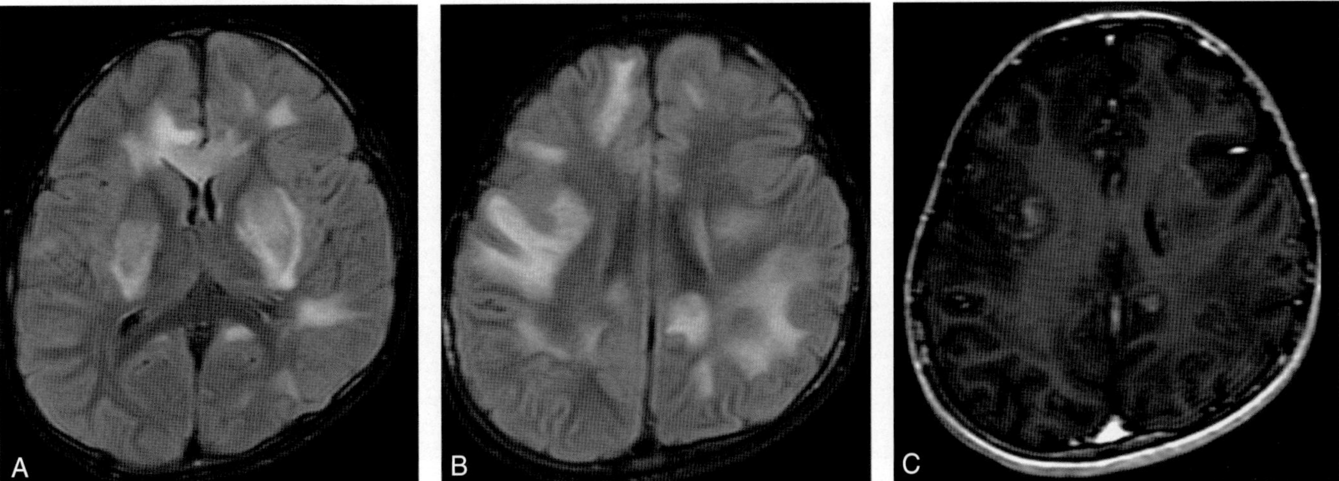

Fig. 6.10 Anti-MOG Demyelination. Encephalitis/leukoencephalopathy patterns. (A to C) A 7-year-old with acute-onset altered dysphagia, drooling, and altered responsiveness. (A and B) Axial FLAIR and (C) axial T1W+C images demonstrate widespread confluent FLAIR hyperintensity in the white matter and basal ganglia with small area of enhancement and no reduced diffusion (not shown). Anti-MOG antibody was positive with titer 1:1000.

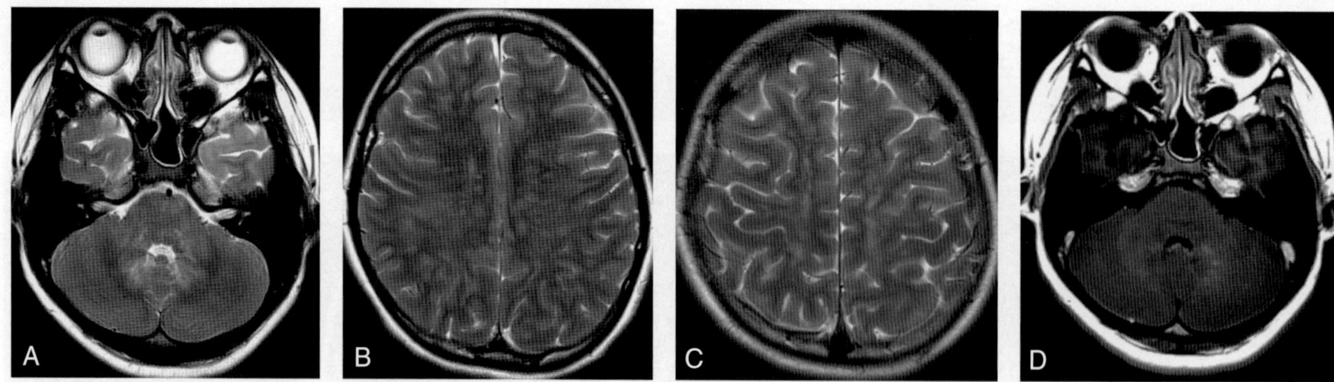

Fig. 6.11 Anti-MOG Demyelination. Encephalitis/leukoencephalopathy pattern. A 4-year-old with lethargy, sleepiness, vomiting, headache, ataxia, and nystagmus for 10 days. (A to C) Axial T2W and (D) axial T1W+C images demonstrate extensive white matter T2W hyperintensities in the supratentorial white matter, brainstem middle cerebellar peduncles, and peridentate cerebellum with mild enhancement in the peridentate cerebellum. Anti-MOG antibody was extremely high (titer 1:10,000) confirming the diagnosis.

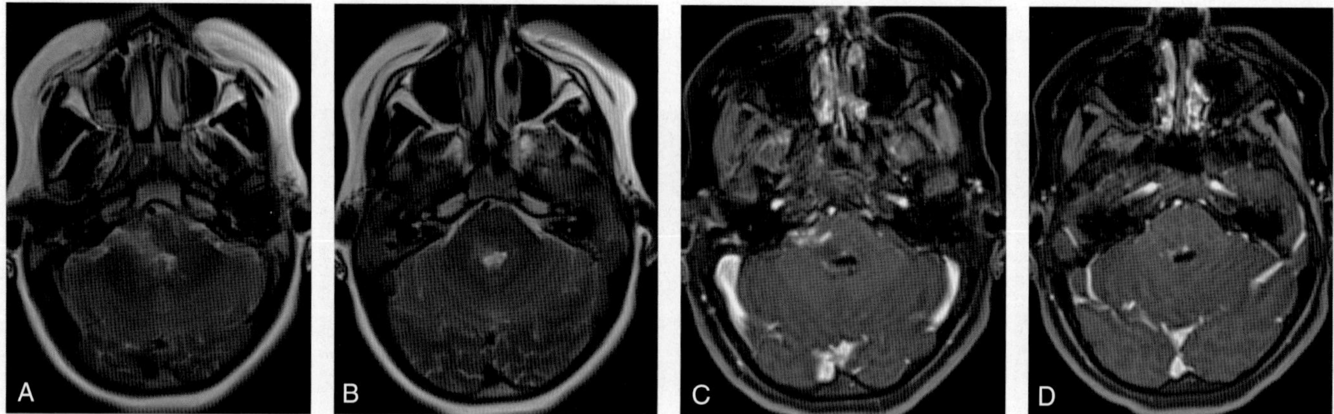

Fig. 6.12 Anti-MOG Demyelination. Isolated brainstem pattern. A 9-year-old with abnormal eye movements and facial weakness. (A and B) Axial T2W and (C and D) axial T1W+C images demonstrate a heterogeneously enhancing focal T2W hyperintense lesion in the right side of the pons and middle cerebellar peduncle with involvement of the cranial nerve 7 and 8 root entry zone. The patient was referred to oncology from an outside institution for tumor evaluation; however, upon review of imaging, a demyelinating lesion was favored and subsequent diagnosis was made following anti-MOG antibody detection (titer 1:100).

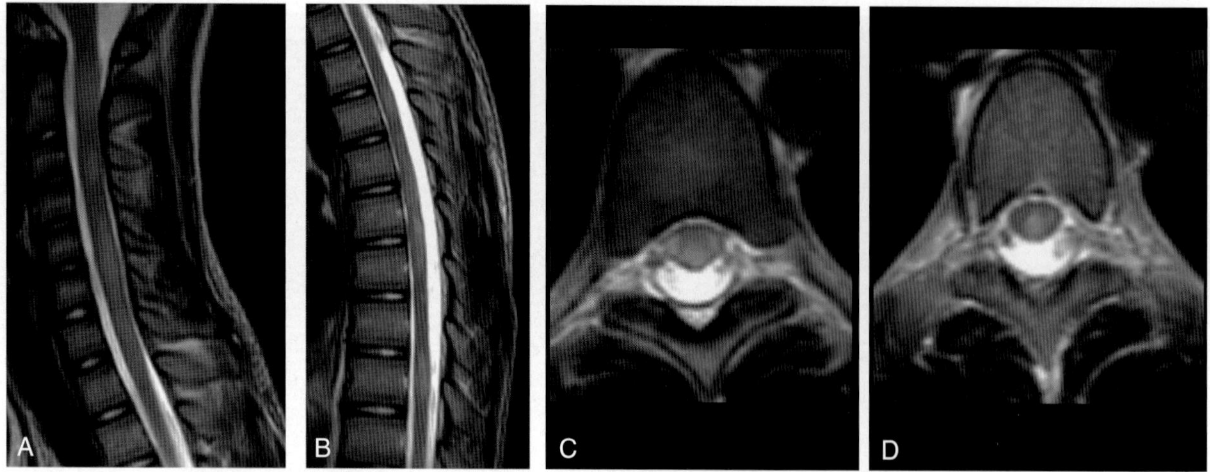

Fig. 6.13 Anti-MOG Demyelination. Longitudinally extensive transverse myelitis. A 15-year-old with numbness in the toes and hands progressing to upper- and lower-extremity weakness. (A to D) Sagittal and axial T2W images demonstrate multiple short and two longitudinally extensive minimally expansile T2W hyperintense spinal cord lesions involving gray and white matter without enhancement (not shown). Anti-MOG antibodies were detected (titer 1:40) while aquaporin-4 antibody was negative.

ANTI- MYELIN OLIGODENDROCYTE GLYCOPROTEIN (MOG) DEMYELINATION

Key Points

Background

- Inflammatory and demyelinating disorder associated with antibodies to myelin oligodendrocyte glycoprotein (MOG).
- Clinicoradiologic patterns include ADEM, ADEM-like, optic neuritis, myelitis, neuromyelitis optica spectrum disorder (NMOSD), and encephalitis
- Clinical presentation depends on CNS region effected and can include altered consciousness, headache, behavioral changes, seizures, neurologic deficits, vision loss, and lower extremity weakness
- Disease course can be monophasic or relapsing remitting
- Young children most often present with ADEM pattern, while children >10 years more frequently present with optic nerve and spinal involvement
- Anti-MOG optic neuritis has good prognosis in >90% of children
- Anti-MOG antibodies are detected in ~20% of aquaporin-4–negative NMOSD. Compared to aquaporin-4–positive NMO, the aquaporin-4–negative anti-MOG–positive NMOSD has more equal male:female ratio, more isolated optic neuritis or myelitis, less severe clinical course, better steroid response, and monophasic disease

Imaging

- Primary imaging patterns are ADEM, optic neuritis, myelitis, and encephalitis
- *ADEM pattern*: Most common pattern; more often monophasic; multifocal subcortical, deep, and periventricular white matter lesions, central gray matter and posterior fossa demyelinating lesions
    - MOG+ ADEM vs. MOG– ADEM: MOG+ ADEM often younger age, greater relapse, more longitudinal extensive transverse myelitis, increased risk of post-ADEM epilepsy
- *Optic neuritis*: Second most common pattern in children; often long segment and bilateral involvement of the intraorbital optic nerves, sparing the chiasm and optic tracts; ~50% have associated perineuritis and adjacent orbital fat inflammation
    - Differential Diagnosis:
        - MS: Typically unilateral and short segment nerve involvement posterior to the globe;
        - NMO: Typically bilateral with involvement of the chiasm
- *Longitudinally extensive transverse myelitis*: ≥2 Vertebral body lengths; may be isolated or have concurrent CNS involvement; clinical and imaging criteria can result in a diagnosis of acute flaccid myelitis in 21%; involvement of the lower spinal cord and conus is more common in anti-MOG (11%–41%) than other CNS demyelinating diseases; {1/3} of cases have multifocal cord lesions; typically gray matter predominant
    - Differential Diagnosis:
        - MS: Less severe; short craniocaudal cord involvement and eccentric location
        - NMO: Worse outcome than anti-MOG; central cord involvement more often cervical and thoracic spinal cord, and more often enhancing (78% compared to 26% with anti-MOG)
- *Encephalitis*: MOG antibodies are commonly found in autoimmune encephalitis (anti-MOG found in 34% of patients versus all other antibodies combined are found in 33%); may coexist with other autoantibodies, particular NMDA receptor antibody
    - Leukodystrophy-like pattern: Extensive confluent T2 FLAIR hyperintensity; more common in young children and possibly related to susceptibility during early stage of myelination
    - FLAIR-hyperintense Lesions in Anti-MOG–associated Encephalitis with Seizure (FLAMES): Unilateral cortical and juxtacortical FLAIR with or without enhancement and reduced diffusion
    - Isolated brainstem involvement: similar appearance to CLIPPERS; seen in 7% to 10% of anti-MOG patients; small nodular foci of enhancement in the pons, middle cerebellar peduncles, and white matter adjacent to the fourth ventricle

REFERENCES

1. Baumann M, Sahin K, Lechner C, et al. Clinical and neuroradiological differences of paediatric acute disseminating encephalomyelitis with and without antibodies to the myelin oligodendrocyte glycoprotein. *J Neurol Neurosurg Psychiatry*. 2015 Mar;86(3):265–272.
2. Gontika MP, Anagnostouli MC. Anti-Myelin Oligodendrocyte Glycoprotein and Human Leukocyte Antigens as Markers in Pediatric and Adolescent Multiple Sclerosis: on Diagnosis, Clinical Phenotypes, and Therapeutic Responses. *Mult Scler Int*. 2018 Nov 22;2018:8487471.
3. Armangue T, Olivé-Cirera G, Martínez-Hernandez E, et al. Spanish Pediatric anti-MOG Study Group. Associations of paediatric demyelinating and encephalitic syndromes with myelin oligodendrocyte glycoprotein antibodies: a multicentre observational study. *Lancet Neurol*. 2020 Mar;19(3):234–246.
4. Salama S, Khan M, Pardo S, et al. MOG antibody-associated encephalomyelitis/encephalitis. *Mult Scler*. 2019 Oct;25(11):1427–1433.
5. Parrotta E, Kister I. The expanding clinical spectrum of myelin oligodendrocyte glycoprotein (MOG) antibody associated disease in children and adults. *Front Neurol*. 2020;11:960.

NEUROMYELITIS OPTICA (NMO)

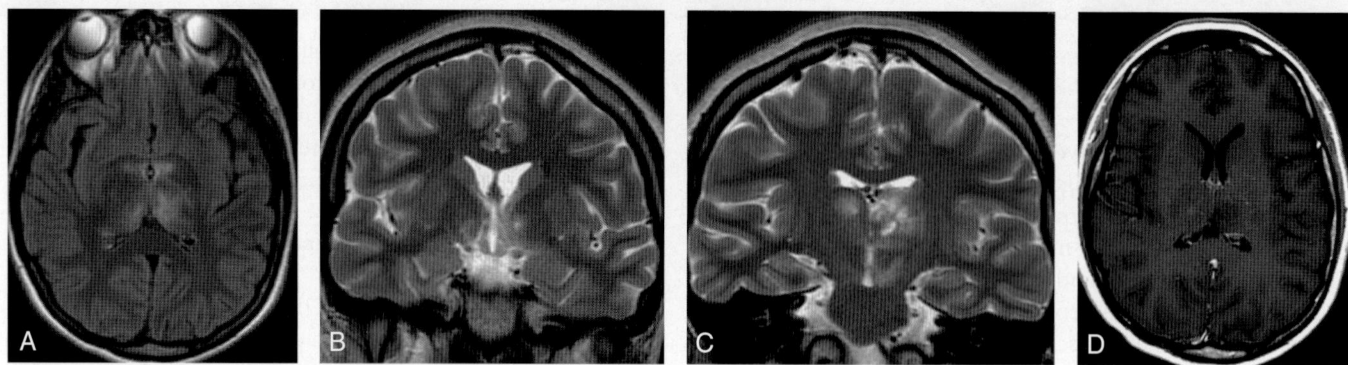

Fig. 6.14 Neuromyelitis Optica (NMO). An 18-year-old with altered mental status, speech, and vomiting lasting longer than 1 month. (A) Axial FLAIR, (B and C) coronal T2W, and (D) axial T1W+C images demonstrate T2W signal hyperintensity in the hypothalamus and thalami with minimal enhancement. Artifact from dental braces is noted, resulting in the hyperintensity of the anterior frontal lobes and orbits on (A). CSF aquaporin-4 antibody was found to be positive.

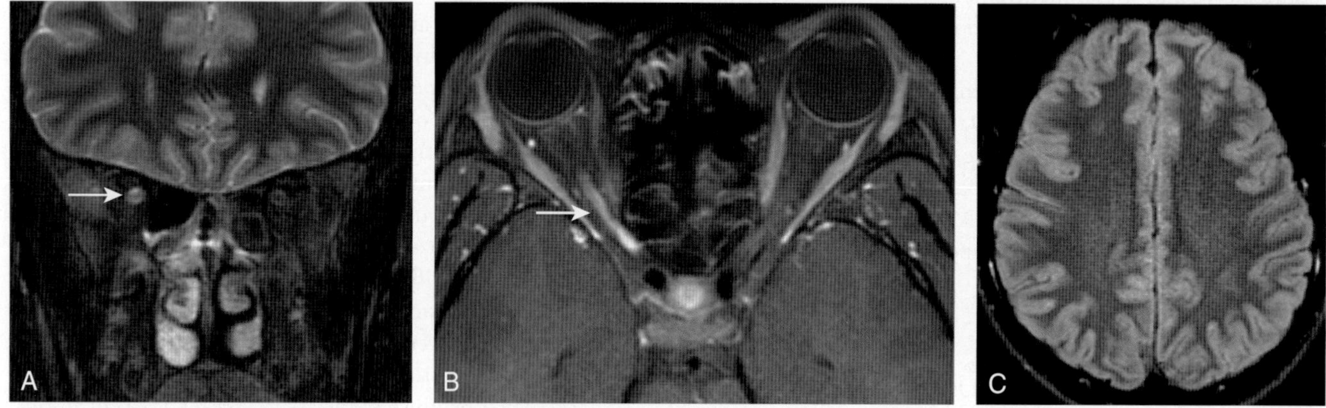

Fig. 6.15 Neuromyelitis Optica (NMO). A 17-year-old with acute onset of right eye vision loss. (A) Coronal STIR, and (B) axial T1W+C images demonstrate nonexpansile T2W signal hyperintensity and enhancement in the right optic nerve consistent with optic neuritis. (C) Axial FLAIR of the brain demonstrates no white matter lesions. CSF aquaporin-4 antibody was found to be positive.

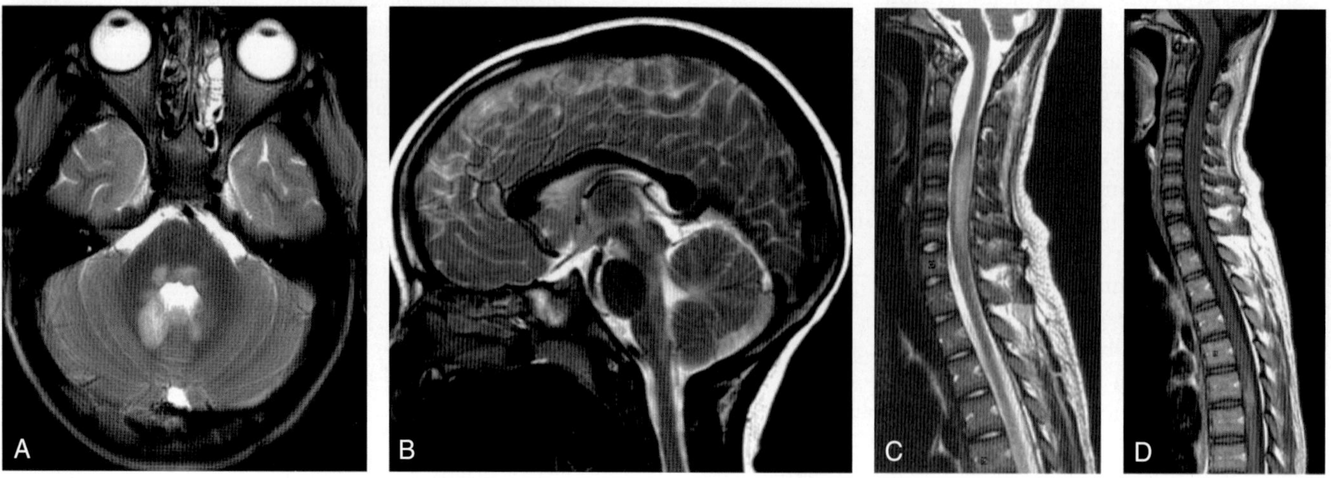

Fig. 6.16 Neuromyelitis Optica (NMO): Two Patients. (A and B) A 7-year-old with acute onset of ataxia and cranial nerve 6 palsy with (A and B) axial and sagittal T2W imaging demonstrating T2W hyperintensity adjacent to the cerebral aqueduct and fourth ventricle within the dorsal midbrain, pons, medulla, right middle cerebellar peduncle, and in the cerebellum. CSF aquaporin-4 antibody was found to be positive. (C and D) A 16-year-old with NMO and longitudinally extensive nonenhancing transverse myelitis that extends from C3 through C7 seen on (C and D) sagittal T2W and T1W+C. An additional area of spinal cord enhancement with spinal cord volume loss is seen from T6 to T8 related to a more chronic area of myelitis.

Key Points

Background

- Formerly known as Devic disease, neuromyelitis optica spectrum disorder (NMOSD) is an autoimmune astrocytopathy due to the aquaporin-4 antibody, which results in astrocyte injury and demyelination
- NMOSD core clinical characteristics include the following:
  - Optic neuritis
  - Acute myelitis
  - Area postrema syndrome: Nausea, vomiting, hiccups due to demyelination in the dorsal medulla
  - Acute brainstem syndrome
  - Symptomatic narcolepsy or acute diencephalic syndrome
  - Symptomatic cerebral syndrome
- Diagnosis of NMOSD can be made with:
  - A positive aquaporin-4 IgG test, one or more core clinical characteristics, and exclusion of alternative diagnosis
  - A negative aquaporin-4 IgG test with at least two core clinical characteristics, with one being optic neuritis (with additional imaging requirement of normal or nonspecific white matter findings or with optic nerve involvement extending over > ½ the optic nerve length or involving the optic chiasm), acute myelitis that is longitudinally extensive (≥3 spinal segments), or area postrema syndrome (with visible lesions in the dorsal medulla/area postrema) and exclusion of alternative diagnoses
- Relapsing remitting course with incomplete recovery between attack episodes
- Occurs across all ethnic groups with strong female predilection (male:female ratio 0.1–0.5)
- Aquaporin-4 IgG is positive in 60% to 80% of patients

Imaging

- Brain
  - T2/FLAIR hyperintense demyelinating lesions with or without enhancement in the brainstem (particularly the periaqueductal gray matter and dorsal medulla), thalamus and hypothalamus, optic chiasm, and limited white matter involvement of periventricular, deep, and subcortical white matter, corpus callosum. Restricted diffusion may occur in acute lesions
- Optic Neuritis
  - T2W hyperintense with or without enhancement of unilateral or bilateral optic nerves
- Longitudinally Extensive Myelitis
  - T2W hyperintensity involving ≥3 spinal segments typically with central gray predominance; enhancement is variable but present to some degree in 78% of patients; entire cross section of the cord may be involved

REFERENCES

1. Patterson SL, Optica Goglin SENeuromyelitis. *Rheum Dis Clin North Am.* 2017 Nov;43(4):579–591.
2. Akaishi T, Nakashima I, Sato DK, et al. Neuromyelitis Optica Spectrum Disorders. *Neuroimaging Clin N Am.* 2017 May;27(2):251–265.
3. Wingerchuk DM, Banwell B, Bennett JL, et al. International panel for NMO diagnosis. International consensus diagnostic criteria for neuromyelitis optica spectrum disorders. *Neurology.* 2015;85:177–189.

TUMEFACTIVE DEMYELINATION

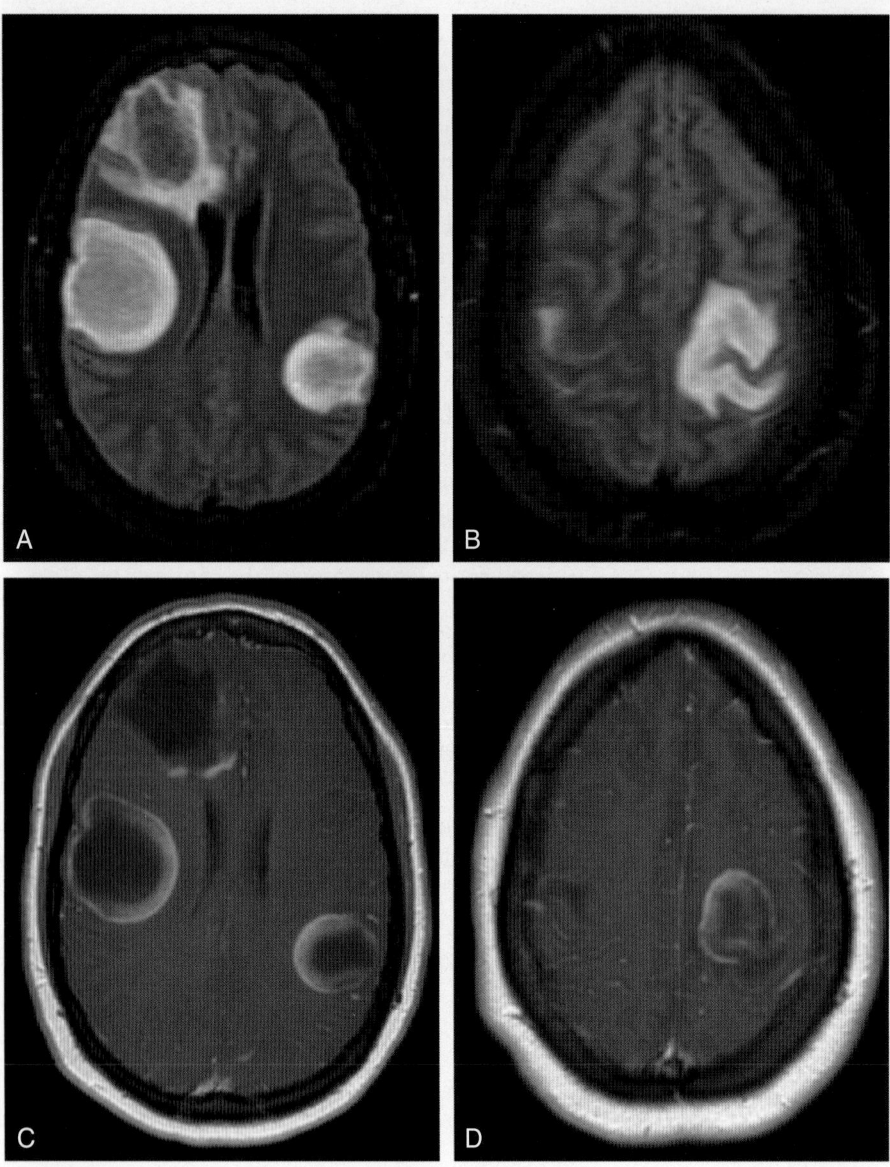

Fig. 6.17 Tumefactive Demyelination. (A and B) Axial FLAIR and (C and D) axial T1W+C images demonstrate large bilateral cerebral tumefactive demyelinating lesion with characteristic incomplete ring of enhancement.

Key Points

Background

- Large, typically >2 cm, demyelinating brain lesions that have resemblance to brain neoplasms, especially high-grade gliomas and CNS lymphoma
- Demyelinating processes that may have this appearance include multiple sclerosis, ADEM, and anti-MOG
- Improves with steroid therapy

Imaging

- Pooled sensitivity and specificity of MR to differentiate tumefactive demyelination from tumor is 89% and 94%, respectively
- Semilunar, incomplete, horseshoe-shaped enhancement has high specificity (98%–100%)
- Tend to be large but with relatively little mass effect and absent or mild surrounding edema
- May show restricted diffusion at margins of acute plaque but lesion otherwise demonstrates facilitated diffusion
- Perfusion weighted imaging (PWI) may help differentiate from neoplasm; cerebral blood volume (CBV) is lower than in tumors

REFERENCES

1. Given CA 2nd, Stevens BS, Lee C. The MRI appearance of tumefactive demyelinating lesions. *AJR Am J Roentgenol.* 2004 Jan;182(1):195–199.
2. Dagher AP, Smirniotopoulos J. Tumefactive demyelinating lesions. *Neuroradiology.* 1996 Aug;38(6):560–565.
3. Suh CH, Kim HS, Jung SC, Choi CG, Kim SJ. MRI Findings in Tumefactive Demyelinating Lesions: A Systematic Review and Meta-Analysis. *AJNR Am J Neuroradiol.* 2018 Sep;39(9):1643–1649.

AUTOIMMUNE ENCEPHALITIS

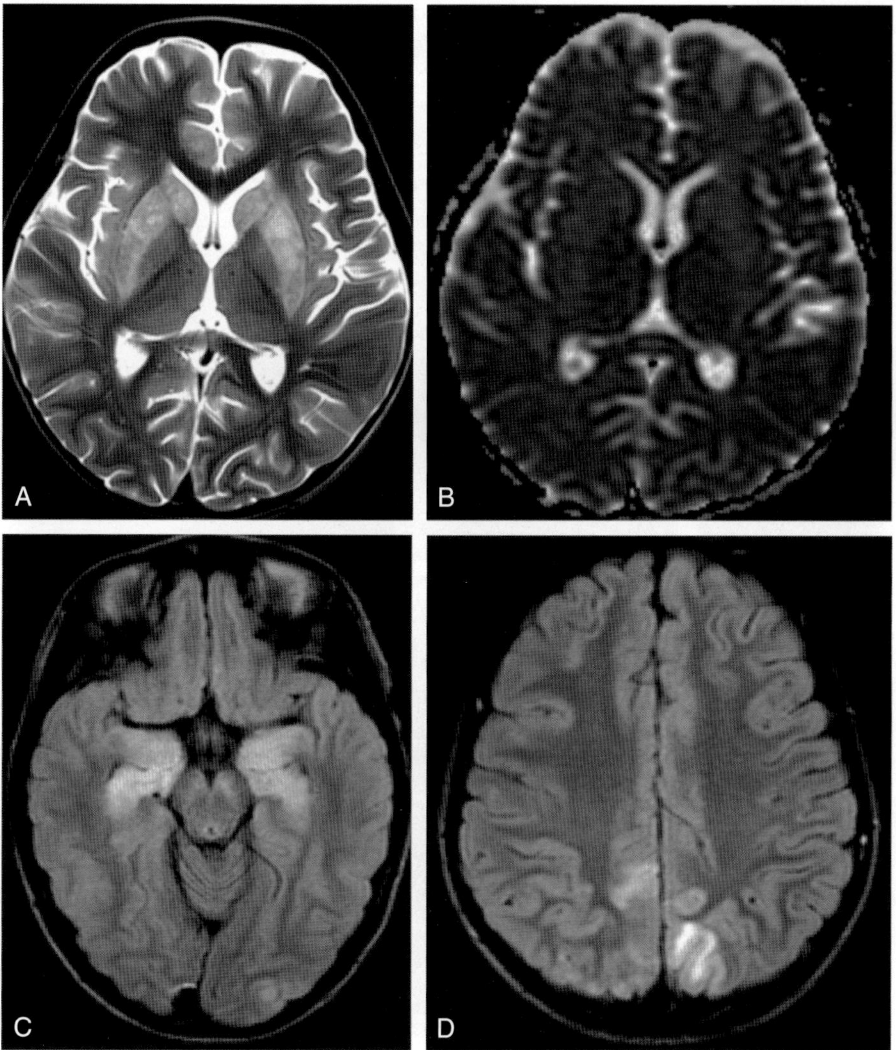

Fig. 6.18 Autoimmune Encephalitis. NMDA receptor auto antibody: (A) Axial T2W and (B) axial ADC images demonstrate T2W and ADC hyperintensity in the bilateral caudate and putamen. Voltage-gated potassium channel auto antibody: (C and D) Axial FLAIR images demonstrates abnormal FLAIR hyperintensity in the bilateral amygdala, hippocampi, and medial parietal lobes.

Key Points

Background

- Auto-antibody mediated attack on intracellular, cell-surface, or extracellular synaptic antigens.
  - Cell-surface include anti-N-methyl-D-aspartate (NMDA) receptor (NMDAR), anti–voltage-gated potassium channel (VGKC), anti-GABA, anti-glycine, and anti-dopamine D2 receptor. NMDAR is the most common autoimmune encephalitis.
  - Intracellular include anti-Hu, anti-Ma, and anti-glutamic acid decarboxylase (GAD).
- May be triggered by infection, vaccination, or occult neoplasm. Herpesvirus is a known trigger of anti-NMDAR.
- May manifest with seizures, movement disorders, cognitive decline, and/or neuropsychiatric symptoms.
- Diagnosed through detection of auto-antibodies in the CSF, although seronegative cases of autoimmune encephalitis exist. Imaging for occult malignancy should be performed.

Imaging

- MRI may be normal.
- MRI is not specific for type of autoimmune encephalitis but can suggest the possibility and need for CSF testing.
- Diffusion restriction and/or T2/FLAIR hyperintensity can involve the basal ganglia, hippocampi, thalami, limbic structures, and other cerebral cortical regions.
- Symmetric bilateral hippocampal pattern is common.
- Can progress to diffuse cerebral and cerebellar atrophy over time such that testing is often performed for unexplained progressive cerebral or atrophy.

REFERENCE

Barbagallo M, Vitaliti G, Pavone P, et al. Pediatric autoimmune encephalitis. *J Pediatr Neurosci*. 2017 Apr-Jun;12(2):130–134.

ACUTE HEMORRHAGIC LEUKOENCEPHALITIS

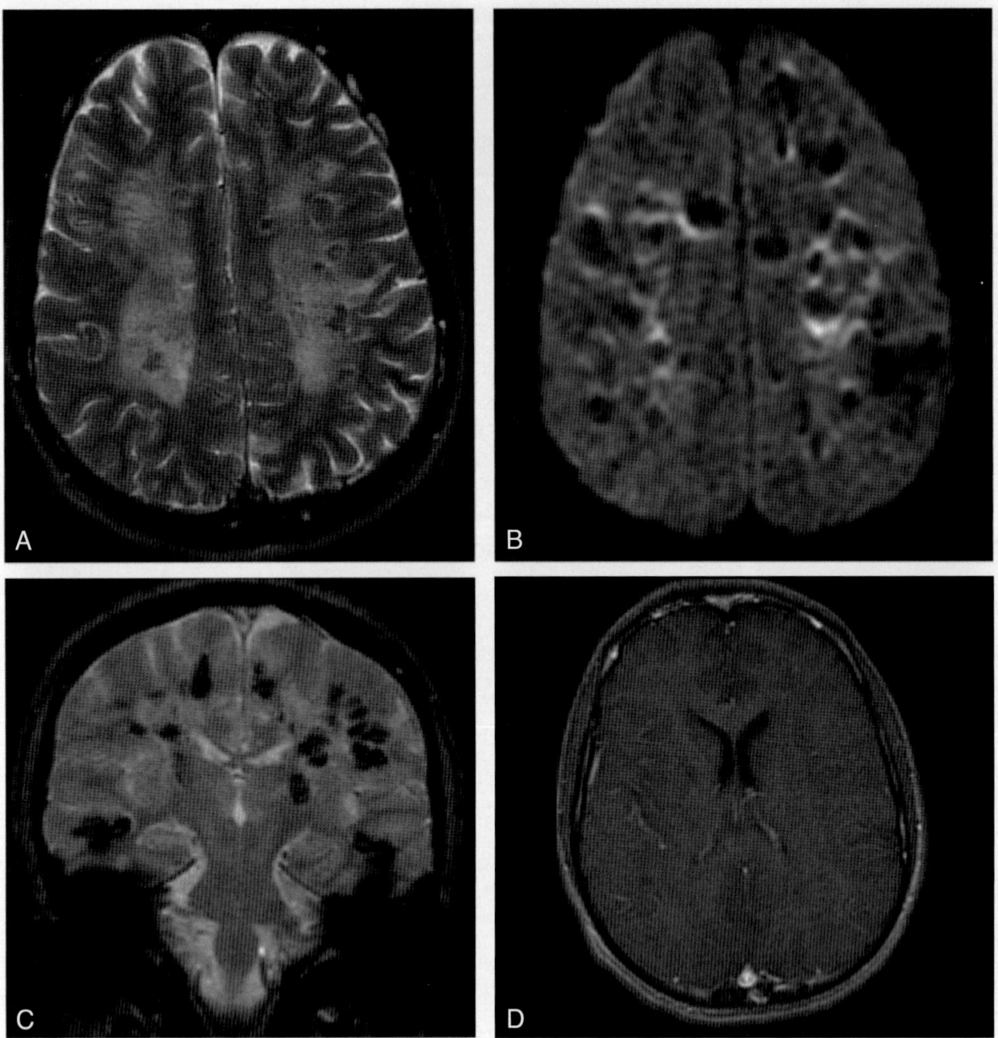

Fig. 6.19 Acute Hemorrhagic Leukoencephalitis. (A) Axial T2W demonstrates diffuse T2W signal abnormality of the cerebral white matter with multifocal T2W shortening from multifocal hemorrhage. (B) Axial DWI demonstrates artifactual heterogeneous restricted diffusion related to susceptibility from multifocal hemorrhage, which is well seen on the (C) coronal GRE. (D) Axial T1W+C image demonstrates no significant enhancement.

Key Points

Background

- Formerly referred to as Weston Hurst syndrome
- Rare, fulminant CNS demyelinating condition usually diagnosed at autopsy
- Considered a variant of ADEM
- AHEM may more commonly occur in young adults, contrary to ADEM, which is more commonly diagnosed in children
- Associated with a variety of viral, and bacterial infections

Imaging

- Predominantly involves supratentorial white matter but may also involve brainstem, cerebellum, and spinal cord
- Large confluent T2W hyperintense lesions to small lesions with associated edema
- Associated focal hemorrhages: Presence of hemorrhage may allow for differentiation from ADEM
- Enhancement may be seen

REFERENCES

1. Geerts Y, Dehaene I, Lammens M. Acute hemorrhagic leukoencephalitis. *Acta Neurol Belg*. 1991;91(4):201–211.
2. Leake JA, Billman GF, Nespeca MP, et al. Pediatric acute hemorrhagic leukoencephalitis: report of a surviving patient and review. *Clin Infect Dis*. 2002 Mar 1;34(5):699–703.
3. Grzonka P, Scholz MC, De Marchis GM, et al. Acute Hemorrhagic Leukoencephalitis: A Case and Systematic Review of the Literature. *Front Neurol*. 2020 Aug 20;11:899.

CEREBELLITIS

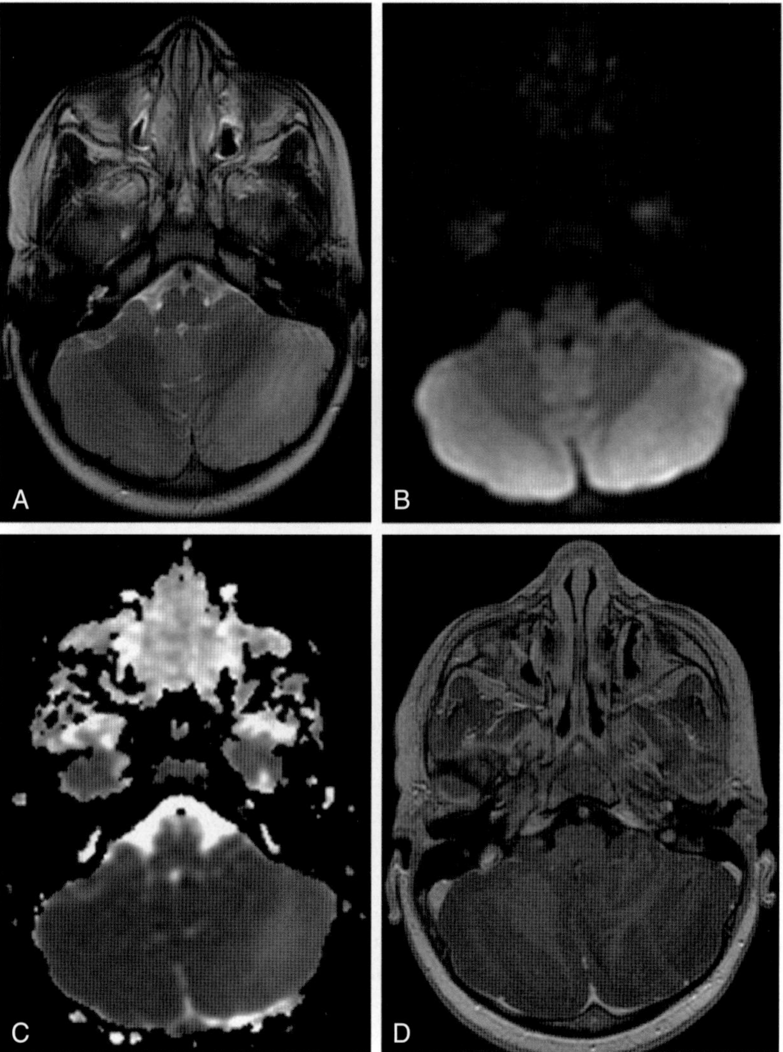

Fig. 6.20 Cerebellitis. (A) Axial T2W, (B) axial DWI, (C) axial ADC map, (D) axial T1W+C images demonstrate cortical and subcortical T2W hyperintensity in the right cerebellum with restricted diffusion and overlying leptomeningeal enhancement.

Key Points

Background

- Rare infectious/parainfectious syndrome characterized by cerebellar dysfunction.
- Most common presenting symptoms are truncal ataxia, dysmetria, fever, headache, nausea, and altered mental status.
- Usually complete neurologic recovery.
- Acute cerebellitis is term used with more severe presentation when imaging is abnormal as opposed to acute cerebellar ataxia which is used when imaging is normal.
- Associated with numerous viruses, *Mycoplasma*, and vaccination.

Imaging

- T2W hyperintense cerebellar cortical, and subcortical signal abnormality involving one or both cerebellar hemispheres, and vermis. Deep white matter may also be involved
- Both diffusion restriction and facilitated diffusion can be seen, but facilitated diffusion is more common.
- Variable enhancement of the cerebellum. Mild leptomeningeal enhancement is uncommon and may be due to vascular congestion.
- Mass effect may be severe, resulting in acute life-threatening hydrocephalus
- Long-term cerebellar atrophy may occur
- Differential Diagnosis: ADEM, Lhermitte-Duclos, diffusely infiltrating glioma or lymphoma, vasculitis, infarct, and drug-related inflammatory processes

REFERENCES

1. De Bruecker Y, Claus F, Demaerel P, et al. MRI findings in acute cerebellitis. *Eur Radiol.* 2004 Aug;14(8):1478–1483.
2. Lancella L, Esposito S, Galli ML, et al. Acute cerebellitis in children: an eleven year retrospective multicentric study in Italy. *Ital J Pediatr.* 2017 Jun 12;43(1):54.

LUPUS

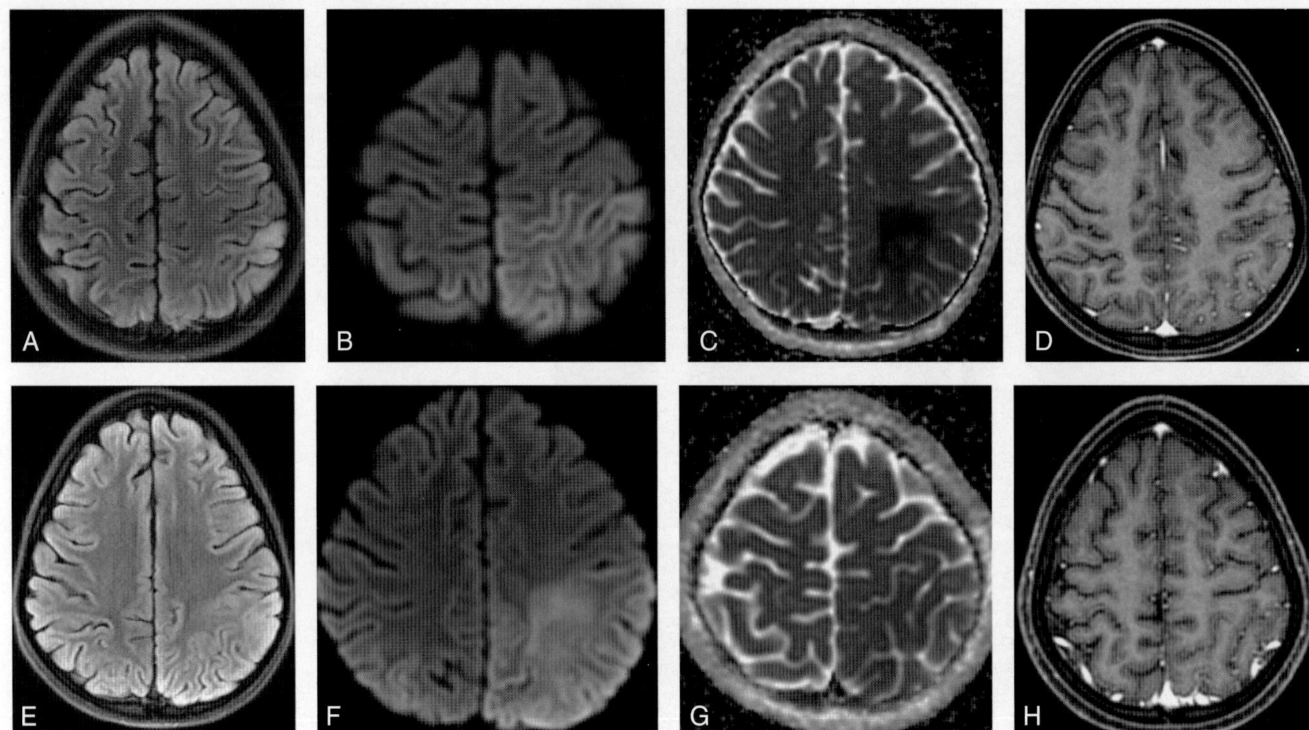

Fig. 6.21 Lupus. A 7-year-old with acute-onset left-sided weakness. (A, E) Axial FLAIR, (B, F) axial DWI, (C, G) axial ADC map, (D, H) axial T1W+C images demonstrate broad region of cortical and white matter reduced diffusion centered in the left precentral and postcentral gyri and adjacent parietal lobe with less conspicuous FLAIR hyperintensity and no associated enhancement.

Key Points

Background

- Lifelong autoimmune disorder with immune dysregulation and chronic multisystem inflammation
- Female predominance, especially after age 10
- Children have more aggressive disease and poorer outcomes compared to adults
- American College of Rheumatology describes central and peripheral nomenclature for neuropsychiatric lupus syndromes
  - Central: Aseptic meningitis, cerebrovascular disease, demyelinating syndromes, headache, movement disorder, myelopathy, seizures, acute confusional state, anxiety disorder, cognitive dysfunction, mood disorder, and psychosis
  - Peripheral: AIDP (Guillain-Barré syndrome), autonomic disorder, mononeuropathy, myasthenia gravis, cranial neuropathy, plexopathy, and polyneuropathy

Imaging

- Brain
  - Infarcts: Large territorial, focal, watershed, or central gray matter patterns can occur
  - Focal white matter T2W hyperintense lesions; tumefactive white matter lesions may occur; enhancement may occur in acute lesions
  - Cortical-subcortical T2W hyperintense regions, which may be numerous; enhancement may occur in acute lesions
  - Other: Parenchymal volume loss, parenchymal hemorrhage, PRES, vasculitis with arterial stenosis, and venous sinus thrombosis
- Spine
  - Myelitis: Longitudinally extensive (>2 vertebral body lengths)

REFERENCES

1. Kaichi Y, Kakeda S, Moriya J, et al. Brain MR findings in patients with systemic lupus erythematosus with and without antiphospholipid antibody syndrome. *AJNR Am J Neuroradiol.* 2014 Jan;35(1):100–105.
2. Lynall M. Neuropsychiatric symptoms in lupus. *Lupus.* 2018 Oct;27(1_suppl):18–20.
3. Tarvin SE, O'Neil KM. Systemic Lupus Erythematosus, Sjögren Syndrome, and Mixed Connective Tissue Disease in Children and Adolescents. *Pediatr Clin North Am.* 2018 Aug;65(4):711–737.

OPHTHALMOPLEGIC MIGRAINE

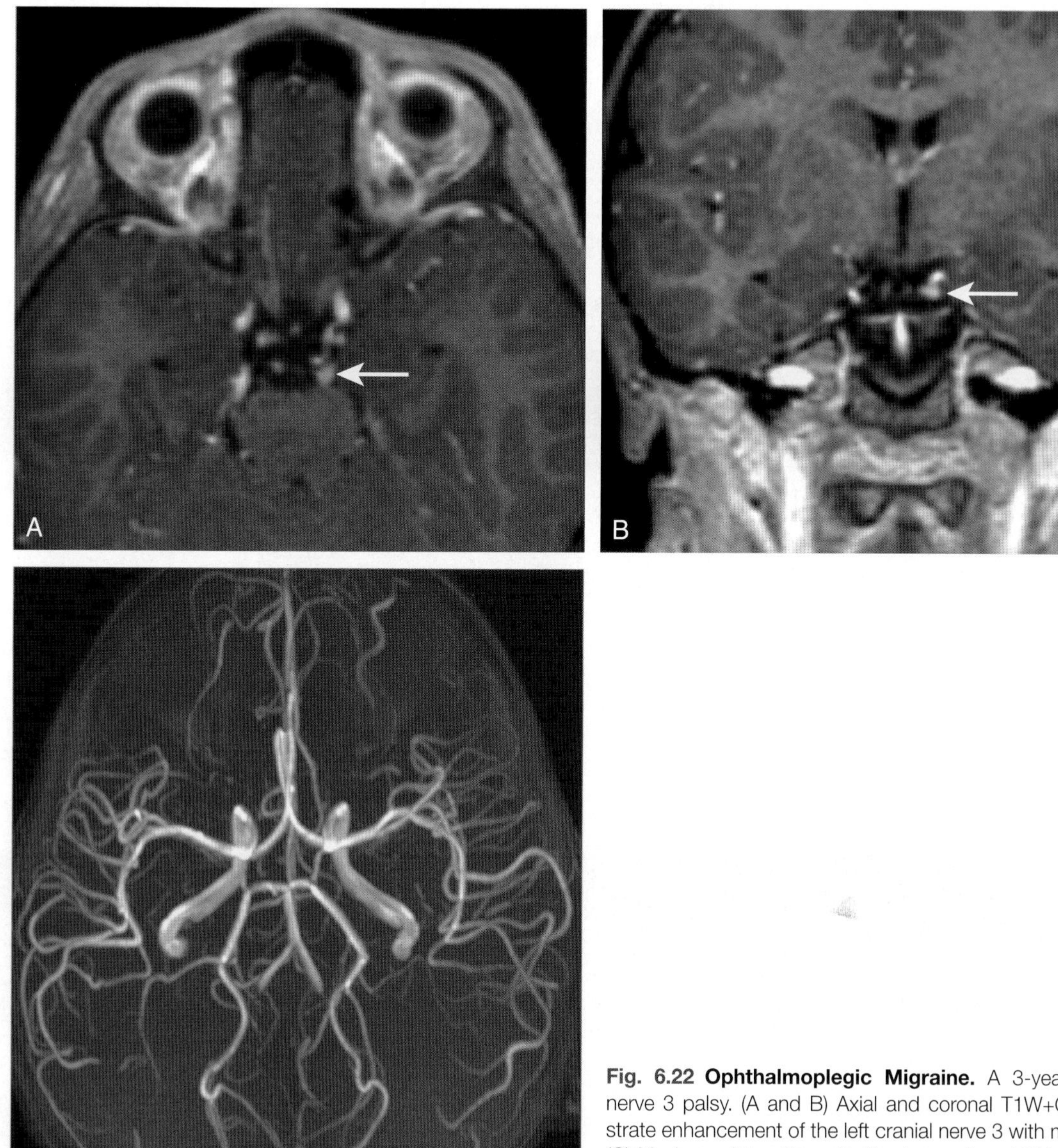

Fig. 6.22 **Ophthalmoplegic Migraine.** A 3-year-old with cranial nerve 3 palsy. (A and B) Axial and coronal T1W+C images demonstrate enhancement of the left cranial nerve 3 with minimal expansion. (C) Maximum intensity projection image from MRA of the brain demonstrates no aneurysms.

Key Points

Background

- Rare entity occurring in children; average age less than 10 years.
- Considered a form of migraine and also a cranial neuralgia.
- Symptoms of recurrent headache with ophthalmoplegia related to paresis of the CN III, IV, or VI. Symptoms can persist for hours to weeks or permanently.
- Etiology is unknown.

Imaging

- Requires thin section T1W+C imaging to demonstrate the homogeneous enhancement of cranial nerve 3
- Enhancement can persist over serial MRIs.
- Important to exclude other causes of third nerve palsy, including aneurysm, and causes of leptomeningeal enhancement, such as infection or tumor.

REFERENCE

1. Bharucha DX, Campbell TB, Valencia I, et al. MRI findings in pediatric ophthalmoplegic migraine: a case report and literature review. *Pediatr Neurol.* 2007 Jul;37(1):59–63.

UNCOMMON INFLAMMATORY DISORDERS

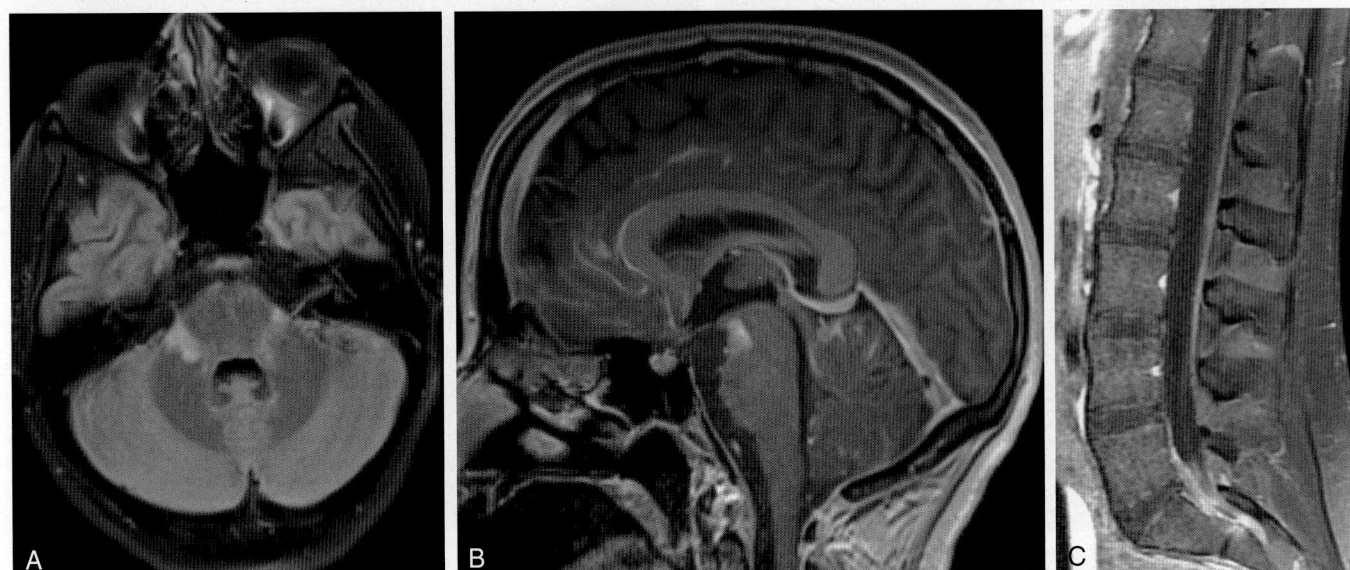

Fig. 6.23 Degos Disease. A 15-year-old with facial numbness, lower extremity rash, gait instability and urinary incontinence. (A) Axial FLAIR demonstrates hyperintensity in the right and left middle cerebellar peduncles. (B) Sagittal T1W+C image demonstrates leptomeningeal enhancement along the brainstem, cerebellar fissures and the anterior frontal and cingulate culci. (C) Sagittal T1W+C image demonstrates abnormal cauda equine enhancement.

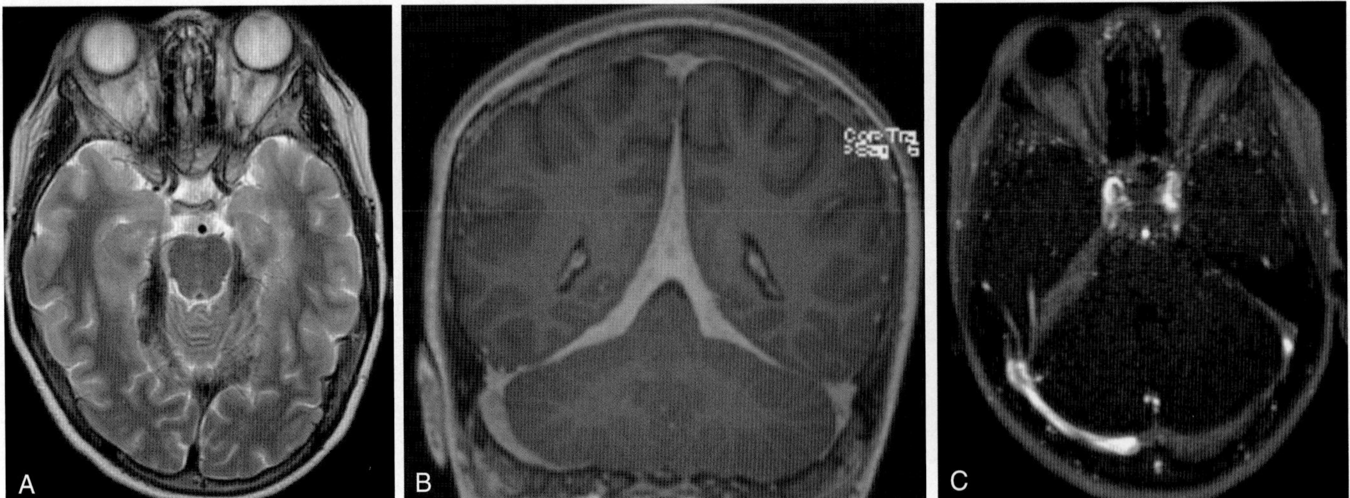

Fig. 6.24 Granulomatosis with Polyangittis. 14-year-old with headache. (A) Axial T2W, (B) coronal T1W+C and (C) axial contrast enhanced MR venogram images demonstrate abnormal T2W hypointensity with homogeneous enhancement along the dura of the tentorium and falx with occlusion of the left transverse sinus and the anterior 1/3 of the superior sagittal sinus (not shown). The T2W hypointensity is a pattern which should alert the radiologist to a potential rare etiology such as granulomatosis with polyangiitis causing fibrosis in the dura.

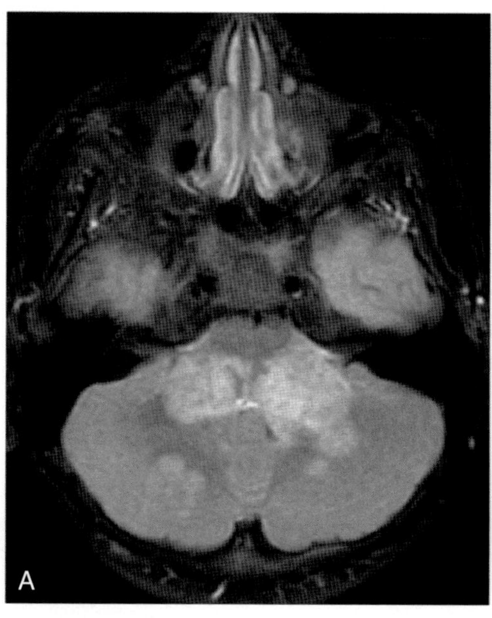

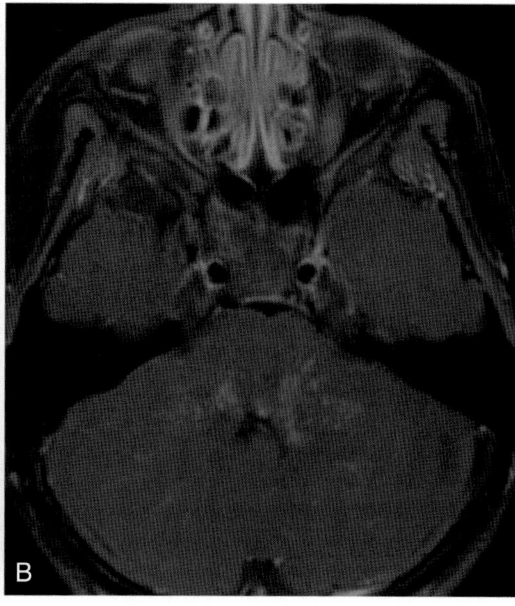

Fig. 6.25 CLIPPERS. An 8-year-old with headache, weakness and diplopia. (A) Axial FLAIR, and (B) axial T1W+C images demonstrate abnormal confluent T2/FLAIR hyperintensity with speckled enhancement in the pons, middle cerebellar peduncles and cerebellum. A brain biopsy demonstrated perivascular and parenchymal lymphocytic inflammatory infiltrate.

Key Points

Background

- Degos:
  - Also known as malignant atrophic papulosis.
  - Degos is a thrombotic microangiopathy of uncertain etiology.
  - Typically involves the skin, internal organs (usually gastrointestinal tract in 50% of patients) and CNS involvement in 20-60% of pateints.
  - Diagnosis can be made with skin biopsy and histopathology that demonstrates small vessel vasculopathy.
  - Neurologic manifestations include cranial nerve deficits and polyradiculopathy.
  - Treated with immunomodulatory medications but has relatively high mortality.
- Granulomatosis with polyangiitis:
  - A necrotizing vasculitis primarily affecting small vessels.
  - Pediatric incidence is ~1:1,000,000.
  - CNS-related symptoms can include headache, diabetes insipidus, and cranial neuropathies.
  - Sinonasal symptoms including rhinosinusitis, and epistaxis, and orbital symptoms including pain, swelling and proptosis.
  - Treated with immunomodulating medications.
- CLIPPERS:
  - Acronym for Chronic Lymphocytic Inflammation with Pontine Perivascular Enhancement Responsive to Steroids.
  - Neuroinflammatory disorder involving the brainstem with a perivascular T-lymphocyte infiltrate on histopathology.
  - Typically occurs in adults in the 4th-5th decade. Pediatric presentation is rare.
  - Presents with progressive symptoms referable to the brainstem and cerebellum.
  - Steroid responsive with a relapsing-remitting course.
  - CSF can show a mild pleiocytosis with lymphocytic predominance. Definitive diagnosis requires biopsy.

Imaging

- Degos:
  - Leptomeningeal enhancement in the brain and spine.
  - Small foci of diffusion restriction and/or T2 FLAIR hyperintensity near the areas of enhancement related to microinfarcts.
- Granulomatosis with polyangiitis:
  - Involvement of the nose and paranasal sinuses is the most common site in the head and neck and can demonstrate nasal septal erosion, mucosal thickening, and paranasal sinus bone erosion and/or sclerosis.
  - Orbital involvement is the next most common and can be in the form of a focal mass.
  - CNS involvement is uncommon but can manifest as pachymeningeal enhancement, particularly along the tentorium, and associated dural sinus thrombosis. Small infarcts due to vasculitis and leptomeningeal enhancement are less common.
- CLIPPERS
  - Punctate foci of enhancement primarily in the pons but can also occur in the middle cerebellar peduncles and cerebellum.
  - Additional lesions can be seen in the basal ganglia, thalami, corpus callosum, cerebral white matter, medulla, and spinal cord.

REFERENCES

1. Moran EJ, Lapin WB, Calame D, et al. Degos disease: A radiological-pathological correlation of the neuroradiological aspects of the disease. *Ann Diagn Pathol.* 2020 Aug;47:151545.
2. Guzman-Soto MI, Kimura Y, Romero-Sanchez G, et al. From Head to Toe: Granulomatosis with Polyangiitis. *Radiographics.* 2021 Nov-Dec;41(7):1973–1991.
3. Nemani T, Udwadia-Hegde A, Keni Karnavat P, Kashikar R, Epari S. CLIPPERS Spectrum Disorder: A Rare Pediatric Neuroinflammatory Condition. *Child Neurol Open.* 2019 Mar 7;6:2329048X19831096.

7 Brain Tumors and Treatment Complications

INTRODUCTION

Background

- Central nervous system (CNS) tumors are the second most common pediatric cancer diagnosed each year, accounting for approximately 25% of childhood cancers. They are responsible for the second most common cause of cancer deaths in children.
- Survival has slowly improved over the years, and overall survival is now approximately 75%.
- Supratentorial tumors predominate during the first 2 years of life and late adolescence, while infratentorial tumors are more common in the remainder of the first decade.
- Presenting signs and symptoms are wide ranging, but common features include headache (especially morning headache), vomiting, lethargy, papilledema, seizure, and neurologic deficit. Some signs and symptoms are more specific to a location of tumor and are emphasized in this chapter.
- Treatment varies, depending on the tumor pathology and location, and is briefly discussed in each section.

Imaging

- Imaging is performed for obtaining a diagnosis or differential diagnosis, determination of tumor extent, and effect on the normal brain. Follow-up imaging is used to assess for recurrence/progression and complications of treatment.
- A general approach for a new pediatric brain tumor for determining the diagnosis or narrow differential diagnosis includes the following:
  - Location and extent of the tumor: This chapter emphasizes a location-based approach
  - Conventional MRI appearance with emphasis on DWI appearance
  - Advanced imaging: MR Spectroscopy (MRS), Arterial Spin Label (ASL) perfusion, Dynamic Contrast Enhanced (DCE) perfusion, and Dynamic Susceptibility Contrast (DSC) perfusion
  - Determination of leptomeningeal disease in the remainder of the brain and spine
- DWI is helpful for determining low grade (WHO grade 1–2) from high grade (WHO grade 3–4). High-grade tumors typically demonstrate DWI hyperintense and ADC hypointense signal relative to normal parenchyma, which is considered a reflection of tumor cellularity (low ADC = high cellularity).
- MR perfusion imaging is helpful for tumors in which the conventional imaging patterns remain inconclusive. Generally, high cerebral blood flow (CBF) and cerebral blood volume (CBV) occur in high-grade tumors and are reflective of tumor microvascular density. An ASL CBF > 50 mL/min/100 g was shown to have sensitivity/specificity for differentiation of low-grade and high-grade pediatric brain tumors at the following locations: cerebral hemisphere (90%/93%), thalamic tumors (100%/80%), and posterior fossa tumors (65%/94%). Determination of specific histopathology remains challenging.
- MRS can be useful when the convention pattern is indeterminate. However, the authors believe the conventional imaging patterns combined with MR perfusion have rendered MRS less favorable in the initial imaging of pediatric brain tumors. Utility may remain in situations of determining radiation necrosis from recurrent tumor.

REFERENCES

1. Rumboldt Z, et al. Apparent diffusion coefficients for a differentiation of cerebellar tumors in children. *AJNR Am J Neuroradiol.* Jun–Jul 2006;27(6):1362–1369.
2. Kralik SF, et al. Diffusion imaging for tumor grading of supratentorial tumors in the first year of life. *AJNR Am J Neuroradiol.* 2014 Apr;35(4):815–823.
3. Dangolouff-Ros V, et al. Arterial spin labeling to predict pediatric brain tumor grading in children: Correlations between histopathologic vascular density and perfusion MR imaging. *Radiology.* 2016 Nov;281(2):553–566.

POSTERIOR FOSSA TUMORS

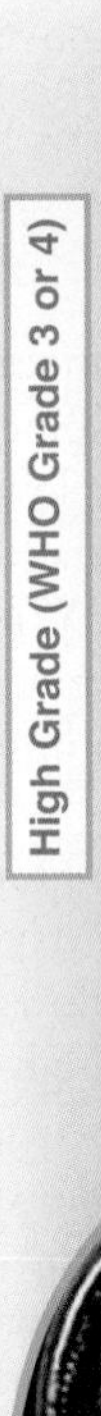

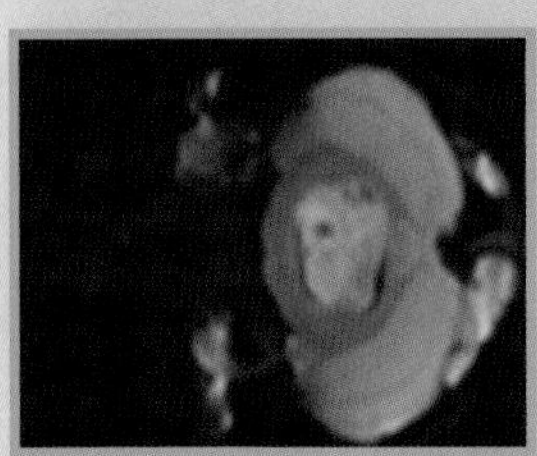

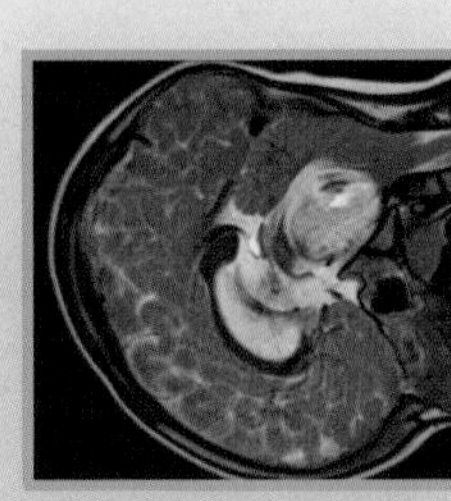

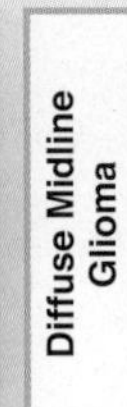

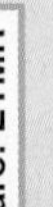

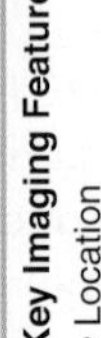

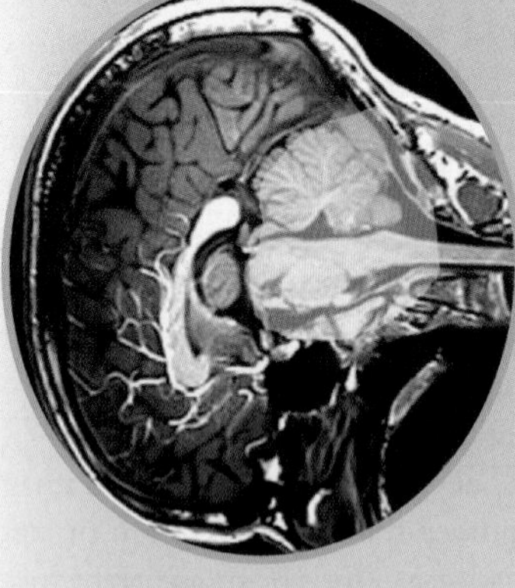

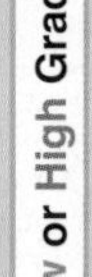

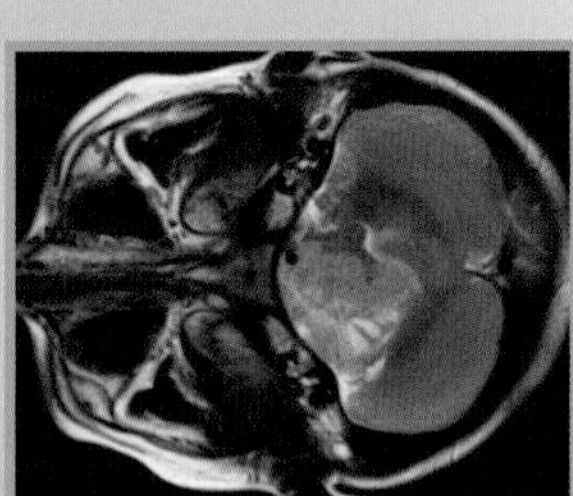

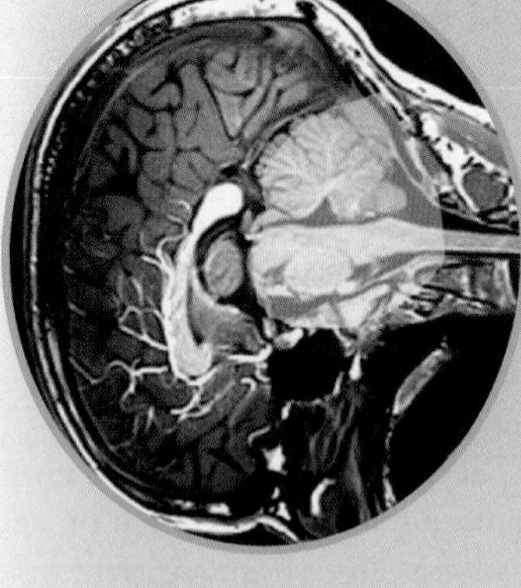

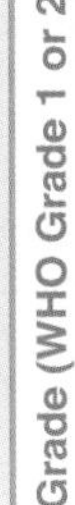

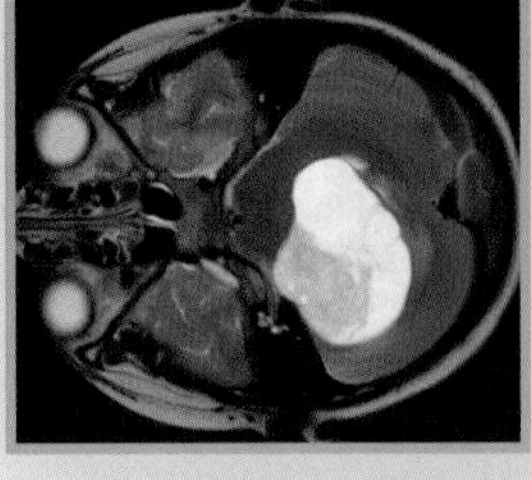

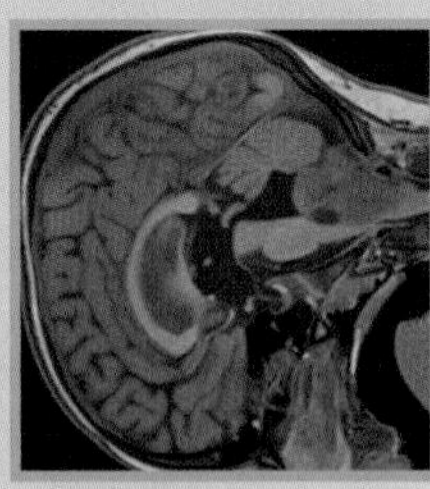

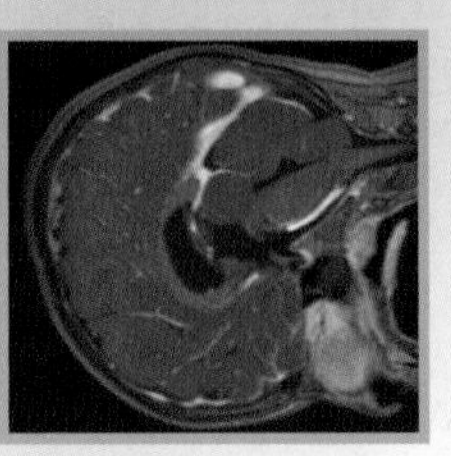

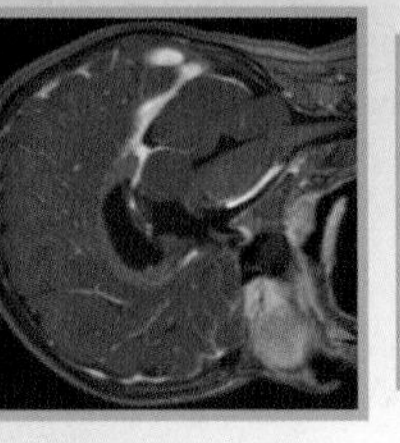

MEDULLOBLASTOMA

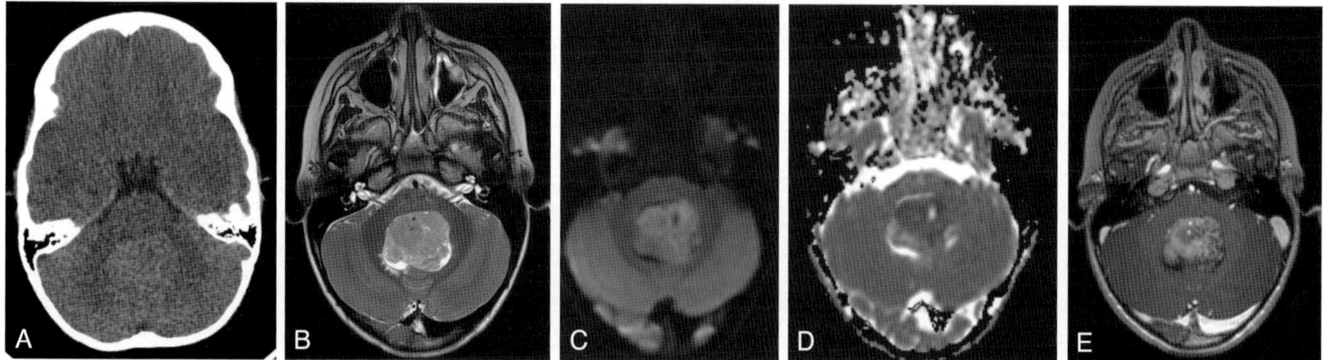

Fig. 7.1 Medulloblastoma. A 4-year-old with headaches and vomiting. (A) Axial CT scan demonstrates a midline posterior fossa mildly hyperdense mass centered in the fourth ventricle. (B) Axial T2W, (C) axial DWI, (D) axial ADC map, and (E) axial T1W+C images demonstrate typical features of a medulloblastoma with mild T2W hyperintensity, reduced diffusion (ADC less than normal parenchyma) and contrast enhancement.

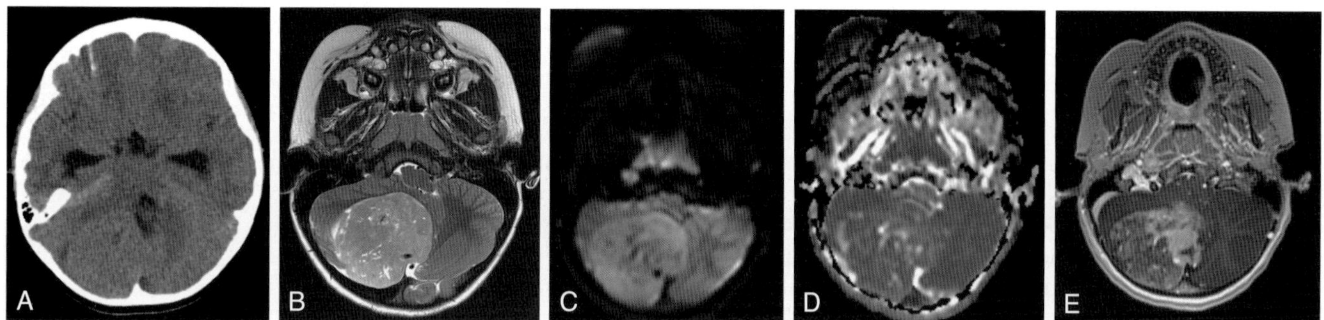

Fig. 7.2 Medulloblastoma. A 3-year-old with lethargy and vomiting. (A) Axial CT scan demonstrates a posterior fossa mildly hyperdense mass centered in the posteromedial right cerebellar hemisphere. (B) Axial T2W, (C) axial DWI, (D) axial ADC map, and (E) axial T1W+C images demonstrate typical features of a medulloblastoma with mild T2W hyperintensity, reduced diffusion (ADC less than normal parenchyma) and contrast enhancement.

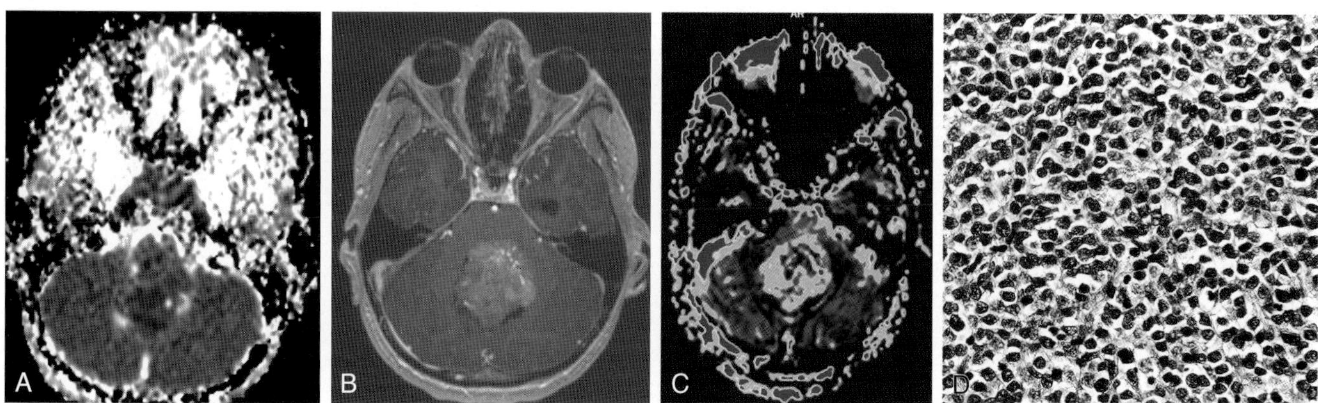

Fig. 7.3 Medulloblastoma: Advanced Imaging and Histopathology. (A) Axial ADC map, and (B) axial T1W+C demonstrate a typical medulloblastoma within the fourth ventricle with reduced diffusion and enhancement. (C) Axial CBV map obtained from DSC perfusion demonstrates typical elevated rCBV. (D) Densely cellular, classic type medulloblastomas are grade 4 tumors, but when the stage and molecular subtype are favorable can have a cure rate of over 80%. (D from Kleinschmidt-DeMasters BK, Rodríguez FJ, Tihan T. *Diagnostic Pathology: Neuropathology*. Elsevier; 2017.)

Key Points

Background

- WHO grade 4
- Account for 30% to 40% of pediatric posterior fossa tumors
- Five histologic subtypes:
    - Classic: Most common (>70%)
    - Desmoplastic/nodular
    - Large cell
    - Anaplastic
    - Medulloblastoma with extensive nodularity
- Molecular subgroups better correlate with demographics, clinical features, and prognostication and may aid development of future molecular targeted therapies
    - Four molecular subgroups—prevalence:
        - Wingless (Wnt): 10%
        - Sonic Hedgehog (SHH): 30%
        - Group 3: 25%
        - Group 4: 35%
- Gorlin syndrome (basal cell nevus syndrome) is associated with increased risk of medulloblastoma and discussed in Chapter 9.

Imaging

CT

- Midline (most common) or cerebellar hemispheric *hyperdense* tumor; commonly cysts or necrotic regions (50% to 90%); calcifications (10% to 40%); significant hemorrhage is uncommon

MRI

- Most commonly arising from the inferior vermis, although location may be variable depending on molecular subtype
- Well-circumscribed; T1W hypointense; T2W isointense to hypointense
- Variable enhancement with majority demonstrating enhancement. Minority may show no enhancement
- *Restricted diffusion* with ADC values <0.9 × 10^3 mm^2/s
    - Metastatic disease at initial diagnosis in 11% to 43%
        - Posterior fossa, intraventricular, subfrontal, and spinal are most common locations for metastases

Advanced Imaging

- MR Perfusion: ↑ CBF and CBV
- MRS: ↑ *Elevated taurine*, choline, and lactate; ↓ NAA and creatine

REFERENCES

1. Partap S, et al. Medulloblastoma incidence has not changed over time: a CBTRUS study. *J Pediatr Hematol Oncol.* 2009;31:970–971.
2. Kijima N, et al. Molecular Classification of Medulloblastoma. *Neurol Med Chir (Tokyo).* 2016 Nov;56(11):687–697.
3. Dangouloff-Ros V, et al. Imaging features of medulloblastoma: Conventional imaging, diffusion-weighted imaging, perfusion-weighted imaging, and spectroscopy: From general features to subtypes and characteristics. *Neurochirurgie.* 2018 Aug 28;S0028-3770(17)30178-9.
4. Rumboldt Z, et al. Apparent Diffusion Coefficients for Differentiation of Cerebellar Tumors in Children AJNR. *Am J Neuroradiol.* 2006 Jun-Jul;27(6):1362–1369.

MEDULLOBLASTOMA: MOLECULAR SUBTYPES

Subgroup	WNT		SHH				Group 3			Group 4		
Subtype	WNT α	WNT β	SHH α	SHH β	SHH γ	SHH δ	Group 3α	Group 3β	Group 3γ	Group 4α	Group 4β	Group 4γ
Subtype proportion												
Subtype relationship												
Clinical data: Age												
Clinical data: Histology			LCA Desmoplastic	Desmoplastic	MBEN Desmoplastic	Desmoplastic						
Clinical data: Metastases	8.6%	21.4%	20%	33%	8.9%	9.4%	43.4%	20%	39.4%	40%	40.7%	38.7%
Clinical data: Survival at 5 years	97%	100%	69.8%	67.3%	88%	88.5%	66.2%	55.8%	41.9%	66.8%	75.4%	82.5%
Copy number: Broad	6^{-}		$9q^{-}$, $10q^{-}$, $17p^{-}$		Balanced genome		7^{+}, 8^{-}, 10^{-}, 11^{-}, i17q		8^{+}, i17q	$7q^{+}$, $8p^{-}$, i17q	i17q	$7q^{+}$, $8p^{-}$, i17q (less)
Copy number: Focal			*MYCN* amp, *GLI2* amp, *YAP1* amp	*PTEN* loss		$10q22^{-}$, $11q23.3^{-}$		*OTX2* gain, *DDX31* loss	*MYC* amp	*MYCN* amp, *CDK6* amp	*SNCAIP* dup	*CDK6* amp
Other events			*TP53* mutations			*TERT* promoter mutations		High *GFI1/1B* expression				

Age (years): 0-3 >3-10 >10-17 >17

Graphical Summary of the 12 Medulloblastoma Subtypes. Schematic representation of key clinical data, copy-number events, and relationship between the subtypes inside each of the four medulloblastoma subgroups. The percentages of patients presenting with metastases and the 5-year survival percentages are presented. The age groups are: infant 0–3 years, child >3–10 years, adolescent >10–17 years, and adult >17 years. (From Cavalli F, Remke M, Rampasek L, et al. Intertumoral heterogeneity within medulloblastoma subgroups. *Cancer Cell*. 2017;31:737–754.e6. https://doi.org/10.1016/j.ccell.2017.05.005)

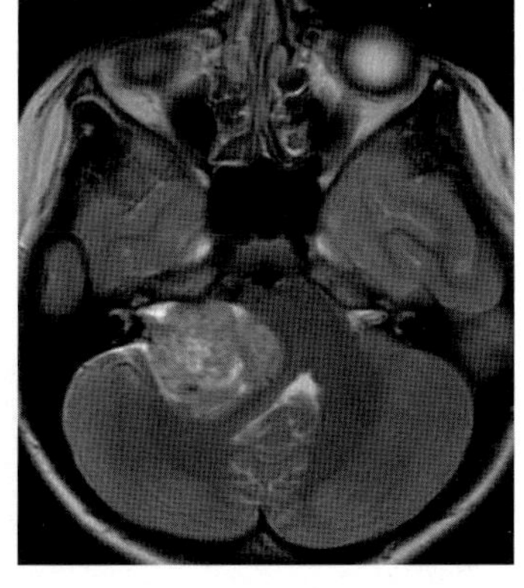

Wnt

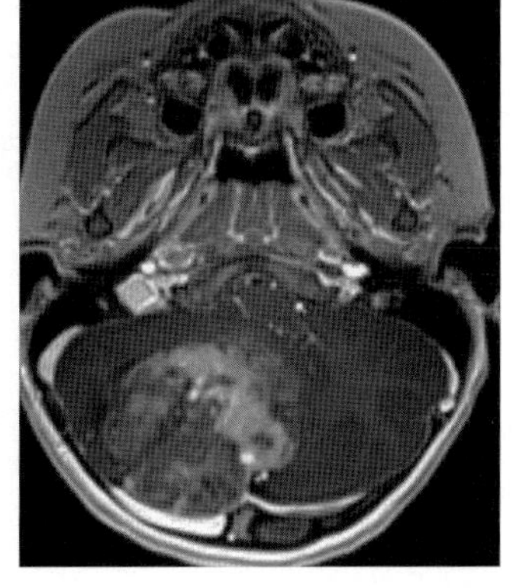

Sonic Hedgehog

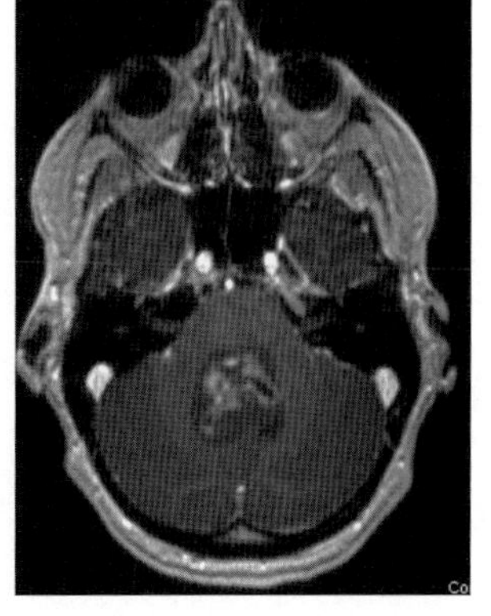

Group 3

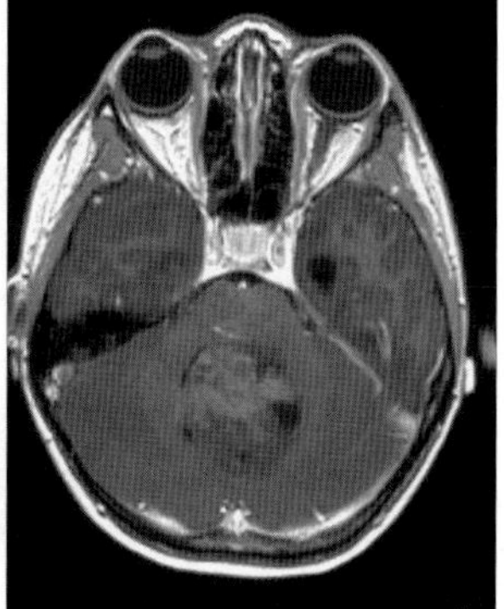

Group 4

MEDULLOBLASTOMA: WNT (WINGLESS)

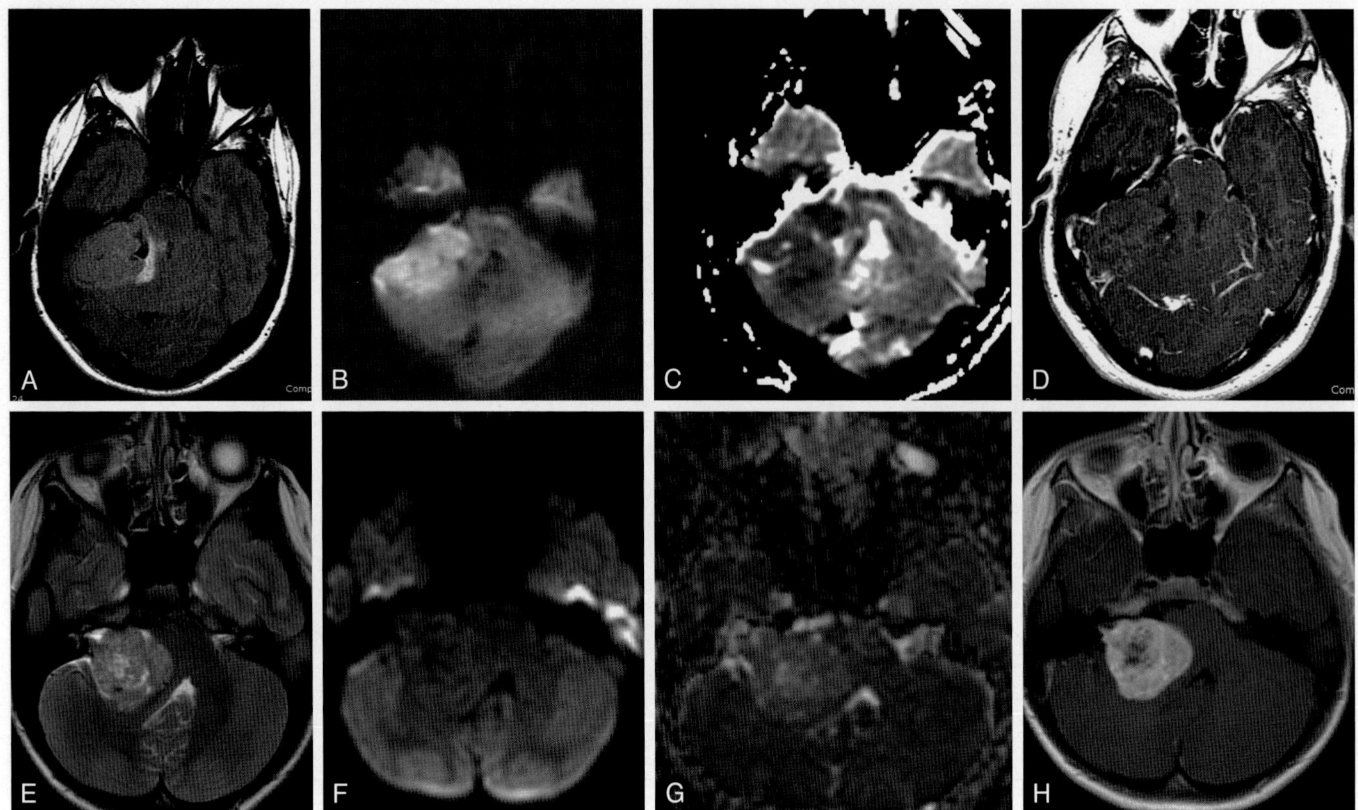

Fig. 7.4 Medulloblastoma WNT Subtype. (A to D) A 16-year-old with medulloblastoma Wnt-subtype. (A) Axial FLAIR, (B) axial DWI, (C) axial ADC map, (D) axial T1W+C demonstrate an off midline mass along the anterolateral margin of the right cerebellar hemisphere with reduced diffusion and minimal enhancement. (E to H) A 9-year-old with wnt-subtype medulloblastoma. (E) Axial T2W, (F) axial DWI, (G) axial ADC map, and (H) axial T1W+C images demonstrate an avidly enhancing mass in the right cerebellopontine angle. Older age and lateral location are typical of the Wnt subtype.

Key Points

Background

- Prevalence: 10% (rarest subgroup)
- Histology: Classic
- Prognosis: 5-year survival 95% *(best prognosis)*
- Demographics: *Older children and teens*; M:F ratio 1:1

Imaging

- Location: *Lateral location (foramen of Luschka, cerebellopontine angle [CPA])*; is most common fourth ventricle, or cisterna magna are less common
- *Rarely presents with metastasis*

REFERENCES

1. Kijima N, et al. Molecular Classification of Medulloblastoma. *Neurol Med Chir (Tokyo)*. 2016 Nov;56(11):687–697.
2. Patay Z, et al. Magnetic resonance imaging characteristics of WNT-subgroup pediatric medulloblastoma. *AJNR Am J Neuroradiol.* 2015 Dec;36(12):2386–2393.
3. Perreault S, et al. MRI surrogates for molecular subgroups of medulloblastoma. *AJNR Am J Neuroradiol.* 2014 Jul;35(7):1263–1269.

MEDULLOBLASTOMA: SONIC HEDGEHOG (SHH)

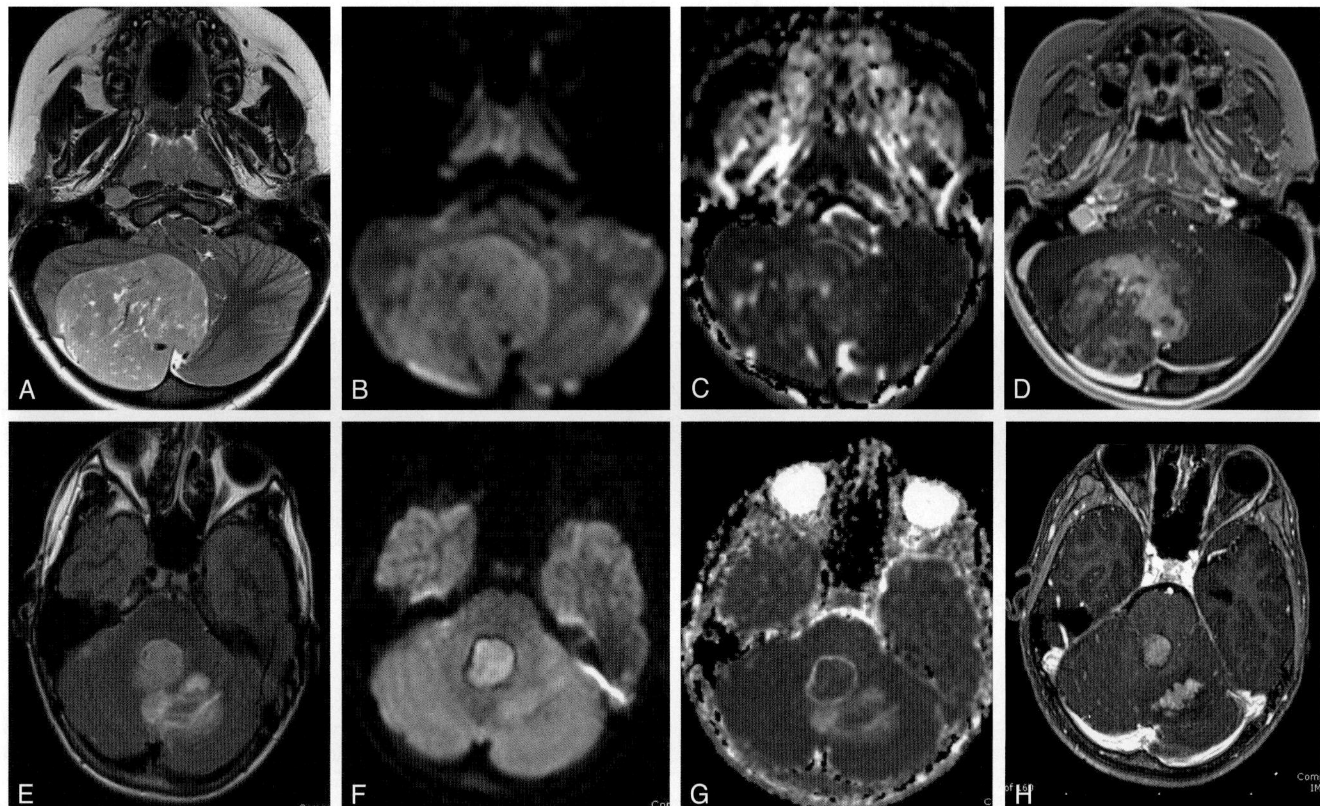

Fig. 7.5 Medulloblastoma: Sonic Hedgehog (SHH) Subtype. (A to E) A 3-year-old with SHH subtype of medulloblastoma and typical MRI appearance. (A) Axial T2W, (B) axial DWI, (C) axial ADC map, and (D) axial T1W+C images demonstrate a large enhancing mass with reduced diffusion in the right cerebellar hemisphere. (E to H) A 13-year-old with SHH subtype of medulloblastoma and atypical imaging pattern. (E) Axial FLAIR, (F) axial DWI, (G) axial ADC map, and (H) axial T1W+C images demonstrate an enhancing fourth intraventricular mass with reduced diffusion and an additional metastatic left cerebellar mass with regional edema. These cases show the common ages and imaging pattern for SHH subtype but also indicate that imaging patterns are not completely reliable for subtype diagnosis.

Key Points

Background

- Prevalence: 30%
- Histology: Desmoplastic/nodular and classic are most common; large cell/anaplastic possible
- Prognosis: 5-year survival 75% (intermediate prognosis)
- Demographics: Infants and teenagers/adults; M:F ratio 1:1

Imaging

- Location: Vermis (infants), or *cerebellar hemisphere* (teenagers/adults)
- Rarely presents with metastasis

REFERENCES

1. Kijima N, et al. Molecular Classification of Medulloblastoma. *Neurol Med Chir (Tokyo).* 2016 Nov;56(11):687–697.
2. Patay Z, et al. Magnetic resonance imaging characteristics of WNT-subgroup pediatric medulloblastoma. *AJNR Am J Neuroradiol.* 2015 Dec;36(12):2386–2393.
3. Perreault S, et al. MRI surrogates for molecular subgroups of medulloblastoma. *AJNR Am J Neuroradiol.* 2014 Jul;35(7):1263–1269.

MEDULLOBLASTOMA: GROUP 3

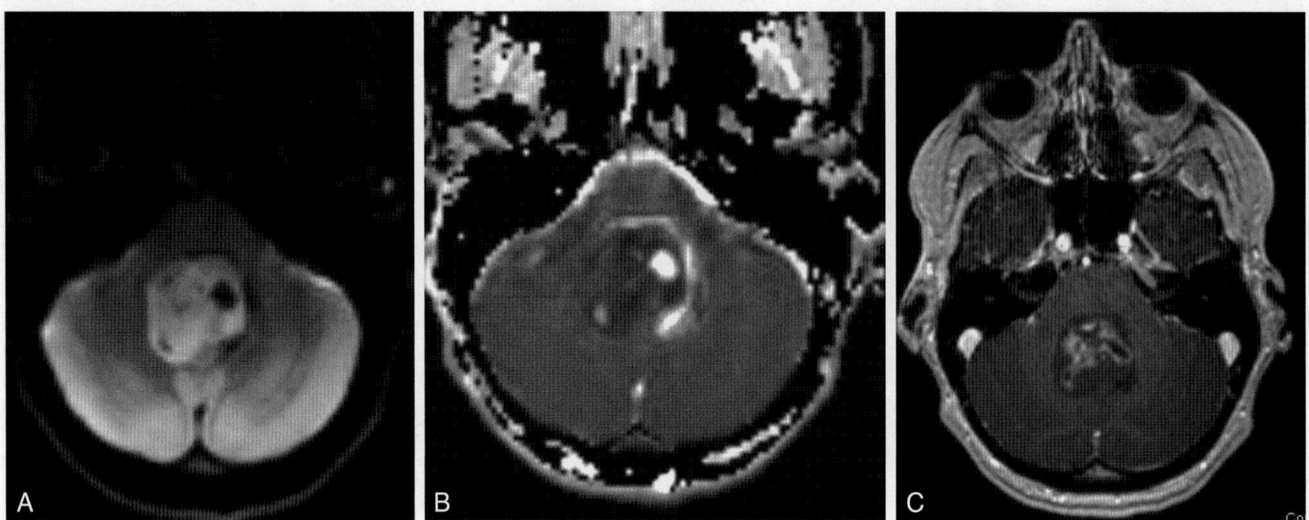

Fig. 7.6 Medulloblastoma Group 3 Subtype. A 14-year-old with medulloblastoma group 3. (A) Axial DWI, (B) axial ADC, and (C) axial T1W+C images demonstrate a midline fourth ventricular solid and cystic mass with restricted diffusion and heterogeneous enhancement typical for the group 3 subtype.

Key Points

Background

- Prevalence: 25%
- Histology: Classic, large cell/anaplastic
- Prognosis: 5-year survival 50% (poor prognosis)
- Demographics: Infants and children; M:F ratio 2:1

Imaging

- Location: *Midline* (vermis, fourth ventricle)
- Enhancement in majority of tumors
- *Higher risk of presentation with metastasis*

REFERENCES

1. Kijima N, et al. Molecular Classification of Medulloblastoma. *Neurol Med Chir (Tokyo)*. 2016 Nov;56(11):687–697.
2. Perreault S, et al. MRI surrogates for molecular subgroups of medulloblastoma. *AJNR Am J Neuroradiol.* 2014 Jul;35(7):1263–1269.

MEDULLOBLASTOMA: GROUP 4

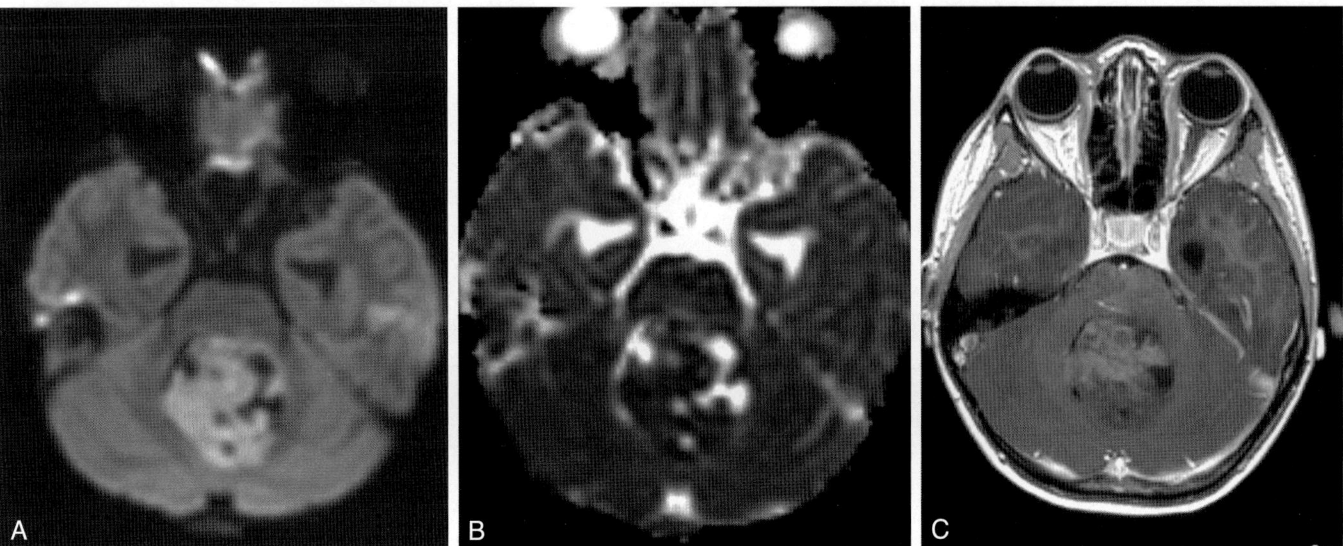

Fig. 7.7 Medulloblastoma Group 4 Subtype. A 10-year-old with medulloblastoma group 4. (A) Axial DWI, (B) axial ADC, and (C) axial T1W+C images demonstrate a midline fourth ventricular solid and cystic mass with restricted diffusion and mild heterogeneous enhancement typical for the group 4 subtype.

Key Points

Background

- Prevalence: 35% *(most common)*
- Histology: Classic, large cell/anaplastic
- Prognosis: 5-year survival 75% (intermediate prognosis)
- Demographics: Infants, children, and adults; M:F ratio 3:1

Imaging

- Location: *Midline* (vermis, fourth ventricle)
- *Less enhancement*
- *Higher risk of presentation with metastasis*

REFERENCES

1. Kijima N, et al. Molecular Classification of Medulloblastoma. *Neurol Med Chir (Tokyo)*. 2016 Nov; 56(11):687–697.
2. Perreault S, et al. MRI surrogates for molecular subgroups of medulloblastoma. *AJNR Am J Neuroradiol.* 2014 Jul;35(7):1263–1269.

PILOCYTIC ASTROCYTOMA

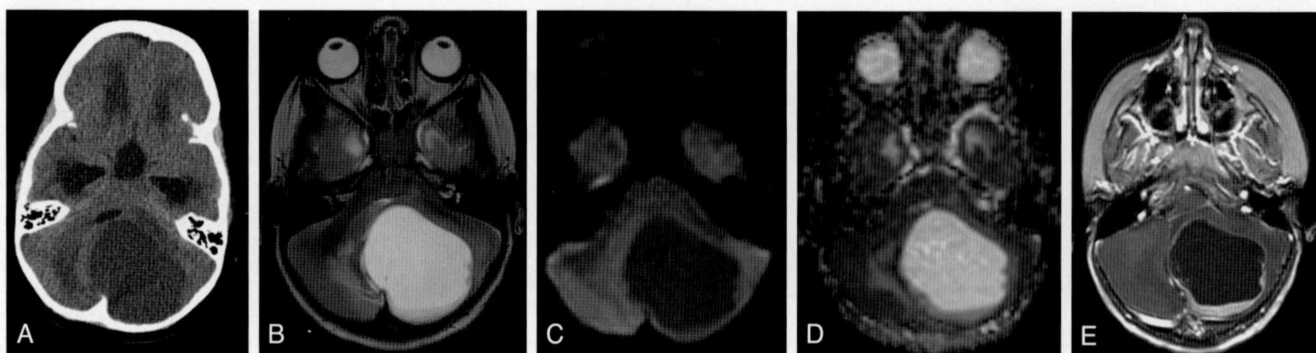

Fig. 7.8 Pilocytic Astrocytoma. A 3-year-old with developmental delay and abnormal gait. (A) Axial CT scan demonstrates a left cerebellar mass with large cystic component and adjacent edema. The large size of the mass is resulting in obstructive hydrocephalus and transependymal edema. (B) Axial T2W, (C) axial DWI, (D) axial ADC map, and (E) axial T1W+C images demonstrate typical features of a pilocytic astrocytoma with T2W hyperintense cyst and peripheral enhancing nodule with increased diffusion (ADC greater than normal parenchyma) of the solid component.

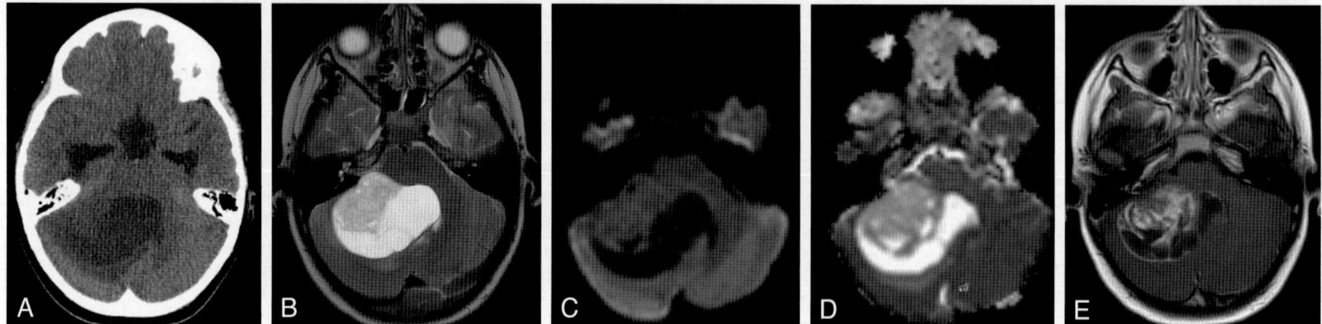

Fig. 7.9 Pilocytic Astrocytoma. A 10-year-old with double vision and headache. (A) Axial CT scan demonstrates a right cerebellar mass with cyst and nodule pattern and obstructive hydrocephalus. The nodule is less dense than normal parenchyma. (B) Axial T2W, (C) axial DWI, (D) axial ADC map, and (E) axial T1W+C images demonstrate typical features of a pilocytic astrocytoma with T2W hyperintense cyst and nodule, increased diffusion, and contrast enhancement of the nodule.

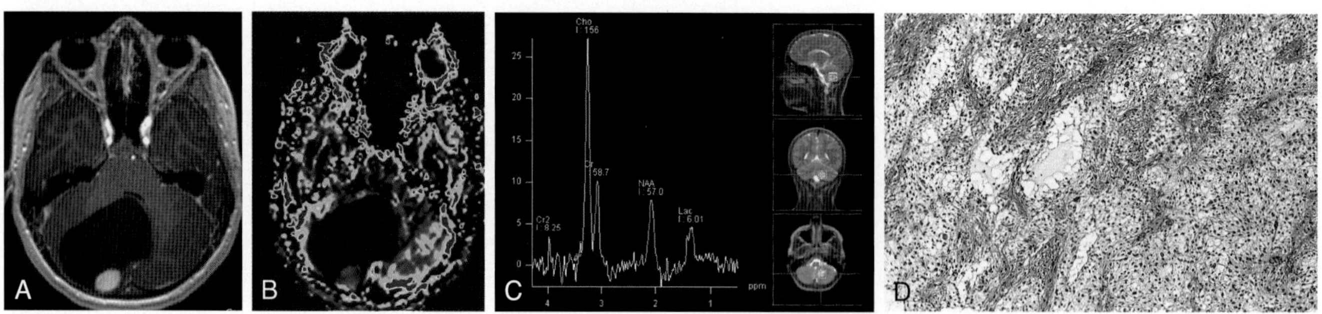

Fig. 7.10 Pilocytic Astrocytoma: Advanced Imaging and Histopathology. (A) Axial T1W+C demonstrate a typical pilocytic astrocytoma with cyst and nodule pattern within right cerebellar hemisphere and axial CBV map (B) obtained from DSC perfusion demonstrates typical low rCBV. (C) MR spectroscopy with long echo in a 13-year-old with a cerebellar juvenile pilocytic astrocytoma demonstrates elevated choline, reduced NAA, and mild elevation of lactate. (D) Pilocytic astrocytoma. The biphasic pattern of pilocytic astrocytoma is commonly observed in tissue sections. Piloid and more stellate astrocytes, associated with microcystic changes, are admixed in different proportions throughout the tumor. Commonly an accentuation of the fibrillary component exists in association with the vascular stroma. (D from Fletcher CDM. *Diagnostic Histopathology of Tumors.* Elsevier; 2021.)

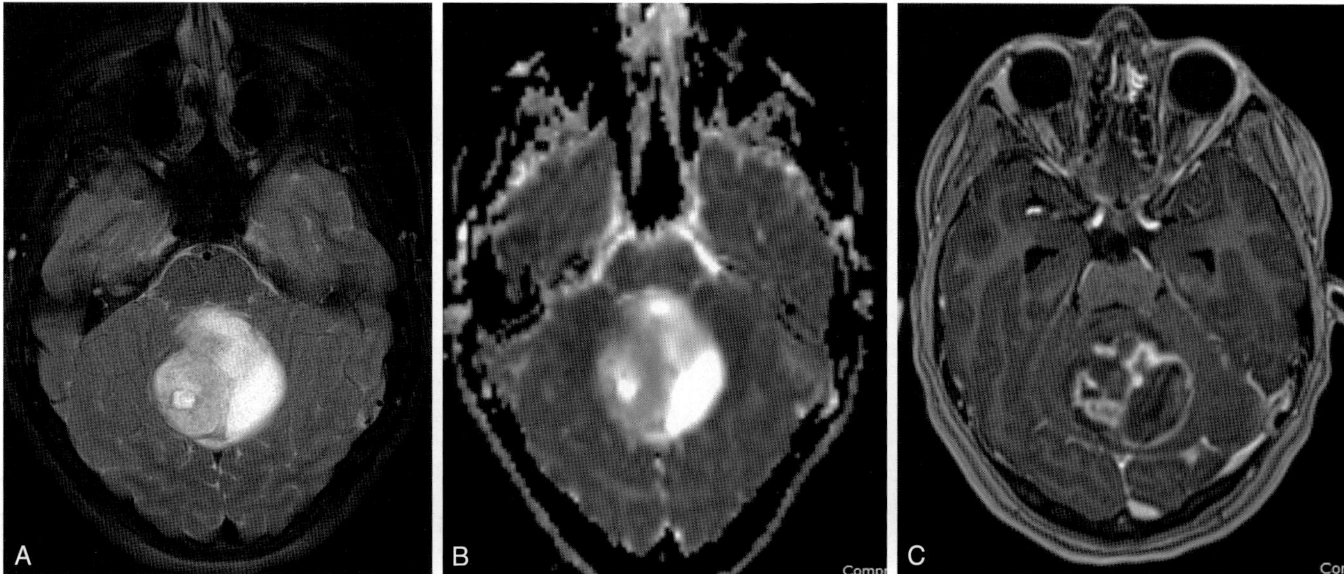

Fig. 7.11 Pilocytic Astrocytoma: Atypical Imaging Pattern. (A) Axial T2W, (B) axial ADC map, and (C) axial T1W+C images demonstrate a midline vermian solid and cystic mass with heterogeneous enhancement. The solid portions have increased ADC, which is useful in reaching the correct diagnosis of pilocytic astrocytoma.

Key Points

Background

- WHO grade 1
- Accounts for 25% to 35% of pediatric posterior fossa tumors
- Most tumors are sporadic in origin. Most tumors have the *BRAF* gene mutation leading to activation of the RAS/ERK/MAPK pathway
- Neurofibromatosis type I associated with increased risk of pilocytic astrocytoma (typically optic gliomas; rarely posterior fossa)
- 95% 5-year survival; prognosis dependent on extent of resection
- Location: Cerebellar hemispheric (most common) or posterior fossa midline, optic pathway/hypothalamus, thalamus and cerebral hemisphere

Imaging

CT

- *Fluid density cysts* and *isodense or hypodense solid* portion; dominant cyst with small iso- to hypodense solid component (most common); may have a small cystic component or entirely solid.
- Calcifications; hemorrhage is uncommon at presentation.

MRI

- *Solid and cystic (commonly a cyst and nodule pattern)*; well-circumscribed; fluid signal intensity or complex fluid signal intensity cystic component; T1W-hypointense, T2W-hyperintense solid component with intense enhancement; cyst wall may enhance but can be reactive rather than indicate tumor presence
- Usually *ADC hyperintense* compared to normal brain; ADC values >1.4 × 10^3 mm^2/s
- Uncommonly metastasize, but possible

Advanced Imaging

- MR perfusion: Variable CBF and CBV; often leaky blood-brain barrier which can lead to a T1 leakage pattern on DSC perfusion images characterized by the signal intensity rising above baseline after the contrast bolus has arrived
- MRS: Aggressive metabolite pattern with ↑ choline and lactate, ↓ NAA and creatine. Can be misleading to diagnosis of a high-grade glioma

REFERENCES

1. Plaza MJ, et al. Conventional and advanced MRI features of pediatric intracranial tumors: posterior fossa and suprasellar tumors. *AJR Am J Roentgenol.* 2013 May200(5):1115–1124.
2. Borja MJ, et al. Conventional and advanced MRI features of pediatric intracranial tumors: supratentorial tumors. *AJR Am J Roentgenol.* 2013 May;200(5):W483–W503.
3. Camilo J, et al. Primary neoplasms of the pediatric brain. *Radiol Clin North Am.* 2019 Nov;57(6):1163–1175.
4. Ohkaki H, et al. Population-based studies on incidence, survival rates, and genetic alterations in astrocytic and oligodendroglial gliomas. *J Neuropathol Exp Neurol.* 2005;64:479–489.
5. Rumboldt Z, et al. Apparent Diffusion Coefficients for Differentiation of Cerebellar Tumors in Children AJNR. *Am J Neuroradiol.* 2006 Jun-Jul;27(6):1362–1369.

EPENDYMOMA

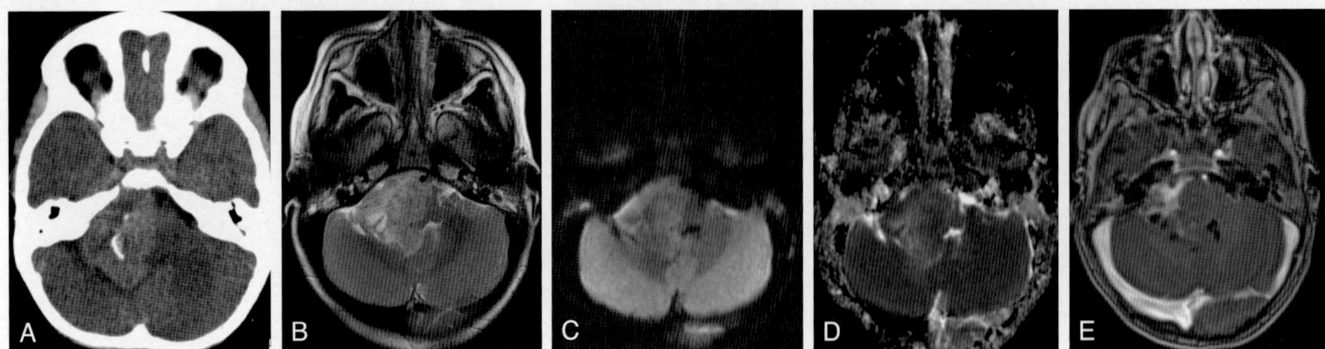

Fig. 7.12 Ependymoma. A 4-year-old with head tilt, morning vomiting, and balance difficulty. (A) Axial CT scan demonstrates a mildly hyperdense mass in the right cerebellopontine and cerebellomedullary angles with internal calcification. There is associated compression of the brainstem and cerebellum. (B) Axial T2W, (C) axial DWI, (D) axial ADC map, and (E) axial T1W+C images demonstrate typical features of an ependymoma located in the right foramen of Luschka with T2W hyperintensity, mixed ADC values, and heterogeneous enhancement. Pathology was a grade 3 anaplastic ependymoma.

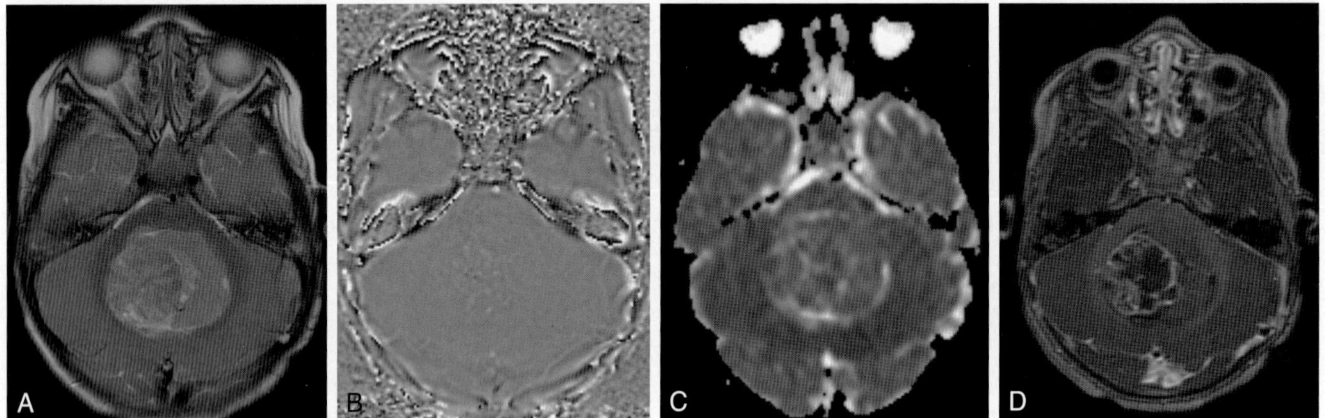

Fig. 7.13 Ependymoma. A 2-year-old with nighttime vomiting, ataxia, and now inability to walk. (A) Axial T2W, (B) axial SWI, (C) axial ADC map phase image, and (D) axial T1W+C images demonstrate a large, mildly T2W hyperintense mass centered within the fourth ventricle with heterogeneous diffusion, small foci of calcification and hemorrhage, and heterogeneous enhancement. Pathology was a grade 3 anaplastic ependymoma.

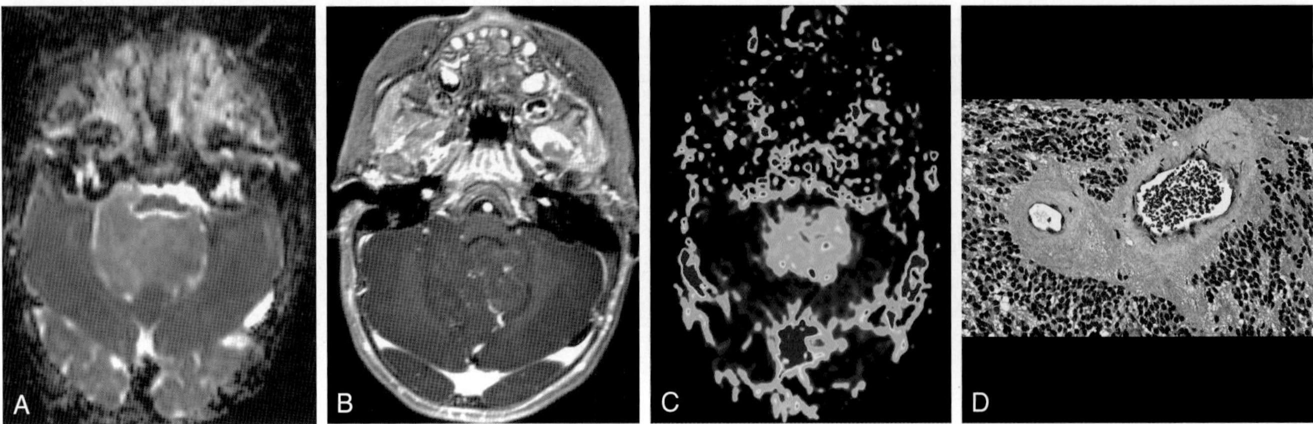

Fig. 7.14 Ependymoma: Advanced Imaging and Histopathology. (A) Axial ADC map and (B) axial T1W+C demonstrate an ependymoma involving the fourth ventricle, right foramen of Luschka, and cerebellomedullary angle with minimal enhancement, and mild elevated ADC. (C) Axial CBV map obtained from DSC perfusion demonstrates typical increased rCBV in the mass. (D) Ependymoma. Perivascular pseudorosette characterized by a fibrillary-appearing perivascular nuclear-free zone (hematoxylin-eosin stain, ×200). (D from Jankovic J, Mazziotta JC, Pomeroy SL, et al. *Bradley and Daroff's Neurology in Clinical Practice*. 8th ed. Elsevier; 2022.)

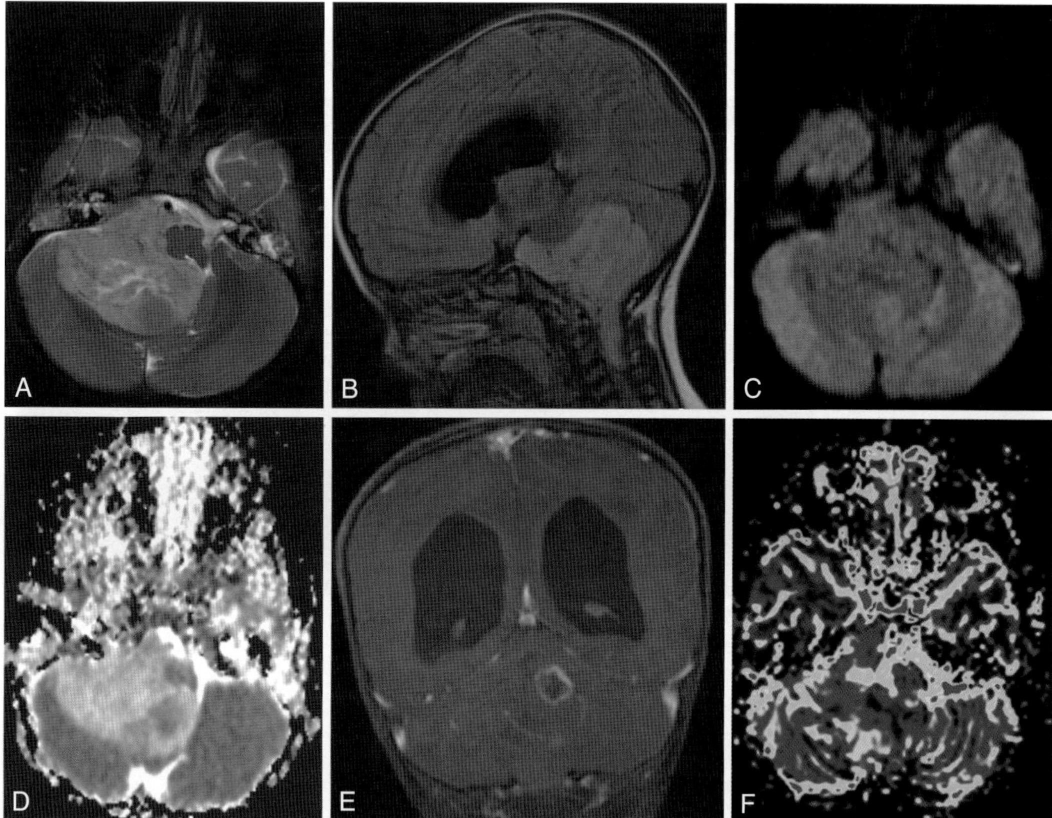

Fig. 7.15 Ependymoma: 3-year-old. (A) Axial T2W, (B) sagittal FLAIR, (C) axial DWI, (D) axial ADC map, (E) coronal T1W+C, and (F) axial CBV color map from DSC perfusion demonstrate an ependymoma involving the fourth ventricle, right foramen of Luschka, cerebellomedullary angle, foramen magnum, and upper cervical canal. Elevated ADC values and low rCBV are predominantly seen. Pathology was a WHO grade 2 ependymoma.

Key Points

Background

- WHO grade 2–3
- Accounts for approximately 20% of pediatric posterior fossa tumors
- Molecular subgroups
    - EPN_PFA (80%): Infants and young children; *poor prognosis*; reduced trimethylation of H3K27
    - EPN_PFB: Older children and adolescents; better prognosis; increased levels of trimethylation of H3K27
    - Subependymoma
- Neurofibromatosis type 2 (NF-2)–associated with increased risk of ependymoma
- 7-year survival is 65%; prognosis dependent on extent of resection, tumor grade, and molecular subtype
- Location: *Floor of the fourth ventricle* with projections of tumor and through the foramen Magendie and *foramina of Luschka*

Imaging

CT

- Isodense-hyperdense; well-defined; *calcifications* more common than any other posterior fossa tumors; small cysts and hemorrhage may occur

MRI

- Well-circumscribed; T1W hypointense, T2W iso- to hyperintense; variable enhancement
- Intermediate ADC signal (usually *isointense compared to normal brain*) between medulloblastoma and pilocytic astrocytomas with ADC values ~1.0-1.3 × 10^3 mm^2/s
- Metastasis uncommon, but increased risk with higher grade, and younger age

Advanced Imaging

- MRS: ↑ *Myoinositol*, choline, and lactate; ↓ NAA
- MR perfusion: ↑ CBF and CBV

REFERENCES

1. Plaza MJ, Borja MJ, Altman N, Saigal G. Conventional and advanced MRI features of pediatric intracranial tumors: posterior fossa and suprasellar tumors. *AJR Am J Roentgenol.* 2013 May;200(5):1115–1124.
2. Camilo J, et al. Primary neoplasms of the pediatric brain. *Radiol Clin North Am.* 2019 Nov;57(6):1163–1175.
3. Rumboldt Z, et al. Apparent Diffusion Coefficients for Differentiation of Cerebellar Tumors in Children. *AJNR Am J Neuroradiol.* 2006 Jun–Jul;27(6):1362–1369.
4. Vijay Ramaswamy, et al. Therapeutic Impact of Cytoreductive Surgery and Irradiation of Posterior Fossa Ependymoma in the Molecular Era: A Retrospective Multicohort Analysis. *J Clin Oncol.* 2016 Jul 20;34(21):2468–2477.
5. Rezai AR, et al. Disseminated ependymomas of the central nervous system. *J Neurosurg.* 1996 Oct;85(4):618–624.

ATYPICAL TERATOID RHABDOID TUMOR

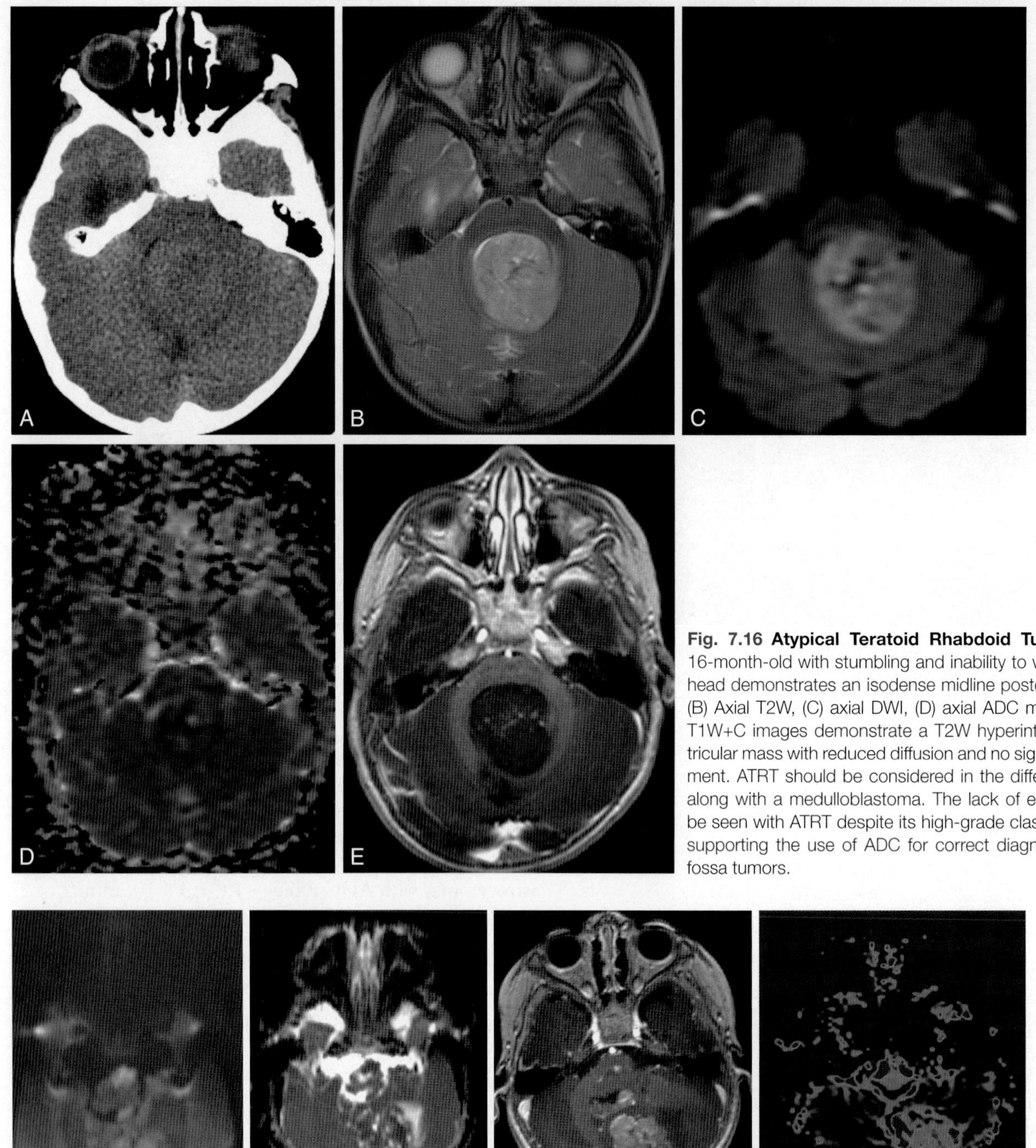

Fig. 7.16 Atypical Teratoid Rhabdoid Tumor (ATRT). A 16-month-old with stumbling and inability to walk. (A) Axial CT head demonstrates an isodense midline posterior fossa mass. (B) Axial T2W, (C) axial DWI, (D) axial ADC map, and (E) axial T1W+C images demonstrate a T2W hyperintense fourth ventricular mass with reduced diffusion and no significant enhancement. ATRT should be considered in the differential diagnosis along with a medulloblastoma. The lack of enhancement can be seen with ATRT despite its high-grade classification, further supporting the use of ADC for correct diagnosis of posterior fossa tumors.

Fig. 7.17 Atypical Teratoid Rhabdoid Tumor (ATRT): Advanced Imaging and Histopathology. A 15-month-old. (A) Axial DWI, (B) axial ADC map, and (C) axial T1W+C images demonstrate a focal left cerebellar mass and two additional posterior fossa nodules with reduced diffusion consistent with CSF metastases. CSF metastases are common with ATRT and the spine should also be imaged. (D) Axial CBV map obtained from DSC perfusion demonstrates increased rCBV in the mass. (E and F) Atypical teratoid/rhabdoid tumor. (E) High-grade, partially necrotic neoplasm composed of rhabdoid cells (*black arrowhead,* hematoxylin-eosin stain, Ã—200). (F) Immunostaining shows loss of nuclear SMARCB1 in tumor cell nuclei with retention in associated vasculature (×100). (E, F from Jankovic J, Mazziotta JC, Pomeroy SL, et al. *Bradley and Daroff's Neurology in Clinical Practice*. 8th ed. Elsevier; 2022.)

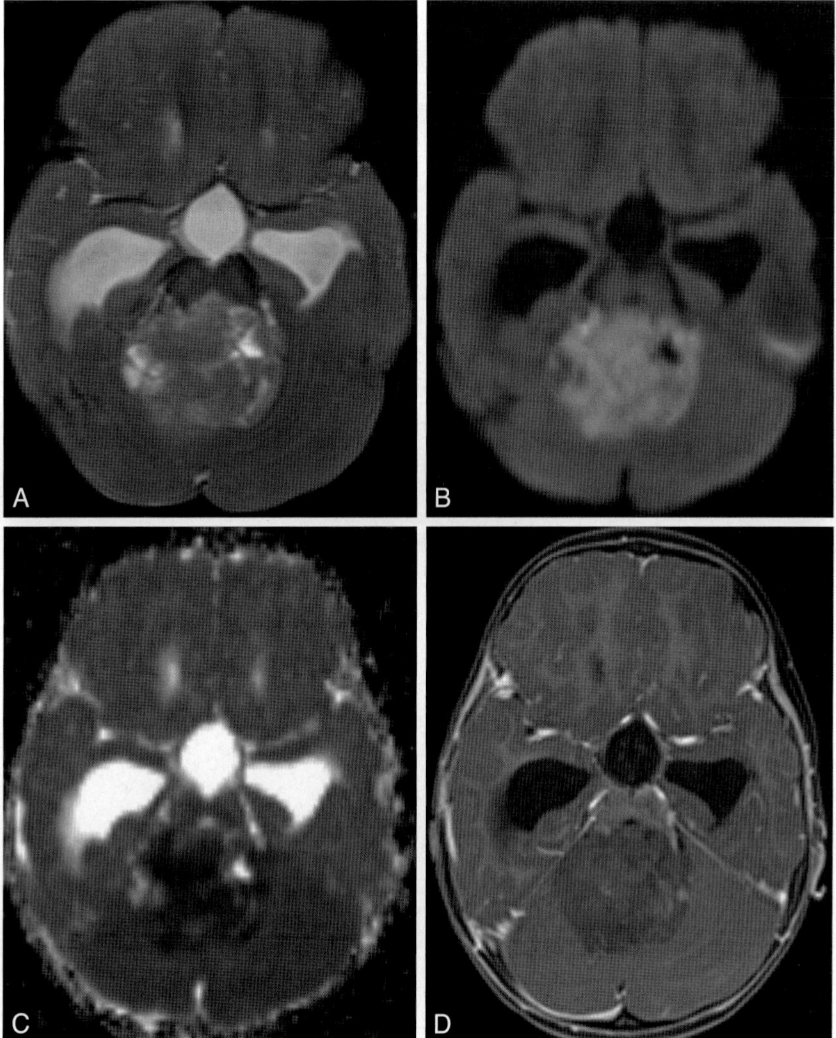

Fig. 7.18 Atypical Teratoid Rhabdoid Tumor (ATRT): 15-month-old. (A) Axial T2W, (B) Axial DWI, (C) axial ADC map, and (D) axial T1W+C images demonstrate a midline enhancing posterior fossa ATRT with reduced diffusion and minimal enhancement.

Key Points

Background

- WHO grade 4
- SMARCB1 mutations
- Rhabdoid tumor predisposition syndrome (RTPS) associated with increased risk of ATRT
- Dismal prognosis in patients <3 years of age *(most common age group is <3 years)*
- Location: Cerebellar, *vermian/fourth ventricular*, supratentorial (older patients)

Imaging

CT

- *Hyperdense* heterogeneous mass, small cysts, necrosis, hemorrhage, and calcification may occur

MRI

- Well-circumscribed heterogeneous mass, T1W isointense, T2W isointense, variable enhancement, small cysts, necrosis, hemorrhage and calcification
- *Restricted diffusion* similar to other embryonal tumors
- Metastasis common at presentation (>20%)

Advanced Imaging

- MR perfusion: ↑ CBF and CBV
- MRS: Aggressive metabolite pattern with ↑ choline, lipid and lactate; ↓ NAA

REFERENCES

1. Plaza MJ, et al. Conventional and advanced MRI features of pediatric intracranial tumors: posterior fossa and suprasellar tumors. *AJR Am J Roentgenol.* 2013 May;200(5):1115–1124.
2. Rumboldt Z, et al. Apparent Diffusion Coefficients for Differentiation of Cerebellar Tumors in Children. *AJNR Am J Neuroradiol.* 2006 Jun-Jul;27(6):1362–1369.
3. Tekautz TM, et al. Atypical Teratoid/Rhabdoid Tumors (ATRT): Improved Survival in Children 3 Years of Age and Older With Radiation Therapy and High-Dose Alkylator-Based Chemotherapy. *J Clin Oncol.* 2005 Mar 1;23(7):1491–1499.
4. Meyers SP, et al. Primary Intracranial Atypical Teratoid/Rhabdoid Tumors of Infancy and Childhood: MRI Features and Patient Outcomes. *AJNR Am J Neuroradiol.* 2006 May;27(5):962–971.

EMBRYONAL TUMOR WITH MULTILAYERED ROSETTES

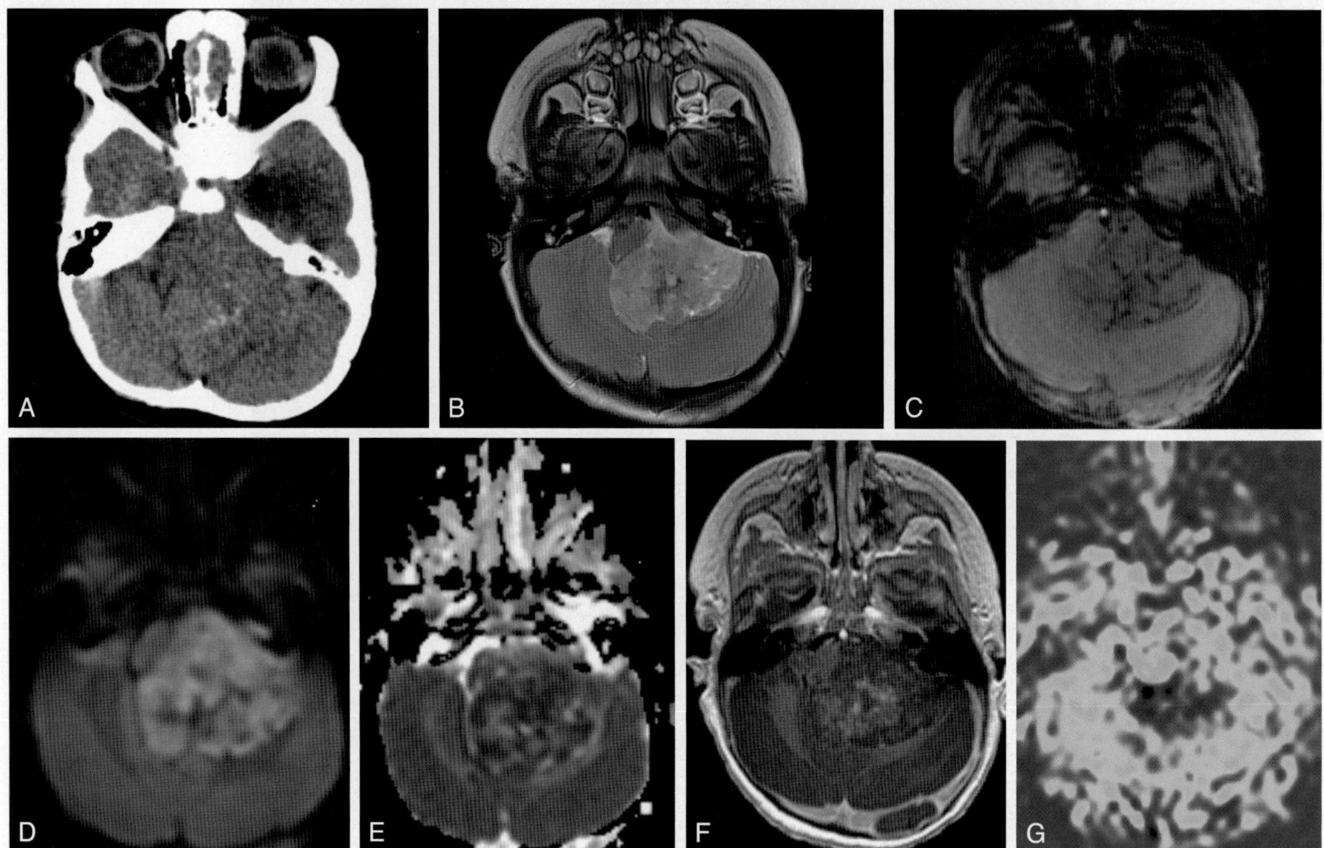

Fig. 7.19 Embryonal Tumor With Multilayered Rosettes (ETMR). A 10-month-old with rapid increase in head circumference. (A) Axial CT image demonstrates an isodense posterior fossa mass with small areas of calcification in the fourth ventricle and left cerebellopontine angle. (B) Axial T2W, (C) axial SWI, (D) axial DWI, (E) axial ADC map, (F) axial T1W+C, and (G) axial ASL CBF color map images demonstrate a posterior fossa mass with reduced diffusion, minimal enhancement, small areas of susceptibility, and low CBF. Pathology confirmed a ETMR. The low CBF is an unusual feature of these tumors and is different from the more common increased CBF in ATRT and medulloblastoma.

Key Points

Background

- Embryonal tumor with multilayered rosettes (ETMR) is a WHO grade 4 tumor recently classified in 2016 as tumors with amplification or gain of the C19MC region on chromosome 19 (19q13.42). This now includes tumors previously known as embryonal tumor with abundant neuropil and true rosettes (ETANTR), ependymoblastoma, and in some cases medulloepithelioma
- Median age at presentation <3 years
- Poor prognosis; median survival is 8 months
- Location: Both supratentorial (cerebral hemisphere) and infratentorial locations (along the tentorium, cerebellar vermis, fourth ventricle, and brainstem)

Imaging

CT

- Variable density with 50% hyperdense; hemorrhage and calcification (67%)

MRI

- Large, well-circumscribed, homogeneous, T2W hyperintense, minimal enhancement, and minimal to no surrounding edema
- *Restricted diffusion* similar to other embryonal tumors (median ADC 728 mm^2/s)
- Leptomeningeal disease uncommon

Advanced Imaging

- MR perfusion:
  - ↓ *CBF (median 30 mL/min/100g; unusual for high-grade tumors* and different than what is seen typically with ATRT and medulloblastoma)
  - ↑ CBV (maximal rCBV 3.5–5.8; mean rCBV 1.7–2.7)
- MRS: Limited data indicate ↑ choline and taurine

REFERENCE

1. Dangouloff-Ros V, Tauziède-Espariat A, Roux CJ, et al. CT and Multimodal MR Imaging Features of Embryonal Tumors with Multilayered Rosettes in Children. *AJNR Am J Neuroradiol.*. 2019 Apr;40(4):732–736.

DYSPLASTIC CEREBELLAR GANGLIOCYTOMA

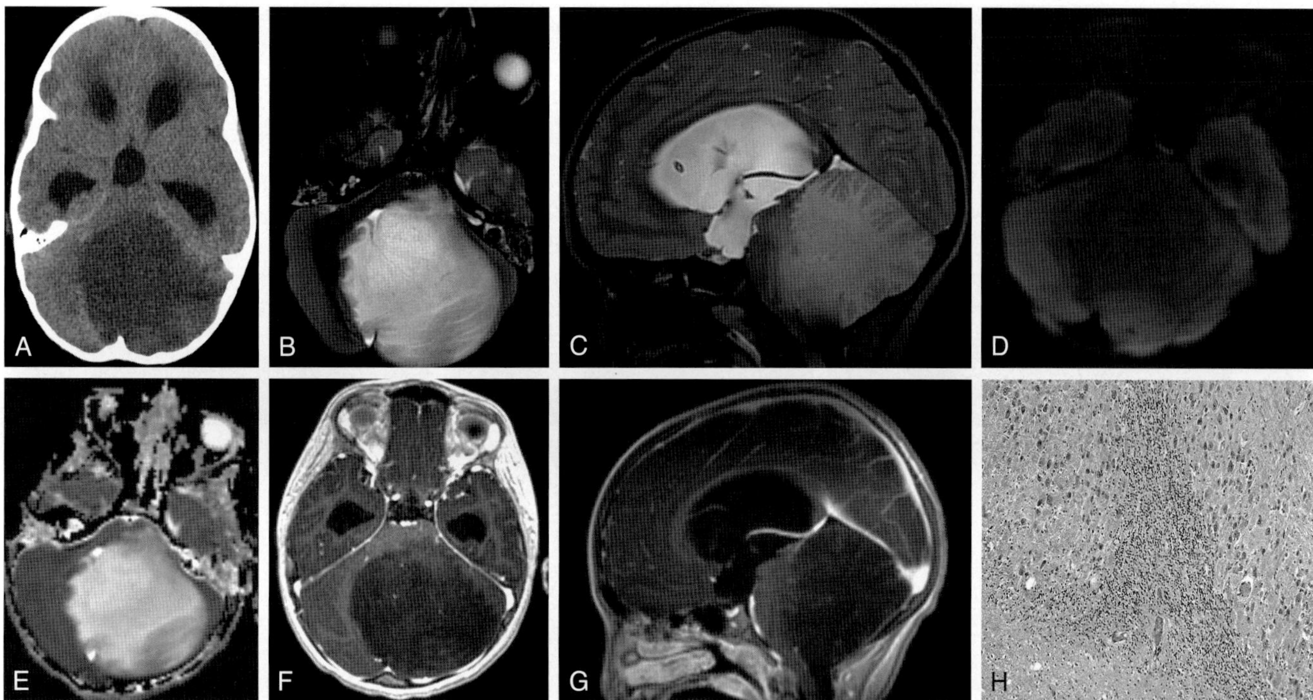

Fig. 7.20 Dysplastic Cerebellar Gangliocytoma. A 1-year-old with ataxia. (A) Axial head CT demonstrates a large low-density mass in the midline and left cerebellar hemisphere. (B and C) Axial and sagittal T2W, (D) axial DWI, (E) axial ADC map, (F and G) axial and sagittal T1W+C images demonstrate T2W hyperintense expansion of the vermis, majority of the left cerebellar hemisphere, and medial right cerebellar hemisphere with "corduroy" appearance, facilitated diffusion, and no enhancement. (H) Dysplastic gangliocytoma of cerebellum. Large, abnormal ganglion cells replace the granular layer in a dysplastic gangliocytoma of the cerebellum, macroscopically corresponding to thickened folia. (G from Fletcher CDM. *Diagnostic Histopathology of Tumors*. Elsevier; 2021.)

Key Points

Background

- Also known as Lhermitte-Duclos. *WHO grade 1*
- May be associated with *hemimegalencephaly* or *hemihypertrophy syndromes*
- *Cowden syndrome* associated with increased risk of dysplastic cerebellar gangliocytoma
- Location: Cerebellar hemisphere; may extend into vermis

Imaging

CT

- Ill-defined hypodense mass; hemorrhage and calcification may occur

MRI

- Well-circumscribed heterogeneous striated mass "enlarging the regional cerebellum," also known as *"corduroy appearance"* with significant mass effect. Bands of alternating T2W hyper- and hypointense signal; areas of cystic change; most do not enhance but may have regions of enhancement; hemorrhage and calcification may occur.
- Lack of restricted diffusion.

Advanced Imaging

- MR perfusion: Regions of ↑ rCBV
- MRS: ↑ Lactate; ↓ NAA and myoI

REFERENCES

1. Klisch J, et al. Lhermitte-Duclos disease: assessment with MR imaging, positron emission tomography, single-photon emission CT, and MR spectroscopy. *AJNR Am J Neuroradiol.* 2001;22:824–830.
2. Dhamija R, et al. Updated Imaging Features of Dysplastic Cerebellar Gangliocytoma. *J Comput Assist Tomogr.* 2019 Mar/Apr;43(2):277–281.

MEDULLARY GLIOMA

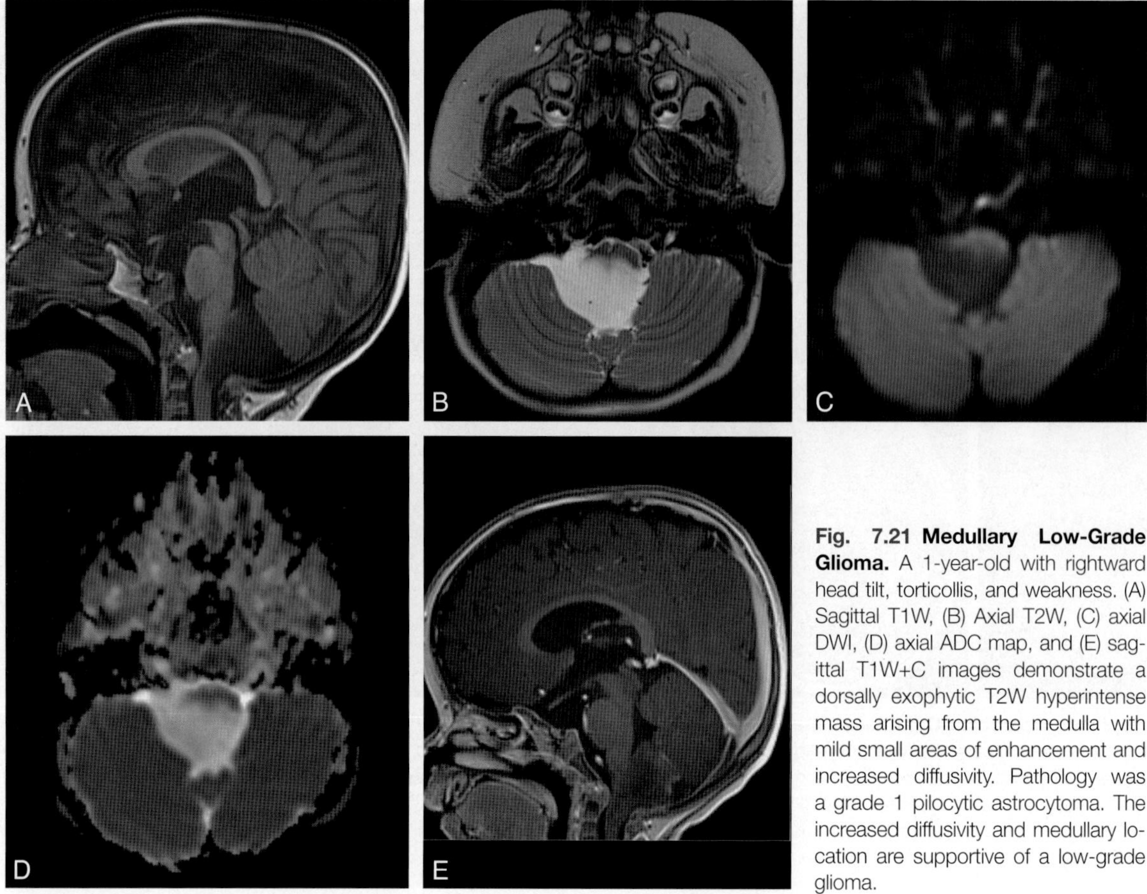

Fig. 7.21 Medullary Low-Grade Glioma. A 1-year-old with rightward head tilt, torticollis, and weakness. (A) Sagittal T1W, (B) Axial T2W, (C) axial DWI, (D) axial ADC map, and (E) sagittal T1W+C images demonstrate a dorsally exophytic T2W hyperintense mass arising from the medulla with mild small areas of enhancement and increased diffusivity. Pathology was a grade 1 pilocytic astrocytoma. The increased diffusivity and medullary location are supportive of a low-grade glioma.

Key Points

Background

- *Low-grade*: WHO grade 1 (dorsally exophytic), WHO grade 2 (diffuse)
- Three subtypes:
  - Dorsally exophytic (pilocytic astrocytoma, ganglioglioma)
  - Diffuse infiltrating (fibrillary astrocytoma)
  - NF-1–associated focal gliomas (pilocytic astrocytoma)
- Prognosis better in dorsally exophytic and NF-1–associated gliomas compared to diffuse infiltrating
- Location: Medulla or cervicomedullary

Imaging

CT

- Hypodense mass

MRI

- Dorsally exophytic
  - Well-circumscribed, multilobulated T1W hypointense, T2W hyperintense, variable enhancement, and small cysts
  - *Lack of restricted diffusion*
  - Dorsally exophytic with *involvement* of the medulla
- Diffuse infiltrating (fibrillary astrocytoma)
  - Less well-defined T1W hypointense, T2W hyperintense, and variable enhancement
  - Lack of restricted diffusion
  - Infiltrative expansion of the medulla
- NF-1–associated focal gliomas (pilocytic astrocytoma)
  - Focal, and usually small; well-defined; T1W hypointense, T2W hyperintense, and variable enhancement

Advanced Imaging

- MR Perfusion: decreased CBV and CBF
- MRS: varies based on histology

REFERENCE

1. McAbee JH, et al. Cervicomedullary tumors in children. *J Neurosurg Pediatr*. 2015 Oct;16(4):357–366.

DIFFUSE MIDLINE GLIOMA (DIFFUSE INTRINSIC PONTINE GLIOMA)

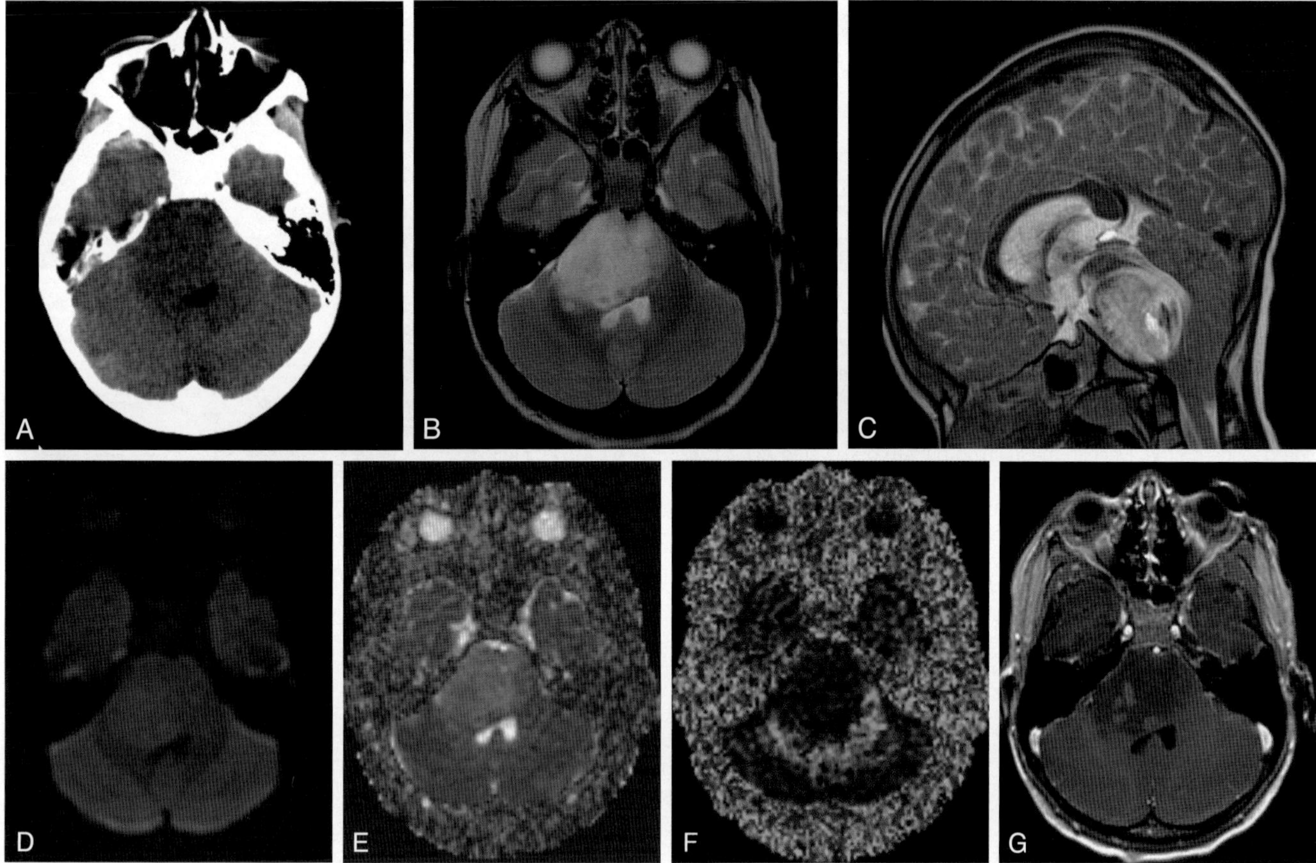

Fig. 7.22 Pontine Glioma. A 6-year-old with cranial nerve 6 and 7 palsy, and truncal ataxia. (A) Axial CT head image demonstrates a low-density mass expanding the pons and extending into the right middle cerebellar peduncle with associated compression of the fourth ventricle. (B and C) Axial and sagittal T2W, (D) axial DWI, (E) axial ADC, (F) axial color FA map, and (G) axial T1W+C images demonstrate a large T2W hyperintense expansile pontine mass infiltrating the brainstem tracts. Pontine gliomas may have foci of enhancement that show hyperperfusion, but the majority of the mass will not enhance and demonstrate hypoperfusion. Regions of enhancement may have restricted diffusion, but the remainder of the mass will demonstrate facilitated diffusion. Biopsy pathology was a high-grade astrocytoma with H3K27M mutation.

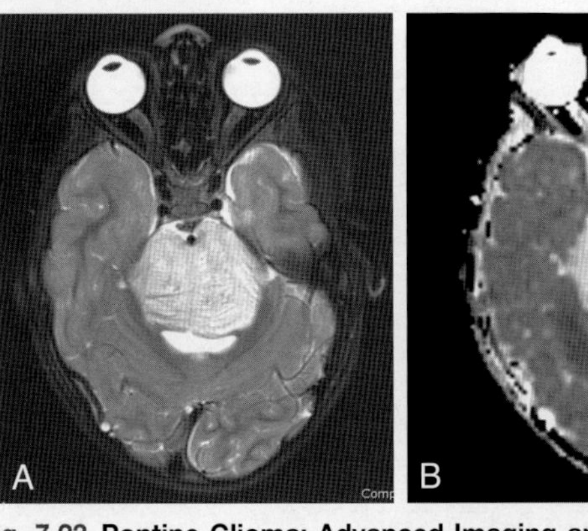

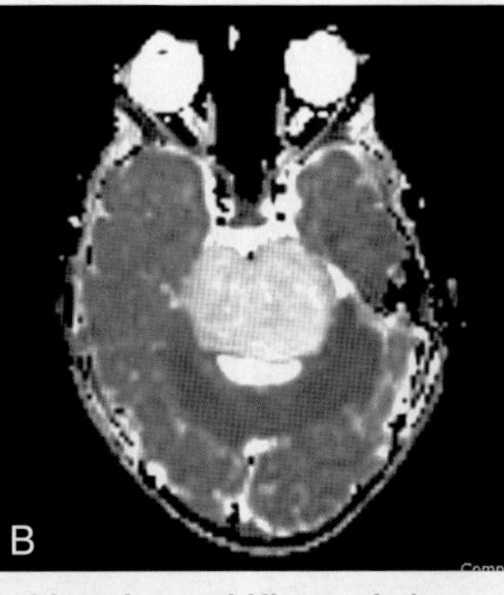

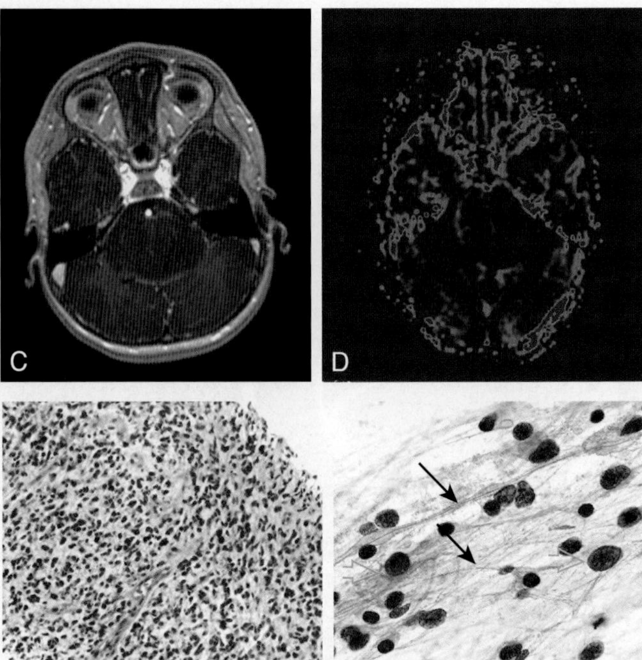

Fig. 7.23 Pontine Glioma: Advanced Imaging and Histopathology. (A) Axial T2W, (B) axial ADC map, and (C) axial T1W+C images demonstrate a typical pontine glioma with nonenhancing T2W hyperintense, elevated ADC expansion of the pons engulfing the basilar artery. (D) Axial CBV map obtained from DSC perfusion demonstrates typical low rCBV in the mass. (E and F) H&E pathology image demonstrates a typical high-grade pontine glioma. Despite the imaging pattern of elevated ADC, low CBV and no enhancement, the location is more important for correct diagnosis of a high-grade tumor. (E) Frozen section from a core needle biopsy of a diffuse intrinsic pontine glioma with anaplastic features, including high cellularity and mitotic activity on frozen section. Necrosis should not be present unless there has been prior radiotherapy. (F) Cytologic appearance: Infiltrating astrocytoma is characterized by irregular, dark, hyperchromatic, ovoid or fusiform nuclei with inconspicuous nucleoli sitting in a fibrillar background. (E, F from Lester SC. *Diagnostic Pathology: Intraoperative Consultation.* 2nd ed. Elsevier; 2018.)

Key Points

Background

- High-grade: WHO grade 3–4
- H3K27M mutation (histone H3 lysine27-to-methionine mutation) is present in 70%
- Term DIPG (diffuse intrinsic pontine glioma) no longer officially is used
- The pons is the most common location of brainstem tumors
- Signs and symptoms include hyperreflexia, ataxia, and cranial neuropathies (particularly abducens palsy). Behavior and cognitive changes also may occur
- Poor prognosis. Median survival is 9 to 11 months
- Location: Midline pons but may extend into the cranial and caudal brainstem and even into the cerebellum and supratentorial brain at end stage

Imaging

CT

- *Hypodense* expansile mass of the pons

MRI

- Poorly circumscribed T1W hypointense, and T2W hyperintense infiltrative expansile mass; *mostly nonenhancing*. May have regions of focal or cystic necrotic peripheral enhancement. Commonly effaces the prepontine cistern and encases or partially *encases the basilar artery*
  - Lack of restricted diffusion, although higher-grade components, which commonly enhance, may have restricted diffusion
  - End stage may metastasize or rarely at presentation

Advanced Imaging

- MR perfusion: Typically, low CBF and CBV at presentation with exception of enhancing areas; postradiotherapy demonstrates increased CBF
- MRS: ↑ Elevated choline, lactate & lipid; ↓ low NAA

REFERENCES

1. Camilo J, et al. Primary neoplasms of the pediatric brain. *Radiol Clin North Am.* 2019 Nov;57(6):1163–1175.
2. Brandão LA. Pediatric brain tumors. *Neuroimaging Clin N Am.* 2013 Aug;23(3):499–525.

TECTAL GIOMA

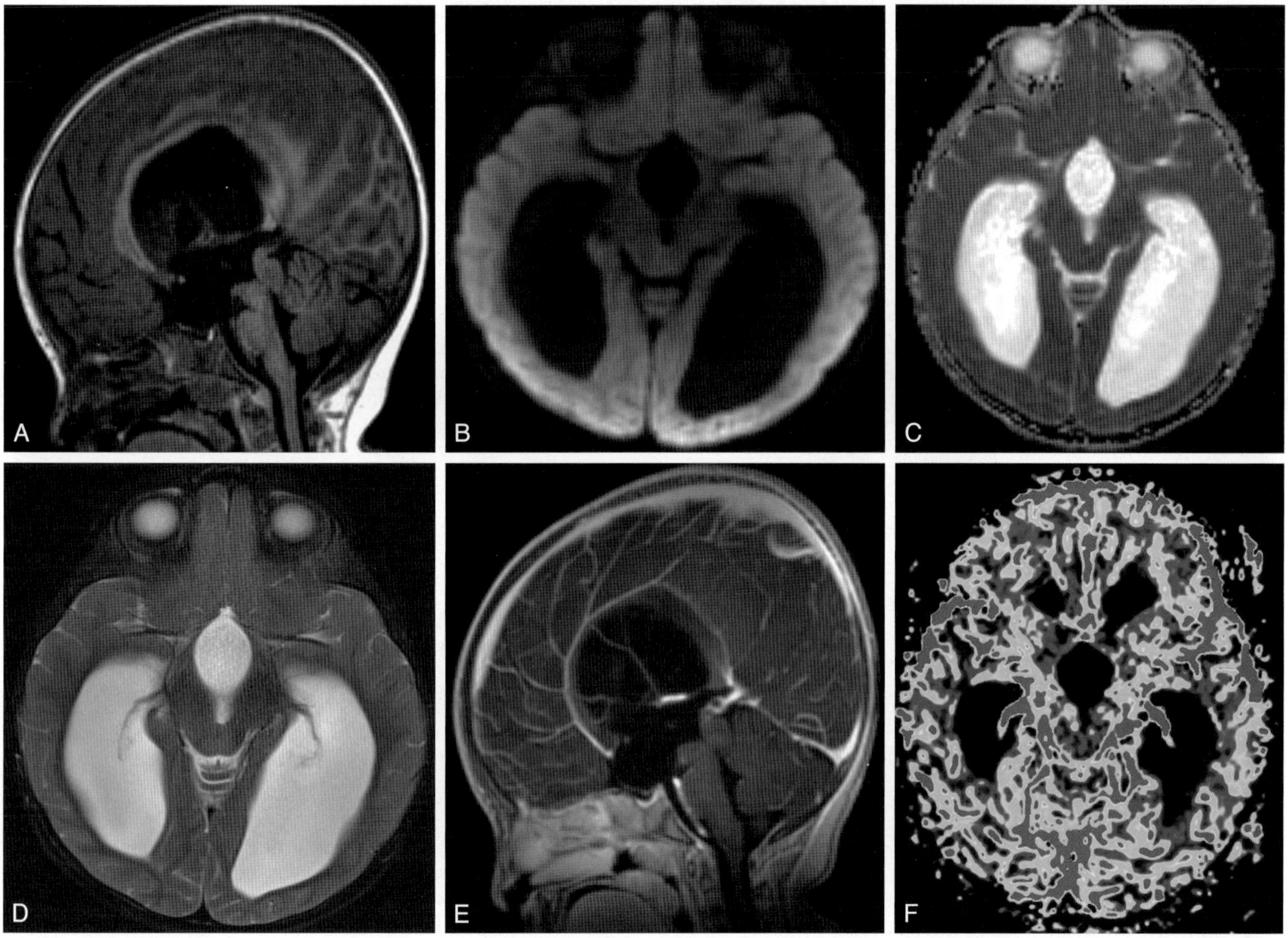

Fig. 7.24 Tectal Glioma. 2-year-old with macrocephaly. (A) Sagittal T1W, (B) axial DWI, (C) axial ADC map, (D) axial T2W, (E) sagittal T1W+C and (F) axial CBV color map from DSC perfusion demonstrate a small T1W and T2W isointense expansile nonenhancing tectal mass without reduced diffusion and with low rCBV, which compresses the cerebral aqueduct and results in obstructive hydrocephalus.

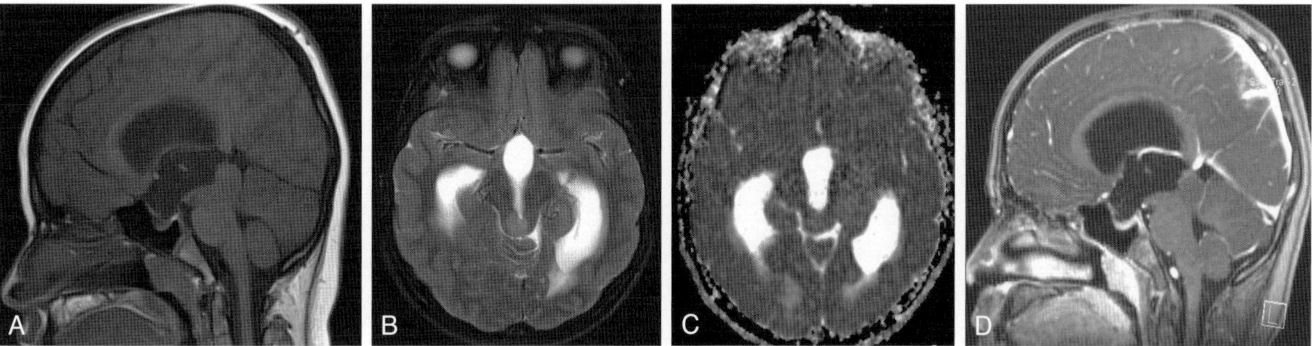

Fig. 7.25 Tectal Glioma. (A) Sagittal T1W, (B) axial T2W, (C) axial ADC map, and (D) sagittal T1W+C demonstrate a small T2W hyperintense expansile nonenhancing tectal mass with isointense diffusion, which compresses the cerebral aqueduct and results in obstructive hydrocephalus with transependymal edema.

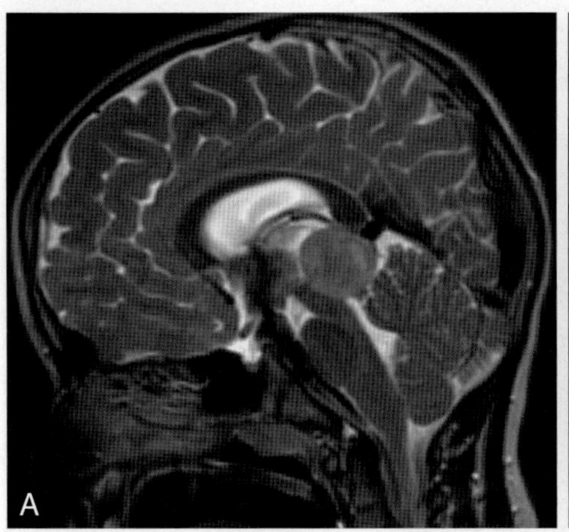

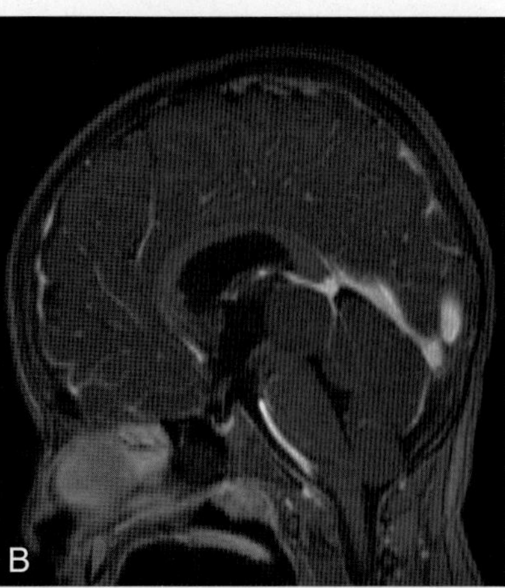

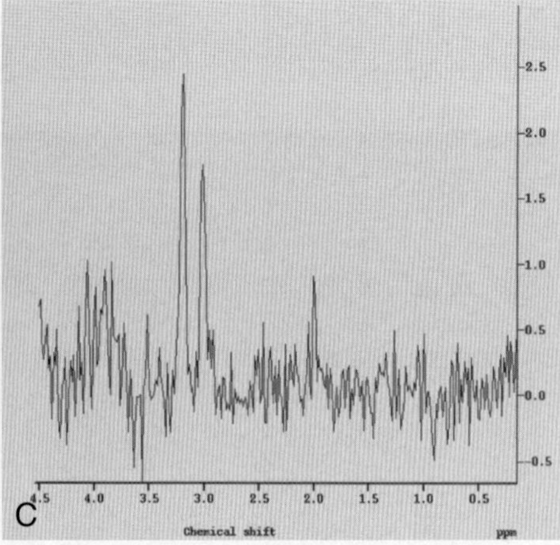

Fig. 7.26 Tectal Glioma. (A) Sagittal T2W and (B) sagittal T1W+C images demonstrate a T2W hyperintense expansile nonenhancing tectal mass compressing the cerebral aqueduct. A third ventriculostomy has been performed resulting in the T2W hypointense flow artifact across the ventriculostomy site which is visible on the T1W image as a small gap. (C) Single voxel proton MR spectroscopy of the mass performed with TE=135 ms demonstrates reduced NAA and elevated choline, which can mimic a high-grade tumor.

Key Points

Background

- *WHO grade 1* (most commonly pilocytic astrocytoma)
- *Obstruction of cerebral aqueduct* leads to hydrocephalus and presentation
- Most managed with third ventriculostomy
- *Excellent prognosis*
- Location: Tectal plate; may extend into the adjacent tegmentum and thalami

Imaging

CT

- Hypodense expansile mass of the tectum

MRI

- Well-defined T1W hypointense, and T2W hyperintense expansile tectal mass; often nonenhancing, but may enhance. Effaces the cerebral aqueduct
- Lack of restricted diffusion

Advanced Imaging

- MR Perfusion: decreased CBV and CBF
- MRS: not routinely performed

REFERENCES

1. Bowers DC, et al. Tectal gliomas: natural history of an indolent lesion in pediatric patients. *Pediatr Neurosurg*. 2000 Jan;32(1):24–29.
2. Liu APY, et al. Tectal glioma as a distinct diagnostic entity: a comprehensive clinical, imaging, histologic and molecular analysis. *Acta Neuropathol Commun*. 2018 Sep 25;6(1):101.

CEREBRAL HEMISPHERE TUMORS

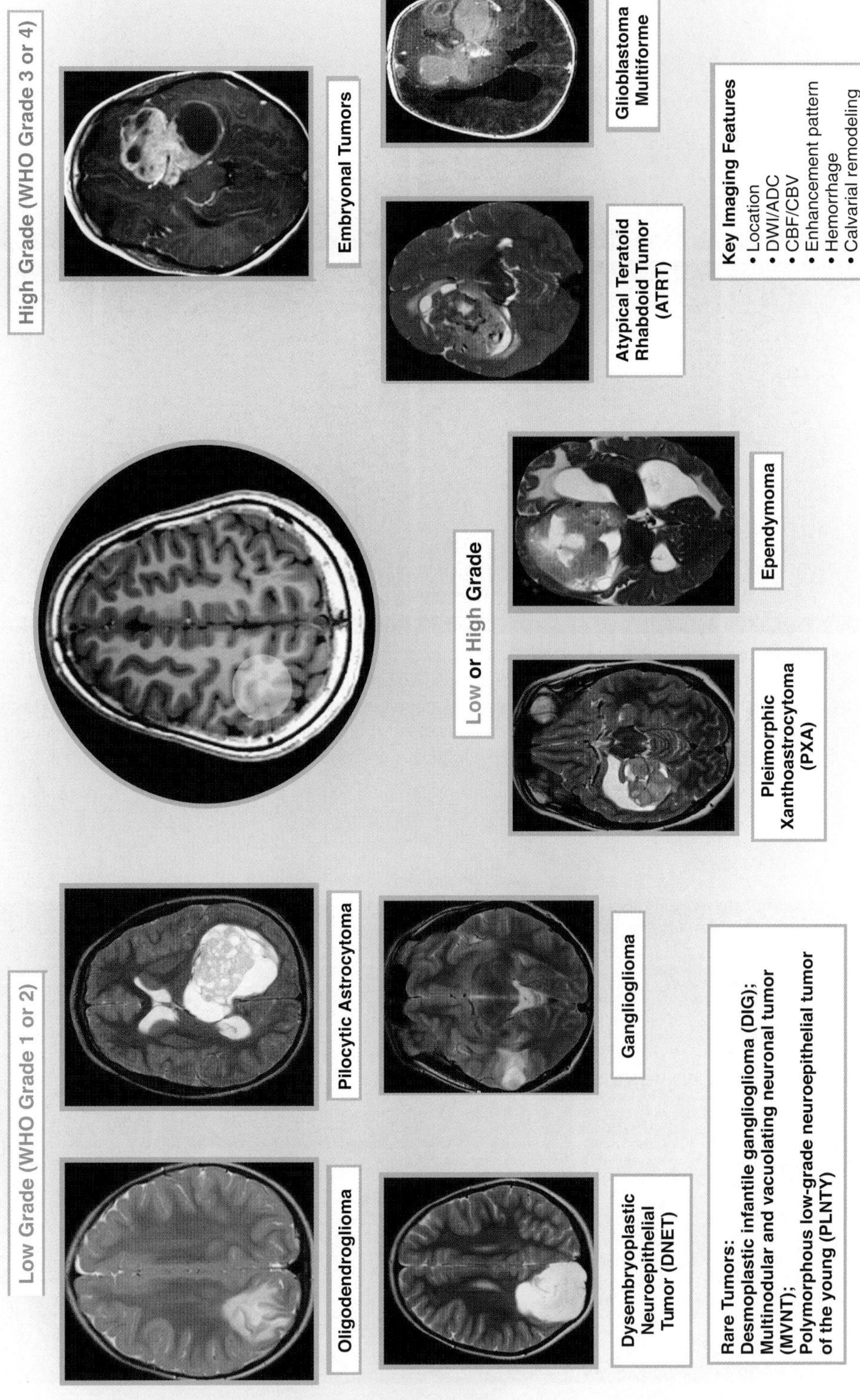

DYSEMBRYOPLASTIC NEUROEPITHELIAL TUMOR

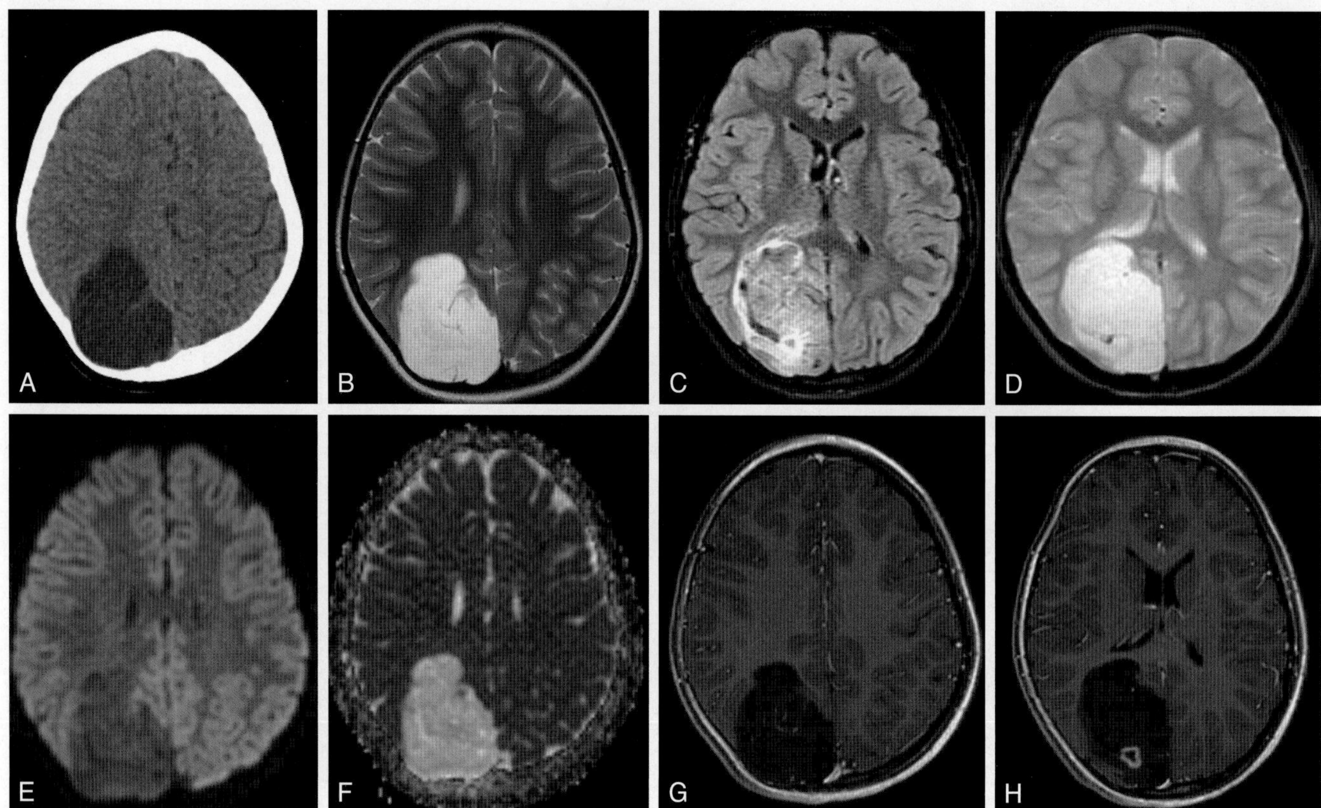

Fig. 7.27 Dysembryoplastic Neuroepithelial Tumor (DNET). A 9-year-old with a seizure. (A) Axial head CT image demonstrates a low-density right parietal mass with adjacent scalloping of the calvarium consistent with long-standing nature of the neoplasm. (B) Axial T2W, (C) axial FLAIR, (D) axial GRE, (E) axial DWI, (F) axial ADC map, and (G and H) axial T1W+C images demonstrate a very T2W hyperintense mass in the cortex and subcortical right parietal lobe with facilitated diffusion and small focus of calcification. The mass is mostly nonenhancing except for a small ring enhancing focus. The key imaging features are the cortical location, very hyperintense T2W signal, elevated ADC, and absence of significant enhancement.

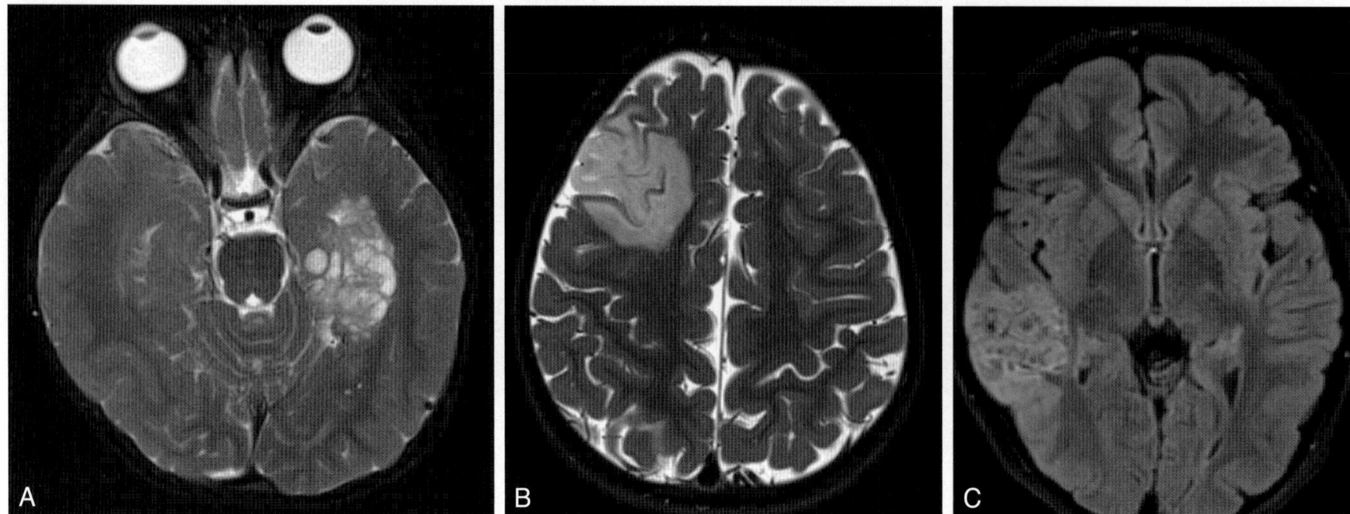

Fig. 7.28 Dysembryoplastic Neuroepithelial Tumor (DNET). Three separate patients. (A) Axial T2W image of a left temporal DNET demonstrating the typical bubbly T2W hyperintense appearance. (B) Axial T2W image demonstrating a right frontal lobe T2W hyperintense cortically based expansile tumor. (C) Axial FLAIR image of a right temporal lobe expansile mass with FLAIR hyperintensity in the cortex and subcortical white matter.

Key Points

Background

- WHO grade 1
- Peak incidence in the second decade of life; affects more M>F
- Presentation with intractable seizures
- Mixed glioneuronal tumor that may be associated with focal cortical dysplasia (type IIIB)
- 5-year survival >95%
- Location
    - Hemispheric tumor in the cortex and subcortical white matter, especially the temporal lobe, but they can occur anywhere. Rarely arise in the brainstem, cerebellum, and basal ganglia.
    - Nearly always solitary; rarely multifocal

Imaging

CT

- Well-defined hypodense mass without hemorrhage. Calcifications may occur. Small lesions may be entirely missed. Scalloping of the overlying calvarium can occur and suggests slow growing and lengthy presence of the mass.

MRI

- T1W hypointense, *T2W hyperintense "bubbly" lesion* due to cystic or microcystic appearance of the tumor. Nodular or diffuse appearance may also be seen. Peripheral rim of T2 FLAIR signal may be present. Some have a triangular configuration, especially larger mass lesions.
- Most commonly nonenhancing but up to one-third will have small areas of nodular, ring-like, or heterogeneous enhancement. Absent peritumoral edema and little to no mass effect.
- Facilitated diffusion.

Advanced Imaging

- MR perfusion: ↓ rCBV
- MRS: normal or ↑ myoI

REFERENCES

1. O'Brien DF, et al. The Children's Cancer and Leukaemia Group guidelines for the diagnosis and management of dysembryoplastic neuroepithelial tumours. *Br J Neurosurg.* 2007;21(6):539–549.
2. Stanescu Cosson R, et al. Dysembryoplastic neuroepithelial tumors: CT, MR findings and imaging follow-up: a study of 53 cases. *J Neuroradiol.* 2001;28(4):230–240.
3. Luzzi S, et al. Dysembryoplastic Neuroepithelial Tumors: What You Need to Know. *World Neurosurg.* 2019;127:255–265.
4. Fellah S, et al. Epileptogenic brain lesions in children: the added-value of combined diffusion imaging and proton MR spectroscopy to the presurgical differential diagnosis. *Childs Nerv Syst.* 2012;28(2):273–282.
5. Zamora C, et al. Supratentorial Tumors in Pediatric Patients. *Neuroimaging Clin N Am.* 2017 Feb;27(1):39–67.
6. Nguyen HS, et al. Dysembryoplastic Neuroectodermal Tumor: An Analysis from the Surveillance, Epidemiology, and End Results Program, 2004-2013. *World Neurosurg.* 2017;103:380–385.

GANGLIOGLIOMA

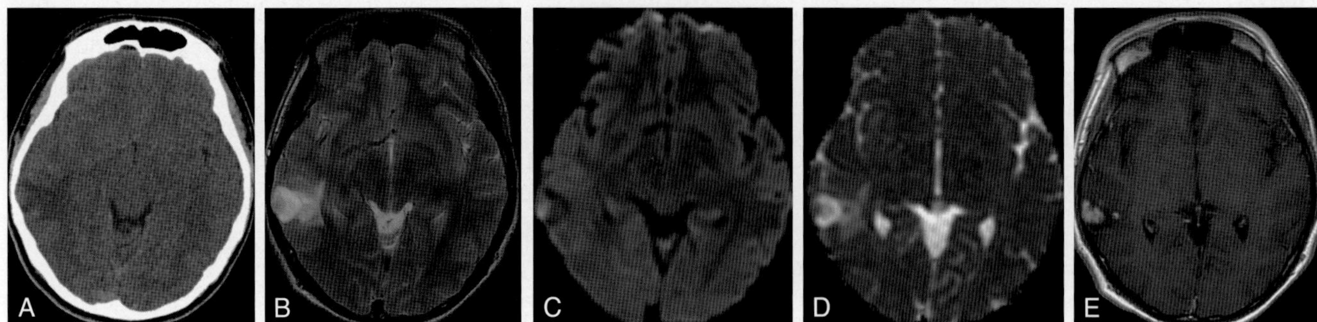

Fig. 7.29 Ganglioglioma. A 15-year-old with seizure. (A) Axial head CT image demonstrates an ill-defined region of low density in the posterolateral right temporal lobe. (B) Axial T2W, (C) axial DWI, (D) axial ADC map, and (E) axial T1W+C images demonstrate a cortical-based cyst and enhancing nodule with surrounding edema in the posterolateral right temporal lobe with increased and intermediate ADC levels.

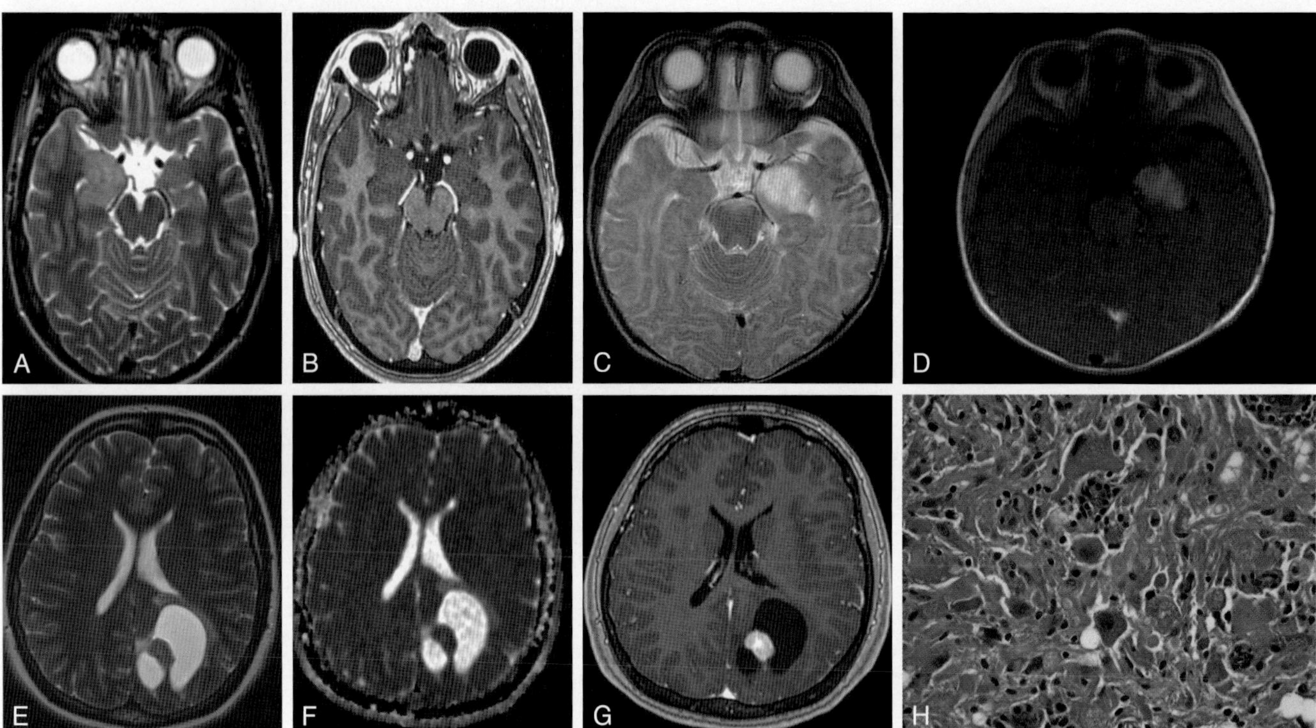

Fig. 7.30 Ganglioglioma: Common Imaging Patterns and Histopathology. (A and B) A 17-year-old with epilepsy with (A) axial T2W, and (B) axial T1W+C images demonstrating a T2W hyperintense expansile nonenhancing mass in the anteromedial right temporal lobe. (C and D) A 4-month-old with new-onset seizure with (C) axial T2W and (D) axial T1W+C images demonstrating a T2W hyperintense homogeneously enhancing mass in the anteromedial left temporal lobe. Both these first two cases demonstrate the common temporal lobe location, seizure presentation, and variable enhancement seen with ganglioglioma. (E to G) Axial T2W, axial ADC map, and axial T1W+C images demonstrate a cyst and nodule pattern, which can occur with ganglioglioma as well as less common extratemporal location. (H) Ganglioglioma. Abnormally clustered neoplastic ganglion cells admixed with eosinophilic granular bodies; perivascular lymphocytic cuffing is also evident (hematoxylin-eosin stain, Ã—200). (H from Jankovic J, Mazziotta JC, Pomeroy SL, et al. *Bradley and Daroff's Neurology in Clinical Practice.* 8th ed. Elsevier; 2022.)

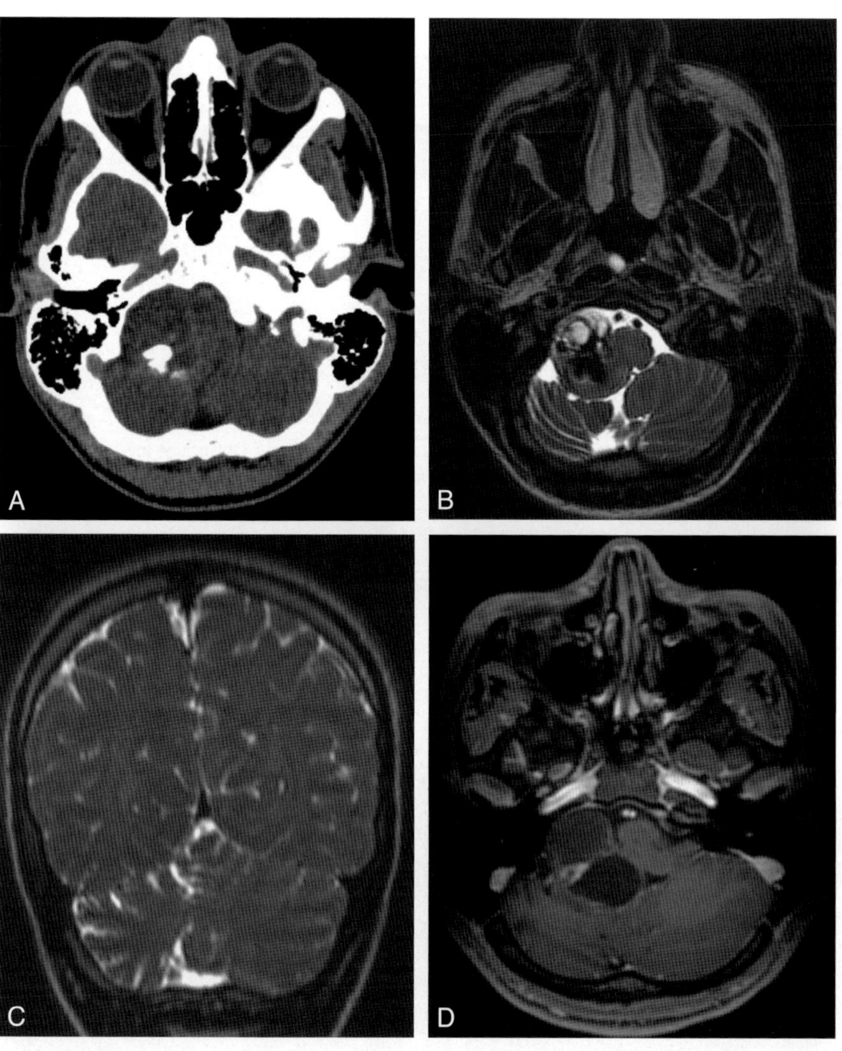

Fig. 7.31 Ganglioglioma: Uncommon Location. A 17-year-old with dizziness and headache. (A) Axial CT, (B and C) axial and coronal 3D T2W, and (D) axial T1W+C images demonstrate solid and cystic mass with large dystrophic calcification arising from the right dorsal medulla and inferior right cerebellar hemisphere with additional findings of scalloping of the right side of the skull base and right cerebellar hemisphere atrophy. The bone scalloping indicates long-term presence of the mass. The cerebellar atrophy is an additional unusual appearance seen with posterior fossa gangliogliomas.

Key Points

Background

- WHO grade 1 (low grade), grade 2 (atypical), and grade 3 (anaplastic). May progress to grade 4.
- Median age of 12 years; male predominance
- Neoplastic neuronal elements and astrocytes
- Similar imaging appearance to gangliocytomas, pilocytic astrocytomas, oligodendrogliomas, and DNETs
- *85% associated with seizures*; reported to be the most common cause of chronic temporal lobe epilepsy
- Survival 98% at 7.5 years
- Location
  - *Temporal*, especially mesial temporal followed by frontal. May rarely occur intraventricular or in brainstem, cerebellum, or spinal cord. Cerebellar gangliogliomas are reported to have unusual associated atrophy of the ipsilateral cerebellar hemisphere.

Imaging

CT

- Small lesions will be easily missed by CT. Hypodense mass; calcification is common; hemorrhage is uncommon

MRI

- Variable appearance
- Typically, T1W hypointense and T2W hyperintense variably enhancing solid mass with or without cysts. Lesions within the mesial temporal lobe; however, may be primarily solid, poorly delineated with little enhancement.
- *Increased ADC*; higher-grade lesions may have lower ADC

Advanced Imaging

- MR perfusion: ↓ CBV and CBF
- MRS: ↓ NAA, ↑ myoI

REFERENCES

1. Zamora C, et al. Supratentorial Tumors in Pediatric Patients. *Neuroimaging Clin N Am.* 2017 Feb;27(1):39–67.
2. Zaky W, et al. Ganglioglioma in children and young adults: single institution experience and review of the literature. *J Neurooncol.* 2018;139(3):739–747.
3. Adachi Y, et al. Gangliogliomas: Characteristic imaging findings and role in the temporal lobe epilepsy. *Neuroradiology.* 2008;50(10):829–834.
4. Raybaud C. Cerebral hemispheric low-grade glial tumors in children: preoperative anatomic assessment with MRI and DTI. *Childs Nerv Syst.* 2016;32(10):1799–1811.

OLIGODENDROGLIOMA

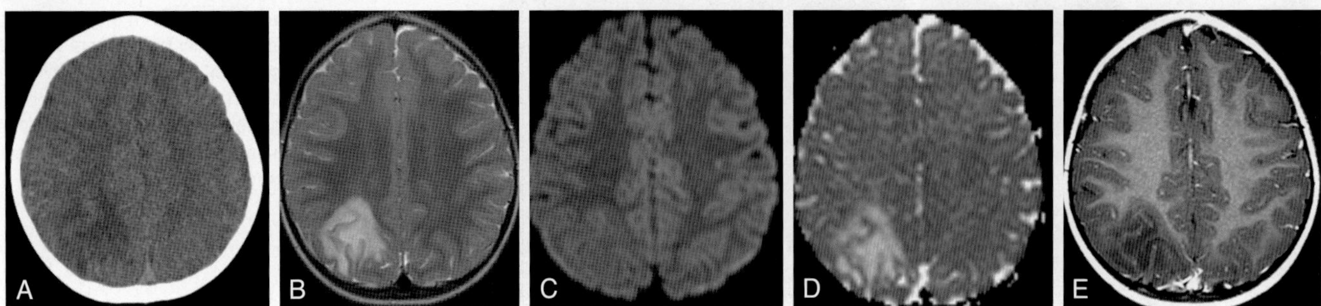

Fig. 7.32 Oligodendroglioma. A 2-year-old with staring spells. (A) Axial head CT image demonstrates an abnormal region of infiltrative low density in the right parietal lobe. (B) Axial T2W, (C) axial DWI, (D) axial ADC map, and (E) axial T1W+C images demonstrate a T2W hyperintense cortical and subcortical mass with facilitated diffusion and no significant enhancement. The imaging pattern favors a low-grade glioma but would be difficult to reach a specific diagnosis.

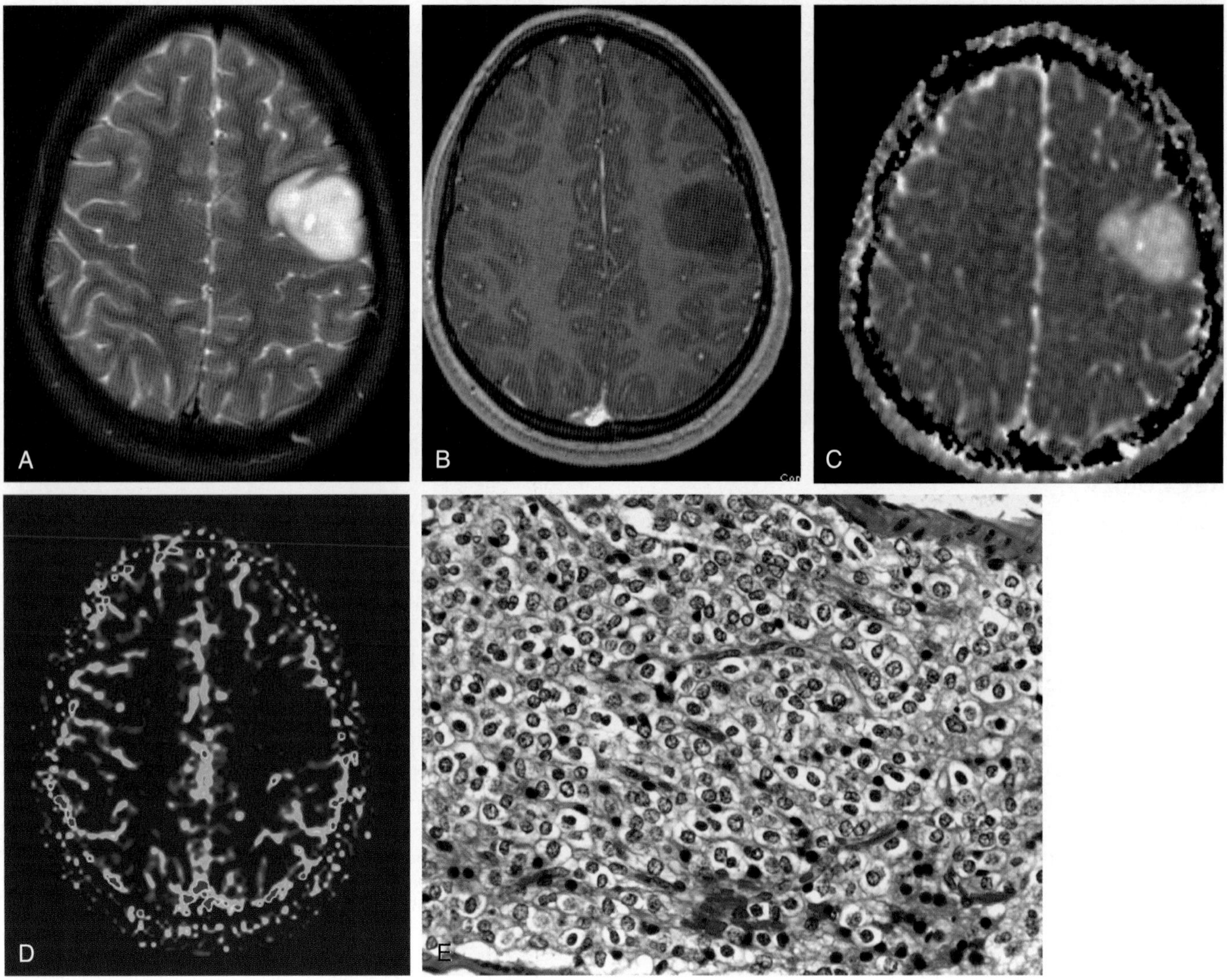

Fig. 7.33 Oligodendroglioma: Advanced Imaging and Histopathology. (A) Axial T2W, (B) axial T1W+C, and (C) axial ADC map demonstrate a left frontal lobe cortical and subcortical T2W hyperintense mass with elevated ADC and no significant enhancement. (D) Axial CBV map obtained from DSC perfusion demonstrates low rCBV in the mass. Some oligodendrogliomas can demonstrate increased CBV despite their low-grade categorization indicating a potential pitfall of the CBV. The ADC signal is more reliable for reaching the correct diagnosis. (E) Cells have uniform round nuclei with bland chromatin and a clear perinuclear halo, producing a "fried-egg" appearance. The rich, branching capillary network has been likened to chicken wire (hematoxylin-eosin stain, Ã—200). (E from Jankovic J, Mazziotta JC, Pomeroy SL, et al. *Bradley and Daroff's Neurology in Clinical Practice.* 8th ed. Elsevier; 2022.)

Key Points

Background

- WHO grade 2 (low grade) and grade 3 (anaplastic)
- 1% to 3% of pediatric CNS neoplasms
- *Rare entity in children compared to adults*; peak incidence is fifth to sixth decade
- *Uncommon to have 1p19q deletion or IDH1 mutation* which is different from adult patients; MGMT promoter methylation is similar to adult patients
- Excellent prognosis; 5-year survival 95%
- Location
  - Typically, hemispheric, cortical and subcortical tumor. Frontal lobe is most common followed by parietal and temporal lobe. Rarer locations include brainstem, cerebellopontine angle, optic nerve, and spinal cord.

Imaging

CT

- Small lesions will be easily missed by CT. Hypodense peripheral mass; calcification may be seen but less common than in adults; hemorrhage is uncommon

MRI

- Well-defined T1W hypointense and T2W hyperintense; nonenhancing to minimally enhancing solid mass with or without cysts; can also be poorly delineated with little enhancement.
- Increased ADC, even in high-grade lesions

Advanced Imaging

- MR perfusion: Variable but potential for ↑ CBV/CBF
- MRS: ↑ Choline, lactate, and lipid in higher-grade lesions and thus may be more helpful than dynamic susceptibility perfusion imaging

REFERENCES

1. Li YX, et al. Oligodendrogliomas in pediatric and teenage patients only rarely exhibit molecular markers and patients have excellent survivals. *J Neurooncol.* 2018;139(2):307–322.
2. Raybaud C. Cerebral hemispheric low-grade glial tumors in children: preoperative anatomic assessment with MRI and DTI. *Childs Nerv Syst.* 2016;32(10):1799–1811.
3. Zamora C, et al. Supratentorial Tumors in Pediatric Patients. *Neuroimaging Clin N Am.* 2017 Feb;27(1):39–67.
4. Brandão LA, et al. Pediatric brain tumors. *Neuroimaging Clin N Am.* 2013 Aug;23(3):499–525.

DESMOPLASTIC INFANTILE GANGLIOGLIOMA

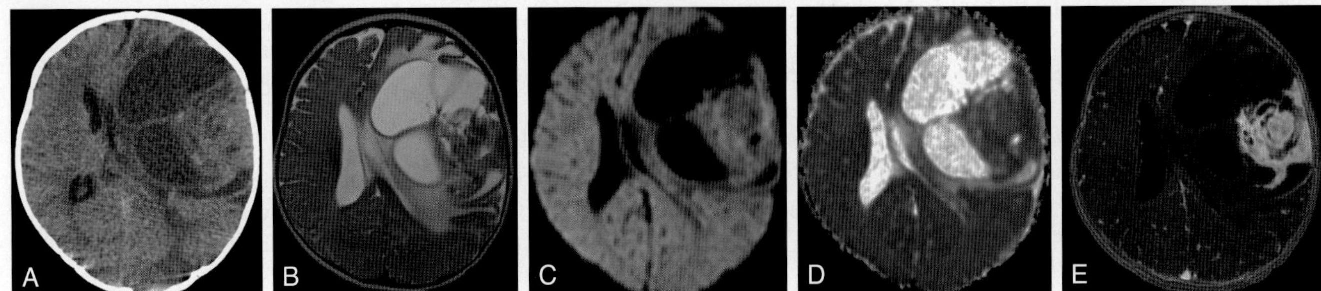

Fig. 7.34 Desmoplastic Infantile Ganglioglioma. A 6-month-old. (A) Axial CT scan demonstrates a large solid and cystic isodense mass occupying majority of the left frontal lobe with adjacent edema and rightward midline shift. (B) Axial T2W, (C) axial DWI, (D) axial ADC map, and (E) axial T1W+C images demonstrate typical features of a DIG with solid and cystic appearance, avid nodular enhancement, leptomeningeal extension simulating an extraaxial location. DWI/ADC are intermediate to mildly reduced in the solid portions, which can lead to misdiagnosis.

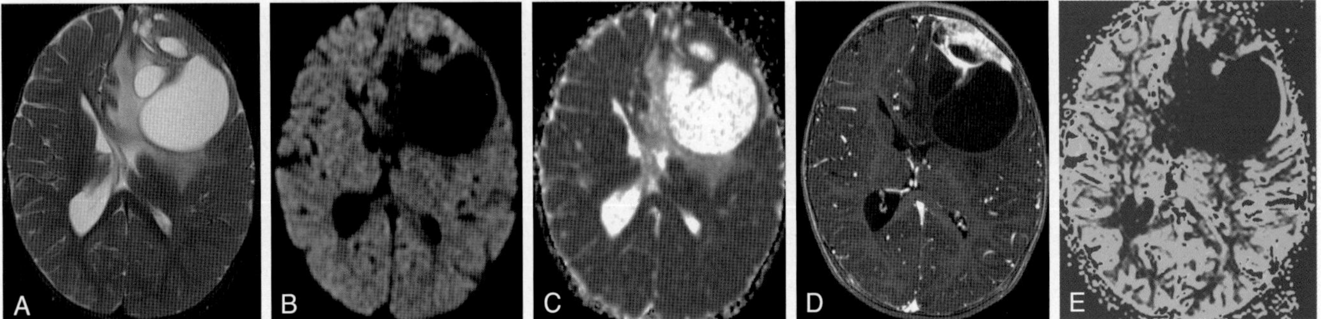

Fig. 7.35 Desmoplastic Infantile Ganglioglioma. A 13-month-old. (A) Axial T2W, (B) axial DWI, (C) axial ADC map, (D) axial T1W+C, and (E) axial CBV color map from DSC perfusion demonstrate a large solid and cystic left frontal lobe mass with adjacent edema and rightward midline shift typical of a DIG. Avid nodular enhancement, leptomeningeal extension simulating an extraaxial location, intermediate to mildly reduced ADC, and some areas of elevated rCBV in the solid portions can lead to misdiagnosis.

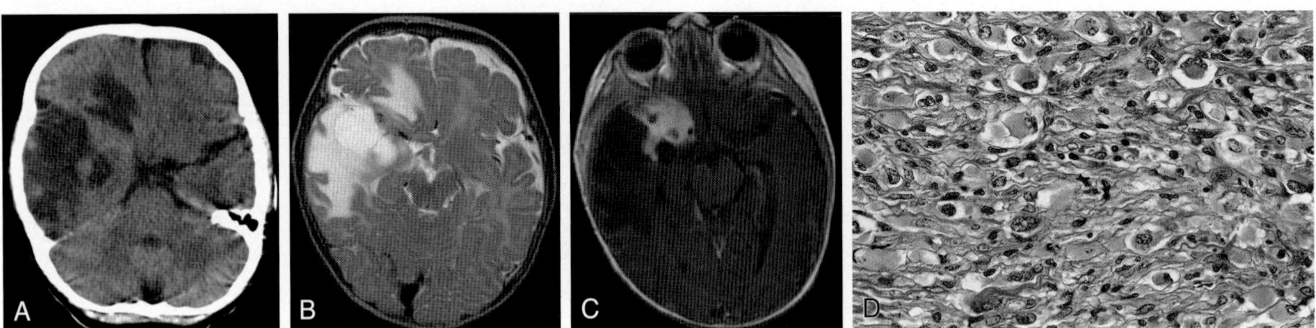

Fig. 7.36 Desmoplastic Infantile Ganglioglioma. A 4-month-old. (A) Axial head CT demonstrates a large low density mass in the right frontal and temporal lobes. (B) Axial T2W, and (C) axial T1W+C images demonstrate and solid and cystic mass in the right frontal and temporal lobes with surrounding edema. (D) Desmoplastic infantile gangliogliomas are composed of a mixed population of heterogeneous glia and globoid neurons in a conspicuous stroma with variable collagen deposition. (D from Fletcher CDM. *Diagnostic Histopathology of Tumors*. Elsevier; 2021.)

Key Points

Background

- WHO grade 1
- Desmoplastic infantile ganglioglioma and desmoplastic astrocytoma of infancy may be referred to as desmoplastic neuroepithelial tumors
- Typical patient age is < 18 months; median age at presentation is 5 months; slight male predominance
- Typical presentation with rapidly progressive macrocephaly, bulging fontanelle, and/or seizures
- Location
    - *Large hemispheric (often multilobar)*, cortical and subcortical tumor with leptomeningeal and dural involvement. Frontal and parietal lobe are most common. Rarer locations include hypothalamus, posterior fossa, and spinal cord.

Imaging

CT

- Variable density, solid and large cystic hemispheric mass lesions; calcification is common

MRI

- Well-defined T1W isointense and T2W isointense to hypointense avidly enhancing cortical based solid mass with large cysts. T2W isointense to hypointense signal differentiates these mass lesions from T2W hyperintense pilocytic astrocytomas
- Leptomeningeal and dural involvement are typical. Cyst walls do not enhance
- Variable peritumoral edema; may be severe
- Solid components may show decreased ADC

Advanced Imaging

- MR perfusion: Can show ↑ CBV despite low grade
- MRS: ↑ myoI

REFERENCES

1. Bianchi F, et al. Supratentorial tumors typical of the infantile age: desmoplastic infantile ganglioglioma (DIG) and astrocytoma (DIA). A review. *Childs Nerv Syst*. 2016;32(10):1833–1838.
2. Zamora C, et al. Supratentorial Tumors in Pediatric Patients. *Neuroimaging Clin N Am*. 2017 Feb;27(1):39–67.
3. Brandão LA, et al. Pediatric brain tumors. *Neuroimaging Clin N Am*. 2013 Aug;23(3):499–525.

RARE LOW-GRADE TUMORS OF THE CEREBRAL HEMISPHERES

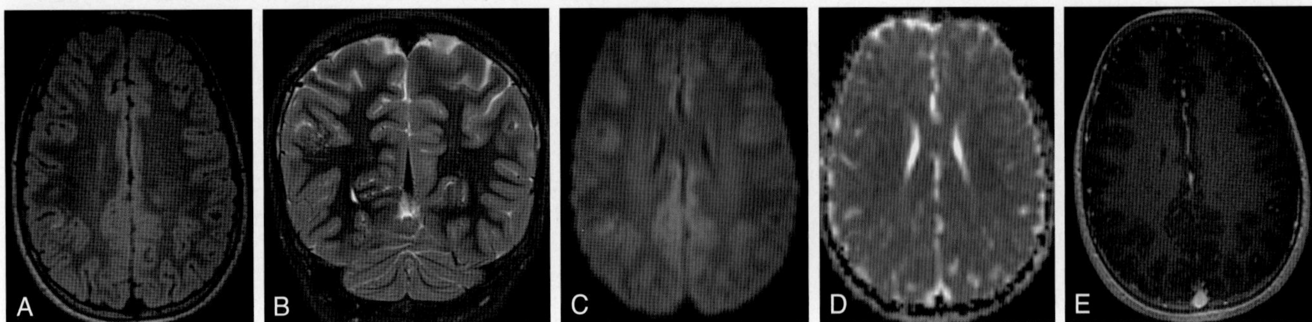

Fig. 7.37 Multinodular and Vacuolating Neuroepithelial Tumor (MVNT). A 10-year-old with seizures. (A) Axial FLAIR, (B) coronal T2W, (C) axial DWI, (D) axial ADC map, and (E) axial T1W+C images demonstrate a cluster of small juxtacortical T2 FLAIR hyperintense nodules without enhancement in the right parietal lobe with mild DWI hyperintensity and ADC isointensity. Histopathology confirmed a diagnosis of MVNT.

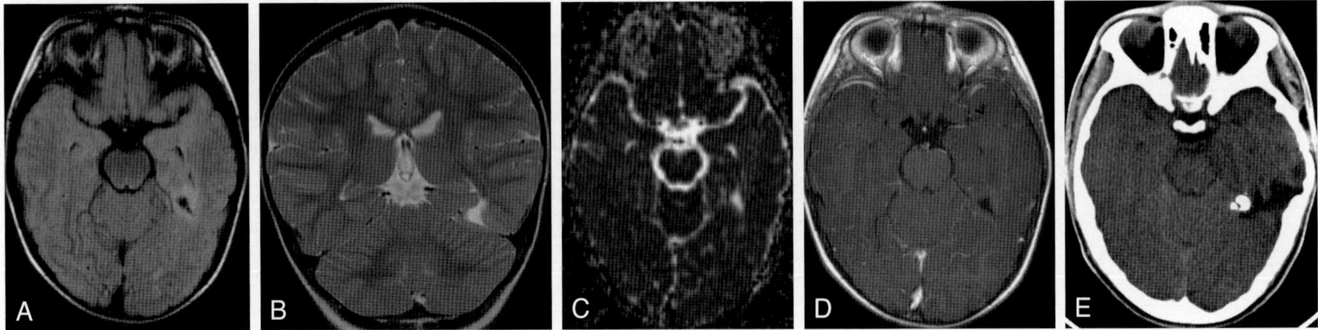

Fig. 7.38 Polymorphous Low-Grade Neuroepithelial Tumor of the Young (PLNTY). A 2-year-old with seizures. (A) Axial FLAIR, (B) coronal T2W, (C) axial ADC map, and (D) axial T1W+C images demonstrate a T2W hyperintense lesion in the left fusiform gyrus, which is partially cystic as indicated by partial attenuation on FLAIR imaging, elevated ADC values, and no associated enhancement. At presentation and time of initial surgery no calcification was visible on imaging; however, 10 years after resection a mass recurred at the resection site with large coarse calcification as seen on axial CT (E). Repeat surgical resection histopathology confirmed a diagnosis of PLNTY.

Multinodular and Vacuolating Neuroepithelial Tumor (MVNT)

Key Points

Background

- Low-grade neuroepithelial tumor described in 2013
- WHO 2016 classification as a unique pattern of gangliocytoma but may be a dysplastic lesion
- May present with seizures or be incidentally detected
- Location: Supratentorial, and juxtacortical

Imaging

- Multiple small (1–5 mm) rounded nonenhancing juxtacortical nodules with T2 FLAIR hyperintensity and no diffusion restriction or susceptibility
- Differential Diagnosis: DNET, perivascular spaces, cortical dysplasia

Polymorphous Low-Grade Neuroepithelial Tumor of the Young (PLNTY)

Key Points

Background

- Rare low-grade neuroepithelial tumor described in 2016
- Usually presents with epilepsy
- Location: Supratentorial, typically temporal lobe (67%), circumscribed, cortical or subcortical location

Imaging

- T2W hyperintense, calcification (89%), cystic (89%), nonenhancing (67%), and no diffusion restriction
- Differential Diagnosis: DNET, ganglioglioma, and oligodendroglioma

REFERENCES

1. Johnson DR, Giannini C, Jenkins RB, et al. Plenty of calcification: imaging characterization of polymorphous low-grade neuroepithelial tumor of the young. *Neuroradiology*. 2019 Nov;61(11):1327–1332.
2. Nunes RH, Hsu CC, da Rocha AJ, et al. Multinodular and Vacuolating Neuronal Tumor of the Cerebrum: A New “Leave Me Alone” Lesion with a Characteristic Imaging Pattern. *AJNR Am J Neuroradiol*. 2017 Oct;38(10):1899–1904.

PLEIOMORPHIC XANTHOASTROCYTOMA

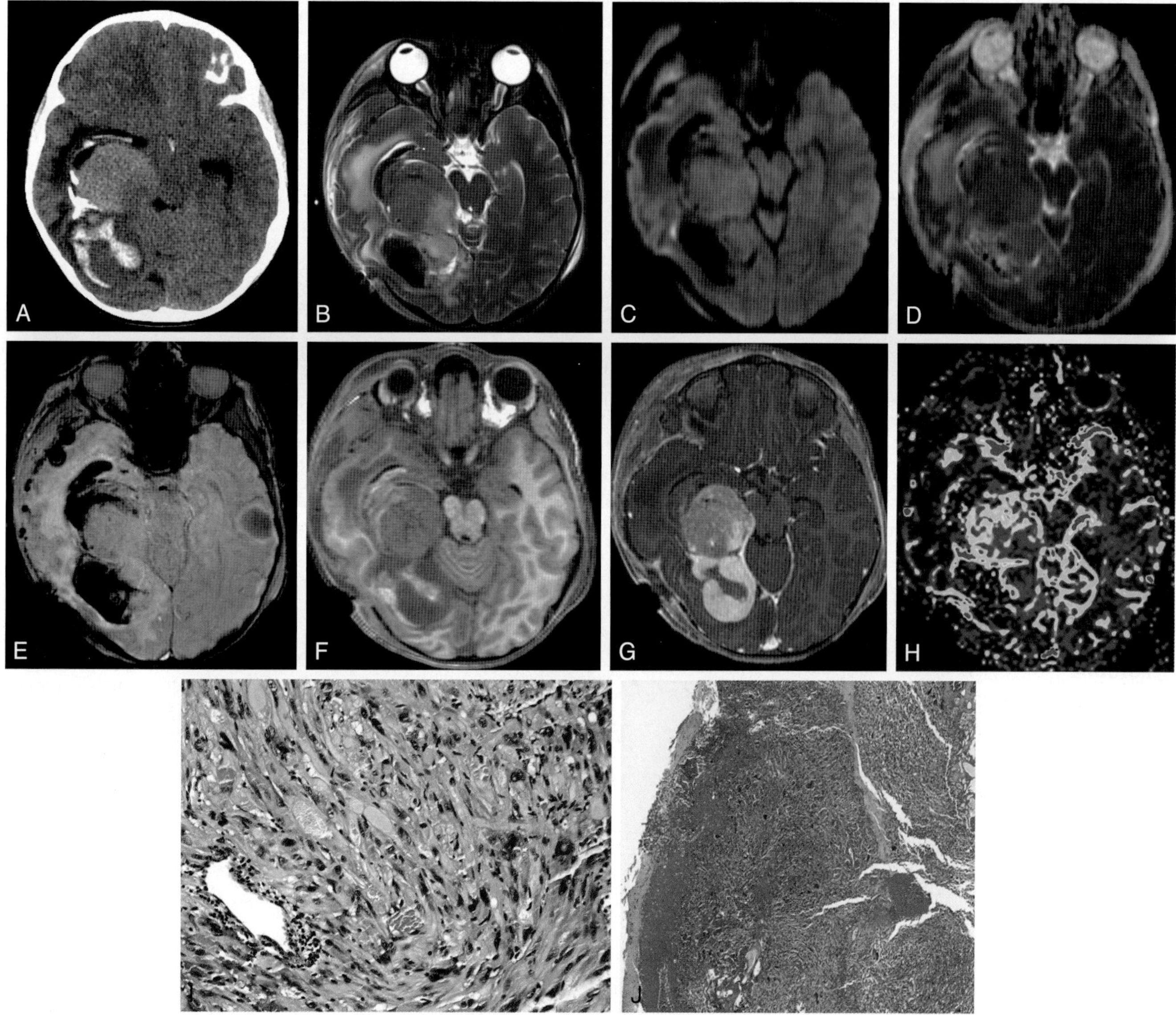

Fig. 7.39 Anaplastic Pleiomorphic Xanthoastrocytoma (PXA). A 6-year-old with altered mental status. (A) Axial head CT images demonstrates a mildly hyperdense right temporal lobe mass with surrounding hemorrhage and obstruction of the temporal horn. (B) Axial T2W, (C) axial DWI, (D) axial ADC, (E) axial SWI, (F) axial T1W, (G) axial T1W+C, and (H) axial CBV map images after emergency decompressive craniotomy resulting from the mass effect from the hemorrhage demonstrate a mixed isointense and mildly T2W hyperintense mass with avid nodular enhancement and curved areas of leptomeningeal enhancement. The mass has isointense DWI signal and ADC similar to normal parenchyma. The rCBV is elevated. (I and J) Histopathology images of a PXA demonstrating the leptomeningeal extension, which is a common feature. PXAs are cortically based tumors and often present with hemorrhage due to the leptomeningeal invasion. Low-grade PXAs often have associated scalloping of the calvarium. (I) Infiltrate of neoplastic astrocytic cells with marked nuclear pleomorphism and xanthomatous changes. Eosinophilic granular bodies are present. (J) Histopathology slide of a PXA demonstrating the leptomeningeal extension surrounding blood vessels which predisposes the tumor to hemorrhage. (I from Reddy VB, David O, Spitz DJ, et al. *Gattuso's Differential Diagnosis in Surgical Pathology.* 4th ed. Elsevier; 2022.)

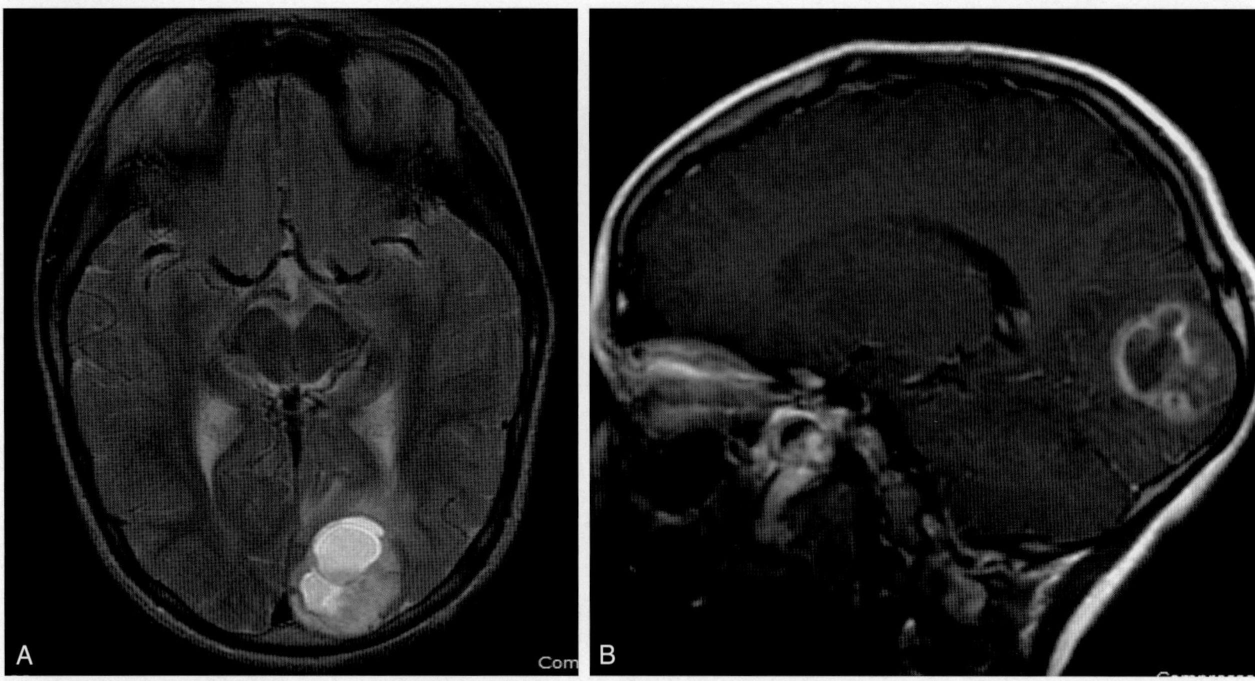

Fig. 7.40 Pleiomorphic xanthoastrocytoma (PXA). (A) Axial T2W and (B) sagittal T1W+C images demonstrate a cortical and subcortical left occipital mass with cyst and nodule pattern.

Key Points

Background

- WHO grade 2 (low grade) and grade 3 (anaplastic)
- Median age at presentation 20 years but wide age presentation from infancy to late adulthood
- Rare tumors; less than 1% of astrocytic tumors
- Commonly present with seizures
- Often associated with focal cortical dysplasia (FCD IIIB)
- BRAF mutation is common
- 5-year survival 75%
- Location
  - Cortical and subcortical tumor abutting the temporal lobe is most common followed by frontal and parietal lobe location.

Imaging

CT

- *Cortical-based* solid or solid and cystic mass lesion. Solid components are isodense to cortex. *Scalloping of the inner table of the calvarium* is typical. Calcifications are rare. *Hemorrhage may occur.*

MRI

- Well-defined T1W hypointense to isointense and T2W isointense to hyperintense *avidly enhancing* cortical-based solid or solid and cystic mass (i.e. cyst and nodule pattern)
- *Leptomeningeal involvement is common.* Dural involvement may occur
- Solid components show mildly decreased ADC
- Peritumoral edema may be significant

Advanced Imaging

- MR perfusion: ↑ CBV and CBF in high-grade PXA
- MRS: ↑ Choline

REFERENCES

1. Zamora C, et al. Supratentorial Tumors in Pediatric Patients. *Neuroimaging Clin N Am.* 2017 Feb;27(1):39–67.
2. Moore W, et al. Pleomorphic xanthoastrocytoma of childhood: MR imaging and diffusion MR imaging features. *AJNR Am J Neuroradiol.* 2014;35(11):2192–2196.
3. Shaikh N, et al. Pleomorphic xanthoastrocytoma: a brief review. *CNS Oncol.* 2019;8(3):CNS39.
4. Perkins SM, et al. Patterns of care and outcomes of patients with pleomorphic xanthoastrocytoma: a SEER analysis. *J Neurooncol.* 2012;110(1):99–104.

CNS EMBRYONAL TUMOR

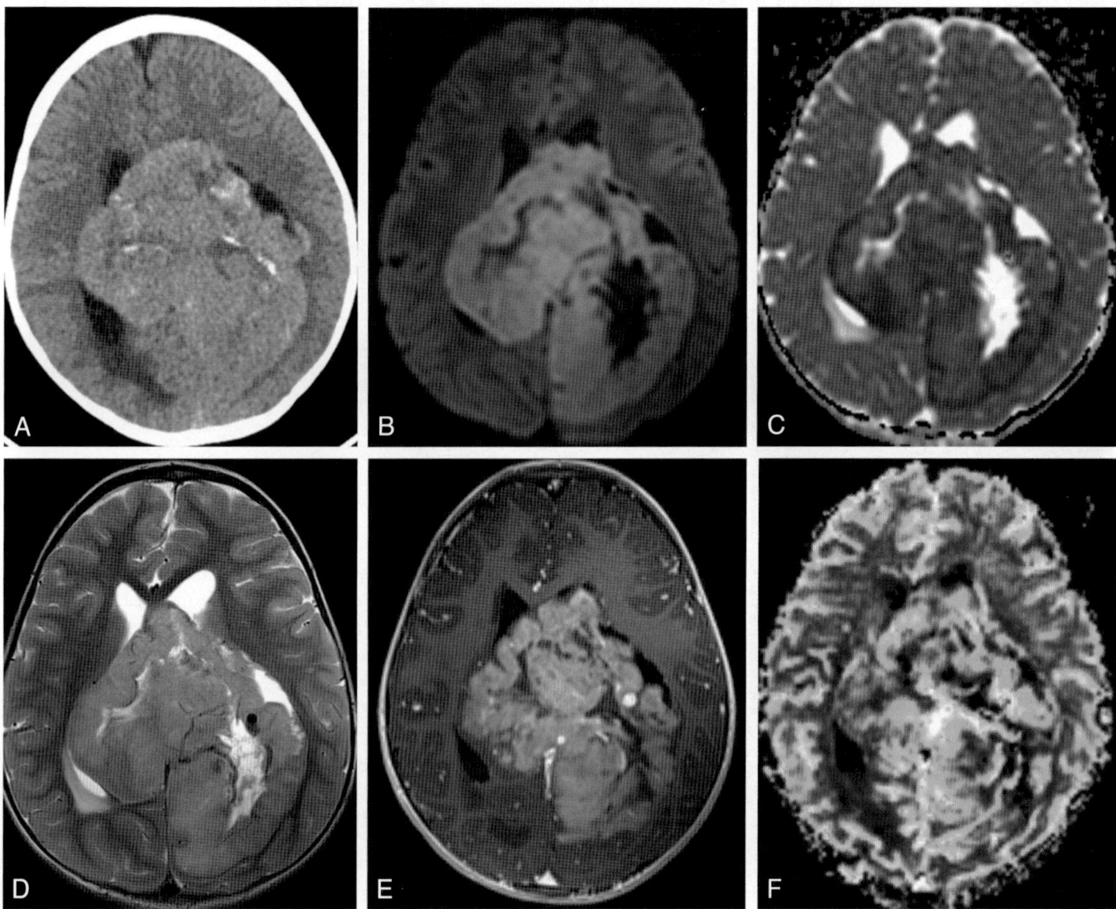

Fig. 7.41 CNS Embryonal Tumor. A 5-year-old with progressive loss of coordination, progressive dragging of the foot over 6 to 8 weeks. (A) Axial head CT image demonstrates a mildly hyperdense mass between the cerebral hemispheres and within the lateral ventricles with areas of internal hemorrhage. (B) Axial DWI, (C) axial ADC, (D) axial T2W, (E) axial T1W+C, and (F) axial rCBV map images demonstrate a mild T2W hyperintense mass with avid enhancement, reduced diffusion, and elevated rCBV, indicative of a high-grade tumor.

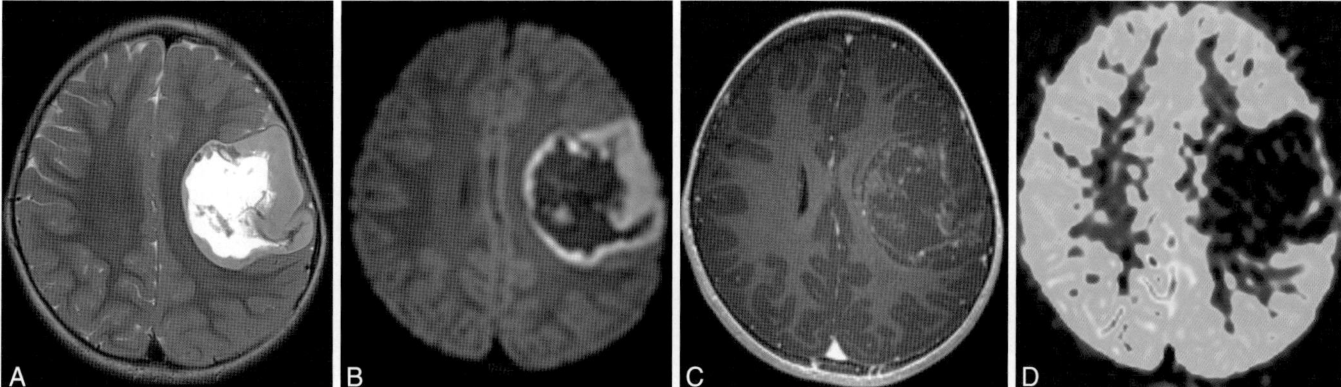

Fig. 7.42 CNS Embryonal tumor. A 2-year-old with acute left sided weakness with pathology proven CNS tumor with BCOR internal tandem duplication. (A) Axial T2W, (B) axial DWI, (C) axial T1W+C, and (D) axial ASL CBF map demonstrate a large left frontal intraparenchymal mass with central necrosis, minimal enhancement (majority of areas were from intrinsic T1W shortening), reduced diffusion (low ADC not shown), low CBF and relative lack of surrounding edema. The tumor extends to the surface but does not invade the dura.

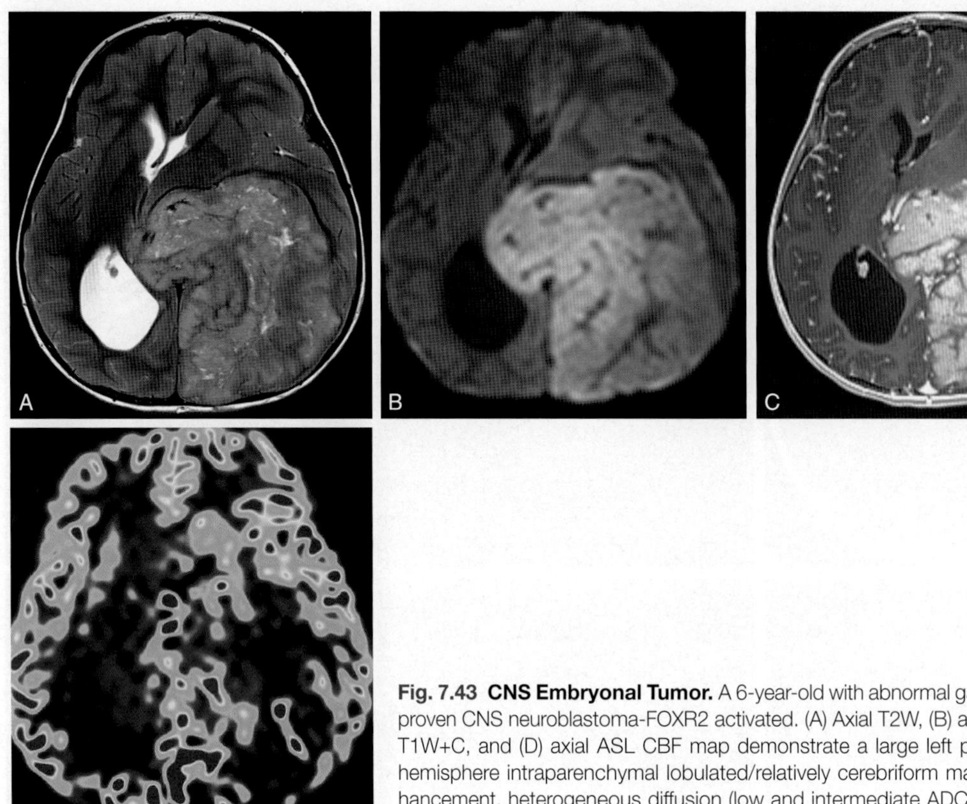

Fig. 7.43 CNS Embryonal Tumor. A 6-year-old with abnormal gait with pathology proven CNS neuroblastoma-FOXR2 activated. (A) Axial T2W, (B) axial DWI, (C) axial T1W+C, and (D) axial ASL CBF map demonstrate a large left posterior cerebral hemisphere intraparenchymal lobulated/relatively cerebriform mass with avid enhancement, heterogeneous diffusion (low and intermediate ADC not shown), low CBF and relative lack of surrounding edema.

Key Points

Background

- WHO grade 4
- Young children <5 years of age; rarely occurs in adults
- 15% of pediatric CNS tumors
- In the most recent revision of the WHO 2021 classification of CNS tumors, embryonal tumors include medulloblastomas and other CNS embryonal tumors. Among the other CNS embryonal tumors are ATRT, Cribriform neuroepithelial tumor, Embryonal tumor with multilayered rosettes (ETMR), CNS neuroblastoma FOXR2 activated, CNS tumor with BCOR internal tandem duplication, and CNS embryonal tumor.
- 5-year survival is approximately 40% to 60%
- Location: Cerebral hemispheres (most common), pineal gland, brainstem, and spinal cord

Imaging

CT

- *Hyperdense* mass resulting from hypercellularity; commonly contains cysts and calcifications; hemorrhage is uncommon

MRI

- As a group, CNS embryonal tumors a typically large heterogeneous solid or solid and cystic/necrotic mass at presentation, often with paucity of regional edema
- Well-circumscribed, heterogeneous mass, T1W hypo to isointense, T2W isointense to hypointense, typically with heterogeneous enhancement, and restricted diffusion
- More specific MRI features described with CNS Neuroblastoma-FOXR2 include large size, multilobulated, reduced diffusion, T2W hyperintensity, minimal to no edema, necrosis, hemorrhage, skull remodeling, and contact with the ventricle.
- More specific MRI features described with CNS neuroepithelial tumor with BCOR mutation include large size, well-circumscribed/sharp borders, minimal edema, necrosis and hemorrhage, calcification, reduced diffusion, low CBF, T2W hyperintensity, and dural contact without invasion.
- Metastatic at presentation is possible → total spine MRI performed at initial presentation to assess for drop metastases

Advanced Imaging

- MR perfusion: ↑ CBV and CBF
- MRS: ↑ *Elevated taurine*, choline, and lactate; ↓ NAA and creatine

REFERENCES

1. Zamora C, et al. Supratentorial Tumors in Pediatric Patients. *Neuroimaging Clin N Am.* 2017 Feb;27(1):39–67.
2. Jakacki RI, et al. Outcome and prognostic factors for children with supratentorial primitive neuroectodermal tumors treated with carboplatin during radiotherapy: a report from the Children's Oncology Group. *Pediatr Blood Cancer.* 2015;62(5):776–783.
3. Reddy AT, et al. Outcome for children with supratentorial primitive neuroectodermal tumors treated with surgery, radiation, and chemotherapy. *Cancer.* 2000;88(9):2189–2193.

GLIOBLASTOMA MULTIFORME

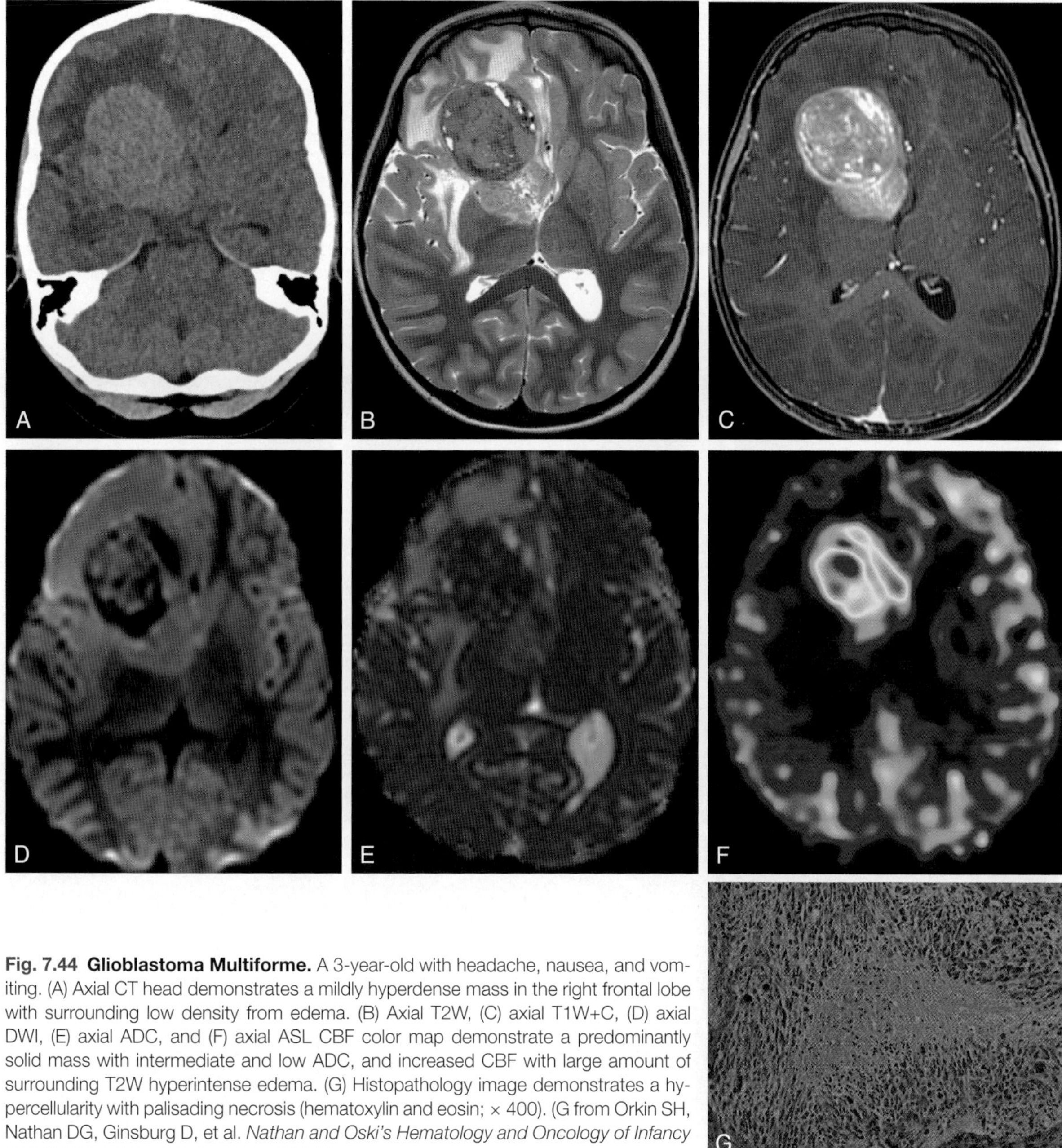

Fig. 7.44 Glioblastoma Multiforme. A 3-year-old with headache, nausea, and vomiting. (A) Axial CT head demonstrates a mildly hyperdense mass in the right frontal lobe with surrounding low density from edema. (B) Axial T2W, (C) axial T1W+C, (D) axial DWI, (E) axial ADC, and (F) axial ASL CBF color map demonstrate a predominantly solid mass with intermediate and low ADC, and increased CBF with large amount of surrounding T2W hyperintense edema. (G) Histopathology image demonstrates a hypercellularity with palisading necrosis (hematoxylin and eosin; × 400). (G from Orkin SH, Nathan DG, Ginsburg D, et al. *Nathan and Oski's Hematology and Oncology of Infancy and Childhood*. 8th ed. Saunders; 2009.)

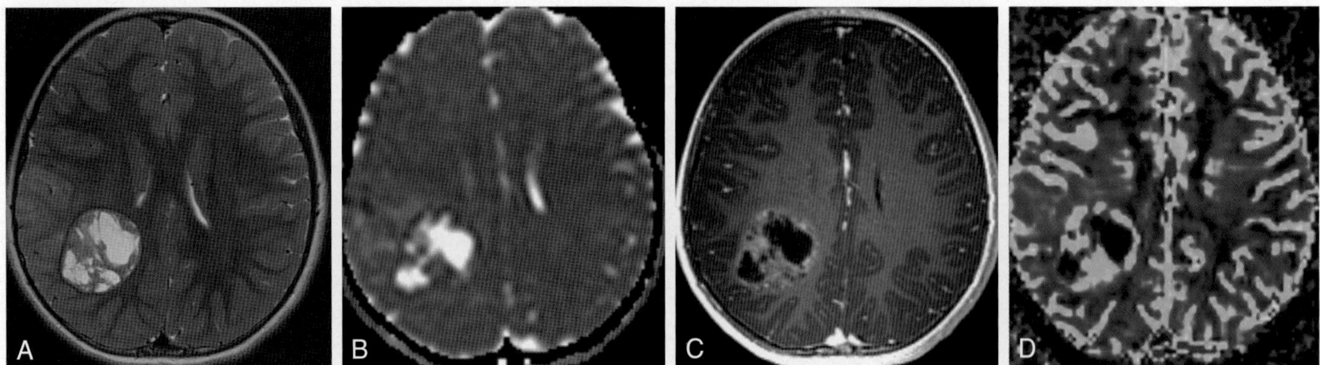

Fig. 7.45 Glioblastoma Multiforme. A 7-year-old with altered mental status, staring spells, headache, and vomiting. (A) Axial T2W, (B) axial ADC map, (C) axial T1W+C, and (D) axial CBV map demonstrate a circumscribed solid and cystic/necrotic right parietal mass with reduced diffusion and elevated rCBV, indicative of a high-grade tumor.

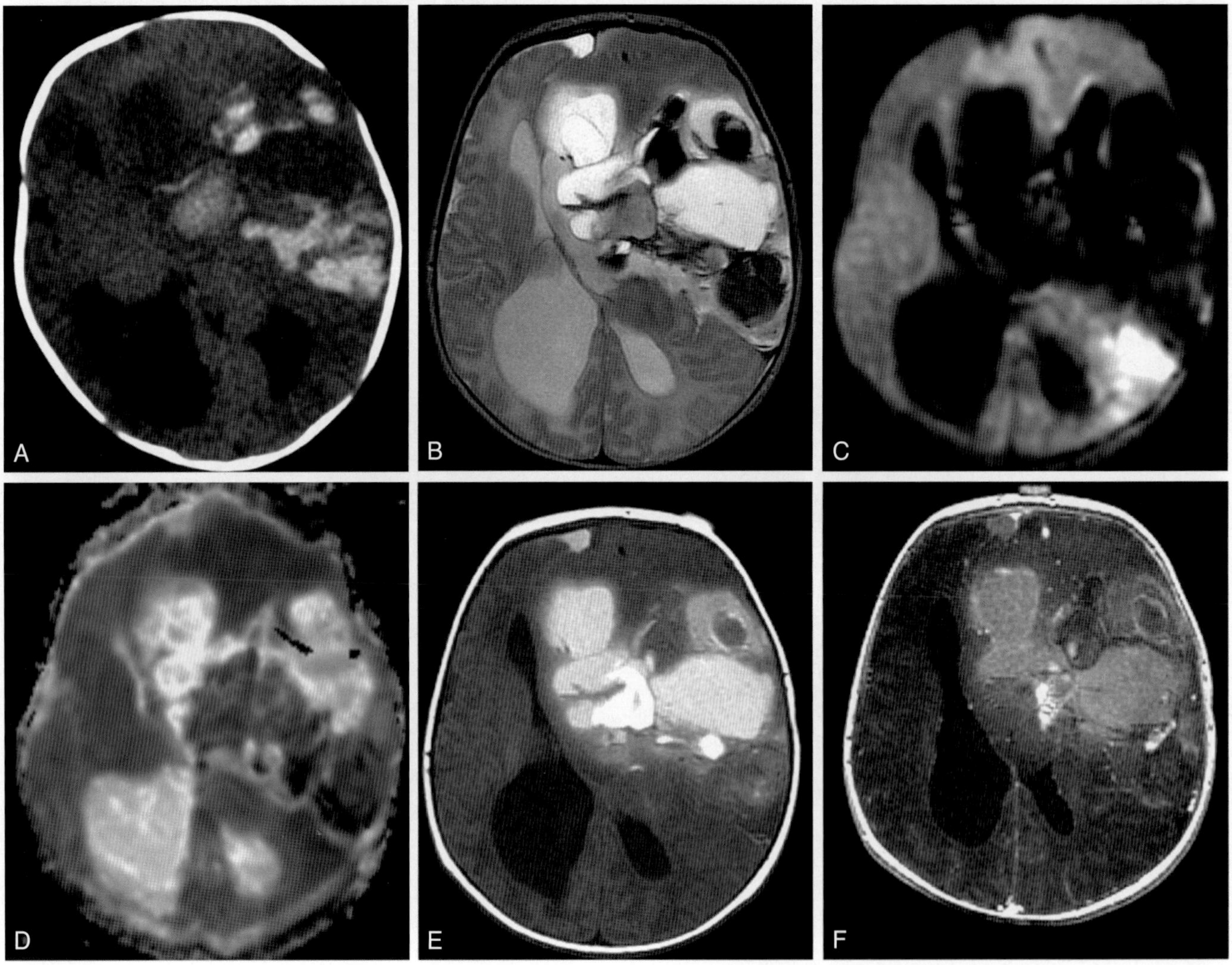

Fig. 7.46 Glioblastoma Multiforme. A 1-month-old with macrocephaly and vomiting. (A) Axial head CT, (B) axial T2W, (C) axial DWI, (D) axial ADC map, (E) axial T1W, and (F) axial T1W+C images demonstrate a large left frontal lobe mass with extensive areas of hemorrhage. Only small areas of enhancement are present because of the extensive hemorrhage. Nonhemorrhagic area at the anterior aspect has reduced ADC. High-grade gliomas are more likely to present with hemorrhage as seen here.

Key Points

Background

- WHO grade 4
- Accounts for less than 5% of pediatric CNS tumors
- Poor prognosis; 5-year survival is 40%, although improved survival compared to adults
- Pediatric glioblastoma multiformes (GBMs) typically are IDH wild type and have p53 mutations. Molecular differences of pediatric GBM compared to adult GBM include low VEGF expression, less EGFR amplification, and less PTEN alteration.
- Location: Cerebral hemispheres (most common) especially frontoparietal parenchyma; may occur in the central gray matter

Imaging

CT

- *Hyperdense* mass due to hypercellularity; may contain hemorrhage and calcifications

MRI

- Solid and cystic/*necrotic mass* at presentation, often with extensive regional T2W signal/edema
- Heterogeneous mass; T1W hypo to isointense, T2W isointense to hypointense, and typically with heterogeneous enhancement
- *Restricted diffusion*

Advanced Imaging

- MR Perfusion: ↑CBV, CBF, and permeability (K-trans)
- MRS: ↓NAA, ↑ choline, lactate, and lipids
- Metastatic at presentation is possible; total spine MRI performed at initial presentation to assess for drop metastases

REFERENCES

1. Zamora C, et al. Supratentorial Tumors in Pediatric Patients. *Neuroimaging Clin N Am.* 2017 Feb;27(1):39–67.
2. Song KS, et al. Long-term outcomes in children with glioblastoma. *J Neurosurg Pediatr.* 2010;6(2):145–149.

CONSTITUTIONAL MISMATCH REPAIR DEFICIENCY

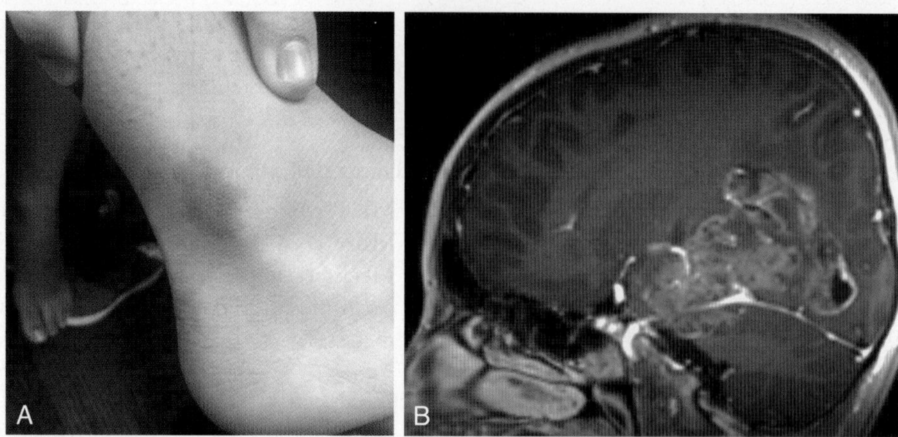

Fig. 7.47 **Constitutional Mismatch Repair Deficiency (CMMRD).** An 8-year-old with vomiting. (A) Café-au-lait spots on examination. (B) Sagittal T1W+C image demonstrates a temporal lobe enhancing mass. Pathology was a WHO grade 4 glioblastoma multiforme.

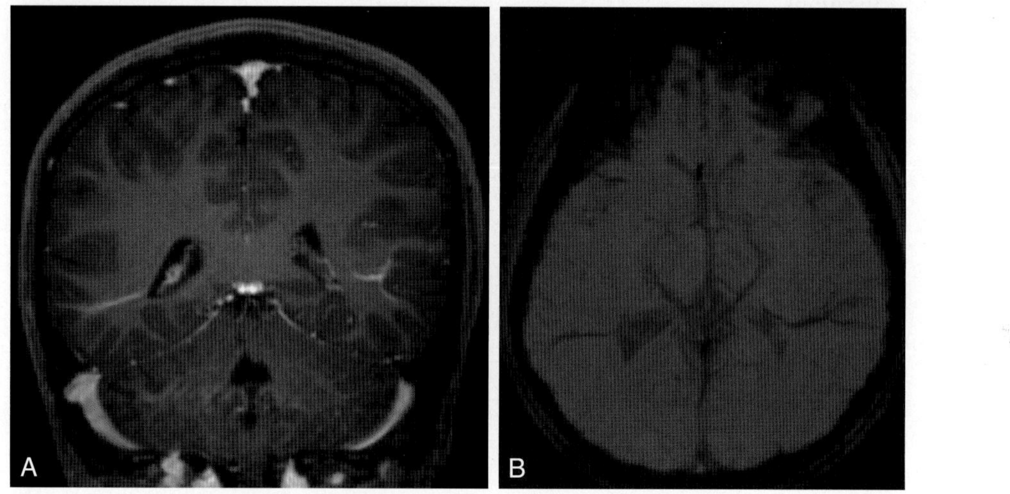

Fig. 7.48 **Constitutional Mismatch Repair Deficiency (CMMRD).** A 16-year-old asymptomatic patient with CMMRD with MRI for tumor surveillance. (A) Coronal T1W+C image and (B) axial SWI image demonstrate bilateral developmental venous anomalies.

Key Points

Background

- Constitutional mismatch repair deficiency (CMMRD) is an autosomal recessive childhood cancer predisposition syndrome characterized by brain, colorectal, and hematologic malignancies.
- The mismatch repair system normally corrects errors that occur during DNA replication.
- Heterozygous mutations in mismatch repair genes lead to Lynch syndrome. Bi-allelic mutations result in CMMRD and typically involve the *MSH6* or PMS2 mutations.
- Brain tumors consisting of gliomas; most commonly high-grade gliomas
- CMMRD should be considered in children with multiple malignancies, café-au-lait spots without NF-1, and family history of Lynch syndrome

Imaging

- Subcortical T2/FLAIR hyperintensities can transform into brain tumors and therefore must be followed routinely.
- DVAs and cavernomas are also more frequent than in normal population.

REFERENCE

1. Kerpel A, et al. Neuroimaging findings in constitutional mismatch repair deficiency syndrome. *AJNR Am J Neuroradiol.* 2020 May; 41(5):904–910.

SUPRATENTORIAL EPENDYMOMA

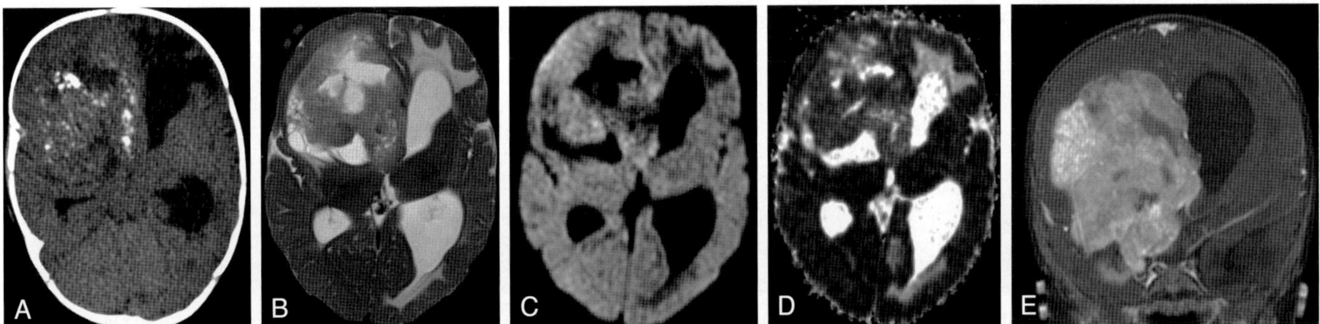

FIGURE 7.49 Supratentorial Ependymoma. A 5-month-old with rapid increase in head circumference. (A) Axial CT head, (B) Axial T2W, (C) axial DWI, (D) axial ADC, and (E) coronal T1W+C images demonstrate a large solid and cystic/necrotic right frontal lobe mass along the right lateral ventricle with low ADC. The findings support a high-grade tumor, but specific diagnosis is challenging. Supratentorial tumors are more common in the first year of life as seen here.

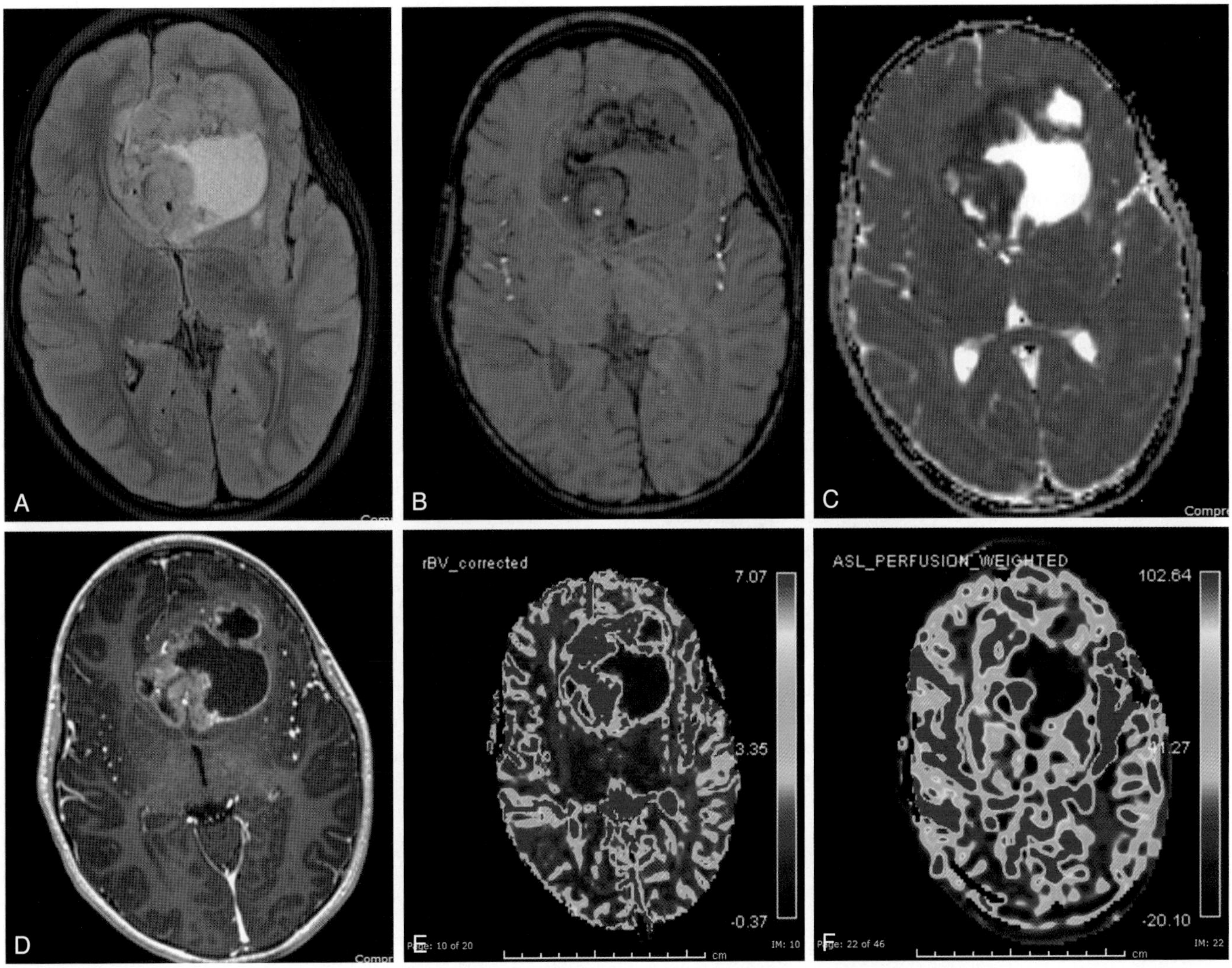

Fig. 7.50 Supratentorial Ependymoma. A 4-year-old with seizures. (A) Axial FLAIR, (B) axial SWI, (C) axial ADC, (D) axial T1W+C, (E) axial rCBV map from DSC perfusion, and (F) axial ASL CBF color map demonstrate a solid and cystic/necrotic left frontal lobe areas of hemorrhage, reduced diffusion, elevated rCBV, and elevated CBF, indicative of a high-grade tumor.

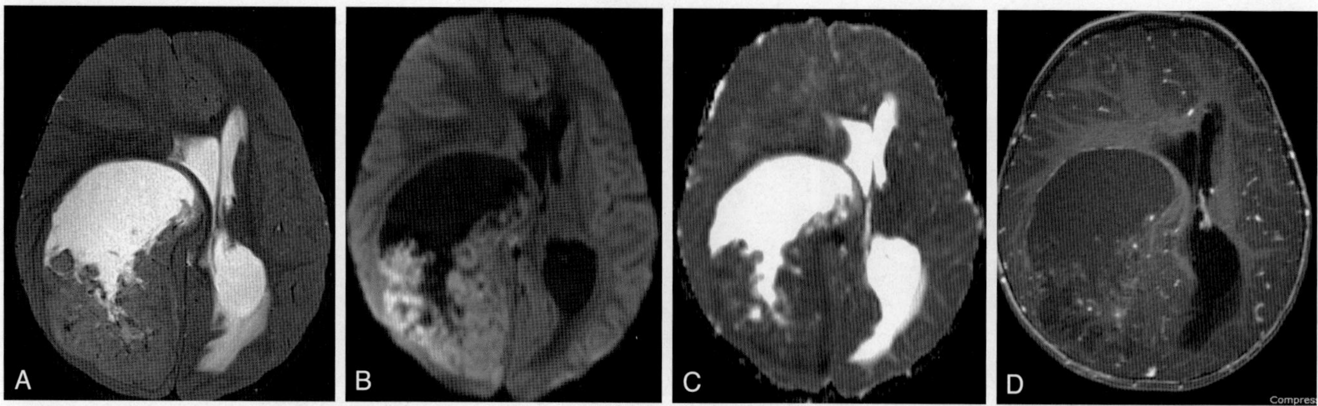

Fig. 7.51 Supratentorial Ependymoma. A 17-month-old with an anaplastic ependymoma. (A) Axial T2W, (B) axial DWI, (C) axial ADC, and (D) axial T1W+C images demonstrate a large solid and cystic/necrotic right parietal lobe mass along the right lateral ventricle with low ADC and associated midline shift, ventricular obstruction with transependymal edema.

Key Points

Background

- WHO grade 2 (differentiated) or 3 (anaplastic)
- Ependymomas account for 6% to 10% of pediatric CNS neoplasms (third most common); 30% to 40% are supratentorial
- Young patients, often less than 10 years of age; affects more M>F
- 5-year survival 70%–80%
- WHO 2021 classification includes molecular subcategories of ZFTA fusion and YAP1 fusion
- Arise from radial glial cells
- Location: Most commonly frontal and parietal

Imaging

CT

- Well-defined solid and cystic mass, solid components are isodense to hypodense, calcifications and hemorrhage are common

MRI

- Variable imaging appearance
  - Large solid and cystic/necrotic periventricular mass is the most common imaging appearance. Cysts may be large, and voluminous at presentation. Typically, significant peritumoral edema is present.
  - Cortical based lesions often smaller, entirely solid, or solid and cystic
  - Intraventricular
- Solid components are T1W hypo to isointense, T2W isointense to hypointense, and typically have heterogeneous enhancement. Restricted diffusion may be seen.
- Metastatic disease at presentation is possible → Total spine MRI performed at initial presentation to assess for drop metastases

Advanced Imaging

- MR perfusion: ↑ CBV and CBF
- MRS: ↓ NAA, Cr, and myoI; ↑ Choline in anaplastic ependymomas; ↑ myoI in differentiated ependymomas

REFERENCES

1. Zamora C, et al. Supratentorial Tumors in Pediatric Patients. *Neuroimaging Clin N Am*. 2017 Feb;27(1):39–67.
2. Lillard JC, et al. Pediatric Supratentorial Ependymoma: Surgical, Clinical, and Molecular Analysis. *Neurosurgery*. 2019;85(1):41–49.
3. Pajtler KW, et al. The current consensus on the clinical management of intracranial ependymoma and its distinct molecular variants. *Acta Neuropathol*. 2017;133(1):5–12.
4. Nowak J, et al. MRI Phenotype of RELA-fused Pediatric Supratentorial Ependymoma. *Clin Neuroradiol*. 2019;29(4):595–604.
5. Castillo M. Stem cells, radial glial cells, and a unified origin of brain tumors. *AJNR Am J Neuroradiol*. 2010;31(3):389–390.
6. Taylor MD, et al. Radial glial cells are candidate stem cells of ependymoma. *Cancer Cell*. 2005;8:323–335.

SUPRATENTORIAL ATYPICAL TERATOID RHABDOID TUMOR

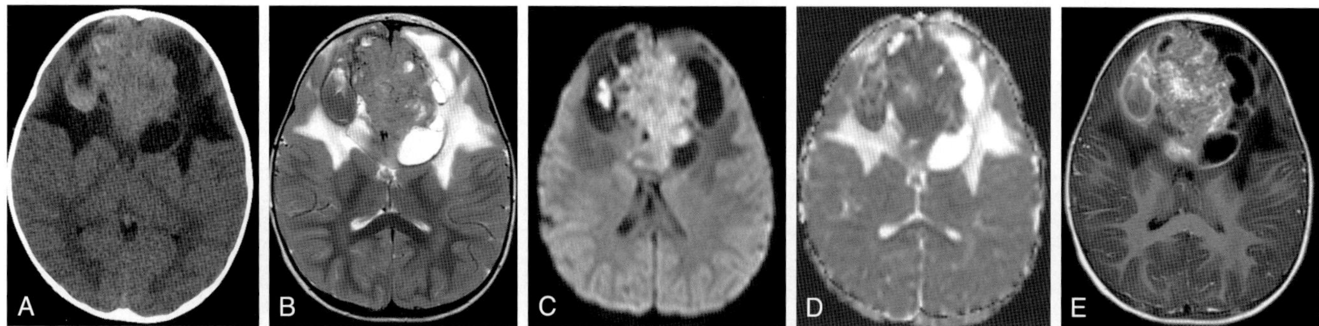

Fig. 7.52 Atypical Teratoid Rhabdoid Tumor (ATRT). A 2-year-old with ATRT. (A) Axial CT scan demonstrates a large bilateral frontal lobe hyperdense mass with large amount of surrounding edema. (B) Axial T2W, (C) axial DWI, (D) axial ADC map, and (E) axial T1W+C images demonstrate typical features of an ATRT with T2W isointensity, avid enhancement and reduced diffusion (low ADC).

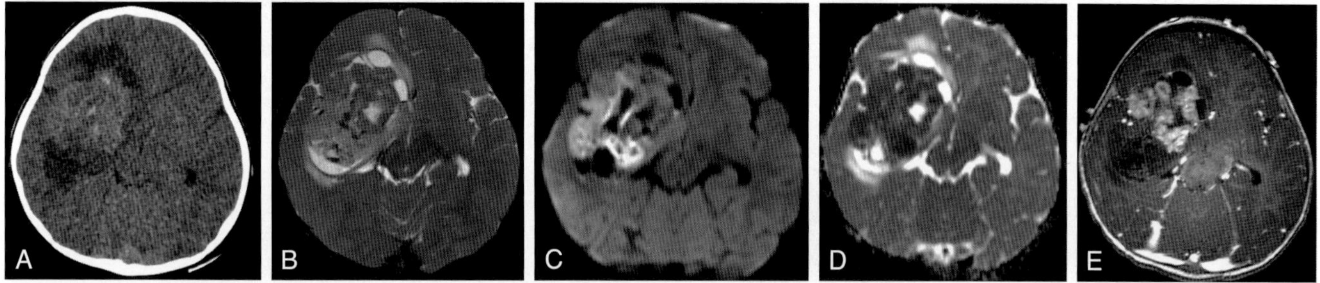

Fig. 7.53 Atypical Teratoid Rhabdoid Tumor (ATRT). An 11-month-old with ATRT. (A) Axial CT head demonstrates a large hyperdense right frontal lobe mass with surrounding edema. (B) Axial T2W, (C) axial DWI, (D) axial ADC map, and (E) axial T1W+C images demonstrate a large mass in the right frontal lobe, right insula, right basal ganglia, and right thalamus with T2W isointensity, reduced diffusion, and heterogeneous enhancement. The hyperdensity and reduced diffusion are typical for high-grade tumors, including ATRT.

Key Points

Background

- Supratentorial location is more common than infratentorial location in older children

Imaging

CT

- *Hyperdense* heterogeneous mass, small cysts, necrosis, hemorrhage and calcification may occur

MRI

- Well-circumscribed heterogeneous mass; T1W isointense, T2W isointense, variable enhancement, small cysts, necrosis, hemorrhage, and calcification
- *Restricted diffusion* similar to other embryonal tumors
- Metastasis common at presentation (>20%)

Advanced Imaging

- MR perfusion: ↑ CBF and CBV
- MRS: Aggressive metabolite pattern with ↑ choline, lipid and lactate ↓ NAA

REFERENCE

1. Meyers SP, et al. Primary Intracranial Atypical Teratoid/Rhabdoid Tumors of Infancy and Childhood: MRI Features and Patient Outcomes. *AJNR Am J Neuroradiol.* 2006 May;27(5):962–971.

SELLA AND SUPRASELLAR TUMORS

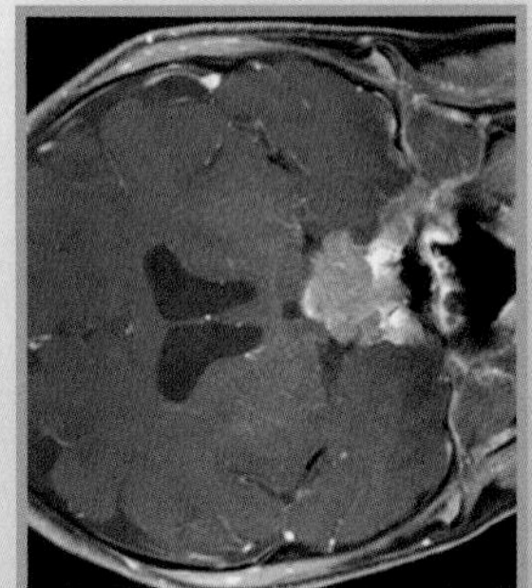

Pituitary Adenoma

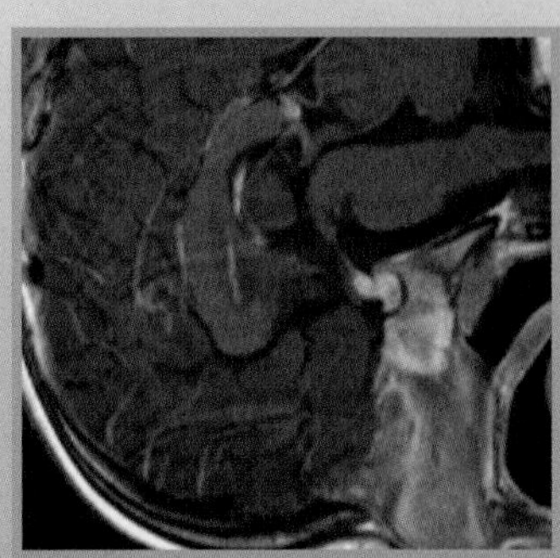

Langerhans Cell Histiocytosis

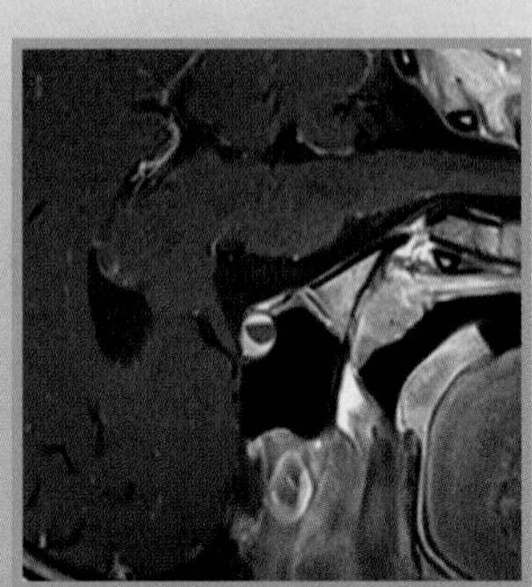

Nontumoral Masses:
Hypothalamic Hamartoma
Rathke Cleft cyst

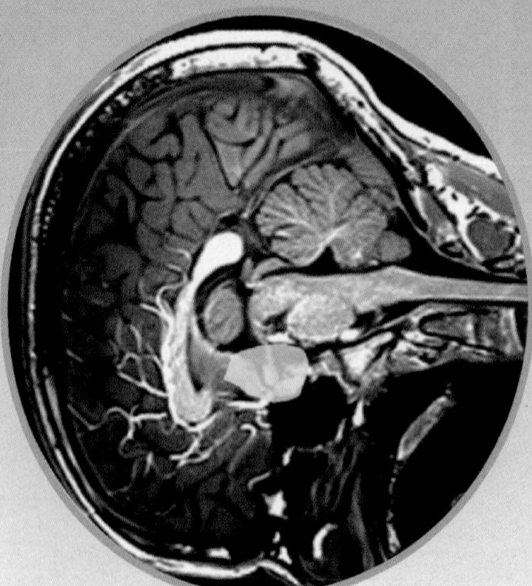

Key Imaging Features
- Location
- Calcification
- Solid versus Cystic

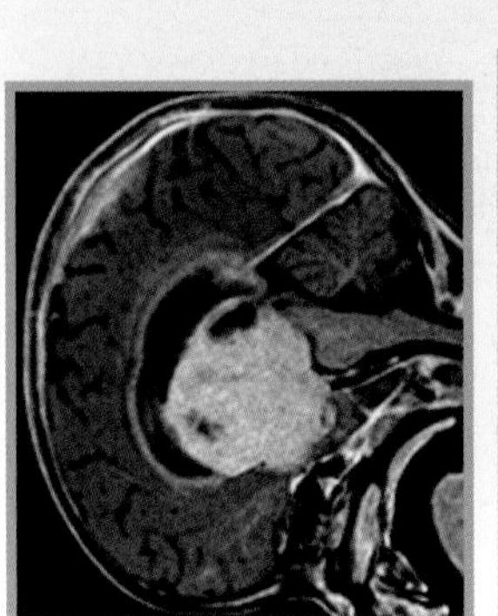

Chiasmatic/Hypothalamic Glioma

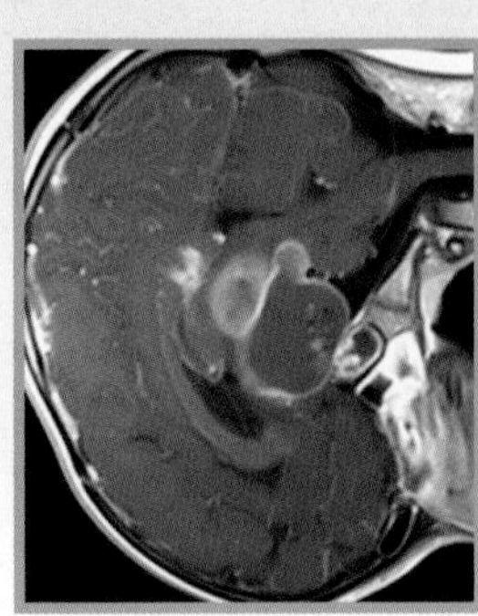

Craniopharyngioma

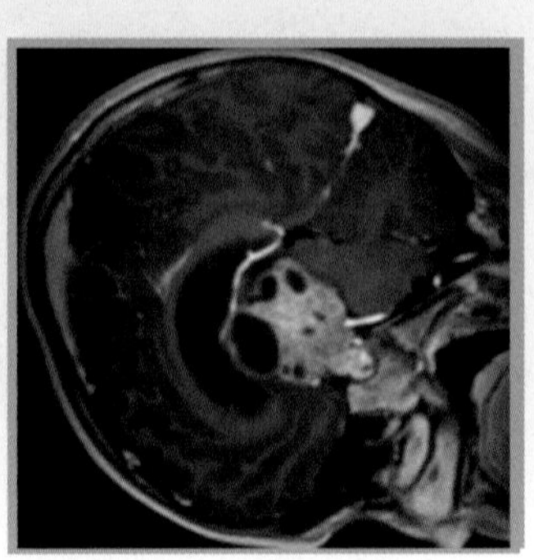

Germinoma

OPTIC NERVE GLIOMA, CHIASMATIC/HYPOTHALAMIC GLIOMA

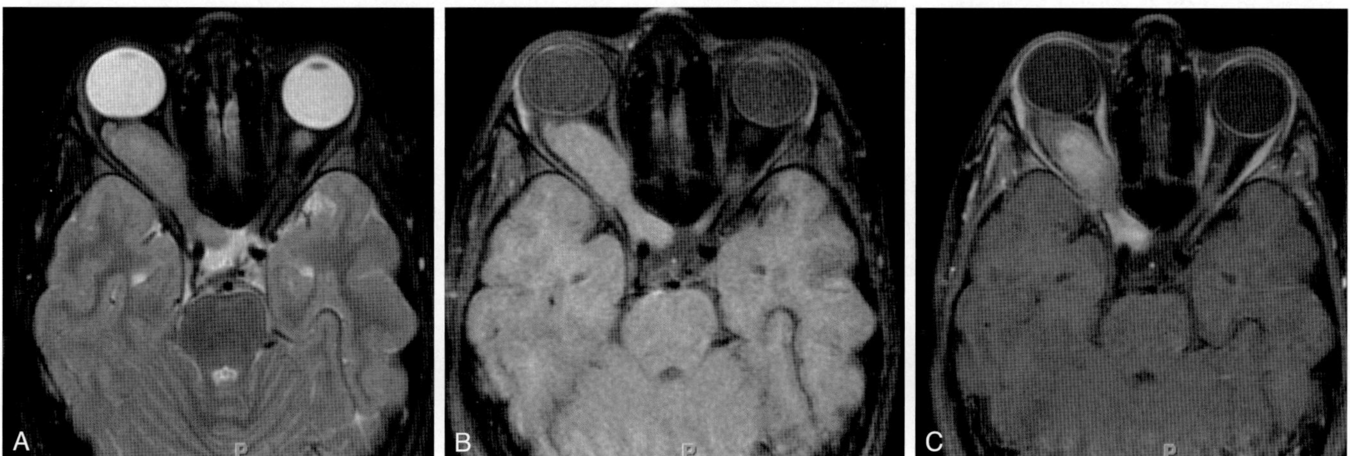

Fig. 7.54 Optic Nerve Glioma. (A) Axial T2W, (B) axial T1W fat saturation, and (C) axial T1W+C fat saturation images demonstrate fusiform enlargement and enhancement of the right optic nerve consistent with a typical optic nerve glioma. Optic pathway gliomas can demonstrate variable enhancement, particularly with NF-1.

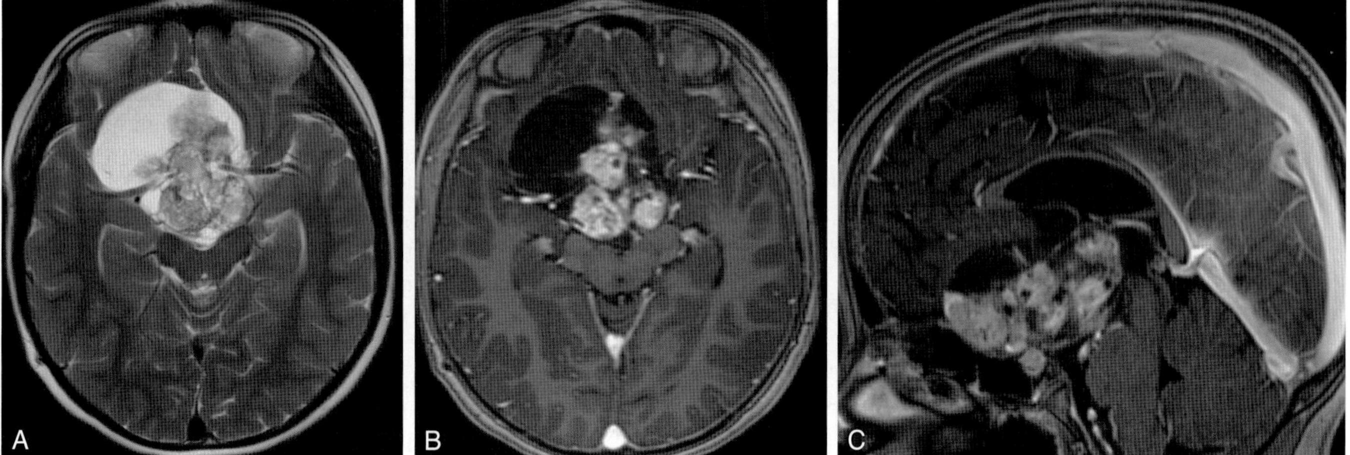

Fig. 7.55 Chiasmatic/Hypothalamic Glioma. A 7-year-old with headache and vision problems. (A) Axial T2W, and (B and C) axial and sagittal T1W+C images demonstrate a solid and cystic mass with nodular enhancement centered in the optic chiasm and hypothalamus with anterior extension along the anterior cranial fossa displacing the medial frontal lobes, and posterior extension causing mass effect on the midbrain.

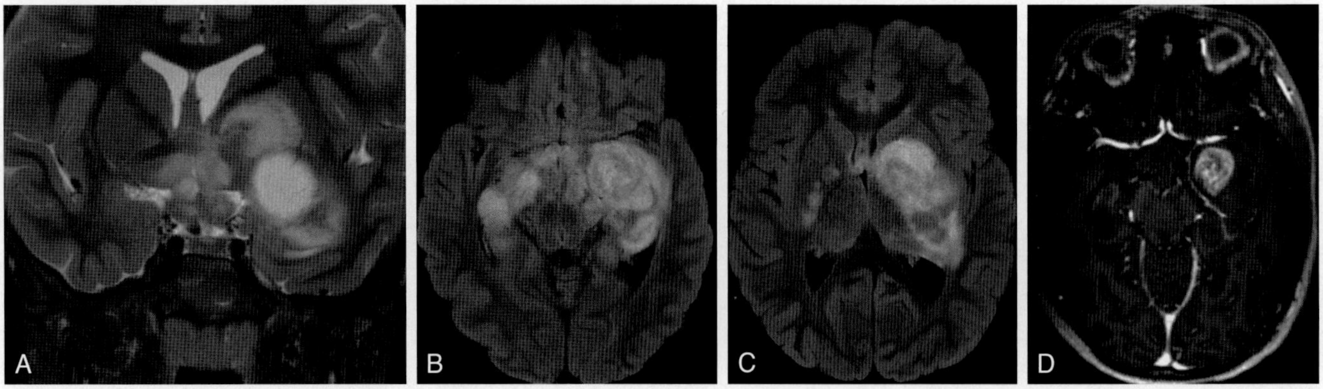

Fig. 7.56 Chiasmatic/Hypothalamic Glioma. A 7-year-old with NF-1. (A) Coronal T2W, (B and C) axial FLAIR, and (D) axial T1W+C images demonstrate an expansile infiltrative optic pathway glioma involving the optic chiasm, optic tracts, internal capsules, basal ganglia, midbrain, left thalamus, and left temporal lobe. Only the left temporal portion demonstrates enhancement, which is typical for these tumors to partially enhance.

Key Points

Background

- WHO grade 1 (pilocytic astrocytoma); malignant (WHO grade 4) optic gliomas may occur in adults
- 70% diagnosed in the first decade; 90% by the second decade
- Majority of patients with optic pathway glioma (OPG), and chiasmatic/hypothalamic glioma have NF-1; up to 20% of NF-1 patients will have OPG
- Bilateral OPG is nearly diagnostic of NF-1
- Common symptoms are *vision loss* and *diencephalic syndrome*
- NF-1–associated OPG is often asymptomatic and without vision loss
- Non-NF-1 OPG (sporadic OPG) is generally more clinically aggressive with up to ~75% experiencing vision loss and ~75% experiencing disease progression
- Imaging screening remains controversial; ophthalmologic screening is, however, widely accepted
- Location: Optic pathway includeing the optic nerve(s), chiasm, tracts and radiations; hypothalamus, basal ganglia, internal capsule, thalamic, and brainstem

Imaging

CT

- Isodense or hypodense optic pathway mass; optic canal remodeling may occur

MRI

- Optic nerve tumors demonstrate fusiform expansion with T2W isointense or hyperintense signal and variable enhancement. Rare pattern of perineural extension into the nerve sheath can be seen as enhancement in the nerve sheath with central expanded nonenhancing optic nerve.
- Chiasmatic/hypothalamic gliomas demonstrate T2W hyperintensity with variable enhancement and variable infiltration of the optic radiations, basal ganglia, thalamus, and internal capsule. Bulky solid and cystic components centered at the chiasm-hypothalamus may occur especially in children without NF-1.
- Enhancement pattern can change on follow-up MRIs and does not indicate regression or progression of the tumor in the absence of a size change. Recent research has also shown that contrast may not be needed to assess tumor size on follow-up MRIs.
- Tumors can have isointense and hyperintense ADC signal
- Pituitary remains visible
- Metastasis are rare but possible

REFERENCES

1. Rasool N, et al. Optic pathway glioma of childhood. *Curr Opin Ophthalmol.* 2017 May;28(3):289–295.
2. Aihara Y, et al. Pediatric Optic Pathway/Hypothalmic Glioma. *Neurol Med Chir (Tokyo).* 2018 Jan 15;58(1):1–9.
3. Campen CJ, et al. Optic Pathway Gliomas in Neurofibromatosis Type 1. *J Child Neurol.* 2018 Jan;33(1):73–81.
4. Fried I, et al. Optic pathway gliomas: a review. *CNS Oncol.* 2013;2(2):143–159.
5. Wan MJ, et al. Long-term visual outcomes of optic pathway gliomas in pediatric patients without neurofibromatosis type 1. *J Neurooncol.* 2016;129:173–178.

CRANIOPHARYNGIOMA

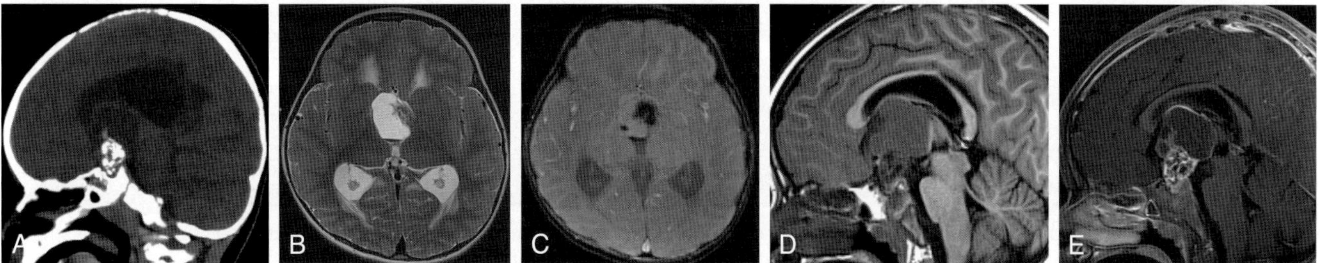

Fig. 7.57 Craniopharyngioma. A 2-year-old with headache, vomiting, and ataxia. (A) Sagittal noncontrast CT, (B) axial T2W, (C) axial SWI, (D) sagittal T1W, and (E) sagittal T1W+C images demonstrate a sellar and suprasellar predominantly cystic and partially calcified mass with thin areas of enhancement.

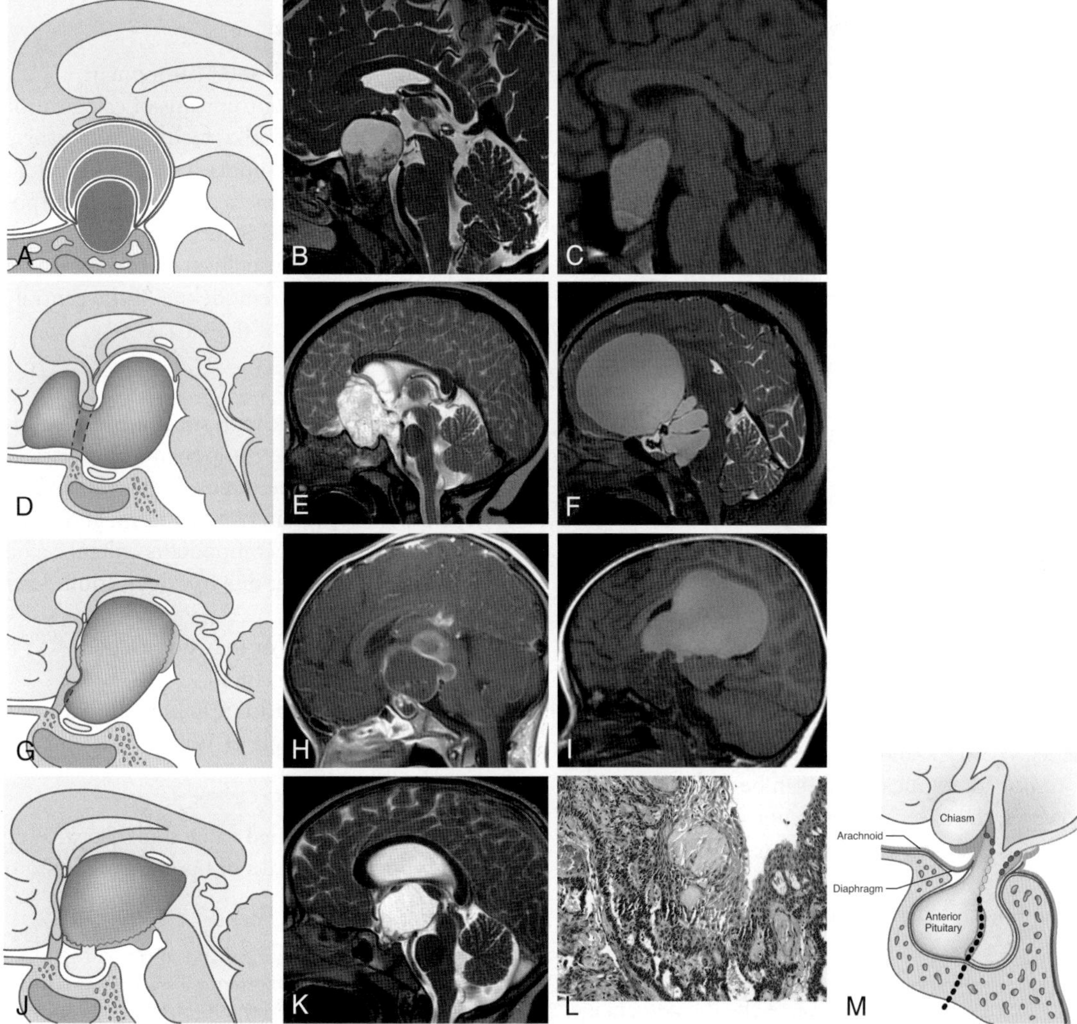

Fig. 7.58 Craniopharyngioma: Origins, Common Locations, and Growth Patterns. (A to C) Infradiaphragmatic craniopharyngioma: tumor centered in an expanded sella; possible inferior extension into the sphenoid or clivus; rounded/oval morphology; superior displacement of the anterior commissure, optic chiasm and anterior communicating artery; mammillary body displaced posteriorly and superiorly. (D to F) Supradiaphragmatic extraventricular: originate in the suprasellar cistern and may extend along anterior cranial fossa; pituitary gland often visible but can extend into the sella; posterior superior displacement of the optic chiasm and anterior communicating artery; no extension into the third ventricle but can displace the third ventricle posteriorly; multilobular morphology. (G to I) Extraventricular and intraventricular: tumor involves suprasellar cistern and third ventricle; optic chiasm and anterior communicating artery displaced superiorly; anterior commissure displaced superiorly; mammillary body displaced posteriorly and inferiorly; and multilobular morphology. (J and K) Intraventricular: centered in the third ventricle; optic chiasm and anterior communicating artery displaced anteriorly; massa intermedia displaced posteriorly; possible retroclival extension; mammillary body displaced posteriorly and inferiorly. (L) Histopathology section shows adamantinomatous squamous epithelium exhibiting keratinization and typical peripherally palisading nuclei. (M) Origins of craniopharyngiomas. Infradiaphragmatic craniopharyngiomas found along the location indicated by a black dotted line, supradiaphragmatic extraventricular arise along the green dotted lines, and the remaining arise from locations with the red dotted lines. (L from Reddy VB, David O, Spitz DJ, et al. *Gattuso's Differential Diagnosis in Surgical Pathology.* 4th ed. Elsevier; 2022.).

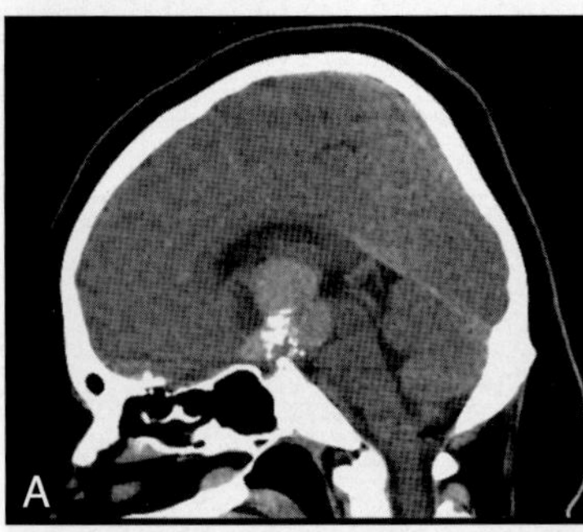
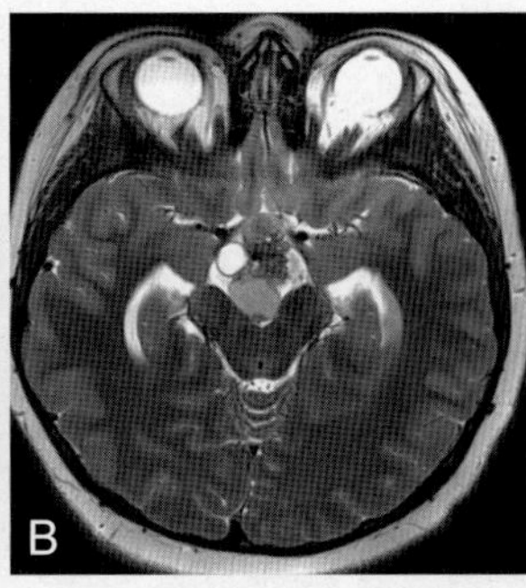
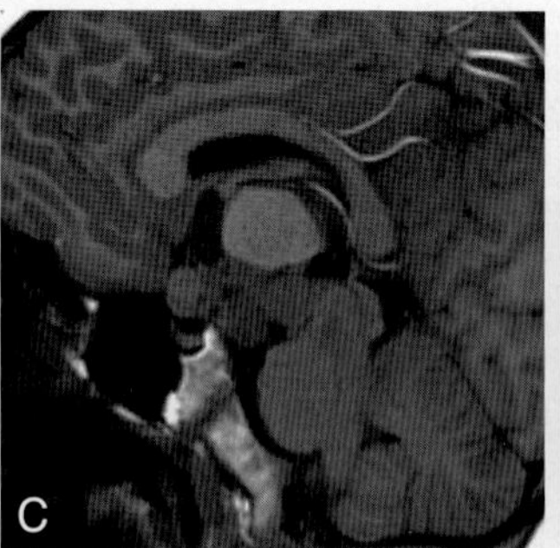
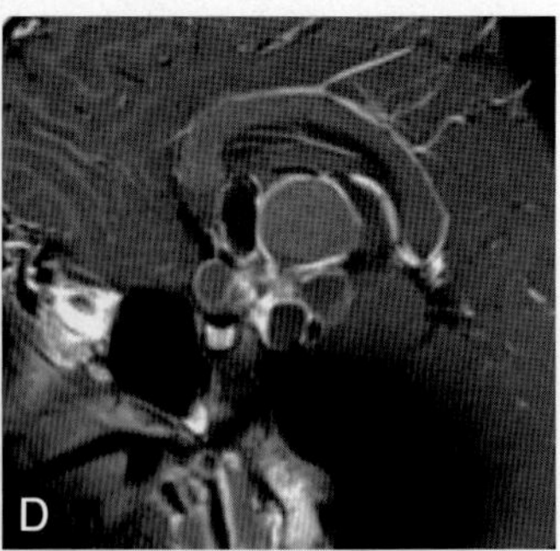

Fig. 7.59 Craniopharyngioma. A 13-year-old with new-onset exotropia and diplopia. (A) Sagittal CT head reformat image demonstrates coarse calcifications and hyperdense proteinaceous cysts in a mass involving the sella and suprasellar cistern. (B) Axial T2W, (C) sagittal T1W, and (D) sagittal T1W+C images demonstrate a multicystic sellar and suprasellar cystic mass with T1 hyperintense cystic fluid from proteinaceous content.

Key Points

Background

- WHO grade 1 histology
- Arise from squamous epithelial, remnants of the Rathke pouch
- Pathologically categorized as adamantinomatous and papillary
    - Adamantinous: bimodal age (5–15 and 45–60 years); CTNNB1 mutations; 90% cystic and contain Ca^{2+}
    - Papillary: 40 to 55 years; BRAF V600E mutations; less commonly cystic or Ca^{2+}
- Account for 50% of suprasellar tumors in children
- Majority diagnosed in the second decade of life
- Presenting symptoms include visual symptoms (60%–80%), *endocrinologic (80%–90%; short stature, delayed puberty, diabetes insipidus)*, headache (50%–70%), and weight gain (10%)
- Location: 90% suprasellar
- Surgically classified as intrasellar, prechiasmatic (anterior to chiasm), and retrochiasmatic (posterior to chiasm)
- Appearance and growth pattern can also be classified as infradiaphragmatic (Inf), supradiaphragmatic extraventricular (S-EV), extraventricular and intraventricular (EV-IV), and intraventricular (IV)
- With large tumors the optic chiasm can be difficult to identify; however, the anterior communicating artery position, which is easier to identify, is a good marker for location of the chiasm
- May encase anterior circulation but does not invade cavernous sinus
- Location affects symptoms and surgical outcome. For Inf, EV, and EV-IV or IV locations, respectively, the percentage of patients with vision changes (89%, 76%, 46%), pituitary dysfunction (87%, 76%, 84%), diabetes insipidus (42%, 13%, 13%), hydrocephalus (8%, 13%, 65%), gross total resection (82%, 96%, 67%), and progression-free 5-year survival (85%, 86%, 63%)
- 10-year survival is >90%, however there is high morbidity (visual and endocrinologic dysfunction) and high recurrence rate. Size and surgical expertise are important factors that affect outcome.

Imaging

CT

- *90% cystic* with small solid component
- *>90% calcified*, either thin rims of calcification or nodular, sometimes bulky foci. CT may play a differential diagnostic role for a suprasellar mass for calcification detection. For the same reason, immediate postoperative CT may be helpful to identify residual calcification/tumor.
- Cystic components usually are hypodense
- CT often will show remodeling of the central skull base, including widening of the sella

MRI

- Predominantly cystic with small areas of solid enhancement. Cystic components have variable signal (hypointense to hyperintense) on T1W and T2W depending on protein concentration and thin wall enhancement. Solid components enhance avidly.
- Susceptibility artifact due to calcification. Lack of restricted diffusion.
- Pituitary gland may or may not visible
- Metastases do not occur
- Higher risk for radiation vasculopathy as a result of location near the circle of Willis

Advanced Imaging

- MR perfusion: Limited value due to cystic appearance
- MRS: Dominant peaks of lipid and cholesterol

REFERENCES

1. Plaza MJ, et al. Conventional and advanced MRI features of pediatric intracranial tumors: posterior fossa and suprasellar tumors. *AJR Am J Roentgenol.* 2013 May;200(5):1115–1124.
2. Mortini P, et al. Neurosurgical treatment of craniopharyngioma in adults and children: early and long-term results in a large case series. *J. Neurosurg..* 2011;114:1350–1359.
3. Müller HL. Craniopharyngioma. *Endocr Rev.* 2014 Jun;35(3):513–543.

GERMINOMA

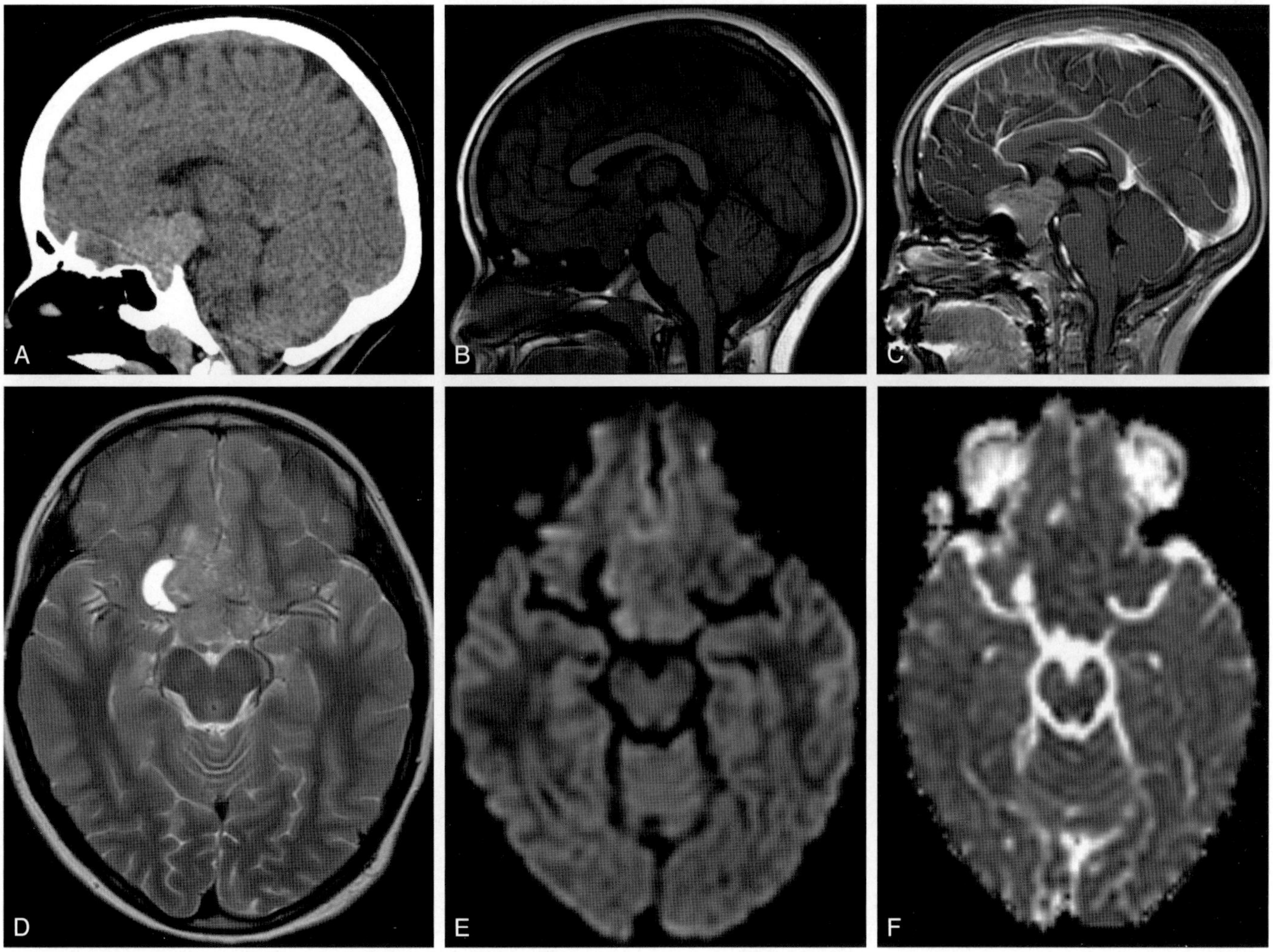

Fig. 7.60 Germinoma. A 10-year-old with bilateral vision loss and afferent pupillary defect. (A) Sagittal reformat head CT demonstrates a solid hyperdense sellar and suprasellar mass. (B) Sagittal T1W, (C) sagittal T1W+C, (D) axial T2W, (E) axial DWI, and (F) axial ADC images demonstrate and solid homogeneously enhancing mass with small right lateral cyst with relative reduced diffusion in the sella and suprasellar cistern.

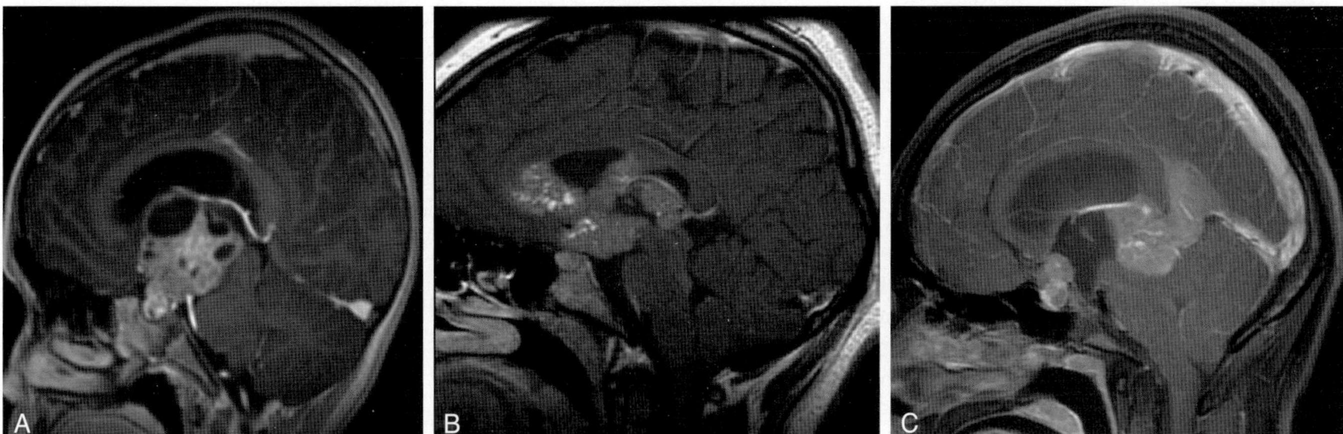

Fig. 7.61 Germinoma: Additional Imaging Patterns in Three Patients. Sagittal T1W+C images in three patients. (A) A solid and cystic sellar and suprasellar germinoma. (B) A suprasellar, pineal, and intraventricular germinoma. (C) A sellar, suprasellar, and pineal germinoma with occluded vein of Galen and proximal straight sinus.

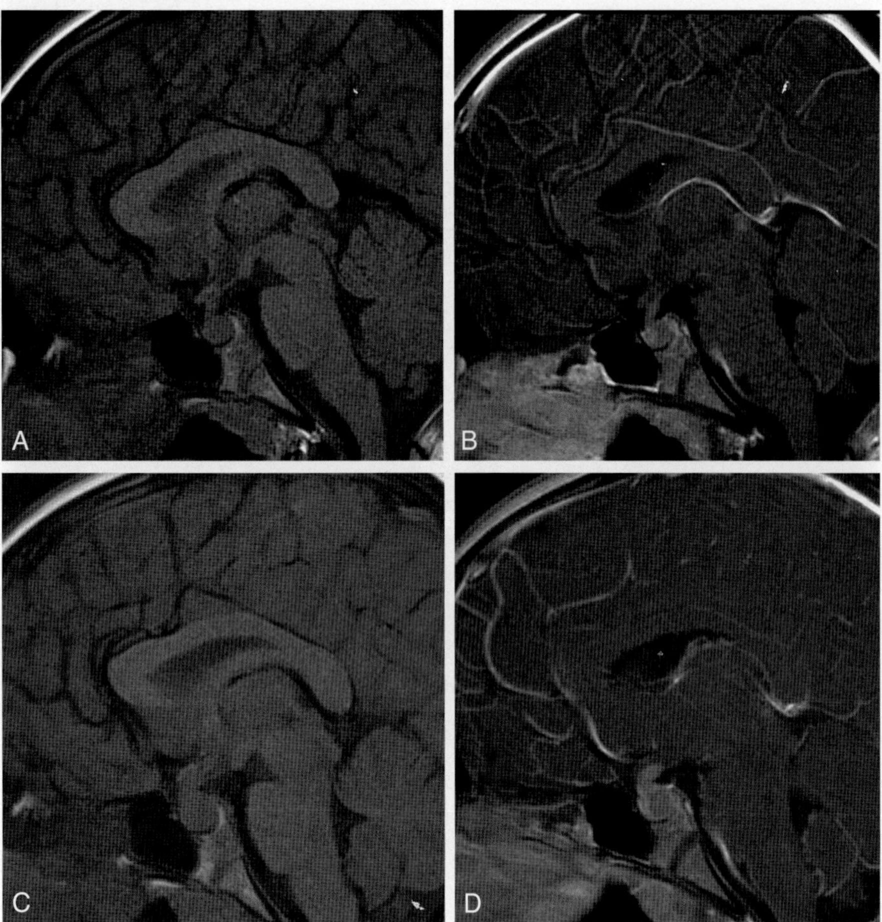

Fig. 7.62 Germinoma: Challenging Presentation. A 10-year-old with urinary frequency, polydipsia, and new diagnosis of diabetes insipidus. Initial MRI (A and B) sagittal T1W and T1W+C images demonstrate loss of the normal posterior pituitary T1W bright spot and vague hypoenhancing nodule in the posterior pituitary gland. A 3-month follow-up MRI (C and D) sagittal T1W and T1W+C images demonstrate enlarging intrasellar nodule and new thickening of the pituitary infundibulum. Differential diagnosis was LCH, germinoma, and lymphocytic hypophysitis. Biopsy pathology was a germinoma.

Key Points

Background

- WHO grade 2. Germ cell tumors (GCTs) are subdivided into germinomas and nongerminomatous germ cell tumors (NGCTs). Germinomas account for two-thirds of intracranial GCTs
- Age <20–30; peak 10 to 12 years with 90% diagnosed by end of second decade; more common in Asians
- All CNS germinomas M:F ratio 1.5-2:1
  - Pineal region germinomas M:F ratio 10:1
  - Suprasellar germinomas F>M
- Increased risk in Klinefelter, Noonan, and Down syndrome
- Presenting symptoms related to location (headache, vision loss, diabetes insipidus)
- *Excellent prognosis*; 5-year survival > 85%; *highly responsive to chemoradiation*
- Location: Predominantly midline; suprasellar or infundibular (49%), pineal (37%), and basal ganglia locations are the three most common locations for germinomas. Because basal ganglia location is rare for CNS tumors, a germinoma should be highly considered in the setting of a mass in the basal ganglia.
- Multifocal and dissemination at presentation is possible

Imaging

CT

- Isodense to *hyperdense* mass; may have engulfed *central calcification* in the pineal region

MRI

- Well-circumscribed, T1W hypointense to isointense, T2W isointense to hypointense, and *homogenously enhancing*
- *Restricted diffusion*
- Classically infiltrates the infundibulum
- Pineal region often presents with obstruction at level of cerebral aqueduct
- Edema in the adjacent brain parenchyma (often thalami)
- Metastatic or multifocal (suprasellar, pineal, basal ganglia) at presentation is possible → Total spine MRI performed at initial presentation to assess for drop metastases

Advanced Imaging

- MR Perfusion: limited data
- MRS: limited data

REFERENCES

1. Osorio DS, et al. Management of CNS germinoma. *CNS Oncol.* 2015;4(4):273–279.
2. Borja MJ, et al. Conventional and advanced MRI features of pediatric intracranial tumors: supratentorial tumors. *AJR Am J Roentgenol.* 2013 May;200(5):W483–W503.

PITUITARY ADENOMA

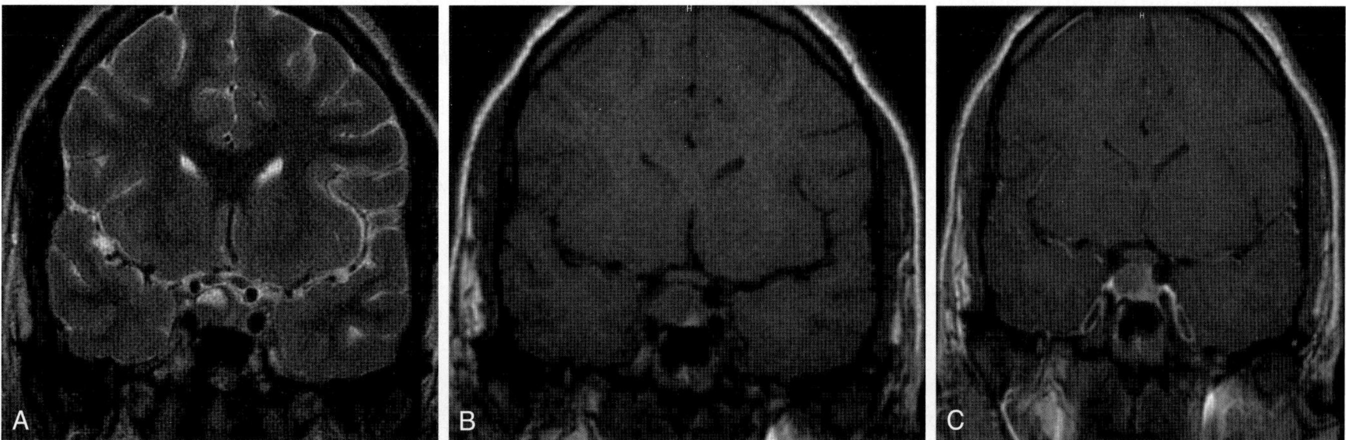

Fig. 7.63 Pituitary Adenoma. An 11-year-old with Cushing's syndrome. (A) Coronal T2W, (B and C) coronal T1W and T1W+C images demonstrate a hypoenhancing right sellar mass measuring less than 1 cm. Pathology was consistent with a microadenoma.

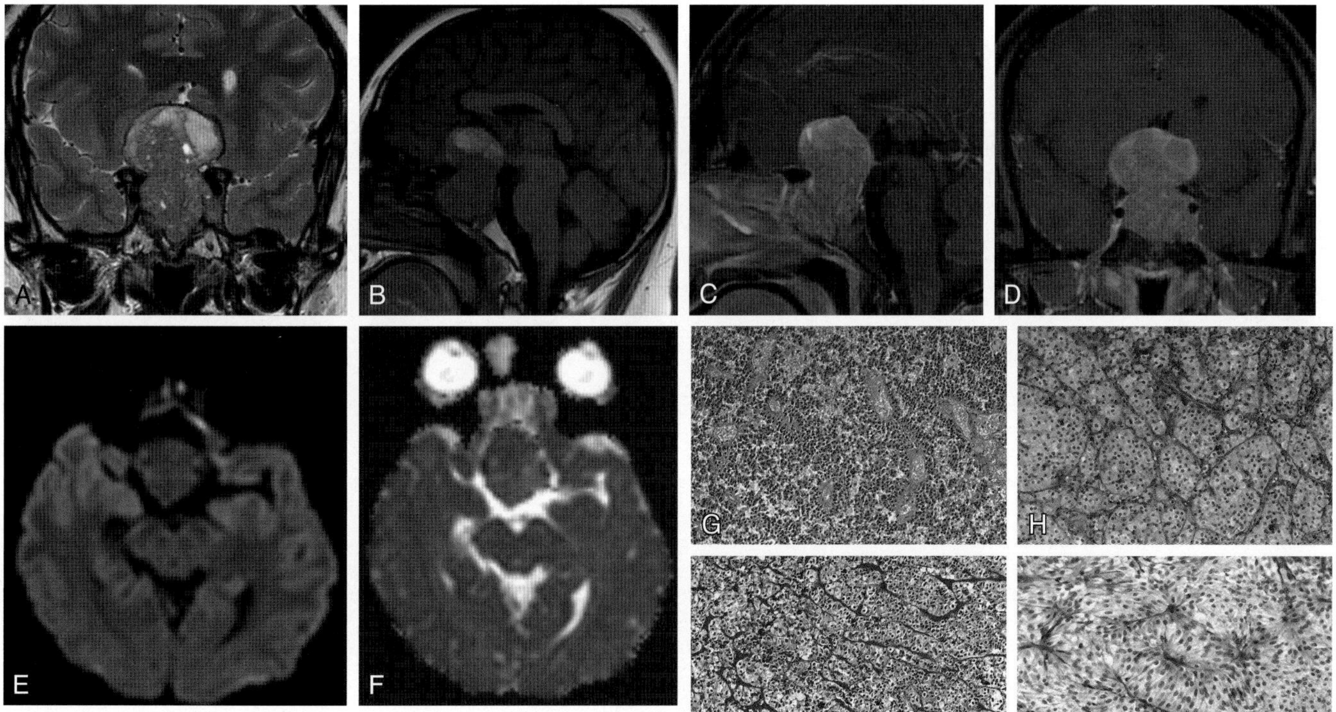

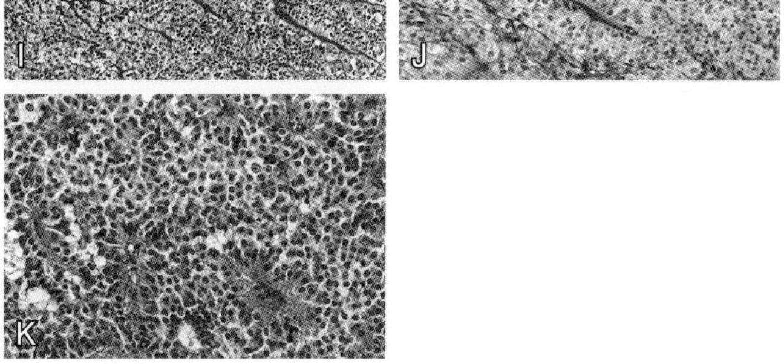

Fig. 7.64 Pituitary Macroadenoma. A 17-year-old with vision loss. (A) Coronal T2W, (B) sagittal T1W, (C and D) sagittal and coronal T1W+C, (E) axial DWI, and (F) axial ADC map images demonstrate a sellar and suprasellar mass with predominantly T2W isointensity, ADC isointensity, solid homogeneous enhancement with exception of areas of hemorrhagic fluid at the superior margin, remodeled and expanded sella, invasion of the central skull base, and invasion of the left cavernous sinus. Optic pathway is not clearly seen but likely stretched by the mass accounting for the vision loss. Serum prolactin was >650 ng/mL and pathology confirmed a prolactinoma. (G to K) Pituitary adenomas may display multiple histologic patterns of growth. (G) Papillary pattern. (H) Alveolar pattern. (I) Trabecular pattern. (J) Spindle cell pattern. (K) High magnification of papillary pattern of pituitary adenoma. (G to K from Fletcher CDM. *Diagnostic Histopathology of Tumors*. Elsevier; 2021.)

Key Points

Background

- Rare neoplasm in pediatric patients of all ages; frequency increases in adolescents and teenagers
- Modifications in oncogenes/tumor suppressor genes common, including *GNAS* (40% of GH secreting adenomas), PTTG, HMGA2, and FGFR4
- Increased risk of pituitary adenomas in MEN1, familial isolated pituitary adenomas, McCune-Albright syndrome and Carney complex
- Presentation is variable and depends on the hormonal imbalance. Nonfunctioning adenomas may present with hormonal deficiency, most commonly growth hormone (GH) deficiency followed by LH/FSH and then ACTH or TSH. Common symptoms include headache, vision disturbance, and cranial nerve palsies with cavernous sinus invasion
- Nonfunctioning adenomas are rare in children; more common in adults. Prolactinomas most common in older children, primarily females, whereas corticotropinomas (ACTH producing) most common in prepubescent patients
- Dopamine agonists are first-line therapy for prolactinoma; surgery is first-line therapy for corticotropinomas; combination pharmacologic and surgery often employed for somatotropinomas
- Location: Sella/suprasellar with or without cavernous sinus invasion; may be locally aggressive with central skull base invasion, or third ventricle extension

Imaging

CT

- Normal appearance with microadenomas. Remodeled expanded sella with large sella/suprasellar mass. No calcifications. Intralesional necrosis or hemorrhage may occur

MRI

- Decreased enhancement compared to native pituitary tissue; isointense or hypointense on T1W and T2W. May be partially or entirely cystic; may contain hemorrhage.
- Macroadenomas may cause compression of the optic apparatus or hydrocephalus secondary to obstruction at the foramina of Monro
- Cavernous sinus or skull base invasion may occur
- Macroadenoma should be distinguished from physiologic pituitary hyperplasia

Advanced Imaging

- MR Perfusion: not routinely performed
- MRS: not routinely performed

REFERENCE

1. Keil MF, et al. Pituitary tumors in childhood: update of diagnosis, treatment and molecular genetics. *Expert Rev Neurother.* 2008 Apr;8(4):563–574.

LANGERHANS CELL HISTIOCYTOSIS

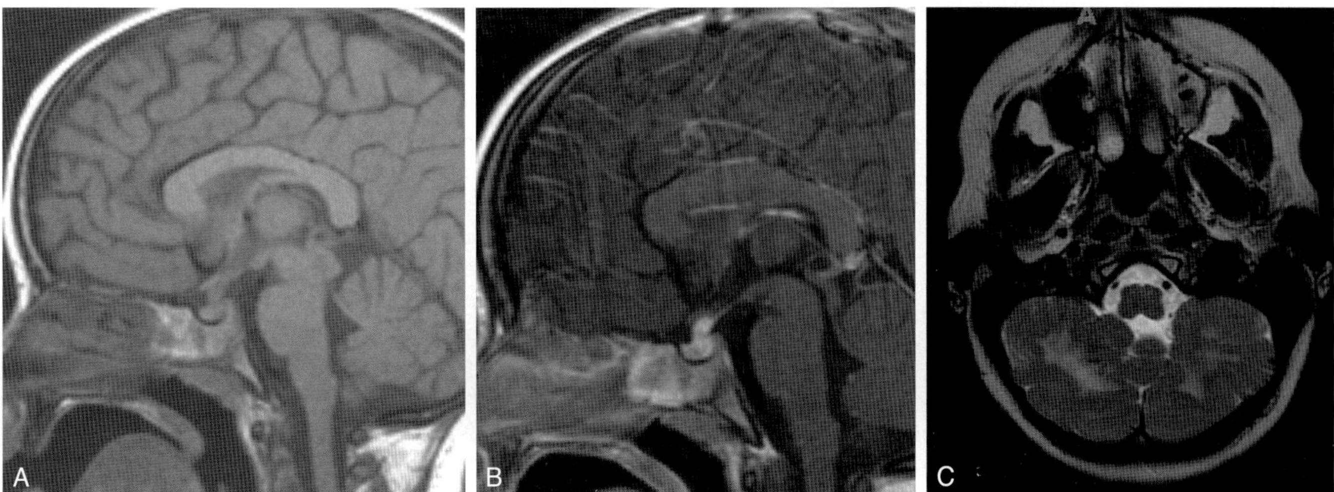

Fig. 7.65 Langerhans Cell Histiocytosis (LCH). A 3-year-old with diabetes insipidus. (A) Sagittal T1W, and (B) sagittal T1W+C, demonstrate homogeneous enhancement and thickening of the pituitary infundibulum and absent posterior pituitary T1 hyperintensity on noncontrast imaging due to LCH involvement. (C) Follow-up axial T2W image demonstrates abnormal T2W hyperintensity in the cerebellar white matter related to LCH neurodegeneration.

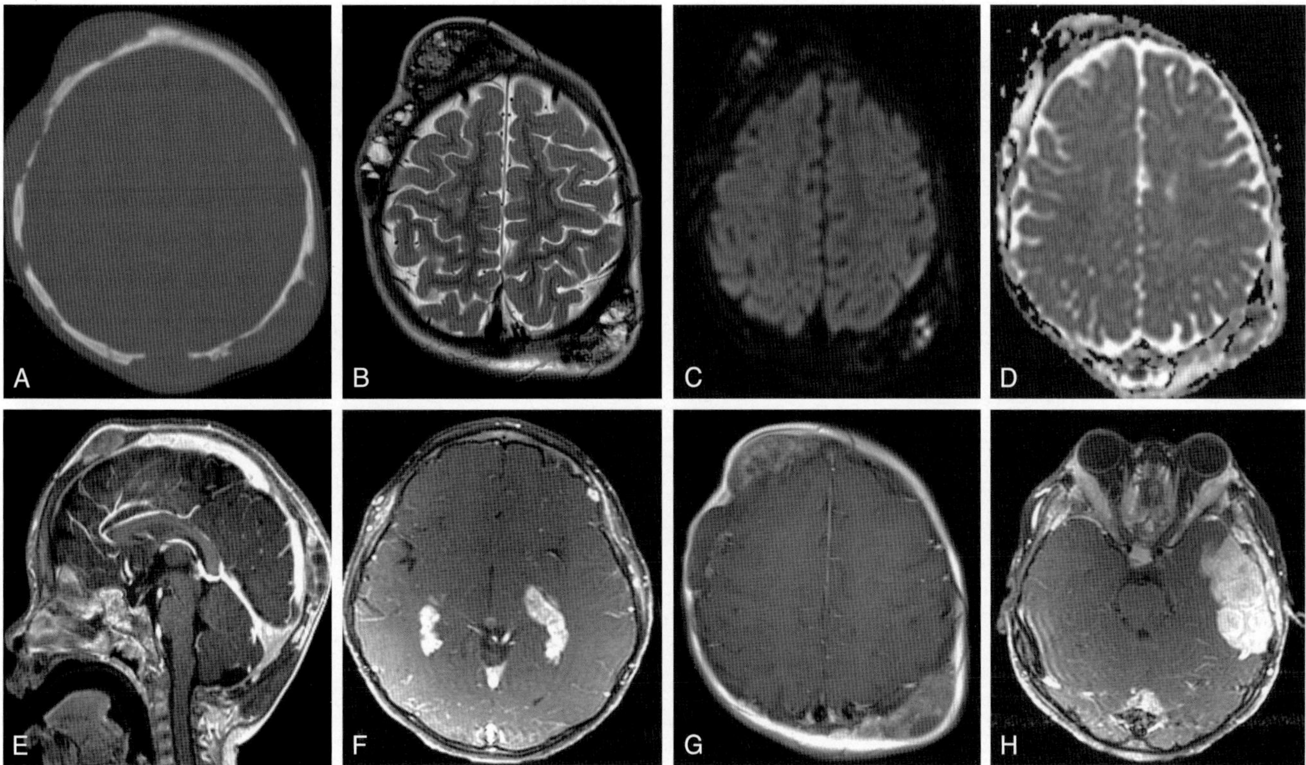

Fig. 7.66 Langerhans Cell Histiocytosis (LCH): Atypical Appearance of Intracranial Disease. A 2-year-old with multiple scalp masses. (A) Axial head CT demonstrates typical multiple lytic bone lesions in the calvarium with beveled edges with greater involvement of the outer cortical bone layer than the inner layer and associated soft tissue masses. (B) Axial T2W, (C) axial DWI, (D) axial ADC map, and (E to H) sagittal and axial T1W+C images demonstrate multiple bone lesions in the calvarium with soft tissue mass as well as homogeneous enhancement in the ventricles in the choroid plexus and a left middle cranial fossa dural-based mass.

Key Points

Background

- Systemic disease accumulation of epidermal dendritic cells (Langerhans cells) involving one or more organs
- In half of patients, oncogenic BRAF mutation is present
- CNS involvement occurs in 4% to 25% of patients, with pituitary infundibulum involvement most common and causing *diabetes insipidus*
- Location:
  - Osseous: Typical mass lesions involve the calvarium, orbit, temporal bone, maxilla, mandible, and vertebrae
  - CNS
    - Tumoral: Pituitary infundibulum is most common lesion with diffuse infiltration. May present as a discrete enhancing mass. Dura and choroid may uncommonly be involved.
    - Neurodegenerative LCH involves the cerebellum, brainstem, basal ganglia, and occasionally the supratentorial white matter. Global atrophy is common.
  - Head and neck soft tissues
    - Lymphadenopathy
    - External auditory canal

Imaging

CT

- Lytic, often described as well marginated or "*beveled edge*" due to greater destruction of the outer cortex compared to the inner cortex of bone. Avidly enhancing mass lesions and can contain hemorrhage and fluid-fluid levels. Soft tissue components may be large with significant regional inflammatory changes, mimicking infection.

MRI

- Osseous: T1W and T2W isointense to muscle, avidly enhancing well-defined masses of variable size with restricted diffusion
- CNS
  - Tumoral: Infiltrative mass lesion of the pituitary infundibulum with similar signal intensity soft tissue as detailed above with or without hypothalamic involvement; *loss of the normal T1W hyperintense posterior pituitary signal.*
  - Neurodegenerative LCH: Nonenhancing patchy T2W signal involving the dentate nuclei, and *peridentate cerebellar parenchyma* is the most common site followed by brainstem (especially pons), middle cerebellar peduncles, and less commonly the basal ganglia (especially globus pallidus). Leukodystrophy has been reported. Risk factors for neurodegenerative LCH include pituitary involvement, skull base or orbit involvement, skin involvement, and BRAF mutation.

Advanced Imaging

- MR Perfusion: not routinely performed
- MRS: not routinely performed

REFERENCES

1. Wang Y, et al. Neuroimaging features of CNS histiocytosis syndromes. *Clin Imaging.* 2020 Mar;60(1):131–140.
2. Héritier S, et al. Incidence and risk factors for clinical neurodegenerative Langerhans cell histiocytosis: a longitudinal cohort study. *Br J Haematol.* 2018 Nov;183(4):608–617.

HYPOTHALAMIC HAMARTOMA

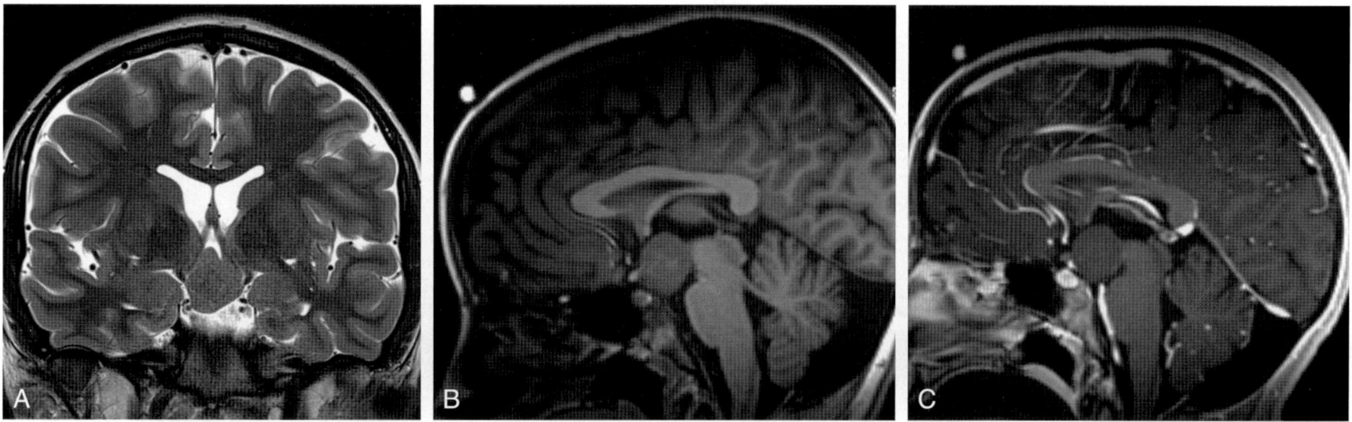

Fig. 7.67 Hypothalamic Hamartoma. A 12-year-old with Pallister Hall syndrome, precocious puberty, and gelastic seizures. (A) Coronal T2W, (B) sagittal T1W, and (C) sagittal T1W+C demonstrate a nonenhancing mass in the hypothalamus/tuber cinereum, which is isointense to cortex on T1W and T2W imaging.

Key Points

- Developmental, malformative *nonneoplastic* grey matter heterotopia of the tuber cinereum (part of the hypothalamus)
- Associated with Pallister Hall syndrome: Polydactyly, hypothalamic hamartoma, bifid epiglottis, imperforate anus, renal anomalies, and genital hypoplasia
- Clinical: More males affected than females; presenting signs and symptoms include *gelastic (laughing) seizures* and *precocious puberty* (GnRH secretion); symptoms often present in infancy and are progressive
- Treatment typically consists of antiepileptic drugs and minimally invasive surgery including endoscopic and laser ablation methodologies
- Classification: Various classification schemes based on location, symptoms, and whether sessile or pedunculated

Imaging

CT

- *Isodense* to grey matter without calcification or hemorrhage

MRI

- Hypothalamic mass that can be sessile or pedunculated; *isointense* to gray matter on T1W and T2W. Less common can have minimal T2W hyperintensity; significant T2W hyperintensity should raise suspicion for hypothalamic glioma or requires evidence of prior treatment with radiotherapy. No enhancement or susceptibility
- High-resolution imaging is needed to evaluate small lesions, which may only be several millimeters in size, and to evaluate the mass with relation to eloquent nearby structures like the mammillary bodies, fornix, mamillothalamic tract, and regional vasculature

Advanced Imaging

- MR Perfusion: not routinely performed
- MRS: not routinely performed

REFERENCES

1. Freeman JL, et al. MR imaging and spectroscopic study of epileptogenic hypothalamic hamartomas: analysis of 72 cases. *AJNR Am J Neuroradiol.* 2004 Mar;25(3):450–462.
2. Shim KW, et al. Endoscopic Treatment of Hypothalamic Hamartomas. *J Korean Neurosurg Soc.* 2017 May;60(3):294–300.

RATHKE CLEFT CYST

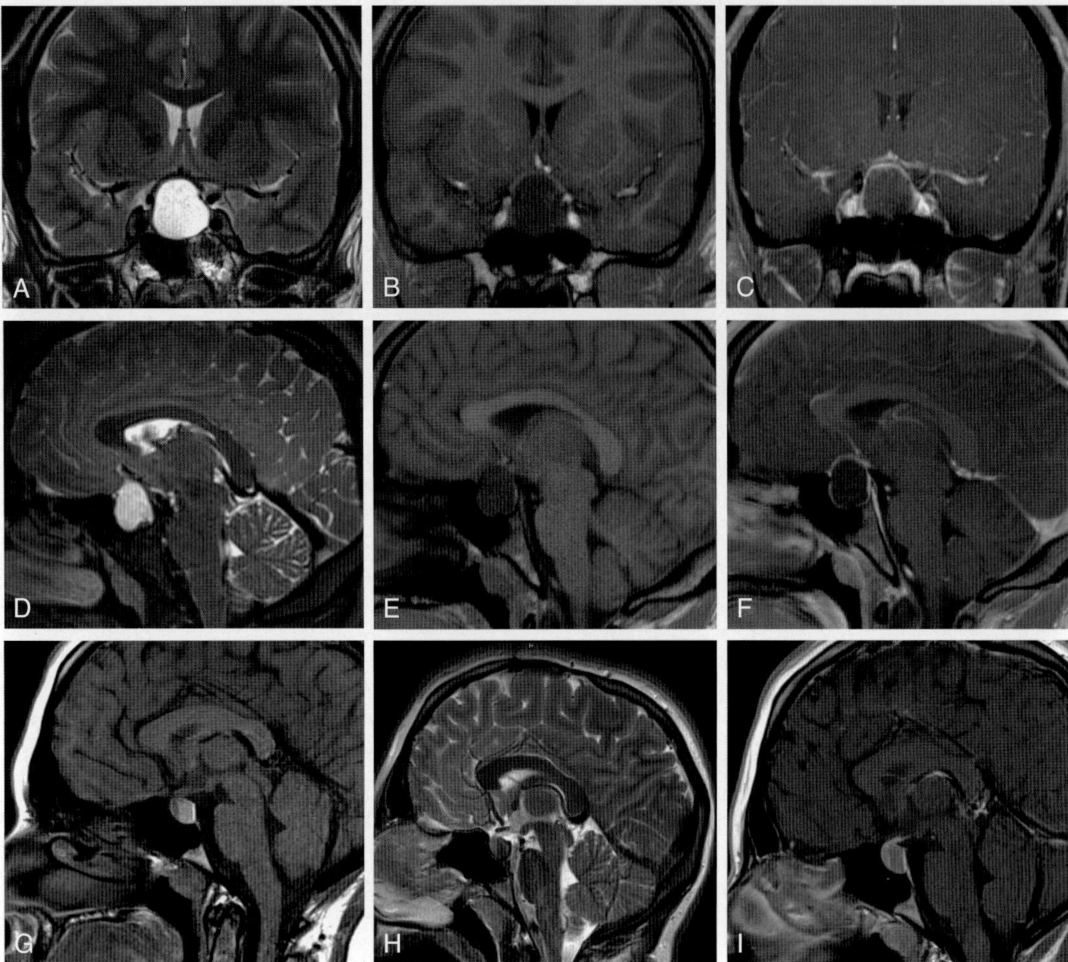

Fig. 7.68 Rathke Cleft Cyst. (A to F) A 14-year-old with headache and blurry vision and pathology proven Rathke cleft cyst. (A and D) Coronal and sagittal T2W, (B and E) coronal and sagittal T1W, and (C and F) coronal and sagittal T1W+C images demonstrate a T2W hyperintense thin-walled nonenhancing cyst in the sella and suprasellar cistern with remodeled/expanded appearance of the sella. A small intracystic nodule is seen at the inferior aspect of the mass. (G to I) A 16-year-old with daily headaches and pathology proven Rathke cleft cyst. (G) Sagittal T1W, (H) sagittal T2W, and (I) sagittal T1W+C images demonstrate a T1W hyperintense, T2W hypointense nonenhancing lesion between the anterior and posterior pituitary gland consistent with a proteinaceous Rathke cleft cyst.

Key Points

Background

- Rathke cleft cysts are nonneoplastic remnants of the Rathke pouch. Embryologically, the Rathke pouch extends dorsally from the oral epithelium to join the pituitary infundibulum. The anterior wall of the pouch forms the anterior pituitary and the posterior wall forms the pars intermedia. The lumen of the pouch forms the Rathke cleft and normally regresses by the 12th week of gestation. The persistence or expansion results in a Rathke cleft cyst.
- Most Rathke cleft cysts are incidentally detected. Large Rathke cleft cysts may cause endocrine dysfunction, headache, and/or changes in vision.

Imaging

CT

- Most commonly hypodense (75%) and difficult to identify when small

MRI

- Nonenhancing cystic lesion in the sella and/or suprasellar cistern typically with T2W hyperintense, and T1W hyperintense signal. Depending on the protein concentration, hypointense, isointense, or hyperintense T1W and T2W signal can be seen. An intracystic nodule is reportedly present in majority of cases.

Advanced Imaging

- MR Perfusion: not routinely performed
- MRS: not routinely performed

PINEAL REGION TUMORS

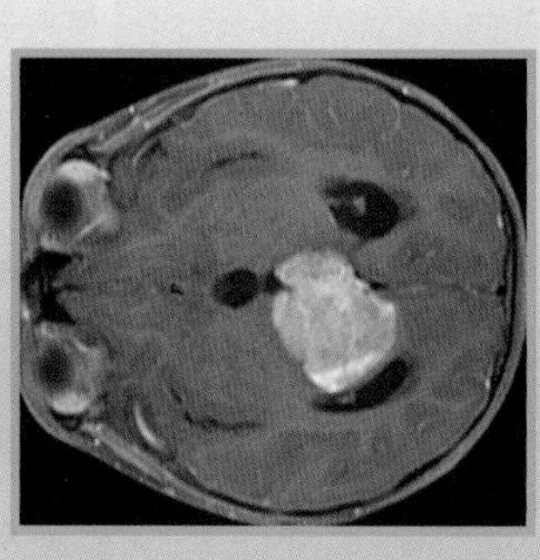

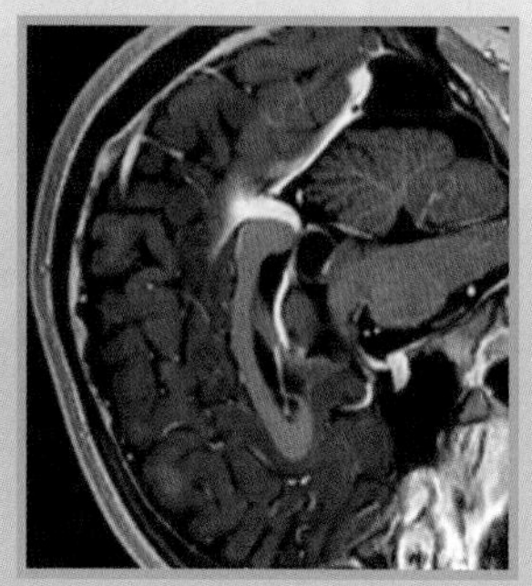

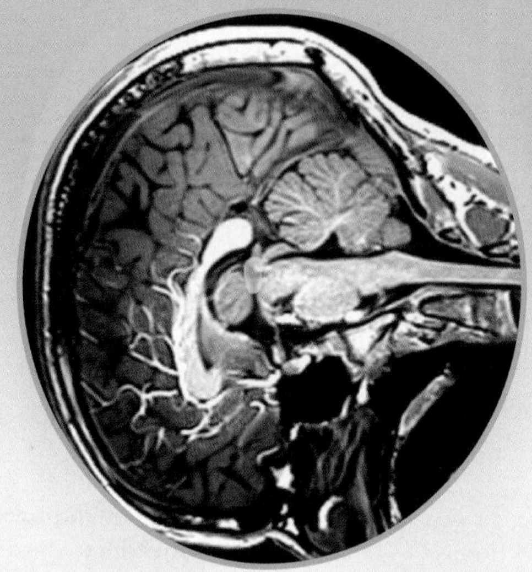

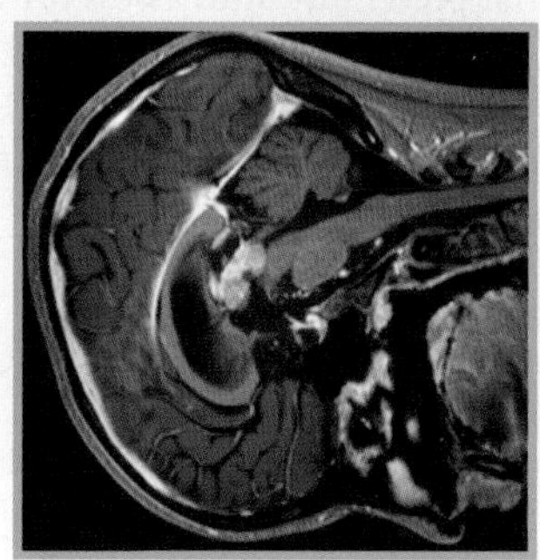

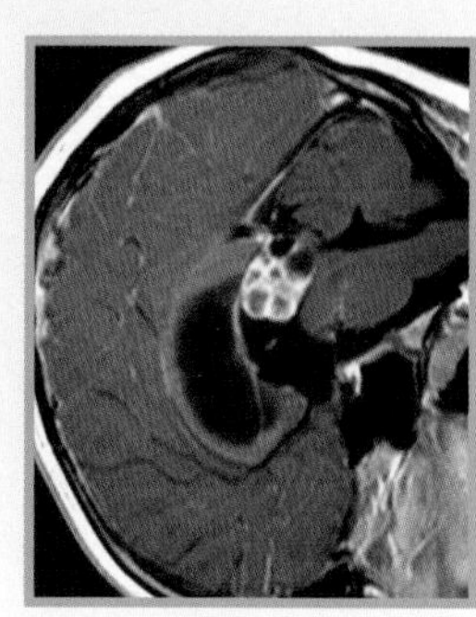

GERMINOMA

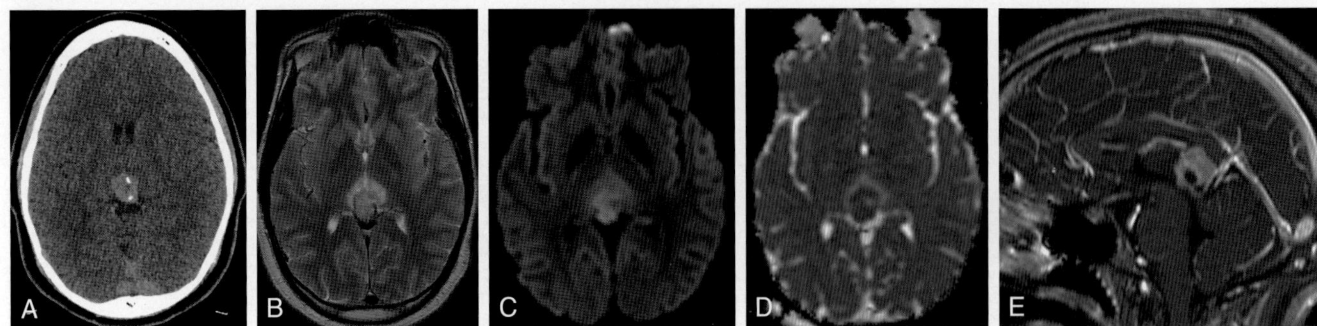

Fig. 7.69 Germinoma. A 17-year-old with progressive ataxia, nausea, and occasional vomiting. (A) Axial CT scan demonstrates a hyperdense pineal mass with central/engulfed calcification. (B) Axial T2W, (C) axial DWI, (D) axial ADC map, and (E) sagittal T1W+C images demonstrate a homogeneously enhancing pineal mass with reduced diffusion and adjacent thalamic edema. The engulfed calcification and age of the patient are more typical of a germinoma than pineoblastoma.

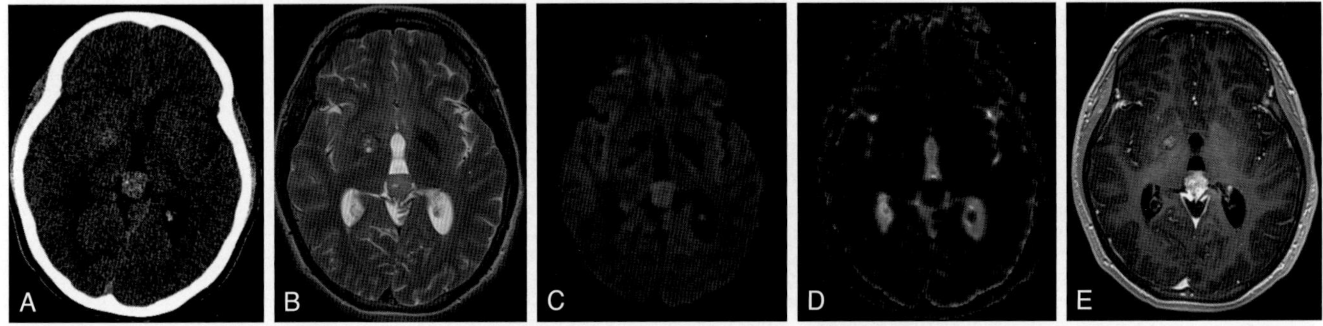

Fig. 7.70 Germinoma. A 16-year-old with progressive ataxia, nausea, and occasional vomiting. (A) Axial CT scan demonstrates a hyperdense pineal mass with small right paracentral calcification and a second hyperdense nodule in the right basal ganglia. (B) Axial T2W, (C) axial DWI, (D) axial ADC map, and (E) axial T1W+C images demonstrate mild T2W hyperintense nodules with homogeneous enhancement. The pineal nodule demonstrates reduced diffusion (low ADC).

Key Points

Background

- WHO grade 2. Germ cell tumors (GCTs) are subdivided into germinomas and nongerminomatous germ cell tumors (NGCTs). Germinomas account for two-thirds of intracranial GCTs
- Age <20 to 30; peak 10 to 12 years with 90% diagnosed by end of second decade; more common in Asians
- M:F ratio of 1.5–2:1 for all CNS germinomas
- Pineal region M:F 10:1
- Suprasellar affects more F>M

Imaging

CT

- Isodense to *hyperdense* mass; may have *engulfed central calcification* in the pineal region

MRI

- Well-circumscribed; T1W hypointense to isointense, T2W isointense to hypointense; *homogenously enhancing*
- *Restricted diffusion*
- Pineal region often presents with obstruction at level of cerebral aqueduct
- Edema in the adjacent brain parenchyma (often thalami)
- Metastatic or multifocal (suprasellar, pineal, basal ganglia) at presentation is possible → Total spine MRI performed at initial presentation to assess for drop metastases

Advanced Imaging

- MR Perfusion: not routinely performed
- MRS: not routinely performed

REFERENCES

1. Osorio DS, et al. Management of CNS germinoma. *CNS Oncol.* 2015;4(4):273–279.
2. Borja MJ, et al. Conventional and advanced MRI features of pediatric intracranial tumors: supratentorial tumors. *AJR Am J Roentgenol.* 2013 May;200(5):W483–W503.

NONGERMINOMATOUS GERM CELL TUMOR

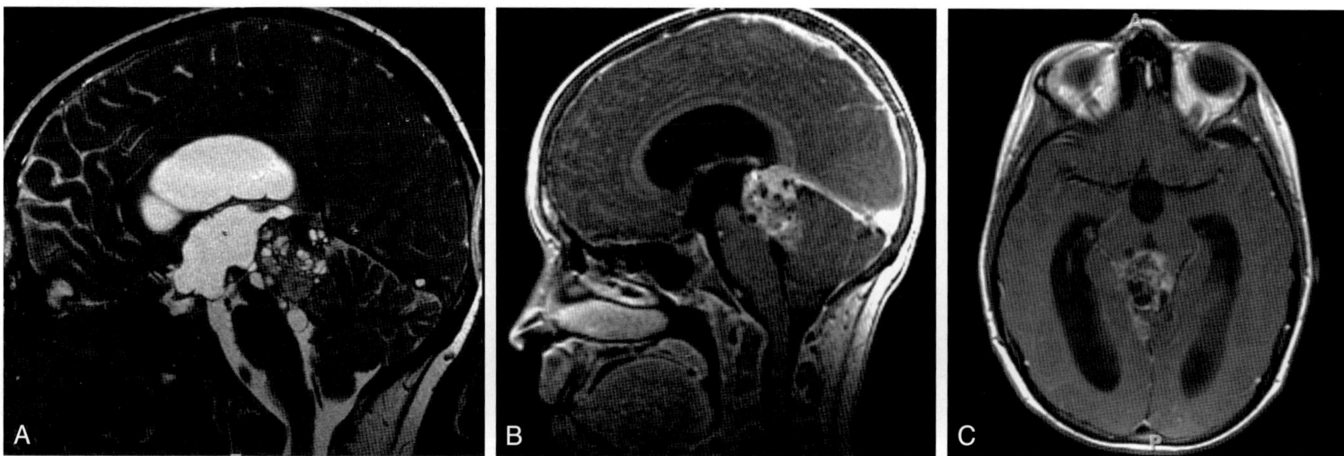

Fig. 7.71 Non-Germinomatous Germ Cell Tumor. (A) Sagittal T2W, and (B and C) sagittal and axial T1W+C images demonstrate a multicystic enhancing pineal region mass compressing the cerebral aqueduct and causing obstructive hydrocephalus.

Key Points

Background

- CNS germ cell tumors are subdivided into germinomas and nongerminomatous germ cell tumors (NGCTs). More than half of NGCTs are mixed germ cell tumors
- NGCTs include embryonal carcinoma, yolk sac tumor, choriocarcinoma, mature teratoma, immature teratoma, and malignant teratoma
- Beta-HCG secretion with choriocarcinoma or malignant teratoma; Alpha fetoprotein (AFP) secretion with yolk sac tumor or malignant teratoma
- Patients with normal B-HCG and AFP require surgical biopsy
- Males more commonly affected than females, most commonly seen in 10- to 20-year-olds; more common in Asians
- Commonly present with signs of increased intracranial pressure due to hydrocephalus from obstruction of the cerebral aqueduct. Symptoms include headache, nausea, vomiting, dyskinesia, and *Parinaud syndrome*; 5-year survival rate of 80%
- Location: Pineal region; may metastasize

Imaging

CT

- Nonspecific soft tissue mass of the pineal region

MRI

- Well-circumscribed, heterogeneous, enhancing, solid, and cystic pineal region mass. Most commonly solid and cystic, more so than germinoma or pineoblastoma
- Compared to germinomas, NGCTs are more heterogeneous in appearance, may be larger at presentation, contain internal foci of T1 shortening (hemorrhage, fat, or calcium), and higher ADC signal ($>1.143 \times 10^{-3}$ mm^2/s) in solid components. NGCTs may also enhance more avidly than germinomas
- Homogenous soft tissue mass with infiltrative margins more commonly seen with germinomas. Bifocal (suprasellar and pineal) mass is typically a germinoma
- Metastatic at presentation is possible → Total spine MRI performed at initial presentation to assess for drop metastases

Advanced Imaging

- MR Perfusion: not routinely performed
- MRS: not routinely performed

REFERENCES

1. Kong Z, et al. Central Nervous System Germ Cell Tumors: A Review of the Literature. *J Child Neurol.* 2018 Aug;33(9):610–620.
2. Wu CC, et al. MRI features of pediatric intracranial germ cell tumor subtypes. *J Neurooncol.* 2017 Aug;134(1):221–230.

TERATOMA

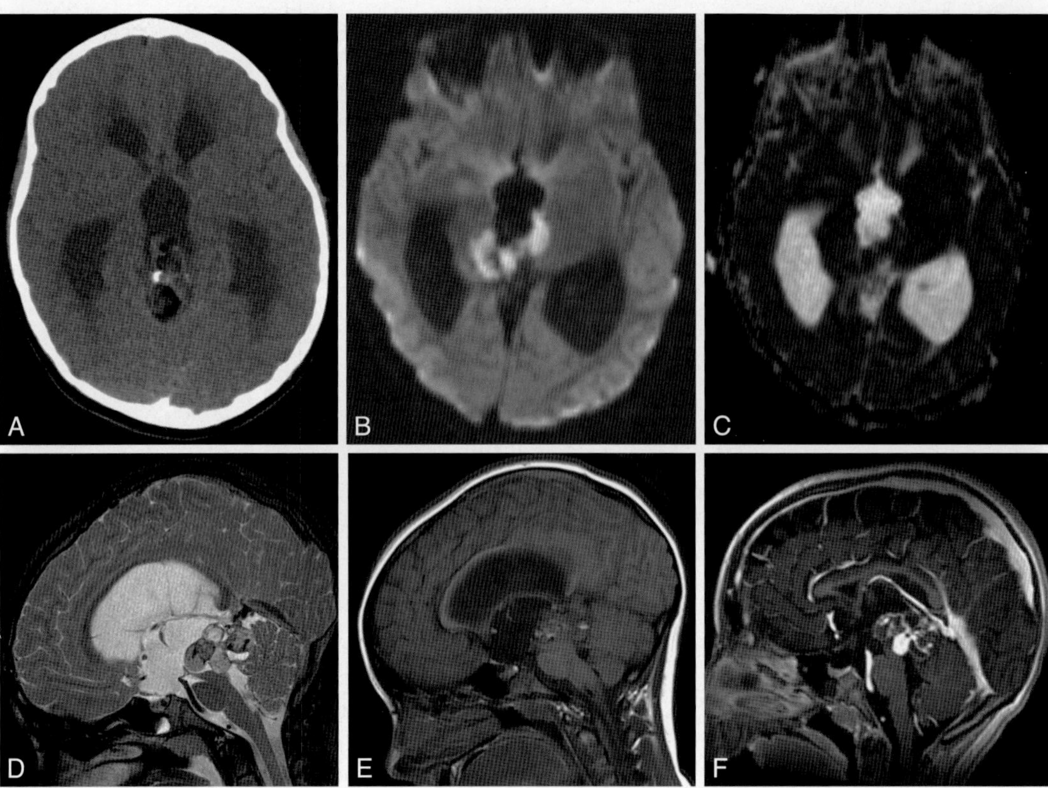

Fig. 7.72 Teratoma. A 7-year-old with right upper extremity tremor and head tilt. (A) Axial CT head, (B) axial DWI, (C) axial ADC map, (D) sagittal T2W, (E) sagittal T1W, and (F) sagittal T1W+C images demonstrate a solid and cystic mass in the pineal gland with macroscopic fat, peripheral areas of reduced diffusion with associated obstructive hydrocephalus due to compression of the cerebral aqueduct.

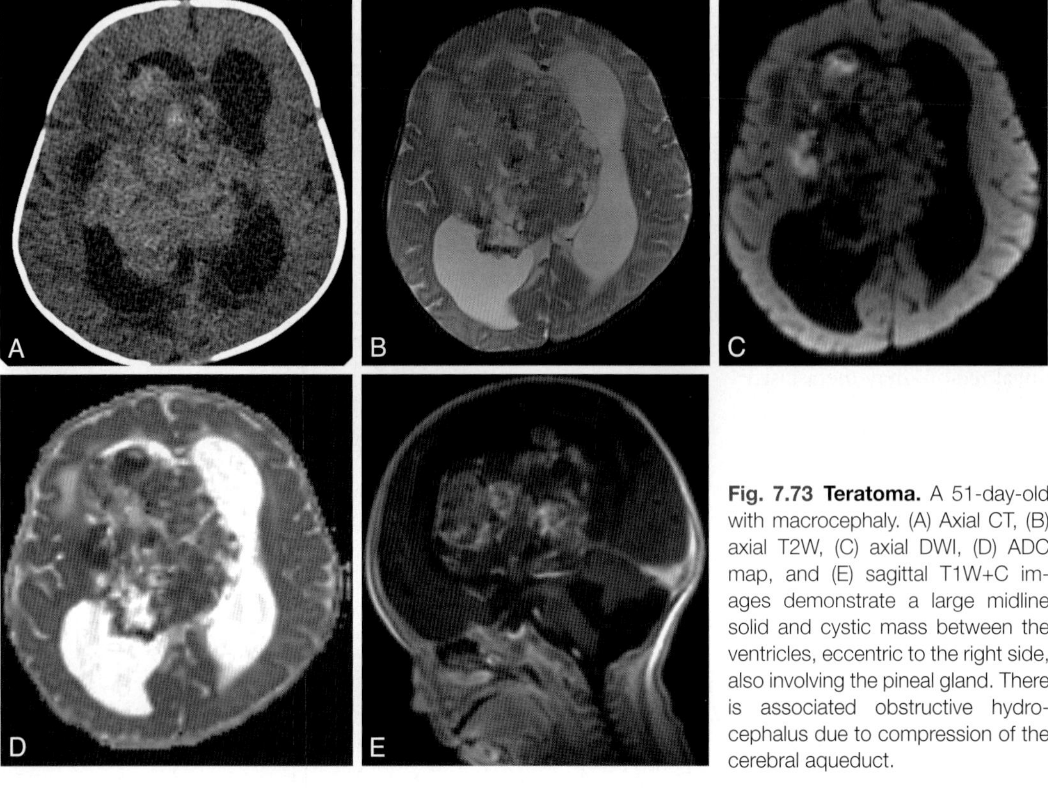

Fig. 7.73 Teratoma. A 51-day-old with macrocephaly. (A) Axial CT, (B) axial T2W, (C) axial DWI, (D) ADC map, and (E) sagittal T1W+C images demonstrate a large midline solid and cystic mass between the ventricles, eccentric to the right side, also involving the pineal gland. There is associated obstructive hydrocephalus due to compression of the cerebral aqueduct.

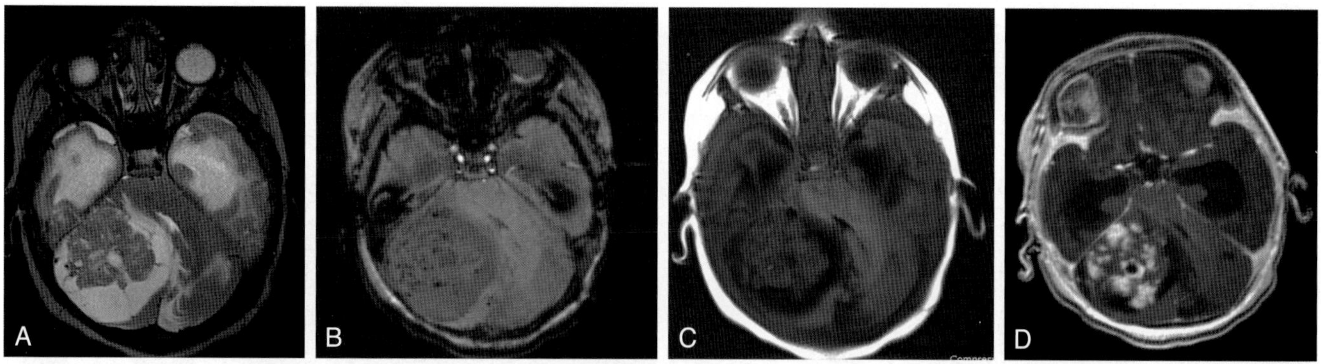

Fig. 7.74 Teratoma: Uncommon Location. A 57-day-old with bulging fontanelle, and sundowning of the eyes (upward-gaze paresis). (A) Axial T2W, (B) axial SWI, (C) axial T1W, and (D) axial T1W+C images demonstrate a solid and cystic mass in the right side of the posterior fossa with small calcifications and heterogeneous enhancement. There is associated obstructive hydrocephalus and cerebral and cerebellar edema. Posterior fossa location is atypical for teratoma.

Key Points

Background

- Teratomas are a subset of nongerminomatous germ cell tumors (NGCTs).
- Includes mature teratoma, immature teratoma, and malignant teratoma
- Teratomas account for 15% of CNS germ cell tumors, second to germinoma. They are the most common nongerminomatous germ cell tumor
- B-HCG and AFP secretion may occur with malignant teratoma
- Males affected more often than females; most commonly seen in 10- to 20-year-olds; more common in Asians
- Commonly present with signs of increased intracranial pressure resulting from hydrocephalus from obstruction of the cerebral aqueduct. Symptoms include headache, nausea, vomiting, dyskinesia, and Parinaud syndrome. May present during fetal screening
- Location: Midline locations including pineal region, suprasellar, and intraventricular; malignant teratoma may metastasize

Imaging

CT

- Solid or solid and cystic mass with calcifications. Adipose tissue is not often present but is a key feature of a teratoma when present. Immature and malignant teratomas are more homogenously solid with fewer calcification and cysts and lack intralesional fat.

MRI

- Well-circumscribed, very heterogenous, multilobulated or multiloculated, solid (enhancing) and cystic midline mass. Immature teratomas and malignant teratomas predominantly solid and commonly do not contain calcification and fat.
- Foci of T1W shortening (fat or calcium), T2W iso- to hypointense soft tissue components, T2W hyperintense cystic components
- Metastatic at presentation is possible with malignant teratomas → total spine MRI performed at initial presentation to assess for drop metastases

Advanced Imaging

- MR Perfusion: not routinely performed
- MRS: not routinely performed

REFERENCES

1. Kong Z, et al. Central Nervous System Germ Cell Tumors: A Review of the Literature. *J Child Neurol.* 2018 Aug;33(9):610–620.
2. Wu CC, et al. MRI features of pediatric intracranial germ cell tumor subtypes. *J Neurooncol.* 2017 Aug;134(1):221–230.
3. Tamrazi B, et al. Pineal Region Masses in Pediatric Patients. *Neuroimaging Clin N Am.* 2017 Feb;27(1):85–97.
4. Fang AS, et al. Magnetic resonance imaging of pineal region tumours. *Insights Imaging.* 2013;4(3):369–382.

PINEOBLASTOMA

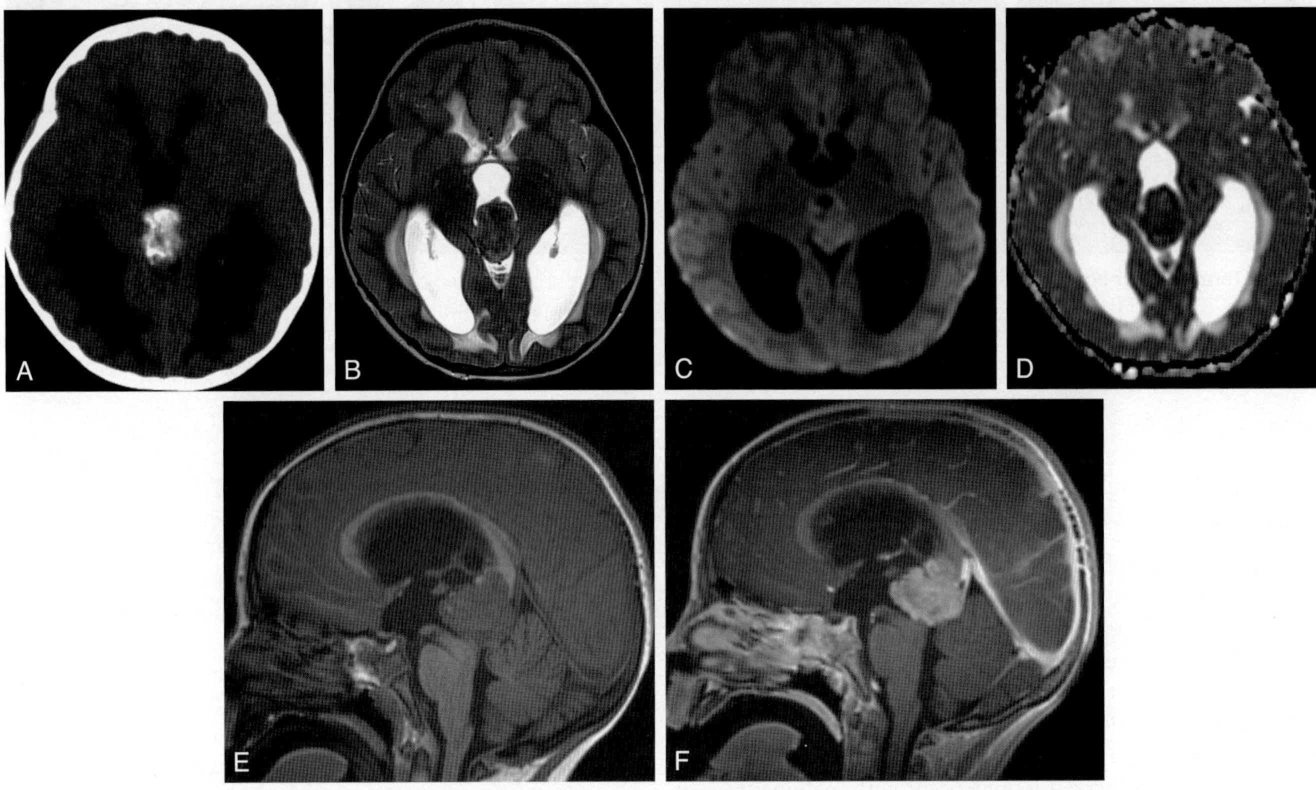

Fig. 7.75 Pineoblastoma. A 4-year-old with papilledema, strabismus and urinary incontinence. (A) Axial CT head, (B) axial T2W, (C) axial DWI, (D) axial ADC map, (E) sagittal T1W, and (F) sagittal T1W+C images demonstrate a diffusely calcified mass in the pineal gland with T2W isointensity, reduced diffusion, and homogeneous enhancement typical of a pineoblastoma.

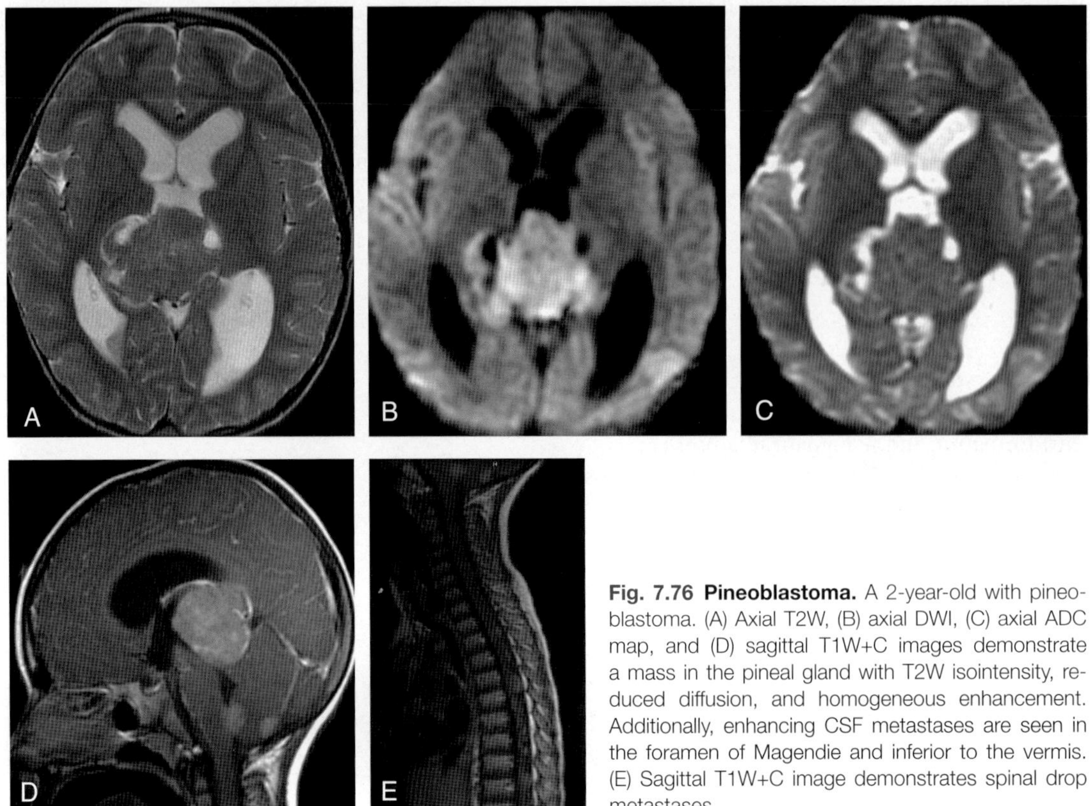

Fig. 7.76 Pineoblastoma. A 2-year-old with pineoblastoma. (A) Axial T2W, (B) axial DWI, (C) axial ADC map, and (D) sagittal T1W+C images demonstrate a mass in the pineal gland with T2W isointensity, reduced diffusion, and homogeneous enhancement. Additionally, enhancing CSF metastases are seen in the foramen of Magendie and inferior to the vermis. (E) Sagittal T1W+C image demonstrates spinal drop metastases.

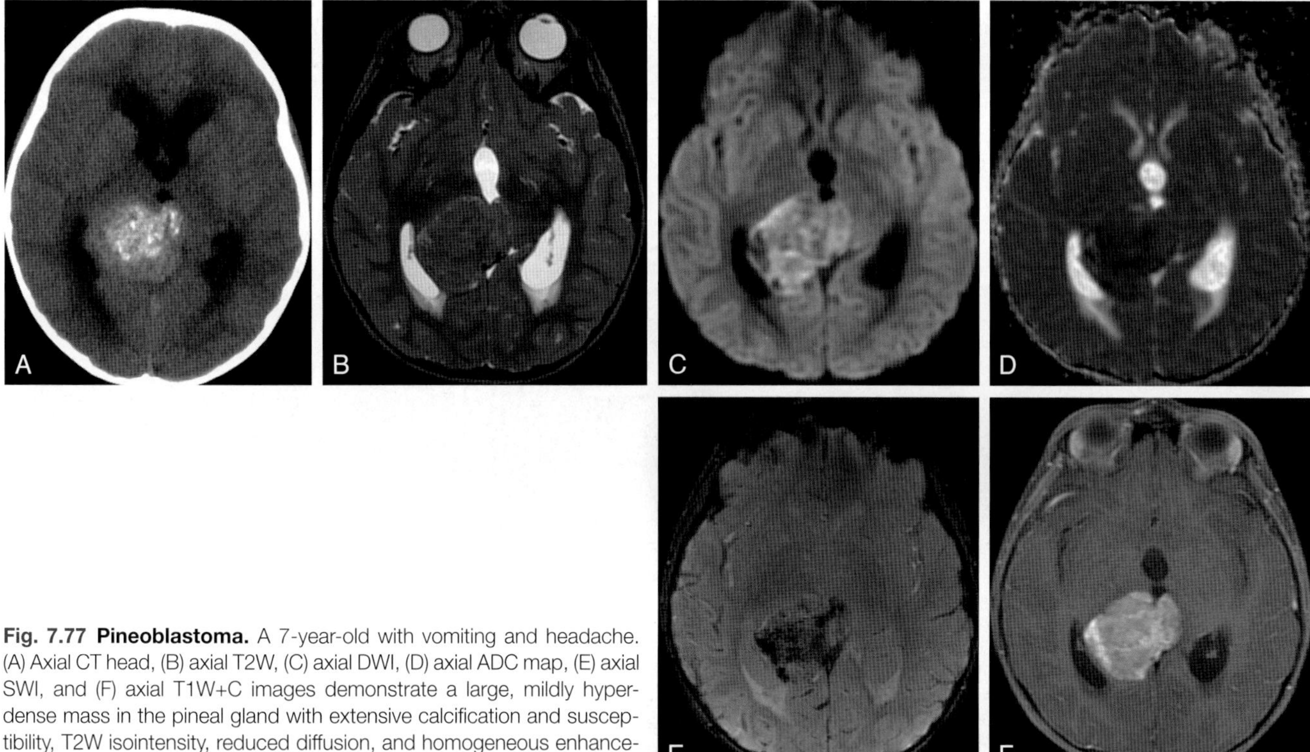

Fig. 7.77 Pineoblastoma. A 7-year-old with vomiting and headache. (A) Axial CT head, (B) axial T2W, (C) axial DWI, (D) axial ADC map, (E) axial SWI, and (F) axial T1W+C images demonstrate a large, mildly hyperdense mass in the pineal gland with extensive calcification and susceptibility, T2W isointensity, reduced diffusion, and homogeneous enhancement typical of a pineoblastoma.

Key Points

Background

- WHO grade 4
- Pineal parenchymal tumors account for 15% to 30% of pineal regional masses, 40% of which are pineoblastomas
- More common in *children <2 years of age*
- M:F ratio 1:1 in contradistinction to male predominance in germ cell tumors
- More common with retinoblastoma gene mutations (trilateral or quadrilateral retinoblastoma), but also occurs in absence of retinoblastoma
- As with other pineal region tumors, pineoblastomas may present with signs of increased intracranial pressure due to hydrocephalus from obstruction of the cerebral aqueduct. Symptoms include headache, nausea, vomiting, dyskinesia, and Parinaud syndrome
- Intermediate prognosis; 5-year survival ~60%
- Location: Pineal region

Imaging

CT

- Soft tissue mass isodense to brain; diffuse or peripheral calcification in contradistinction to germ cell tumors (GCTs), which have central calcifications

MRI

- Well-circumscribed, T1W hypointense to isointense, T2W isointense to hypointense, avid homogenous or heterogeneous enhancing solid components. Restricted diffusion
- Metastatic or multifocal (trilateral or quadrilateral retinoblastoma) at presentation is possible → total spine MRI performed at initial presentation to assess for drop metastases

Advanced Imaging

- MR Perfusion: not routinely performed
- MRS: not routinely performed

REFERENCES

1. Tamrazi B, et al. Pineal Region Masses in Pediatric Patients. *Neuroimaging Clin N Am*. 2017 Feb;27(1):85–97.
2. Smith AB, et al. From the archives of the AFIP. Lesions of the pineal region: radiologic-pathologic correlation. *Radiographics*. 2010;30:2001–2020.

THALAMIC TUMORS

Low Grade (WHO Grade 1 or 2)

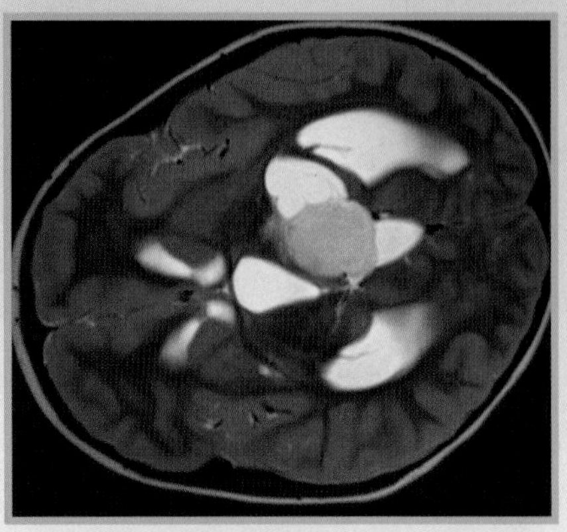

Low Grade Glioma

Key Imaging Features
- Imaging patterns overlap

High Grade (WHO Grade 3 or 4)

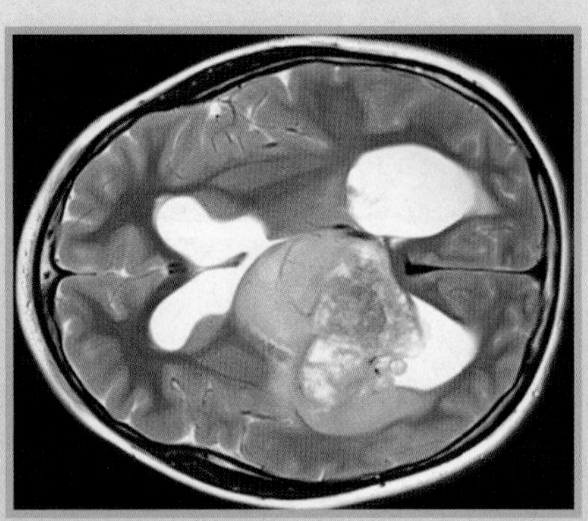

Midline High Grade Glioma

THALAMIC HIGH-GRADE GLIOMA

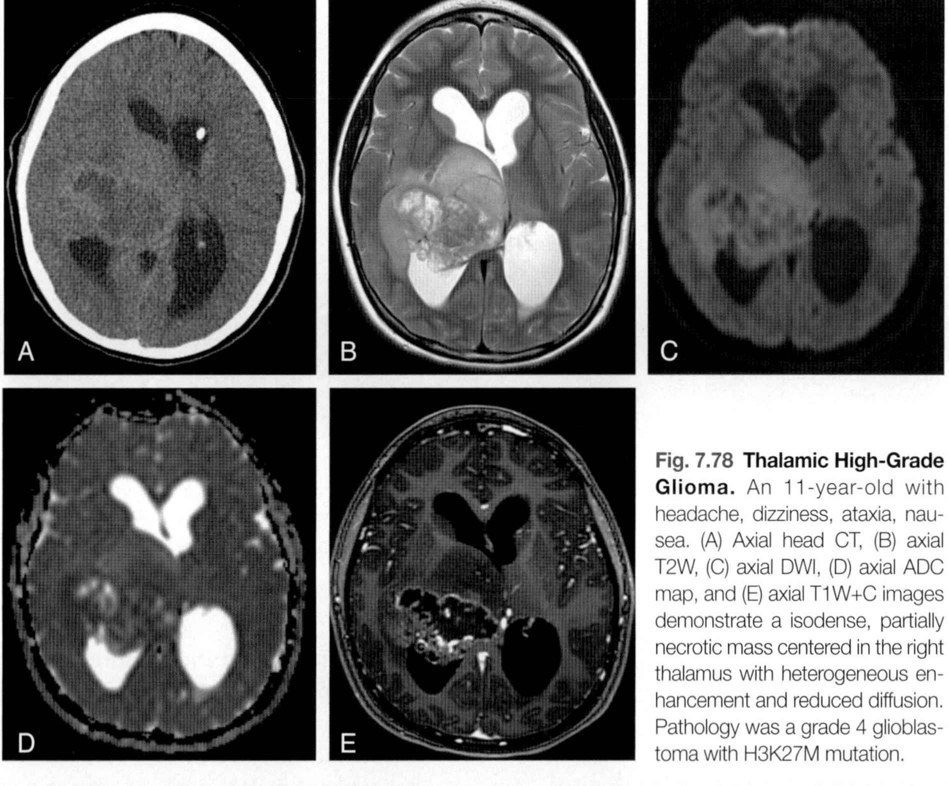

Fig. 7.78 Thalamic High-Grade Glioma. An 11-year-old with headache, dizziness, ataxia, nausea. (A) Axial head CT, (B) axial T2W, (C) axial DWI, (D) axial ADC map, and (E) axial T1W+C images demonstrate a isodense, partially necrotic mass centered in the right thalamus with heterogeneous enhancement and reduced diffusion. Pathology was a grade 4 glioblastoma with H3K27M mutation.

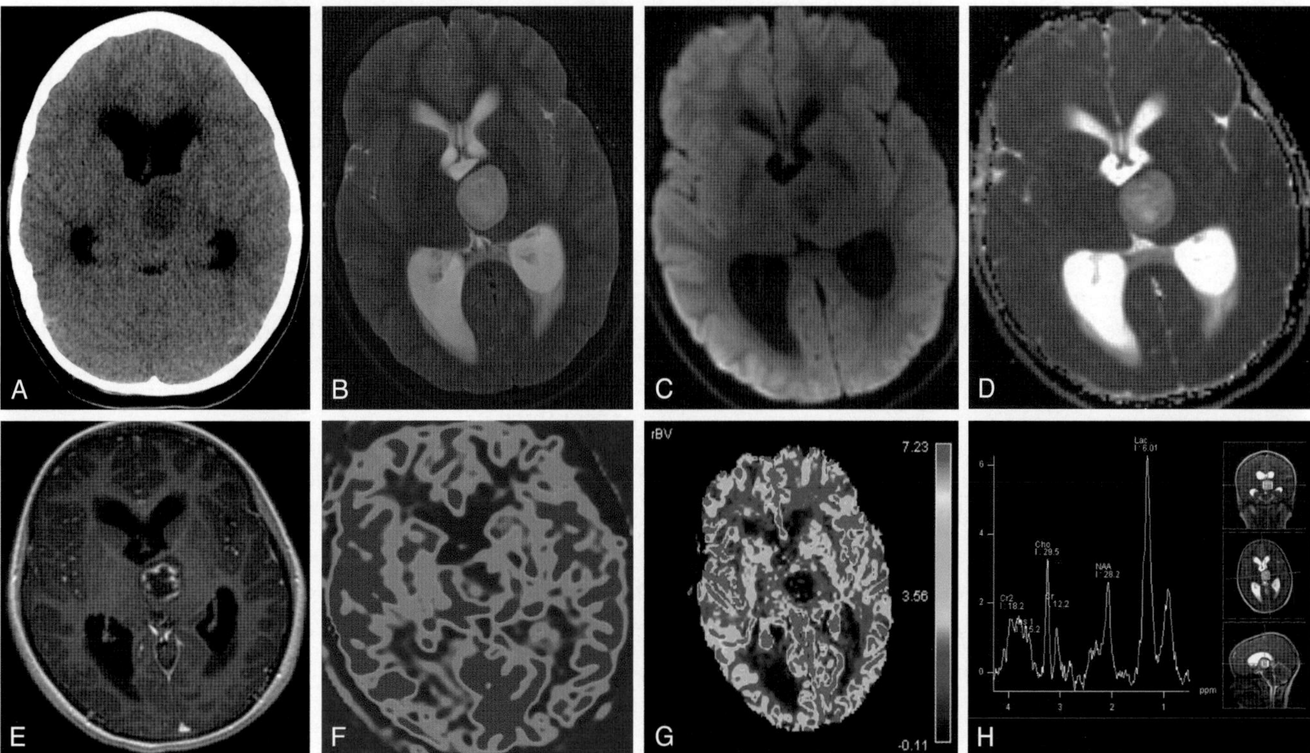

Fig. 7.79 Thalamic High-Grade Glioma: Advanced Imaging. An 11-year-old with headache. (A) Axial CT images demonstrates an ovoid circumscribed low-density mass in the left thalamus. (B) Axial T2W, (C) axial DWI, (D) axial ADC map, and (E) axial T1W+C images demonstrate a homogenous T2W hyperintense ovoid mass in the left thalamus with elevated ADC values and irregular peripheral enhancement. (F) Axial ASL CBF color map demonstrates low CBF in the mass. (G) Axial DSC perfusion rCBV color map demonstrates low rCBV in the mass. (H) Proton MR spectroscopy with short echo demonstrates reduced NAA, increased choline, and increased lactate.

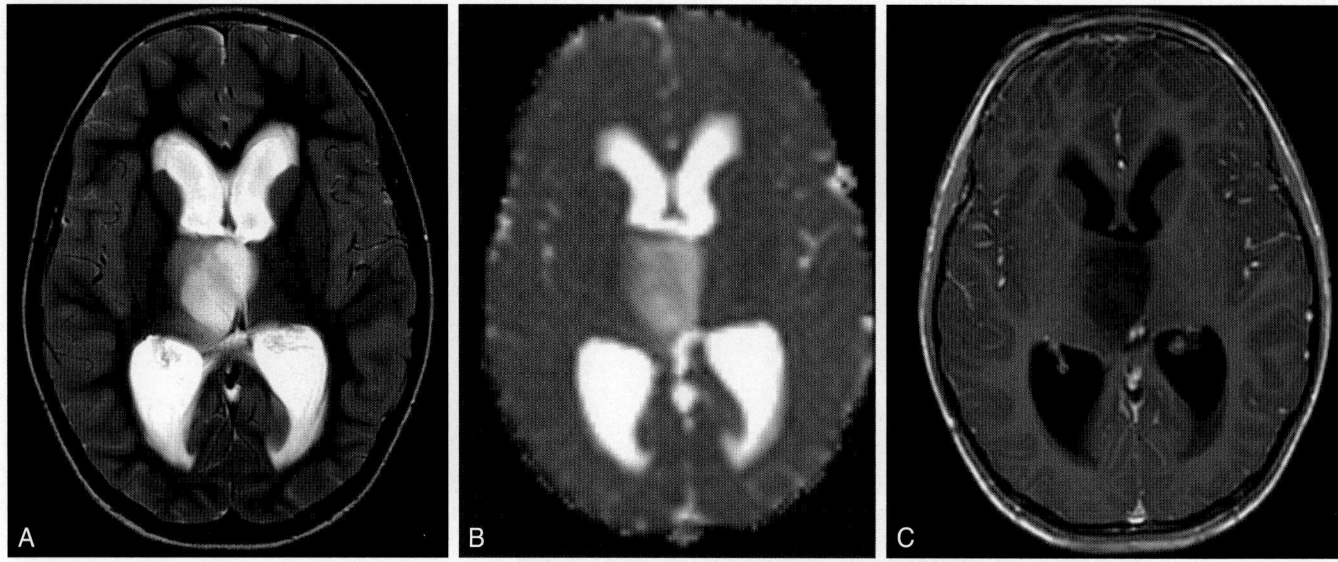

Fig. 7.80 Thalamic High-Grade Glioma. A 9-year-old with morning headaches, nausea, and vomiting. (A) Axial T2W, (B) axial ADC map, and (C) axial T1W+C images demonstrate a circumscribed T2W hyperintense nonenhancing mass with elevated ADC involving majority of the right thalamus and obstructing the third ventricle, resulting in hydrocephalus and mid transependymal edema. Pathology was a WHO grade 4 diffuse midline glioma with H3K27M mutation. Despite the appearance that is more consistent with a low grade, the thalamic location should always raise concern for high-grade glioma.

Key Points

Background

- WHO grades 3 to 4
- *H3K27* mutation versus wild-type histone H3; limited series suggest that imaging cannot reliably differentiate these subtypes
- 5% of pediatric brain tumors arise from the thalamus with up to *50% with high-grade* histology; thalamic high-grade gliomas account for 13% of pediatric high-grade gliomas
- Fatal/extremely poor prognosis with 5-year survival 10% to 15%. Poorer prognosis in patients with H3K27 mutation
- Location: Unilateral or bilateral thalamus, may extend into adjacent structures such as the brainstem, internal capsule, basal ganglia, and cerebral hemispheres (e.g., temporal lobe). May involve a portion or the entire thalamus

Imaging

CT

- Hypodense expansile infiltrative diffuse or focal mass, typically without calcification. May have areas of necrosis and hemorrhage

MRI

- *Difficult to distinguish low-grade from high-grade gliomas in the thalamus due to overlapping conventional and advanced MRI appearances*
- Large solid or solid and necrotic infiltrative, expansile T1W hypointense and T2W hyperintense mass (higher-grade portions will have lower T2W signal). Smaller masses may only partially involve the thalamus. Foci of hemorrhage may be seen. May have nodular or patchy heterogeneous foci of enhancement or peripheral enhancement of necrotic portions
- Typically does not demonstrate restricted diffusion although foci of restricted diffusion, especially corresponding to foci of enhancement may be seen
- Peritumoral edema is usually but not always absent
- Metastasis at presentation is rare

Advanced Imaging

- MR Perfusion: Typically low CBF and CBV
- MRS: unknown whether MR spectroscopy can differentiate low-grade and high-grade thalamic gliomas

REFERENCES

1. Kramm CM, et al. Thalamic high-grade gliomas in children: a distinct clinical subset? *Neuro Oncol.* 2011;13(6):680–689.
2. Aboian MS, et al. Imaging Characteristics of Pediatric Diffuse Midline Gliomas with Histone H3 K27M Mutation. *AJNR Am J Neuroradiol.* 2017;38(4):795–800.

INTRAVENTRICULAR TUMORS

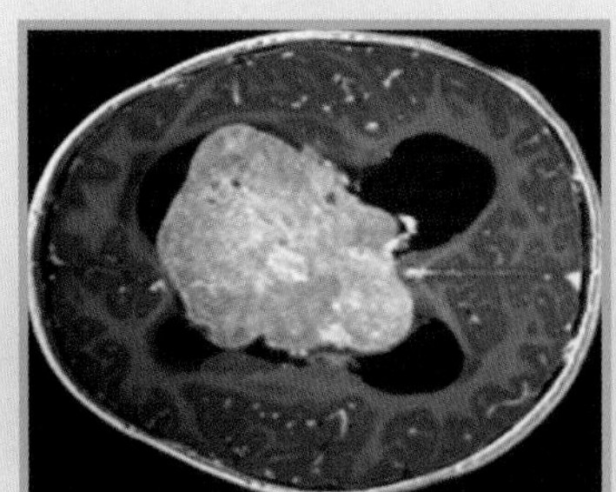

Rare: Meningioma, Langerhans Cell Histiocytosis, ATRT, CNS Embryonal Tumor, Central Neurocytoma

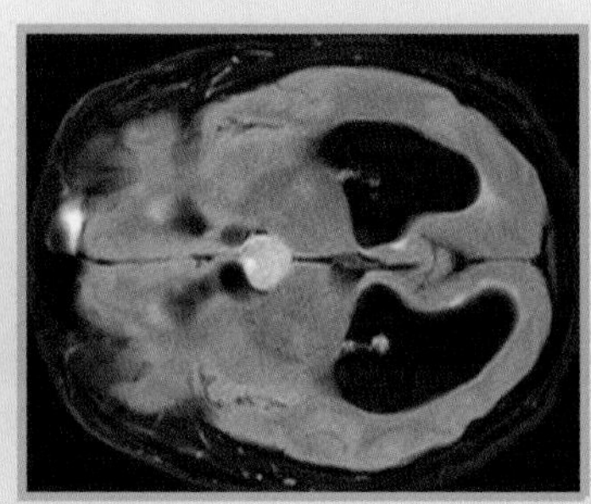

Non-tumor Masses: Colloid Cyst, Arachnoid Cyst

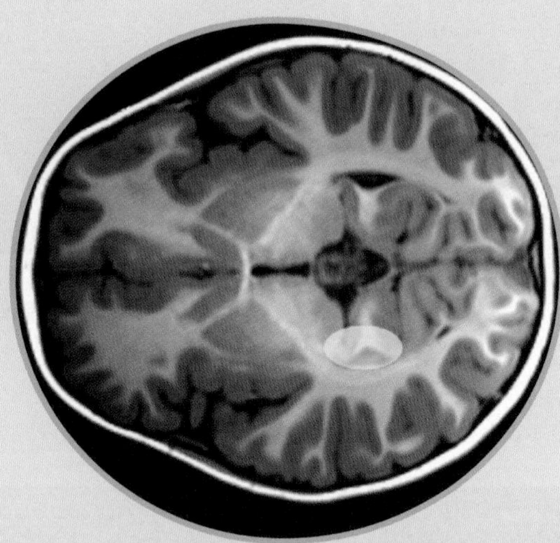

Key Imaging Features
- Location
- Enhancement pattern

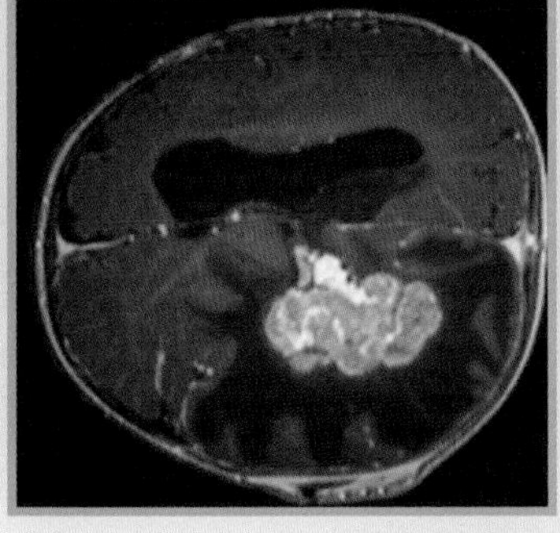

Choroid Plexus Papilloma Carcinoma

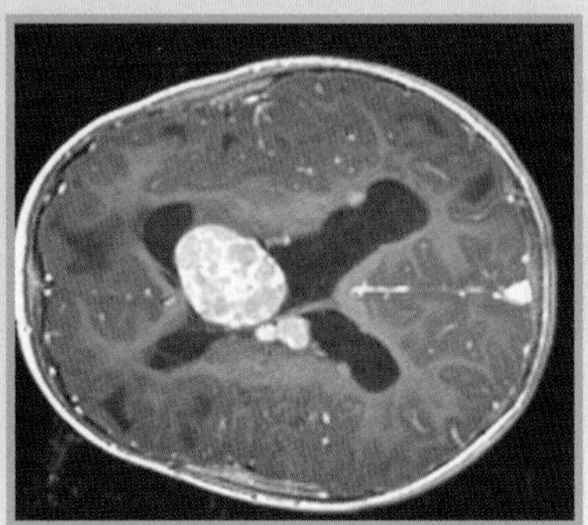

Subependymal Giant Cell Astrocytoma

CHOROID PLEXUS PAPILLOMA AND CARCINOMA

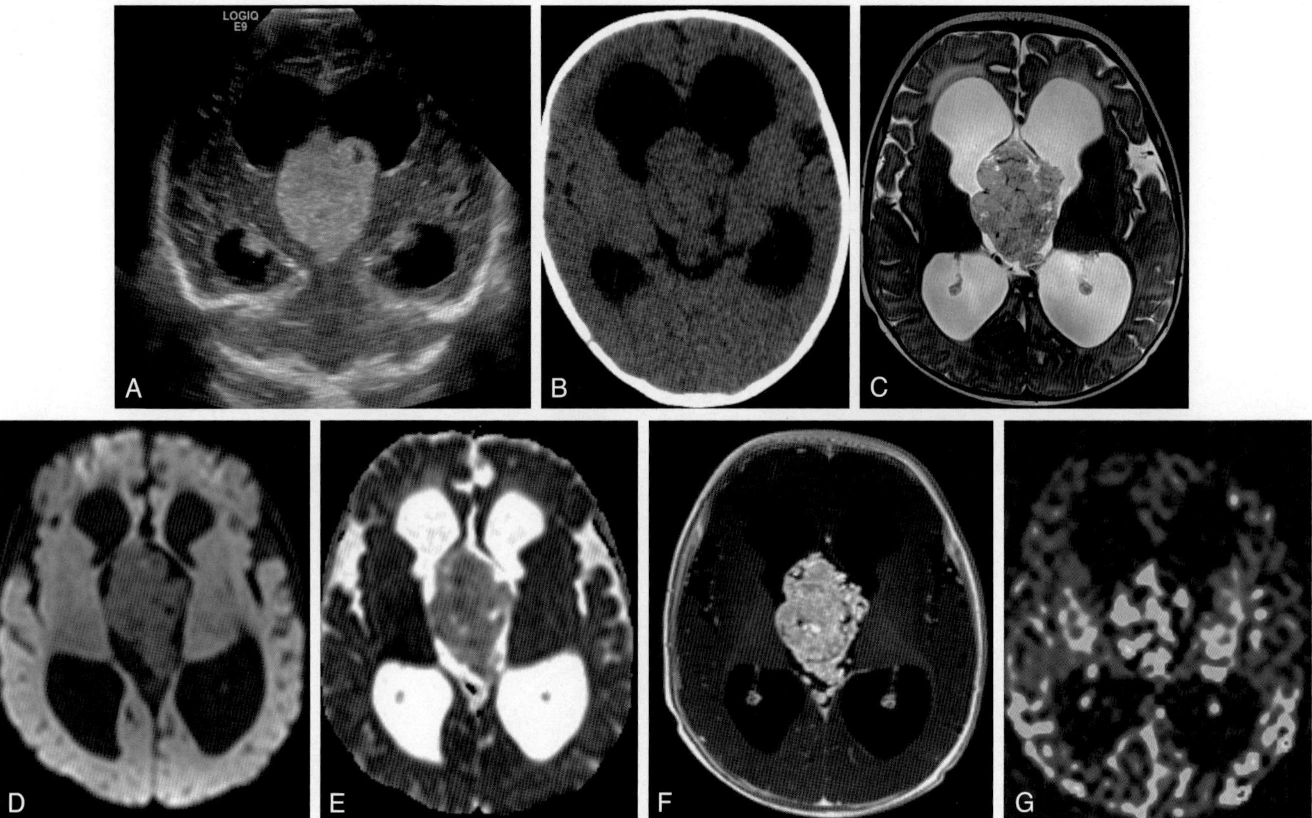

Fig. 7.81 Choroid Plexus Papilloma. A 4-month-old with rapidly increasing head circumference. (A) Coronal head ultrasound, (B) axial CT head, (C) axial T2W, (D) axial DWI, (E) axial ADC map, (F) axial T1W+C, and (G) axial ASL CBF color map images demonstrate a hyperechoic, isodense mass in the third ventricle with elevated ADC, homogeneous enhancement, and areas of increased CBF indicative of a choroid plexus papilloma. There is associated hydrocephalus of the lateral ventricles.

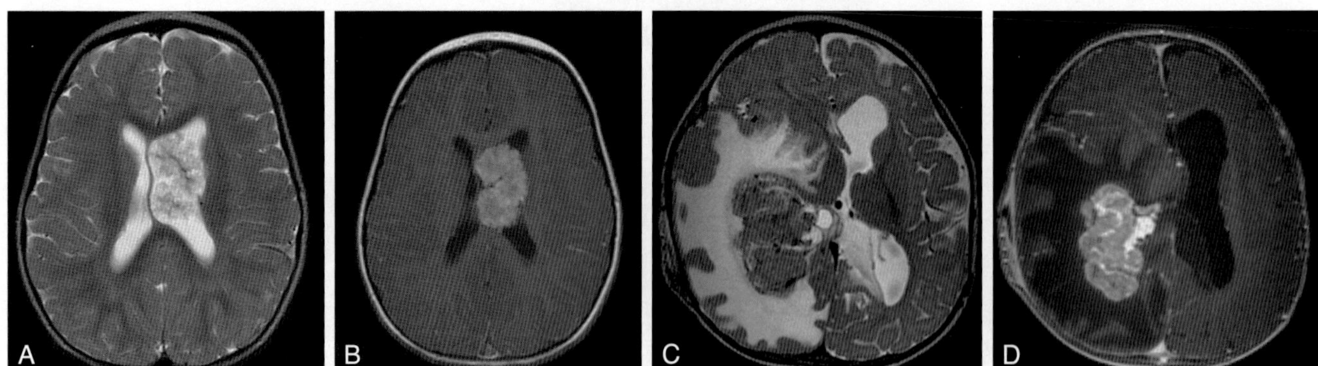

Fig. 7.82 Choroid Plexus Papillomas in Two Patients. (A and B) Axial T2W and axial T1W+C images in a 12-month-old with a choroid plexus papilloma in the left lateral ventricle with typical appearance with frond-like homogeneously enhancing T2W hyperintense mass. (C and D) Axial T2W and axial T1W+C images in a 6-month-old with increasing head circumference and abnormal eye movements with less common appearance with T2W isointense homogeneous enhancing right intraventricular/atrial mass and large amount of adjacent edema from ventricular obstruction and possibly CSF overproduction.

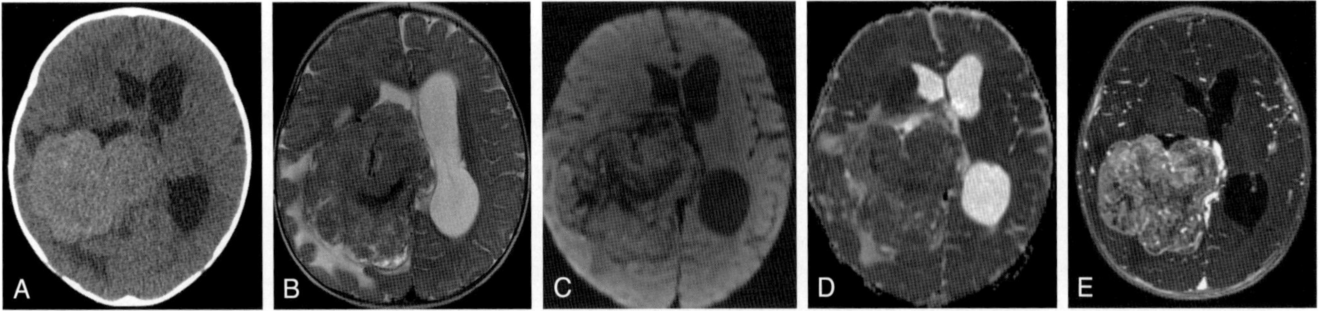

Fig. 7.83 Choroid Plexus Carcinoma. A 12-month-old with macrocephaly and vomiting. (A) Axial CT head, (B) axial T2W, (C) axial DWI, (D) axial ADC map, (E) axial T1W+C images demonstrate a hyperdense mass with T2W isointensity, isointense diffusion, and homogeneous enhancement in the posterior body and atrium of the right lateral ventricle with adjacent parenchyma edema.

Key Points

Background

- WHO grade 1 (papillomas), grade 2 (atypical papillomas), and grade 3 (carcinomas)
- 2% to 4% of all brain tumors in children; 20% to 40% of choroid plexus tumors are choroid plexus carcinomas
- *Young age (median age 1.5 years)*; slight male predominance
- Presentation with hydrocephalus from ventricular obstruction and/or CSF overproduction, focal neurologic deficits and seizures
- Arise from epithelium of the choroid plexus
- Choroid plexus papilloma (CPP) 5-year survival 90% to 100%; choroid plexus carcinoma (CPC) overall survival rate is 26% to 41%
- Location: *Trigone lateral ventricles* most common; less common fourth ventricle

Imaging

CT

- Isodense to hyperdense mass lesions with frond-like margins, often with calcification

MRI

- Well-defined, hypervascular frond-like T1W isointense to hypointense and T2W hypointense to hyperintense mass with avid enhancement. ADC signal may be isointense to brain parenchyma, typically lower than pilocytic astrocytoma, but higher than embryonal tumors. Peritumoral edema can be significant
- Imaging features that favor papilloma over carcinoma include lack of parenchyma invasion, no parenchymal edema, no internal necrosis, preserved cauliflower margin, T2W hyperintensity, and solid enhancement
- Metastatic at presentation is possible for both CPPs and CPCs → Total spine MRI performed at initial presentation to assess for drop metastases

Advanced Imaging

- MR perfusion: ↑ CBV and CBF
- MRS
  - CPP: ↑ myoI, ↓ Cr, Choline
  - CPC: ↓ myoI compared with CPPs, ↓ Cr; ↑ Lac and Lip

REFERENCES

1. Brandão LA, et al. Pediatric brain tumors. *Neuroimaging Clin N Am.* 2013 Aug;23(3):499–525.
2. Lam S, et al. Choroid plexus tumors in children: a population-based study. *Pediatr Neurosurg.* 2013;49(6):331–338.
3. Wolff JE, et al. Choroid plexus tumours. *Br J Cancer.* 2002;87(10):1086–1091.
4. Krieger MD, et al. Differentiation of choroid plexus tumors by advanced magnetic resonance spectroscopy. *Neurosurg Focus.* 2005;18(6A):E4 Published 2005 Jun 15.
5. Bull JG, et al. Discrimination of paediatric brain tumours using apparent diffusion coefficient histograms. *Eur Radiol.* 2012;22(2):447–457.

SUBEPENDYMAL GIANT CELL ASTROCYTOMA

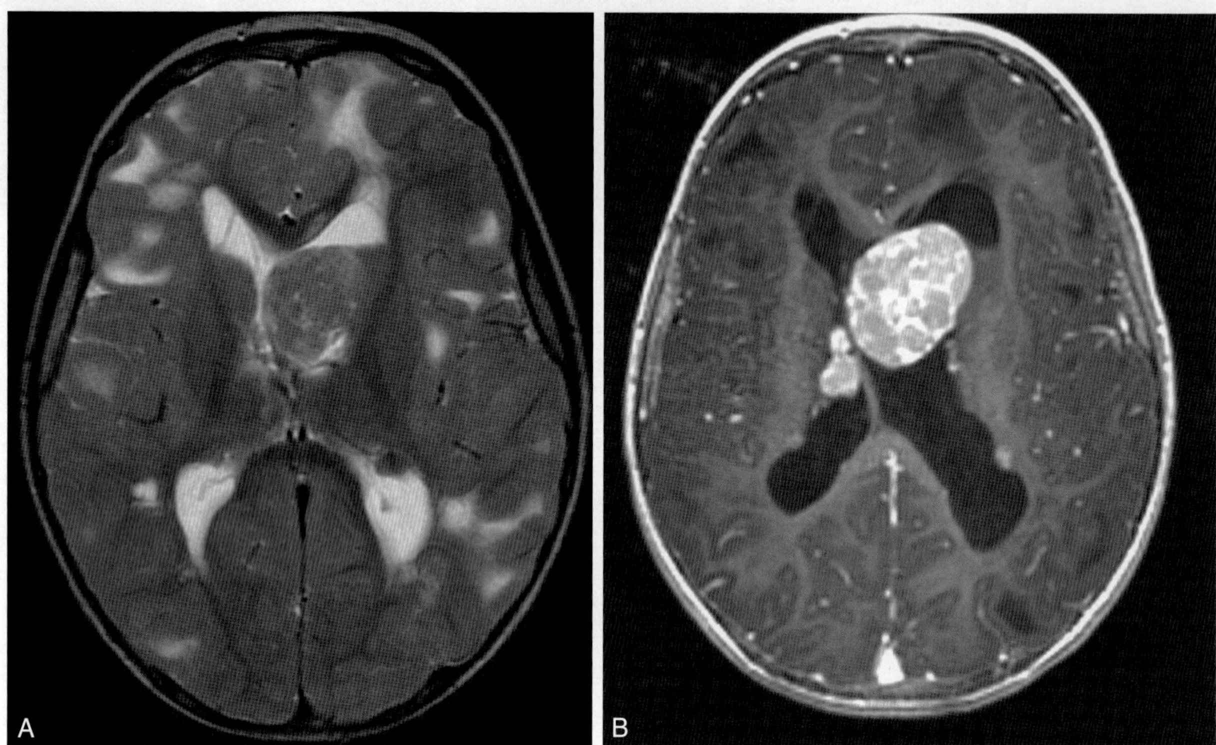

Fig. 7.84 Subependymal Giant Cell Astrocytoma. A 7-year-old with tuberous sclerosis. (A and B) Axial T2W and axial T1W+C images demonstrate a large homogeneously enhancing intraventricular mass in the left lateral ventricle. Additional MRI findings of tuberous sclerosis are present, including numerous cortical tubers and subependymal nodules.

Key Points

Background

- WHO grade 1
- 1% to 2% of all pediatric brain tumors
- Highly associated with *tuberous sclerosis*, occurring in 5% to 20% of patients with tuberous sclerosis (TS)
- Mean age at diagnosis: 16 years; males affected more often than females
- Mixed glioneuronal lineage. Arises from subependymal nodules
- Enlargement over time is the only definitive discriminator from subependymal nodule. An enlarging nodule at the foramen of Monro despite the size should be considered a subependymal giant cell astrocytoma (SEGA). If no prior imaging is available, a subependymal nodule at the foramen of Monro measuring greater than 1 cm is considered suspicious for a SEGA and requires follow-up imaging.
- Hydrocephalus, neurologic deficits, or seizures at presentation
- Treatment is surgical or mTOR inhibitor (rapamycin)
- 5-year survival: 92%
- Location: Lateral ventricle at the level of *foramen of Monro* is most common; may occur in other intraventricular locations

Imaging

CT

- Hypodense to isodense mass lesion often with calcification. Obstructive hydrocephalus of the lateral ventricles when large

MRI

- Well-defined, T1W isointense to hypointense and T2W isointense to hyperintense mass with avid enhancement. ADC isointense to brain parenchyma

Advanced Imaging

- MR Perfusion: not typically performed
- MRS: not typically performed

REFERENCES

1. Brandão LA, et al. Pediatric brain tumors. *Neuroimaging Clin N Am.* 2013 Aug;23(3):499–525.
2. Nguyen HS, et al. Subependymal Giant Cell Astrocytoma: A Surveillance, Epidemiology, and End Results Program-Based Analysis from 2004 to 2013. *World Neurosurg.* 2018;118:e263–e268.
3. Jóźwiak S, et al. Natural History and Current Treatment Options for Subependymal Giant Cell Astrocytoma in Tuberous Sclerosis Complex. *Semin Pediatr Neurol.* 2015;22(4):274–281.

COLLOID CYST

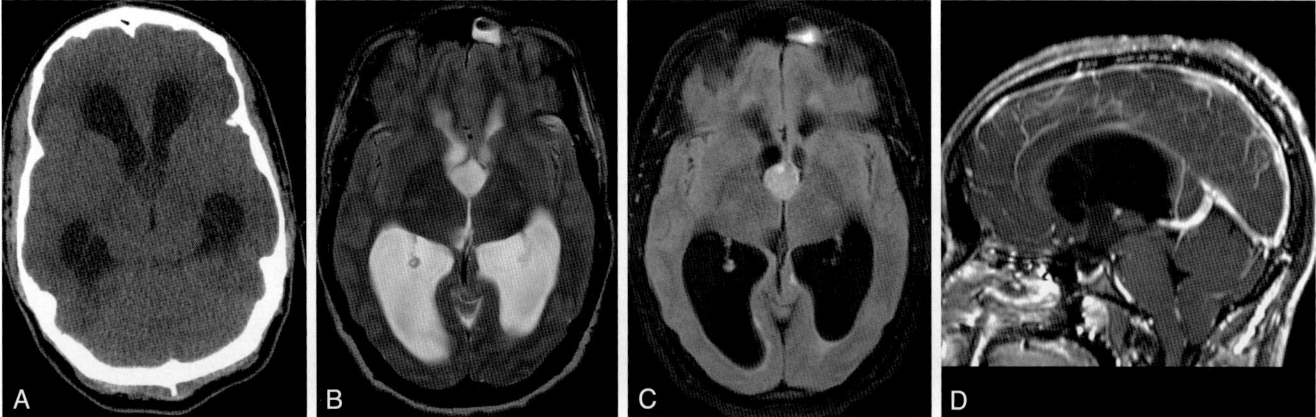

Fig. 7.85 Colloid Cyst. A 16-year-old with headache and vomiting. (A) Axial head CT, (B) axial T2W, (C) axial FLAIR, and (D) sagittal T1W+C images demonstrate a nonenhancing, well-defined cystic lesion at the foramen of Monro with secondary hydrocephalus. Colloid cysts may have variable density and signal intensity related to the protein concentration.

Key Points

Background

- Nonneoplastic, pseudostratified epithelial lined lesion with mucin producing goblet cells and interspersed ciliated cells
- Possibly endodermal origin lesion, similar to Rathke cleft cysts, versus neuroepithelial origin versus origin from the diencephalic vesicle or persistence of embryonic paraphysis
- Rarely presents in childhood
- Presentation with hydrocephalus, including sudden death from acute hydrocephalus, and/or headaches
- Increased size, volume, and increased extension into the third ventricle have increased risk of hydrocephalus, although smaller lesions may still present in an acute fashion
- Location: Anterior superior third ventricle

Imaging

CT

- Variable; often hyperdense due to high protein concentration; rarely calcified

MRI

- Highly variable T1W and T2W signal; absent or peripheral wall enhancement

Advanced Imaging

- MR Perfusion: not typically performed
- MRS: not typically performed

REFERENCES

1. Samadian M, et al. Colloid Cyst of the Third Ventricle: Long-Term Results of Endoscopic Management in a Series of 112 Cases. *World Neurosurg*. 2018;111:e440–e448.
2. Beaumont TL, et al. Natural history of colloid cysts of the third ventricle. *J Neurosurg*. 2016;125(6):1420–1430.
3. Sribnick EA, et al. Neuroendoscopic colloid cyst resection: a case cohort with follow-up and patient satisfaction. *World Neurosurg*. 2014;81(3-4):584–593.
4. Armao D, et al. Colloid cyst of the third ventricle: imaging-pathologic correlation. *AJNR Am J Neuroradiol*. 2000;21(8):1470–1477.

MULTIFOCAL CNS TUMORS

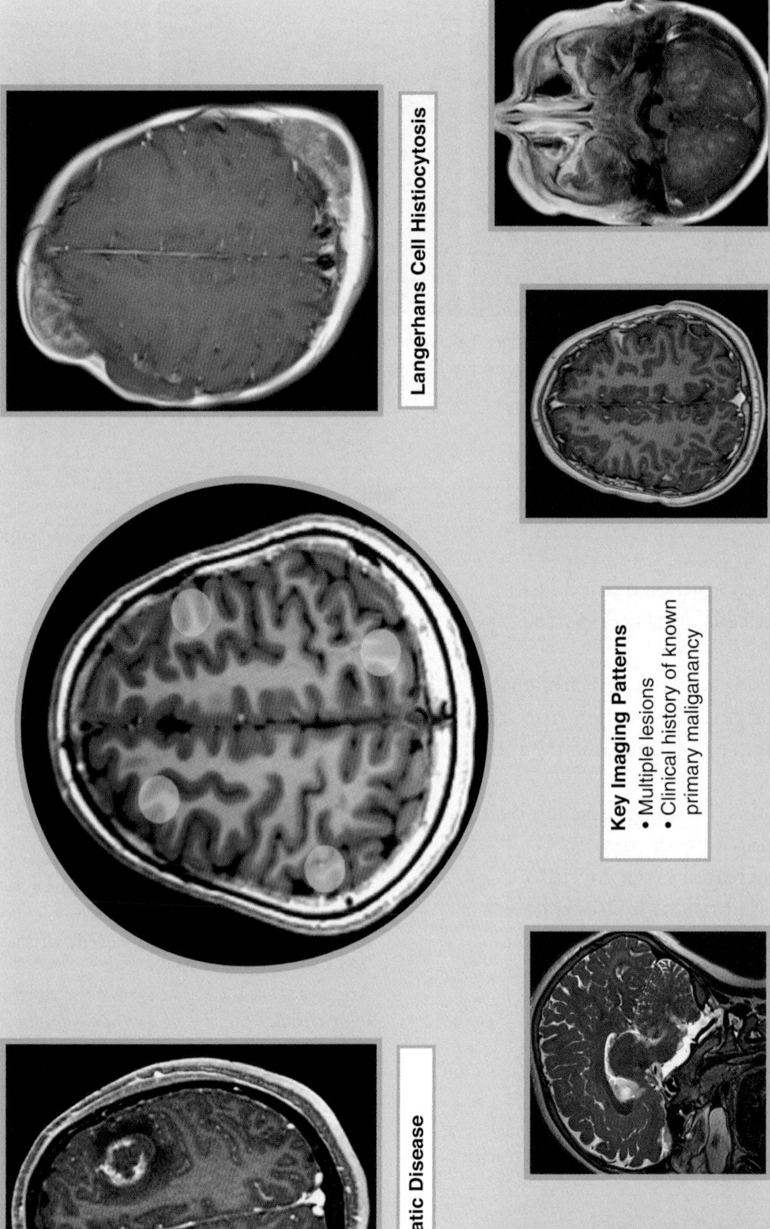

SYSTEMIC METASTASES

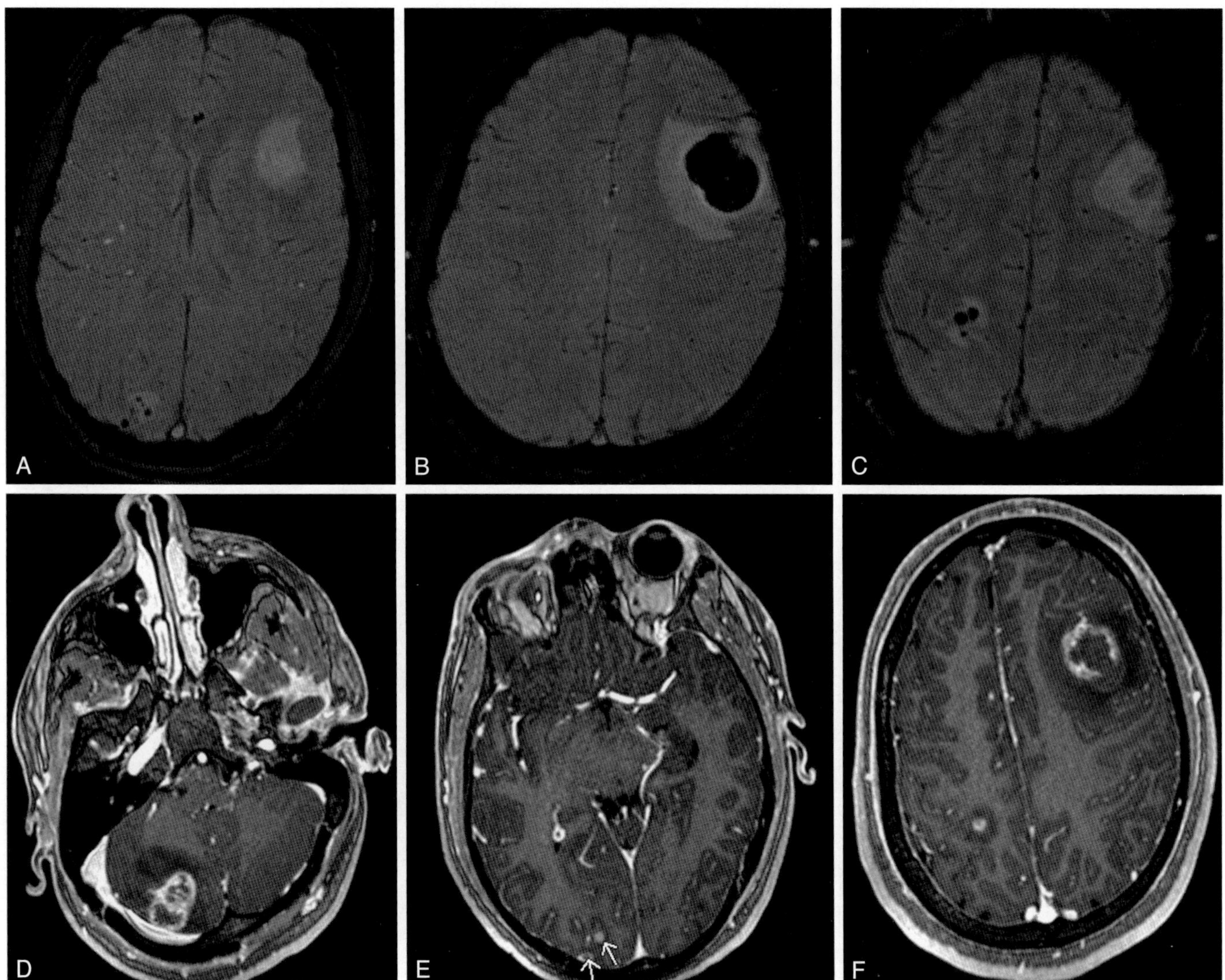

Fig. 7.86 Metastatic Disease. A 15-year-old with testicular cancer and hemorrhagic brain metastases. (A to C) Axial SWI, and (D to F) axial T1W+C images demonstrate numerous enhancing intraparenchymal lesions, many of which have associated susceptibility from hemorrhage and surrounding T1W hypointensity from edema.

Key Points

Background

- Metastases to the brain parenchyma from a solid tumor are uncommon in children compared to adults.
- Most common tumors with brain metastases are Ewing sarcoma, neuroblastoma, and osteosarcoma.

Imaging

- Solid or ring-enhancing intraparenchymal lesions with or without hemorrhage.

REFERENCE

1. Bouffet E, Doumi N, Thiesse P, et al. Brain metastases in children with solid tumors. *Cancer*. 1997 Jan 15;79(2):403–410.

DIFFUSE LEPTOMENINGEAL GLIONEURONAL TUMOR

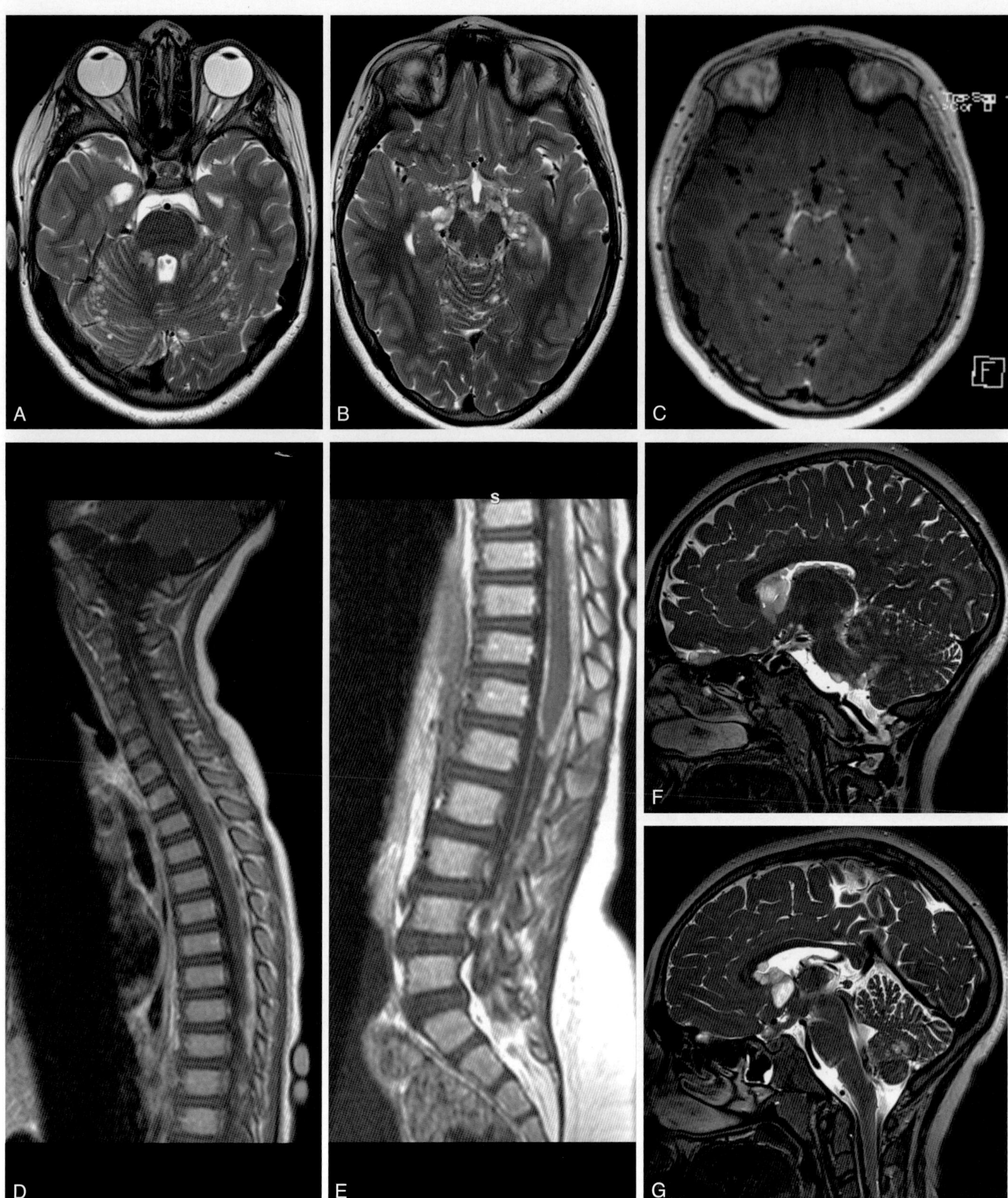

Fig. 7.87 Diffuse Leptomeningeal Glioneuronal Tumor. (A and B) Axial T2W, (C) axial T1W+C, (D and E) sagittal T1W+C spine, and (F and G) sagittal 3D T2W images demonstrate numerous enhancing and nonenhancing T2W hyperintense nodules along the cerebellar fissures, basal cisterns, ventricles, and spinal cord surface. 3D T2W imaging is particularly useful for these types of tumors as shown here.

Key Points

Background

- Entity appears in WHO 2016. Previously known as disseminated oligodendroglial-like leptomeningeal tumor (DOLT)
- Rare CNS neoplasm with oligodendrocyte-like cells, astrocytic cells, and neurons scattered in glial cells within desmoplastic or myxoid leptomeningeal stroma
- Pediatric presentation is most common; slight male predominance
- 5-year survival variable, depending on the grade of tumor, with some patients experiencing an aggressive clinical course
- Important to first exclude infectious or granulomatous disease (TB, sarcoid, fungal)
- Location: *Superficial parenchymal, and leptomeningeal location.* May occur anywhere in the neuroaxis, including supratentorial, but more commonly posterior fossa and spinal cord with secondary spread to the supratentorial with advanced disease. Central gray matter and intraventricular involvement may occur with advanced disease.

Imaging

CT

- Hypodense cystic foci along the periphery of the involved brain parenchyma

MRI

- Well-defined T1W hypointense and T2W hyperintense cystic foci along the surface of the parenchyma with mixed nonenhancing and enhancing foci
- Increased ADC signal
- Coexisting, potentially extensive, leptomeningeal enhancement especially along the cerebellum, basal cisterns, and spinal canal
- Early disease may reportedly begin as a single mass lesion with dissemination over time
- Total spine MRI performed at initial presentation

Advanced Imaging:

- MR Perfusion: not typically performed
- MRS: not typically performed

REFERENCES

1. Deng MY, et al. Molecularly defined diffuse leptomeningeal glioneuronal tumor (DLGNT) comprises two subgroups with distinct clinical and genetic features. *Acta Neuropathol.* 2018;136(2):239–253.
2. Kang JH, et al. A Diffuse Leptomeningeal Glioneuronal Tumor Without Diffuse Leptomeningeal Involvement: Detailed Molecular and Clinical Characterization. *J Neuropathol Exp Neurol.* 2018;77(9):751–756.

JUVENILE XANTHOGRANULOMA

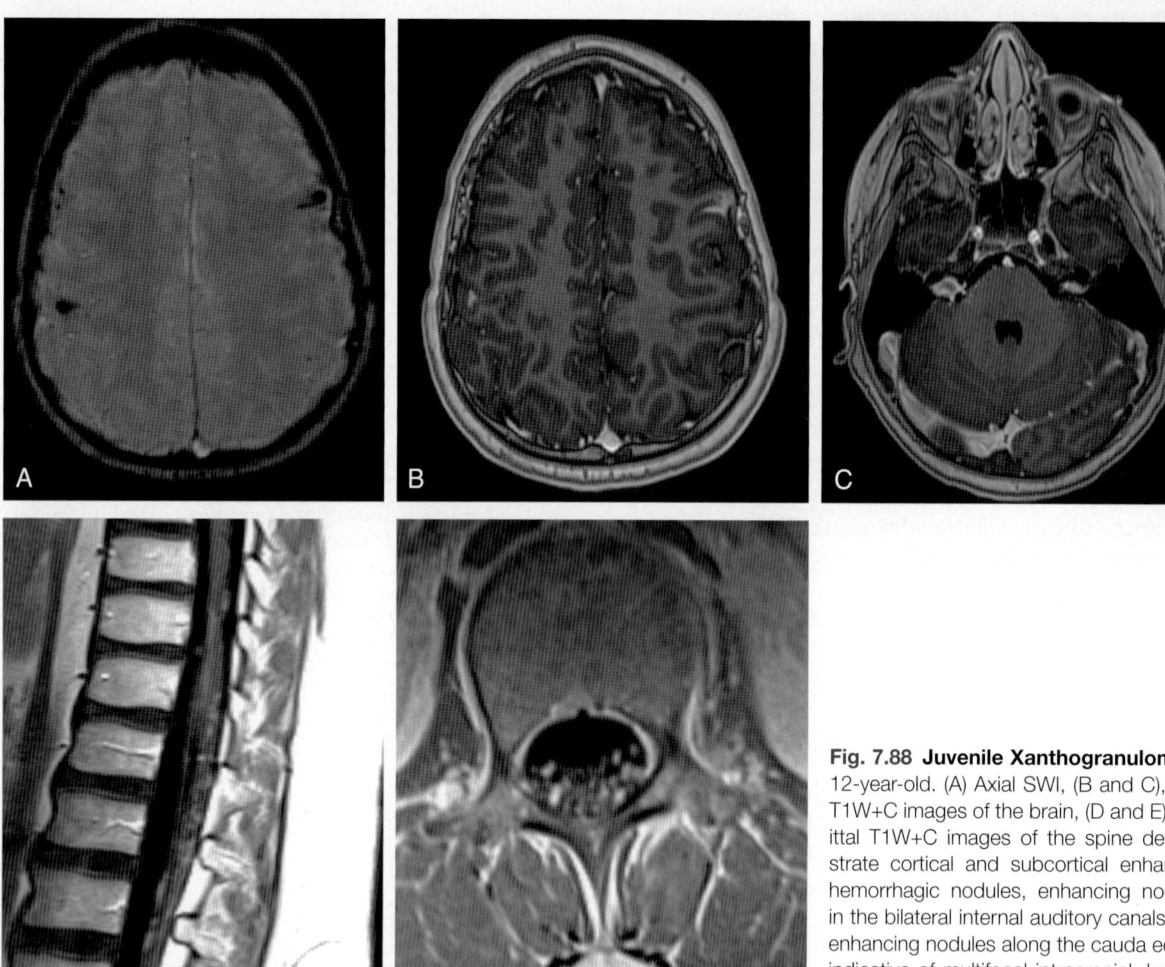

Fig. 7.88 Juvenile Xanthogranuloma. A 12-year-old. (A) Axial SWI, (B and C), axial T1W+C images of the brain, (D and E) sagittal T1W+C images of the spine demonstrate cortical and subcortical enhancing hemorrhagic nodules, enhancing nodules in the bilateral internal auditory canals, and enhancing nodules along the cauda equina indicative of multifocal intracranial Juvenile Xanthogranulomas.

Key Points

Background

- Rare, non-Langerhans cell histiocytosis
- Majority diagnosed in the first year of life
- Cutaneous lesions common but in approximately 10% of patients it can involve = a variety of other organ systems, including the central and peripheral nervous system and the head and neck
- Can be solitary or multifocal, dural, leptomeningeal, and/or parenchymal

Imaging

CT

- Hypodense mass lesions without hemorrhage or calcification

MRI

- Well-defined T1W isointense to hyperintense and T2W isointense to hypointense *avidly enhancing masses* with decreased ADC. Peritumoral edema may be present.

Advanced Imaging

- MR Perfusion: not typically performed
- MRS: ↑ taurine and glutamate

REFERENCES

1. Höck M, et al. The various clinical spectra of juvenile xanthogranuloma: imaging for two case reports and review of the literature. *BMC Pediatr*. 2019;19(1):128 Published 2019 Apr 24.
2. Lalitha P, et al. Extensive intracranial juvenile xanthogranulomas. *AJNR Am J Neuroradiol*. 2011;32(7):E132–E133.
3. Dehner LP. Juvenile xanthogranulomas in the first two decades of life: a clinicopathologic study of 174 cases with cutaneous and extracutaneous manifestations. *Am J Surg Pathol*. 2003;27(5):579–593.
4. Matsubara K, et al. Elevated taurine and glutamate in cerebral juvenile xanthogranuloma on MR spectroscopy. *Brain Dev*. 2016;38(10):964–967.
5. Ginat DT, et al. Imaging Features of Juvenile Xanthogranuloma of the Pediatric Head and Neck. *AJNR Am J Neuroradiol*. 2016;37(5):910–916.

HEMOPHAGOCYTIC LYMPHOHISTIOCYTOSIS

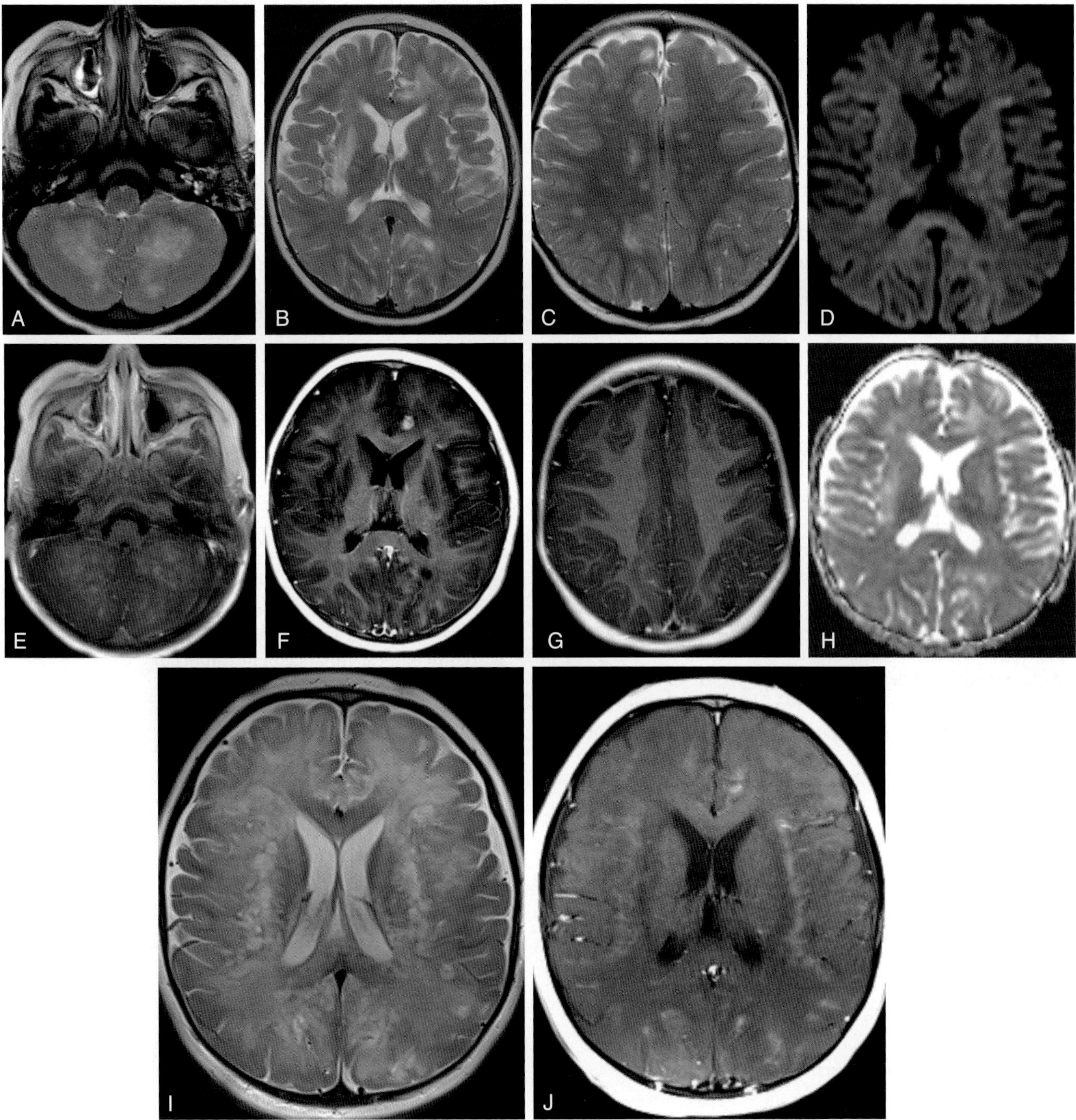

Fig. 7.89 Hemophagocytic Lymphohistiocytosis. A 14-month-old with encephalopathy. (A to C) Axial T2W, (D) axial DWI, (E to G) axial T1W+C, and (H) axial ADC at initial presentation demonstrates focal and confluent areas of T2W hyperintensity with elevated ADC and partial enhancement. A 3-month follow-up MRI (I and J) axial T2W and axial T1W+C images demonstrate confluent T2W hyperintensity, focal areas of white matter cavitation, extensive loss of myelin, continued multifocal parenchymal enhancement.

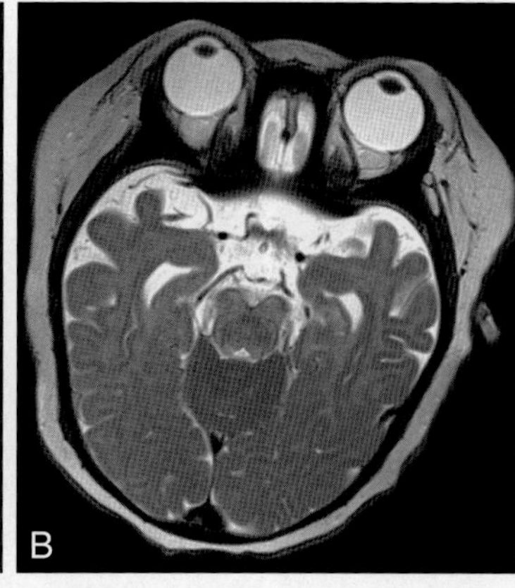

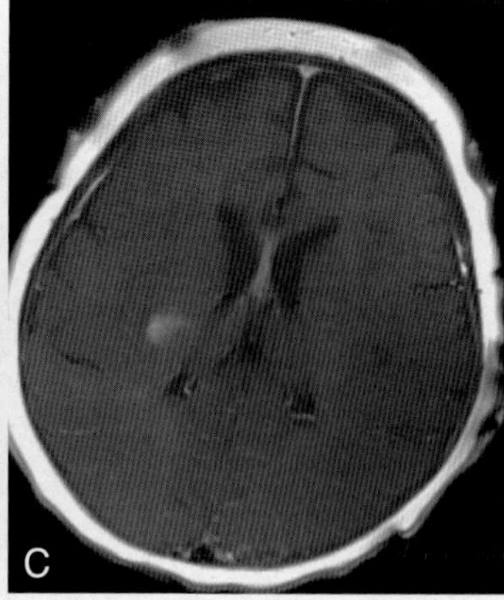

Fig. 7.90 Hemophagocytic Lymphohistiocytosis. (A and B) Axial T2W, and (C) axial T1W+C demonstrate T2W hyperintensity in the brainstem, cerebellum, and periventricular white matter. Note the enhancing lesion in the right corona radiata and the fornix.

Key Points

Background

- Primary or familial hemophagocytic lymphocytic histiocytosis (HLH) is autosomal recessive or X-linked presenting in infancy. Genetic basis involve multiple genes in the perforin-dependent granule exocytosis pathway.
- Secondary HLH, often presenting in adults, is associated with immune activation or immune deficiency including viral infections such as cytomegalovirus (CMV) and Epstein-Barr virus (EBV) and other organisms, including bacteria, and fungi as well as T cell malignancy and prolonged immunosuppression
- Pathogenesis includes hemophagocytosis in bone marrow, with persistent uncontrolled T lymphocyte and natural killer and macrophage activation, and overproduction of inflammatory cytokines
- Presentation with fever, hepatosplenomegaly, lymphadenopathy, neurologic manifestations, including encephalopathy, seizures, irritability, cranial nerve and motor deficits
- Involvement of multiple organs, including marrow, spleen, liver, lymph nodes, liver, and CNS
- In the CNS, infiltration by T-cell lymphocytes and histiocytes results in perivascular and meningeal infiltration and inflammation
- Location: Periventricular white matter, cortical/subcortical white matter, cerebellum, brainstem, and central gray matter are potential sites of involvement

Imaging

- Neuroimaging may be normal even in patients with neurologic symptoms in early stages or conversely can be abnormal in asymptomatic patients.

CT

- Periventricular white matter hypodensity, and parenchymal calcifications may occur

MRI

- Broad confluent or patchy regions of T2W signal hyperintensity in the affected parenchyma, especially in periventricular white matter, cerebellum, and brainstem
- Parenchymal volume loss
- Enhancing focal, diffuse or multifocal lesions, often small with perilesional T2W signal abnormality
- Lesions may show restricted diffusion
- Leptomeningeal enhancement can occur

Advanced Imaging

- MR Perfusion: not typically performed
- MRS: not typically performed

REFERENCES

1. Fitzgerald NE, et al. Imaging characteristics of hemophagocytic lymphohistiocytosis. *Pediatr Radiol.* 2003;33(6):392–401.
2. Al-Samkari H, et al. Hemophagocytic Lymphohistiocytosis. *Annu Rev Pathol.* 2018;13:27–49.
3. Niece JA, et al. Hemophagocytic lymphohistiocytosis in Texas: observations on ethnicity and race. *Pediatr Blood Cancer.* 2010;54(3):424–428.
4. Deiva K, et al. CNS involvement at the onset of primary hemophagocytic lymphohistiocytosis. *Neurology.* 2012;78(15):1150–1156.
5. Guandalini M, et al. Spectrum of imaging appearances in Australian children with central nervous system hemophagocytic lymphohistiocytosis. *J Clin Neurosci.* 2014;21(2):305–310.

SUMMARY OF BRAIN TREATMENT-RELATED COMPLICATIONS

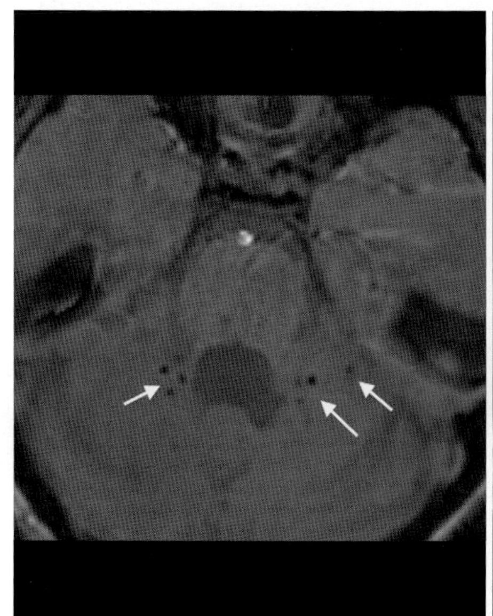

Microhemorrhages and Cavernous malformations.

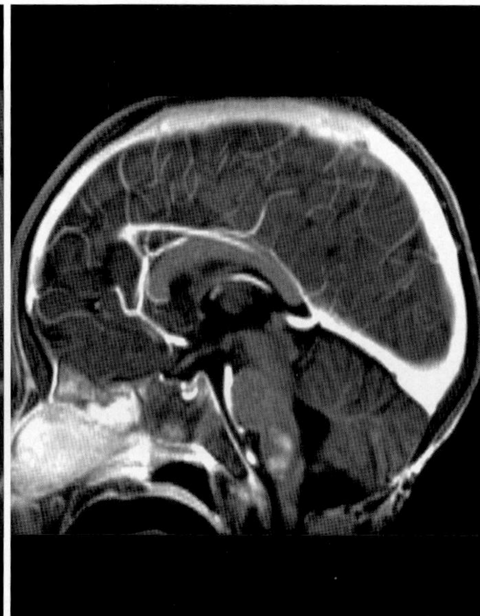

Radiation Necrosis.

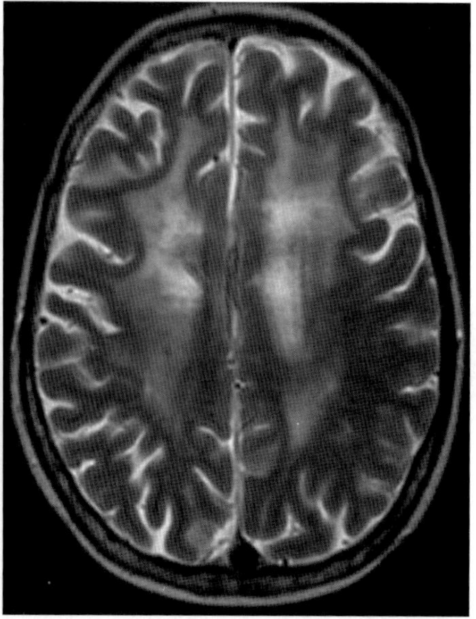

White Matter Injury.

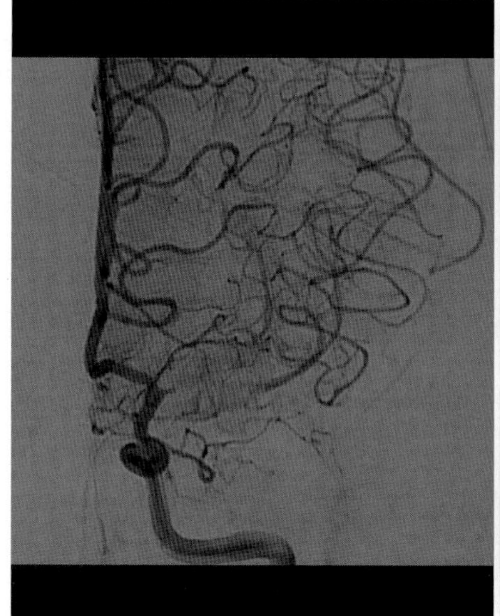

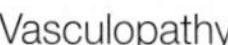

Vasculopathy.

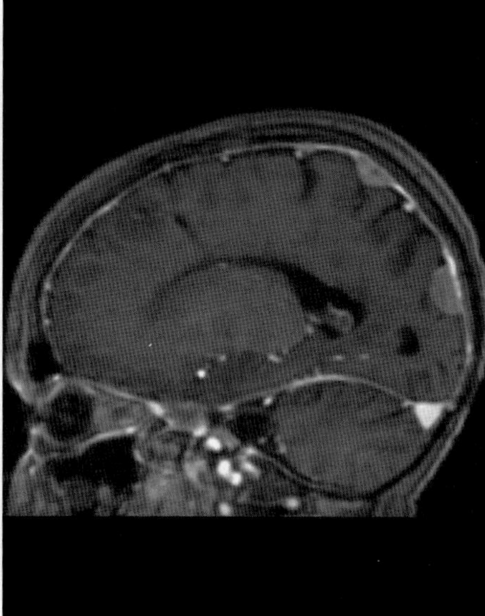

Tumors.

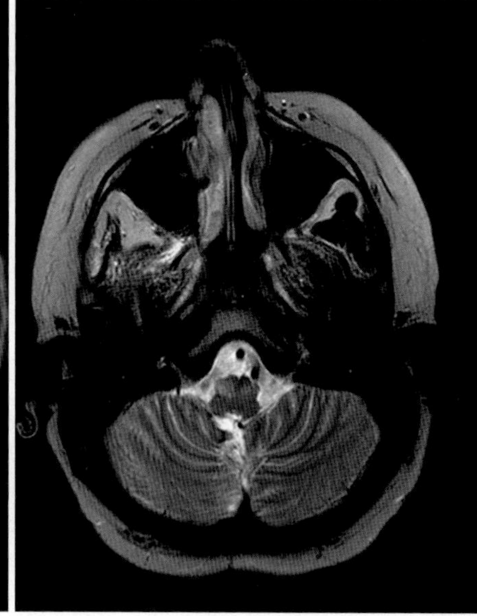

Hypertrophic Inferior Olivary Nuclear Degeneration.

RADIATION MICROHEMORRHAGES AND CAVERNOUS MALFORMATIONS

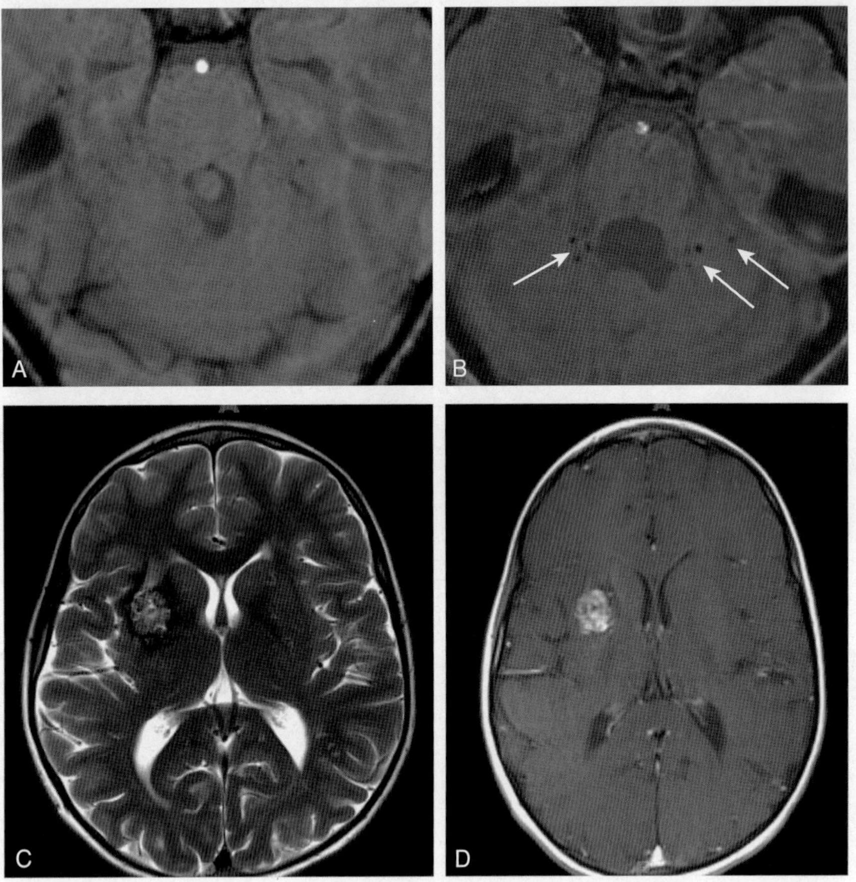

Fig. 7.91 Radiotherapy Microhemorrhages and Cavernoma. (A and B) A 3-year-old with medulloblastoma s/p resection, chemotherapy, and radiotherapy with (A) pre-radiotherapy and (B) post radiotherapy SWI images demonstrate new punctate foci of susceptibility (*arrows*) in the superior cerebellar hemispheres consistent with radiotherapy-related microhemorrhages. (C) Axial T2W and (D) axial T1W+C images demonstrate a cavernous malformation in the right putamen and corona radiata in a patient previously treated with radiotherapy.

Key Points

Background

- Median time to development of microhemorrhages is 8 months postradiation. Microhemorrhages accumulate over time. Presumed etiology is endarterial or capillary injury.
- Risk factors for proton radiation–induced microhemorrhages include percentage and volume of brain exposed to >30 Gy, maximum radiation dose, and younger age at irradiation.
- Radiotherapy-related cavernous malformations are associated with higher follow-up age, longer follow-up since diagnosis and since irradiation, whole brain irradiation, higher whole brain doses. Patients with cavernous malformations have a higher risk of suffering from neurologic symptoms (headache, seizure, history of stroke or TIA) and disability.
- Location: Irradiated brain parenchyma

Imaging

CT

- Microbleeds: Not identified by CT
- Cavernous malformations: Can be difficult to identify; Ill-defined or well-defined; mild hyperdensity; may present with acute hemorrhage with surrounding edema

MRI

- Microbleeds: Small (usually < 5 mm) foci of susceptibility on SWI or GRE T2* without T1W hyperintensity
- Cavernous malformations: Foci of variable size (usually > 5 mm) with T1W and T2W signal, typically T1W and T2W hyperintensity centrally with peripheral T2W hypointensity due to hemosiderin deposition. Larger lesions typically have enhancement. Perilesional edema suggests recent hemorrhage.

REFERENCES

1. Kralik SF, et al. Radiation-Induced Cerebral Microbleeds in Pediatric Patients With Brain Tumors Treated With Proton Radiation Therapy. *Int J Radiat Oncol Biol Phys*. 2018;102(5):1465–1471.
2. Gastelum E, et al. Rates and characteristics of radiographically detected intracerebral cavernous malformations after cranial radiation therapy in pediatric cancer patients. *J Child Neurol*. 2015;30(7):842–849.
3. Neu MA, et al. Susceptibility-weighted magnetic resonance imaging of cerebrovascular sequelae after radiotherapy for pediatric brain tumors. *Radiother Oncol*. 2018;127(2):280–286.

RADIATION NECROSIS

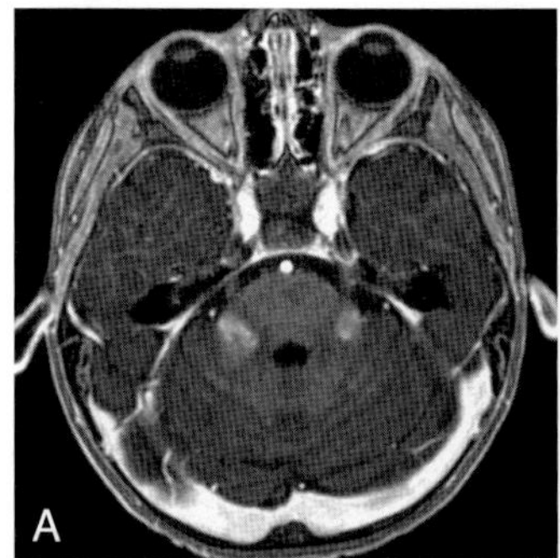

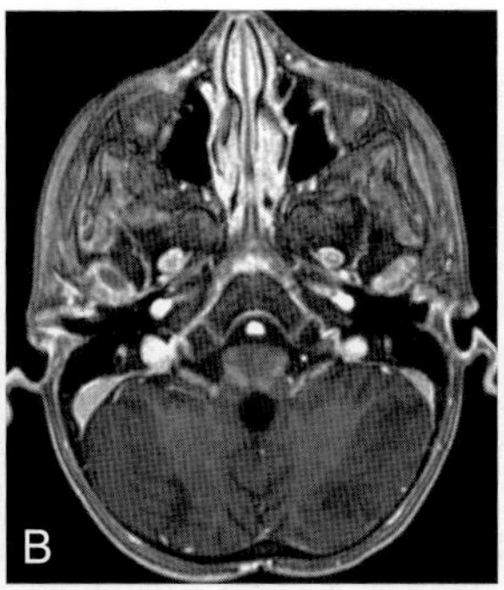

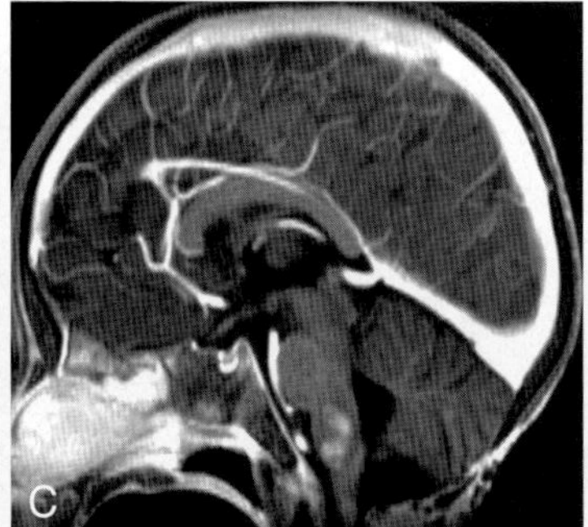

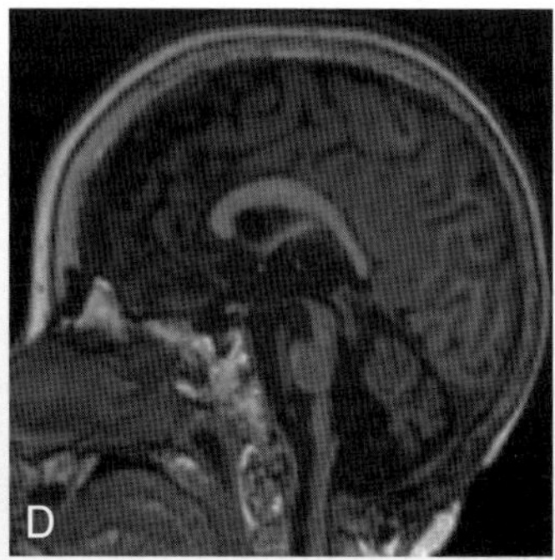

Fig. 7.92 Radiation Necrosis. A 23-month-old with history of posterior fossa ATRT who developed radiation necrosis 4 months after proton radiotherapy. (A to C) Axial and sagittal T1W+C images demonstrate multifocal non-mass-like areas of enhancement in the brainstem, and brachium pontis. (D) Follow-up sagittal T1W image demonstrates resolution of enhancement but significant brainstem and cerebellar atrophy.

Key Points

Background

- The incidence of radiation necrosis is ~5% with photon radiotherapy with median time to onset 1.2 months after completion of radiotherapy in a single series.
- The incidence of radiation necrosis on imaging is 17% to 31% with proton with median time to onset 5 months after completion of radiotherapy. Symptomatic radionecrosis occurs in ~7% of patients treated with proton radiotherapy. When Dmax (maximum point dose) and V55 (volume of brainstem receiving >55 Gy) are kept <55.8 Gy relative biologic equivalent (RBE) and <= 6% respectively, the, 5-year incidence of symptomatic radiation brainstem injury is <2%. However it is important to realize the percentage of brainstem radionecrosis detected by imaging is higher as this includes patients who may not have overt neurologic injury or that which is uncovered through rigorous testing.
- Exposure to chemotherapy has been associated with increased risk of radiation necrosis
- Children may have an increased risk of radiation necrosis compared to adults
- Location
  - Irradiated brain parenchyma. In children, given the dominance of posterior fossa neoplasms, radiation necrosis is often seen in the brainstem and cerebellar parenchyma

Imaging

- CT: May not be identifiable. Larger lesions appear as a region of hypodensity
- MRI
  - Subcentimeter enhancing foci in the irradiated volume that develop and regress spontaneously is the classical appearance. Restricted diffusion may occur
  - Classical radiation necrosis findings in adults of T2W signal abnormality with "lacy," "soap-bubble" enhancement are not typically seen in children except when a large residual tumor is treated such as for high grade gliomas of the pons and thalami.

REFERENCES

1. Kralik SF, et al. Radiation Necrosis in Pediatric Patients with Brain Tumors Treated with Proton Radiotherapy. *AJNR Am J Neuroradiol.* 2015;36(8):1572–1578.
2. Plimpton SR, et al. Cerebral radiation necrosis in pediatric patients. *Pediatr Hematol Oncol.* 2015;32(1):78–83.
3. Bojaxhiu B, et al. Radiation Necrosis and White Matter Lesions in Pediatric Patients With Brain Tumors Treated With Pencil Beam Scanning Proton Therapy. *Int J Radiat Oncol Biol Phys.* 2018;100(4):987–996.

RADIATION-INDUCED INTRACRANIAL VASCULOPATHY

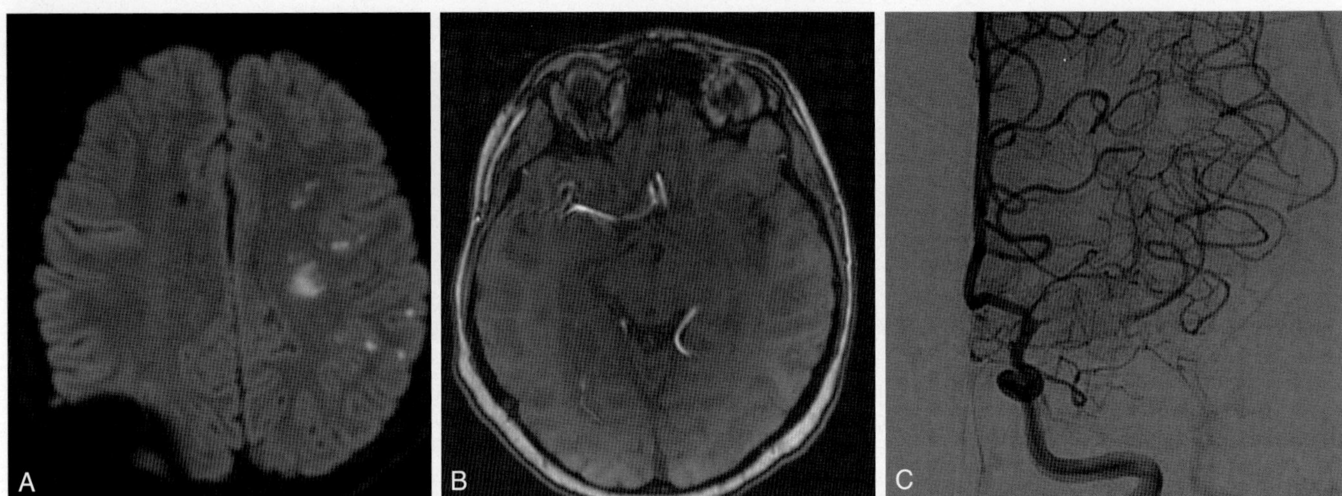

Fig. 7.93 Radiation-Induced Intracranial Vasculopathy. (A) Axial DWI image demonstrates multifocal DWI-hyperintense ischemic lesions in the central and subcortical left hemispheric white matter secondary to a radiation induced left middle cerebral artery vasculopathy. (B) Axial time-of-flight MRA demonstrates no flow-related signal in the left middle cerebral artery. (C) Coronal digital subtraction angiography after left ICA injection shows the M1 segment of the left middle cerebral artery is occluded.

Key Points

- Therapeutic cranial radiation may result in endothelial vessel wall damage resulting in focal thrombosis, dilatation, stenosis, and fibrosis.
- The radiation-induced vasculopathy (moyamoya pattern) increases the risk for ischemic lesions to the brain on top of radiation induced white and gray matter injury (demyelination, necrosis), development of cavernomas and capillary telangiectasia, and can be complicated by multifocal intracranial microhemorrhages.
- On CT/CTA and MRI/MRA, contour irregularity of the radiation exposed vasculature is noted with areas of stenosis and poststenotic dilatation. On contrast-enhanced black blood MR imaging, the thickened vessel wall typically shows contrast enhancement.
- Within the cerebral hemispheric gray and white matter, multifocal acute and/or chronic ischemic lesions can be noted, either within the vascular territory of the affected artery or in watershed distribution if the entirety of the circle of Willis is involved.
- Further research is needed to better understand risk factors and timing for development of radiation-induced intracranial vasculopathy. In one study, the mean time to development was 3 years (range 1–7.5 years). Tumors near the circle of Willis, particularly craniopharyngioma, appear to be more often associated with radiation vasculopathy.

REFERENCES

1. Murphy ES, Xie H, Merchant TE, Yu JS, et al. Review of cranial radiotherapy-induced vasculopathy. *J Neurooncol.* 2015;12293:421–429.
2. Kralik SF, Watson GA, Shih CS, Ho CY, et al. Radiation-induced large vessel cerebral vasculopathy in pediatric patients with brain tumors treated with proton radiation therapy. *Int J Radiat Oncol Biol Phys.* 2017 Nov 15;99(4):817–824.

RADIATION THERAPY-RELATED WHITE MATTER INJURY

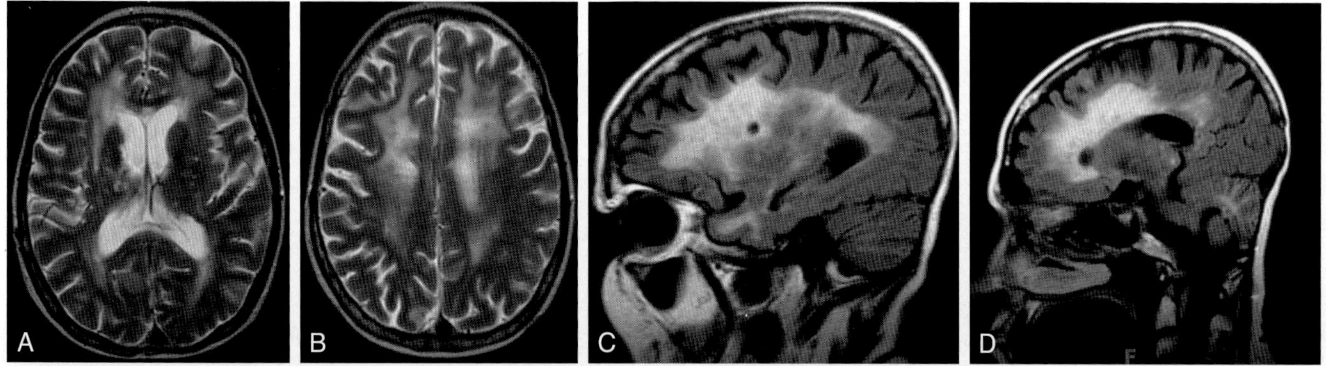

Fig. 7.94 Radiation Therapy–Related White Matter Injury. (A and B) Axial T2W and (C and D) sagittal FLAIR images demonstrate diffuse T2/FLAIR white matter hyperintensity associated with reduced white matter volume and mild ex vacuo enlargement of the lateral ventricles.

Key Points

Background

- Acute brain injury (days to weeks) postirradiation is rare in the modern era. Early delayed injury is seen 1 to 6 months postirradiation. Both are typically asymptomatic reversible and resolve spontaneously
- Late delayed injury (>6 months) postirradiation are irreversible and progressive. Multifactorial injury to the brain is likely to blame including a complex interplay between vascular and parenchymal injury phenomena. A proposed vascular etiology suggests that vascular damage leads to ischemia and white matter injury/necrosis. A proposed parenchymal etiology injury to the oligodendrocyte progenitors, astrocytes, activated microglial and neuron injury.
- Location: Periventricular and deep white matter

Imaging

CT

- White matter hypodensity

MRI

- Confluent T2W signal abnormality. Areas of enhancement and decreased ADC signal may occur. Decreased white matter volume occurs over time.
- Diffusion tensor imaging (DTI) has been used to assess white matter injury in adults and children and may be used to correlate with neurocognitive function. DTI is able to identify microstructural abnormalities even without abnormalities on conventional T1W and T2W sequences as evidenced by decreased fractional anisotropy (FA).

REFERENCES

1. Nieman BJ, et al. White and Gray Matter Abnormalities After Cranial Radiation in Children and Mice. *Int J Radiat Oncol Biol Phys*. 2015;93(4):882–891.
2. Greene-Schloesser D, et al. Radiation-induced brain injury: A review. *Front Oncol*. 2012;2:73. Published 2012 Jul 19.
3. Khong PL, et al. White matter anisotropy in post-treatment childhood cancer survivors: preliminary evidence of association with neurocognitive function. *J Clin Oncol*. 2006;24(6):884–890.
4. Khong PL, et al. Diffusion-tensor imaging for the detection and quantification of treatment-induced white matter injury in children with medulloblastoma: a pilot study. *AJNR Am J Neuroradiol*. 2003;24(4):734–740.

RADIATION THERAPY-RELATED TUMOR

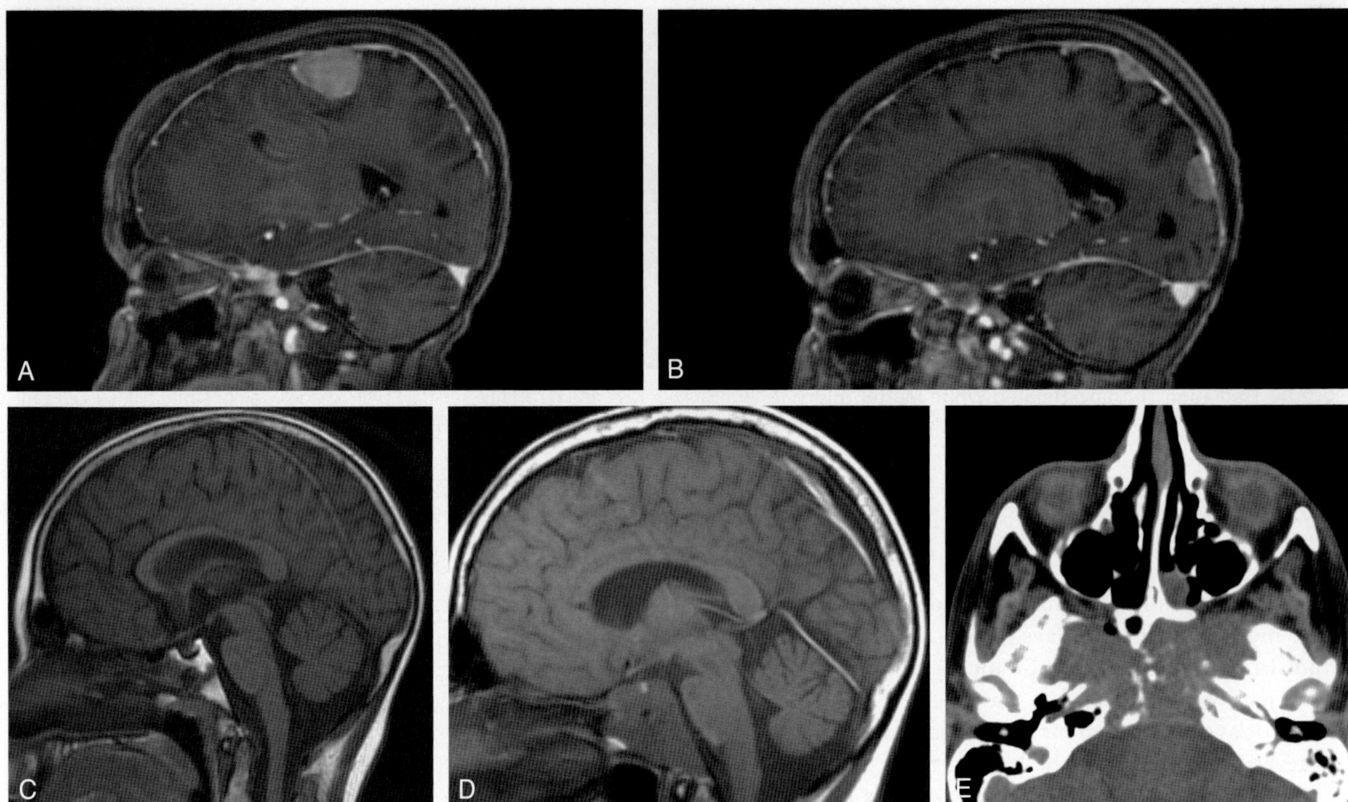

Fig. 7.95 Radiation Therapy–Related Tumors. (A and B) Sagittal T1W+C images of a 21-year-old patient who at age 4 was diagnosed with medulloblastoma and treated with surgery and chemoradiation. Multiple dural-based homogeneous enhancing tumors were identified and pathology confirmed multiple meningiomas. (C to E) A 16-year-old patient who at age 6 was diagnosed with a PNET and treated with surgery and chemoradiation. (C) Baseline sagittal T1W image 10 years after treatment demonstrates normal hyperintense T1W signal in the clivus related to fatty marrow; however, 6 months later a (D) sagittal T1W image now demonstrates T1W isointense signal infiltrating the clivus and (E) axial CT image demonstrates lytic destruction of the skull base. Pathology confirmed a high-grade undifferentiated sarcoma.

Key Points

Background

- Radiation-induced brain tumor criteria
  - Tumor must occur in the irradiated field
  - Sufficient latency period between radiation and occurrence of the tumor
  - Different histologic type than the original tumor irradiated
  - Absence of a tumor predisposition syndrome for said tumor
- Meningiomas are the most common brain tumor after cranial radiation, followed by gliomas
- Grade 1 to 3 meningiomas have been reported in the literature
- One or multiple meningiomas may occur
- Aggressive and multiple meningiomas are more common with higher radiation doses
- Latency period: 22.9± 11.4 years
- Imaging appearance of meningiomas is no different than nonirradiated patients

REFERENCES

1. Yamanaka R, et al. Radiation-Induced Meningiomas: An Exhaustive Review of the Literature. *World Neurosurg*. 2017;97:635–644.e8.
2. Ron E, et al. Tumors of the brain and nervous system after radiotherapy in childhood. *N Engl J Med*. 1988;319(16):1033–1039.
3. Cahan WG, et al. Sarcoma arising in irradiated bone: report of eleven cases. 1948. *Cancer*. 1998;82(1):8–34.

HYPERTROPHIC OLIVARY NUCLEAR DEGENERATION

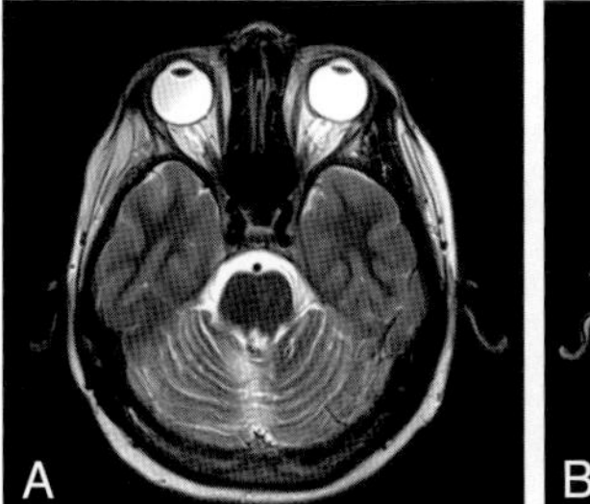

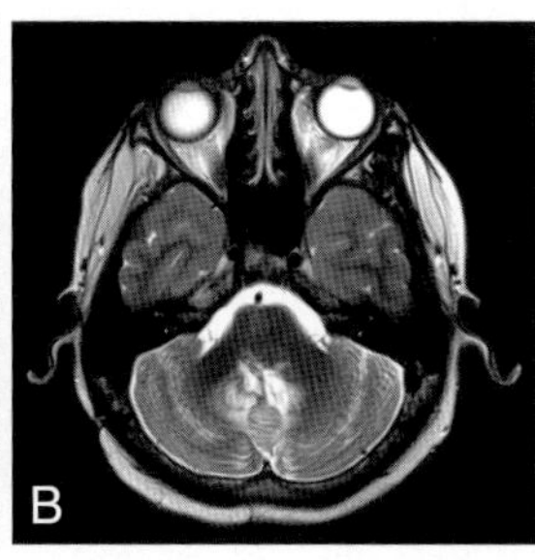

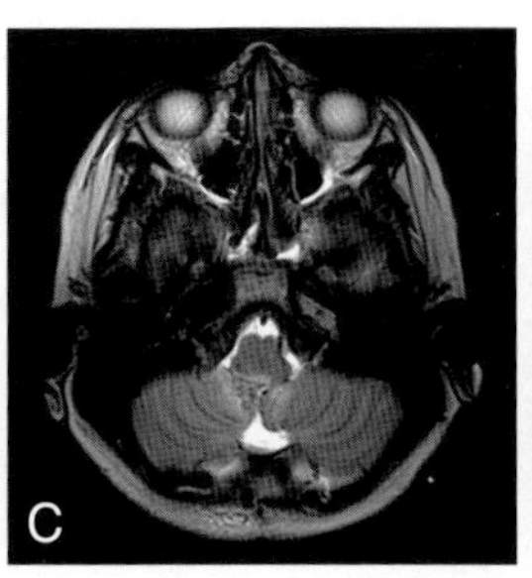

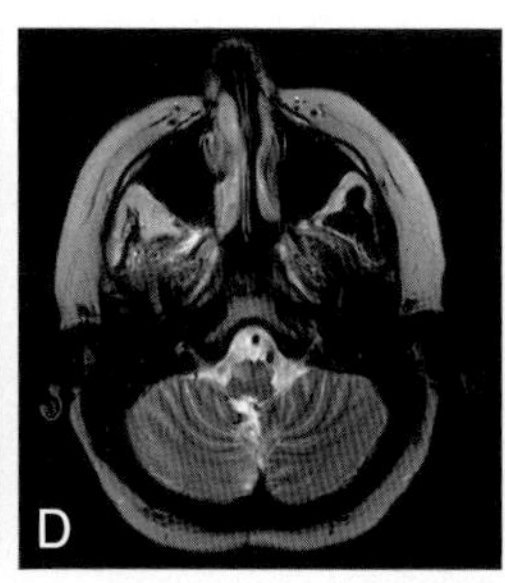

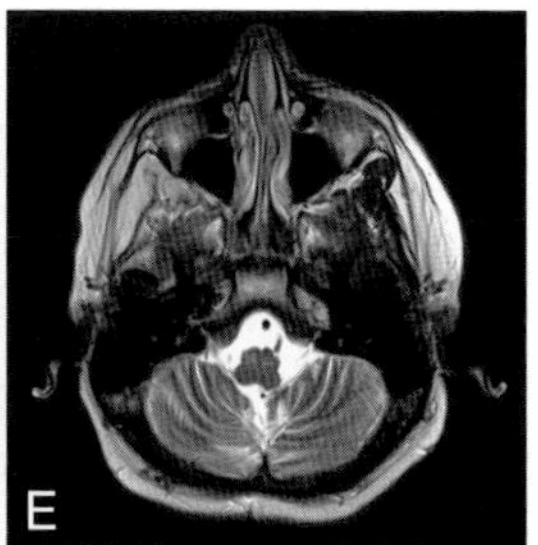

Fig. 7.96 Hypertrophic Olivary Nuclear Degeneration. A 9 year-old boy s/p gross total resection of posterior fossa medulloblastoma. (A and B) Axial T2W images demonstrate a midline resection cavity involving the bilateral superior cerebellar peduncles, right greater than left central tegmental tract, and gliosis of the dentate and peridentate parenchyma. (C) Axial T2W image of the immediate postoperative appearance of the medulla. (D) Axial T2W image at 1 year demonstrates right greater than left T2W hyperintensity in the inferior olivary nuclei with mild swelling. (E) Axial T2W image at 4 years demonstrates resolution of swelling and minimal residual T2W signal in the inferior olivary nuclei.

Key Points

Background

- A lesion within in the triangle of Guillain and Mollaret manifests with palatal tremor
- Transsynaptic degeneration resulting in neuronal vacuolation, increased glial cells, and demyelination
- Three anatomic structures and pathways in the triangle of Guillain and Mollaret (Fig. 7.97)
  - Dentate nucleus (contralateral)
  - Red nucleus
  - Inferior olivary nucleus
  - Superior cerebellar peduncle (red nucleus to contralateral dentate nucleus)
  - Inferior cerebellar peduncle (contralateral dentate nucleus to inferior olivary nucleus)
  - Central tegmental tract (red nucleus to inferior olivary nucleus)

Imaging

CT

- Difficult to identify

MRI

- MRI: T2W hyperintensity with or without hypertrophy of the inferior olivary nucleus depending on the stage of degeneration. Absence of enhancement. Increased ADC signal.
  - Three dynamic stages
    - Increased T2W signal of the inferior olivary nucleus (first 6 months)
    - Increased T2W signal and olivary hypertrophy (6 months to 3–4 years)
    - Increased T2 signal of the inferior olivary nucleus (>3–4 years)

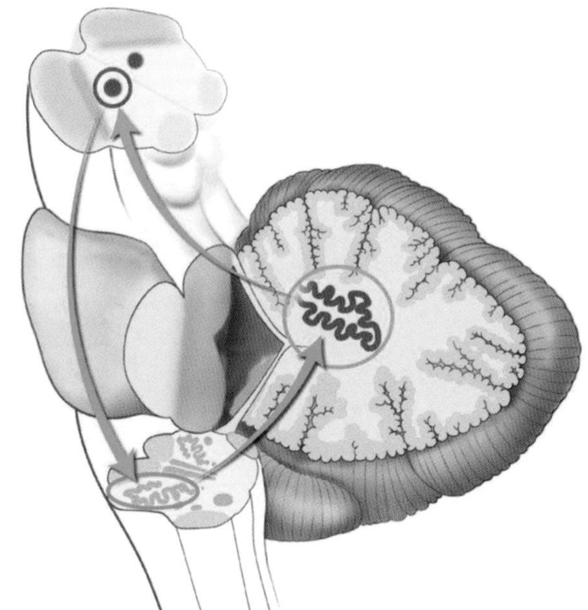

Fig. 7.97 Guillain-Mollaret Triangle (Dentato-Rubro-Olivary Pathway). This functional circuit is responsible for modulating spinal cord motor activity. It is composed of the ipsilateral red nucleus (RN) *(red circle)* of the midbrain, the ipsilateral inferior olivary nucleus (ION) *(green oval)* of the medulla, and the contralateral dentate nucleus (DN) *(orange circle)* of the cerebellum. The RN communicates with the ipsilateral ION via the central tegmental tract (CTT). The ION communicates with the contralateral DN via the inferior cerebellar peduncle. The DN communicates with the contralateral red nucleus via the superior cerebellar peduncle (SCP). The lesions that affect the afferent pathways to the olive result in hypertrophic olivary degeneration (HOD). Therefore lesions resulting in HOD of the right ION would involve the right RN, the right CTT, the left DN, or the left SCP. Lesions affecting efferent pathways to the olive (inferior cerebellar peduncle lesions) are less likely to cause HOD. (From Small JE, Noujam DL, Ginat DT, Kelly HR, Schaefer PW. *Neuroradiology: Spectrum and Evolution of Disease.* Elsevier; 2019.)

REFERENCES

1. Goyal M, et al. Hypertrophic olivary degeneration: metaanalysis of the temporal evolution of MR findings. *AJNR Am J Neuroradiol.* 2000;21(6):1073–1077.
2. Meoded A, et al. Diffusion tensor imaging in a child with hypertrophic olivary degeneration. *Cerebellum.* 2013;12(4):469–474.

8 Epilepsy

INTRODUCTION

Background

Epilepsy is a chronic seizure condition in which abnormal excessive or uncoordinated neuronal activity leads to abnormal brain function. About 1% of children in the United States have epilepsy. Approximately 66% to 75% of children with epilepsy will become seizure free with anticonvulsant medication. Intractable epilepsy is defined as failure of two or more appropriate antiepileptic drugs and more than one seizure per month over an 18-month period.

Common testing used in the evaluation of epilepsy includes electroencephalogram (EEG), CT, MRI, PET, single-photon emission computerized tomography (SPECT), and magnetoencephalography (MEG). Epilepsy can be nonlesional or lesional depending on whether a structural abnormality can be detected by standard anatomic imaging. If a structural lesion can be identified, the odds of becoming seizure free are at least 2.5 times higher than nonlesional epilepsy. Although there is value in lesion detection, epilepsy is a network disorder, and remote areas of the brain are affected by the epileptogenic focus.

Imaging can lead to further invasive monitoring with depth electrodes as well as surgical treatment. A variety of surgical treatment options are available, depending on seizure and presence of a lesion. Options include lesion resection or ablation, lobectomy, hemispherectomy, corpus callosotomy, vagal nerve stimulation, and responsive neurostimulation (RNS).

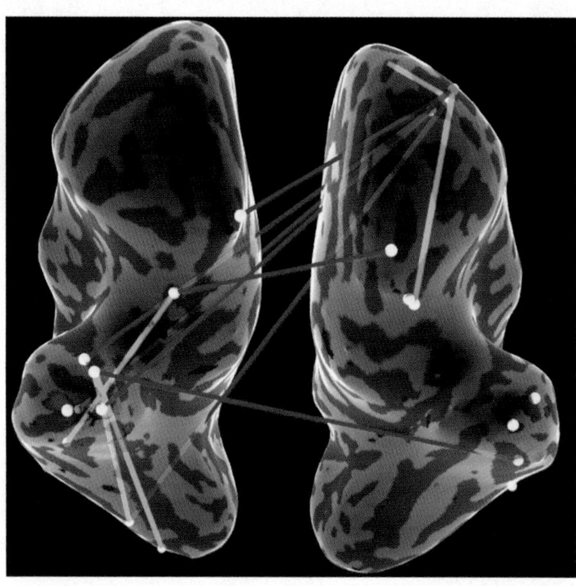

Fig. 8.1 Epilepsy. Effective connectivity derived from magnetoencephalography (MEG) between a seizure focus and other brain locations, demonstrating the principle of epilepsy as a network disorder. (Image courtesy of Dr. Noam Peled, created using the Multi-Modal Neuroimaging Analysis and Visualization Tool (MMVT) https://doi.org/10.48550/arXiv.1912.10079).

Imaging

The primary imaging modality for epilepsy is MRI. High-resolution MRI at 3.0T using 32 to 64 channel head coils provides exquisite anatomic detail necessary for detection of lesions, particularly cortical dysplasias. To maximize chances of detecting subtle lesion such as cortical dysplasias, MRI protocols should include the following sequences: a 3D T1W with 1-mm slice thickness, a 3D FLAIR with 1-mm slice thickness, coronal oblique T2W and FLAIR imaging through the hippocampi, axial T2W, axial susceptibility-weighted imaging (preferred over gradient echo), and axial DWI/DTI. Contrast not typically recommended unless a mass is identified or acute presentation with first-time seizure, necessitating investigation for various acute neurologic emergencies such as meningitis.

Fluorodeoxyglucose positron emission tomography (FDG PET) CT is commonly used in the evaluation of epilepsy. FDG is distributed to the brain by cerebral blood flow, but subsequent distribution reflects glucose utilization and neuronal function. The majority of epileptogenic lesions are hypometabolic, and the region of hypometabolism often extends beyond the lesion, indicating the effects are broader than the lesion itself but also limiting precise lesion localization. FDG PET is approximately 85% sensitive for temporal lobe epilepsy and 33% to 55% sensitive for extratemporal lobe epilepsy.

Single-photon emission computerized tomography (SPECT) is used for identifying epileptogenic lesions based on the principle that there is increased ictal regional cerebral blood flow and decreased interictal regional blood flow. There is greater sensitivity of ictal SPECT versus interictal SPECT because there is a larger increase in ictal perfusion (~50%) compared to the interictal perfusion reduction, typically 0 to 10% and at most 40% reduction. The accuracy of SPECT is improved by subtraction ictal SPECT coregistered to MRI (SISCOM), which subtracts the ictal SPECT and interictal SPECT and coregisters this to MRI. False localization with SPECT can be caused by propagation of ictal activity and/or rapid switch from ictal hyperperfusion to postictal hypoperfusion. Injection time of the radiotracer ^{99}Tc-HMPAO is critical for accuracy, and an injection time <20 seconds from time of seizure reduces false localization.

Functional MRI (fMRI) can be used to localize the motor and language networks for surgical candidates. Determination of language lateralization in relationship to the lesion is helpful in predicting postoperative language function. Children present more challenges in performing fMRI compared with adult patients due to issues of patient motion, cooperation, and sedation requirements. Because of this, there is significant need for development of resting state fMRI as a tool for localizing motor and language

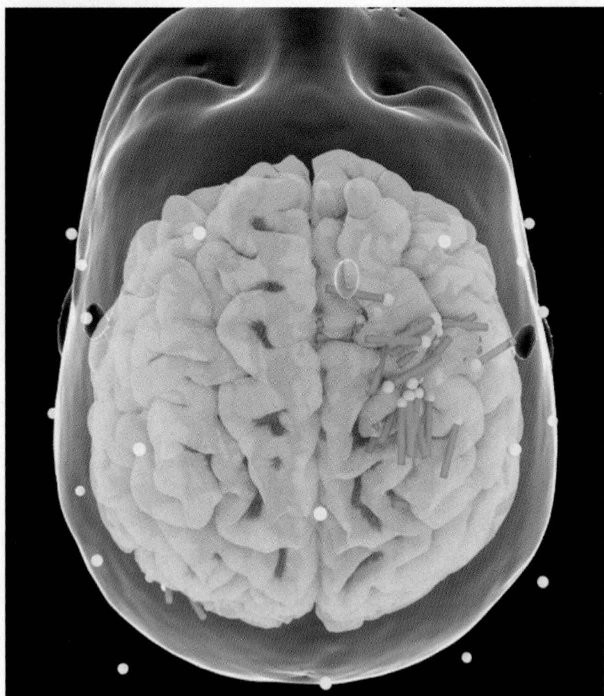

Fig. 8.2 MEG clusters overlaid on volumetric MRI localize to the epileptogenic region. (Image courtesy of Dr. Noam Peled, created using the Multi-Modal Neuroimaging Analysis and Visualization Tool (MMVT) https://doi.org/10.48550/arXiv.1912.10079).

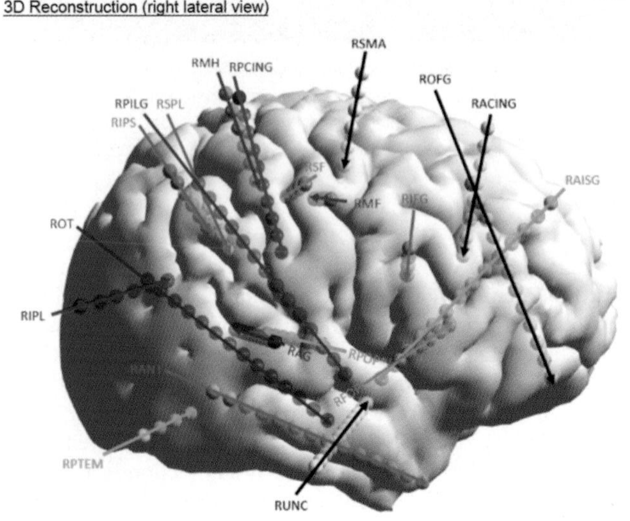

Fig. 8.3 Epilepsy depth electrodes visualized on a 3D MRI of the brain in a patient with epilepsy.

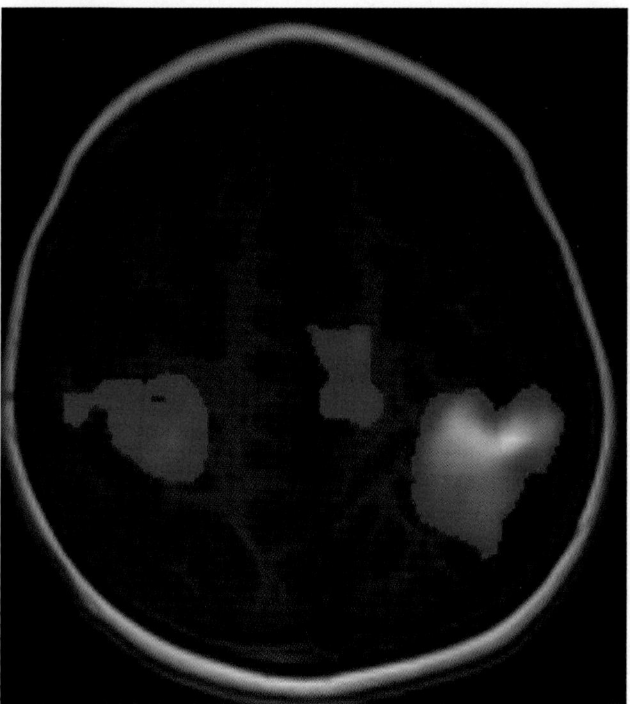

Fig. 8.4 Epilepsy. A 2-year-old with epilepsy. Resting state fMRI bilateral sensorimotor networks from independent component analysis were obtained despite the patient being unable to complete a motor task because of young age and need for sedation.

regions in children with epilepsy. A greater percentage of atypical language lateralization is seen in children with epilepsy, and epilepsy medications can alter the fMRI networks.

The ability of diffusion tensor imaging (DTI) to depict major white matter tracts, such as corticospinal tracts or optic radiations, is useful for planning surgical approaches to lesions. DTI has also shown value differences in regional and whole-brain white matter microstructure in epilepsy patients, further supporting the notion of epilepsy as a network disorder.

This chapter illustrates common and uncommon causes of epilepsy, imaging patterns seen with acute seizures, and postsurgical appearances of the brain following epilepsy surgery.

REFERENCE

1. Felsenstein O, Peled N, Hahn E, et al. Multi-Modal Neuroimaging Analysis and Visualization Tool (MMVT). arXiv.org. https://doi.org/10.48550/arXiv.1912.10079. Published June 2, 2022. Accessed September 8, 2022.

SUMMARY: EPILEPTOGENIC LESIONS

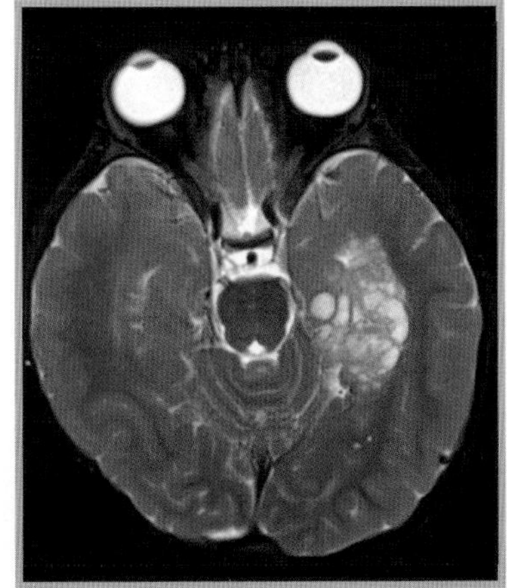

Tumors

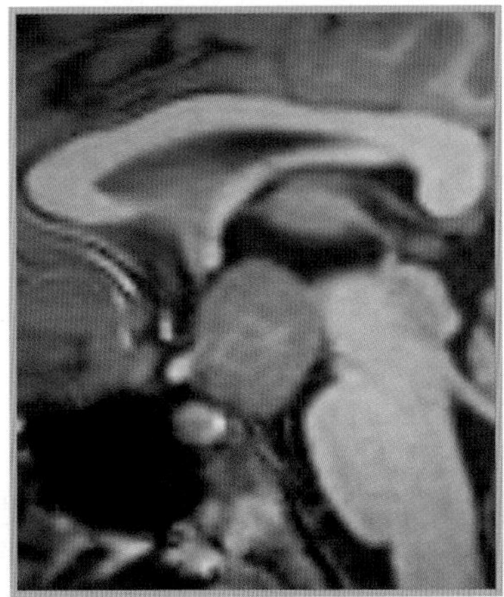

Hamartoma

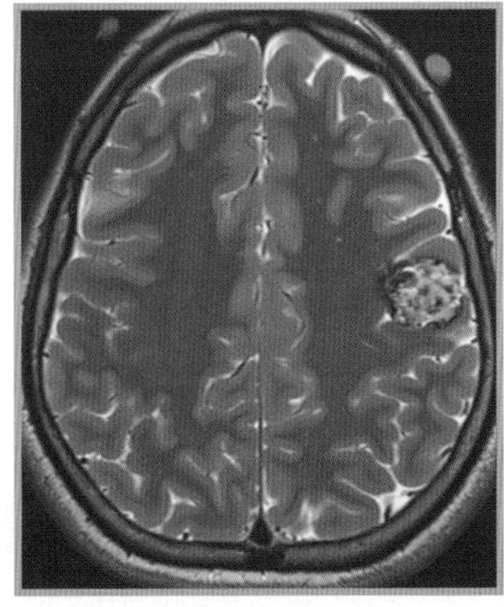

Cavernous Malformation

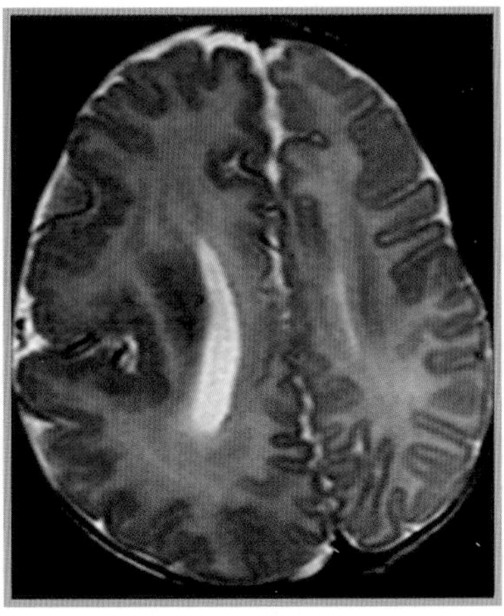

Cortical Malformation

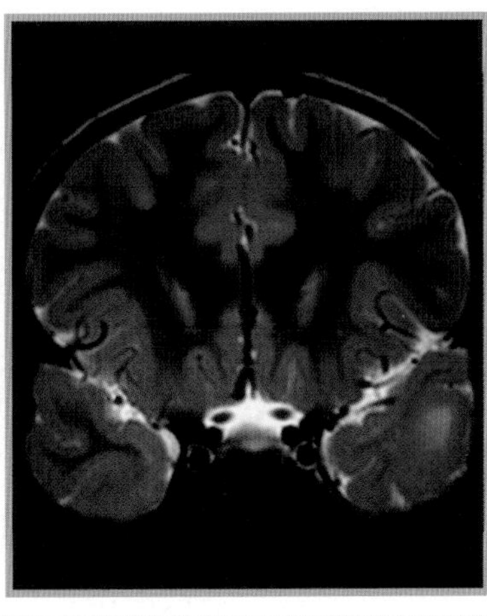

Cortical Dysplasia

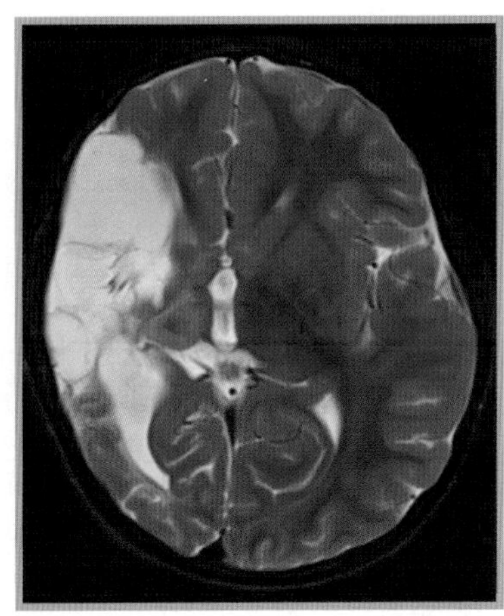

Encephalomalacia

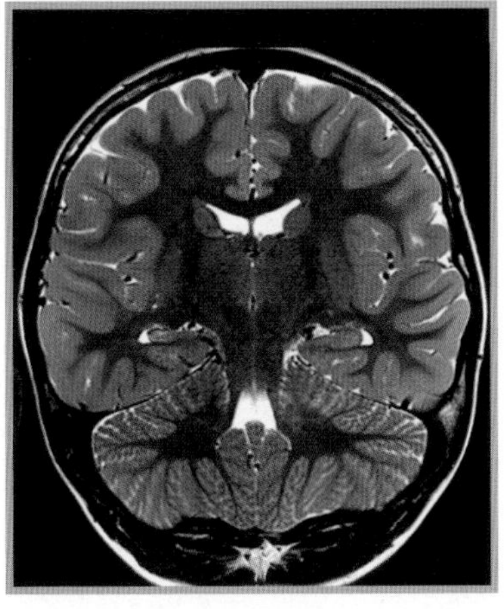

Mesial Temporal Sclerosis

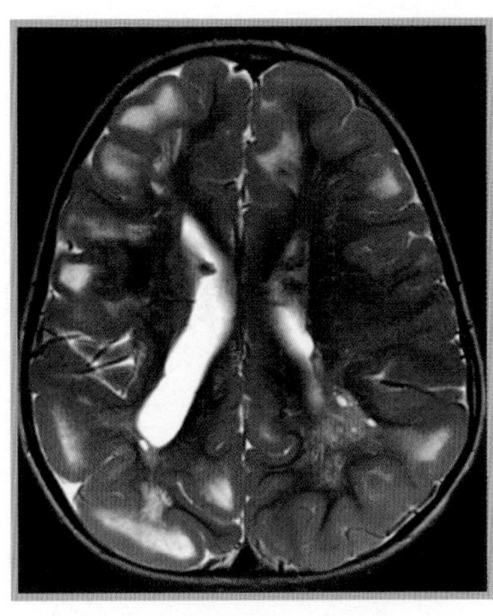

Tuberous Sclerosis

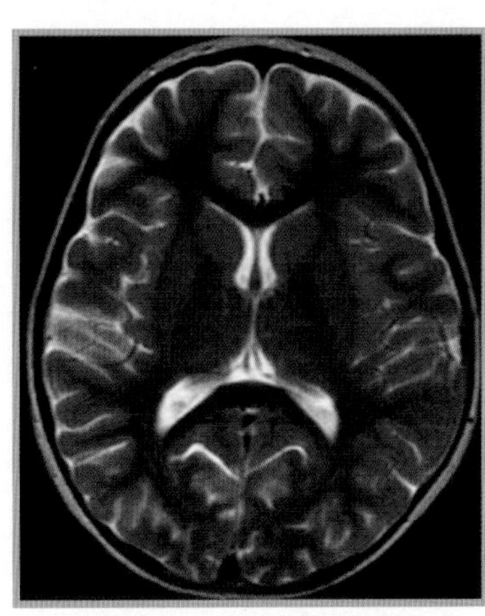

Rasmussen Encephalitis

FOCAL CORTICAL DYSPLASIAS

TABLE 8.1 Histopathologic Classification of Focal Cortical Dysplasias.

FCD Type 1	
1a	Abnormal radial cortical lamination
1b	Abnormal tangential cortical lamination
1c	Abnormal radial and tangential cortical lamination
FCD Type 2	
2a	Dysmorphic neurons
2b	Dysmorphic neurons and balloon cells
FCD Type 3	
3a	Cortical lamination abnormalities in the temporal lobe associated with hippocampal sclerosis
3b	Cortical lamination abnormalities adjacent to a glial or glioneuronal tumor
3c	Cortical lamination abnormalities adjacent to a vascular malformation
3d	Cortical lamination abnormalities adjacent to any other lesion acquired during early life (e.g., perinatal ischemia, trauma, hemorrhage, encephalitis)

Key Points

- Focal cortical dysplasia was originally described by Taylor in 1971 in patients with localized seizures. Current classification by the International League Against Epilepsy (ILAE) divides focal cortical dysplasias as shown in Table 8.1.
- Focal cortical dysplasias occur in an estimated prevalence of 10% of all patients with epilepsy and 50% of children undergoing surgery for intractable epilepsy.
- FCD type 1 is classified as a malformation due to abnormal post migrational development while FCD type 2 represents a malformation due to abnormal proliferation or apoptosis.
- Recent genetic findings have shown that mutations in genes involved in the MTOR pathway can lead to FCD type 2 as well as tuberous sclerosis, hemimegalencephaly and megalencephaly. The MTOR pathways regulates cell proliferation, growth, metabolism and survival and mutations associated with these disorders cause an upregulation of the MTOR pathway. The timing of a somatic mutation during cortical development leading to mosaicism explains how these mutations can lead to a large region of malformation as seen in hemimegalencephaly (early somatic mutation) versus a small region of malformation seen in FCD (late mutation). In addition, disorders can be caused by a combined germline and somatic mutation (two hit mutation) and the timing of the somatic mutation again can lead to this phenotypic difference.

REFERENCE

1. Najm IM, Sarnat HB, Blümcke I, et al. Review: The international consensus classification of Focal Cortical Dysplasia - a critical update 2018. *Neuropathol Appl Neurobiol.* 2018 Feb;44(1):18–31.

FOCAL CORTICAL DYSPLASIA TYPE 1

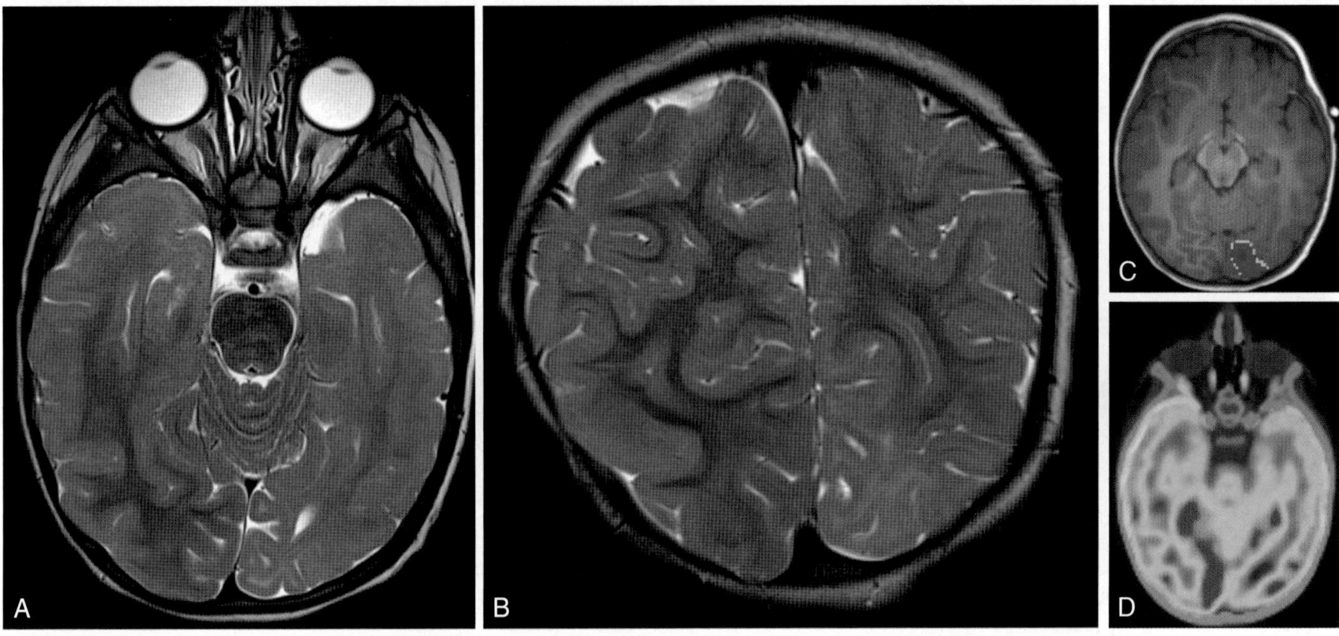

Fig. 8.5 Focal Cortical Dysplasia Type 1. A 2-year-old with epilepsy. (A and B) Axial and coronal T2W images demonstrate asymmetric left occipital juxtacortical T2W hyperintense signal with slight volume loss. (C) Subtraction ictal SPECT coregistered to MRI (SISCOM) image demonstrates corresponding increased flow to the area of dysplasia. (D) FDG PET CT demonstrates hypometabolism in the area of the dysplasia. Pathology was an FCD type 1B.

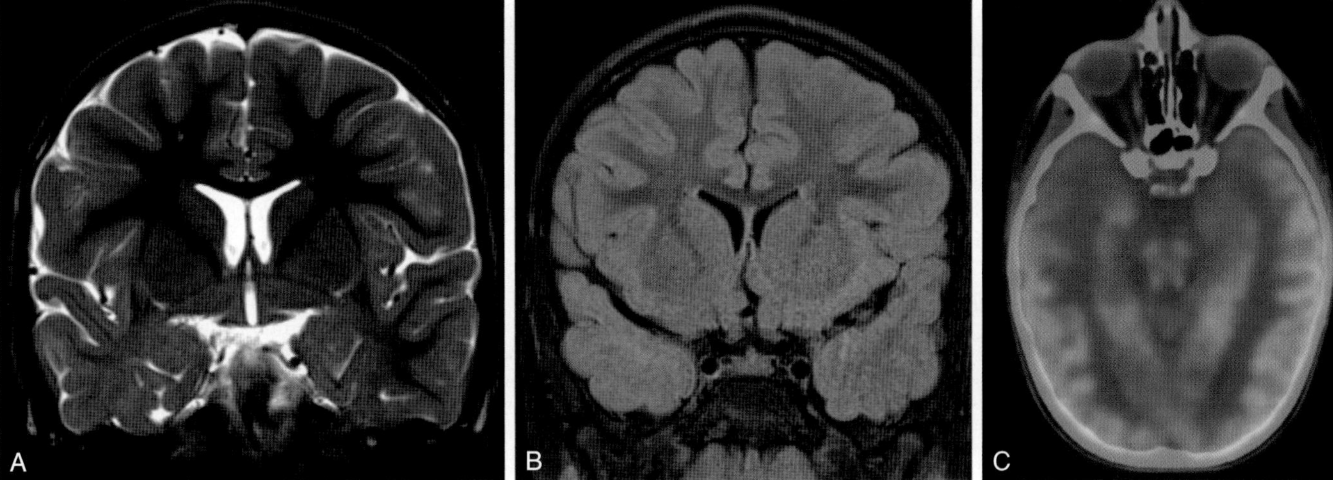

Fig. 8.6 Focal Cortical Dysplasia Type 1. (A) Coronal T2W and (B) coronal FLAIR images demonstrate asymmetric right anterior temporal juxtacortical and subcortical T2/FLAIR hyperintense signal with slight volume loss. (C) FDG PET CT demonstrates decreased FDG uptake in the anterior right temporal lobe.

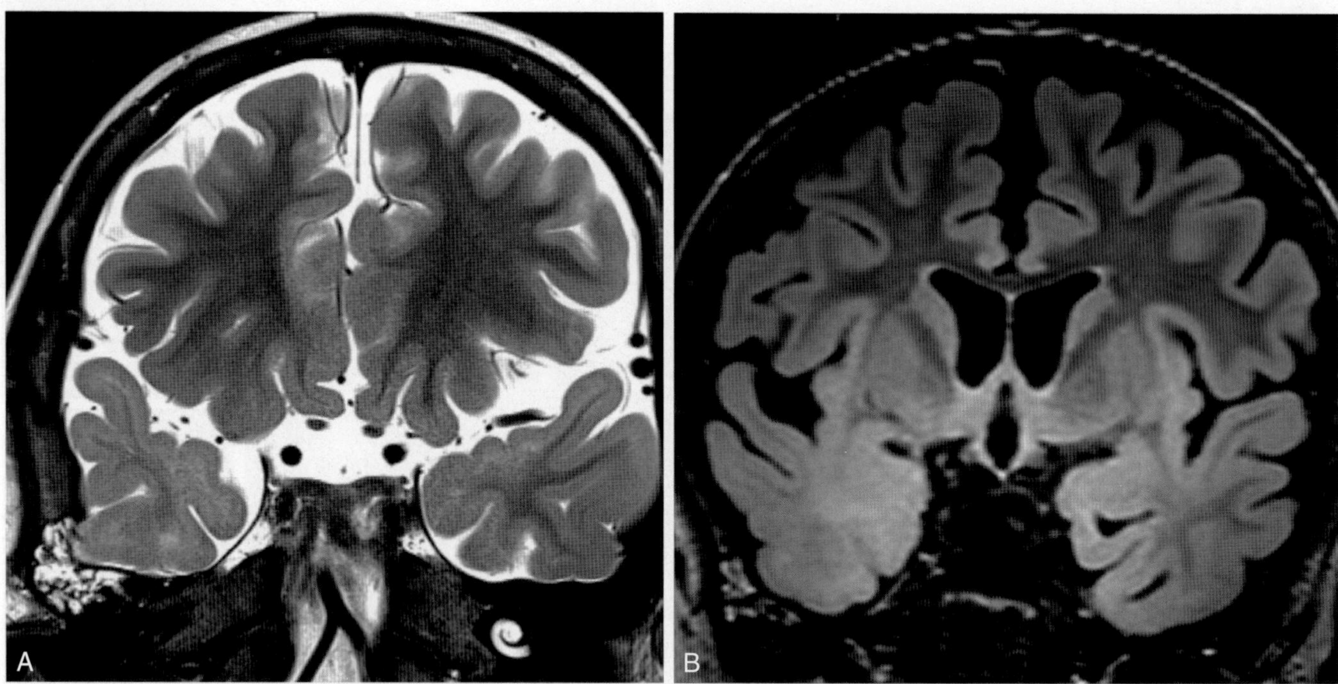

Fig. 8.7 Focal Cortical Dysplasia Type 1. (A) Coronal T2W and (B) coronal FLAIR images demonstrate asymmetric right anterior temporal subcortical T2/FLAIR hyperintense signal with slight volume loss.

Key Points

Background

- Dyslamination and disorganization of tissue architecture with normal glial cells and neurons
  - Focal cortical dysplasia (FCD) type 1a: Disturbance of radial neuronal arrangement, most common
  - FCD type 1b: Disturbance of horizontal/tangential neuronal arrangement
  - FCD type 1c: Disturbance of radial and horizontal neuronal arrangement
- FCD type 1 with additional pathology is classified as FCD type 3
- Less common than FCD type 2
- Outcome after surgery: 21% of children have seizure freedom (worse than FCD type 2)

Imaging

- More often temporal lobe or multilobar than FCD type 2
- *Overlapping imaging appearances with FCD type 2* prevents specificity of MRI findings for diagnosis of FCD type 1
- Imaging findings may be very subtle; conventional MRI may be normal
- More often associated with mesial temporal sclerosis than FCD type 2
- MRI findings
  - Mild to moderate decreased T1W and increased T2W signal with blurring of gray-white matter differentiation (less discrete blurring than with FCD type 2) appearing as hypomyelination
  - Cortical, subcortical volume loss
  - Abnormal gyral folding pattern

REFERENCES

1. Najm IM, Sarnat HB, Blümcke I, et al. Review: The international consensus classification of Focal Cortical Dysplasia - a critical update 2018. *Neuropathol Appl Neurobiol.* 2018 Feb;44(1):18–31.
2. Mata-Mbemba D, Iimura Y, Hazrati LN, et al. MRI, Magnetoencephalography, and Surgical Outcome of Oligodendrocytosis versus Focal Cortical Dysplasia Type I. *AJNR Am J Neuroradiol.* 2018 Dec;39(12):2371–2377.
3. Oguz Cataltepe GIJ, Jallo George I. *Pediatric Epilepsy Surgery: Preoperative Assessment and Surgical Treatment.* 2nd Edition: Thieme; 2019.
4. Kresk P, Karlmeier A, Hildebrandt M, et al. Different presurgical characteristics and seizure outcomes in children with focal cortical dysplasia type 1 or 2. *Epilepsia.* 2009 Jan; 50(1):125–137.

FOCAL CORTICAL DYSPLASIA TYPE 2

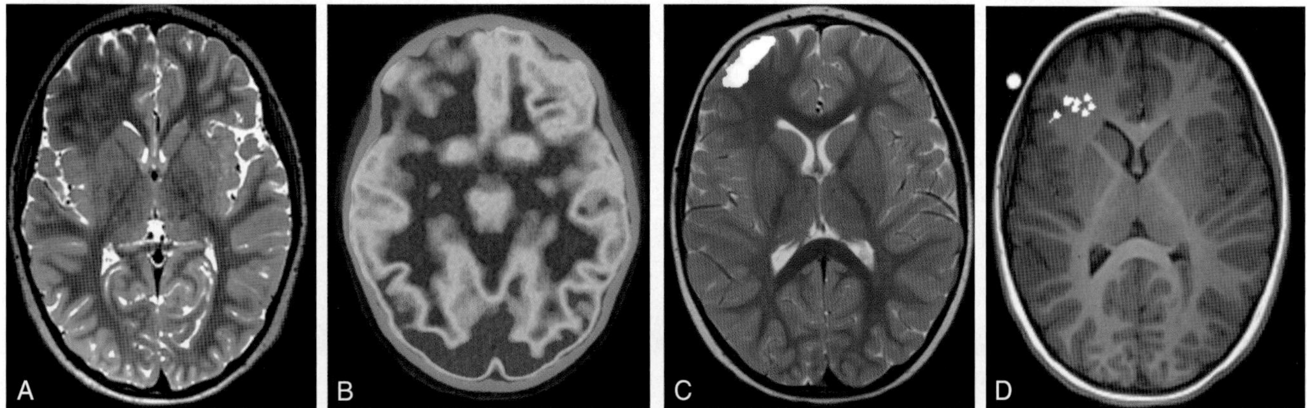

Fig. 8.8 Focal Cortical Dysplasia Type 2. (A) Axial T2W image demonstrates abnormal region of decrease right frontal lobe cortical and subcortical T2W signal intensity. (B) Axial FDG PET CT image demonstrating decreased FDG uptake in the right frontal lobe. (C) SISCOM overlayed onto T2W image demonstrating increased ictal uptake in the right frontal lobe. (D) MEG dipoles localize to the right frontal cortical dysplasia. Pathology was an FCD type 2A.

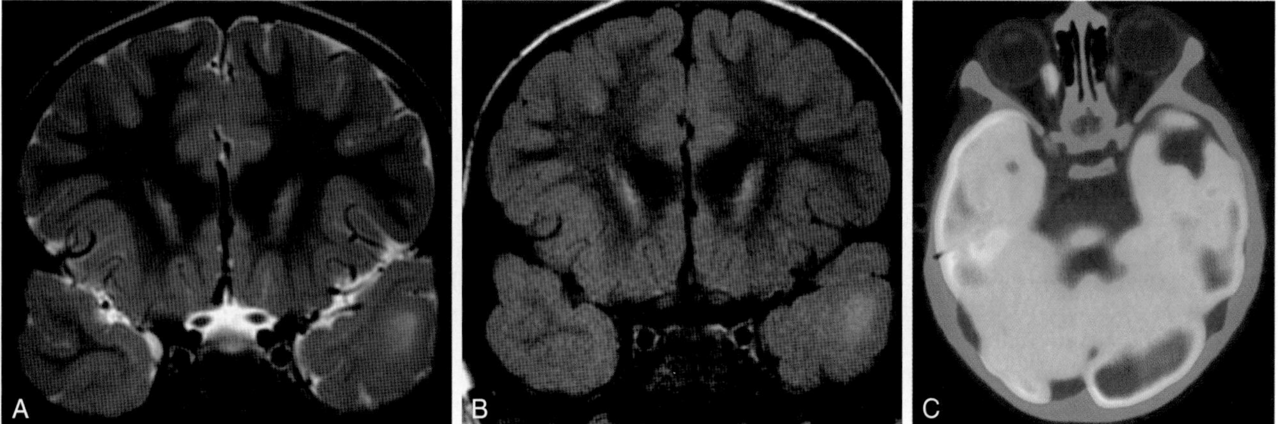

Fig. 8.9 Focal Cortical Dysplasia Type 2. A 4-year-old with epilepsy. (A) Coronal T2W and (B) coronal FLAIR images demonstrate asymmetric left anterior temporal juxtacortical T2/FLAIR hyperintense signal. (C) Axial FDG PET CT demonstrates hypometabolism in the left anterior temporal lobe in the region of the dysplasia. Pathology was an FCD type 2B.

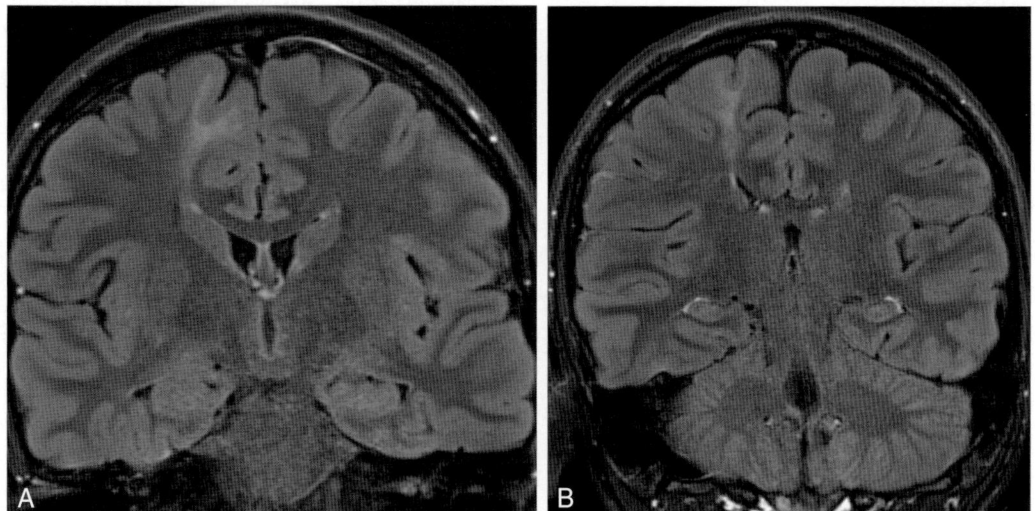

Fig. 8.10 Focal Cortical Dysplasia Type 2. An 8-year-old with epilepsy. (A and B) Coronal FLAIR images demonstrate triangular FLAIR hyperintense signal extending from the right superior frontal gyrus to the ventricle indicative of a transmantle dysplasia. Pathology was an FCD type 2B.

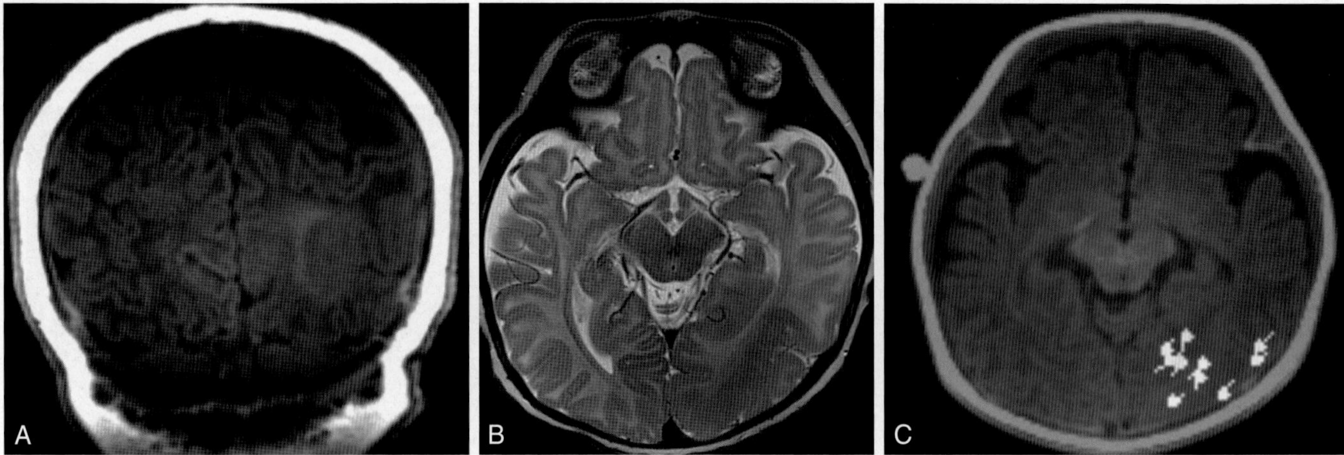

Fig. 8.11 Focal Cortical Dysplasia Type 2. A 2-month-old with seizures. (A) Coronal T1W image demonstrating asymmetric accelerated myelination seen as T1 hyperintense signal in the left parietooccipital junction white matter. (B) Axial T2W image through the left occipital lobe demonstrates abnormal T2 hypointense juxtacortical signal. (C) MEG dipoles localize to the left occipital lobe dysplasia. Pathology was an FCD 2B.

Key Points

Background

- Dysplastic neurons intermixed with normal neurons without balloon cells (FCD type 2a) or with balloon cells (FCD type 2b)
  - Glial cells are dysplastic and enlarged, and presence of phosphorylated tau protein in mTOR mutations including hemimegalencephaly, and tuberous sclerosis.
- Typically younger age of onset of seizures and shorter seizure duration compared to FCD type 1
- Variables associated with seizure freedom:
  - Outcome after surgery: 75% of children with FCD type 2 have seizure freedom (higher likelihood of seizure freedom compared to FCD type 1)
  - Complete resection of an FCD
  - Presence of auras
  - Single type of seizure

Imaging

- FCD 2 are common in extratemporal locations, especially frontal lobe
- FCD 2 may be isolated to a depth of a sulcus
- No consistent features that differentiate FCD type 2a from FCD type 2b with the exception of the transmantle sign
- MRI findings:
  - Cortical thickening
  - Blurring of gray-white matter differentiation, more distinct than FCD type 1
  - Triangular shaped T2/FLAIR hyperintensity from cortex to ependymal margin known as the "transmantle sign" corresponds with an FCD type 2b
  - In the unmyelinated brain, the FCD can show a pattern of abnormal T1W hyperintensity and T2W hypointensity

REFERENCES

1. Atlas SW. *Magnetic Resonance Imaging of the Brain and Spine*. Fifth Edition: LWW; September 28, 2016.
2. Oguz Cataltepe GIJ, Jallo George I. *Pediatric Epilepsy Surgery: Preoperative Assessment and Surgical Treatment*. 2nd Edition: Thieme; September 23, 2019:2019.
3. Jayalakshmi S, Nanda SK, Vooturi S, et al. Focal Cortical Dysplasia and Refractory Epilepsy: Role of Multimodality Imaging and Outcome of Surgery. *AJNR Am J Neuroradiol*. 2019 May;40(5): 892–898.
4. Colombo N, Tassi L, Deleo F, et al. Focal cortical dysplasia type IIa and IIb: MRI aspects in 118 cases proven by histopathology. *Neuroradiology*. 2012 Oct;54(10):1065–1077.
5. Kresk P, Karlmeier A, Hildebrandt M, et al. Different presurgical characteristics and seizure outcomes in children with focal cortical dysplasia type 1 or 2. *Epilepsia*. 2009 Jan;50(1):125–137.

FOCAL CORTICAL DYSPLASIA TYPE 3

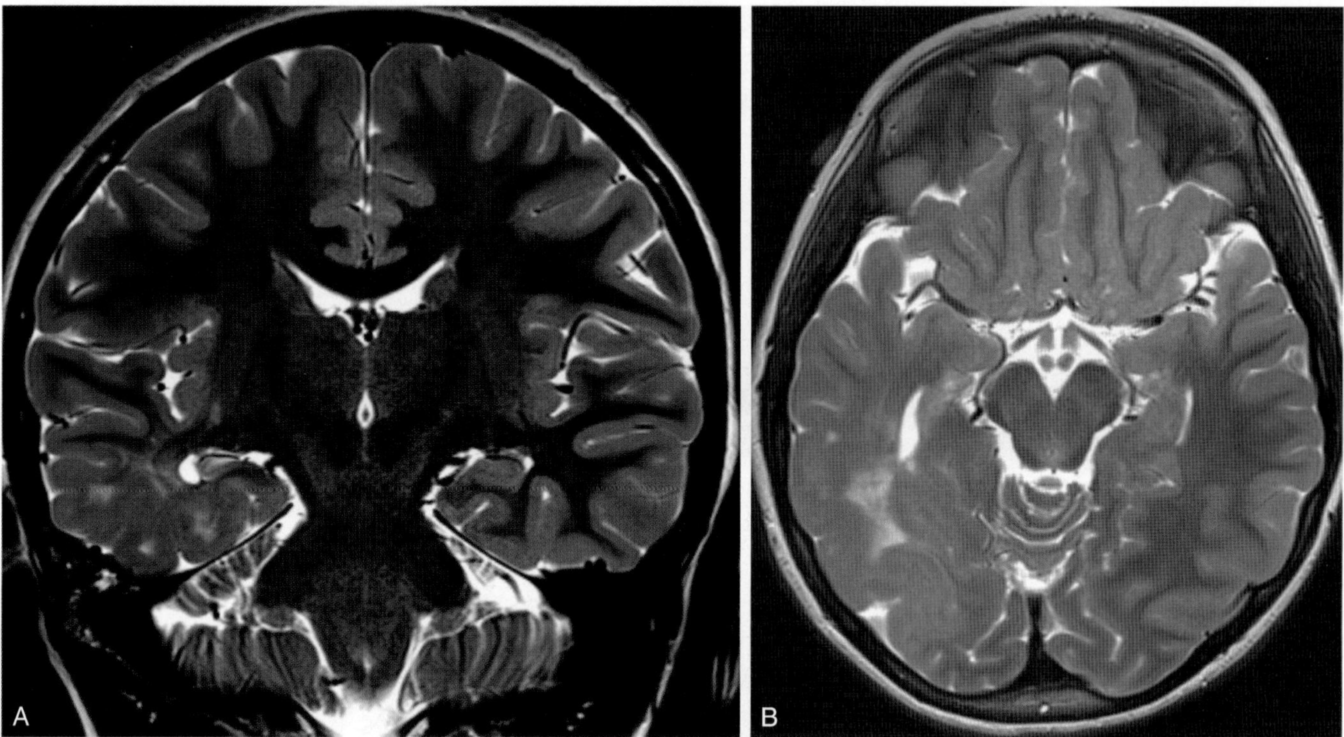

Fig. 8.12 Focal Cortical Dysplasia Type 3. An 8-year-old with epilepsy. (A and B) Coronal and axial T2W images demonstrate abnormal juxtacortical T2W hyperintensity in the right temporal lobe white matter and abnormal sulcation in the right posterior temporal lobe associated with right hippocampal volume loss and T2W hyperintensity indicative of dysplasia with hippocampal sclerosis. Pathology was an FCD type 3A.

Key Points

Background

- FCD 3 is an FCD 1 adjacent/associated with another primary lesion as follows:
  - FCD type 3a: Hippocampal sclerosis with FCD in the temporal lobe
  - FCD type 3b: Adjacent to a glial or glioneuronal tumor (ex. DNET, or ganglioglioma)
  - FCD type 3c: Adjacent to a vascular malformation
  - FCD type 3d: Early childhood insult, including gliosis from ischemia (large or small territory), hemorrhage, and others

Imaging

- Important to detect the primary lesion (tumor, vascular malformation, hemorrhage, encephalomalacia) as well as realize there can be associated dysplasia.
- The FCD associated with lesions often demonstrates a confluent T2/FLAIR hyperintensity. This can be difficult to distinguish however from edema or gliosis caused by the lesion and final determination is performed by histopathology assessment.

REFERENCE

1. Najm IM, Sarnat HB, Blümcke I, et al. Review: The international consensus classification of Focal Cortical Dysplasia - a critical update 2018. *Neuropathol Appl Neurobiol.* 2018 Feb;44(1):18–31.

BOTTOM OF SULCUS DYSPLASIA

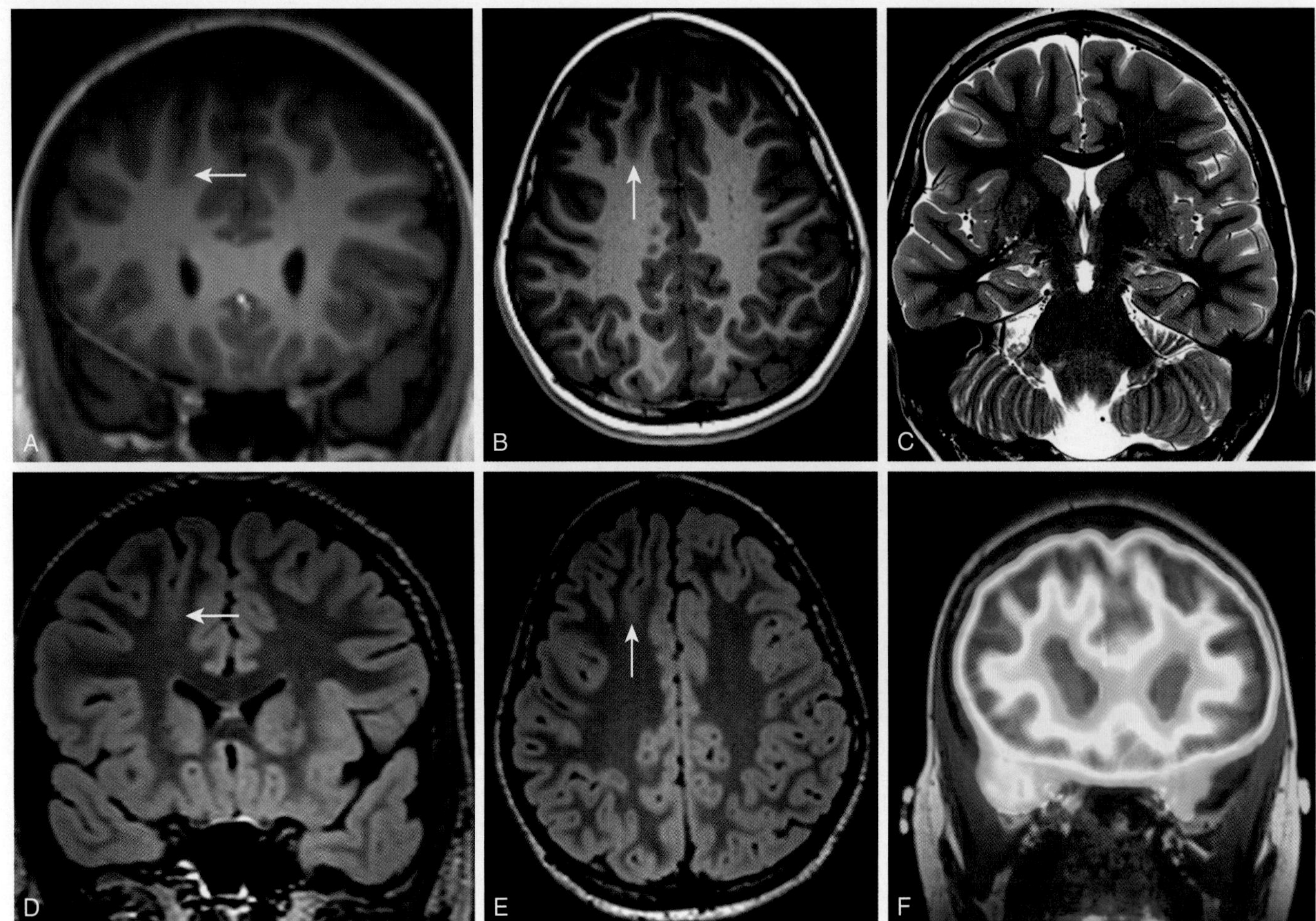

Fig. 8.13 Bottom of Sulcus Dysplasia. (A and B) Coronal and axial T1W, (D and E) coronal and axial FLAIR, and (C) coronal T2W images demonstrate decreased signal intensity in the cortex and blurring of the gray-white matter junction in the right parasagittal frontal lobe at the bottom of the right superior frontal sulcus. (F) Coronal FDG PET CT image demonstrates subtle decreased metabolism of the lesion.

Key Points

Background

- Subtype of FCD 2 located at the bottom of the sulcus
- Highly epileptogenic; high rate of seizure freedom (90%) if completely resected
- Due to deeper location, MEG dipoles may not accurately localize to the bottom of sulcus dysplasia

Imaging

- Imaging appearance includes blurring of gray-white matter interface, transmantle dysplasia, cortical T2/FLAIR hyperintensity, and/or straightening and elongation of the sulcus
- Typically found in the frontal lobe, insula, or parietal lobes
- Hypometabolic on FDG PET

REFERENCES

1. Hofman PA, Fitt GJ, Harvey AS, et al. Bottom of sulcus dysplasia: imaging features. *AJR Am J Roentgenol*. 2011 Apr;196(4):881–885.
2. Nakajima M, Widjaja E, Baba S, et al. Remote MEG dipoles in focal cortical dysplasia at bottom of sulcus. *Epilepsia*. 2016 Jul;57(7):1169–1178.

MESIAL TEMPORAL SCLEROSIS

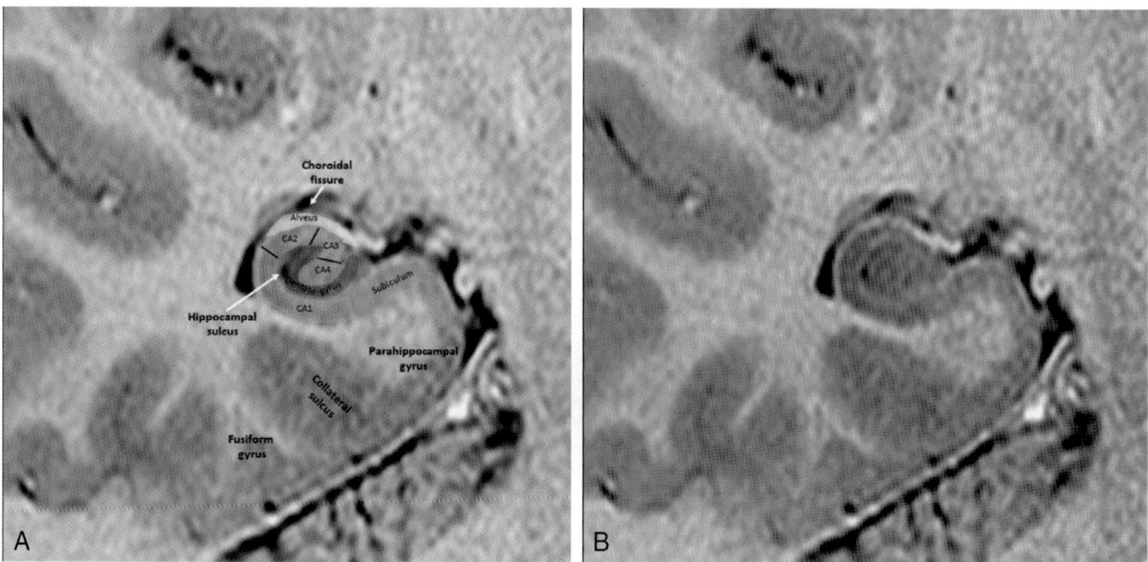

Fig. 8.14 Hippocampal Anatomy. (A) Illustration of the subparts of the mesial temporal lobe. The hippocampus is composed of CA1-4 (green) and the dentate gyrus (red). Additional structures in proximity to the hippocampus include the alveus (yellow) which is the white matter extension of the fornix, and the subiculum (blue). The parahippocampal gyrus which is inferomedial to the hippocampus is separated from the fusiform gyrus by the collateral sulcus. The hippocampal sulcus is between the dentate gyrus and the CA, while the choroidal fissure is superior to the alveus and forms the medial border of the temporal horn and is an attachment site for choroid plexus. (B) Coronal T1W image demonstrating the corresponding MRI appearance of a normal mesial temporal lobe.

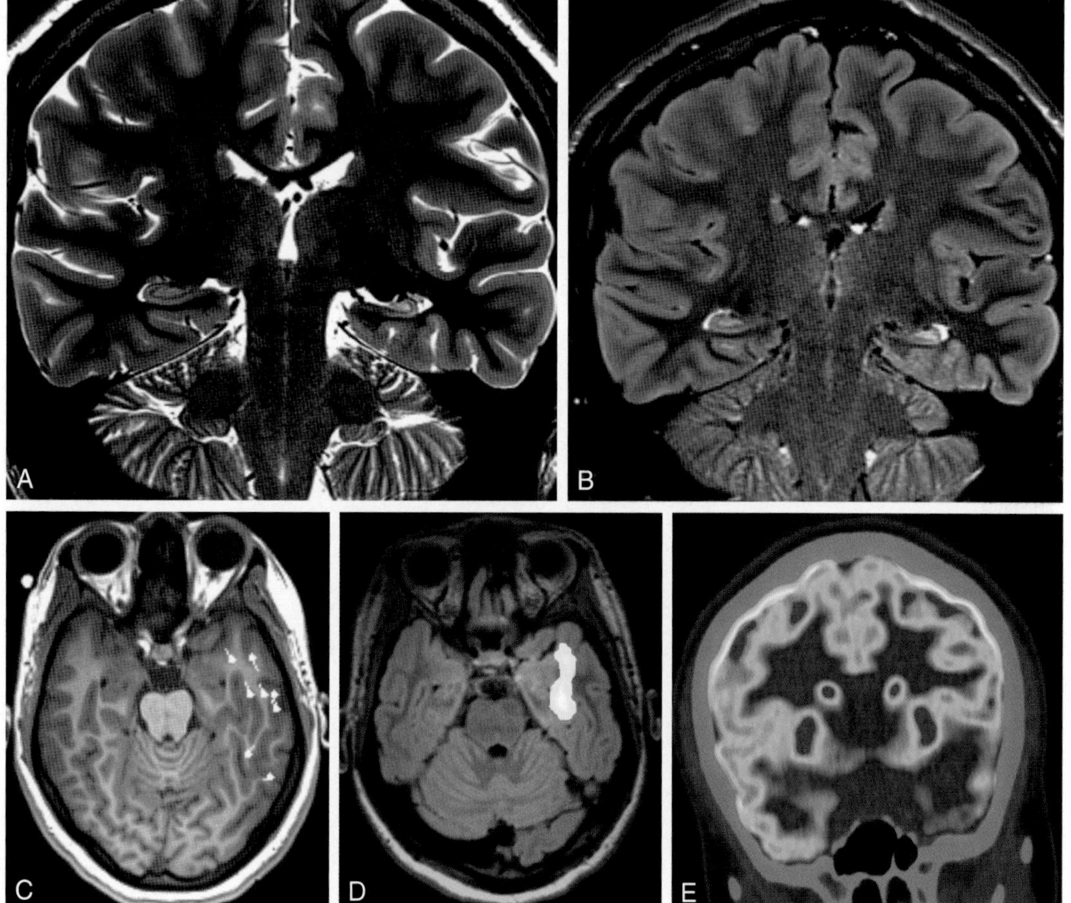

Fig. 8.15 Mesial Temporal Sclerosis. (A and B) Coronal T2W and FLAIR images demonstrate left hippocampal body volume loss and T2/FLAIR hyperintensity. (C) MEG dipole clusters are present in the left temporal lobe. (D) SISCOM SPECT demonstrates hyperperfusion in the anterior left temporal lobe. (E) FDG PECT CT coronal image demonstrate hypometabolism in the anterior left temporal lobe.

Key Points

Background

- Most common lesion in adults with intractable temporal lobe epilepsy but less common cause of epilepsy in children
- Patients may have a history of complicated childhood febrile seizures or febrile status epilepticus, and onset of recurrent medically intractable seizures during the first decades of life
- Neuropathology characterized by neuronal loss, gliosis of the hippocampus with axonal reorganization; dentate gyrus, cornu ammonis CA 1, and CA 4 are principally involved
- Mesial temporal sclerosis (MTS) may be isolated or may be seen with other extrahippocampal pathology such as cortical malformations
- Most commonly unilateral; less common bilateral
- Treatment for refractory temporal lobe epilepsy in MTS is surgical (anterior temporal lobectomy or selective resection or selective laser ablative)

Imaging

- Coronal high-resolution 2D T2W/ T2 FLAIR is best to qualitatively diagnose MTS
- Primary findings in the hippocampus
  - Volume loss
  - T2/FLAIR hyperintensity
  - Internal architectural distortion
- Additional findings
  - Enlarged ipsilateral temporal horn
  - Volume loss and/or signal abnormality can occur in the ipsilateral temporal lobe, fornix, mammillary bodies, white matter in parahippocampal gyrus (collateral white matter), amygdala, insula, basal frontal cortex, and ipsilateral hemisphere (rare)
  - Loss of gray-white matter differentiation of the ipsilateral temporal lobe, especially anteriorly
- Quantification of hippocampal volume has been shown to be more sensitive for detection of hippocampal volume loss compared to qualitative assessment.

REFERENCES

1. Chan S, Erickson JK, Yoon SS. Limbic system abnormalities associated with mesial temporal sclerosis: a model of chronic cerebral changes due to seizures. *Radiographics*. 1997;17:1095–1110.
2. Bronen RA, Cheung G, Charles JT, et al. Imaging findings in hippocampal sclerosis: correlation with pathology. *AJNR Am J Neuroradiol*. 1991;12:933–940.
3. Ng YT, McGregor AL, Duane DC, et al. Childhood mesial temporal sclerosis. *J Child Neurol*. 2006 Jun;21(6):512–517.
4. Guzmán Pérez-Carrillo GJ, Owen C, Schwetye KE, et al. The use of hippocampal volumetric measurements to improve diagnostic accuracy in pediatric patients with mesial temporal sclerosis. *J Neurosurg Pediatr*. 2017 Jun;19(6):720–728.
5. Wieser HG; ILAE Commission on Neurosurgery of Epilepsy. ILAE Commission Report. Mesial temporal lobe epilepsy with hippocampal sclerosis. Epilepsia. 2004 Jun;45(6):695-714.
6. Mettenburg JM, Branstetter BF, Wiley CA, et al. Improved Detection of Subtle Mesial Temporal Sclerosis: Validation of a Commercially Available Software for Automated Segmentation of Hippocampal Volume. *AJNR Am J Neuroradiol*. 2019 Mar;40(3):440–445.

ACUTE SEIZURE AND STATUS EPILEPTICUS

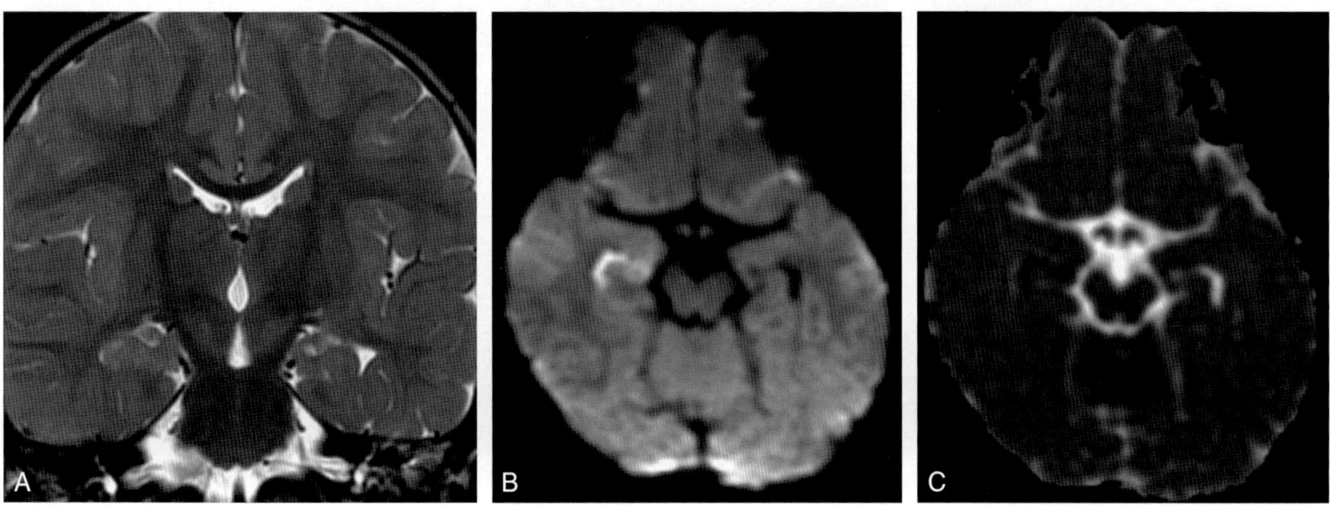

Fig. 8.16 Status Epilepticus. (A) Coronal T2W, (B) axial DWI, and (C) axial ADC images demonstrate abnormal T2W hyperintensity in the right hippocampus associated with abnormal diffusion restriction.

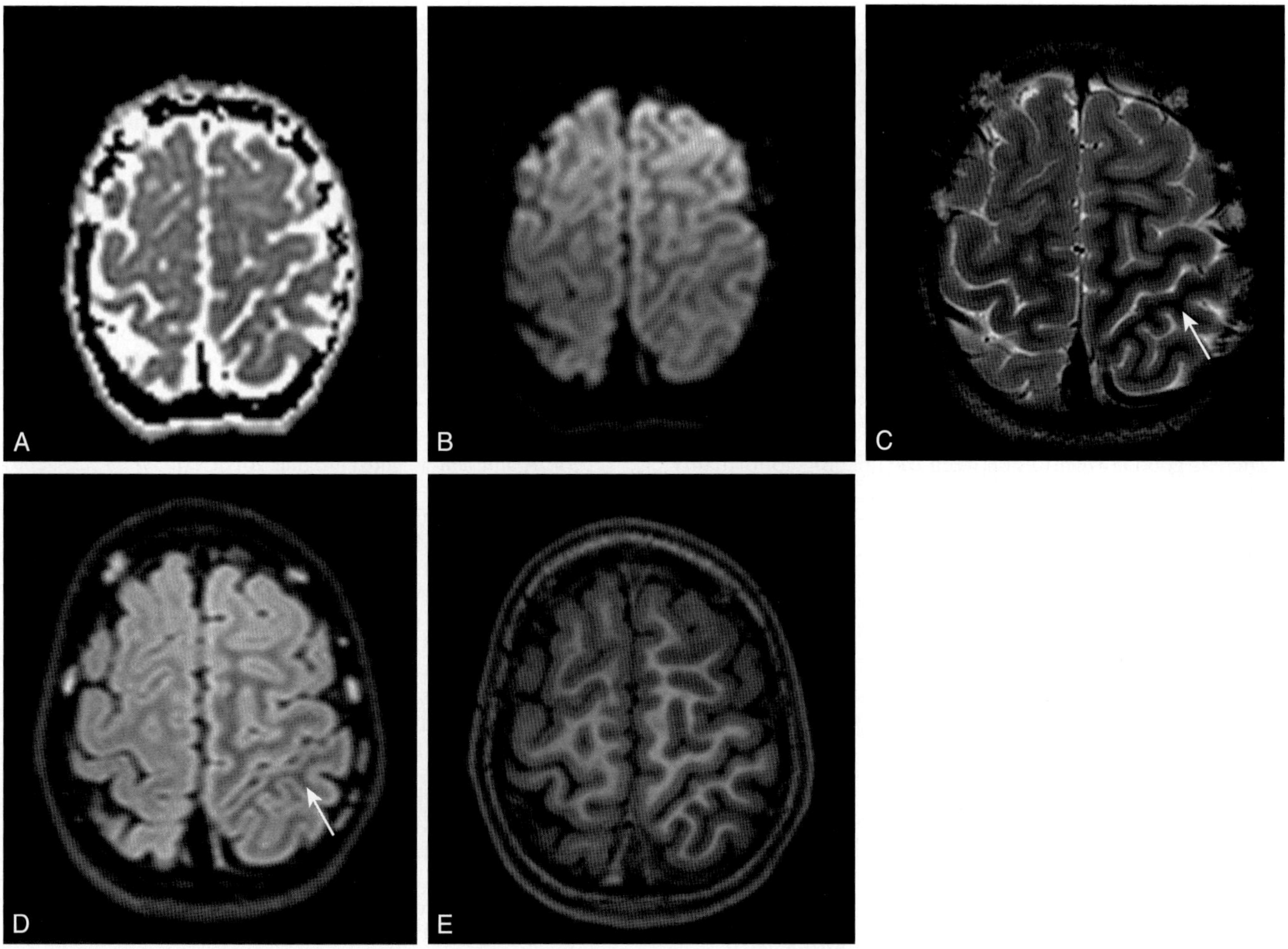

Fig. 8.17 Status Epilepticus. (A) Axial ADC, (B) axial DWI images demonstrate decreased ADC signal without diffusion signal abnormality in the left perirolandic parenchyma. (C) Axial T2W, (D) axial FLAIR, and (E) axial T1W demonstrate subcortical T2W and T1W shortening with exaggerated gray-white matter differentiation.

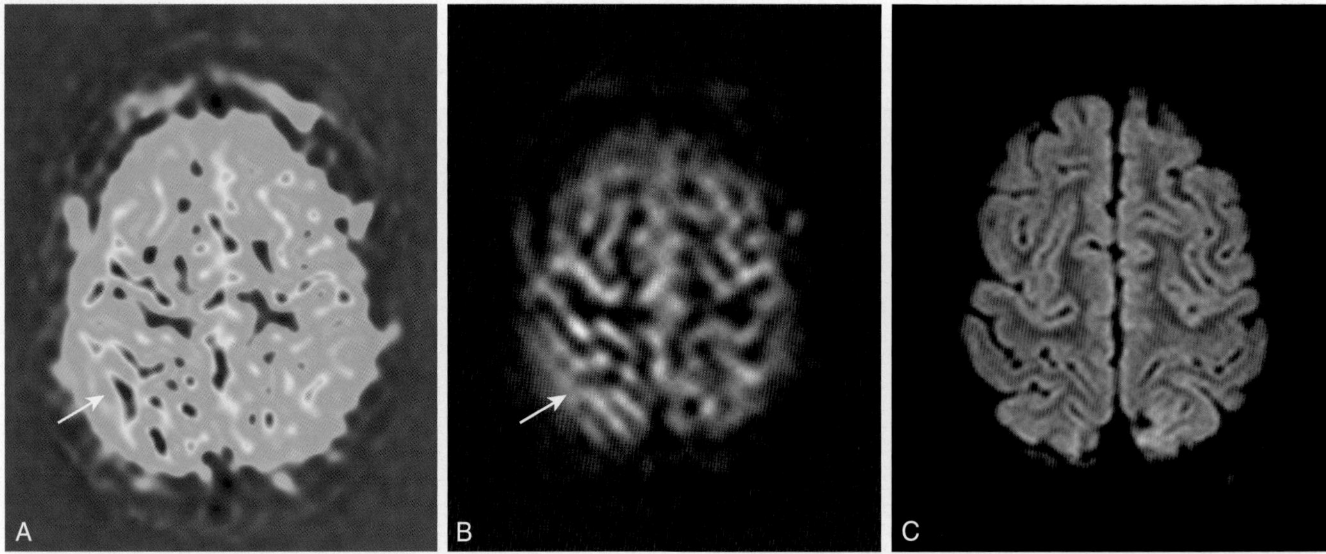

Fig. 8.18 New-Onset Seizures With Left-Sided Todd's Paralysis. (A and B) Axial color and gray scale ASL images demonstrate hyperperfusion of the right parietal and posterior frontal lobe. No abnormality is seen on the (C) axial FLAIR sequence.

Key Points

Background

- During status epilepticus, increased metabolic demand is met with increased cerebral blood flow
- Persistent seizure activity results in further oxygen and glucose demand that cannot be met with augmented CBF, resulting in energy depletion, tissue hypoxia, and anaerobic metabolism
- Depending on the severity and persistence of ictal activity, cytotoxic edema may occur with the potential for permanent injury, resulting in long-term volume/neuronal loss
- Vasogenic edema is reversible and without restricted diffusion. Regions of vasogenic and cytotoxic may coexist in status epilepticus
- There is good correlation between the imaging abnormality and EEG activity

Imaging

- Within 24 hours, majority of patients with status epilepticus will demonstrate some imaging abnormality. Imaging findings are transient and may resolve before imaging.
- T2W/T2 FLAIR hyperintensity is most common
- Subcortical T2W hypointensity has also been reported of uncertain etiology
- Variable presence or absence of diffusion restriction
- Leptomeningeal enhancement from vascular congestion
- Perfusion-weighted imaging (e.g., arterial spin label (ASL), dynamic susceptibility contrast (DSC))
    - ASL demonstrated a perfusion abnormality in 58% of children with new-onset seizure and a normal MRI
    - Hyperperfusion in affected brain parenchyma in the ictal or periictal phase. Hyperperfusion may be seen in regions of DWI abnormality, as well as the ipsilateral thalamus and contralateral cerebellum
    - Hypoperfusion pattern is seen in the postictal period.
- Abnormalities on MRI can be seen in a regional or diffuse cortical and subcortical distribution, thalami (especially pulvinar) due to cortical-subcortical interaction, hippocampi, splenium of the corpus callosum, and basal ganglia (uncommon)

REFERENCES

1. Chan S, Chin SS, Kartha K, et al. Reversible signal abnormalities in the hippocampus and neocortex after prolonged seizures. *AJNR Am J Neuroradiol.* 1996;17:1725–1731.
2. Kim JA, Chung JI, Yoon PH, et al. Transient MR signal changes in patients with generalized tonicoclonic seizure or status epilepticus: periictal diffusion-weighted imaging. *AJNR Am J Neuroradiol.* 2001 Jun-Jul;22(6):1149–1160.
3. Kim SE, Lee BI, Shin KJ, et al. Characteristics of seizure-induced signal changes on MRI in patients with first seizures. *Seizure.* 2017 May;48:62–68.
4. Cianfoni A, Caulo M, Cerase A, et al. Seizure-induced brain lesions: a wide spectrum of variably reversible MRI abnormalities. *Eur J Radiol.* 2013 Nov;82(11):1964–1972.
5. Meletti S, Monti G, Mirandola L, et al. Neuroimaging of status epilepticus. *Epilepsia.* 2018 Oct;59(Suppl 2):113–119.
6. Williams JA, Bede P, Doherty CP, et al. An exploration of the spectrum of peri-ictal MRI change; a comprehensive literature review. *Seizure.* 2017 Aug;50:19–32.
7. Nicholson P, Abdulla S, Alshafai L, et al. Decreased Subcortical T2 FLAIR Signal Associated with Seizures. *AJNR Am J Neuroradiol.* 2020 Jan;41(1):111–114.
8. Lee SM, Kwon S, Lee YJ, et al. Diagnostic usefulness of arterial spin labelingin MR negative children with new onset seizures. *Seizure.* 2019 Feb;65:151–158.

TRANSIENT SPLENIAL LESION

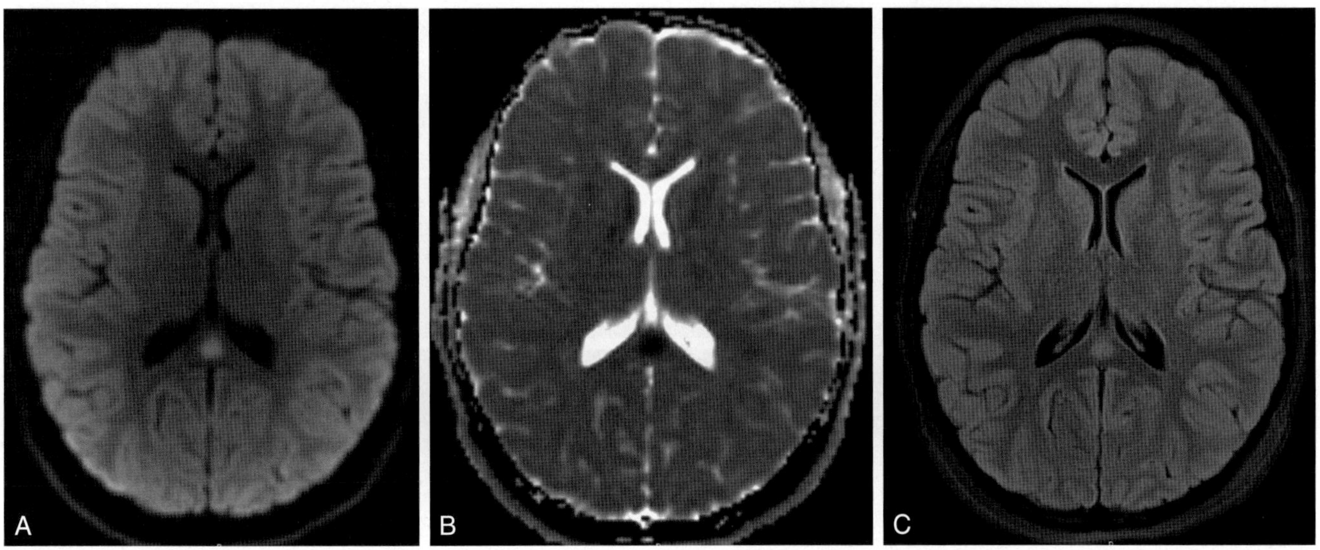

Fig. 8.19 Transient Splenial Lesion. (A) Axial DWI, (B) axial ADC, and (C) axial FLAIR images demonstrate abnormal diffusion restriction and mild FLAIR hyperintensity in the splenium of the corpus callosum.

Key Points

Background

- Mechanism of this imaging abnormality is not certain. An intramyelinic excitotoxic mechanism has been proposed.
- Site predilection may be due to functional relationship with the temporal lobes and limbic system with inherent vulnerability.
- Etiologies
  - Epilepsy related: Seizures, antiepileptic drug (AED) toxicity, and AED withdrawal
  - Infection: Viral encephalitis, bacterial, and atypical bacterial
  - Metabolic: Hypoglycemia, Wernicke encephalopathy, hypernatremia, hepatic encephalopathy, and extrapontine myelinolysis
  - Drugs: Numerous including antidepressants, and antipsychotics; toxic chemicals like methyl bromide
  - Other: Hemolytic-uremic syndrome, altitude brain injury, and axonal injury

Imaging

- Well-delineated round, oval, or boomerang shape
- Reversible, nonenhancing T2W hyperintensity typically with restricted diffusion

REFERENCES

1. Garcia-Monco JC, Cortina IE, Ferreira E, et al. Reversible splenial lesion syndrome (RESLES): what's in a name? *J Neuroimaging*. 2011 Apr;21(2):e1–14.
2. Gallucci M, Limbucci N, Paonessa A, et al. Reversible focal splenial lesions. *Neuroradiology*. 2007 Jul;49(7):541–544.
3. Starkey J, Kobayashi N, Numaguchi Y, et al. Cytotoxic Lesions of the Corpus Callosum That Show Restricted Diffusion: Mechanisms, Causes, and Manifestations. *Radiographics*. 2017 Mar-Apr;37(2):562–576.

FEBRILE INFECTION-RELATED EPILEPSY SYNDROME (FIRES)

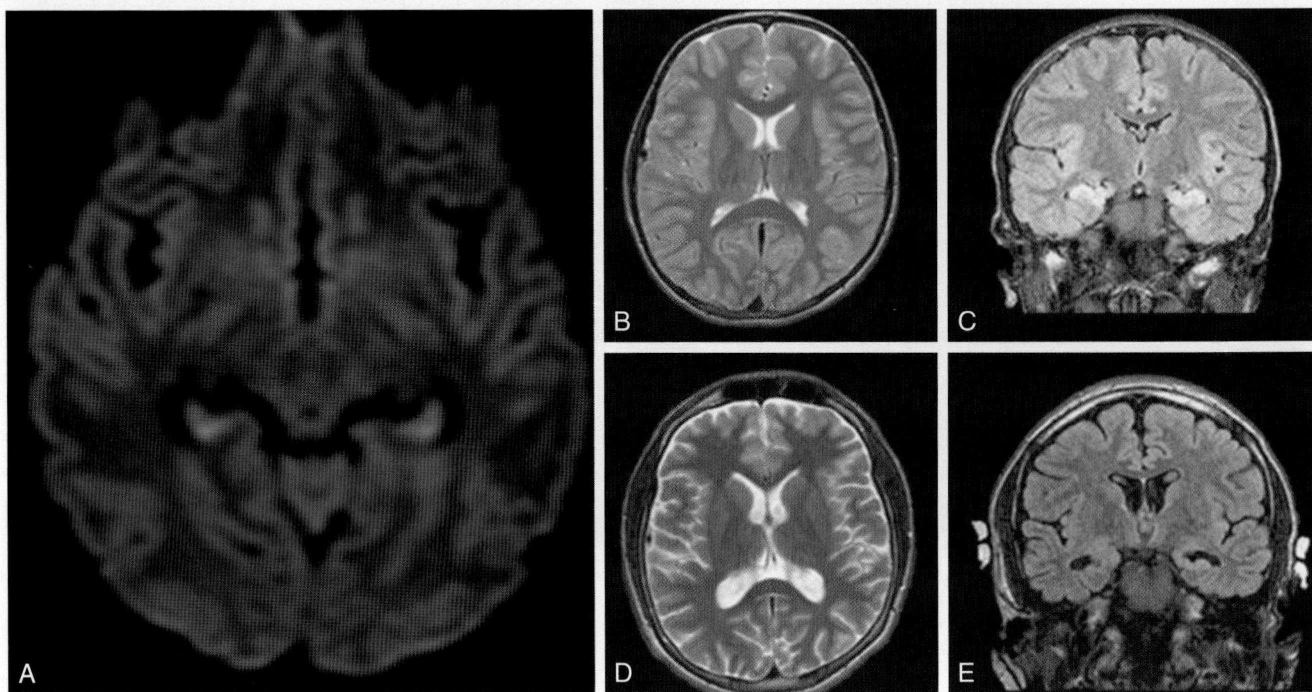

Fig. 8.20 Febrile Infection–Related Epilepsy Syndrome (FIRES). (A) Axial DWI in a 2-year-old with FIRES demonstrating symmetric diffusion restriction in the bilateral hippocampi (ADC hypointensity not shown). (B and C) Axial T2W and coronal FLAIR at presentation in a different patient with FIRES demonstrates normal cerebral volume and abnormal FLAIR hyperintensity in the bilateral hippocampi. Follow-up imaging with (D and (E) axial T2W and coronal FLAIR demonstrate interval cerebral volume loss, and resolution of FLAIR hyperintensity in the hippocampi but with bilateral hippocampal volume loss.

Key Points

Background

- Severe epileptic encephalopathy of uncertain pathogenesis occurring in a minority of patients with status epilepticus. FIRES is a subcategory of new-onset refractory status epilepticus (NORSE)
- Diagnosis requires febrile illness 24 hours to 2 weeks prior to onset of status epilepticus with or without fever at the time of status epilepticus.
- Absence of any identified infectious agent; etiology may be an autoimmune postinfectious process
- Outcome of FIRES is poor, with a death rate of up to 30%. Outcomes also include typical development of drug-resistant epilepsy and neurocognitive impairment.
- No specific diagnostic biomarkers

Imaging

- MRI can be normal.
- If abnormal, MRI findings include T2W hyperintense signal in the bilateral hippocampi, and/or periinsular region.
- Follow-up MRI demonstrates diffuse atrophy and some cases demonstrate mesial temporal sclerosis.

REFERENCES

1. Kramer U, Chi CS, Lin KL, et al. Febrile infection-related epilepsy syndrome (FIRES): pathogenesis, treatment, and outcome: a multicenter study on 77 children. *Epilepsia*. 2011;52:1956–1965.
2. Howell KB, Katanyuwong K, Mackay MT, et al. Long-term follow-up of febrile infection-related epilepsy syndrome. *Epilepsia*. 2012;53:101–110.
3. Serino D, Santarone ME, Caputo D, et al. Febrile infection-related epilepsy syndrome (FIRES): prevalence, impact and management strategies. *Neuropsychiatr Dis Treat*. 2019 Jul 9;15:1897–1903.

HEMICONVULSION-HEMIPLEGIA EPILEPSY SYNDROME

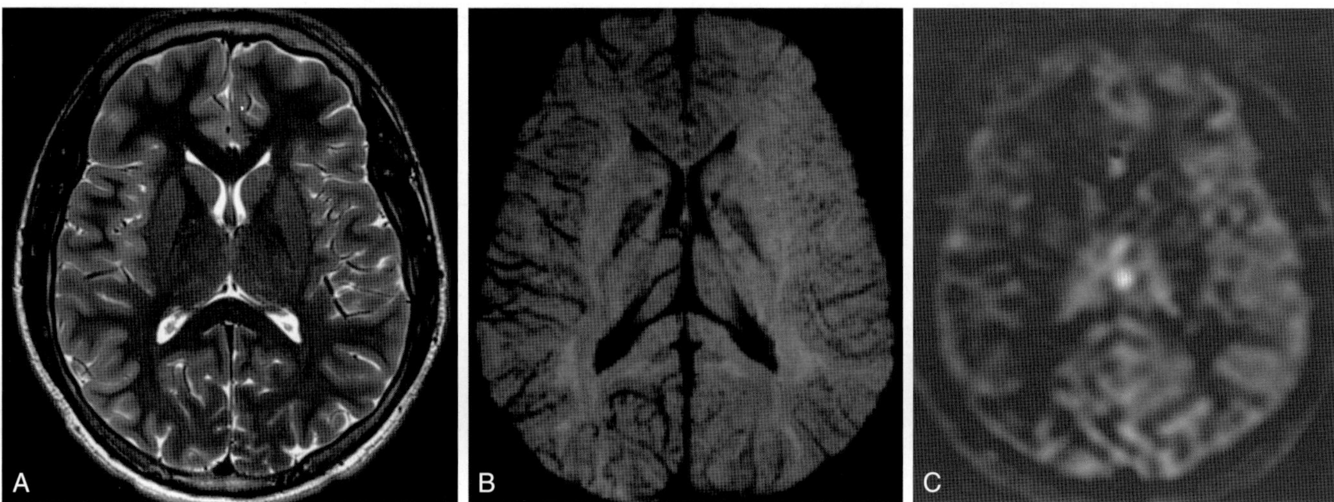

Fig. 8.21 Hemiconvulsion-Hemiplegia Epilepsy Syndrome. (A) Axial T2W image demonstrates mild right hemicerebral cortical T2W hyperintensity. (B) Axial SWI demonstrates increased susceptibility in the vessels of the right cerebral hemisphere. (C) Axial ASL cerebral blood flow (CBF) image demonstrates decreased flow to the right cerebral hemisphere.

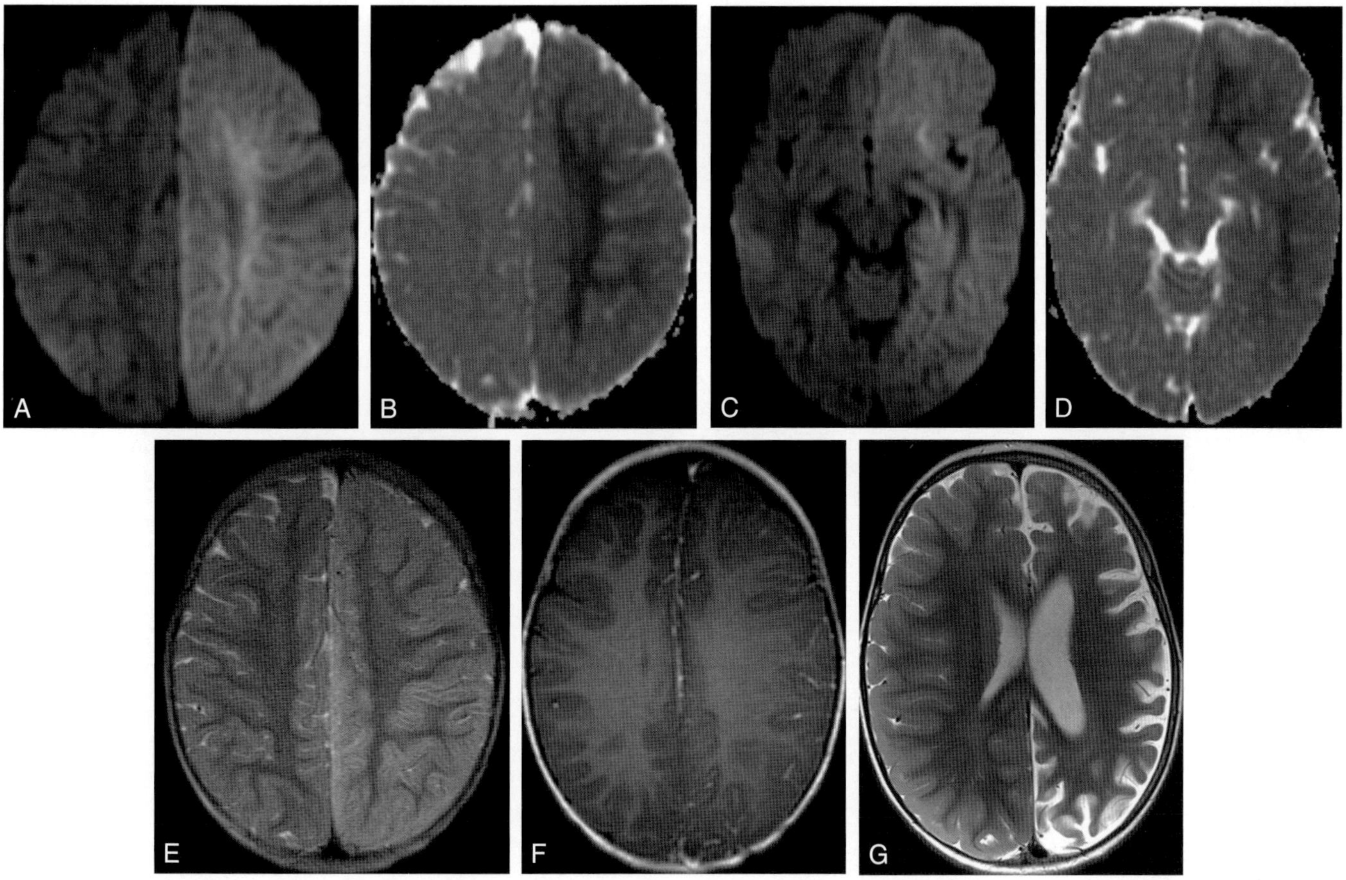

Fig. 8.22 Hemiconvulsion-Hemiplegia Epilepsy Syndrome. Acute presentation. (A and C) Axial DWI, (B and D) axial ADC, (E) axial T2W, and (F) axial T1W+C images demonstrate diffusion restriction in the left cerebral white matter, cortical T2 hyperintensity, and mild sulcal vessel prominence. The 6-month follow-up (G) axial T2W image demonstrates left hemisphere volume loss.

Key Points

Background

- Occurs in children typically less than 2 years of age
- Prolonged unilateral, clonic seizure during the course of a febrile illness and is followed by transient or permanent hemiplegia ipsilateral to the side of convulsions. Contralateral seizures may occur.
- Two subgroups
  - Idiopathic: Fever and presumed extracranial infection
  - Symptomatic: Fever and an identified predisposing factor like intracranial infection, cerebrovascular disease, or head trauma
- Likely a multifactorial process involving an inflammatory encephalopathy and seizures similar to FIRES, and NORSE

Imaging

- Diffuse unilateral hemispheric cortical and central gray and white matter T2 hyperintensity with restricted diffusion
- T2/FLAIR hyperintensity may occur in the ipsilateral or bilateral hippocampi
- Areas of contralateral signal abnormality may occur
- Ipsilateral leptomeningeal enhancement and greater prominence of vessels on SWI presumably from venous congestion
- Hyperperfusion in the acute phase and hypoperfusion in subacute or the chronic phase
- Volume loss on follow-up imaging

REFERENCES

1. Auvin S, Bellavoine V, Merdariu D, et al. Hemiconvulsion-hemiplegia-epilepsy syndrome: current understandings. *Eur J Paediatr Neurol.* 2012;16:413–421.
2. Tenney JR, Schapiro MB. Child neurology: hemiconvulsion-hemiplegia-epilepsy syndrome. *Neurology.* 2012;79:e1–e4.
3. Barcia G, Desguerre I, Carmona O, et al. Hemiconvulsion-hemiplegia syndrome revisited: longitudinal MRI findings in 10 children. *Dev Med Child Neurol.* 2013 Dec;55(12):1150–1158.

RASMUSSEN ENCEPHALITIS

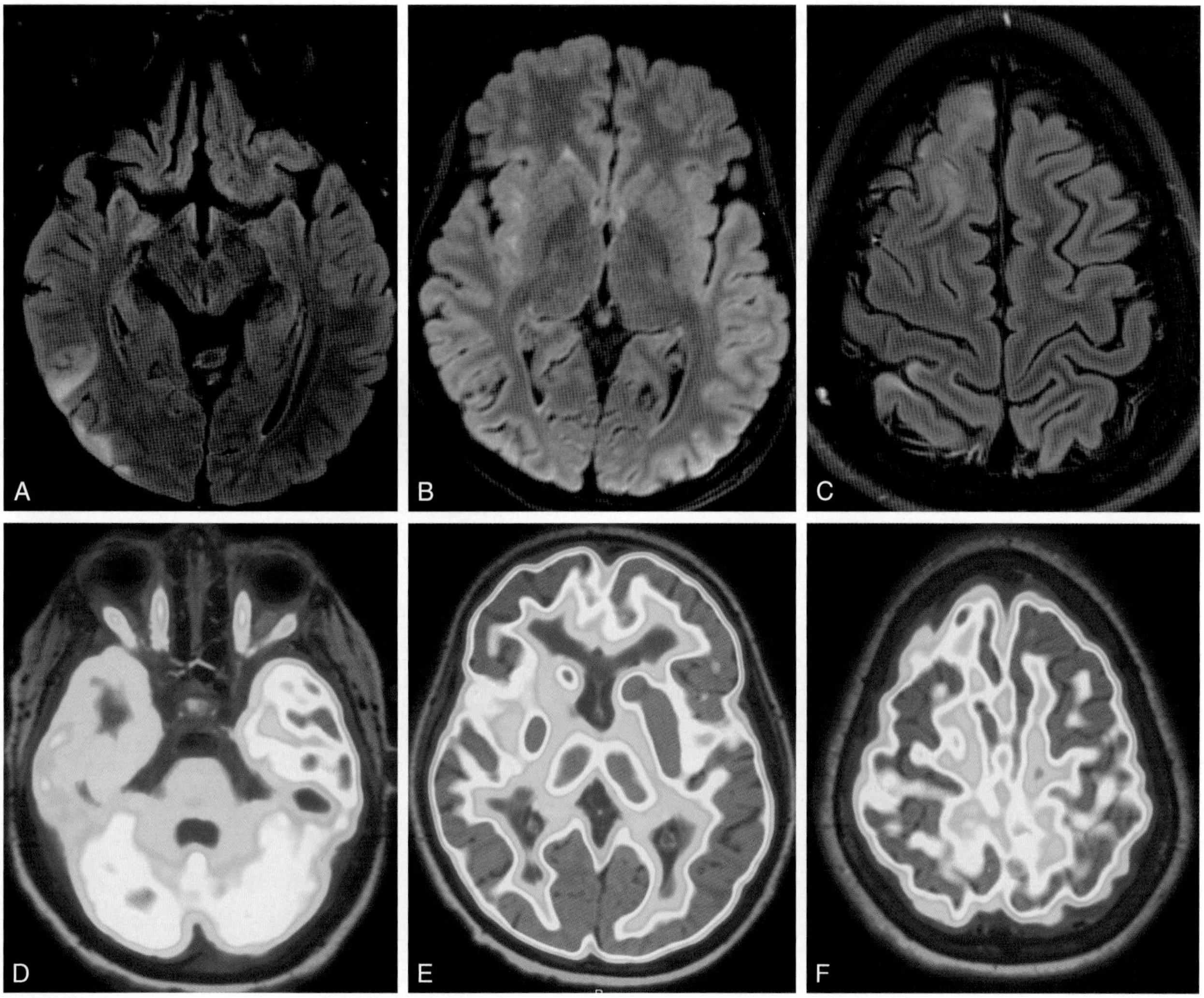

Fig. 8.23 Rasmussen Encephalitis. (A to C) Axial FLAIR images demonstrate abnormal FLAIR hyperintensity in the right subinsular white matter, right frontal cortex and juxtacortical white matter, right parietal cortex, and right posterolateral temporal and occipital cortex. (D–F) FDG PET images fused to MRI demonstrate broad regions of hypometabolic cortex in the right cerebral hemisphere and basal ganglia.

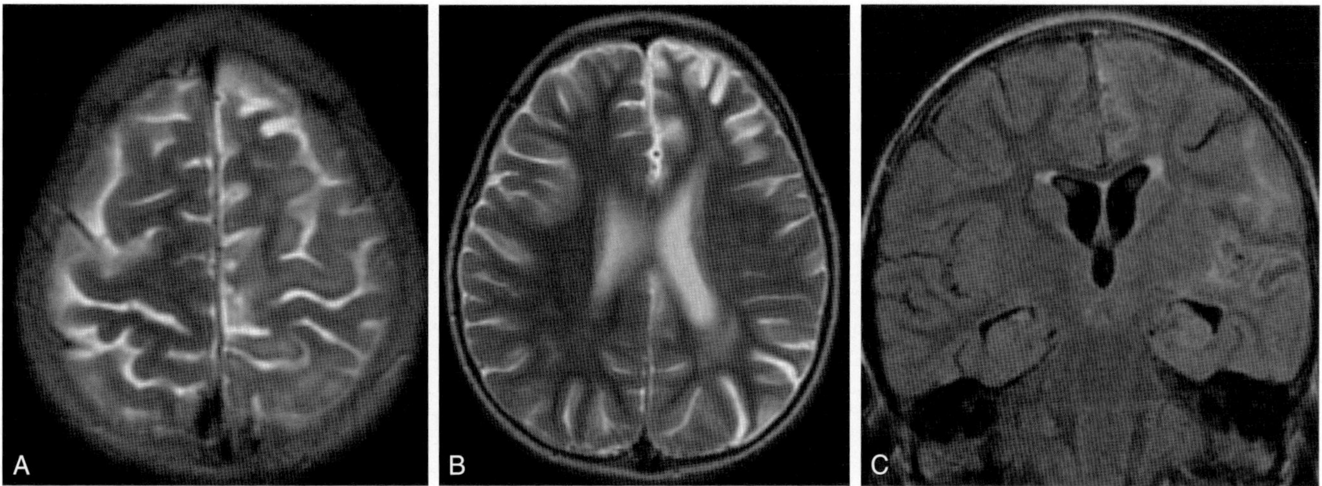

Fig. 8.24 Rasmussen Encephalitis. (A and B) Axial T2W and (C) coronal FLAIR images demonstrate abnormal volume loss and T2/FLAIR hyperintensity in the left frontal and parietal cortex and juxtacortical white matter, left insula, and superior temporal gyrus.

Key Points

Background

- Sporadic drug-resistant focal epilepsy with progressive hemiplegia, neurocognitive decline with unilateral hemispheric atrophy
  - Viral etiologies have been historically suggested, but this has not been proven and consistently supported in the literature
  - Most likely an autoimmune, inflammatory process mediated by humoral (autoantibodies) and T lymphocytes (especially cytotoxic T cells)
- Multiphasic
  - Prodromal stage: Low seizure frequency with occasionally mild hemiparesis
  - Acute stage
    - Initial presentation may be in the acute phase in a subset of patients
    - Frequent seizures, mostly simple partial seizures often epilepsia partialis continua
    - Progressive hemiparesis, hemianopia, neurocognitive impairment and possibly aphasia with involvement of the language dominant hemisphere
  - Residual stage
    - Frequent seizures but less than in the acute phase
    - Stable, permanent neurologic deficits, although not all are hemiplegic
- Surgical options (functional hemispherectomy and functional hemispherotomy) are the only curative treatments to avoid progression

Imaging

- Initially may be normal
- Progressive cortical and subcortical T2 signal with progressive atrophy (atrophy most significant in the first 8 months)
  - Predilection for the frontal and temporal lobes, insular/periinsular parenchyma, and basal ganglia (especially caudate nucleus and putamen)
- MRS: Low NAA, low Cr, elevated Glu/Gln
- Perfusion-weighted imaging will demonstrate hyperperfusion during ictus followed by hypoperfusion corresponding to atrophy on MRI
- FDG-PET demonstrates unilateral cerebral hypometabolism that may be more striking than early MRI findings

REFERENCES

1. Tien RD, Ashdown BC, Lewis DVJ, et al. Rasmussen's encephalitis: neuroimaging findings in four patients. *AJR Am J Roentgenol.* 1992;158:1329–1332.
2. Rasmussen T, Olszewski J, LLoydsmith D, et al. Focal seizures due to chronic localized encephalitis. *Neurology.* 1958;8:435–445.
3. Bien CG, Granata T, Antozzi C, et al. Pathogenesis, diagnosis and treatment of Rasmussen encephalitis: a European consensus statement. *Brain.* 2005 Mar;128(Pt 3):454–471.
4. Varadkar S, Bien CG, Kruse CA, et al. Rasmussen's encephalitis: clinical features, pathobiology, and treatment advances. *Lancet Neurol.* 2014 Feb;13(2):195–205.
5. Cendes F, Andermann F, Silver K, et al. Imaging of axonal damage in vivo in Rasmussen's syndrome. *Brain.* 1995 Jun;118(Pt 3):753–758.
6. Kumar S, Nagesh CP, Thomas B, et al. Arterial spin labeling hyperperfusion in Rasmussen's encephalitis: Is it due to focal brain inflammation or a postictal phenomenon? *J Neuroradiol.* 2018 Feb;45(1):6–14.

MALIGNANT MIGRATING PARTIAL SEIZURES IN INFANCY

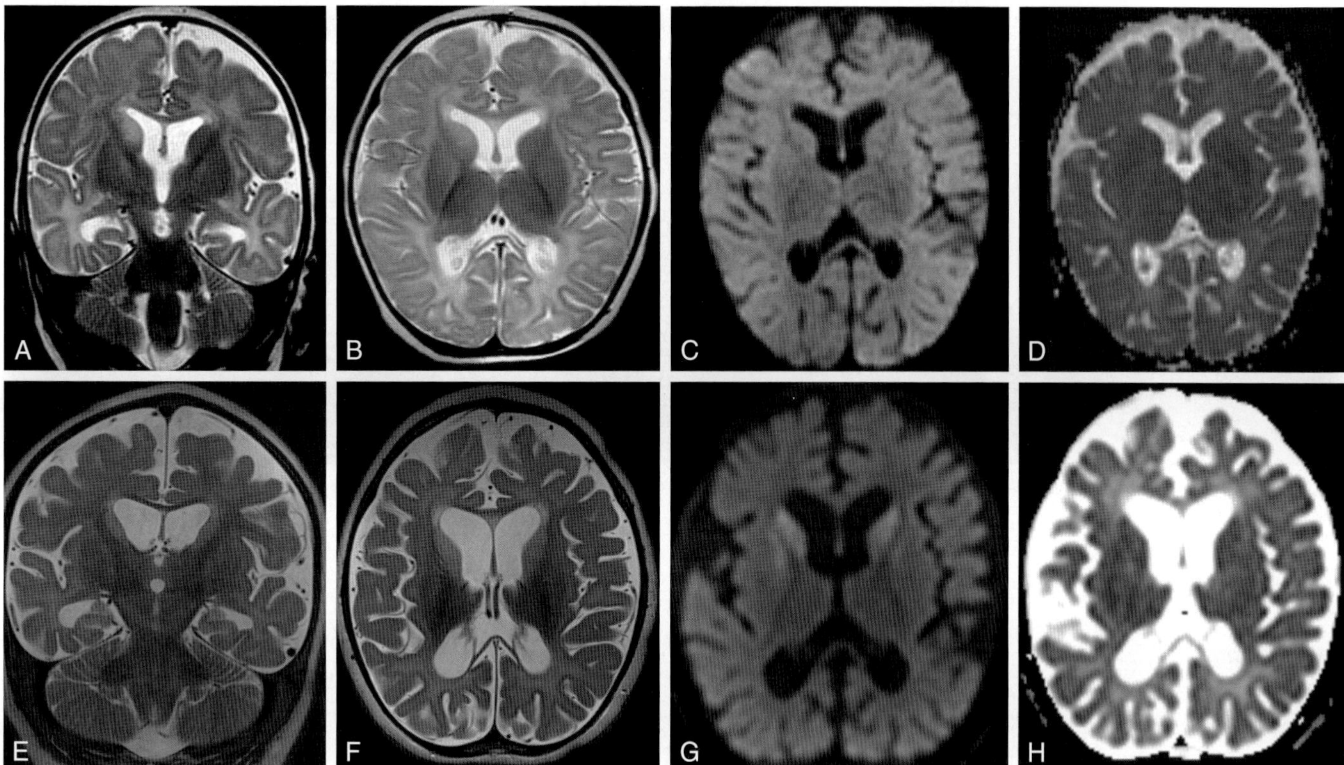

Fig. 8.25 Malignant Migrating Partial Seizures in Infancy. (A and B) Initial MRI coronal and axial T2W images and (C and D) axial DWI and ADC demonstrate mild volume loss and T2W hyperintensity in the right caudate head without diffusion restriction. (E to H) Follow-up MRI coronal and axial T2W, and DWI and ADC images demonstrate progression of volume loss particularly in the basal ganglia, and T2 hyperintensity and reduced diffusion in the bilateral caudate heads.

Key Points

Background

- Rare epilepsy syndrome with drug-resistant polymorphous focal bilateral seizure onset in the first 6 months of life with abnormal psychomotor development
- Etiology resulting from sodium or potassium channel genetic mutation. Malignant migrating partial seizures in infancy (MMPSI) can occur with mutations in KCNT1, which encodes a sodium-activated potassium channel, mutations in SCN1A, a sodium voltage-gated channel alpha subunit 1, and mutations in PLCB1, phospholipase C-1. Mutations in SCN1A can also lead to Dravet syndrome which is characterized by frequent prolonged seizures triggered by high body temperature, and epileptic encephalopathy causing developmental delay, speech impairment, ataxia, and hypotonia.
- Seizures in MMPSI are drug resistant. Outcome is poor with children often left with severe psychomotor impairment.

Imaging

- Initial imaging can be normal
- Progressive atrophy and delayed myelination delay with ex vacuo ventriculomegaly
- T2 signal abnormality with or without diffusion restriction in caudate nuclei, putamen, and hippocampi

REFERENCES

1. Coppola G. Malignant migrating partial seizures in infancy. *Handb Clin Neurol.* 2013;111:605–609.
2. Barcia G, Fleming MR, Deligniere A, et al. De novo gain-of-function KCNT1 channel mutations cause malignant migrating partial seizures of infancy. *Nat Genet.* 2012 Nov;44(11):1255–1259.
3. Kuchenbuch M, Barcia G, Chemaly N, et al. KCNT1 epilepsy with migrating focal seizures shows a temporal sequence with poor outcome, high mortality and SUDEP. *Brain.* 2019 Oct 1;142(10):2996–3008.
4. Freilich ER, Jones JM, Gaillard WD, et al. Novel SCN1A mutation in a proband with malignant migrating partial seizures of infancy. *Arch Neurol.* 2011 May;68(5):665–671.

EPILEPSY SURGERY: CORPUS CALLOSOTOMY

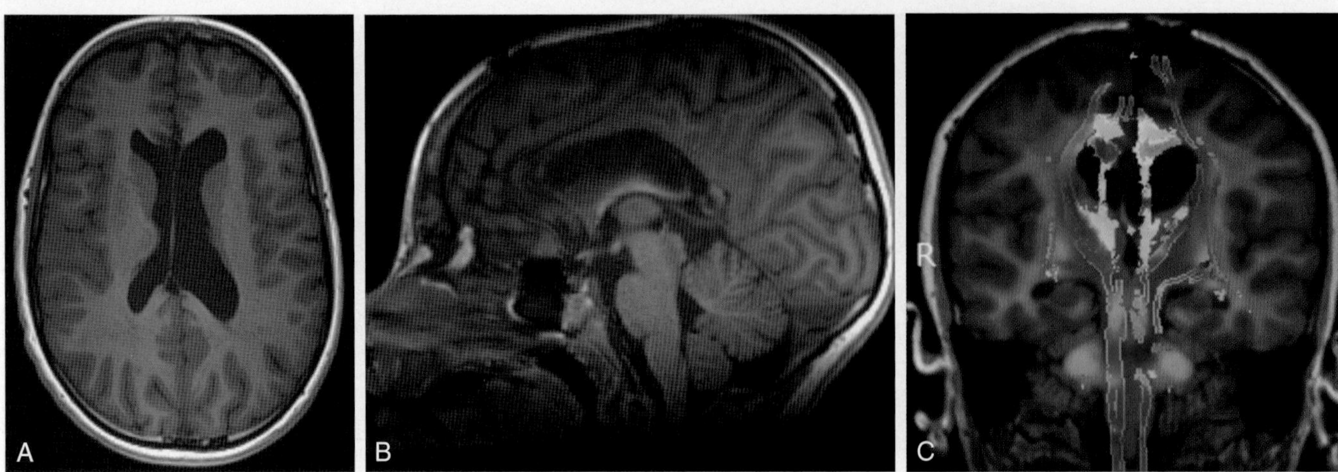

Fig. 8.26 Corpus Callosotomy. (A and B) Axial and sagittal T1W images and (C) DTI tractography image demonstrate disconnection of the corpus callosum.

Key Points

Background

- The corpus callosum is composed of 180 million axons connecting each cerebral hemisphere.
- Corpus callosotomy is a useful palliative procedure for children with drug-resistant generalized or multifocal refractory epilepsy and drop attack seizures.
- Partial or complete callosotomy aims to block interhemispheric spread of epileptic discharges.
- Complete callosotomy results in a greater reduction in seizures than partial callosotomy but with increased risk of permanent disconnection syndrome.
- Improvement occurs in 65% to 85% of patients after total corpus callosotomy, especially in patients with drop attacks.
- Callosotomy may be performed with open and endoscopic surgical techniques and by laser ablation.
- Disconnection syndromes can complicate the clinical outcome. These include SMA syndrome, alien hand syndrome, dichotic listening suppression, tactile dysnomia, hemispatial neglect, nondominant hand agraphia, alexia without agraphia, and tachistoscopic visual suppression.

Imaging

- Disconnected fibers/portions of the corpus callosum can be better evaluated with DTI in addition to 3D T1 and 3D T2 imaging.

REFERENCES

1. Oguz Cataltepe GIJ. Pediatric Epilepsy Surgery: Preoperative Assessment and Surgical Treatment. Thieme; 2nd Edition (September 23, 2019); 2019
2. Graham D, Tisdall MM, Gill D, et al. Corpus callosotomy outcomes in pediatric patients: A systematic review. *Epilepsia*. 2016 Jul;57(7):1053–1068.
3. Roland JL, Akbari SH, Salehi A, et al. Corpus callosotomy performed with laser interstitial thermal therapy. *J Neurosurg*. 2019 Dec 13:1–9.
4. Smyth MD, Vellimana AK, Asano E, et al. Corpus callosotomy-Open and endoscopic surgical techniques. *Epilepsia*. 2017 Apr;58(Suppl 1):73–79.
5. Jea A, Vachhrajani S, Widjaja E, et al. Corpus callosotomy in children and the disconnection syndromes: a review. *Childs Nerv Syst*. 2008;24:685–692.

EPILEPSY SURGERY: POSTERIOR QUADRANT DISCONNECTION

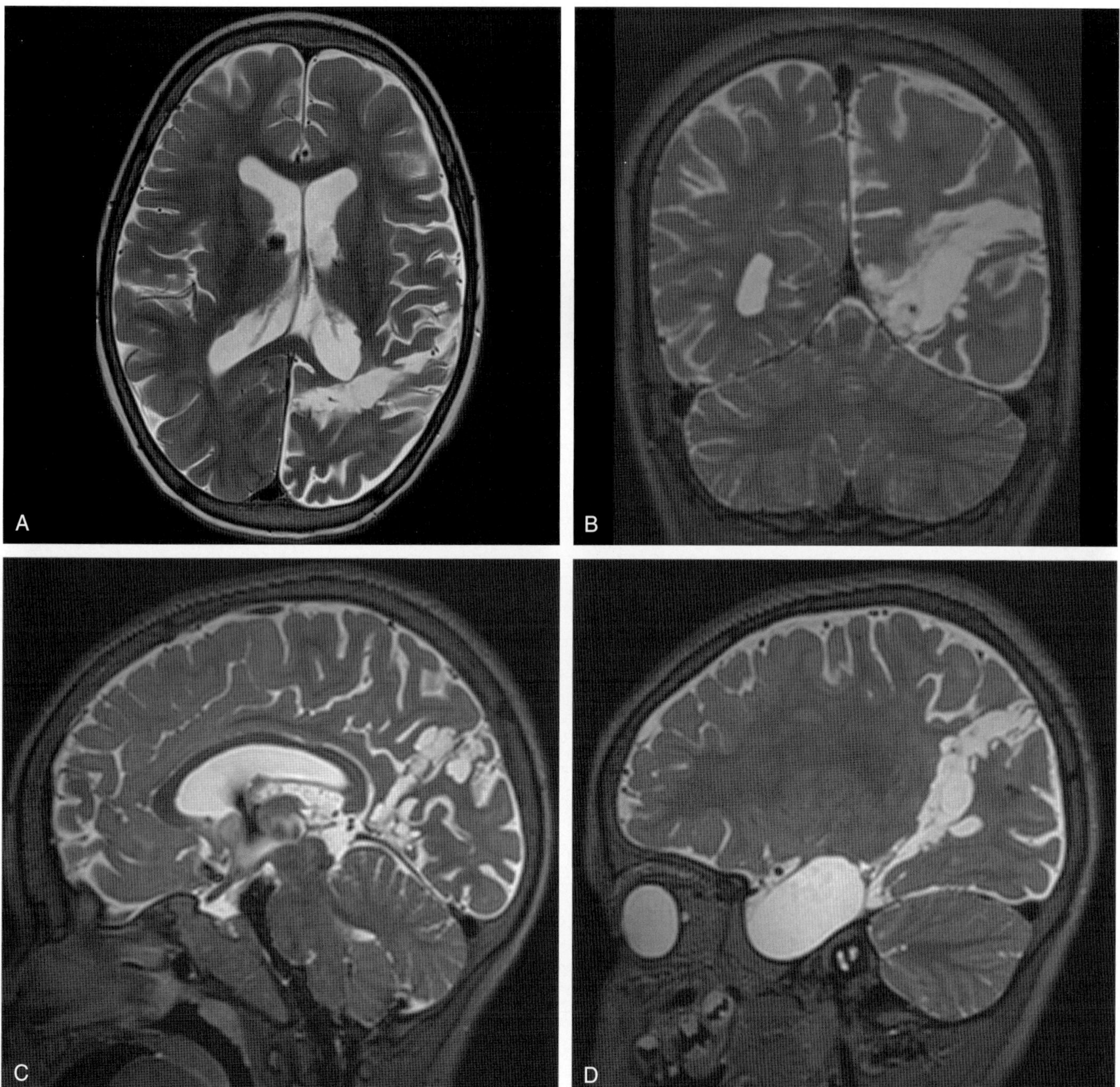

Fig. 8.27 Posterior Quadrant Disconnection. (A to D) Multiplanar T2W, images demonstrate the expected appearance of a posterior quadrant disconnection.

Key Points

Background

- Surgical procedure for refractory unilateral temporoparieto-occipital epilepsy
- Surgical procedure consists of the following:
  - Exposure of the insular cortex
  - Disconnection of the temporal stem at the inferior periinsular cortex
  - Extension of disconnection from limen insulae to the atrium of the lateral ventricle
  - Amygdalohippocampectomy
  - Disconnection of the parietal lobe at the postcentral sulcus to the atrium of the lateral ventricle; medial parietal lobe disconnection to the corpus callosum
  - Disconnection of the splenium of the corpus callosum
  - Division of the fornix at the atrium of the lateral ventricle

Imaging

- Imaging of a posterior quadrant disconnection includes an oblique parenchymal defect separating the occipital lobe from the remainder of the cerebral hemisphere, defect through the temporal stem, disconnection of the splenium, and resection of the medial temporal lobe.

REFERENCES

1. Oguz Cataltepe GIJ, George I. Jallo. Pediatric Epilepsy Surgery: Preoperative Assessment and Surgical Treatment. Thieme; 2nd Edition (September 23, 2019); 2019.
2. Kalbhenn T, Cloppenborg T. Wörmann FG et al Operative posterior disconnection in epilepsy surgery: Experience with 29 patients. *Epilepsia*. 2019 Sep;60(9):1973–1983.
3. Umaba R, Uda T, Nakajo K, et al. Anatomic Understanding of Posterior Quadrant Disconnection from Cadaveric Brain, 3D Reconstruction and Simulation Model, and Intraoperative Photographs. *World Neurosurg*. 2018 Dec;120:e792–e801.
4. Daniel RT, Meagher-Villemure K, Farmer JP, et al. Posterior quadrantic epilepsy surgery: technical variants, surgical anatomy, and case series. *Epilepsia*. 2007 Aug;48(8):1429–1437.

EPILEPSY SURGERY: HYPOTHALAMIC HAMARTOMA ABLATION

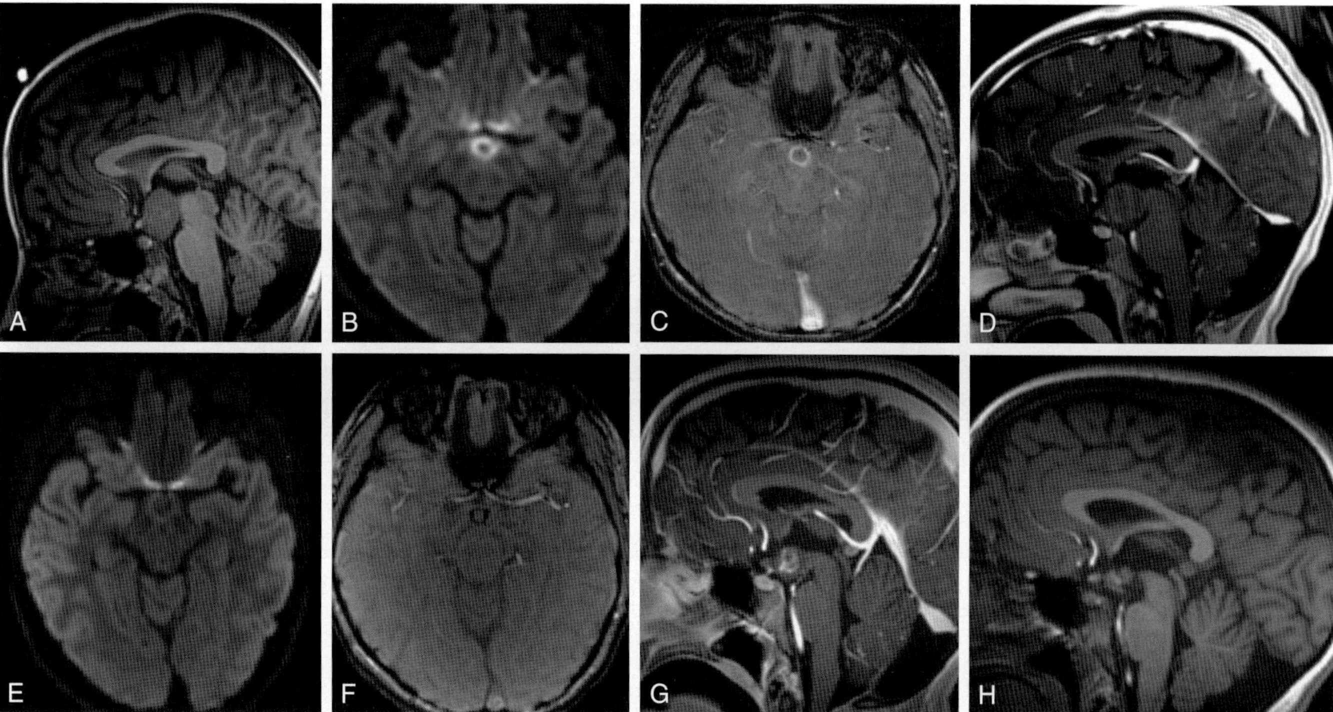

Fig. 8.28 Hypothalamic Hamartoma Ablation: Evolution of Appearance. (A) Sagittal T1W image at initial presentation demonstrating a T1W isointense mass in the tuber cinereum. (B to D) Intraoperative imaging with axial DWI, axial SWI, and sagittal T1W+C images demonstrate diffusion restriction and linear enhancement at the ablation site. (E to G) The 3-month follow-up axial DWI, axial SWI, and sagittal T1W+C images demonstrate less diffusion restriction, new hypointense SWI signal, and greater linear enhancement. (H) The 10-month follow-up sagittal T1W image demonstrates significant reduction in size compared to initial presentation.

Key Points

Background

- Nonneoplastic heterotopic tissue containing neurons and glia (astrocytes and oligodendrocytes)
- Patients may have a variety of different types of seizures, most commonly gelastic; seizures typically begin in infancy but may have onset later in life.
- Associated with central precocious puberty, behavioral disorders, and neurocognitive delay
- Variable size; size of the lesion may correlate with symptoms and seizure severity
- Open and endoscopic surgical options have historically been employed; stereotactic laser ablation is a modern, minimally invasive technique with high safety profile.
  - 93% of patients are free of gelastic seizures at 1 year after laser ablation

Imaging

- Sessile and pedunculated morphologies can be seen
- Isointense to gray matter on T1W and T2W imaging. May have mild T1 hypointensity and mild T2 hyperintiensity. No enhancement and no diffusion restriction unless treated.
- Rarely contains cystic foci
- Laser ablation cavity
  - Acute: T2 hyperintense with restricted diffusion, peripheral enhancement, microhemorrhage, restricted diffusion
  - Chronic: Hamartoma shrinkage

REFERENCES

1. Oguz Cataltepe GIJ, George I. Jallo. Pediatric Epilepsy Surgery: Preoperative Assessment and Surgical Treatment. Thieme; 2nd Edition (September 23, 2019); 2019.
2. Curry DJ, Raskin J, Ali I, et al. MR-guided laser ablation for the treatment of hypothalamic hamartomas. *Epilepsy Res.* 2018;142:131–134.
3. Alomari SO, Houshiemy MNE, Bsat S, et al. Hypothalamic hamartomas: A comprehensive review of the literature - Part 1: Neurobiological features, clinical presentations and advancements in diagnostic tools. *Clin Neurol Neurosurg.* 2020 Oct;197:106076.
4. Alomari SO, El Houshiemy MN, Bsat S, et al. Hypothalamic Hamartomas: A comprehensive review of literature - Part 2: Medical and surgical management update. *Clin Neurol Neurosurg.* 2020 Aug;195:106074.

EPILEPSY SURGERY: HEMISPHERECTOMY

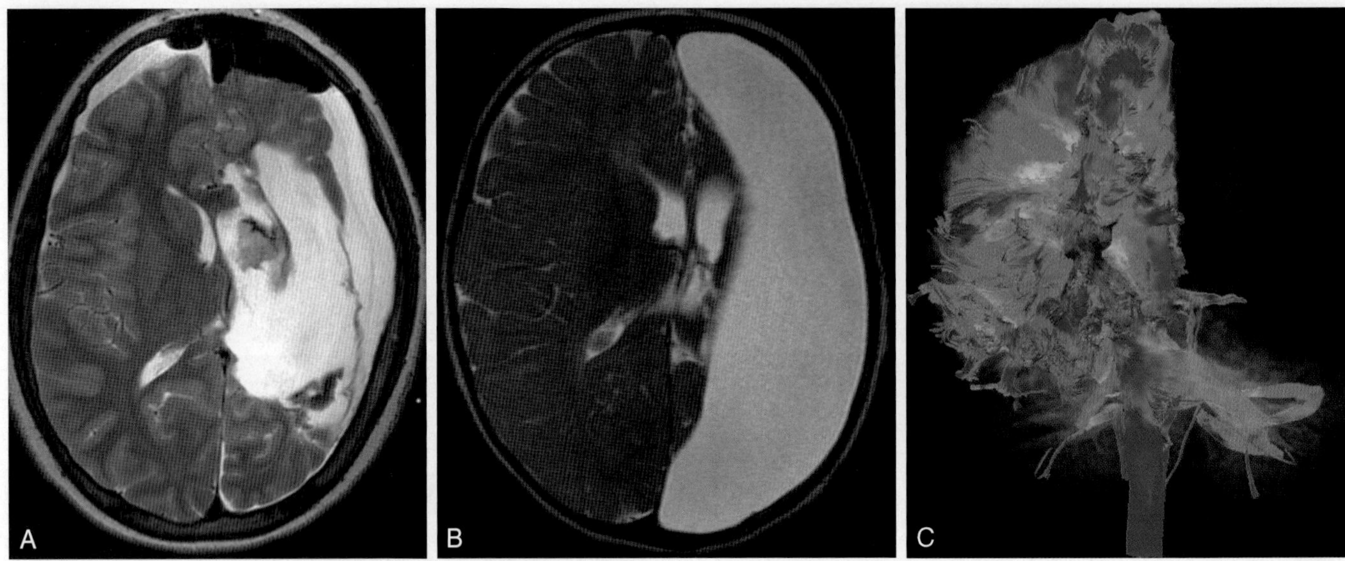

Fig. 8.29 Hemispherectomy. (A and B) Axial T2W images demonstrate early and late appearances of a left hemispherectomy. Early postoperative appearance demonstrates extra-axial air and fluid, resection of the majority of the left cerebral hemisphere and disconnection of the corpus callosum. Follow-up imaging demonstrates majority of the left hemicranium is fluid filled. (C) Tractography demonstrates no crossing fibers in the remaining left cerebral hemisphere.

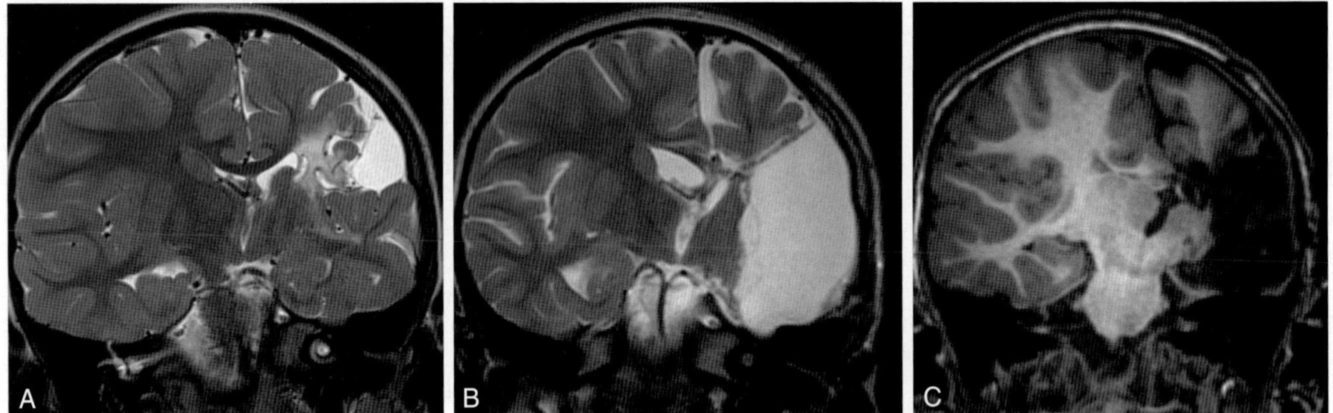

Fig. 8.30 Functional Hemispherectomy. (A) Preoperative coronal T2W image prior to surgery demonstrates a large region of encephalomalacia in the left cerebral hemisphere due to a perinatal infarct. (B and C) Postoperative coronal T2W and T1W images demonstrate functional hemispherectomy surgical changes with resection of the encephalomalacia, left temporal lobectomy, and disconnection of the left cerebral hemisphere.

Key Points

Background

- Hemispherectomy is a neurosurgical procedure to treat children with intractable seizures that start in childhood and arise diffusely from a single hemisphere.
- These include congenital (e.g., hemimegalencephaly and prenatal stroke) or postnatally acquired (e.g., Rasmussen encephalitis and traumatic brain injury) lesions.
- Seizure freedom achieved in 61% to 80% of patients. Causes of failure from surgical technique include incomplete disconnection of the corpus callosum, frontobasal cortex, or insula.

Imaging

- Two types of hemispherectomy
  - Anatomic
    - Resection of the entirety of the cortical parenchyma with retention of the central gray matter
    - Increased risk for postoperative hydrocephalus
    - Uncommonly performed
  - Functional (hemispherotomy) including:
    - Frontoparietal topectomy
    - Frontal disconnection
    - Posterior disconnection
    - Temporal lobectomy
  - Callosotomy
    - Advanced neuroimaging can evaluate for reorganization/neuroplasticity of the remaining hemisphere. DTI metrics may add information about Wallerian and/or transneuronal degeneration of the white matter tracts within the remaining hemisphere.

REFERENCES

1. Vining EP, Freeman JM, Pillas DJ, et al. Why would you remove half a brain? The outcome of 58 children after hemispherectomy-the Johns Hopkins experience: 1968 to 1996. *Pediatrics.* 1997;100:163–171.
2. Meoded A, Faria AV, Hartman AL, et al. Cerebral Reorganization after Hemispherectomy: A DTI Study. *AJNR Am J Neuroradiol.* 2016;37:924–931.
3. Baumgartner JE, Blount JP, Blauwblomme T et al. Technical descriptions of four hemispherectomy approaches: From the Pediatric Epilepsy Surgery Meeting at Gothenburg 2.

9 Phakomatoses

INTRODUCTION

TABLE 9.1 Summary of Findings in the Common Phakomatoses

Disorder	CNS	Globe and Orbit	Skin	Other
Neurofibromatosis type 1	Myelin vacuolization Gliomas Sphenoid wing dysplasia Moyamoya Aneurysms Short, thickened corpus callosum	Optic nerve glioma Lisch nodules Buphthalmos	Café-au-lait spots Axillary/inguinal freckling	Neurofibromas Malignant peripheral nerve sheath tumor Meningocele Dural ectasia Arachnoid cysts Scoliosis Gibbus deformity
Neurofibromatosis type 2	Meningioma Ependymoma Schwannoma	Optic nerve sheath meningioma Cataracts	Café-au-lait spots	Schwannomas
Tuberous sclerosis	Cortical tubers Radial migration lines Subependymal nodules Subependymal giant cell adenoma Moyamoya	Retinal hamartoma	Ash leaf spot Facial angiofibroma Shagreen patch Dental pits	Angiomyolipoma Cardiac rhabdomyoma Pulmonary Lymphangiomyomatosis Rectal polyps Bone cysts
Sturge-Weber syndrome	Pial angiomatosis Ipsilateral choroid plexus hyperplasia Cortical atrophy Cortical calcification Calvarial hypertrophy	Choroidal/scleral angiomatosis Glaucoma	Port-wine stain	
Von Hippel-Lindau syndrome	Hemangioblastomas Endolymphatic sac tumor	Retinal hemangioblastoma	Capillary malformations (uncommon)	Kidney: Renal cell carcinoma and renal cysts Pancreas: Cysts, microcystic serous adenomas, islet cell tumors Pheochromocytoma Epididymal or broad ligament cystadenoma

Phakomatoses are a group of neurocutaneous disorders that involve structures arising from the embryologic ectoderm, resulting in abnormalities of the skin, nervous system, retina, and globe.

There are approximately 30 different phakomatoses; however, the main phakomatoses include neurofibromatosis type 1 (NF-1), neurofibromatosis type 2 (NF-2), tuberous sclerosis, Sturge-Weber syndrome, and Von Hippel-Lindau disease. Table 9.1 highlights the CNS, globe and orbit, skin, and other abnormalities seen with these phakomatoses. A few other rare disorders also are discussed in this chapter. Cowden disease and Gomez-Lopez-Hernandez syndrome are discussed briefly in the brain tumor and brain malformation Chapter 2, Brain Malformations, and Chapter 7, Brain Tumors and Treatment Complications, respectively.

Because tumors are associated with the phakomatoses, serial imaging is often performed in these patients. MRI is the primary modality in which abnormalities of the phakomatoses are best identified.

NEUROFIBROMATOSIS TYPE 1

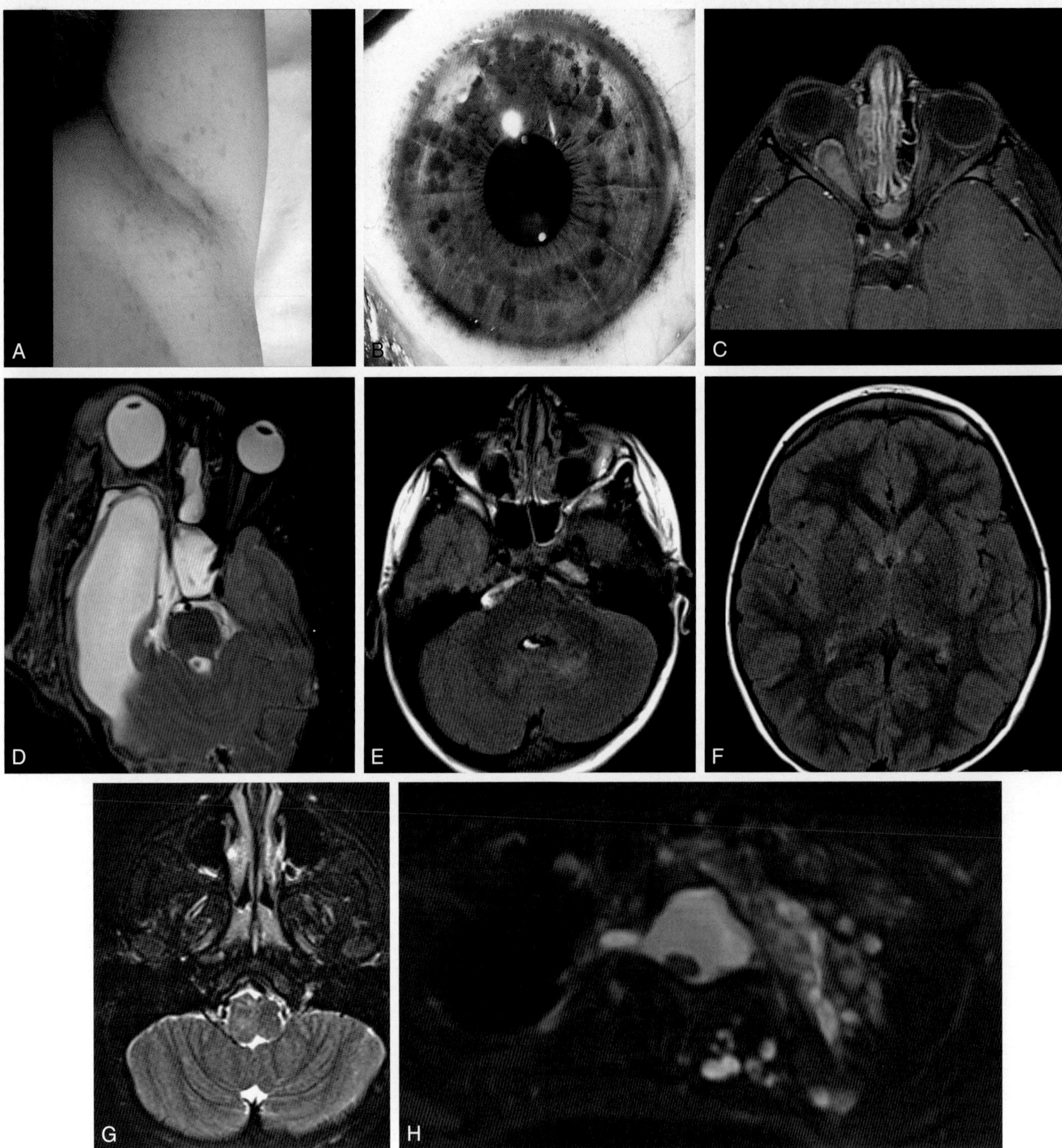

Fig. 9.1 Neurofibromatosis Type 1. (A) Café-au-lait spots in the axillary region in neurofibromatosis type 1. (B) Pigmented hamartomas of the iris (Lisch nodules). (C) Axial T1W+C fat saturation image of the orbits demonstrating fusiform enlargement and enhancement of the right optic nerve consistent with an optic nerve glioma. (D) Axial T2W fat saturation image demonstrates buphthalmos of the right globe, right sphenoid wing dysplasia, and dural ectasia resulting in an expanded fluid-filled sella and anterior cranial fossa adjacent to the right ethmoid sinus. (E and F) Axial FLAIR images demonstrate FLAIR hyperintense non-mass-like lesions in the dentate nuclei and globus pallidi consistent with myelin vacuolization. (G) Axial T2W fat saturation image demonstrates T2 hyperintensity in the right side of the medulla with mild expansion. This could represent a glioma as well as myelin vacuolization. (H) Axial T2W fat saturation image demonstrates dural ectasia and a plexiform neurofibroma. (A from Passeron T, Mantouz F, Ortonne JP. Genetic disorders of pigmentation. *Clin Dermatol*. 2005;23[1]:56–67. B from Zitelli BJ, McIntire SC, Nowalk AJ, eds. *Zitelli and Davis' Atlas of Pediatric Physical Diagnosis*. 7th ed. Elsevier; 2018.)

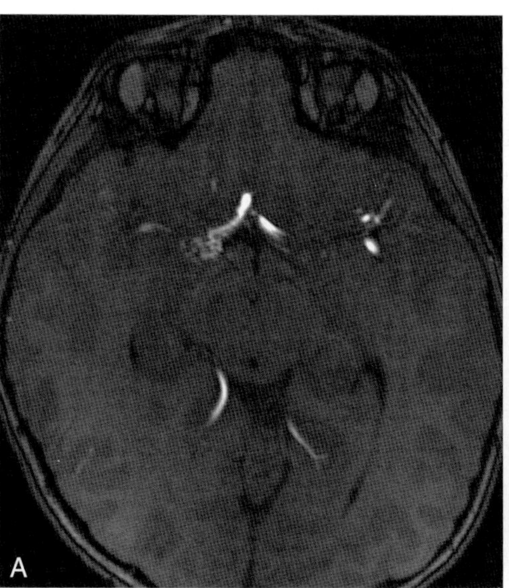

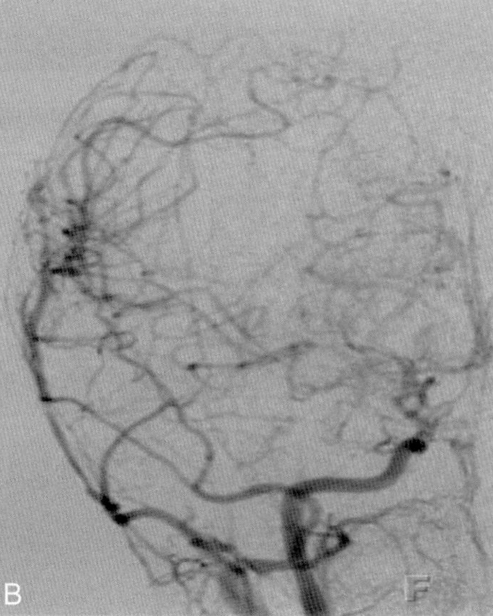

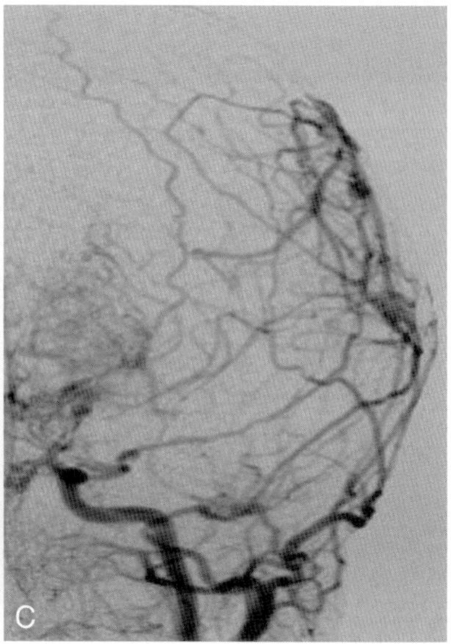

Fig. 9.2 Neurofibromatosis Type 1. (A) Axial MR angiography image demonstrates bilateral occlusions of the ICA terminus and collateral vessels on the right side. (B and C) Catheter angiography AP images from ICA injections demonstrate bilateral ICA occlusions, collateral vessels consistent with moyamoya vasculopathy, and prior bilateral dural synangiosis.

Key Points

Background

- Also known as von Recklinghausen disease; NF-1 is a tumor suppressor gene encoded by chromosome 17q11.2; NF-1 encodes neurofibromin, which is an inhibitor of RAS-MAPK pathway, a regulatory pathway of cellular growth and differentiation. Autosomal dominant (first-degree relative)

Clinical

- Diagnostic Criteria
  - Clinical diagnosis made when at least two of the following are present: six or more café-au-lait spots, at least two neurofibromas or one plexiform neurofibroma, axillary or inguinal freckling, optic glioma, at least two Lisch nodules, a distinctive bone lesion such a sphenoid wing dysplasia or long bone cortical thickening with or without pseudoarthrosis, first-degree relative with NF-1
- Skin: Café-au-lait spots, axillary/inguinal freckling
- Orbit and globe: Lisch nodules, which are melanocytic hamartomas and have increasing incidence with age in NF-1 (5% in age <3 years, 55% at age 5–6 years, and 100% in age >21 years); optic pathway glioma, which are associated with decreased visual acuity and visual field defects in <50% of patients; buphthalmos; glaucoma
- Other: Learning disability (30%–65%)

Imaging

- *Gliomas*: Optic pathway (1.5% to 15% incidence, median age 4.9 years) > brain (1%–3% incidence) and spinal cord. Usually low-grade glioma pathology (pilocytic astrocytoma). Appearance: T2W hyperintense, well-defined masses with variable enhancement. Optic pathway gliomas in NF-1 usually involve the anterior optic pathway.
- *Myelin vacuolization:* Occurs in 60% to 80% of NF-1 patients. Typical locations: basal ganglia (the primarily globus pallidus), internal capsule, brainstem, and around the cerebellar dentate nuclei. Appearance: transient nonenhancing, ill-defined T2W hyperintense foci begin appearing around age 3, peaking at approximately age 12 years, and uncommonly seen after 20 years of age. If an area demonstrates enhancement or mass effect, a glioma should be considered. Some small, confined areas such as the brainstem can be difficult to determine whether the signal abnormality is from myelin vacuolization or glioma, and follow-up imaging should be performed. Additionally, MRS can help differentiate vacuolization from glioma as vacuolization demonstrates elevated choline, reduced creatine, and normal NAA, while glioma demonstrates choline:creatine ratio > 2 and reduced NAA.
- *Neurofibromas, plexiform neurofibroma*, and rarely malignant peripheral nerve sheath tumor. Plexiform neurofibromas are multispatial, infiltrative T2 hyperintense avidly enhancing lesions.
- Sphenoid wing dysplasia
- Orbit: *Buphthalmos* (large globe)
- Vascular: *Moyamoya* syndrome, cerebral aneurysms
- Spine: *Dural ectasia, meningoceles*, arachnoid cysts, gibbus deformity, and scoliosis
- Short, thickened corpus callosum

REFERENCES

1. Rodriguez D, Young Poussaint T. Neuroimaging findings in neurofibromatosis type 1 and 2. *Neuroimaging Clin N Am*. 2004 May;14(2):149–170.
2. Borofsky S, Levy LM. Neurofibromatosis: types 1 and 2. *AJNR Am J Neuroradiol*. 2013 Dec;34(12):2250–2251.

NEUROFIBROMATOSIS TYPE 2

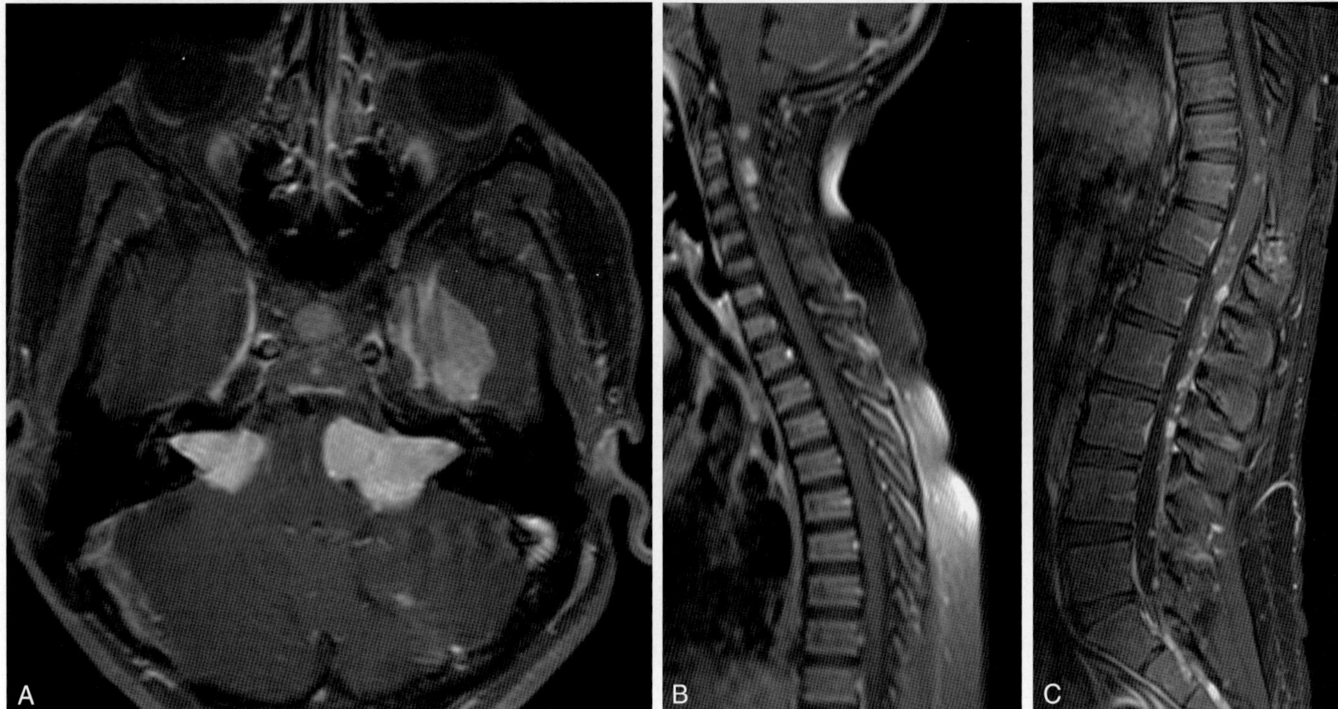

Fig. 9.3 Neurofibromatosis Type 2. (A) Axial T1W+C fat saturation image demonstrates nodular enhancement in the bilateral internal auditory canals and left Meckel's cave consistent with multiple schwannomas, and extra-axial enhancement in the left middle cranial fossa enhancement consistent with a meningioma. (B and C) Sagittal T1W+C fat saturation images demonstrate intramedullary enhancing nodules consistent with ependymomas and multiple enhancing nodules along the cauda equina consistent with schwannomas.

Key Points

Background

- Autosomal dominant disorder. NF-2 encodes tumor suppressor gene on chromosome 22q12.2, which encodes merlin, a cell growth regulator
- *"MISME" acronym:* Multiple inherited schwannomas, meningiomas, and ependymomas

Clinical

- Clinical diagnosis of NF-2 is made in the presence of any of the following:
  - Bilateral vestibular schwannomas
  - Unilateral vestibular schwannoma and first-degree relative with NF-2
  - Any two of the following: meningioma, nonvestibular schwannoma, ependymoma, cataract, AND first-degree relative with NF-2 or unilateral vestibular schwannoma and negative LZTR1 testing
  - Multiple meningiomas and unilateral vestibular schwannoma or any two of the following: nonvestibular schwannoma, ependymoma, cataract
- Probable NF-2 diagnosis: Family history of NF-2 and unilateral vestibular schwannoma plus a meningioma, glioma, juvenile cortical cataract
- Skin: Café-au-lait spots (far less common than NF-1), and cutaneous schwannomas
- Orbit and globe: Cataracts, and optic nerve sheath meningioma

Imaging

- *Schwannomas*: Vestibular schwannomas occur in 95% of adult patients. Other cranial nerves, intramedullary and extramedullary spinal involvement, and peripheral nerve schwannomas commonly occur. Schwannomas are classically T1 hypointense, T2 hyperintense with avid enhancement.
- *Meningiomas*: Dural-based lesions with T1 and T2 isointense signal with avid enhancement
- Ependymomas: enhancing lesion in the center of the spinal cord
- Meningioangiomatosis: Cortical-subcortical heterogeneous lesion(s) with variable enhancement and calcification; overlying leptomeninges may be involved

REFERENCE

1. Rodriguez D, Young Poussaint T. Neuroimaging findings in neurofibromatosis type 1 and 2. *Neuroimaging Clin N Am*. 2004 May;14(2):149–170.

TUBEROUS SCLEROSIS

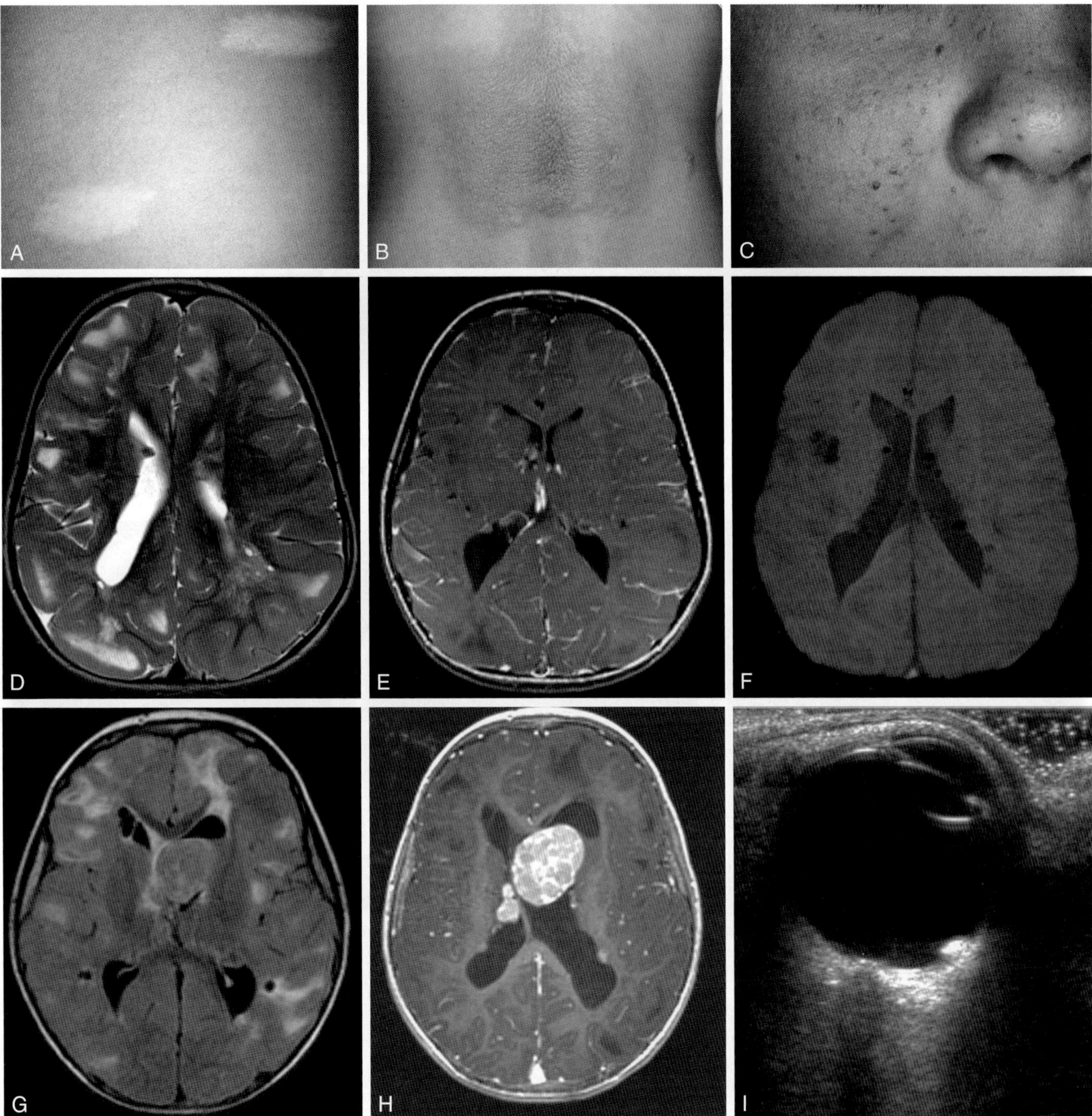

Fig. 9.4 Tuberous Sclerosis. (A) Ash leaf spots: hypopigmented macules in tuberous sclerosis. (B) Shagreen patch. The shagreen patch is characteristically found at the lumbosacral area and has a peau d'orange texture. (C) Facial angiofibromas. These pink to red, dome-shaped smooth papules occur most commonly on the cheeks, nasolabial folds, and chin. They may occasionally be confused with lesions of acne vulgaris. (D) Axial T2W, (E) axial T1W+C, (F) axial SWI images demonstrate multiple nonenhancing juxtacortical T2 hyperintensities in the cerebral hemispheres consistent with cortical tubers and dysplasias as well as nodular foci of susceptibility in the periventricular white matter due to calcified subependymal nodules. (G) Axial FLAIR, and (H) axial T1W+C images demonstrate multiple cortical tubers, dysplasias and a large enhancing mass in the left lateral ventricle consistent with a subependymal giant cell astrocytoma. (I) Ultrasound image of a retinal hamartoma seen as a hyperechoic nodule. (A from Dinulos JGH, Habif TP. *Habif's Clinical Dermatology: A Color Guide to Diagnosis and Therapy.* 7th ed. Elsevier; 2021. B and C from Paller AS, Mancini AJ: *Hurwitz clinical pediatric dermatology: a textbook of skin disorders of childhood and adolescence*, ed 6, Philadelphia, 2022, Elsevier.)

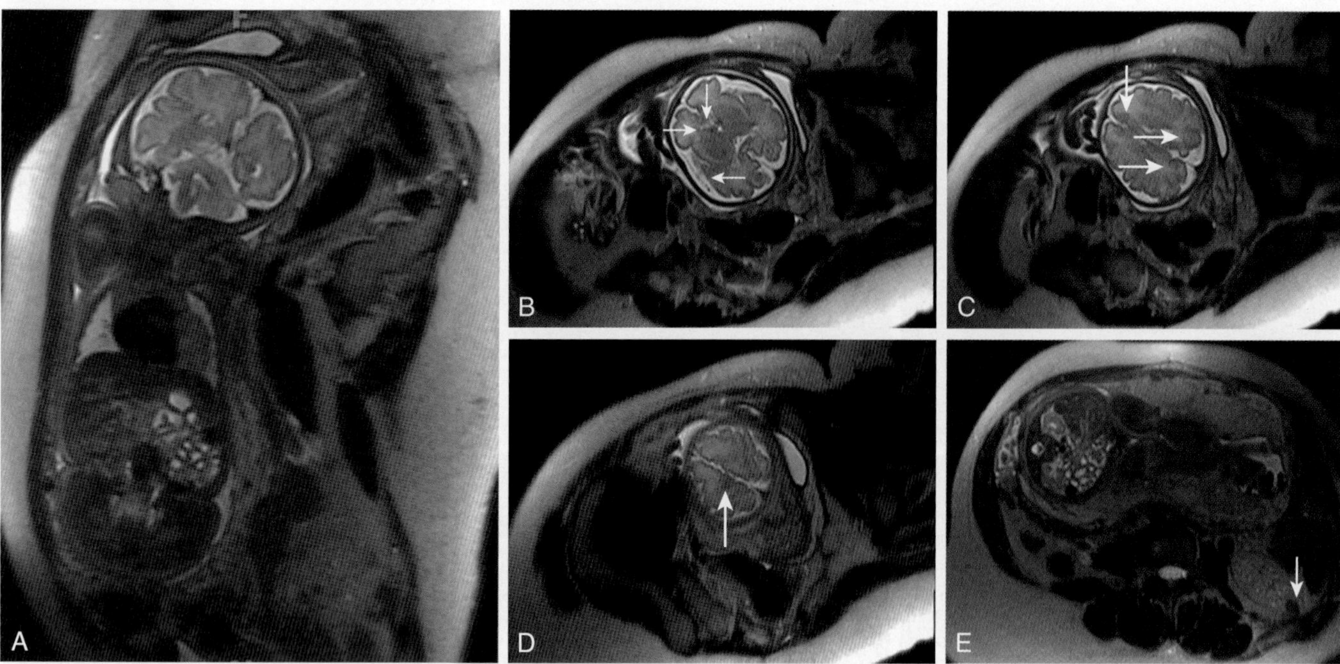

Fig. 9.5 Tuberous Sclerosis. (A to E) Multiplanar T2W fetal MR images demonstrate a fetal cardiac rhabdomyoma (A), and arrows indicating subependymal nodules near the foramen of Monro (B), subtle T2 hypointense cortical tubers (C and D), and maternal renal angiomyolipoma (E).

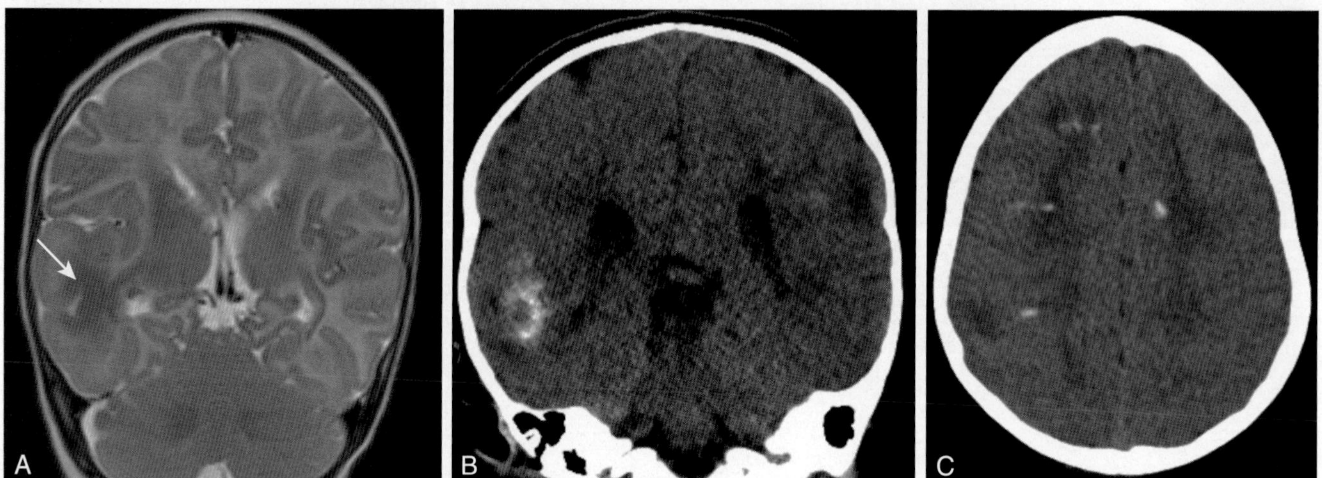

Fig. 9.6 Tuberous Sclerosis. (A) Coronal T2W image demonstrates a neonatal brain with a T2 hypointense right temporal cortical and juxtacortical lesion consistent with a tuber (*arrow*). (B and C) Coronal and axial CT images demonstrate calcification of the temporal lobe tuber as well as additional calcified tubers in the frontal lobes and more typical hypodense tubers without calcification.

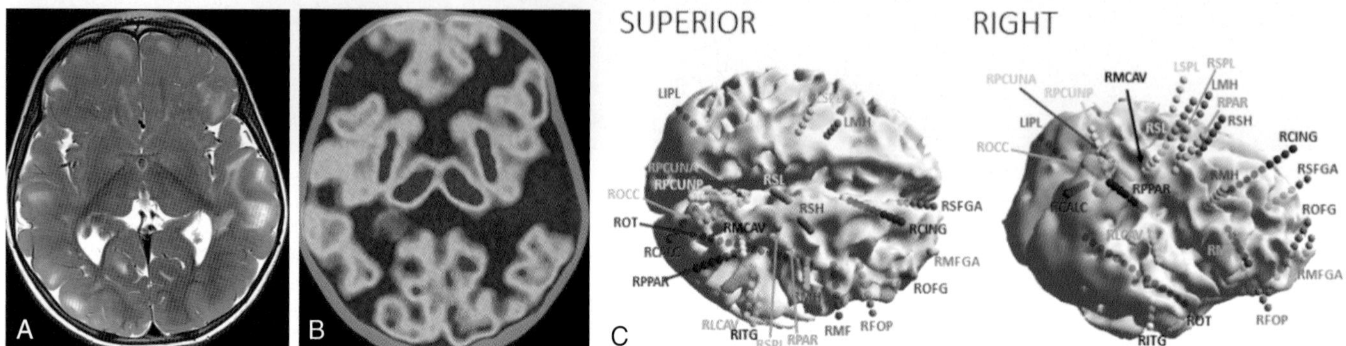

Fig. 9.7 Tuberous Sclerosis: Epilepsy Workup. (A) Axial T2W image demonstrates multiple cortical tuberous in a patient with tuberous sclerosis. (B) Axial FDG PET CT image demonstrating multiple hypometabolic regions corresponding to the tubers. This presents a challenge in determining whether one or multiple tubers is the primary seizure generator. (C) A 3D fused image of color-coded depth electrodes on the brain of a tuberous sclerosis patient. Invasive monitoring with depth electrodes is often necessary for more precise seizure localization prior to any attempted resection or ablation of a tuber.

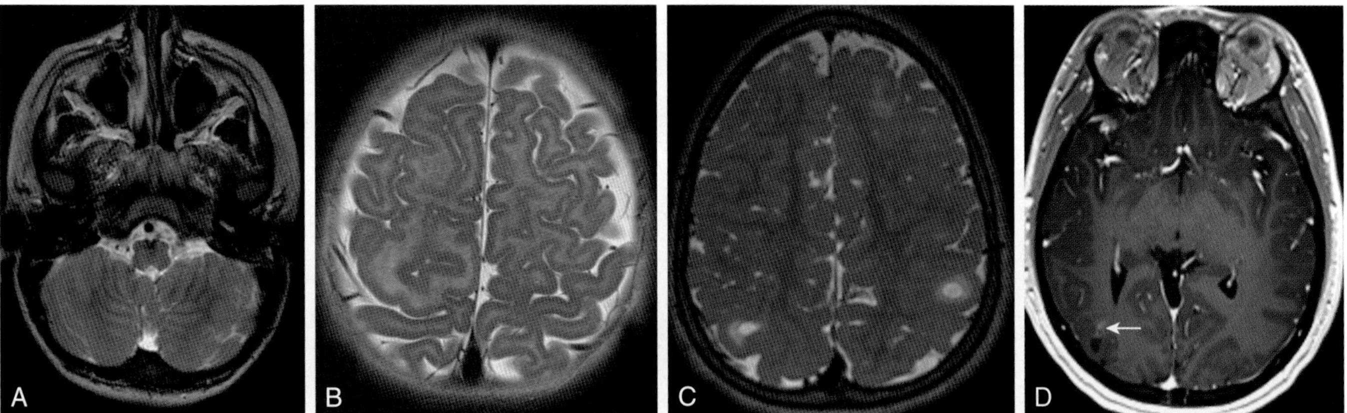

Fig. 9.8 Tuberous Sclerosis: Uncommon Appearances. (A) Axial T2W image demonstrating abnormal sulcation of the left cerebellar hemisphere. (B) Axial T2W image demonstrating focal broad gyrus in the right superior frontal gyrus (pachygyria). (C) Axial T2W image demonstrates cystic degeneration in two tubers. (D) Axial T1W+C image demonstrates enhancement of a right occipital tuber (*arrow*).

Key Points

Background

- Also known as Bourneville-Pringle disease; autosomal dominant mutations in TSC1 (chromosome 9q34) and TSC2 (chromosome 16p13.3) tumor suppressor genes involved in the PI3K/AKT/mTOR pathway
- TSC2 mutations are far more common than TSC1 mutations

Clinical

- Diagnostic Criteria
    - Diagnosis made by genetic testing identifying TSC1 or TSC2 mutation or through clinical criteria with two major criteria or one major and two or more minor criteria as follows:
        - Major criteria: Hypomelanotic macules (≥3, at least 5 mm in diameter), angiofibromas (≥3), ungual fibromas (≥2), shagreen patch, multiple retinal hamartomas, cortical dysplasias (tubers and radial migration lines), subependymal nodules, subependymal giant cell astrocytoma (SEGA), cardiac rhabdomyoma, lymphangioleiomyomatosis (LAM), angiomyolipomas
        - Minor criteria: Confetti skin (1- to 2-mm hypomelanotic macules), dental enamel pits (≥3), intraoral fibromas (≥2), retinal achromic patch, multiple renal cysts, nonrenal hamartomas
- Skin: Ash leaf spots, facial angiofibroma, shagreen patch, "confetti" skin lesions, and nontraumatic ungual/periungual angiofibroma
- Orbit and globe: Retinal astrocytic hamartomas
- Other: Dental pits and gingival angiofibromas, hamartomatous rectal polyps, bone cysts, mental retardation, and *epilepsy*

Imaging

- *Cortical tubers* and dysplasias (focal cortical dysplasia type 2b): Variable appearance based on the degree of myelination of brain. Transitions from T1 hyperintense and T2 hypointense in the immaturely myelinated brain to T1 hypointense and T2 hyperintense in the maturely myelinated brain. Less commonly may enhance and/or calcify. Common in the supratentorium, most commonly in the frontal and parietal lobes but may occur in the cerebellum. Magnetization transfer and T2 FLAIR sequences are optimal for identification of cortical tubers.
- *Radial migration lines:* T2 hyperintense, nonenhancing lines extending from ependymal surface to cortex to ventricular margin, typically associated with a cortical tuber.
- *Subependymal nodules:* Well-defined nodules, most commonly caudothalamic in location that progressively calcify with age. Variable enhancement. Well seen on 3D T1 sequence without contrast and SWI when lesional calcification is present.
- *Subependymal giant cell astrocytoma (SEGA):* Arise from a subependymal nodule at the foramen of Monroe. A subependymal nodule at the foramen of Monroe that is greater than 10 mm without documented stability on serial imaging or an enlarging nodule < 10 mm should raise concern for a SEGA. A SEGA will typically demonstrate avid enhancement and when large can cause ventricular obstruction, progressive increase in size. Typically demonstrate avid enhancement.
- Moyamoya syndrome.
- Other: Cardiac rhabdomyomas, lymphangiomyomatosis, renal angiomyolipomas and cysts

REFERENCES

1. Smirniotopoulos JG. Neuroimaging of phakomatoses: Sturge-Weber syndrome, tuberous sclerosis, von Hippel-Lindau syndrome. *Neuroimaging Clin N Am.* 2004 May;14(2):171–183.
2. Nandigam K, Mechtler LL, Smirniotopoulos JG. Neuroimaging of neurocutaneous diseases. *Neurol Clin.* 2014 Feb;32(1):159–192.

STURGE-WEBER SYNDROME

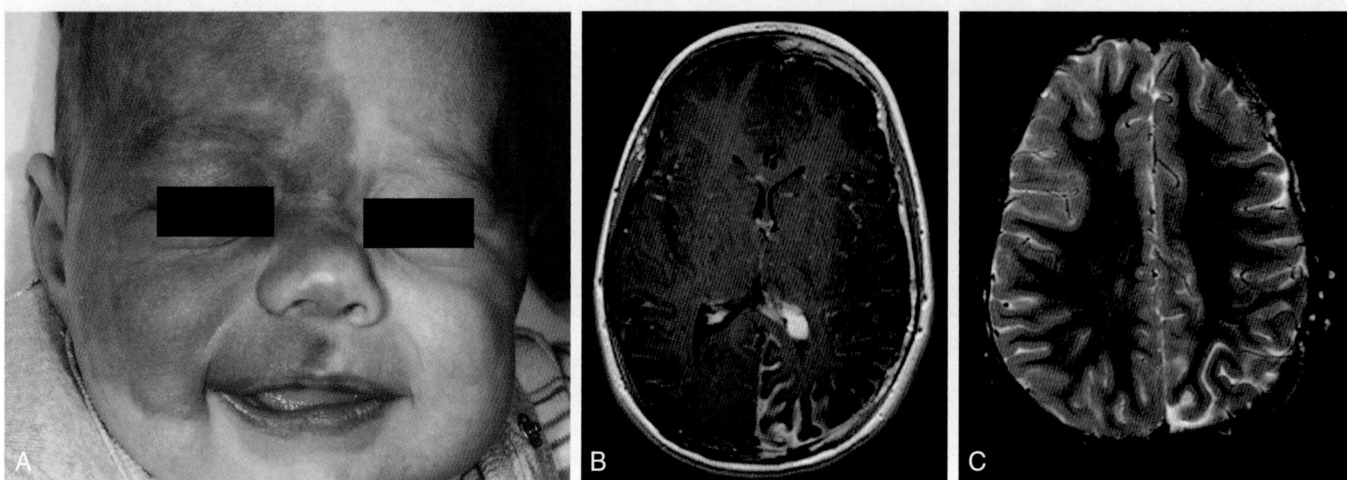

Fig. 9.9 Sturge-Weber Syndrome: Classic Findings. (A) Port-wine stain involving both the right V1 and V2 trigeminal dermatomes in this infant with Sturge-Weber syndrome. (B) Axial T1W+C and (C) axial T2W images in a different patient demonstrate abnormal leptomeningeal enhancement of the left parietal and occipital lobe, ipsilateral enlarged choroid plexus, and parenchymal volume loss. (A from Paller AS, Mancini AJ. *Hurwitz Clinical Pediatric Dermatology.* 4th ed. Saunders; 2011. Courtesy Annette Wagner, MD. In Goljan EF. *Rapid Review Pathology.* 5th ed. Elsevier; 2019.)

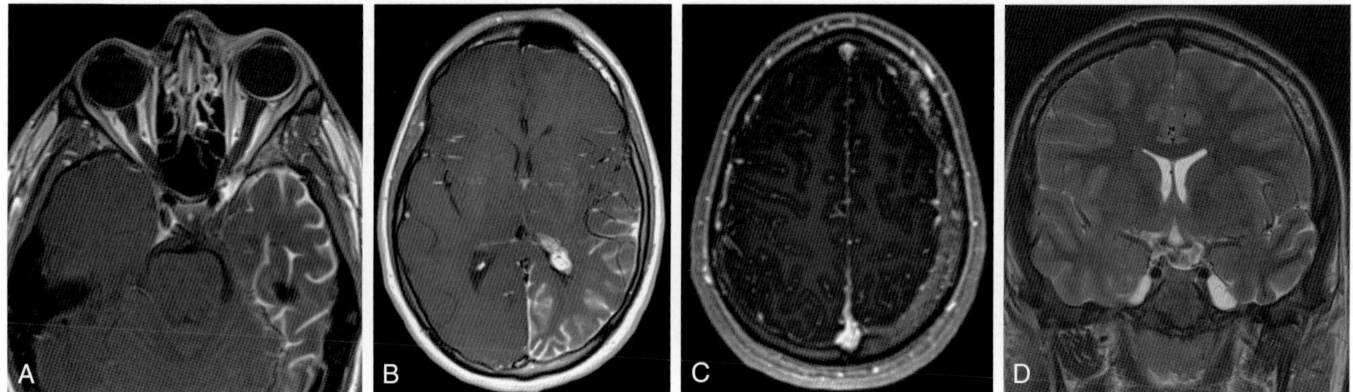

Fig. 9.10 Sturge-Weber Syndrome: Classic Findings. (A to C) Axial T1W+C and (D) coronal T2W images demonstrate abnormal leptomeningeal enhancement along the left temporal, parietal, and occipital lobes, thickened and enhancing left choroidal layer of the globe due to an angioma, left choroid plexus enlargement, left calvarial thickening, left hemisphere atrophy, absent left septal vein, and dilated left Meckel's cave.

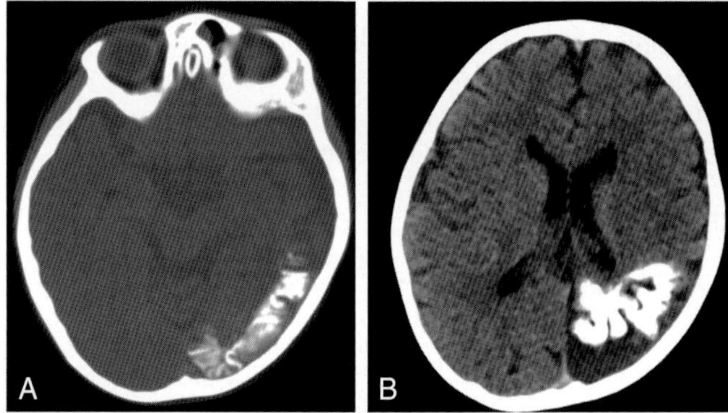

Fig. 9.11 Sturge-Weber Syndrome: CT Findings. (A and B) Axial CT images demonstrate cortical calcification in the left parietal and occipital lobes associated with volume loss.

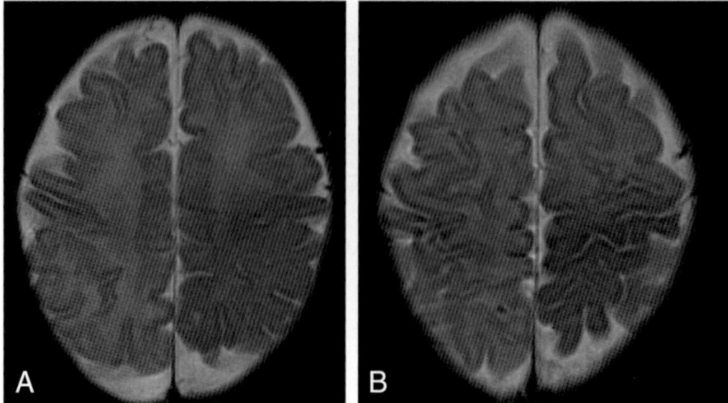

Fig. 9.12 Sturge-Weber Syndrome: Infant Findings. (A and B) Axial T2W images demonstrate hypointense signal in the left parietal lobe, presumably from venous congestion and/or accelerated myelination.

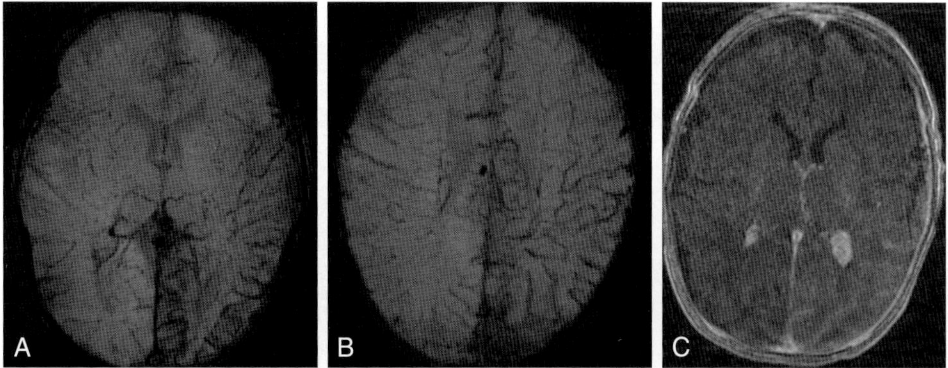

Fig. 9.13 Sturge-Weber Syndrome: SWI Findings. (A and B) Axial SWI and (C) axial T1W+C images demonstrate increased susceptibility in the left parietal and occipital lobe sulci from pial angiomatosis, mild enhancement of the leptomeninges, and enlarged left choroid plexus.

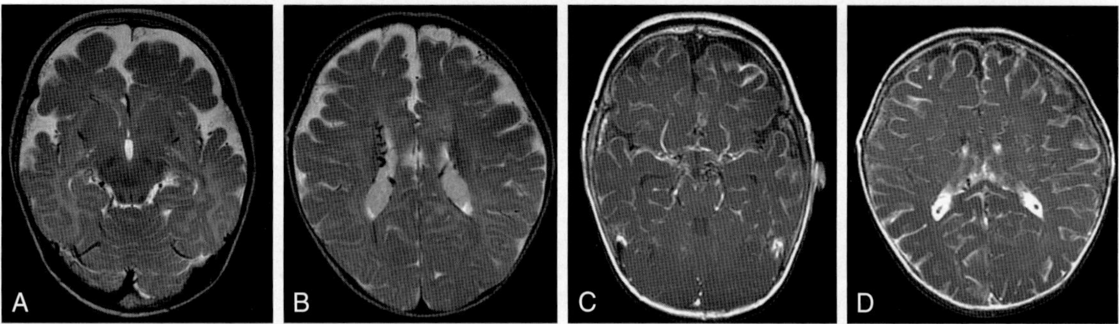

Fig. 9.14 Sturge-Weber Syndrome: Atypical Diffuse Involvement. (A and B) Axial T2W and (C and D) axial T1W+C images demonstrate cerebral volume loss, diffuse leptomeningeal enhancement, and enlarged bilateral choroid plexus. Tortuous and dilated perimedullary veins are noted along the lateral ventricles.

Key Points

Background

- Also known as encephalotrigeminal angiomatosis
- Sporadic neurocutaneous disorder with somatic mutation in *GNAQ* gene. Characterized by facial cutaneous capillary malformation (port wine stain), choroidal/scleral angiomatosis with glaucoma and leptomeningeal angiomatosis with impaired cerebral venous drainage. Chronic venous ischemia with eventual parenchymal hypoperfusion results in parenchymal injury with secondary volume loss and dystrophic calcification

Clinical

- Diagnosis made by detection of facial capillary malformation and leptomeningeal angiomatosis
- Skin: Facial port-wine stain (nevus flammeus)
- Orbit and globe: Choroidal/scleral angioma occurring in 20% to 70% of patients; glaucoma occurring in 30% to 70% of patients
- Other: Seizures commonly in first 2 years of life, hemiparesis and stroke-like events, intellectual disability, behavioral problems, and growth hormone deficiency

Imaging

- Brain
    - *Leptomeningeal angiomatosis* (excessive tortuous, leptomeningeal vasculature) manifests as avid leptomeningeal enhancement, often ipsilateral to the facial port wine stain best identified by T2 FLAIR postcontrast imaging.
    - *Ipsilateral enlarged choroid plexus* due to venous engorgement.
    - Underdeveloped cortical venous drainage with secondary recruitment of deep medullary venous outflow.
    - Asymmetric T2 hypointensity in young patients is presumedly due to hypermyelination underlying regions of angiomatosis.
    - Chronic venous ischemia results in progressive *parenchymal volume loss, and cortical dystrophic calcification.*
- Skull.
    - *Calvarial hypertrophy* and paranasal sinus expansion. Commonly, avid enhancement of the ipsilateral calvarial regional to the pial angiomatosis is observed.
- Eye.
    - *Choroidal/scleral angiomatosis* may be seen as thickening and enhancement of the globe margin.

REFERENCES

1. Smirniotopoulos JG. Neuroimaging of phakomatoses: Sturge-Weber syndrome, tuberous sclerosis, von Hippel-Lindau syndrome. *Neuro-imaging Clin N Am.* 2004 May;14(2):171–183.
2. Pinto AL, Chen L, Friedman R, et al. Sturge-Weber Syndrome: Brain Magnetic Resonance Imaging and Neuropathology Findings. *Pediatr Neurol.* 2016 May;58:25–30.

VON HIPPEL-LINDAU SYNDROME

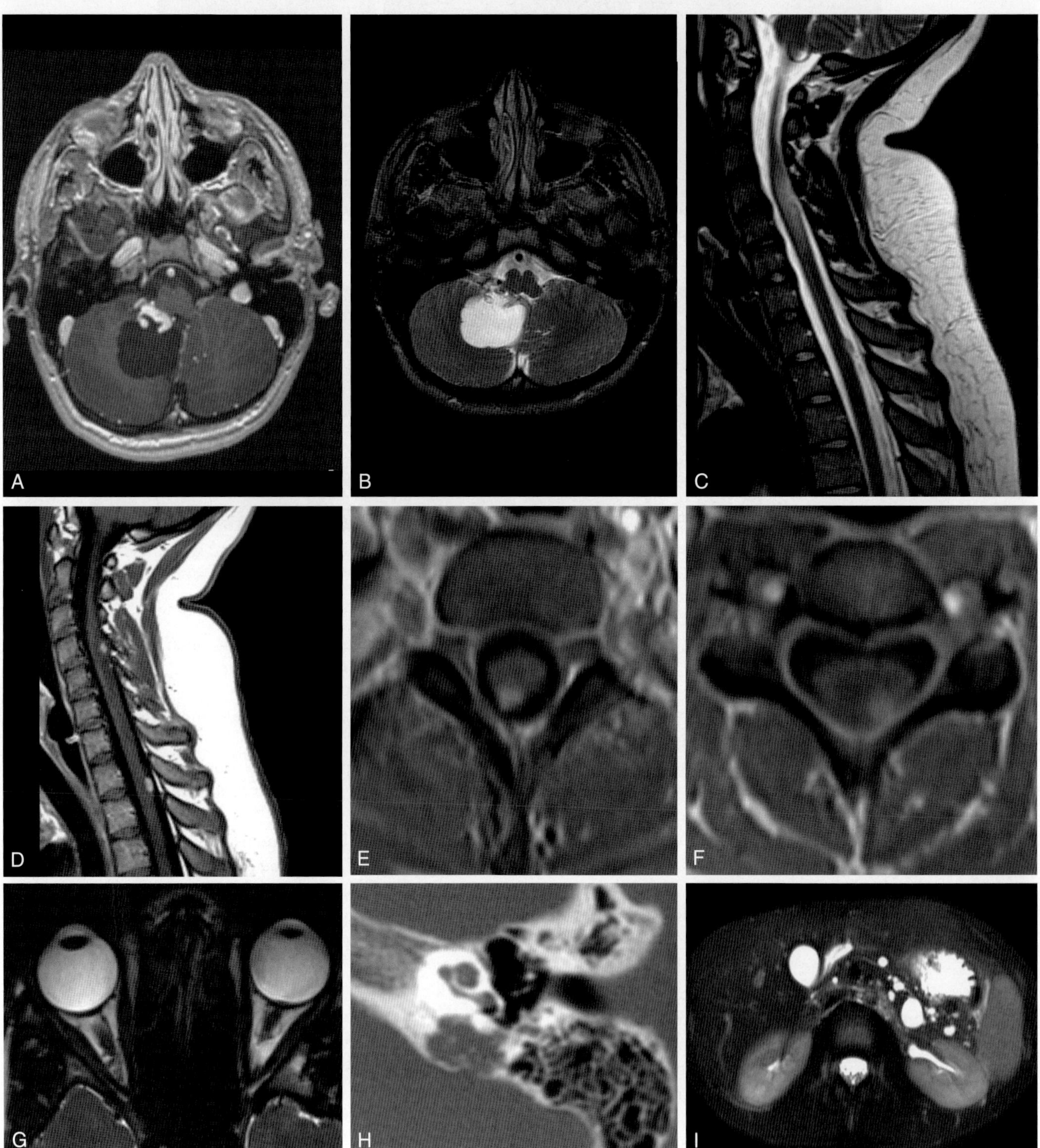

Fig. 9.15 Von Hippel-Lindau (VHL): Classic Findings. (A) Axial T1W+C and (B) axial T2W images demonstrate a right cerebellar hemisphere mass with cyst and nodule pattern consistent with a hemangioblastoma. (C) Sagittal T2W, (D to F) sagittal and axial T1W+C images demonstrate multiple enhancing nodules consistent with hemangioblastomas along the pial surface of the spinal cord with associated region of intramedullary spinal cord T2 hyperintensity consistent with edema in the cervical cord. (G) Axial T2W image demonstrating abnormal T2 isointense thickening of the left posterior retina. Fundoscopy confirmed a retinal angioma. (H) Axial CT demonstrates an expansile lytic bone lesion along the vestibular aqueduct consistent with an endolymphatic sac tumor in a patient with VHL. (I) Axial T2W fat saturation image demonstrating multiple pancreatic cysts. Renal cell carcinoma is not seen in this patient but should be evaluated for in patients with VHL.

Key Points

Background

- Mutations in the tumor suppressor gene, VHL gene on chromosome 3p25.3; autosomal dominant disorder

Clinical

- Diagnostic Criteria
  - Clinical diagnosis made by either of the following:
    - A positive family history and one of the following tumors: CNS hemangioblastoma, clear cell renal cell carcinoma, or pheochromocytoma
    - A negative family history with two CNS hemangioblastomas or one CNS hemangioblastoma and either a clear cell renal cell carcinoma, or pheochromocytoma
- Orbit and globe: Retinal hemangioblastoma occurring in 43% to 85% of patients

Imaging

- *Hemangioblastoma:* Most common in the cerebellum (65%) followed by the spine (25%) and brainstem (10%). Supratentorial lesions are very rare, but possible. Lesions are typified by cyst and mural nodule. Cystic component may be large or small or entirely absent. T2 hyperintense solid component avidly enhance and classically are superficial, presenting to a pial surface. Regional flow voids about the solid components may be seen in contradistinction to pilocytic astrocytomas, where such flow voids are absent (angiographically occult).
- Endolymphatic sac tumor: Locally aggressive, highly vascular low-grade adenocarcinomas in patients presenting with hearing loss, tinnitus, and vertigo. Heterogeneous T1 and T2 (but mostly T2 hyperintense) signal with heterogeneous enhancement. Regional flow voids may be seen. CT will demonstrate regional bony erosion centered at the vestibular aqueduct of the temporal bone with intralesional calcifications.
- Other
  - Kidney: *Renal cell carcinoma* (~25%–60% of patients), and renal cysts
  - Pancreas: Pancreatic microcystic serous adenomas, pancreatic islet cell tumors, and pancreatic cysts
  - Adrenal and extraadrenal *pheochromocytoma* (10%–20% of patients)
  - Epididymal cystadenoma (25% to 60% of males); broad ligament cystadenoma (10% of females)

REFERENCES

1. Smirniotopoulos JG. Neuroimaging of phakomatoses: Sturge-Weber syndrome, tuberous sclerosis, von Hippel-Lindau syndrome. *Neuroimaging Clin N Am.* 2004 May;14(2):171–183.
2. Nandigam K, Mechtler LL, Smirniotopoulos JG. Neuroimaging of neurocutaneous diseases. *Neurol Clin.* 2014 Feb;32(1):159–192.
3. Wick CC, Manzoor NF, Semaan MT, et al. Endolymphatic sac tumors. *Otolaryngol Clin North Am.* 2015 Apr;48(2):317–330.

PHACES

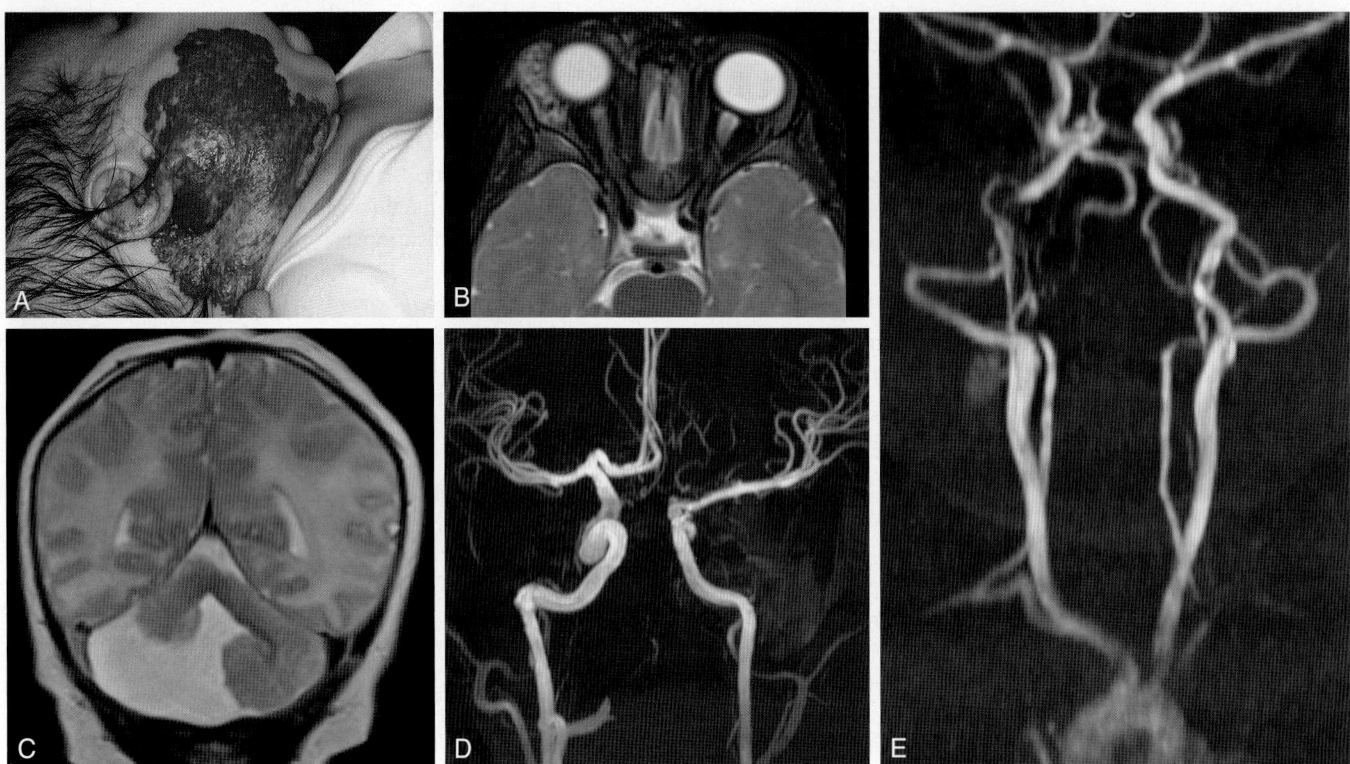

Fig. 9.16 PHACES Syndrome. (A) Large facial hemangioma commonly seen in PHACES syndrome. (B and C) Axial and coronal T2W images demonstrate right orbital hemangioma and a right cerebellar hypoplasia. (D and E) MRA volumetric images demonstrate fusiform dilatation and ectasia of the right internal carotid artery and tortuosity of bilateral cervical internal carotid arteries. (A from Paller AS, Mancini AJ. *Hurwitz Clinical Pediatric Dermatology: A Textbook of Skin Disorders of Childhood and Adolescence.* 6th ed. Elsevier; 2022.)

Key Points

Background

- PHACES acronym consists of the following abnormalities and major criteria:
    - **P**osterior fossa (30%–80%): Dandy-Walker malformation, cerebellar hypoplasia, arachnoid cyst
    - **H**emangiomas: Large and segmental typically on the face, head, or neck
    - **A**rterial (83%–91%): Intracranial and/or extracranial arterial tortuosity or absence
    - **C**ardiovascular (41%–67%): Coarctation of the aorta, aneurysm, aberrant subclavian artery
    - **E**ye: Microphthalmia, optic nerve hypoplasia, cataract
    - **S**upraumbilical raphe and sternal cleft, defect, or deformity
- PHACES syndrome includes a segmental infantile hemangioma larger than 5 cm on the face, scalp, or cervical region with one major or two minor criteria
- Possible PHACES syndrome includes an infantile hemangioma with one minor criteria
- Vascular abnormalities increase the risk of stroke in PHACES, particularly severe arterial narrowing or absent vessel without collateral vessels
- Etiology is unknown. Occurs sporadically.

Imaging

- MRI and MRA of the brain and MRA of the neck are performed to evaluate the hemangiomas and the arterial and brain abnormalities
- Most common arterial abnormalities involve the carotid arteries and include dysgenesis, abnormal origin and course, narrowing and absence of the vessels

REFERENCE

1. Rotter A, Samorano LP, Rivitti-Machado MC, et al. PHACE syndrome: clinical manifestations, diagnostic criteria, and management. *An Bras Dermatol.* 2018 Jun;93(3):405–411.

NEUROCUTANEOUS MELANOSIS

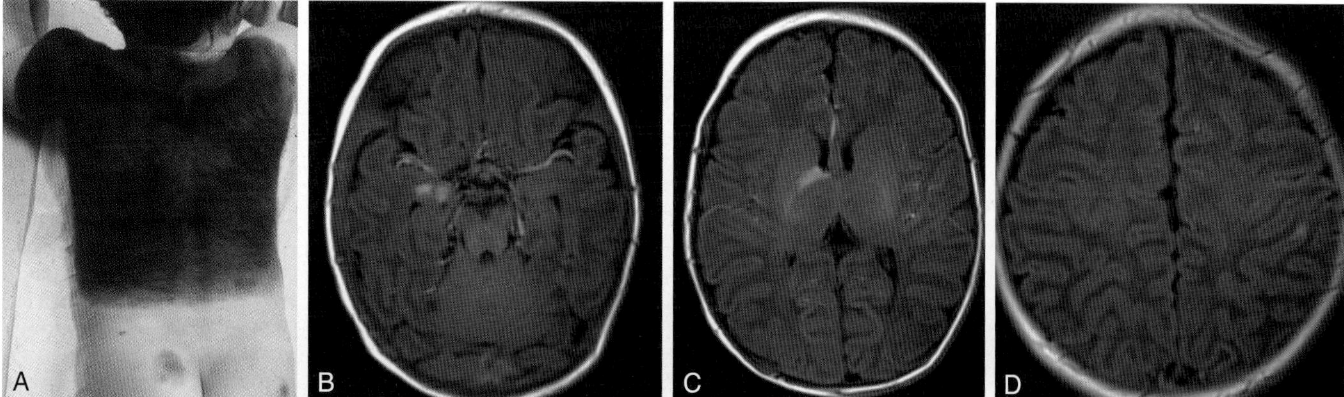

Fig. 9.17 Neurocutaneous Melanosis. (A) Large, dark hairy nevus covering most of the back of an infant with neurocutaneous melanosis. (B to D) Axial T1W images demonstrate focal T1 hyperintense lesions in the left postcentral gyrus, right caudothalamic groove, and right amygdala. (A from Jankovic J, Mazziotta JC, Pomeroy SL, et al. *Bradley and Daroff's Neurology in Clinical Practice*. 8th ed. Elsevier; 2022.)

Key Points

Background

- Mutations in codon 61 on chromosome 1p13 leading to activation of mosaic RASopathies with the mutation thought to occur in developing neuroectoderm

Clinical

- Rare neuroectodermal phakomatosis characterized by proliferation of melanocytes in the CNS (meningeal and brain) in association with giant congenital melanocytic nevi (disorder of embryologic ectoderm affecting nervous system, skin, eyes).
- Diagnostic criteria have been published by Kadanoaga and Frieden in 1991.
    - One large congenital nevus (20 cm or more in adults; 9 cm on the head or 6 cm on the trunk of an infant) or three or more smaller congenital nevi, together with either melanoma or melanosis of the meninges.
    - No cutaneous melanoma except when examined areas of meningeal lesions are benign.
    - No melanoma of the meninges except when examined areas of the cutaneous lesions are histologically benign.
- Patients may present with signs/symptoms of increased intracranial pressure/hydrocephalus, seizures, motor deficits, myeloradiculopathy, bowel and bladder symptoms.

Imaging

- Imaging is best performed with MRI 3D T1 imaging of the brain and spine with and without contrast with initial screening before 4 months of age.
- CNS lesions demonstrate *T1 hyperintense (melanin) foci* in the leptomeninges of the brain and spine. Brain parenchyma involvement may also occur especially at the level of the cerebellum and *anterior temporal lobes* including the amygdala and brainstem. T1 hyperintense foci in the brain may be less well seen when myelination has occurred. Hydrocephalus may occur with extensive melanin deposition or with malignant degeneration to melanoma.
- Hindbrain malformations may occur to include cerebellar, pontine hypoplasia, and Dandy-Walker.
- Leptomeningeal enhancement suggests malignant degeneration.

REFERENCES

1. Bekiesińska-Figatowska M, Sawicka E, Żak K, et al. Age related changes in brain MR appearance in the course of neurocutaneous melanosis. *Eur J Radiol.* 2016 Aug;85(8):1427–1431.
2. Barkovich AJ, Frieden IJ, Williams ML. MR of neurocutaneous melanosis. *AJNR Am J Neuroradiol.* 1994 May;15(5):859–867.
3. Kadonaga JN, Frieden IJ. Neurocutaneous melanosis: definition and review of the literature. *J Am Acad Dermatol.* 1991 May;24(5 Pt 1):747–755.
4. Waelchli R, Aylett SE, Atherton D, et al. Classification of neurological abnormalities in children with congenital melanocytic naevus syndrome identifies magnetic resonance imaging as the best predictor of clinical outcome. *Br J Dermatol.* 2015 Sep;173(3):739–750.

BASAL CELL NEVUS SYNDROME

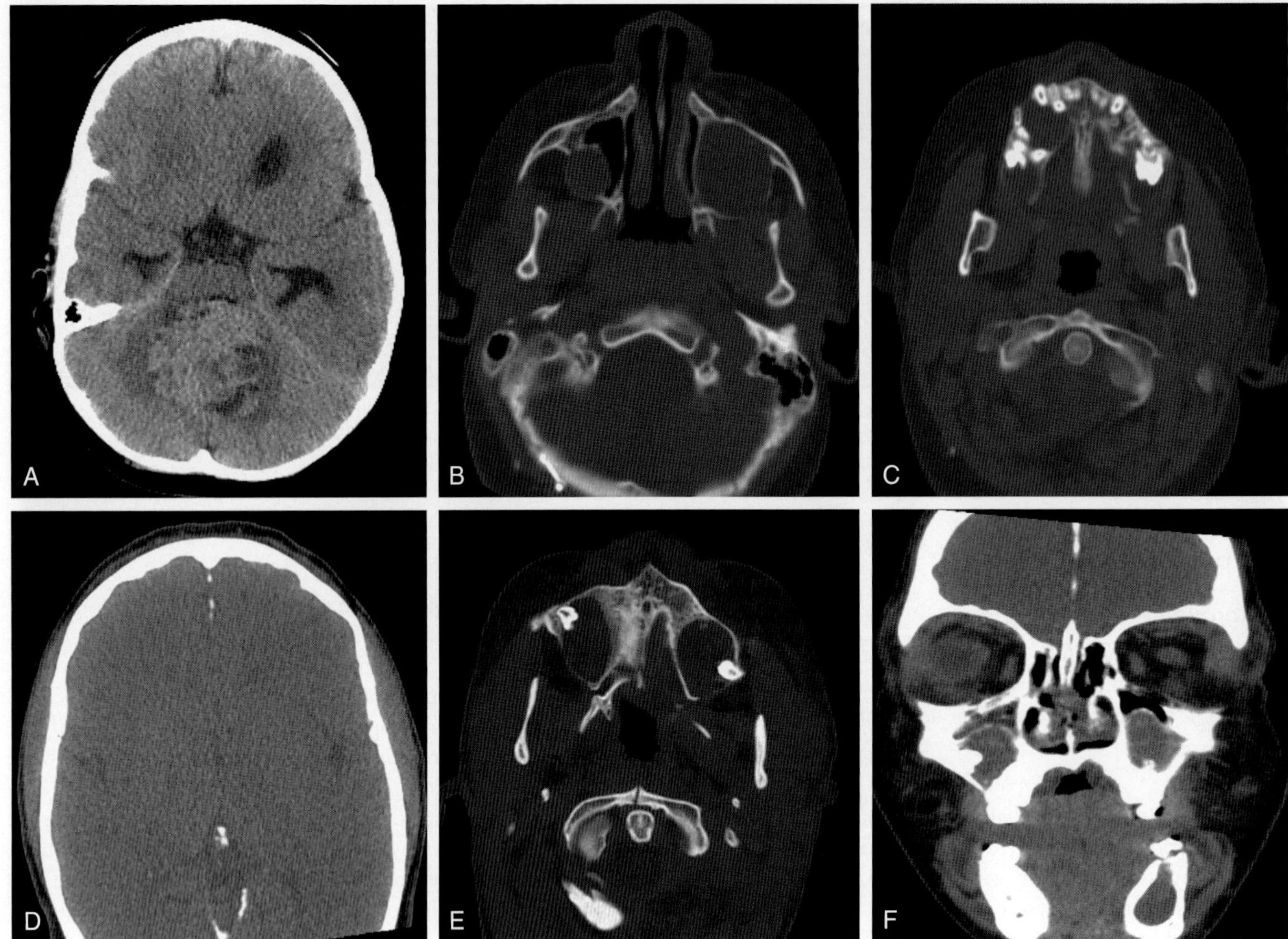

Fig. 9.18 Basal Cell Nevus Syndrome. (A to F) Axial and coronal CT images demonstrate a midline posterior fossa mildly hyperdense mass consistent with a medulloblastoma, cystic lesions of the maxilla consistent keratocystic odontogenic tumors, and calcifications of the falx and tentorium.

Key Points

Background

- Also known as Gorlin-Goltz syndrome
- Rare, autosomal dominant disorder. Loss of function mutation in *PTCH1*, a tumor suppressor gene on chromosome 9q22.3 or mutations in *SUFU* gene

Clinical

- Cutaneous basal cell carcinomas, often clinically aggressive beginning at about the time of puberty. Most commonly occurs on the face but may occur elsewhere. More common in light-pigmented individuals.
- Characteristic facial features include frontal bossing, hypertelorism, macrocephaly, and cleft lip/palate deformities.
- Dyskeratotic palmar and plantar pitting.
- Susceptible to a variety of neoplasms, including desmoplastic medulloblastomas, meningiomas, keratocystic odontogenic tumors, ovarian and cardiac fibromas, mesenteric keratocysts, and rhabdomyosarcomas.

Imaging

- Radiation sensitivity in these patients should preclude exposure to ionizing radiation.
- Brain
  - *Early calcification of the dura* (up to 77% in patients between the ages of 20 and 40) and ligaments (petroclinoid, nuchal)
  - *Medulloblastoma*, especially desmoplastic (overall 5% lower risk with *PTCH1* gene mutation, significantly higher with *SUFU* gene mutation)
  - Meningiomas (rare)
  - Corpus callosum abnormalities (10%)
  - Macrocephaly

- Head and Neck
  - *Keratocystic odontogenic tumors* (70%–80%): Unilocular lesions associated with the crown of an unerupted tooth
  - Cleft lip/palate
- Spine
  - Scoliosis, segmentation anomalies
- Other
  - Bifid, absent, rudimentary, or splayed ribs; flame-shaped lucent bony lesions; polydactyly

REFERENCES

1. Bresler SC, Padwa BL, Granter SR. Nevoid Basal Cell Carcinoma Syndrome (Gorlin Syndrome). *Head Neck Pathol.* 2016 Jun;10(2):119–124.
2. Kimonis VE, Mehta SG, Digiovanna JJ, et al. Radiological features in 82 patients with nevoid basal cell carcinoma (NBCC or Gorlin) syndrome. *Genet Med.* 2004 Nov-Dec;6(6):495–502.
3. Smith MJ, Beetz C, Williams SG, et al. Germline mutations in SUFU cause Gorlin syndrome-associated childhood medulloblastoma and redefine the risk associated with PTCH1 mutations. *J Clin Oncol.* 2014 Dec 20;32(36):4155–4161.

ENCEPHALOCRANIOCUTANEOUS LIPOMATOSIS

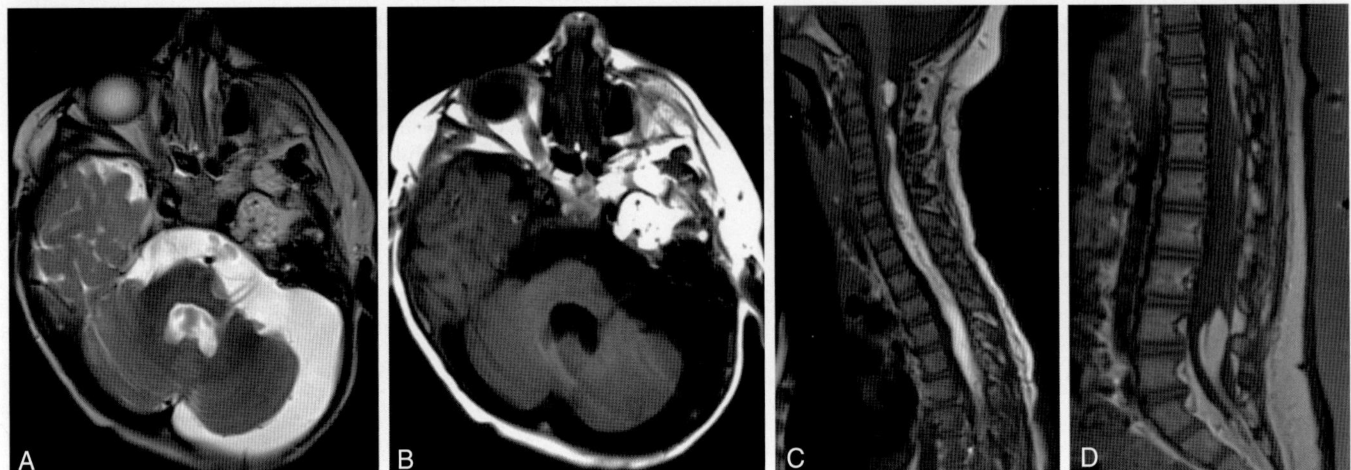

Fig. 9.19 Encephalocraniocutaneous Lipomatosis. (A) Axial T2W and (B) axial T1W images demonstrate absent left globe, and dysplasia of the left middle cranial fossa with lipomatosis. (C and D) Sagittal T1W images of the spine demonstrate T1 hyperintense fat along the posterior spinal cord and distal thecal sac.

Key Points

Background

- Sporadic neurocutaneous syndrome with mosaic activation of FGFR1

Clinical

- Skin: Nevus psiloliparus characterized by alopecia with regional excessive scalp adipose tissue; nonscarring alopecia
- Orbit: eye choristomas (dermoid, lipodermoid), with or without associated eye anomalies (corneal, anterior chamber anomalies); ocular and eyelid colobomas; globe calcification
- Other: seizures, intellectual disability, hemiplegia, facial palsy, sensorineural hearing loss, and behavioral abnormalities

Imaging

- Brain
  - Lipomas
  - Parenchymal ischemic injury: Volume loss, porencephalic cysts, and calcifications
  - Arachnoid cysts, ventriculomegaly, corpus callosum dysgenesis, and/or volume loss
  - Vascular dysplasia, and leptomeningeal angiomatosis
- Head and Neck
  - Maxillary/mandibular lesions: Osteoma, odontoma, ossifying fibromas, and bone cysts
- Spine: Lipomas
- Other: Aortic coarctations

REFERENCES

1. Bavle A, Shah R, Gross N, et al. Encephalocraniocutaneous Lipomatosis. *J Pediatr Hematol Oncol.* 2018 Oct;40(7):553–554.
2. Siddiqui S, Naaz S, Ahmad M, et al. Encephalocraniocutaneous lipomatosis: A case report with review of literature. *Neuroradiol J.* 2017 Dec;30(6):578–582.

OCULOCEREBROCUTANEOUS SYNDROME

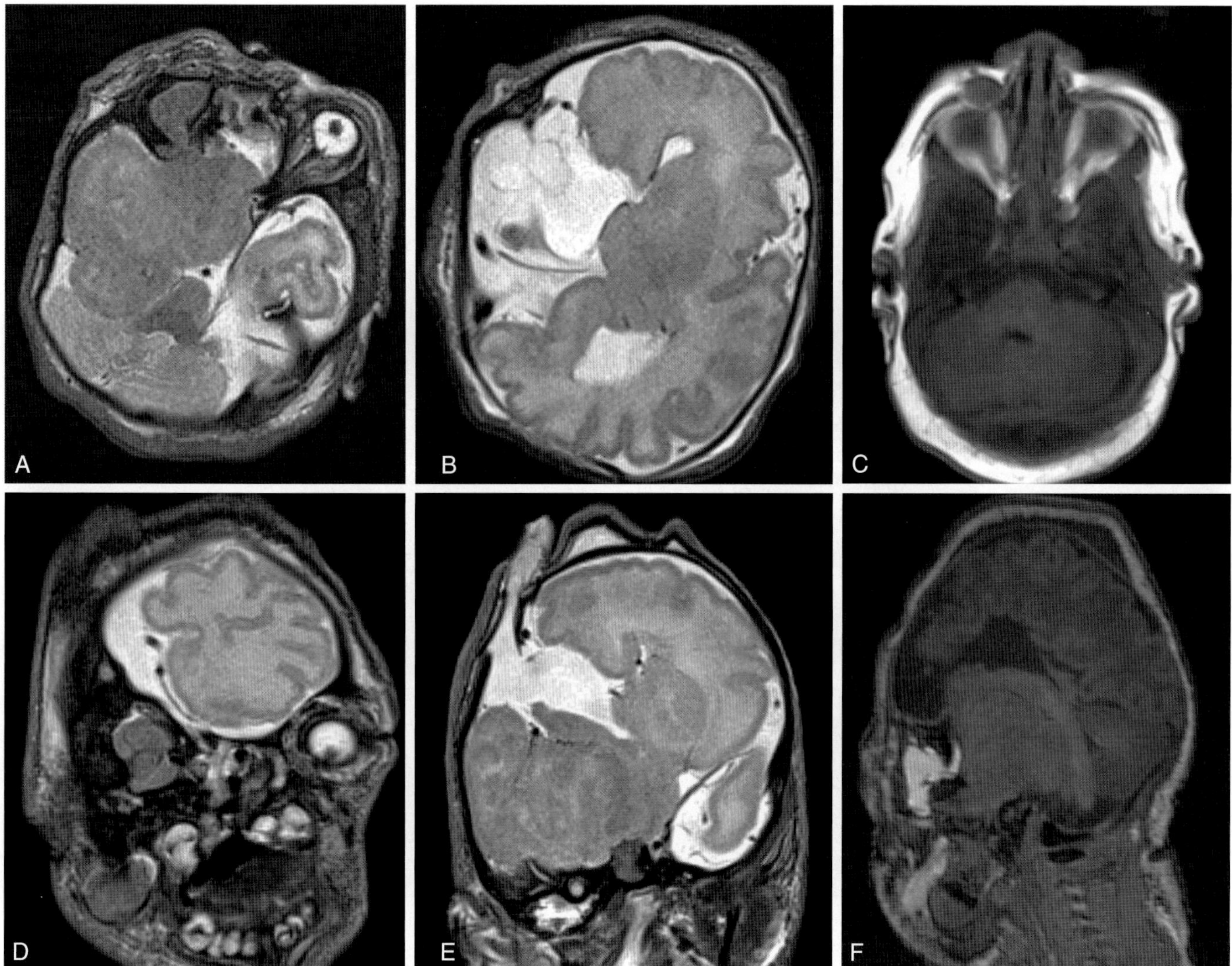

Fig. 9.20 Oculocerebrocutaneous Syndrome. (A and B) Axial T2W and (C) Axial T1W, (D and E) coronal T2W, and (F) sagittal T1W images demonstrate dysplastic right cerebral hemisphere, absent right globe, let globe microphthalmia, right periorbital skin tag, right frontal meningocele, cleft lip and palate, and dysplastic and elongated midbrain.

Key Points

Background

- Also known as Delleman syndrome; etiology is unknown; occurs sporadically

Clinical

- *Triad of eye* (cyst; microphthalmia; anophthalmia; coloboma), *brain malformations*, and *skin findings* (appendages; focal dermal hypoplasia or aplasia; punch-like defects; crescent hypoplasia)

Imaging

- Malformations include frontal polymicrogyria, periventricular heterotopia, callosal malformation +/− interhemispheric cyst, ventriculomegaly, *large dysplastic tectum* with absent vermis (reported to be pathognomonic), and cerebellar hypoplasia

REFERENCE

1. Bosemani T, Huisman TA, Poretti A. Pediatric Neurocutaneous Syndromes with Cerebellar Involvement. *Neuroimaging Clin N Am.* 2016 Aug;26(3):417–434.

PARRY-ROMBERG SYNDROME

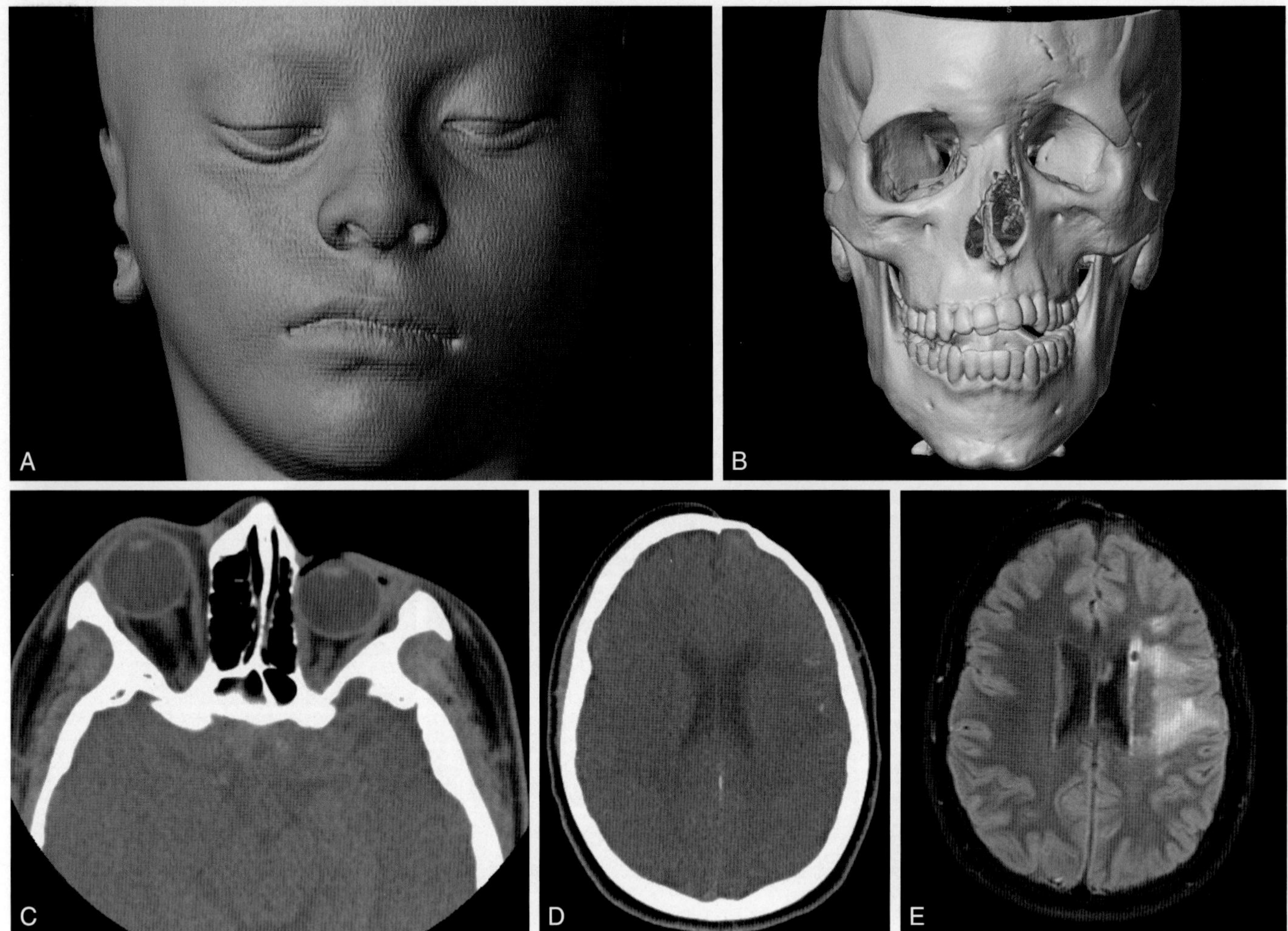

Fig. 9.21 Parry-Romberg Syndrome. (A and B) 3D volumetric CT images demonstrate decreased left facial soft tissue and bone causing facial asymmetry. (C and D) Axial CT images demonstrate decreased left orbit fat, enophthalmos, thin left frontal scalp fat, thin left frontal bone, and dystrophic calcification in the left frontal lobe. (E) Axial FLAIR image demonstrates a confluent region of FLAIR hyperintensity in the region of parenchymal calcification.

Key Points

Background

- Etiology unknown

Clinical

- *Progressive facial hemiatrophy,* involving skin, subcutaneous tissue, muscle, and bone.
- Neurologic symptoms in 15% to 20%.
- Ophthalmology symptoms in 10% to 35%.
- Onset in first or second decade. Slow progression over 2 to 20 years.

Imaging

- *Unilateral facial atrophy,* including skin, muscle, bone, and salivary gland.
- *20% have intracranial findings*: Ipsilateral frontal lobe subcortical calcification, ipsilateral brain atrophy, and white matter gliosis. Less commonly demonstrate ventriculomegaly, leptomeningeal enhancement, abnormal cortical thickening or gyral pattern, hamartoma, microhemorrhage, aneurysm, vascular malformation, and arterial stenoses.

REFERENCE

1. Wong M, Phillips CD, Hagiwara M, et al. Parry Romberg Syndrome: 7 Cases and Literature Review. *AJNR Am J Neuroradiol.* 2015 Jul;36(7):1355–1361.

OTHER RARE PHAKOMATOSES

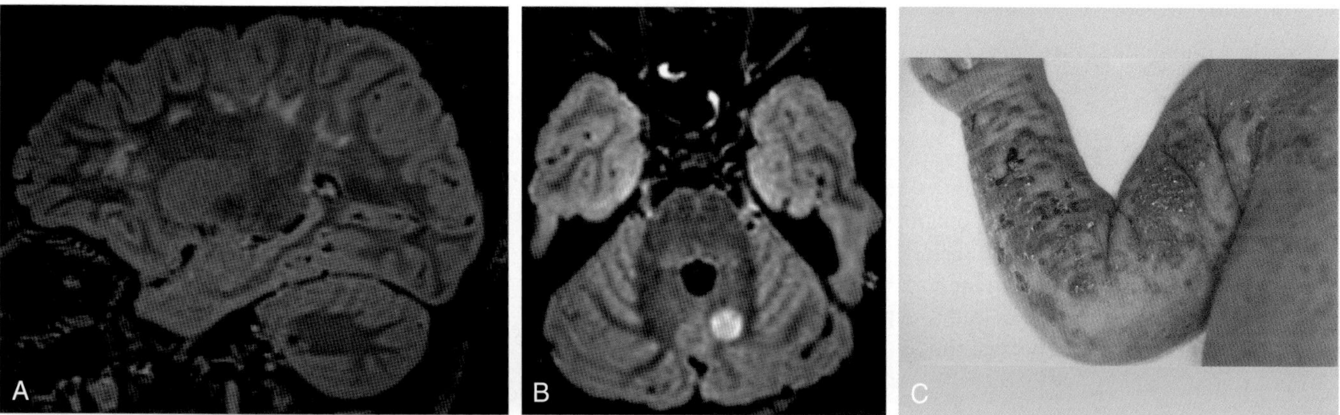

Fig. 9.22 Incontinentia Pigmenti. (A and B) Sagittal and axial FLAIR demonstrate periventricular FLAIR hyperintensities and left cerebellar rounded hyperintensity. (C) Early skin appearance in Incontinentia Pigmenti. (From James WD, Elston DM, Treat J, Rosenbach M, Neuhaus IM. *Andrews' Diseases of the Skin: Clinical Dermatology.* 13th ed. Elsevier; 2020.)

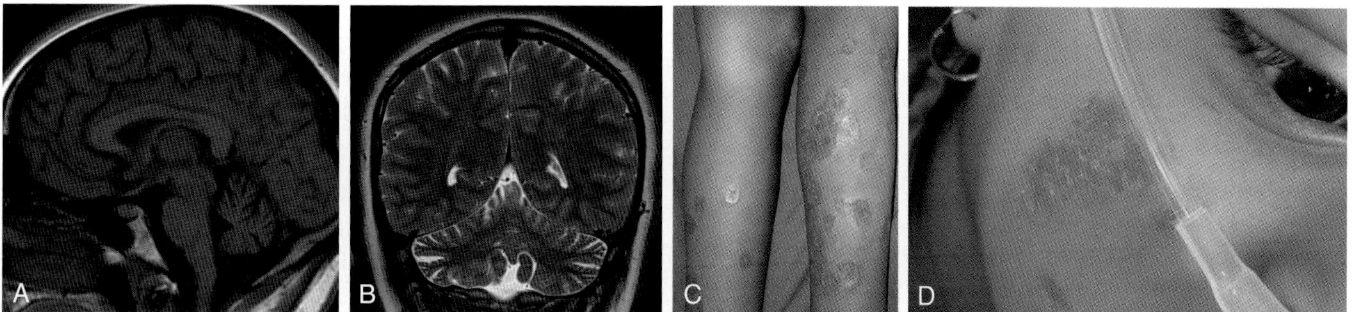

Fig. 9.23 Ataxia Telangiectasia. (A) Sagittal T1W and (B) coronal T2W images demonstrate cerebellar volume loss. Skin Granulomatous Lesions in a Child With Ataxia-Telangiectasia. (C) Multiple granulomas of the legs. (D) Granulomas of the face. (From Sullivan KE, Stiehm ER. *Stiehm's Immune Deficiencies: Inborn Errors of Immunity*. 2nd ed. Elsevier/Academic Press; 2020.)

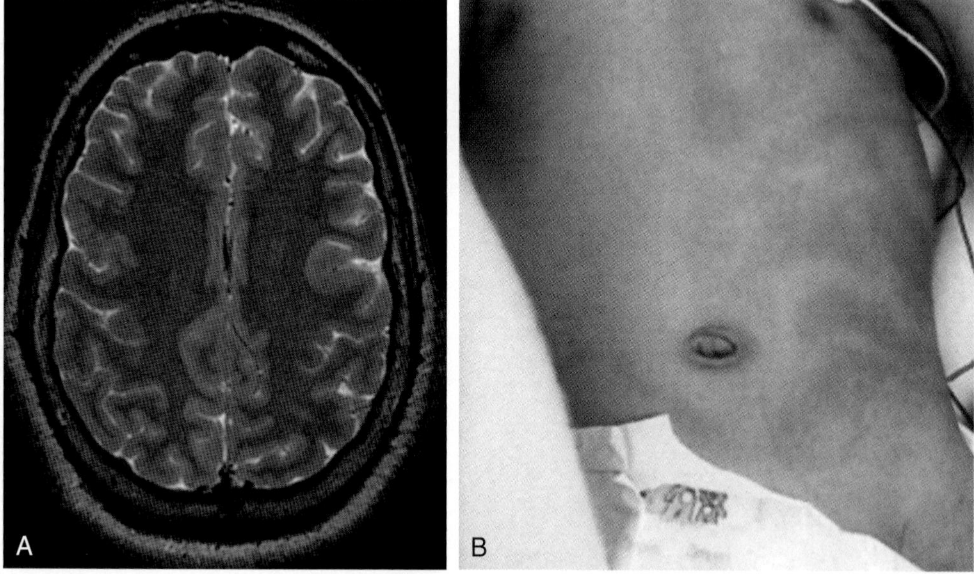

Fig. 9.24 Hypomelanosis of Ito. (A) Axial T2W image demonstrates focal bilateral frontal polymicrogyria. (B) Characteristic swirling pigmentation of the trunk of a 4-month-old infant with hypomelanosis of Ito. This patient also had seizures and cataracts. (B from Daroff RB. *Bradley's Neurology in Clinical Practice.* 7th ed. Elsevier; 2016.)

Key Points

Incontinentia Pigmenti

Background

- X-linked mutation in the *NEMO* gene. Nearly always fatal in males

Clinical

- Skin lesions in four stages; vesicular → verrucous → hyperpigmented → atrophic/hypopigmented.
- CNS symptoms in 30% to 50% include seizures, quadriplegia, intellectual deficit, and ataxia.
- Retinal vascular anomalies can lead to retinal fibrosis
- Other: Alopecia; tooth abnormalities.

Imaging

- *Findings include periventricular and/or watershed T2/FLAIR hyperintensity*, hypoplasia of the corpus callosum, multiple cerebral infarcts, progressive cortical and white matter atrophy, cerebellar lesions, and hemorrhagic foci in the parenchyma

Ataxia Telangiectasia (Louis-Bar Syndrome)

Background

- Autosomal recessive disorder of the ataxia telangiectasia mutated *(ATM)* gene, which is involved in response to DNA double strand breaks, oxidative stress, and cell cycle checkpoint. Cerebellar atrophy primarily affects the Purkinje cells and lesser extent the granule neurons

Clinical

- Immune deficiency leading to infections (usually sinus and lung), cancer predisposition (10%–15% develop malignancy), radiation sensitivity, and progressive cerebellar ataxia.
- Ataxia presentation as a toddler and may be mistaken for ataxic cerebral palsy due to slow changes at this time period, until age 5 to 10, when there is a decline in function.
- Neurodegeneration progresses to dysarthria, chorea, and oculomotor abnormalities.
- Skin telangiectasias are seen at age 3 to 6 years.

Imaging

- *Cerebellar cortical atrophy* and infarcts and hemorrhage due to telangiectasias and systemic emboli

Hypomelanosis of Ito

Background

- Likely multifactorial genetic causes

Clinical

- Cutaneous hypopigmented zone with irregular streaks, whorls, and patches.
- Seizures, developmental delay, and low IQ

Imaging

- Spectrum of findings from normal or enlarged perivascular spaces to cerebral *malformations* including heterotopia, polymicrogyria, focal cortical dysplasia, hemimegalencephaly, and lissencephaly

REFERENCE

1. Rothblum-Oviatt C, Wright J, Lefton-Greif MA, et al. Ataxia telangiectasia: a review. *Orphanet J Rare Dis*. 2016 Nov 25;11(1):159.

10 Brain Trauma

INTRODUCTION

Background

Trauma is the most common cause of death and a significant cause of morbidity in children. Both accidental and nonaccidental trauma are common in children.

Several anatomic differences in younger children should be highlighted to understand why younger children are more susceptible to certain types of injury. First, the skull of young children is thin and pliable and thickens during the first 2 years of life. Second, a skull with fused sutures transfers the force of an impact throughout the skull and is more prone to fracture compared to a skull with unfused sutures. Third, an infant's head weighs about 10% to 15% of the total body weight compared to only 2% to 3% in an adult. Fourth, the infant brain has a softer consistency because of higher water content, immature glial cells, immature myelination, and smaller axons. Consequently, the unmyelinated brain has a lower threshold for injury than an adult. Last, the neck muscles of a child are less developed and provide less protection from acceleration-deceleration trauma.

Accidental head trauma includes injuries from birth trauma, motor vehicle accidents, drowning, crush injury, and falls. Short falls that occur in and around the home from a distance of less than 6 feet are associated with focal contact injuries such as scalp contusion or laceration. About 1% to 3% of short falls in young children cause a skull fracture. The majority of these skull fractures are simple linear fractures without associated intracranial hemorrhage or neurologic deficit. The minority of fractures are associated with an epidural hemorrhage or, less commonly, a subdural hemorrhage. With short falls there is no diffuse brain injury, however falls from heights greater than 10 feet, such as those from a building, lead to greater head injury and are similar to crush injuries. Crushing head injury is relatively common in children compared to adults. Examples of crush injuries include heavy objects, such as a television falling onto the head. Crush injuries cause parenchymal contusions, lacerations, and fractures.

Epidural hemorrhages require an impact to the head and are associated with skull fractures in 85% of cases. Epidural hemorrhages usually occur from falls in young children, rather than an inflicted blow to the head, which is more likely to cause acceleration of the head and more diffuse injury. Clinical significance of an epidural hemorrhage depends on the size and rate of enlargement.

Subdural hemorrhages can result from both impact injuries as well as from inertial forces. The most common cause of subdural hemorrhage in young children is abusive head injury.

Parenchymal contusions are commonly seen adjacent to a skull fracture. However, coup and countercoup contusions are rare in children less than 4 years of age because of the soft consistency of young brains. Because a young child is already near the ground, a fall does not accelerate the head sufficiently to cause a countercoup contusion.

Abusive head trauma (AHT) accounts for the majority of head injury in children less than 1 year, and head injury is the leading cause of death from child abuse. A multidisciplinary approach is necessary as the diagnosis involves clinical history, physical examination, laboratory results, radiological findings, and scene investigation and interviews with other family members by child protective services and police. AHT has a multitude of possible imaging findings, which are demonstrated in this chapter.

Imaging

Head trauma findings seen on imaging include soft tissue contusions, lacerations, fracture, epidural hemorrhage, subdural hemorrhage, subarachnoid hemorrhage, parenchymal contusion, parenchymal laceration, axonal injury, edema, and ischemia. Radiographs, ultrasound, CT, and MRI are imaging modalities commonly used to evaluate pediatric trauma patients. Radiographs are quick and useful for determination of fractures but have become less commonly used in the acute trauma patient. CT imaging is often the initial neuroimaging study performed for assessment of head trauma due to the fast acquisition, and excellent detection of fractures and intracranial hemorrhage. MRI is more sensitive than CT for extent of intracranial trauma, particularly diffuse axonal injury and ischemia but has longer acquisition time compared to CT and may require sedation so CT is currently the initial imaging study of choice. This section illustrates the imaging findings of head trauma and related diagnoses in children seen on radiographs, ultrasound, CT, and MRI.

REFERENCES

1. Case ME. Accidental traumatic head injury in infants and very young children. *Brain Pathol.* 2008 Oct;18(4):583–589.
2. Case ME. Inflicted traumatic brain injury in infants and young children. *Brain Pathol.* 2008 Oct;18(4):571–582.
3. Orman G, Kralik SF, Meoded A, et al. MRI findings in pediatric abusive head trauma: a review. *J Neuroimaging.* 2019:1–13.

SCALP TRAUMA

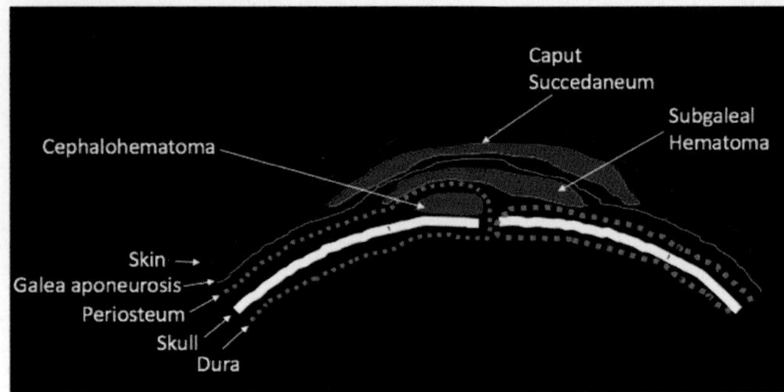

Fig. 10.1 Locations of Scalp Hemorrhage. Layers of the scalp are the skin, galea aponeurosis, and periosteum. Caput succedaneum is between the skin and galea aponeurosis and can cross sutures. Subgaleal hematoma is between galea aponeurosis and periosteum and can cross sutures. Cephalohematoma is between the periosteum and the bone and does not cross sutures.

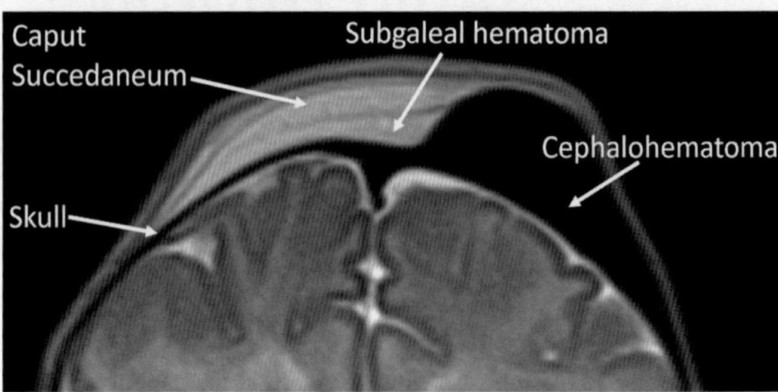

Fig. 10.2 Scalp Hemorrhage. Coronal T2W images demonstrating a caput succedaneum, subgaleal hematoma, and cephalohematoma.

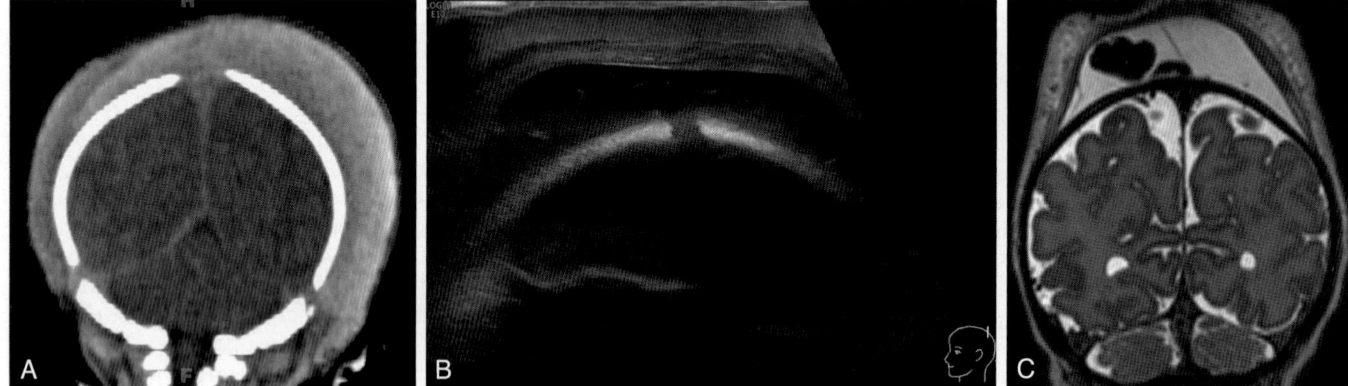

Fig. 10.3 Subgaleal Hematoma: Multiple Patients. (A) Coronal CT image demonstrating hyperdense scalp hematoma from a subgaleal hematoma that crosses the sagittal suture and left lambdoid suture. (B) Transverse ultrasound image across the sagittal suture demonstrates a mixed echogenic subgaleal collection crossing the sagittal suture. (C) Coronal 3D T2W image of the same patient in (B) demonstrates the subgaleal hematoma with areas of T2 hypointense and hyperintense signal.

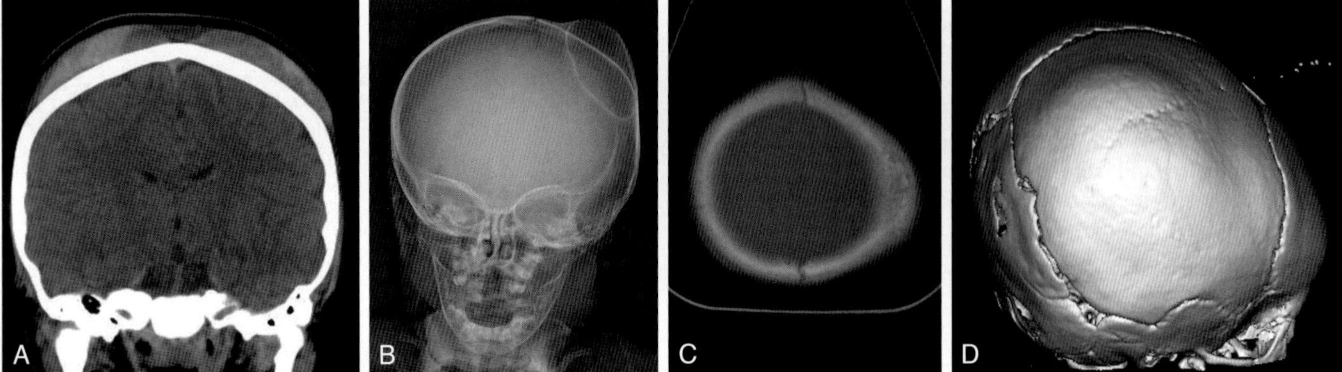

Fig. 10.4 Cephalohematoma: Multiple Patients. (A) Coronal CT image demonstrating bilateral hyperdense cephalohematomas that do not cross the sagittal suture. (B) AP skull radiograph demonstrating peripheral calcification of a left parietal cephalohematoma. (C) Axial head CT image demonstrating ossification of a left parietal cephalohematoma. (D) 3D volumetric image demonstrating a bulge in the skull caused by a calcified cephalohematoma.

Key Points

Caput Succedaneum

- Serosanguinous, transudative fluid between the skin and galea aponeurosis typically located at the vertex that occurs during normal birth.
- Crosses sutures.
- Secondary to high pressure on the infant's head during labor. Typically seen in primigravidas, prolonged deliveries, and premature rupture of membranes (due to reduced amniotic fluid).
- Typically diffuses quickly and becomes stable or rapidly resolves within 24 to 48 hours. Consequently, treatment is rarely necessary.
- Imaging may be performed to exclude subgaleal hematoma (SGH).

Subgaleal Hematoma

- Many small emissary veins traverse the loose connective tissue of the subgaleal space. A tear or tears of these emissary veins is believed to be the cause of an SGH.
- External force such as use of vacuum extraction (associated with SGH in 60% to 89% of cases) can result in rupture of veins in the subgaleal space and subsequent hemorrhage that crosses the sutures.
- A SGH can result in significant blood loss. A 1-cm increase in depth of the subgaleal space can contain 40 to 260 mL of blood. The circulating blood volume in a neonate is approximately 90 mL/kg body weight such that in a 3-kg neonate, a blood loss of 54 mL is a 20% loss of circulating blood volume.
- Signs and symptoms: Boggy head with pitting edema, increasing head circumference, jaundice, eye and ear swelling. A drop in hemoglobin is a late sign of severe hemorrhage because of insufficient time for fluid shift to cause the hemodilution.
- Severity criteria: Approximately 6% are asymptomatic, 15% to 20% are mild (<1-cm increase in head circumference, no jaundice, no hypovolemia), 40% to 50% are moderate (1–3 cm increase in head circumference, jaundice, mild hypovolemia), and 25% to 33% are severe (>3 cm increase in head circumference, jaundice, severe hypovolemia).
- Hypoxic ischemic injury occurs in 62% to 72% of subgaleal hematomas, and brain trauma (edema or hemorrhage) occurs in 33% to 40%.

Cephalohematoma (Also Known as a Subperiosteal Hematoma)

- Localized hemorrhage between bone and periosteum
- More common in primigravidas, fetal macrocephaly, instrument-assisted delivery, prolonged and/or difficult labor, premature rupture of membranes, and with oligohydramnios (can occur in utero)
- Aspiration is not performed because typically the blood has clotted and there is risk for causing infection
- Hemorrhage can take weeks to months to resorb and can calcify to result in skull asymmetry
- Associated skull fracture in 5% to 18%
- Does not cross sutures and not a risk for serious blood loss due to the containment
- Unilateral or bilateral
- May coexist with subgaleal hematoma and caput succedaneum
- Calcification may occur in 3% to 5% of subperiosteal hematomas. Calcified subperiosteal hematomas have been subclassified as type 1 (nondepressed inner cortex) and type 2 (depressed inner cortex)

REFERENCES

1. Huisman TAGM, Phelps T, Bosemani T, et al. Parturitional injury of the head and neck. *J Neuroimaging*. 2015 Mar–Apr;25(2):151–166.
2. Colditz MJ, Lai MM, Cartwright D, et al. Subgaleal haemorrhage in the newborn. *Journal of Pediatric and Child Health*. 2015;51:14–146.
3. Wong CH, Foo CL, Seow WT. Calcified cephalohematoma: classification, indications for surgery and techniques. *J Craniofac Surg*. 2006 Sep;17(5):970–979.

BIRTH-RELATED SUBDURAL HEMORRHAGE

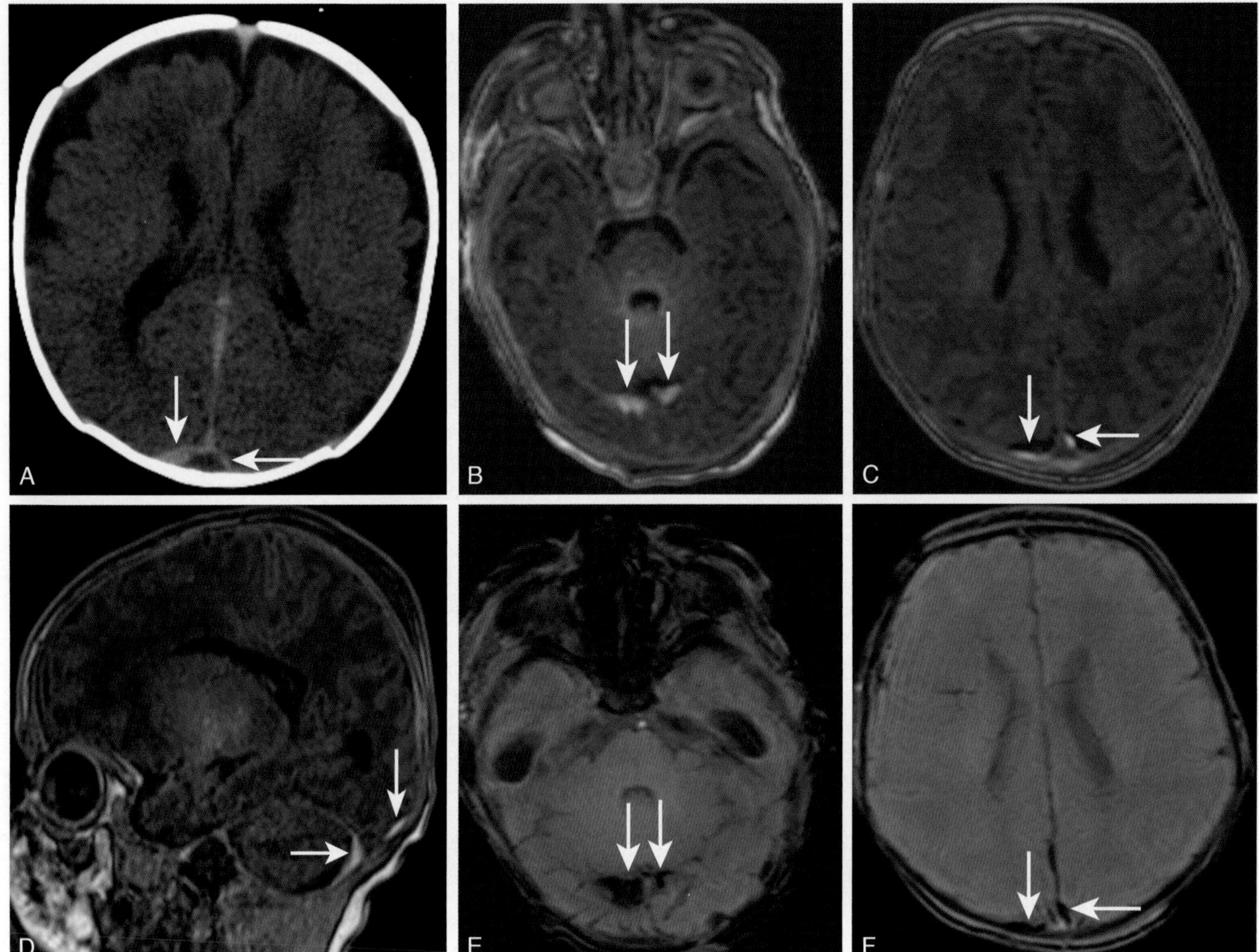

Fig. 10.5 Birth-Related Subdural Hemorrhage. (A) Axial head CT demonstrating hyperdense subdural hemorrhage along the right and left sides of the posterior falx (*arrows*). (B, C, D) Axial and sagittal T1W images demonstrating T1W hyperintense subdural hemorrhage along the tentorium, occipital lobes and posterior to the cerebellar hemispheres with associated susceptibility on (E and F) axial SWI images (*arrows*).

Key Points

Background

- Occurs in approximately 50% births
- No intervention or follow-up imaging in vast majority

Imaging

- Usually small (<4 mm in thickness)
- T1W hyperintense signal on MRI and hyperdense on CT
- No significant mass effect, and located posterior fossa, tentorium, posterior falx, posterior occipital (<4 mm in thickness)
- Most resolve by 1 month. All resolve by approximately 3 months
- In addition to subdural hemorrhage (SDH), can also see small amounts of subarachnoid hemorrhage (SAH) and intraventricular hemorrhage (IVH) from birth trauma

REFERENCE

1. Rooks VJ, Eaton JP, Ruess L, et al. Prevalence and evolution of intracranial hemorrhage in asymptomatic term infants. *AJNR Am J Neuroradiol.* 2008 Jun;29(6):1082–1089.

VENOUS SINUS HEMOCONCENTRATION

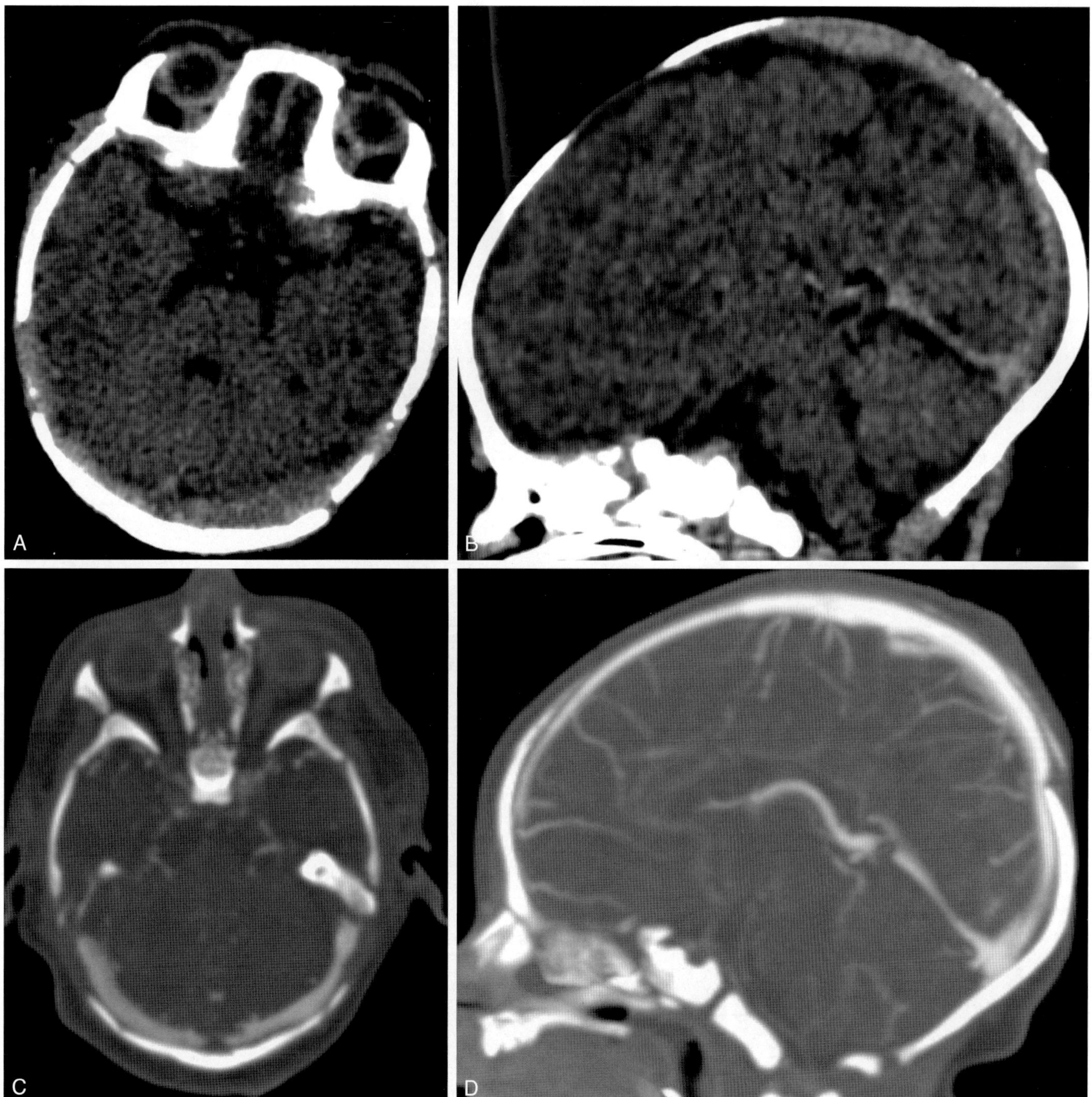

Fig. 10.6 Venous Hemoconcentration. (A and B) Axial and sagittal head CT images with mild hyperdensity along transverse sinuses, sagittal sinus, and straight sinus, which was indeterminate for thrombosis requiring a CT venogram (C and D), which confirmed patency and hyperdensity due to hemoconcentration.

Key Points

- Hyperdense dural sinuses can be seen on head CTs of neonates and accentuated by the relative lower density of the immature brain. Differentiation from thrombus can be difficult and result in potential pitfall.
- Mean Hounsfield units (HU) demonstrate a correlation with hemoglobin levels (correlation coefficient $r = 0.411$). The mean sinus density in normal pediatric population is 44 to 47 HU.
- Thrombosed venous sinuses measured 66 HU; however, the neonatal population has not been adequately studied.

REFERENCE

1. Yurtturan N, Kizildag B, Sarica MA, et al. Effect of hemoconcentration on dural sinus computed tomography density in a pediatric population. *Neuropediatrics*. 2016 Oct;47(5):327–331.

SUBPIAL HEMORRHAGE

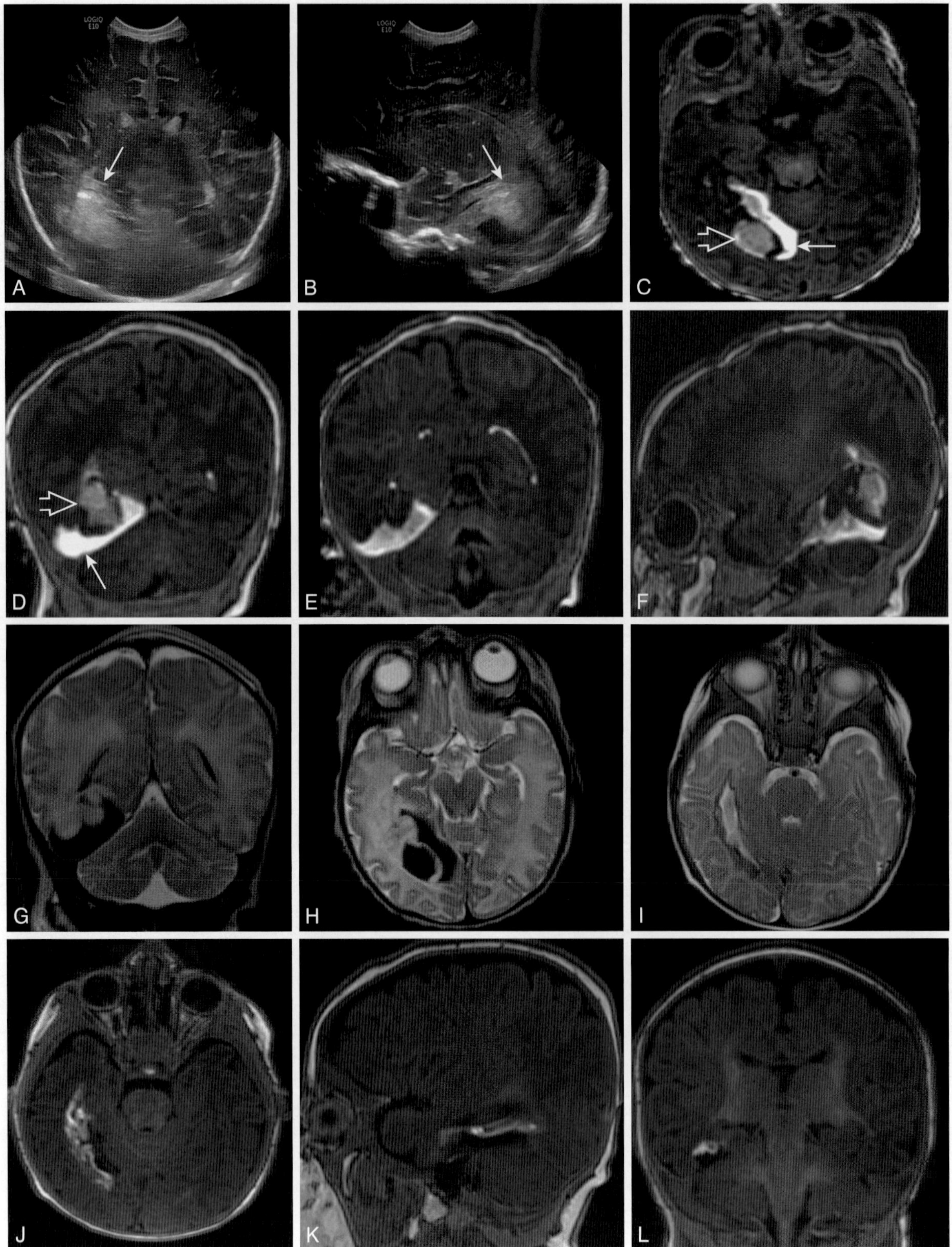

Fig. 10.7 Subpial Hemorrhage. (A and B) Coronal and sagittal head ultrasound demonstrating ill-defined asymmetric right temporal lobe hyperechogenicity (*arrows*). (C to F) Axial, coronal, and sagittal T1W images with T1W hyperintense subpial (*thin arrow*) and parenchymal hemorrhage (*wide arrow*) in the right temporal and occipital lobes. (G and H) Coronal and axial T2W images show T2 hypointense signal in the hemorrhage and parenchymal edema. (I to L) Follow up axial T2 and multiplanar T1 weighted images demonstrate decreasing subpial and parenchymal hemorrhage with associated parenchymal volume loss.

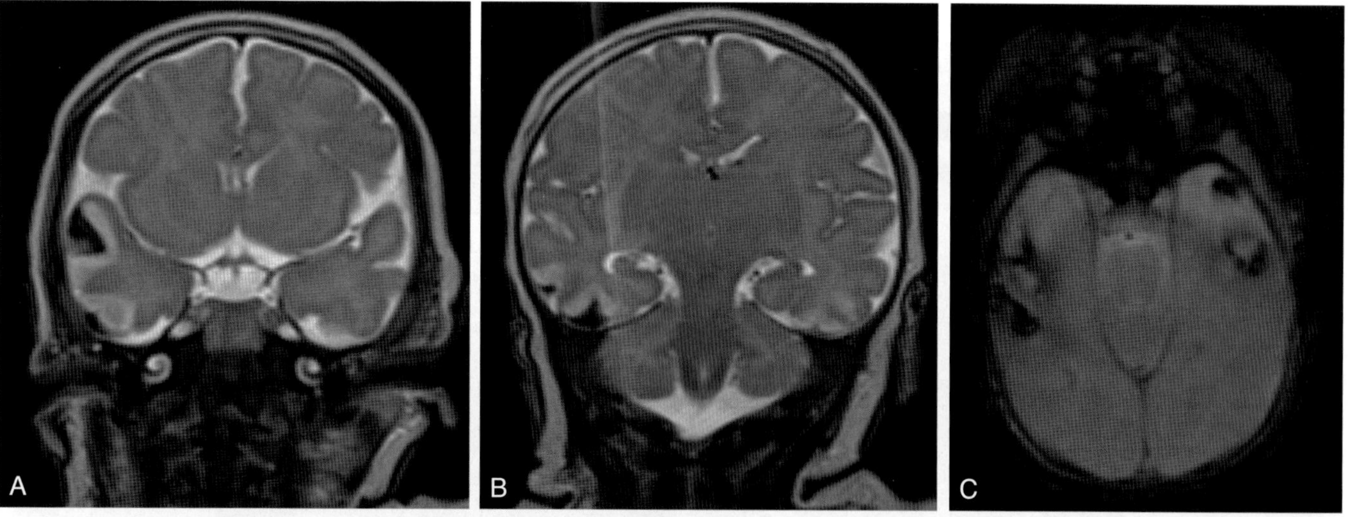

Fig. 10.8 Subpial Hemorrhage. (A and B) Coronal T2W and (C) axial GRE demonstrating characteristic subpial hemorrhages in the temporal lobes as areas of T2 hypointense signal and GRE susceptibility in a triangular configuration as well as evidence of parenchymal edema.

Key Points

Background

- Etiology unknown; possibly birth-related trauma or venous compression, injury, or venous thrombosis
- Potential explanation is that the pia mater is more easily separated from the brain in neonates than older children; therefore this may account for the relative low frequency of detection of this type of hemorrhage in older infants and children
- Typical presentation is a term neonate with apnea or seizure following spontaneous vaginal delivery
- Relatively uncommon but frequently occur in the temporal lobes
- Limited data suggest good prognosis

Imaging

- At time of imaging the hemorrhage is usually T2 hypointense and T1 hyperintense and demonstrates susceptibility. The hemorrhage has a characteristic triangular shape due to the extension into the sulcus and covering of the outer cortex.
- Intraparenchymal and intraventricular hemorrhage can coexist in continuity with a subpial hemorrhage.
- Follow-up imaging can demonstrate encephalomalacia, gliosis, and laminar necrosis.

REFERENCE

1. Huang AH, Robertson RL. Spontaneous superficial parenchymal and leptomeningeal hemorrhage in term neonates. *AJNR Am J Neuroradiol.* 2004 Mar;25(3):469–475.

ACCIDENTAL TRAUMA

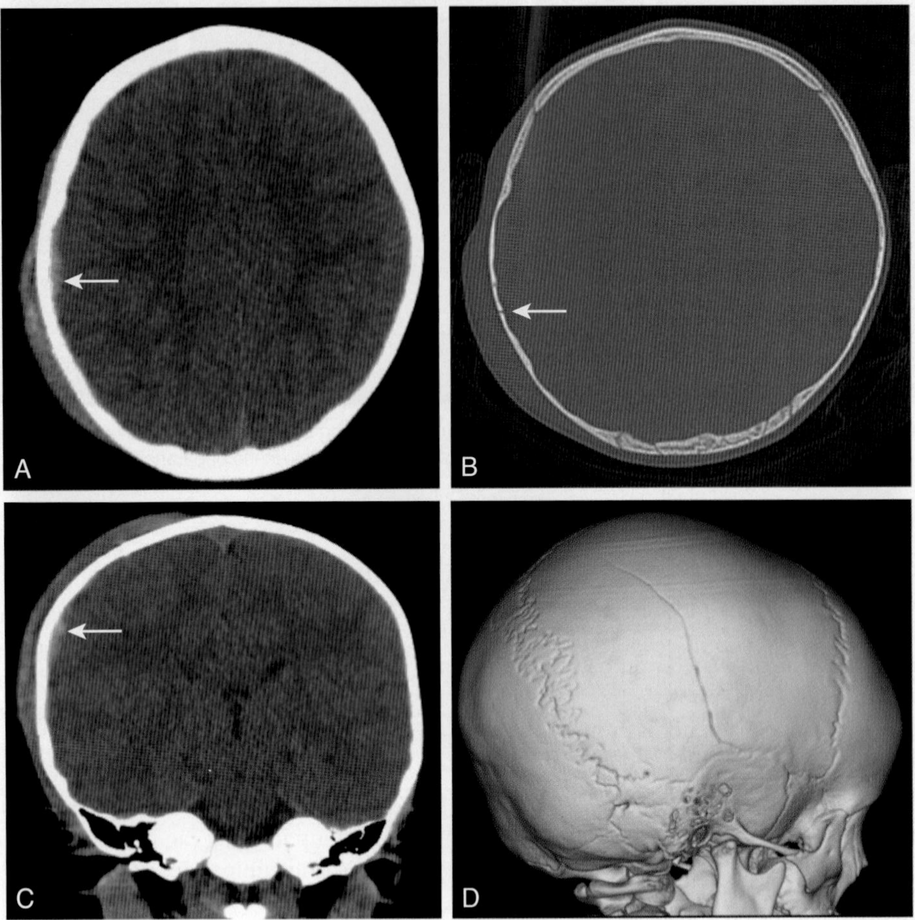

Fig. 10.9 Accidental Trauma. A 1-year-old with fall from high chair. (A and B) Axial head CT, (C) coronal head CT reformat, and (D) 3D volumetric CT images demonstrate and right parietal scalp subgaleal hematoma, a nondisplaced right parietal skull fracture (*arrow*, image B), and a hyperdense/acute epidural hemorrhage (*arrow*, images A and C) along the lateral right parietal lobe adjacent to the fracture.

Key Points

- Head trauma findings in order of most common to least common are: scalp hematoma > scalp hematoma with skull fracture > scalp hematoma with skull fracture and epidural hemorrhage.
- Skull fractures most commonly involve the parietal bone. Fractures can also be seen as suture diastasis rather than fracture lucency through the bone.
- Most epidural hematomas are small but require consultation with neurosurgery for conservative versus surgical management.
- Epidural hematomas are more likely from accidental rather than nonaccidental trauma.
- Subdural hemorrhage can occur in accidental trauma but should raise suspicion of nonaccidental trauma in young children.
- Fractures crossing a venous sinus are associated with sinus thrombosis in 20% to 40% of cases and external compression in approximately 30%.

REFERENCES

1. Kemp AM, Jaspan T, Griffiths, et al. Neuroimaging: what neuroradiological features distinguish abusive from non-abusive head trauma? A systematic review. *Arch Dis Child*. 2011;96:1103–1112.
2. Piteau SJ, Ward MGK, Barrowman NJ, et al. Clinical and Radiographic Characteristics Associated With Abusive and Nonabusive Head Trauma: A Systemic Review. *Pediatrics*. 2012;130(2):315–323.
3. Hersh DS, Shimony N, Groves ML, et al. Pediatric cerebral venous sinus thrombosis or compression in the setting of skull fractures from blunt head trauma. *J Neurosurg Pediatr*. 2018 Mar;21(3):258–269.

FRACTURE-RELATED DURAL SINUS COMPRESSION AND THROMBUS

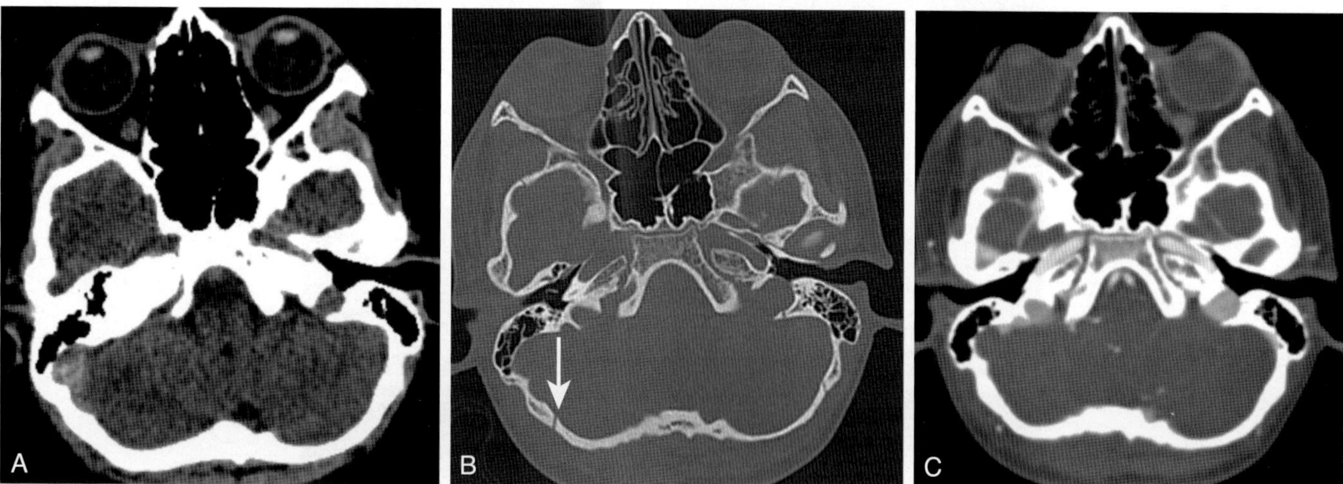

Fig. 10.10 Fracture-Related Dural Sinus Thrombus. A 13-year-old with backward fall onto concrete, subsequent vomiting, headache, and scalp swelling. (A) Axial head CT demonstrates a hyperdensity in the right sigmoid sinus. (B) Axial bone filter image demonstrates a subtle asymmetrically widened diastatic fracture of the right lambdoid suture (*arrow*). (C) Axial CT venogram demonstrates a filling defect with abrupt cutoff in the right sigmoid sinus due to thrombus.

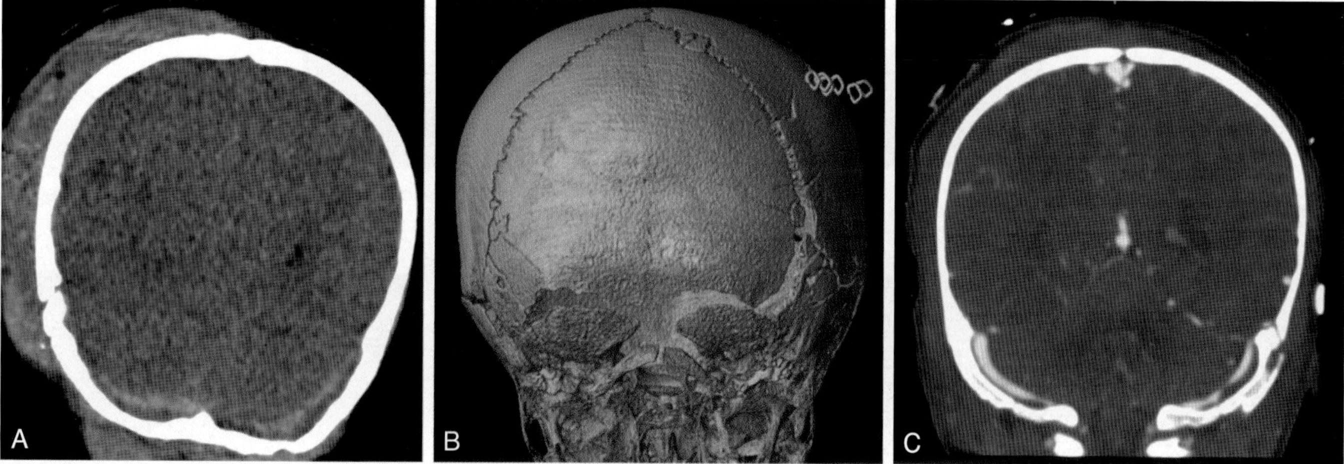

Fig. 10.11 Fracture-Related Dural Sinus Compression. A 2-year-old hit by a car. (A) Coronal reformat head CT demonstrates acute extraaxial hemorrhage in the posterior fossa. (B) A 3D reformat head CT demonstrates bilateral diastatic fractures of the occipital bone. (C) Coronal reformat CT venogram image demonstrates compression and narrowing of the right and left sigmoid sinuses.

Key Points

Background

- Acute fractures of the calvarium can result in focal epidural hematomas that compress and narrow or occlude the dural venous sinus or cause endothelial injury and subsequent thrombus formation.
- Most often involves the transverse and/or sigmoid sinuses from a fracture of the occipital bone, diastatic fracture of the lambdoid suture, or petrous temporal bone.
- The decision to anticoagulate for trauma-induced sinus thrombosis is controversial.

Imaging

- CT demonstrates hyperdense epidural hemorrhage and/or intraluminal thrombus. CT venogram confirms the dural sinus compression and/or thrombus but at times the differentiation of the two can remain difficult.
- Associated hemorrhagic venous infarcts are uncommon.

REFERENCE

1. Delagado Almandoz JE, Kelly HR, Schaefer PW, et al. Prevalence of traumatic dural venous sinus thrombosis in high-risk acute blunt head trauma patients evaluated with multidetector CT venography. *Radiology*. 2010 May;255(2):570–577.

PING PONG FRACTURE

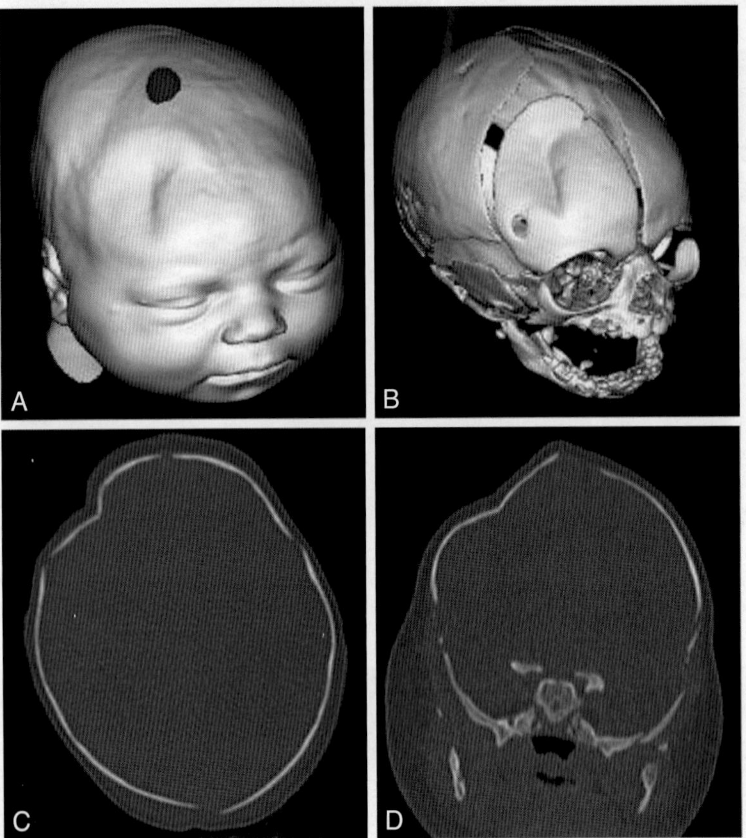

Fig. 10.12 Ping Pong Fracture. (A and B) 3D volumetric CT images, and (C and D) axial and coronal head CT images demonstrate a ping pong fracture of the right frontal bone with characteristic internal depression and angulation.

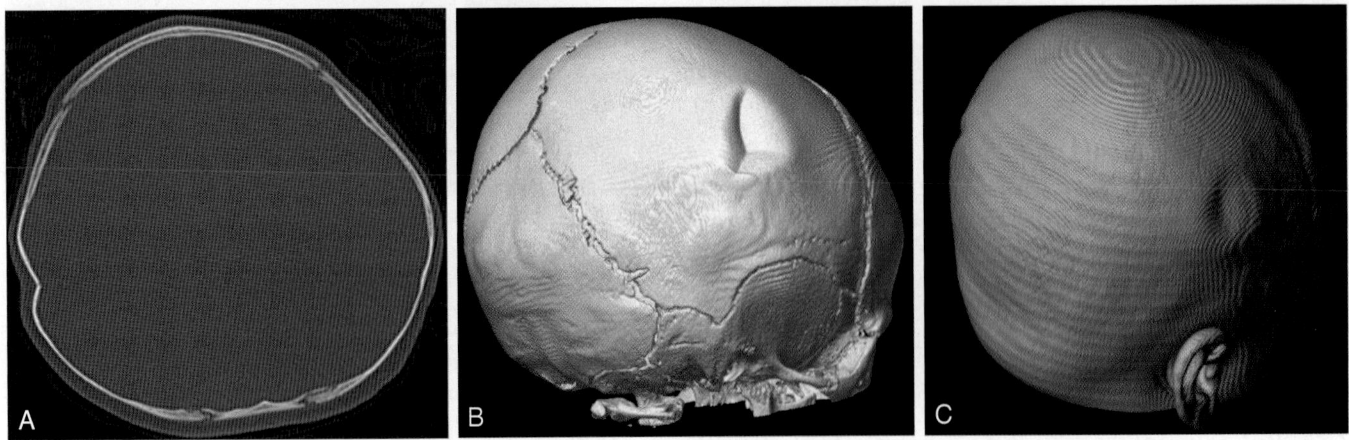

Fig. 10.13 Ping Pong Fracture. (A) axial head CT and (B and C) 3D volumetric CT images demonstrate a ping pong fracture of the right parietal bone with characteristic internal depression and angulation and noticeable contour deformity of the scalp.

Key Points

- Uncommon fracture pattern demonstrating focal concave fracture
- Occurs in newborns and young infants due to the calvarium being more soft and resilient to fracturing at this age
- Has been reported in both accidental and nonaccidental trauma
- Can be treated surgically and nonsurgically, depending on the severity

REFERENCE

1. Silva JB, Joao A, Miranda N. Ping-pong fracture in newborn: a rare diagnosis. *Acta Med Port*. 2019 Jul–Aug 1;32(7-8):549.

LEPTOMENINGEAL CYST

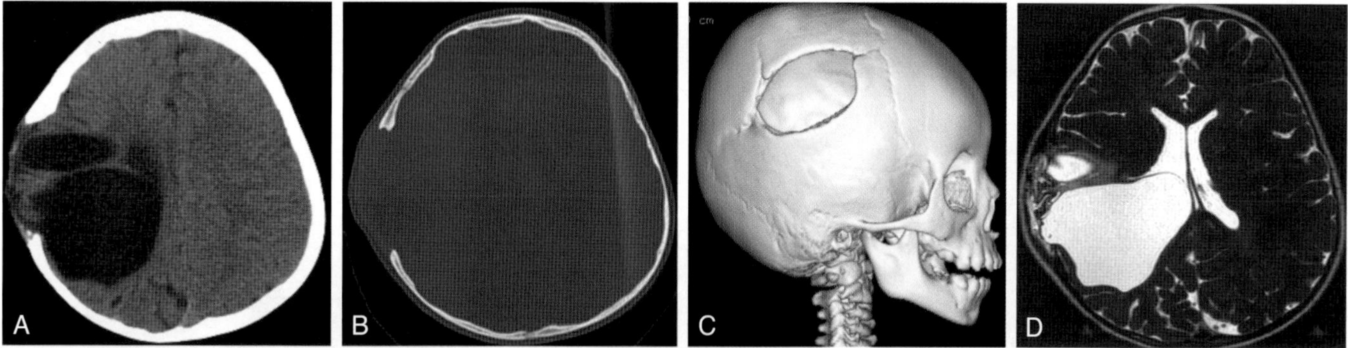

Fig. 10.14 Leptomeningeal Cyst. (A to C) Axial CT and 3D volumetric CT images demonstrate an ovoid defect in the right parietal bone and adjacent linear fractures. The right frontal and parietal lobes herniate into the fracture site, and there is cystic encephalomalacia of the herniated parenchyma. (D) Axial 3D T2W image better demonstrates the encephalomalacia and gliosis of the right frontal and parietal lobe parenchyma.

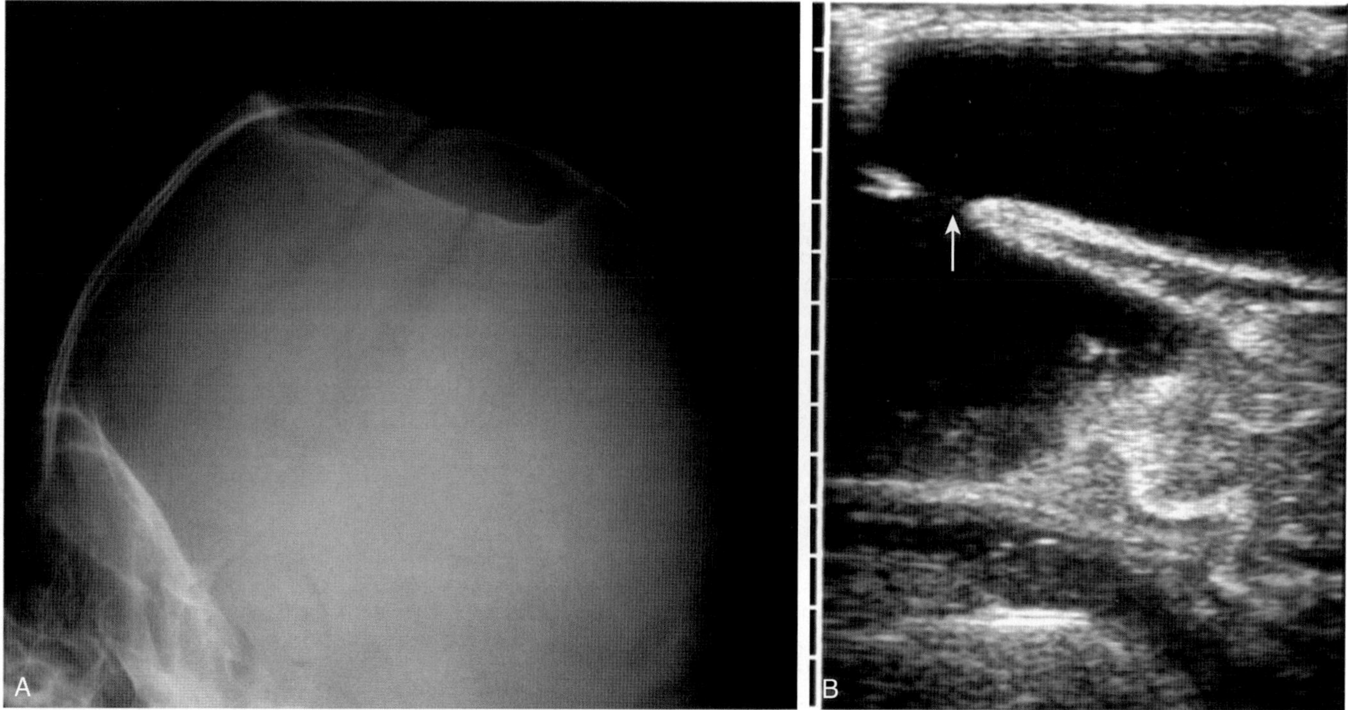

Fig. 10.15 Leptomeningeal Cyst: Radiograph and Ultrasound Appearance. (A) Sagittal skull radiograph demonstrating a large ovoid lucency in the skull. (B) Focused ultrasound image demonstrating a scalp fluid collection extending and communicating with the intracranial extraaxial space through a skull defect (arrow).

Key Points

- Rare complication from trauma that results from a fracture and herniation of meninges through a dural tear into the fracture site resulting in widening of the fracture and frequently encephalomalacia of the brain
- Surgical repair with duraplasty and cranioplasty is needed to repair the defect

REFERENCE

1. Scarfo GB, Mariottini A, Tomaccini D, et al. Growing skull fractures: progressive evolution of brain damage and effectiveness of surgical treatment. *Childs Nerv Syst.* 1989 Jun;55(3):163–167.

ACCESSORY SUTURE

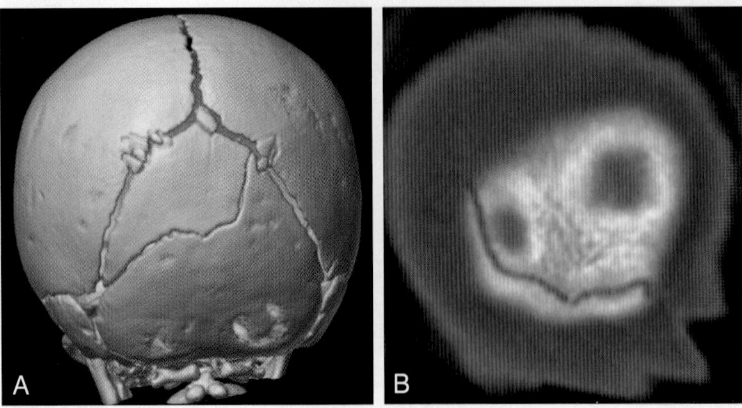

Fig. 10.16 Accessory Suture. (A) 3D Volumetric CT image and (B) coronal reformat head CT image demonstrate an accessory suture in the occipital bone, differentiated from a fracture by the zigzag appearance. Axial images could mimic a fracture, which is why there is value in multiplanar and volumetric images.

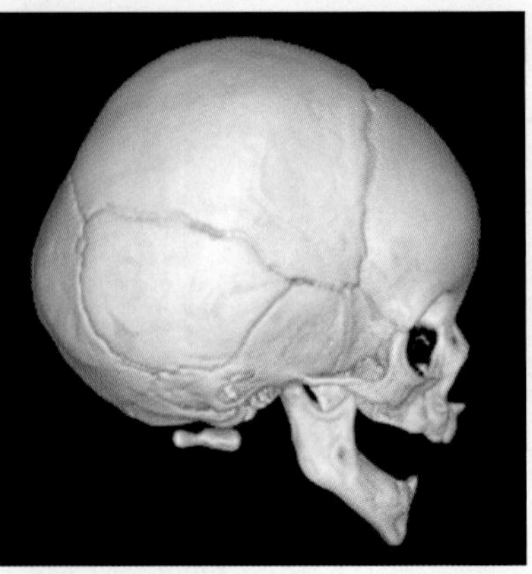

Fig. 10.17 Accessory Suture. A 3D Volumetric CT image demonstrates an accessory suture in the lateral aspect of the parietal bone.

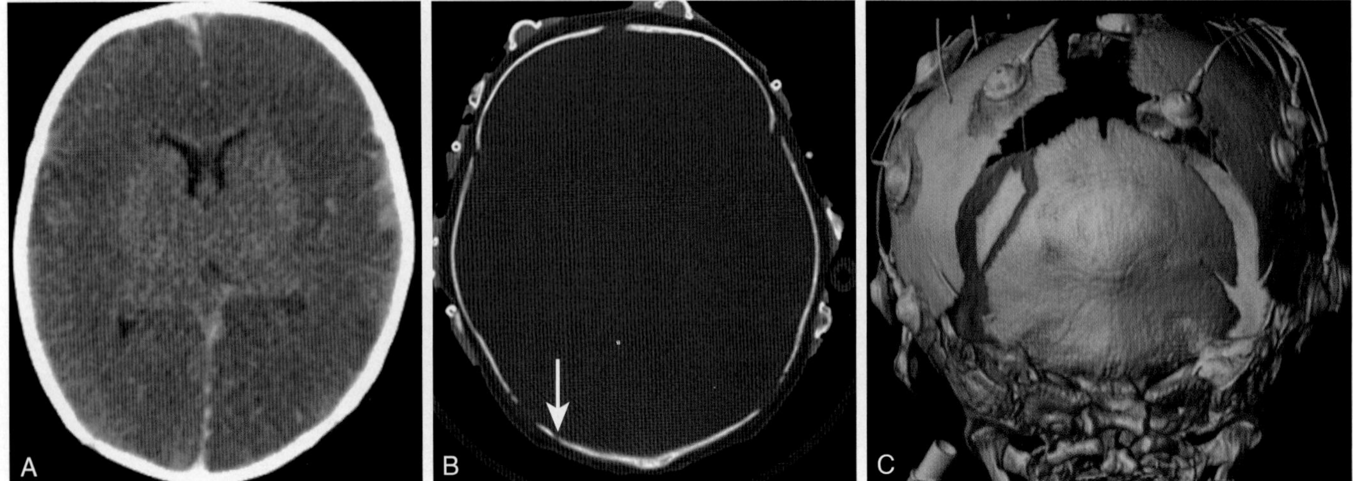

Fig. 10.18 Accessory Suture. (A and B) Axial CT images demonstrate large regions of parenchymal edema, hyperdensities in the subarachnoid spaces concerning for hemorrhage, and a lucency in the right side of the occipital bone concerning for a fracture (*arrow*). These findings were concerning for potential abusive head trauma. (C) 3D volumetric CT image, however, shows the sutures are widened and the right occipital lucency is a widened accessory suture. The infant was found to have bacterial meningitis. Autopsy confirmed an accessory suture.

Key Points

- Accessory sutures and intrasutural ossicles are common along the lambdoid suture.
- These can mimic fractures on axial CT imaging and radiographs.
- 3D reformatted images and multiplanar reformatted images are helpful in determining if an accessory suture is present based on the zigzag appearance along the margins.

REFERENCES

1. Sanchez T, Stewart D, Walvick M, et al. Skull fracture vs. accessory sutures: how can we tell the difference? *Emerg Radiol.* 2010 Sep;17(5):413–418.
2. Orman G, Wagner MW, Seeburg D, et al. Pediatric skull fracture diagnosis: should 3D CT reconstructions be added as routine imaging? *J Neurosurg Pediatr*. 2015;16:426–431.

PARENCHYMAL CONTUSION

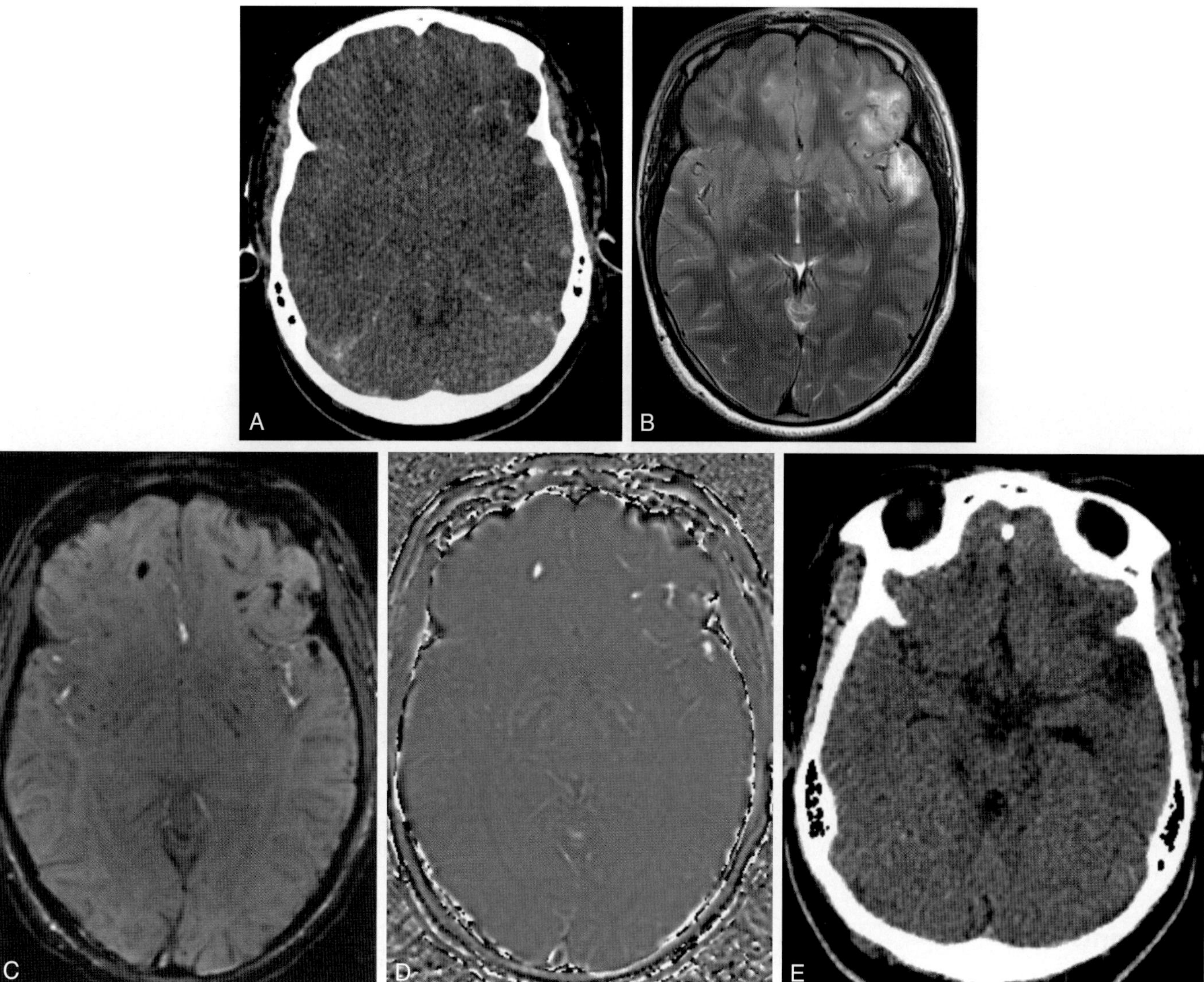

FIG. 10.19 Parenchymal Contusion. (A) Axial head CT demonstrating foci of acute hemorrhage in the bilateral frontal lobes and left temporal lobe with surrounding edema. (B) Axial T2W image demonstrating areas of hemorrhage see as T2 hypointense signal and surrounding edema. (C) Axial SWI and (D) axial SWI phase image demonstrate multifocal susceptibility in the parenchyma consistent with hemorrhage as indicated on the phase map hyperintense signal similar to veins. (E) Follow-up axial head CT, demonstrating parenchymal volume loss and low density indicative of encephalomalacia and gliosis at sites of previous contusions.

Key Points

- Parenchymal contusions can be from accidental or nonaccidental trauma.
- CT demonstrates hyperdense blood in the acute phase with surrounding low density from edema.
- MRI in the acute setting will demonstrate hypointensity on SWI with surrounding edema. Often additional traumatic findings are present such as diffuse axonal injury (DAI), SAH, and SDH.
- SWI phase images can be used to confirm blood products from calcification. Blood is paramagnetic while calcification is diamagnetic, resulting in difference on phase images. Because SWI phase images are dependent on the scanner, the internal cerebral veins are a useful internal reference for whether blood is bright or dark on phase images.
- Follow-up imaging months later will demonstrate volume loss consistent with encephalomalacia and gliosis.

REFERENCE

1. Suskauer SJ, Huisman TAGM. Neuroimaging in pediatric traumatic brain injury: current and future predictors of functional outcome. *Dev Disabil Res Rev*. 2009;15(2):117–123.

DIFFUSE AXONAL INJURY

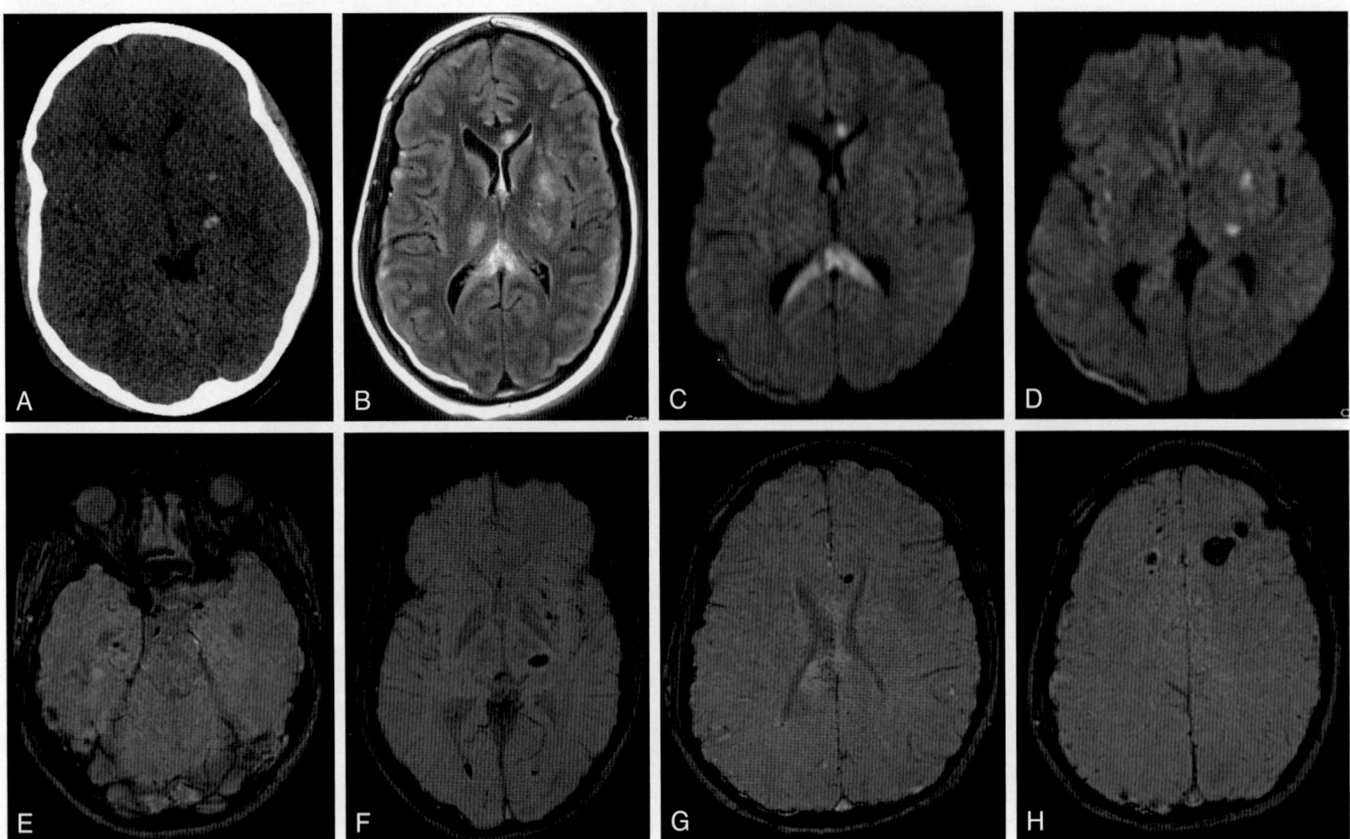

Fig. 10.20 Diffuse Axonal Injury. (A) Axial head CT demonstrating foci of acute hemorrhage in the left putamen and thalamus. (B) Axial FLAIR image demonstrating areas of hyperintensity in the corpus callosum, bilateral thalami, and left putamen in addition to a right occipital subdural hemorrhage. A small subdural hematoma is also prersent posterior to the right occipital lobe. (C and D) Axial DWI images demonstrate hyperintense signal in the corpus callosum, left thalamus, left putamen, and right subinsular white matter. The right occipital subdural hemorrhage is also seen. (E to H) Axial SWI images demonstrate multifocal susceptibility in the parenchyma consistent with hemorrhage from diffuse axonal injury.

Key Points

Background

- Severe rotational acceleration-deceleration mechanism
- Increased number of diffuse axonal injury (DAI) lesions is associated with lower Glascow coma score, prolonged coma, and moderate or severe disability or vegetative state

Imaging

- Typical locations: Corpus callosum, subcortical white matter, and brainstem
- Children can also demonstrate DAI in basal ganglia and thalami > adults
- Usually less than 10 mm in diameter; usually seen in conjunction with other trauma findings such as skull fracture, SAH, contusion and/or SDH
- Hemorrhagic and nonhemorrhagic on imaging seen as foci of susceptibility, diffusion restriction, and T2/FLAIR hyperintensity
- SWI sequence is recommended over GRE because of higher sensitivity for detection of hemorrhage

REFERENCE

1. Tong KA, Ashwal S, Holshouser BA, et al. Diffuse axonal injury in children: clinical correlation with hemorrhagic lesions. *Ann Neurol.* 2004 Jul;56:36–50.

RETROCLIVAL HEMATOMA

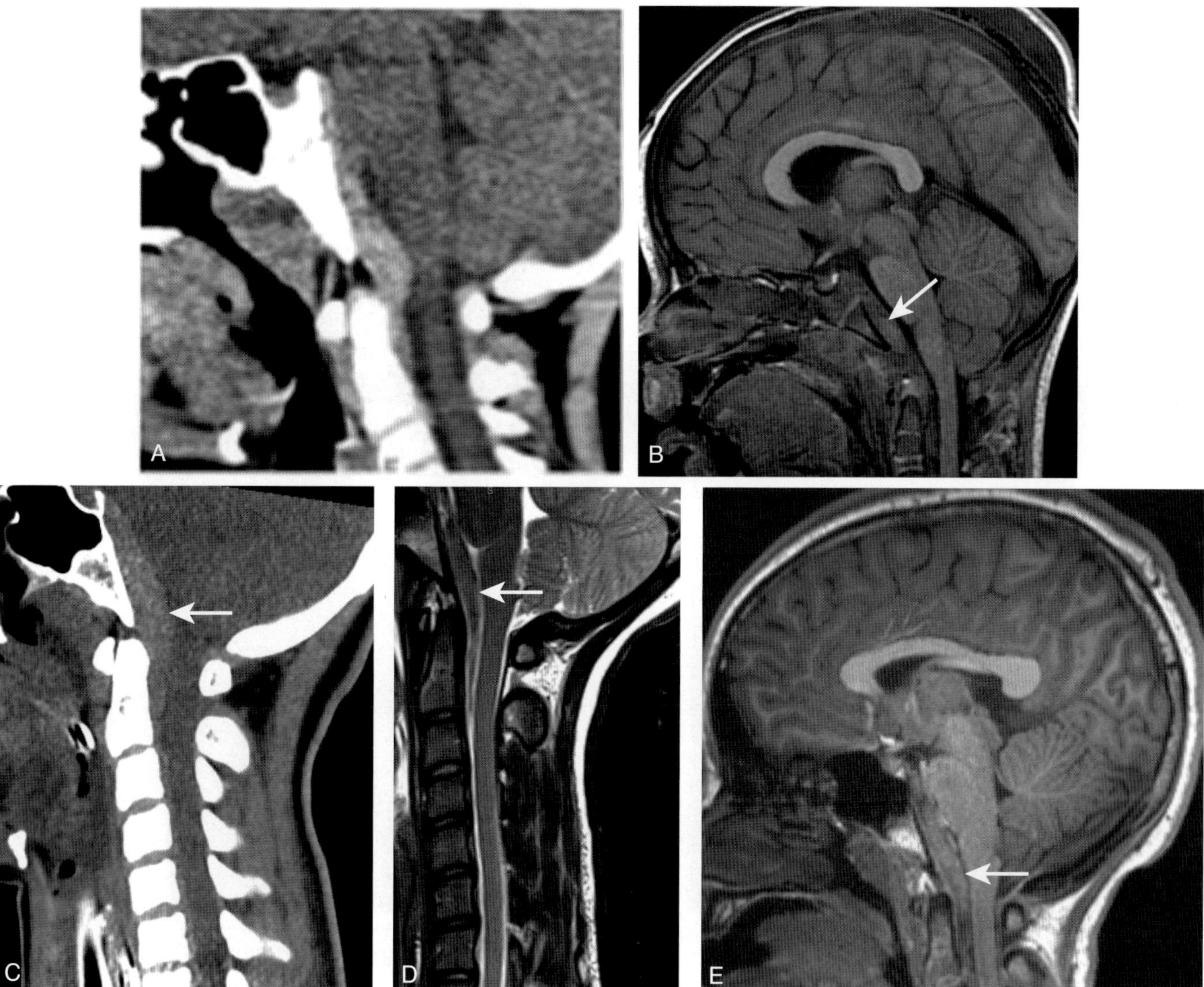

Fig. 10.21 Retroclival Hematoma. (A) Sagittal reformat head CT image demonstrating hyperdense hemorrhage posterior to the clivus. (B) Sagittal T1W image demonstrating isointense and mild hyperintense T1W signal posterior to the clivus due to hemorrhage (*arrow*). (C) Sagittal reformat CT image demonstrating hyperdense hemorrhage posterior to the clivus (*arrow*). (D) Sagittal T2W and (E) Sagittal T1W images demonstrate T2W hypointense and T1W isointense to mild hyperintense signal due to hemorrhage posterior to the clivus (*arrows*).

Key Points

- Can be seen with both accidental and nonaccidental trauma
- Retroclival collections were found in 32% of children with abusive head trauma
- Retroclival collections were visible on CT in 38% and on MRI in 85%
- In one research study, 48% were subdural, 14% epidural, 10% both, and 28% indeterminate in location

REFERENCES

1. Koshy J, Scheurkogel MM, Clough L, et al. Neuroimaging findings of retroclival hemorrhage in children: a diagnostic conundrum. *Childs Nerv Syst.* 2014 May;30:835–839.
2. Silvera VM, Danehy AR, Newton AW, et al. Retroclival collections associated with abusive head trauma in children. *Pediatr Radiol.* 2014 Dec;44(Suppl 4):5621–5631.

ABUSIVE HEAD TRAUMA: COMMON FINDINGS

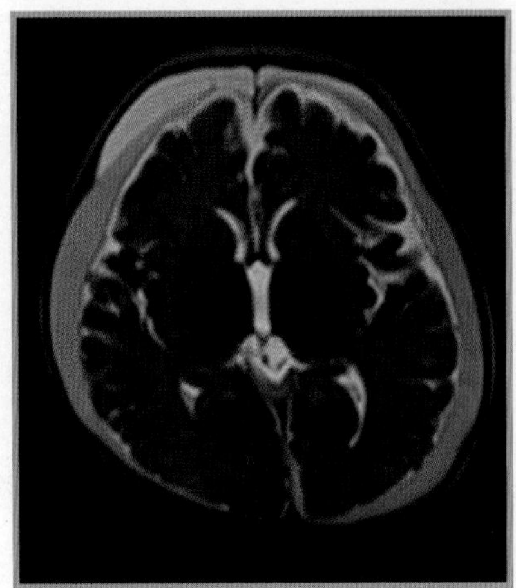

Subdural Hemorrhage

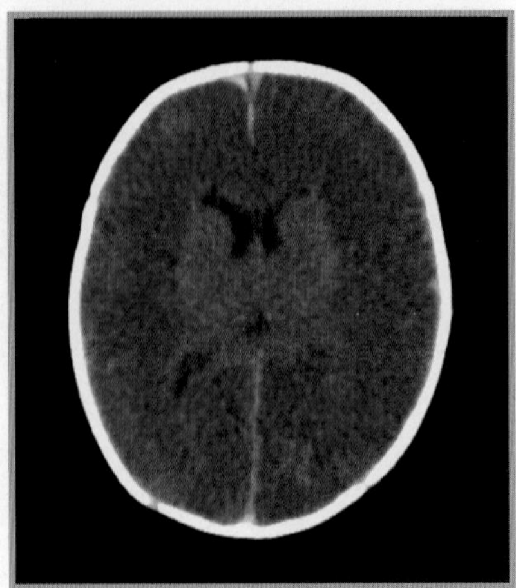

Ischemia

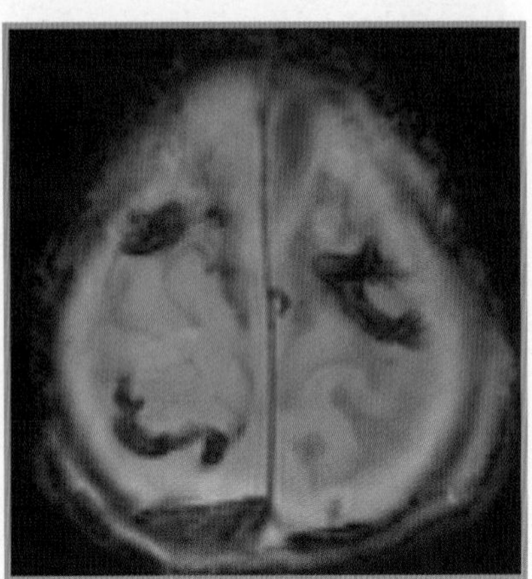

Venous Injury

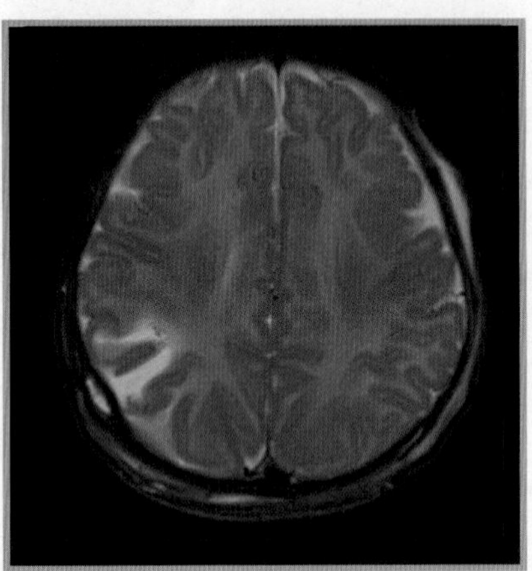

Parenchymal Laceration

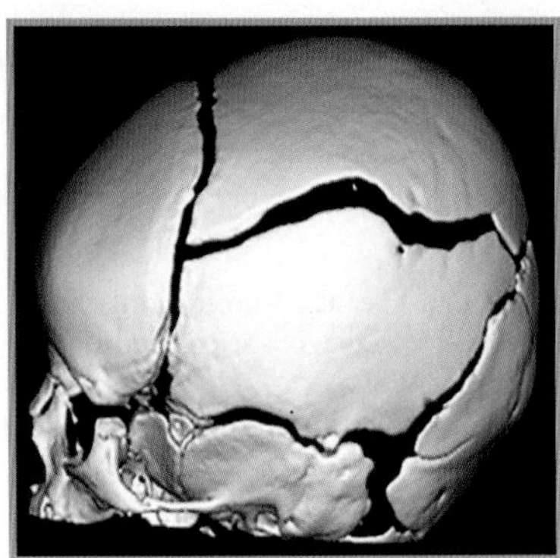

Skull Fracture

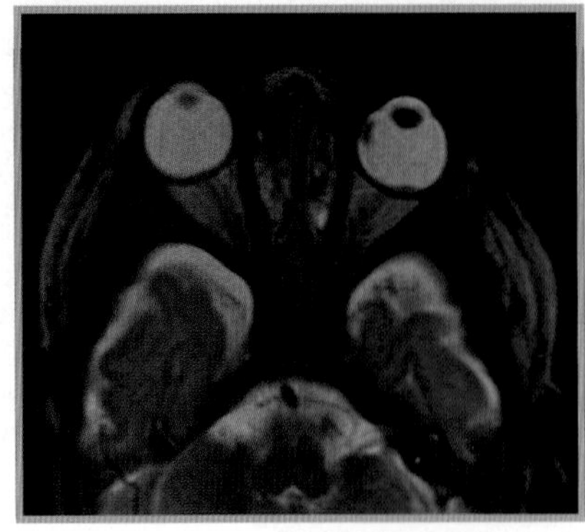

Retinal Hemorrhage

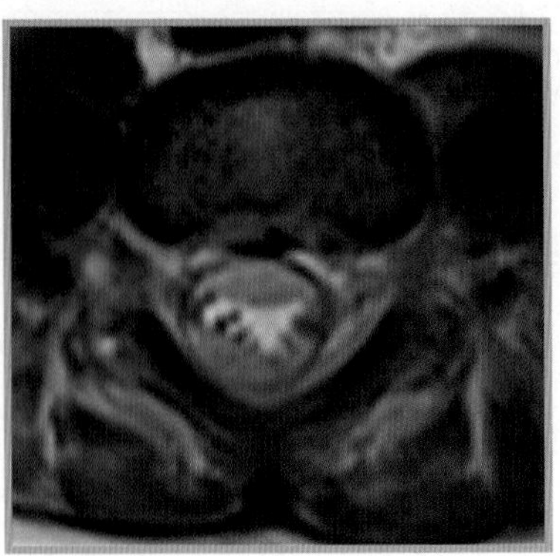

Spinal Hemorrhage

ABUSIVE HEAD TRAUMA: OVERVIEW

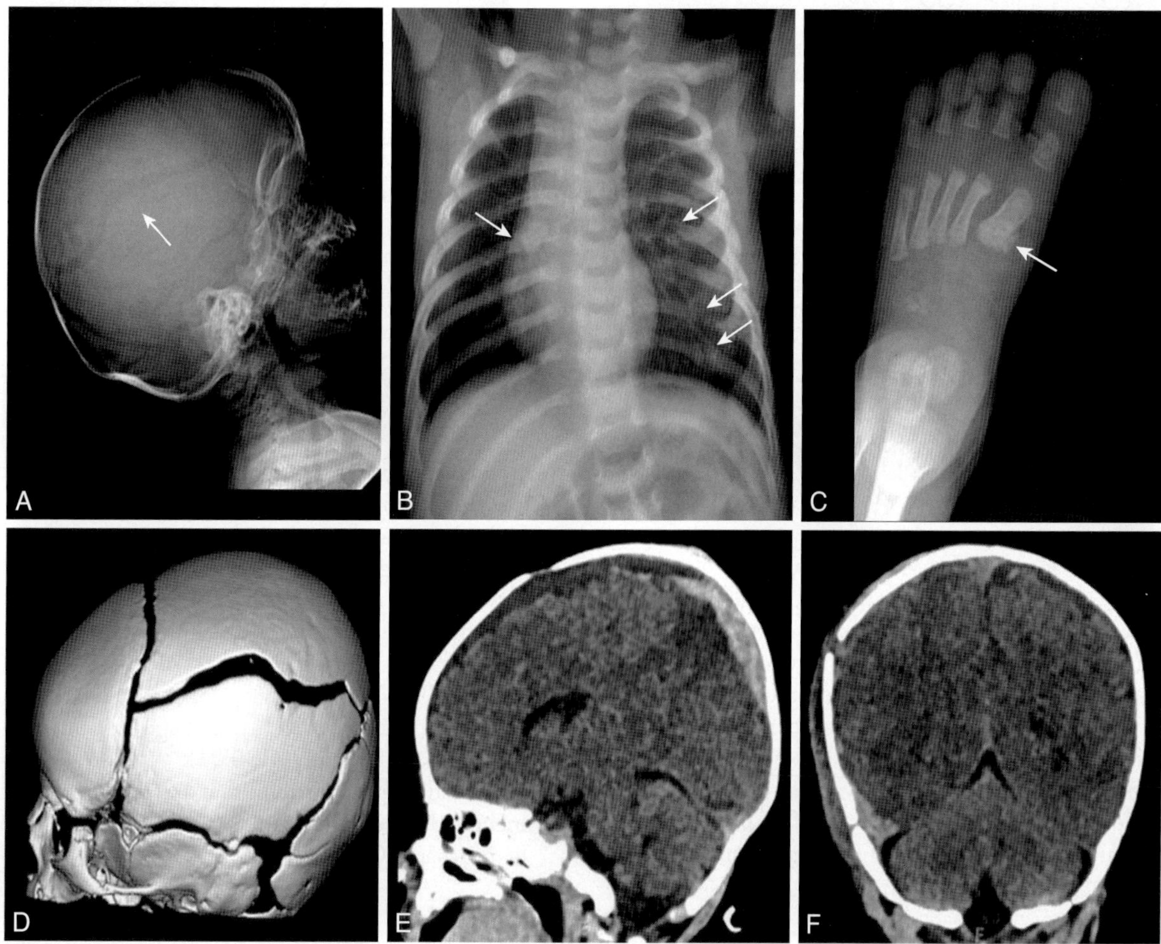

Fig. 10.22 Abusive Head Trauma. (A) Lateral skull radiograph demonstrates a linear parietal bone lucency due to a fracture (*arrow*). (B) AP chest radiograph demonstrates bilateral healing rib fractures (*arrows*). (C) AP foot radiograph demonstrates a healing first metatarsal fracture (*arrow*). (D) 3D volumetric CT demonstrates the parietal bone fracture. (E and F) Sagittal and coronal head CT reformat images demonstrate mixed density subdural hemorrhage along the right cerebral hemisphere and right temporal scalp edema.

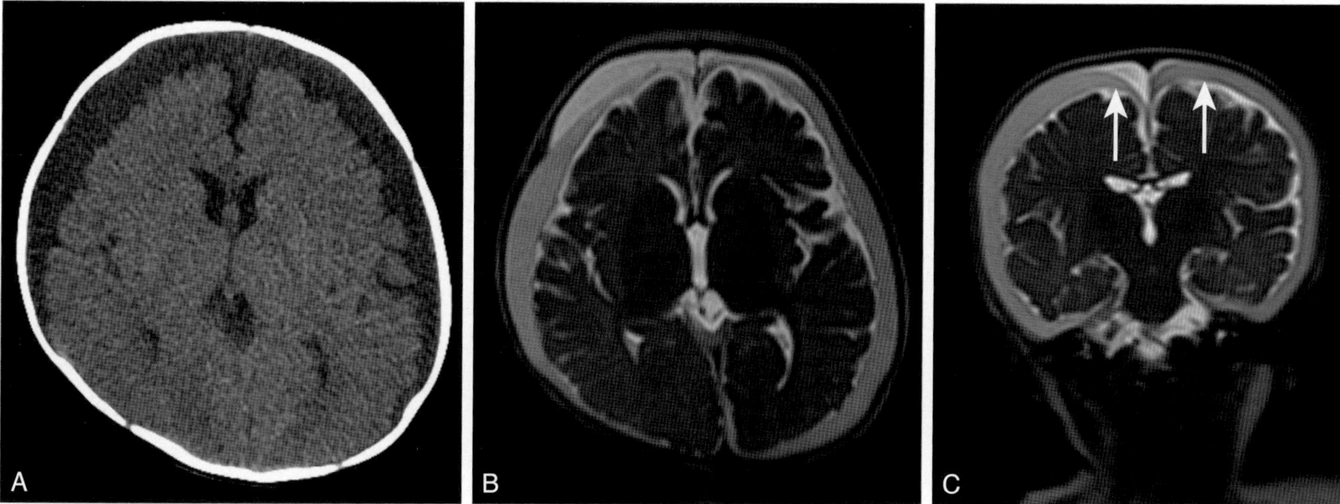

Fig. 10.23 Abusive Head Trauma. (A) Axial head CT demonstrates enlarged bilateral frontoparietal low-density extraaxial spaces. No vessels traverse these spaces, which should raise concern for subdural fluid collections. (B and C) Axial and coronal ultrafast T2W images confirm bilateral subdural fluid collections and presence of internal septations. The dura is delineated by the *arrows*.

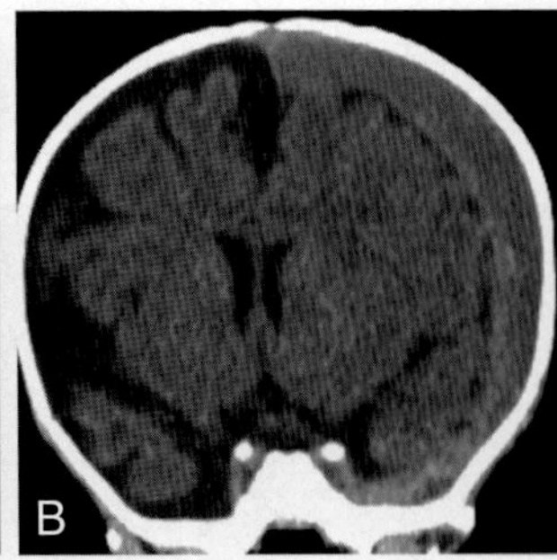
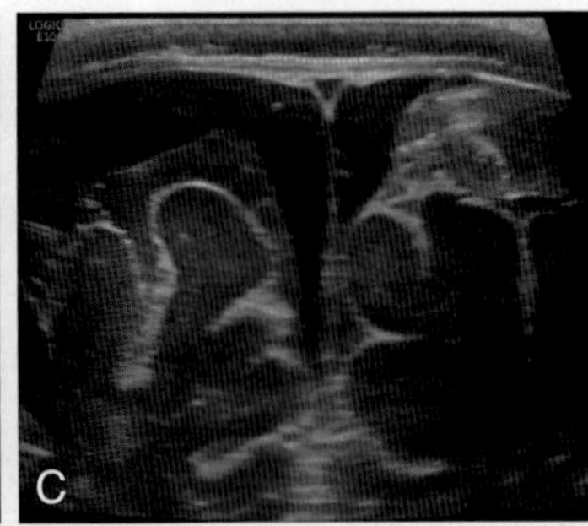
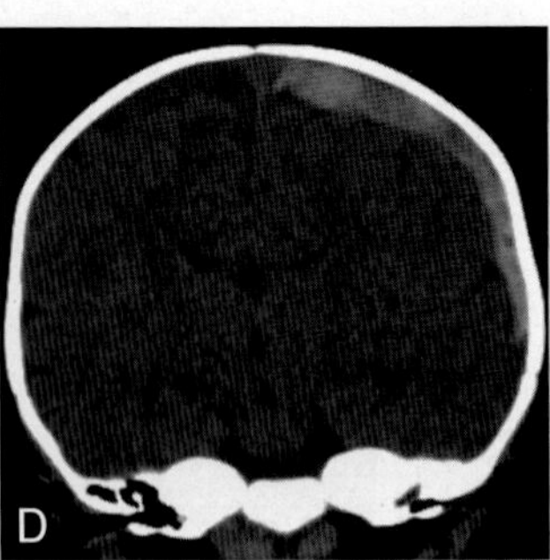

Fig. 10.24 Abusive Head Trauma: Ultrasound Appearance. (A) Coronal head ultrasound image demonstrates a mild hyperechoic subdural hematoma along the left vertex. (B) Coronal noncontrast reformat CT image correlate for image A demonstrates an isodense subdural hematoma along the left cerebral hemisphere. (C) Coronal head ultrasound image demonstrates a hypoechoic right vertex subdural fluid collection displacing the subarachnoid space and a left sided hyperechoic subdural hematoma along the left vertex. (D) Coronal reformat noncontrast CT image confirms bilateral subdural fluid collections of different densities.

Key Points

Clinical

- Abusive head trauma (AHT) is the leading cause of fatal head injuries in children less than 2 years of age.
- AHT diagnosis is missed in 31% of cases at initial presentation. Reasons include children are too young to provide adequate history, perpetrators are unlikely to provide truthful account of trauma, and clinicians may not consider a diagnosis of AHT because of a nontraumatic clinical presentation such as lethargy or seizure.
- A higher mortality rate and higher rate of neurologic impairment is associated with AHT victims compared to accidental head trauma.
- A multidisciplinary approach is necessary and diagnosis includes clinical history, physical examination, laboratory results, radiological findings, and scene investigation and interviews with other family members by child protective services and police.

Imaging

- Head CT and MRI are necessary for diagnosis in addition to skeletal survey and retinal examination.
- MRI technique should include multiplanar thin section T2W, T1W, FLAIR, and SWI sequences to maximize accuracy for detection of intracranial injury.
- Common neuroimaging findings include subdural hemorrhage, subarachnoid hemorrhage, ischemia, fractures, bridging vein injury, and spine trauma including ligamentous injury and hematomas.
- Uncommon neuroimaging findings include parenchymal laceration, parenchymal contusion, subpial hemorrhage, focal infarct, and venous ischemia.
- Neuroradiological findings with odds ratio (OR) favoring AHT include subdural hemorrhage(s) (SDH) (OR 8.92), skull fracture(s) with intracranial injury (OR 7.76), cerebral ischemia (OR 4.79), and cerebral edema (OR 2.2).
- Neuroradiological findings favoring accidental head trauma include epidural hemorrhage(s) (OR 0.15), and isolated skull fracture (OR 0.01).
- Neuroradiological findings that are equivocal for AHT include diffuse axonal injury (OR 1.47), and subarachnoid hemorrhage (OR 1.42).

REFERENCES

1. Orman G, Kralik SF, Meoded A, et al. MRI findings in pediatric abusive head trauma: a review. *J Neuroimaging*. 2019;00:1–13.
2. Duhaime AC, Christian C, Moss E, et al. Long-term outcome in infants with the shaking-impact syndrome. *Pediatr Neurosurg*. 1996;24(6):292–298.
3. Piteau SJ, Ward MGK, Barrowman NJ, et al. Clinical and Radiographic Characteristics Associated with Abusive and Nonabusive Head Trauma: A Systemic Review. *Pediatrics*. 2012;130(2):315–323.
4. Kemp AM, Jaspan T, Griffiths J, et al. Neuroimaging: what neuroradiological features distinguish abusive from non-abusive head trauma? A systematic review. *Arch Dis Child*. 2011;96:1103–1112.
5. Parks SE, Sugerman D, Xu L, et al. Pediatric Abusive Head Trauma: Recommended Definitions for Public Health Surveillance and Research. Atlanta, GA: Centers for Disease Control and Prevention; 2012.
6. Barlow KM, Minns RA. Annual incidence of shaken impact syndrome in young children. *Lancet*. 2000;356:1571–1572.

ABUSIVE HEAD TRAUMA: SUBDURAL HEMORRHAGE

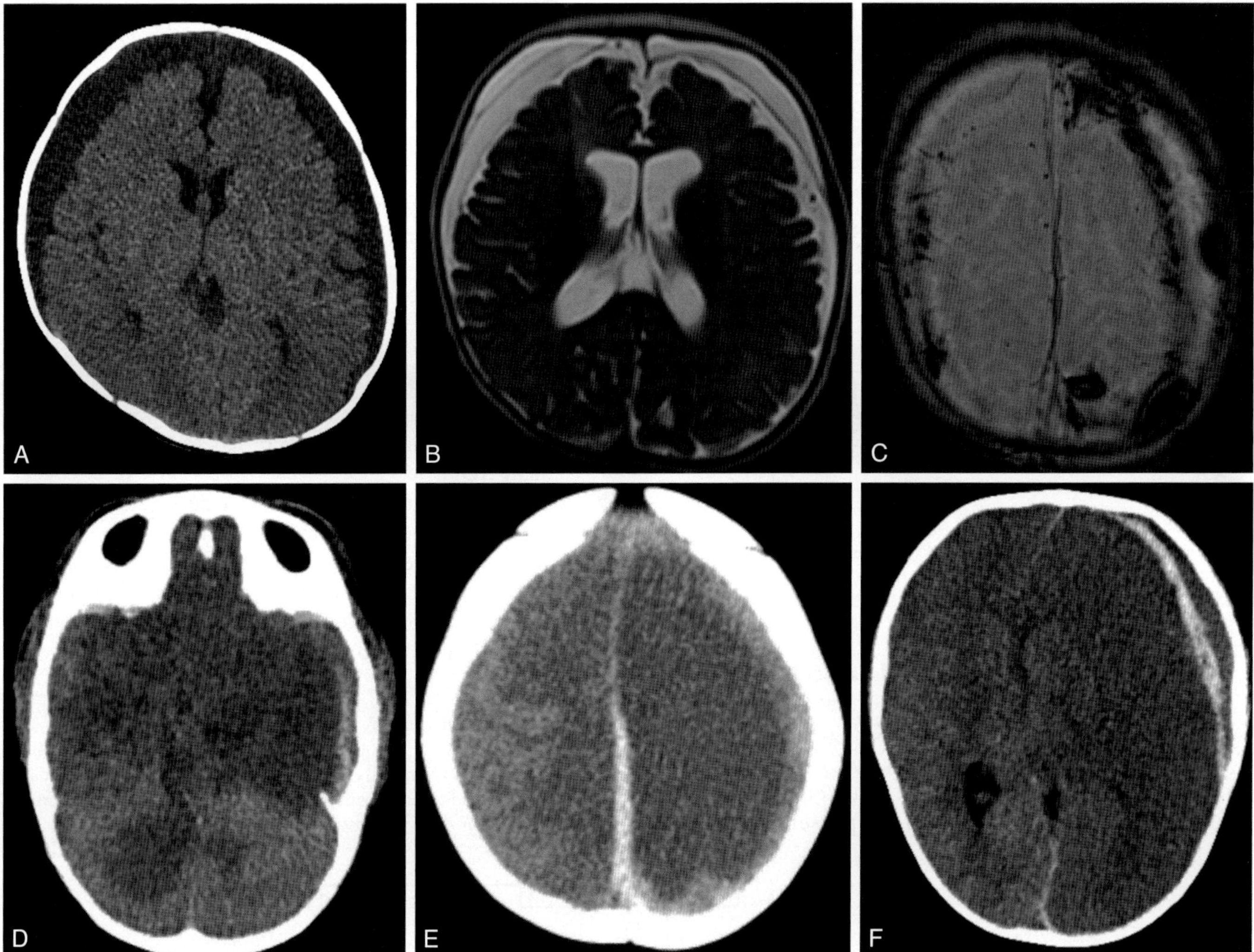

Fig. 10.25 Abusive Head Trauma: Subdural Hemorrhage Patterns. (A) Axial head CT demonstrates bilateral frontoparietal low-density extraaxial spaces. No vessels traverse these spaces, which should raise concern for subdural fluid collections. (B) Axial T2W images demonstrate bilateral frontal subdural fluid collections with septations. (C) Axial SWI image shows susceptibility from hemorrhage in the bilateral subdural spaces. (D and E) Axial head CT demonstrating hyperdense subdural hemorrhage along the falx and left cerebral hemisphere in addition to large regions of parenchymal ischemia. (F) Axial head CT demonstrating a mixed density subdural hematoma along the lateral left frontal lobe with associated large region of loss of gray and white matter differentiation, midline to the right, and subfalcine herniation of the frontal lobe.

Key Points

Background

- The dura is composed of fibroblasts and extracellular collagen. The inner layer of the dura is known as the dural border cell layer and is characterized by flattened fibroblasts with limited intracellular junctions, no extracellular collagen, and prominent extracellular spaces. The dural border cell layer is continuous with the arachnoid outer barrier cell layer. A subdural space can be created by blood entering the dura-arachnoid junction and dissecting open the dural border cell layer. The dural border cell layer is the weakest plane and dissects open with trauma. The dura is attached to the inner table of the skull, while the arachnoid is attached to the pia on the surface of the brain. The walls of the bridging veins are attached to the dural border cell layer and to the arachnoid cells. The attachment of the bridging veins to the arachnoid is stronger than the attachment to the dural border cell layer. With sufficient strain, the dura moves with the skull and the arachnoid moves with the brain, causing a strain on the bridging veins. A tear of a bridging vein then causes blood to enter the intradural space between the dural border cells and meningeal dura and is called a subdural hemorrhage (SDH).
- Only a few acute subdural hemorrhages evolve into chronic subdural hemorrhages. The majority of posttraumatic subdural hemorrhages develop from subdural hygromas (SDHys). A subdural hygroma forms from an arachnoid tear, allowing CSF into the subdural space as the subdural hemorrhage is resolving. The tear in the dural border zone

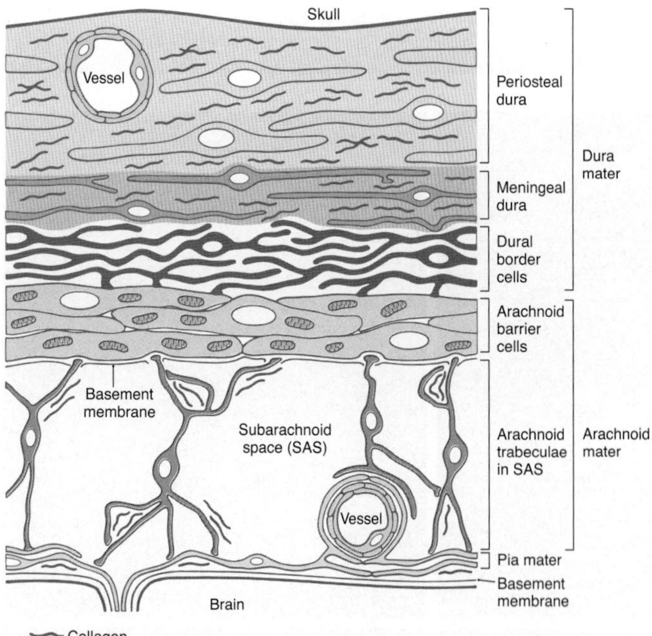

Fig. 10.26 The Structure of the Meninges. Layers of the dura are shown in shades of gray, the arachnoid in shades of pink, and the pia in green. (From Haines DE, Mihailoff GA. *Fundamental Neuroscience for Basic and Clinical Applications.* 5th ed. 2019; Elsevier.)

tissues can lead to proliferation of dural border cells and production of a neomembrane. The cleaved membrane may remain a persistent space, and CSF or fluid from the acute subdural hemorrhage can pass into the space and create a hygroma. If there is a return of normal pressure, the hygroma resolves. If low pressure persists, the hygroma can expand and form more neomembranes and neovascularization. These new vessels are more prone to tearing and result in microhemorrhage with minimal trauma. Repetitive microhemorrhages and resolution of the hemorrhage lead to enlarging subdural hygroma and transformation to a chronic subdural hematoma.

Imaging

- Subdural hemorrhage can be hypodense, isodense, or hyperdense.
- SDH can be compartmentalized/septated.
- Timing of subdural hemorrhage is imprecise and should be avoided.
  - The exact time frames for different densities may vary considerably from patient to patient.
  - Layering does not indicate traumatic injury separated in time.
  - Membranes suggest trauma older than a week.
  - Active bleeding may cause a mixed attenuation in an acute SDH.
  - Disruption of arachnoid membrane during trauma may create a mixed density hemorrhage and hygroma, or dilute the hemorrhage and causing a hypoattenuating collection.
- Mass effect can result in midline shift, mass effect, and herniation. Herniation and elevated intracranial pressure can result in infarct from arterial compression.

REFERENCES

1. Case ME. Inflicted traumatic brain injury in infants and young children. *Brain Pathol.* 2008 Oct;18(4):571–582.
2. Wittschieber D, Karger B, Niederstadt T, et al. Subdural hygromas in abusive head trauma: pathogenesis, diagnosis, and forensic implications. *AJNR Am J Neuroradiol.* 2015 Mar;36(3):432–439.

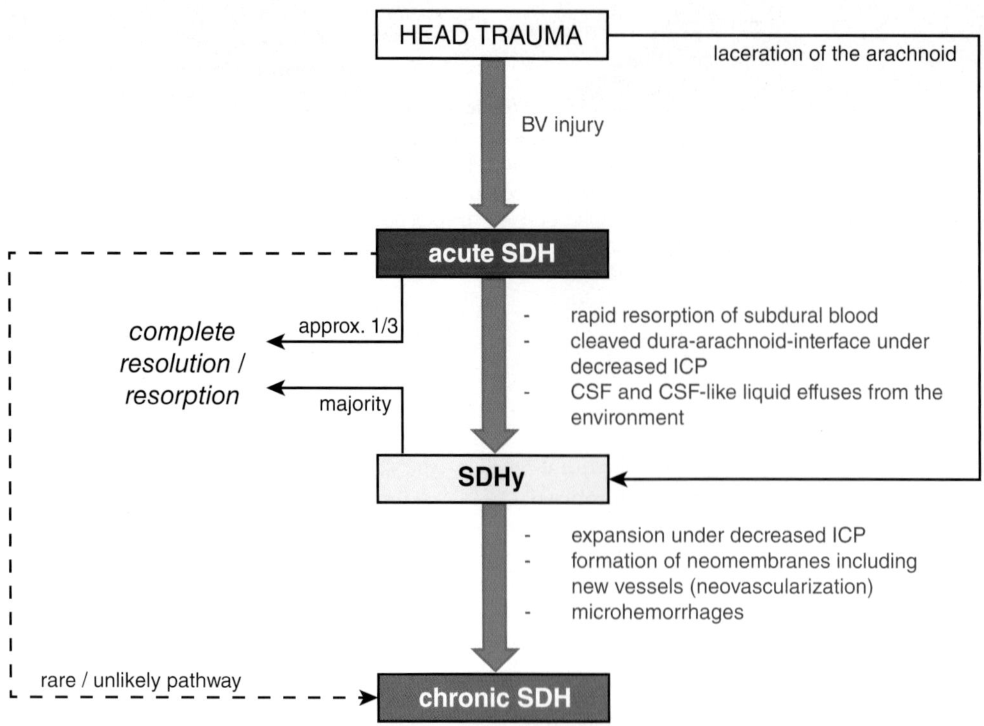

Fig. 10.27 Simplified Schematic Drawing of the Pathogenetic Pathways of the Origin and Fate of Subdural Hygromas (SDHys). *ICP*, Intracranial pressure; *SDH*, subdural hematoma. (From Wittschieber D, Karger B, Niederstadt T, Pfeiffer H, Hahnemann ML. Subdural hygromas in abusive head trauma: pathogenesis, diagnosis, and forensic implications. *Am J Neuroradiol.* 2014;36[3]:432–439. https://doi.org/10.3174/ajnr.a3989)

ABUSIVE HEAD TRAUMA: ISCHEMIA

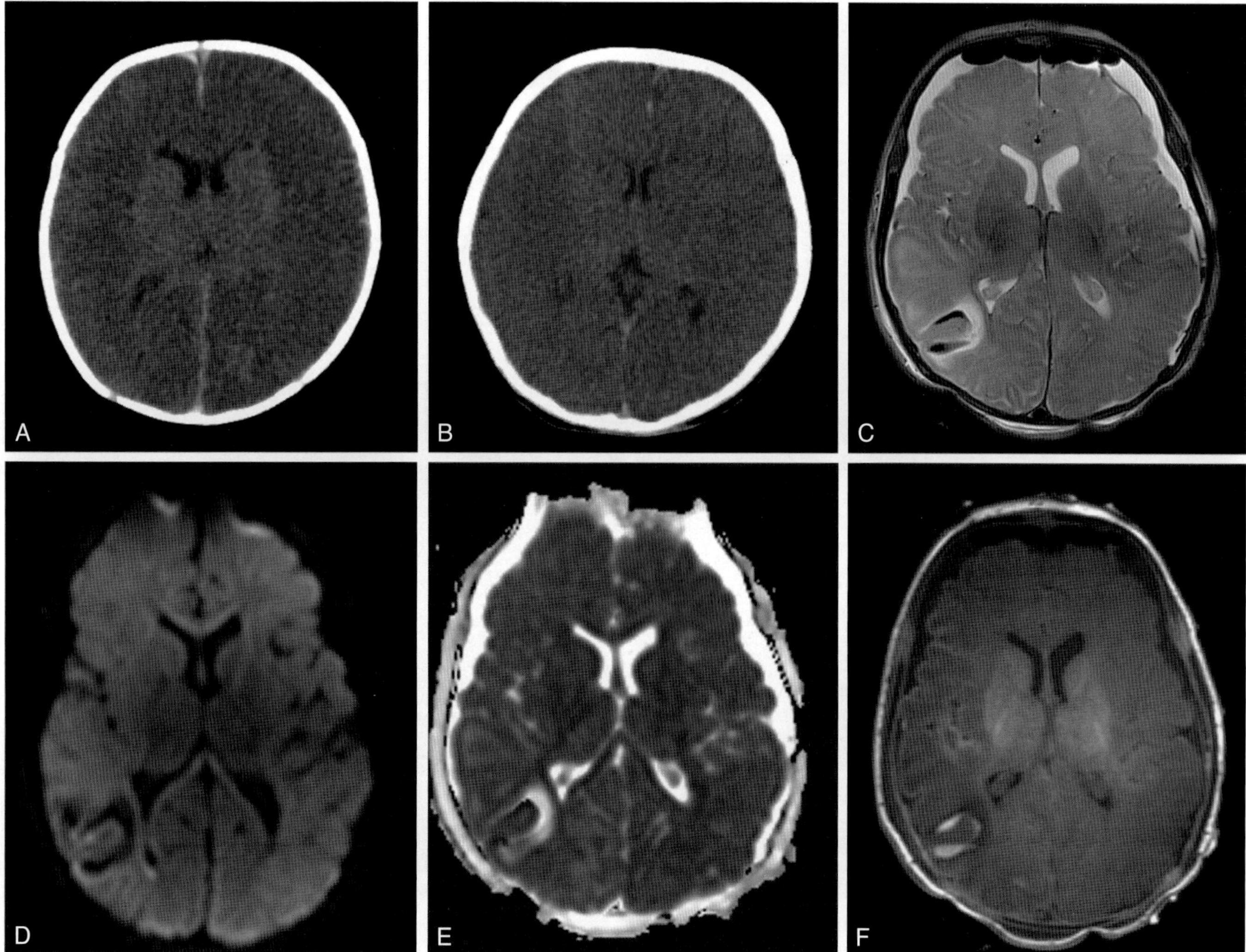

Fig. 10.28 Abusive Head Trauma: Ischemia. (A and B) Axial head CT images demonstrate diffuse low density and loss of gray-white differentiation in bilateral cerebral hemispheres consistent with diffuse ischemia. (C) Axial T2W, (D) Axial DWI, (E) axial ADC, and (F) axial T1W images show diffuse parenchymal T2 hyperintensity and diffusion restriction from ischemia in addition to bilateral T2 hyperintense subdural fluid collections (with air anteriorly from recent surgical drainage) and a right temporo-occipital hemorrhage with T1W hyperintensity and T2W hypointensity with surrounding edema. Combination of subdural fluid collections, ischemia, and parenchymal hemorrhage is highly concerning for abusive head trauma. Diffuse ischemia can be challenging on MRI due to the symmetry.

Key Points

- Patterns of ischemia can include diffuse cortical, watershed, deep gray matter, and focal infarct. Unilateral hypoxic ischemic injury is a less common pattern.
- Incidence of hypoxic ischemic injury in abusive head trauma (AHT) is 31% to 39%.
- Detection of ischemia on head CT can be difficult in neonates and infants due to the hypodense appearance of the white matter, but with standard CT techniques, the radiologist should always be able to see density of the deep gray matter similar to cortex, and a preserved cortical-white matter differentiation in normal patients.
- MRI is recommended in these patients to assess full extent of injury. Because diffuse or symmetric ischemia is often encountered, the radiologist should find an internal reference for signal intensity such as the cerebellum or brainstem, which are less frequently affected.

REFERENCES

1. Orman G, Kralik SF, Meoded A, et al. MRI findings in pediatric abusive head trauma: a review. *J Neuroimaging*. 2019;00:1–13.
2. McKinney AM, Thompson LR, Truwit CL, Velders S, Karagulle A, Kiragu A. Unilateral hypoxic-ischemic injury in young children from abusive head trauma, lacking craniocervical vascular dissection or cord injury. *Pediatr Radiol*. 2007;38(2):164–174.

ABUSIVE HEAD TRAUMA: VENOUS INJURY

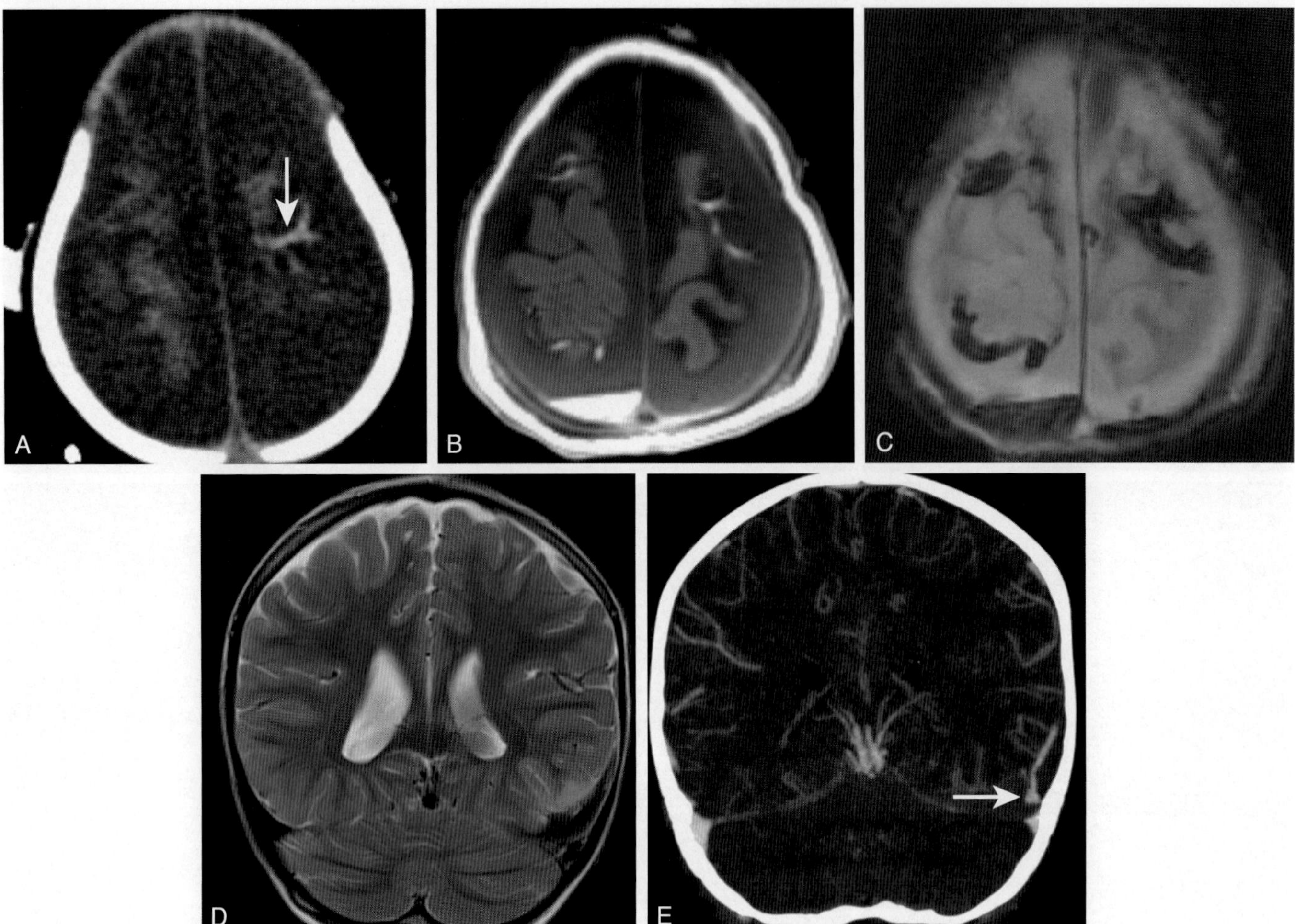

Fig. 10.29 Abusive Head Trauma: Venous Injury. (A) Axial head CT image demonstrates linear hyperdensity from thrombosed bridging vein. (B) Axial T1W and (C) axial SWI images confirm vein thrombosis by the T1W hyperintense signal and susceptibility. (E) Coronal T2W image demonstrates a left occipital T2W hypointense subdural hemorrhage and adjacent parenchymal edema. (E) Coronal reformat CT venogram image demonstrates a tear of the left vein of Labbe and a "tadpole" sign from the retracted vein.

Key Points

- Injury can include bridging vein tear or thrombosis
- Bridging vein thrombosis leads to a linear hyperdensity on CT and susceptibility on MRI
- Bridging vein thrombosis is seen in 44% of AHT patients

REFERENCES

1. Orman G, Kralik SF, Meoded A, et al. MRI findings in pediatric abusive head trauma: a review. *J Neuroimaging*. 2019;00:1–1.
2. Choudhary A, Bradford R, Dias MS, et al. Venous injury in abusive head trauma. *Pediatr Radiol*. 2015 Nov;45(12):1803–1813.

ABUSIVE HEAD TRAUMA: PARENCHYMAL LACERATION

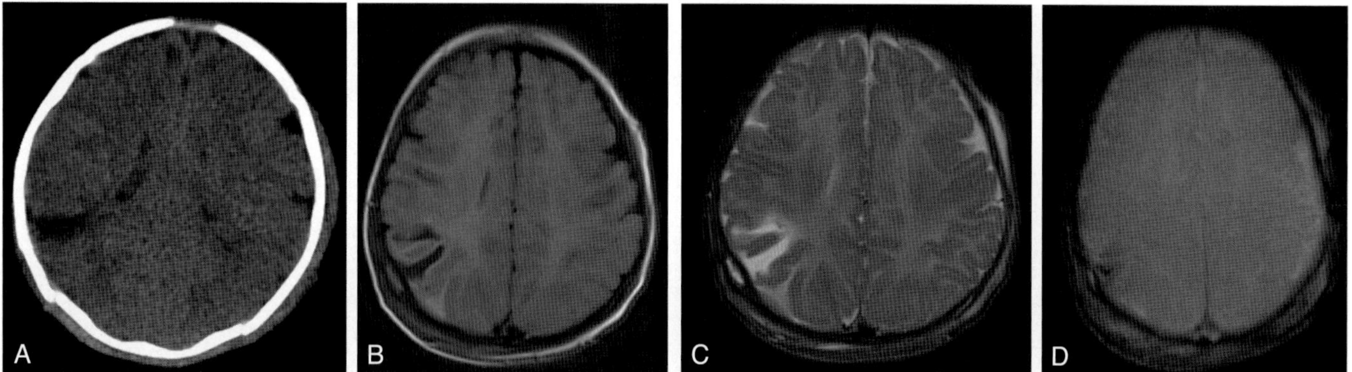

Fig. 10.30 Abusive Head Trauma: Parenchymal Laceration. (A) Axial CT head demonstrates a triangular low density in the right parietal lobe. (B) Axial FLAIR, (C) axial T2W, and (D) axial SWI images demonstrate a right parietal laceration with cleft-like fluid signal and hemorrhage.

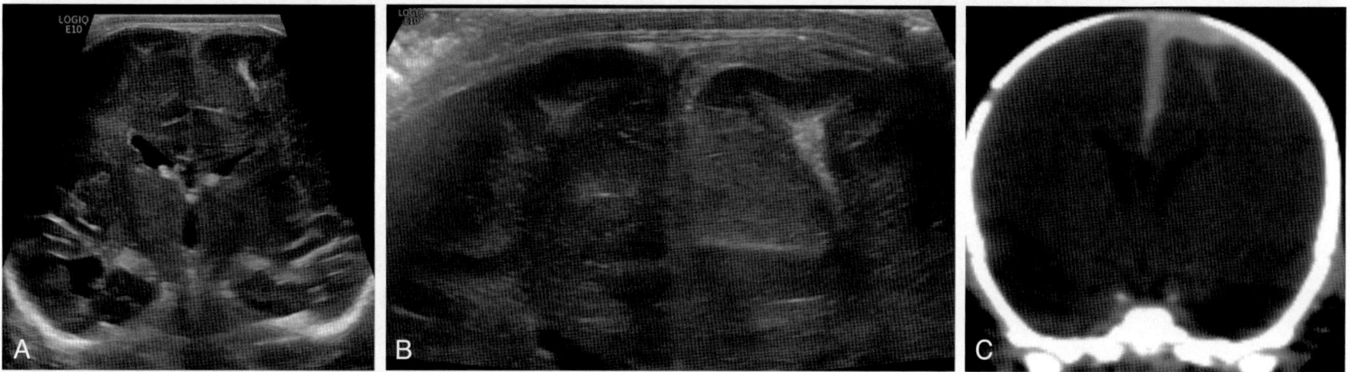

Fig. 10.31 Abusive Head Trauma: Parenchymal Laceration. (A and B) Coronal ultrasound images demonstrate a triangular hyperechoic area in the left medial frontal lobe resulting from a laceration. Hyperechoic subdural hemorrhage along the left vertex, hypoechoic regions in the temporal lobes, and poor cortical differentiation are also present. (C) Coronal reformat CT head correlate demonstrates a triangular low density in the right parietal lobe related to the laceration. Hyperdense subdural hemorrhage is present along the falx and left vertex. Abnormal low densities in the temporal lobes and loss of cortical distinction are due to diffuse ischemia. This case shows how multiple parenchymal injuries are often present in abusive head trauma.

Key Points

- Also known as contusional tear, subcortical contusion, or subcortical cleft
- May occur in young infants due to the poorly myelinated brain
- The same inertial deformation that causes diffuse axonal injury causes these tears in young infants
- Uncommon but relatively specific finding in AHT
- Appears as linear cleft or cavity in the subcortical white matter

REFERENCES

1. Orman G, Kralik SF, Meoded A, et al. MRI findings in pediatric abusive head trauma: a review. *J Neuroimaging*. 2019;00:1–13.
2. Palifka LA, Frasier LD, Metzger RR, et al. Parenchymal brain laceration as a predictor of abusive head trauma. *AJNR Am J Neuroradiol*. Jan 2016;37(1):163–168.

ABUSIVE HEAD TRAUMA: SPINAL TRAUMA

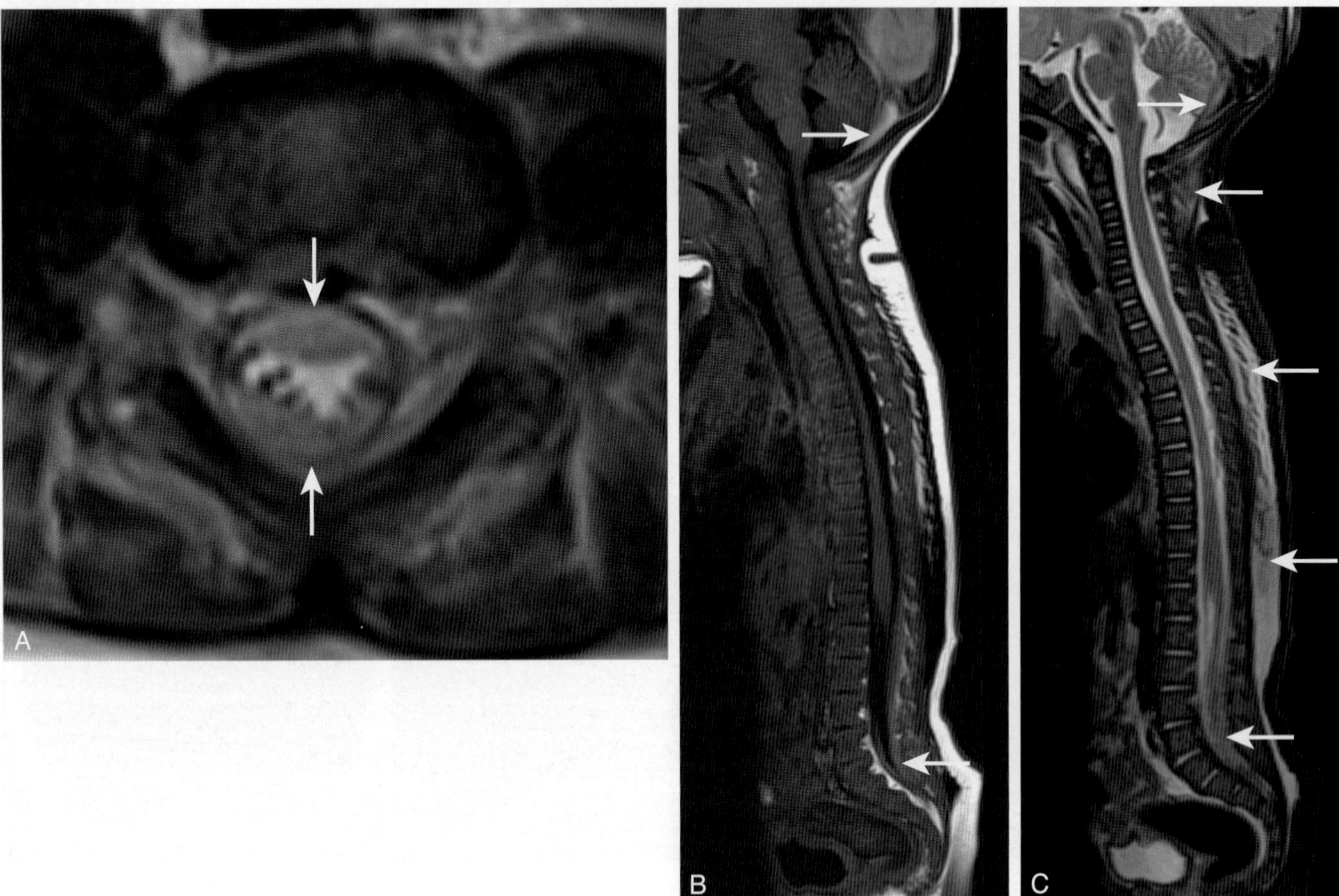

Fig. 10.32 Abusive Head Trauma: Spinal Trauma. (A) Axial T2W, (B) sagittal T1W, and (C) sagittal STIR images demonstrate abnormal T2W signal less than CSF and T1W signal greater than CSF along the periphery of the thecal sac in a configuration consistent with subdural hemorrhage. Large region of subcutaneous edema in the spine, edema along the nuchal ligament, and posterior fossa and falcine subdural hemorrhages are also seen.

Key Points

- Traumatic findings can include ligamentous injury, cord injury, muscular injury, and spinal hematoma.
- Spinal subdural hemorrhage is suspected to be due to gravitational movement of intracranial subdural blood. Imaging demonstrates an intrathecal fluid collection with distinct boundary with sites of adherence often in a V-shaped configuration posteriorly.
- Retroclival hematoma found in 32% of AHT.
- Ligamentous injury typically from hyperflexion and include injury to the nuchal ligament and atlanto-occipital and atlantoaxial ligaments.

REFERENCES

1. Choudhary AK, Bradford RK, Dias MS, et al. "Spinal Subdural Hemorrhage in Abusive Head Trauma: A Retrospective Study." *Radiology*. 2012, Jan;262(1):216–223.
2. Choudhary AK, Ishak R, Zacharia TT, et al. "Imaging of spinal injury in abusive head trauma: a retrospective study." *Pediatr Radiol.* 2014 Sep;44(9):1130–1140.

ABUSIVE HEAD TRAUMA: RETINAL HEMORRHAGE

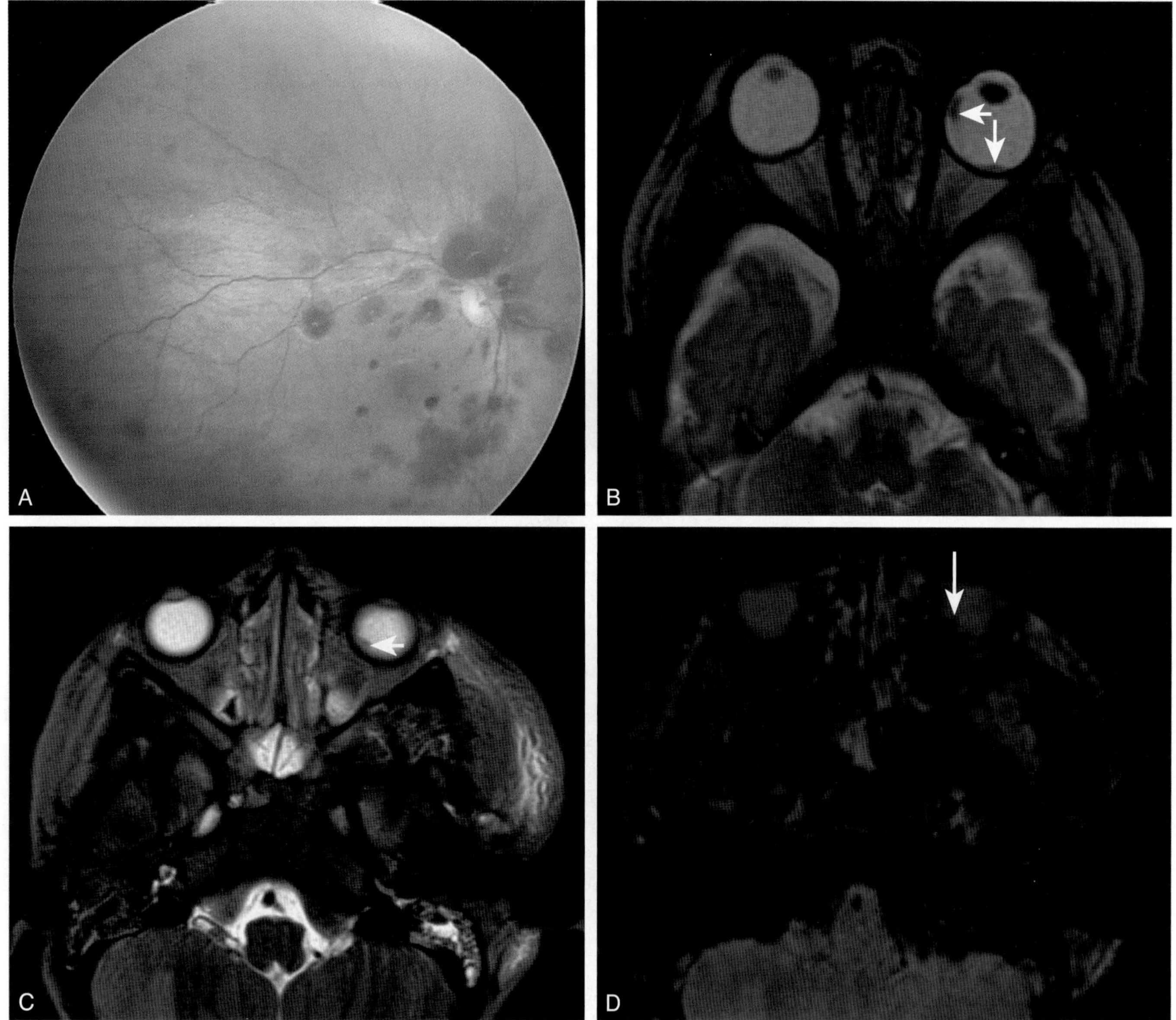

Fig. 10.33 Abusive Head Trauma: Retinal Hemorrhage. (A) RetCam photograph of preretinal, intraretinal, and subretinal hemorrhages, extending to the periphery. (B and C) Axial T2W and (D) axial SWI images demonstrate hypointense foci in the posterior globes and right media globe consistent with retinal hemorrhage. MRI should not be the primary diagnostic tool to identify retinal hemorrhages. (A Courtesy Tineke Chan, MD, Children's Hospital of Pittsburgh, University of Pittsburgh Medical Center, Pittsburgh, PA. In Zitelli B, McIntire S, Nowalk A. *Zitelli and Davis' Atlas of Pediatric Physical Diagnosis*. 7th ed. Elsevier; 2018.)

Key Points

- Retinal hemorrhages occur in approximately 85% of AHT. Retinal hemorrhages can also occur with very severe accidental head trauma, particularly motor vehicle collisions, sepsis, coagulopathy, meningitis, and in some newborns but tend to be fewer in number and confined to the posterior pole of the retina.
- Retinal hemorrhages from AHT are typically seen as numerous, multilayered hemorrhages extending in the periphery of the retina.
- MRI is less sensitive than dilated fundoscopic examination (DFE).
- Standard SWI and high-resolution orbital SWI were 75% and 83% sensitive for detection of retinal hemorrhage using DFE as the gold standard.

REFERENCES

1. Zuccoli G, Panigrahy A, Haldipur A, et al. Susceptibility weighted imaging depicts retinal hemorrhages in abusive head trauma. *Neuroradiology*. 2013 Jul;55(7):889–893.
2. Case ME. Inflicted traumatic brain injury in infants and young children. *Brain Pathol*. 2008 Oct;18(4):571–582.

ABUSIVE HEAD TRAUMA: RARE TRAUMATIC FINDINGS AND NEW TECHNIQUES

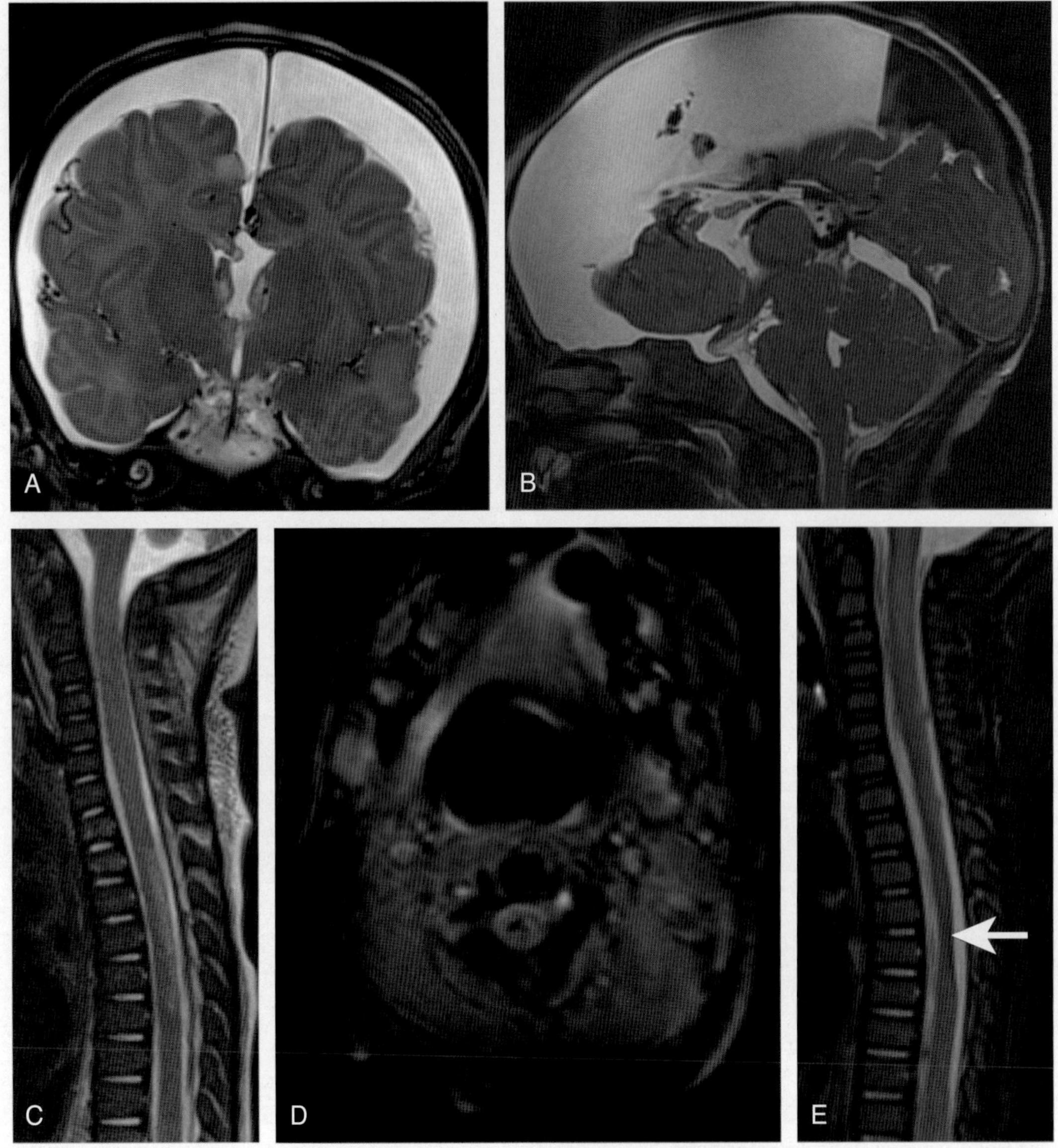

Fig. 10.34 Abusive Head Trauma: Rare Traumatic Findings of Corpus Callosum and Spinal Cord Injury. (A and B) A 2-month-old with abusive head trauma (AHT) and coronal and sagittal T2W images demonstrating disruption of the corpus callosum with adjacent hyperintense signal along the margins in addition to bilateral subdural fluid collections along the cerebral and cerebellar hemispheres. (C to E) A 4-month-old with AHT with initial spine sagittal T2W (C) and axial GRE (D) demonstrating abnormal intramedullary T2W hyperintensity from T2-T6, subtle trabecular microfractures at T1W and T2W with marrow T2W hyperintensity, spinal cord hemorrhage indicated by the hypointensity on GRE image, and (E) follow-up spine MRI T2W image demonstrating segmental cord volume loss from T2-T5.

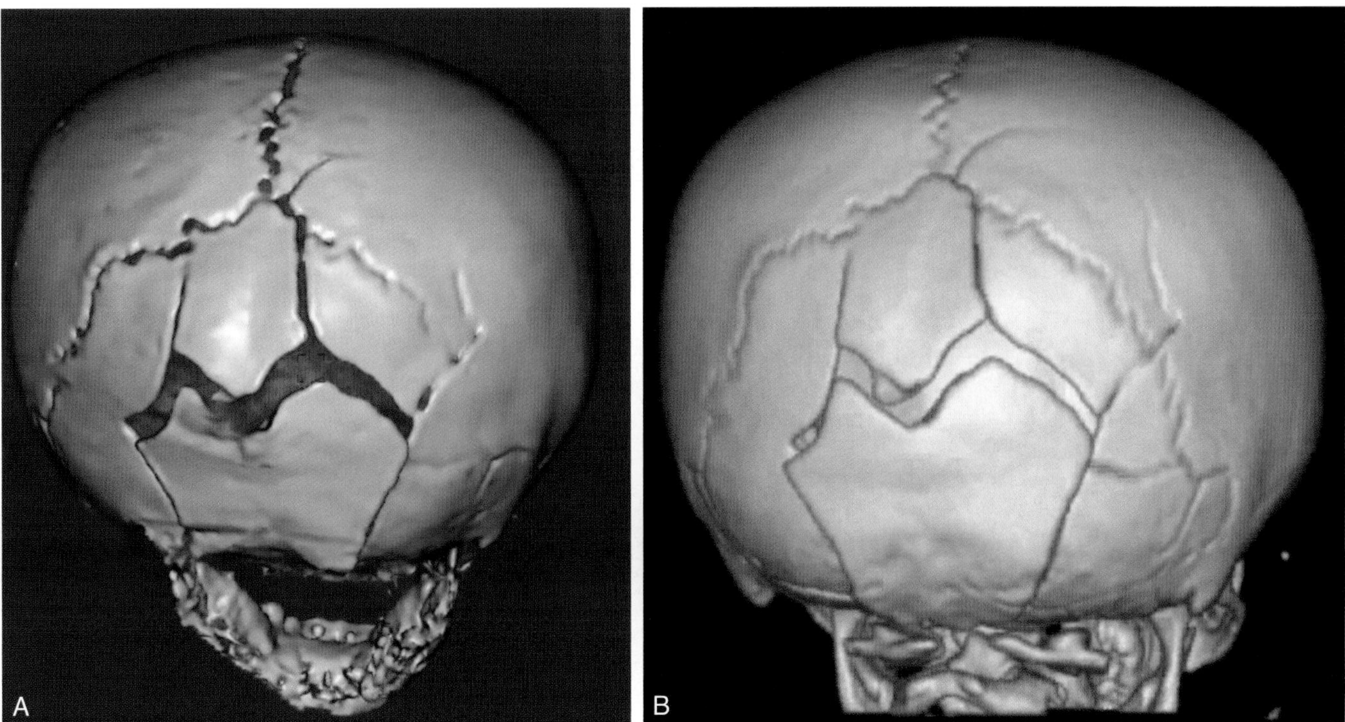

Fig. 10.35 Abusive Head Trauma: Rare Traumatic Findings. (A) 3D volumetric black bone MRI obtained with postprocessing of an ultrashort TE MRI sequence shows similar fracture representation compared to (B) 3D volumetric CT. The ultrashort TE allows for thin (1-mm) slice images, which can render 3D volumetric images similar to CT. Further research is needed to determine potential for this technique to be clinically implemented.

REFERENCES

1. Kralik SF, Supakul N, Wu IC, et al. Black bone MRI with 3D reconstruction for the detection of skull fractures in children with suspected abusive head trauma. *Neuroradiology*. 2019 Jan;61(1):81–87.
2. Dremmen MHG, Wagner MW, Bosemani T, et al. Does the addition of a "Black Bone" sequence to a fast multisequence trauma MR protocol allow for MRI to replace CT after traumatic brain injury in children. *AJNR Am J Neuroradiol*. 2017 Nov;38(11):2187–2192.

11 Hydrocephalus and Other Cerebrospinal Fluid Disorders

INTRODUCTION

Embryology

The ventricles arise from the lumen of the forebrain, midbrain, and hindbrain. At approximately the sixth week of gestation, the lateral ventricles arise as extensions from the anterior-superior aspect of the third ventricle and communicate through the foramen of Monro. The lumen of the hindbrain expands to become the fourth ventricle. The cerebral aqueduct persists in the midbrain and allows communication between the third and fourth ventricles.

Cerebrospinal Fluid Physiology

Cerebrospinal fluid (CSF) is produced in the choroid plexuses as well as the vascular ependymal cells and pia mater (Fig. 11.1). The CSF circulates from the lateral ventricles → foramen of

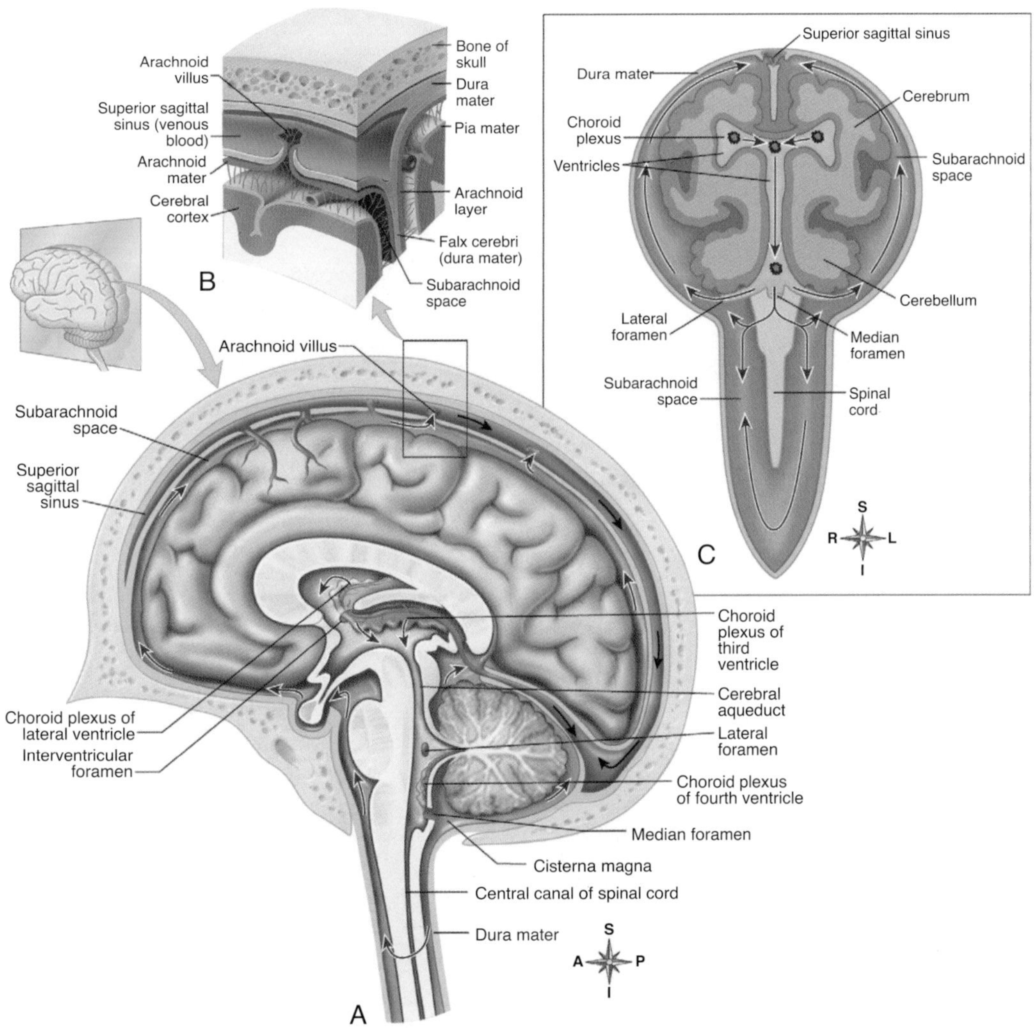

Fig. 11.1 Flow of Cerebrospinal Fluid. (A) Fluid produced by filtration of blood by the choroid plexus of each ventricle flows inferiorly through the lateral ventricles, interventricular foramen, third ventricle, cerebral aqueduct, fourth ventricle, and subarachnoid space and to blood. (B) *Inset* showing arachnoid villus, where CSF is reabsorbed into the blood of the superior sagittal sinus. (C) Simplified diagram showing flow of CSF. (From Patton KT. *Anatomy and Physiology*. 10th ed. Elsevier; 2019.)

Monro → third ventricle → cerebral aqueduct → foramina of Magendie and Luschka → subarachnoid spaces along the brain and spinal cord. CSF drains through the arachnoid villi and at the spinal nerve sheaths.

The CSF volume in the CNS is approximately 50 mL in neonates, 60 to 100 mL in children, and 130 to 150 mL in adults.

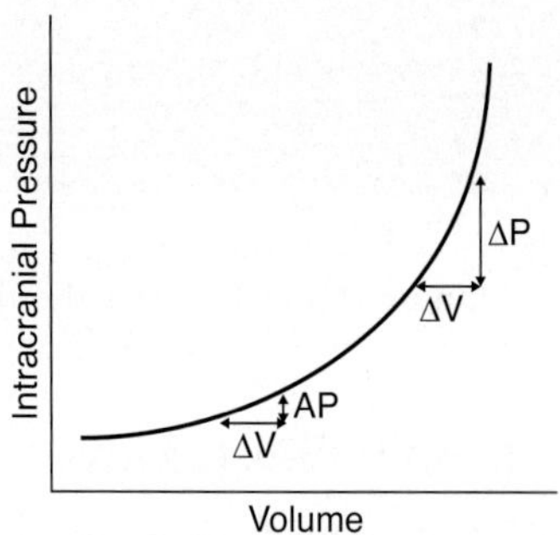

Fig. 11.2 Relationship of Intracranial Pressure and Volume.

CSF is produced at a rate of 0.35 mL/min, and in children the daily turnover is 10 to 15 mL/kg compared to 500 mL in adults. CSF pressure is affected by age, positioning, elasticity of the brain, skull, and meninges, and arterial and venous pressure. CSF pressure is approximately 3 to 7 mm/Hg in neonates, 6 to 15 mm Hg in infants, and 10 to 20 mm/kg in adults.

There is a monoexponential relationship between the change in CSF volume and intracranial pressure (Fig. 11.2). The same added volume of fluid at a lower total CSF volume causes a smaller change in intracranial pressure versus a larger change in intracranial pressure when the total CSF volume is high. Disorders affecting CSF physiology discussed in this chapter will include hydrocephalus, idiopathic intracranial hypertension, intracranial hypotension, and benign enlaregment of subarachnoid spaces.

REFERENCES

1. Tortori-Donati P. *Pediatric Neuroradiology*: Springer; 2005.
2. Barkovich AJ, Raybaud C. *Pediatric Neuroradiology*. 6th edition Philadelphia: Wolters-Kluwer; 2019.

HYDROCEPHALUS

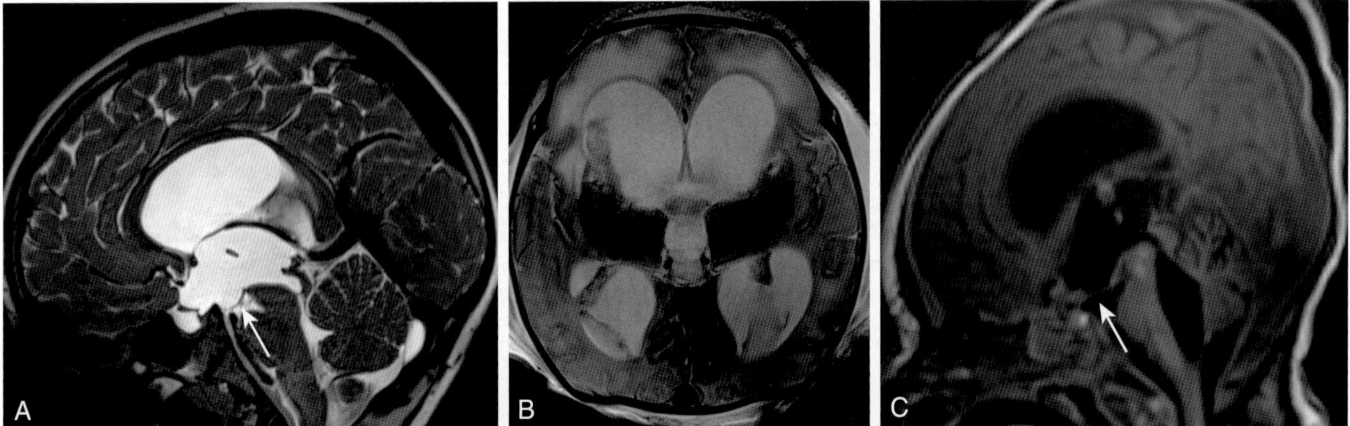

Fig. 11.3 Hydrocephalus Imaging Findings. (A) Sagittal T2W image in a patient with inferior aqueductal stenosis demonstrates inferior bowing of the third ventricle (*arrow*) with dilatation of the recesses of the third ventricle and stretching of the corpus callosum. (B) Axial T2W image in a patient with meningitis demonstrates disproportionate enlargement of the lateral and third ventricles relative to the sulci and parenchymal edema. (C) Sagittal T1W image demonstrating hydrocephalus findings of inferior bowing of the third ventricle with dilatation of the recesses of the third ventricle, stretching of the corpus callosum, enlarged fourth ventricle, and an adhesion at the foramen of Magendie obstructing CSF outflow.

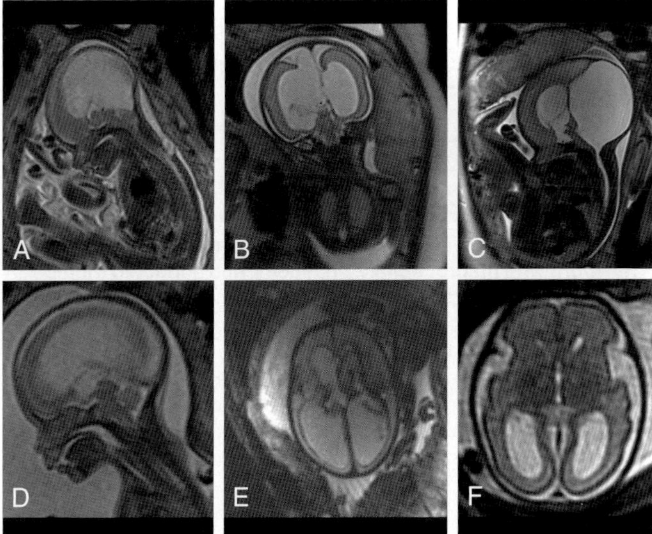

Fig. 11.4 Fetal Ventriculomegaly. Among the many causes for fetal ventriculomegaly include (A) myelomeningocele and Chiari II, (B) callosal agenesis with interhemispheric cyst, (C) Dandy-Walker malformation, (D) aqueductal stenosis, (E) intraventricular hemorrhage, and (F) isolated bilateral ventriculomegaly (when no additional abnormalities are present).

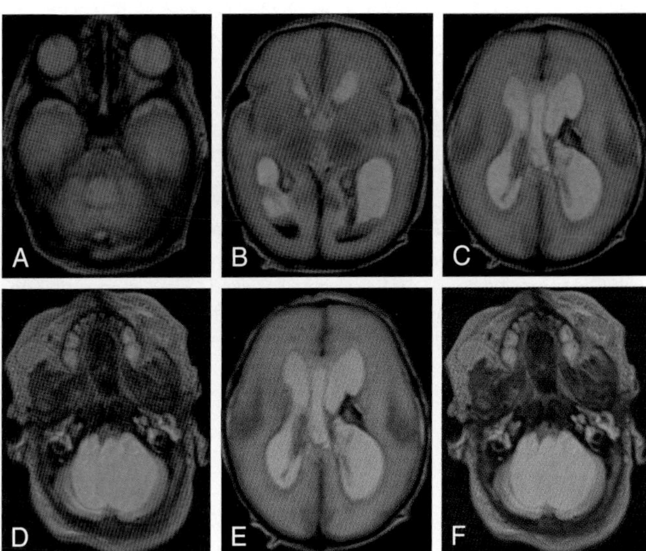

Fig. 11.5 Hydrocephalus Secondary to Hemorrhage. A 26-week premature infant with germinal matrix and intraventricular hemorrhage. (A to C) Axial T2W images demonstrate hypointense areas of hemorrhage within the ventricles, left caudothalamic groove, and periventricular white matter and mild enlargement of the ventricles. (D to F) Axial T2W images on 2-month follow-up MRI demonstrate hydrocephalus of all the ventricles, compressed subarachnoid spaces, intraventricular adhesions, and ventricular diverticulations from the lateral ventricles.

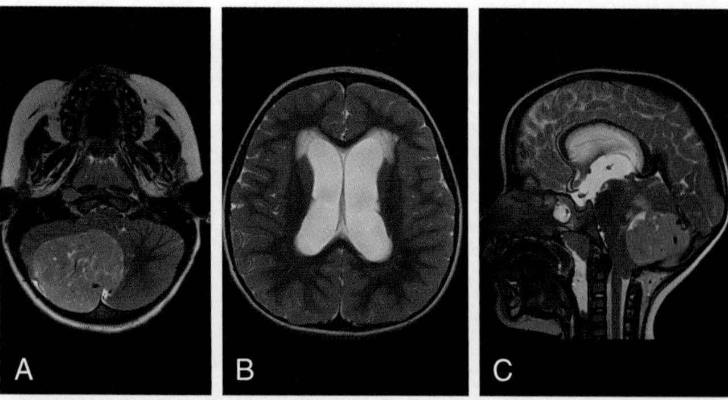

Fig. 11.6 Hydrocephalus Secondary to Tumor Obstruction. (A to C) Axial and sagittal T2W images in a 3-year-old with medulloblastoma with tumor compressing the fourth ventricle and obstructing CSF outflow resulting in acute obstructive hydrocephalus of the lateral ventricles and third ventricle with periventricular edema.

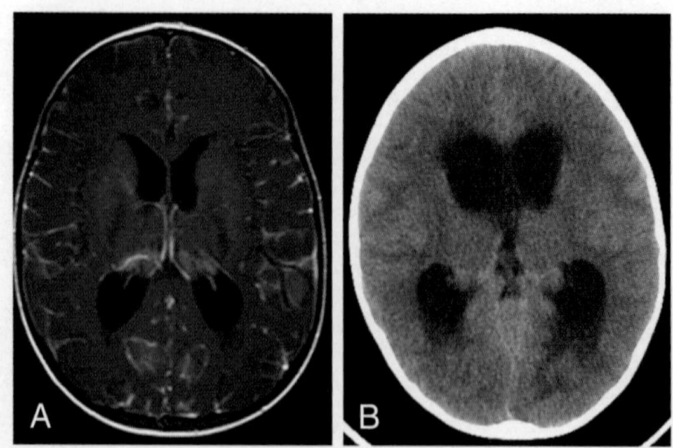

Fig. 11.7 Hydrocephalus Secondary to Leptomeningeal Carcinomatosis. A 3-year-old with medulloblastoma found to have abnormal leptomeningeal enhancement on axial T1W+C (A) and 7 days later developed enlarged ventricles with interstitial edema seen on (B) axial head CT.

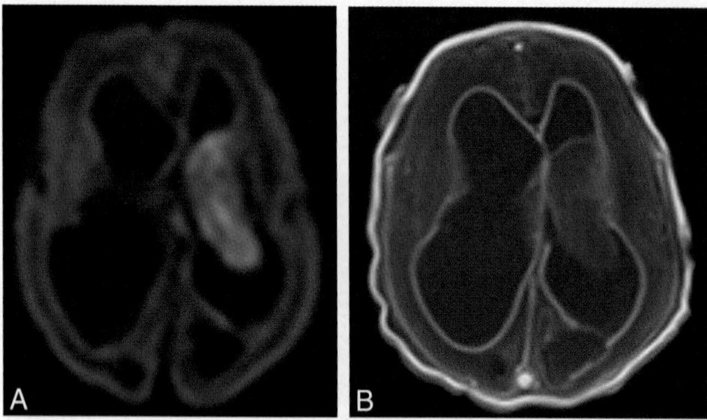

Fig. 11.8 Hydrocephalus Secondary to Meningitis. A 1-month-old with *E. coli* meningitis. (A) Axial DWI and (B) axial T1W+C images demonstrate intraventricular purulent material, ependymal enhancement, intraventricular adhesion in the posterior left lateral ventricle, and hydrocephalus of the lateral ventricles.

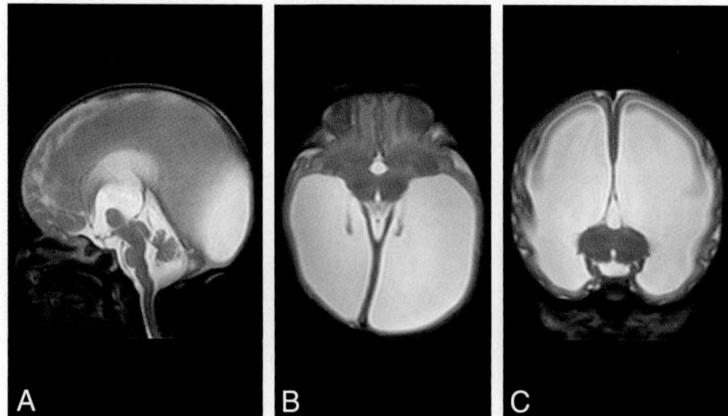

Fig. 11.9 X-linked Hydrocephalus/CRASH Syndrome/L1 Syndrome. A newborn with macrocephaly, spasticity, and adducted thumbs. (A to C) Sagittal, axial, and coronal T2W images demonstrate enlarged lateral ventricles, compressed subarachnoid spaces, fused thalami, dysmorphic midbrain, and aqueductal stenosis. This is a rare syndrome affecting 1 in 30,000 males caused by genetic mutations of the *L1CAM* gene and presents with prenatal hydrocephalus, aqueductal stenosis, corpus callosum hypoplasia/agenesis, adducted thumbs, spasticity, and mild to moderate intellectual disability. Additional findings can include fused thalami, abnormal brainstem, and small corticospinal tracts.

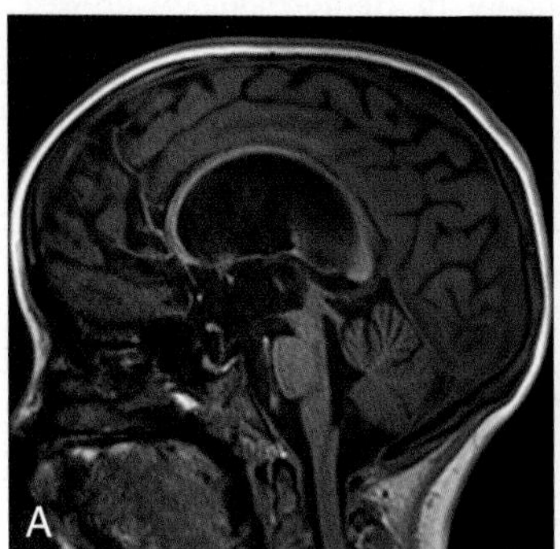

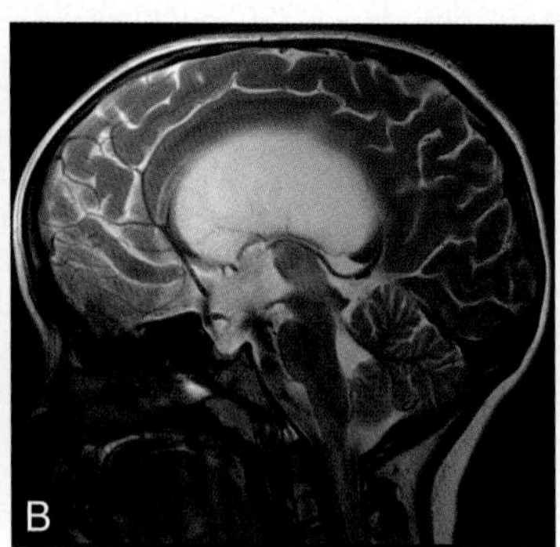

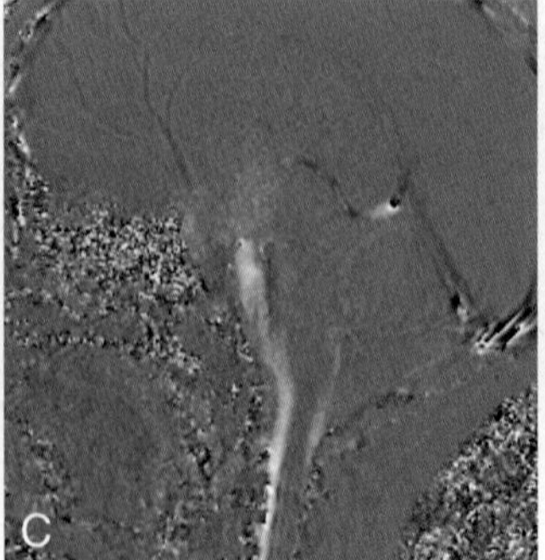

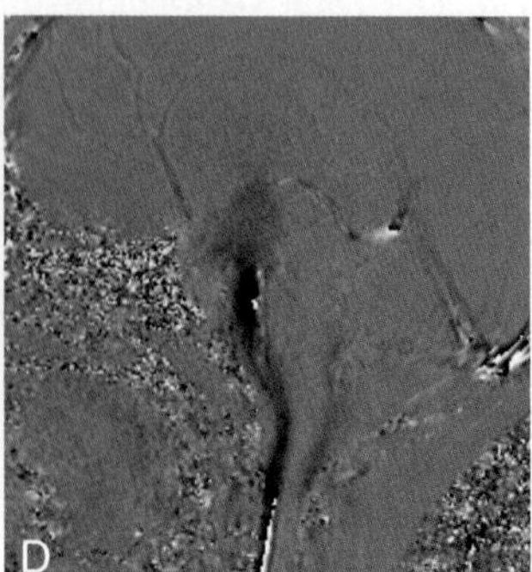

Fig. 11.10 Third Ventriculostomy Findings. (A) Sagittal T1W image demonstrates occlusion of the cerebral aqueduct due to a tectal glioma and associated obstructive hydrocephalus. (B) Sagittal T2W image demonstrates a flow jet across the third ventriculostomy, indicating patency. (C and D) Sagittal phase contrast CSF flow images demonstrate flow across the third ventriculostomy site with white signal representing cranial to caudal direction flow and black signal indicating caudal to cranial flow.

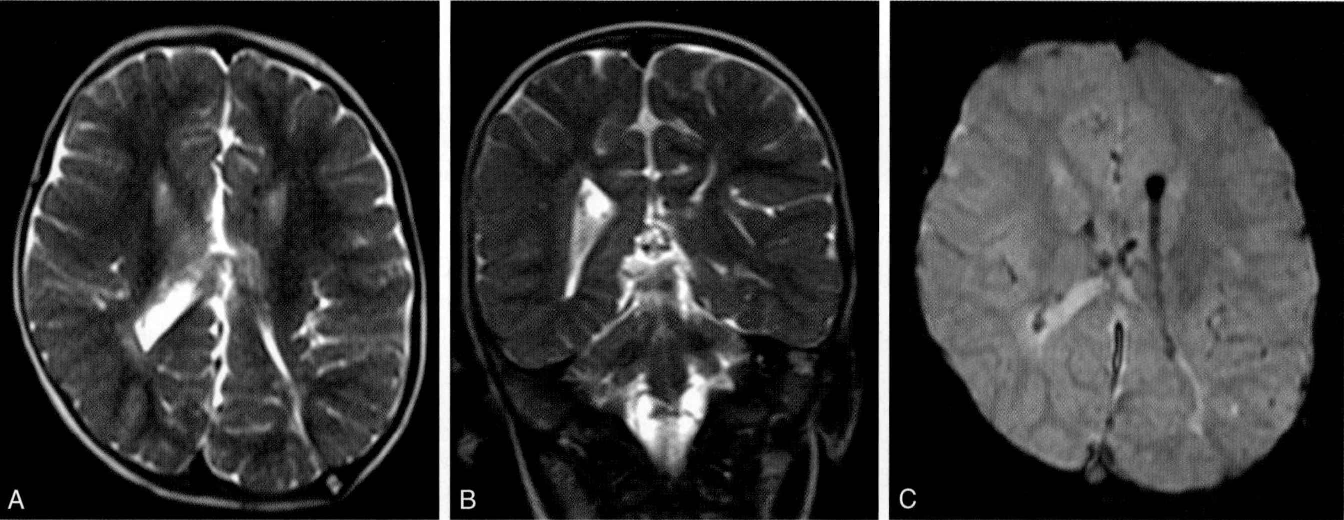

Fig. 11.11 Ultrafast MRI for Shunt Evaluation. (A and B) Ultrafast axial and coronal T2 HASTE images of the brain demonstrate the decompressed ventricles and (C) echo-planar T2* image demonstrates the catheter position. Ultrafast MRI can reduce the use of CT for evaluating ventricle size and are faster than standard MRI sequences, which can reduce need for sedation.

Key Points

Background

- Hydrocephalus refers to increased CSF volume in the ventricles and subarachnoid spaces.
- Current understanding of the pathogenesis of hydrocephalus is explained by the bulk flow model and the hemodynamic model. The bulk flow model is the classic explanation, in which hydrocephalus is caused by CSF overproduction, obstruction of CSF flow, or abnormal CSF resorption at the arachnoid granulations. The hemodynamic model proposed by Greitz et al suggests that pathologic processes reduce the normal arterial pulsations → greater pressure transmitted to the brain → larger transmantle cerebral pressure → ventricular dilatation.
- Most common etiologies of hydrocephalus include intraventricular hemorrhage, infection, myelomeningocele, aqueductal stenosis, tumor, and others. Rare causes of hydrocephalus can include CSF overproduction from a choroid plexus papilloma and hydrocephalus from a spinal tumor possibly through increased CSF protein causing high CSF viscosity, tumoral obstruction of the foramen magnum, or subarachnoid spaces in the thecal sac.
- Categorization: Hydrocephalus is divided into noncommunicating (obstructive) and communicating hydrocephalus.
  - Obstructive hydrocephalus occurs when there is obstruction of the CSF pathways. The CSF pathways proximal to the obstruction become distended and the elevated intracranial pressure leads to periventricular interstitial edema. Etiology can be due to tumors, cysts, adhesions from infection or hemorrhage, and malformations.
  - Communicating hydrocephalus occurs when there is no visible obstruction of the CSF pathways and is presumed to be caused by a failure of CSF absorption typically at the arachnoid granulations. Etiologies include meningitis, hemorrhage, leptomeningeal carcinomatosis, and venous hypertension. Communicating hydrocephalus demonstrates enlargement of the lateral, third, and fourth ventricles, although the fourth ventricle may only be mildly enlarged.
- Enlarged ventricles in a fetus may not be associated with macrocephaly and instead are termed ventriculomegaly. Causes of fetal ventriculomegaly include malformations (most commonly myelomeningoceles, aqueductal stenosis, callosal anomalies), hemorrhage, and isolated ventriculomegaly when no etiology is found. Ventriculomegaly in a fetus is defined as measuring >10 mm at the level of the atrium of the lateral ventricles. Between a 10- and 12-mm diameter is defined as mild ventriculomegaly, and the outcome is normal in 93%. Between 12 and 15 mm is defined as moderate ventriculomegaly and has a 21% to 25% probability of resulting in developmental delay. More than 15 mm is defined as severe ventriculomegaly and has a 40% probability of developmental delay.
- For infants younger than age 2, hydrocephalus is associated with macrocephaly, abnormal rate of increase in head circumference, and abnormal eye movement. Children older than age 2 present with morning headache, vomiting, and papilledema.
- Hydrocephalus can ultimately lead to histopathologic changes of choroid plexus degeneration and sclerosis, ependymal cell loss and microlacerations, subependymal fibrosis, white matter gliosis, and axonal degeneration.

With shunting, axons can regenerate and lead to improved white matter volume after shunting.

Treatment

- Prior to the 1950s, before shunting was performed, the prognosis of hydrocephalus was poor: 49% of patients died by the end of a 20-year observation period, and only 38% of survivors had an IQ greater than 85.
- Treatment includes addressing the cause of ventricular obstruction and potential placement of a temporary or permanent ventricular catheter(s), depending on the long-term requirement for CSF shunting. Shunts result in reduced morbidity and mortality.
- Long-term shunting typically drains CSF distally into the peritoneal cavity or less commonly the right atrium of the heart or pleura.
- Third ventriculostomy is an alternate treatment of hydrocephalus when there is obstruction at the cerebral aqueduct but is less effective in children younger than 2 years of age due to immature arachnoid granulations.
- There is no consensus regarding the management of obstructive hydrocephalus in children with posterior fossa tumors before, during, or after surgery. Approximately 30% of children with posterior fossa tumors will require shunting. Children with symptom duration less than 3 months, larger Evan's index (>0.33), and larger frontal occipital horn ratio (>0.46) were found to correlate with need for postoperative shunting. Children with midline tumors, medulloblastomas, and ependymomas were more likely to require shunting.

Imaging

- Imaging of hydrocephalus can be performed with ultrasound, CT, and MRI.
- Imaging findings indicative of hydrocephalus include disproportionate enlargement of the ventricles relative to the sulci, inferior bowing of the third ventricle, enlarged anterior or posterior recess of the third ventricle, and periventricular interstitial edema/transependymal edema.
- Imaging is also helpful in conjunction with the clinical history for determining the cause of hydrocephalus through identification of additional findings such as evidence of hemorrhage, malformation, tumor, or infection.
- Ultrasound of the head is the modality of choice for following ventricular size in neonates as it is fast, widely available, does not require sedation, and does not have ionizing radiation. Ultrasound can also measure the resistive index, which has shown value in hydrocephalus:
  - The resistive index (RI) = (peak systolic velocity – end diastolic velocity)/peak systolic velocity and is increased with increased intracranial pressure (>0.8 in neonates and >0.65 in infants). The change in RI between compression and noncompression at the anterior fontanelle (ΔRI = 100 × (compression RI – baseline RI) / baseline RI) showed the best correlation with elevated intracranial pressure ($\underline{r}$ = 0.8), and infants with a ΔRI > 45% required ventricular drainage.
- MRI is often performed for better assessment of the etiology of the hydrocephalus, including infections, malformations, and tumors. Specific MRI additions to help diagnosis include the following:
  - Thin section (1 mm) 3D T2W is useful for assessing stenosis or web at the cerebral aqueduct and patency of a third ventriculostomy.
  - Phase contrast CSF flow imaging is useful for demonstration of flow across the cerebral aqueduct and third ventriculostomy.
  - Ultrafast MRI using T2W and T2* sequences can allow for imaging of the ventricles and shunt catheter in approximately 30 seconds per sequence. This allows for reduction in CT imaging and may reduce the need for sedation.
  - New areas of MRI research into hydrocephalus include measuring cerebral blood flow with arterial spin label perfusion (ASL), assessment of white matter with diffusion tensor imaging (DTI), and measurement of the venous sinus diameter. Hydrocephalus decreases the cerebral blood flow, and ASL has shown that CBF increases after alleviation of obstructive hydrocephalus. DTI has shown axonal degeneration with hydrocephalus and changes in fractional anisotropy and perpendicular and parallel diffusion within white matter lateral to the ventricles.
- CT of the head has been a mainstay for imaging hydrocephalus because it is fast, widely available, and generally free from artifacts. Because of the ionizing radiation involved, reducing radiation dose for head CTs evaluating shunts is recommended.
- Several measurements for hydrocephalus that can be performed, although most assessments for hydrocephalus can be done qualitatively. The frontal occipital horn ratio (FOHR) is one measurement that can be used to assess ventricular enlargement. FOHR = (frontal horn distance + atrium distance)/(2 × biparietal distance). The normal FOHR value is 0.37 and is independent of age.

REFERENCES

1. Tortori-Donati P. *Pediatric Neuroradiology*: Springer; 2005.
2. Taylor GA, Madsen JR. Neonatal hydrocephalus: hemodynamic response to fontanelle compression-correlation with intracranial pressure and need for shunt placement. *Radiology*. 1996;201(3): 685–689.
3. Del Bigio MR. Neuropathological changes caused by hydrocephalus. *Acta Neuropathol*. 1993;85(6):573–585.
4. Yeom KW, Lober RM, Alexander A, et al. Hydrocephalus decreases arterial spin-labeled cerebral perfusion. *AJNR Am J Neuroradiol*. 2014 Jul;35(7):1433–1439.
5. Gopalakrishnan CV, Dhakoji A, Menon G, et al. Factors predicting the need for cerebrospinal fluid diversion following posterior fossa tumor surgery in children. *Pediatr Neurosurg*. 2012;48:93–101.
6. Greitz D. Radiological assessment of hydrocephalus: new theories and implications for therapy. *Neurosurg Rev*. 2004 Jul;27(3):145–165; discussion 166–167.

SHUNT MALFUNCTION AND COMPLICATIONS

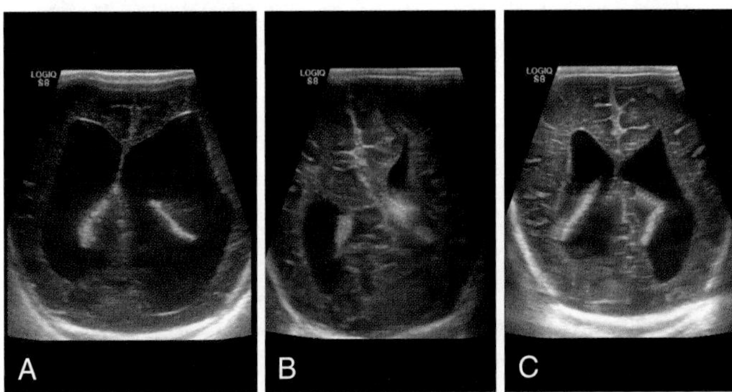

Fig. 11.12 Shunt Malfunction. (A) Coronal head ultrasound image of a newborn with Chiari II malformation and hydrocephalus. (B) Follow-up head ultrasound following shunt placement *(arrow)* shows smaller ventricles. (C) Follow-up head ultrasound at 1 month of age shows interval enlargement of the ventricles, indicating a shunt malfunction.

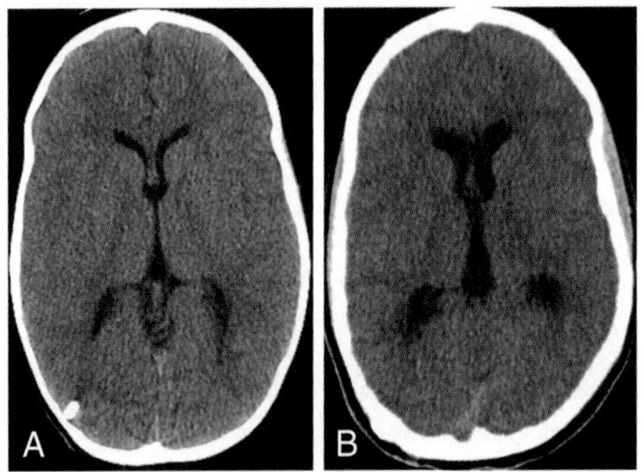

Fig. 11.13 Shunt Malfunction. (A) Baseline axial head CT image at 4 years of age shows a right posterior approach shunt catheter and normal ventricular size. (B) At age 10 the patient presented with headache and vomiting for 3 days. Head CT image shows interval enlargement of the ventricles and mild transependymal edema, indicating a shunt malfunction.

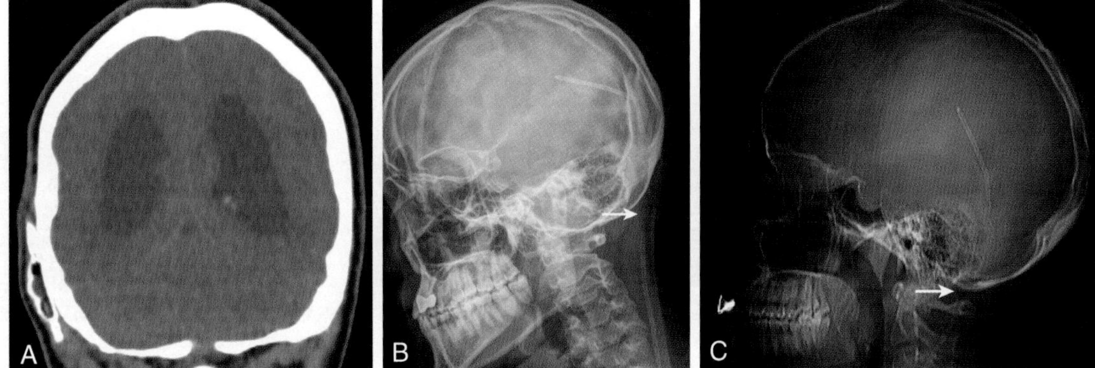

Fig. 11.14 Shunt Malfunction. An 18-year-old with past history of prematurity, germinal matrix and intraventricular hemorrhage, and shunted hydrocephalus. (A) Coronal head CT demonstrates enlarged ventricles and disconnected shunt tubing, which is also confirmed on (B) lateral shunt radiograph *(arrow)*. (C) The disconnection is also seen on the localizer image of the CT, which is a reminder to view the localizer images for additional findings not covered in the CT dataset.

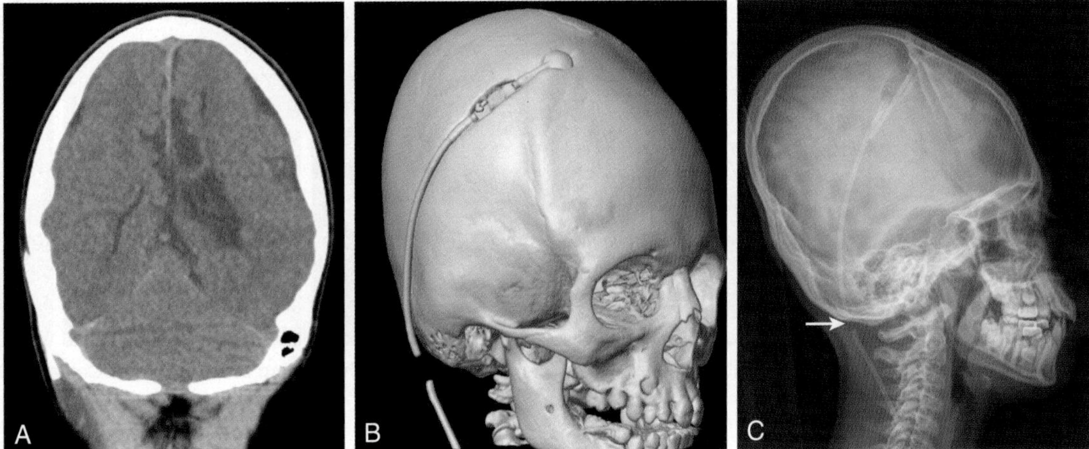

Fig. 11.15 Shunt Malfunction. (A) Coronal head CT, (B) 3D CT volume reconstruction, and (C) lateral shunt radiograph demonstrating shunt tubing fracture and separation *(arrow)*.

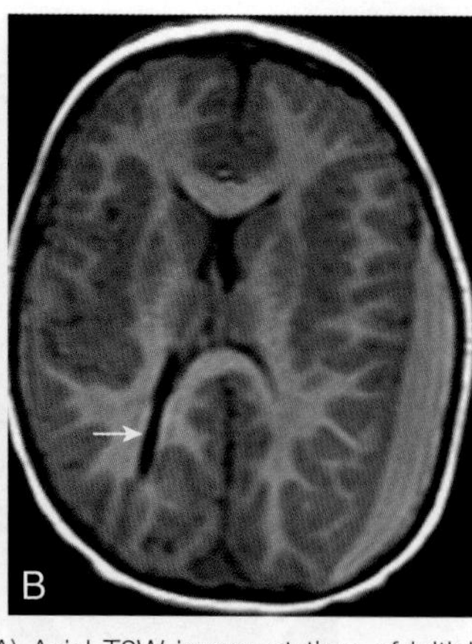

Fig. 11.16 Shunt Complication. (A) Axial T2W image at time of initial shunt placement. Air in the frontal horn of the left lateral ventricle is related to the shunt placement. (B) Follow-up MRI axial T1W image demonstrates an interval decrease in ventricular size, nearly slit-like, and development of a T1W hyperintense left lateral subdural hematoma caused by over shunting of CSF.

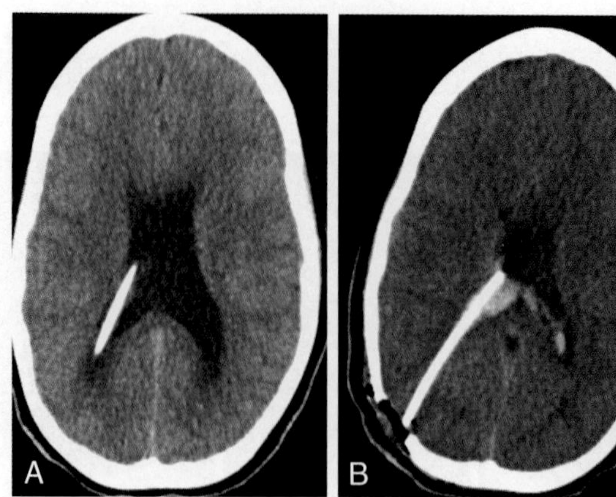

Fig. 11.17 Shunt Revision Complication. (A) Axial CT head prior to shunt revision. (B) Axial CT head with revision of the shunt and new intraventricular hemorrhage.

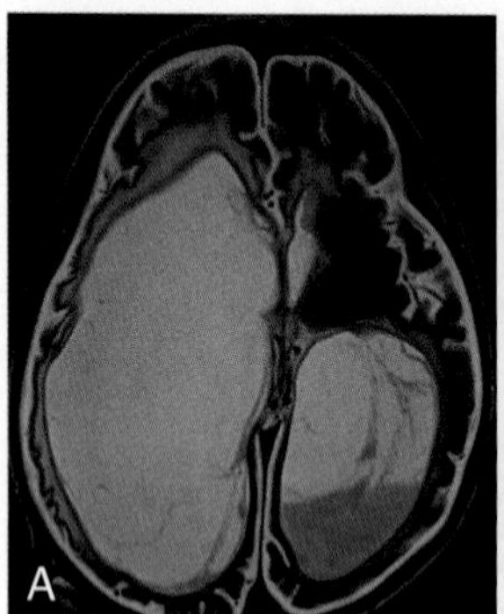

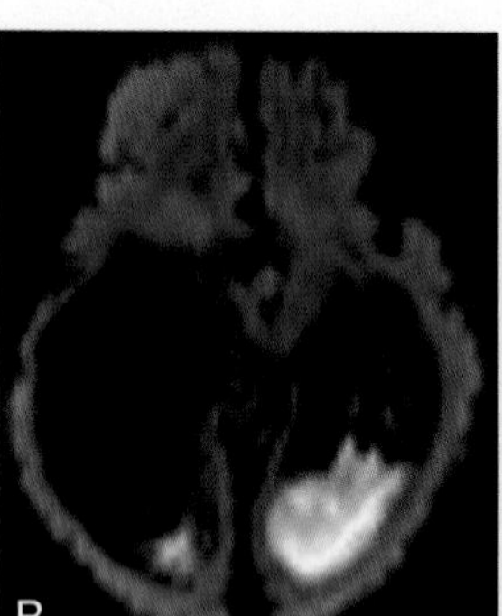

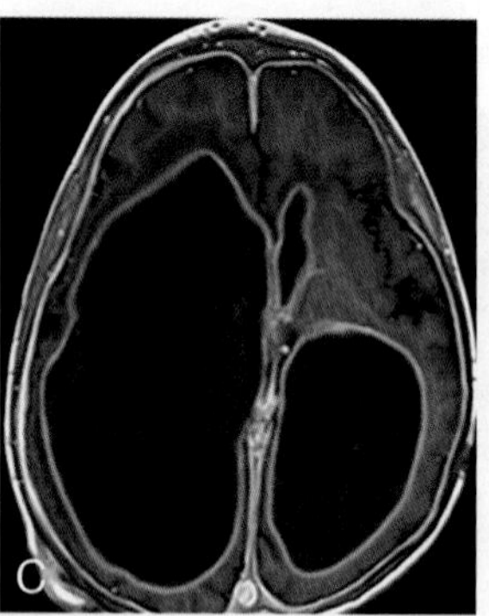

Fig. 11.18 Shunt Infection. (A) Axial T2W, (B) axial DWI, and (C) axial T1W+C images demonstrate disproportionate ventricular enlargement, ependymal enhancement, intraventricular septations, diffusion restricting purulent material in the atria of the ventricles, and periventricular edema.

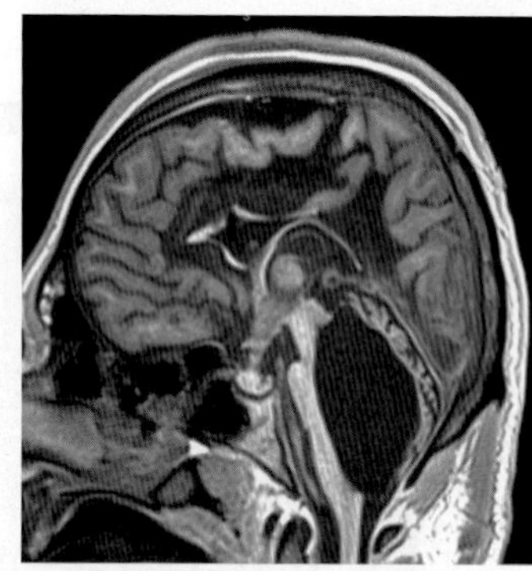

Fig. 11.19 Trapped Fourth Ventricle. An 18-year-old with prematurity and shunted hydrocephalus. Sagittal T1W image demonstrates a distended fourth ventricle following decompression of the lateral ventricles. The fourth ventricle compresses the brainstem and cerebellum.

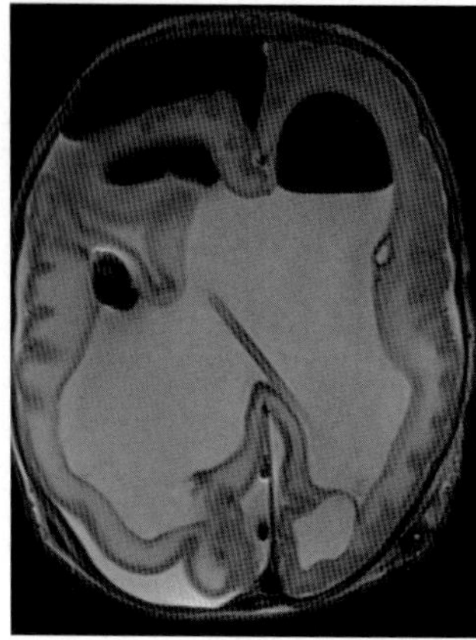

Fig. 11.20 Cortical Mantle Infolding Following Shunt Placement. Axial T2W image demonstrates cortical infolding in the right cerebral hemisphere.

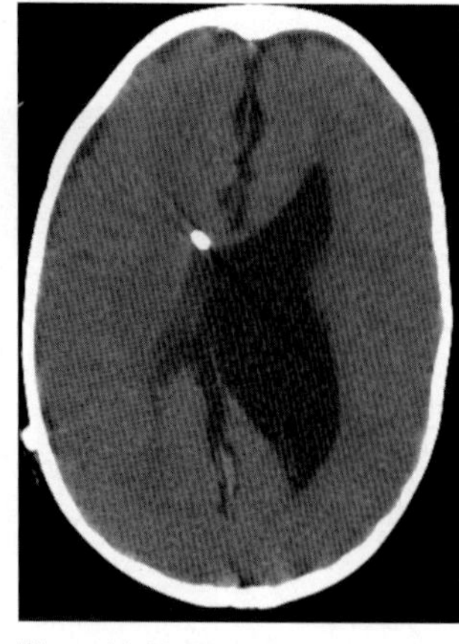

Fig. 11.21 Slit-Like Ventricle Syndrome. Axial CT head demonstrates a slit-like right lateral ventricle and an enlarged left lateral ventricle.

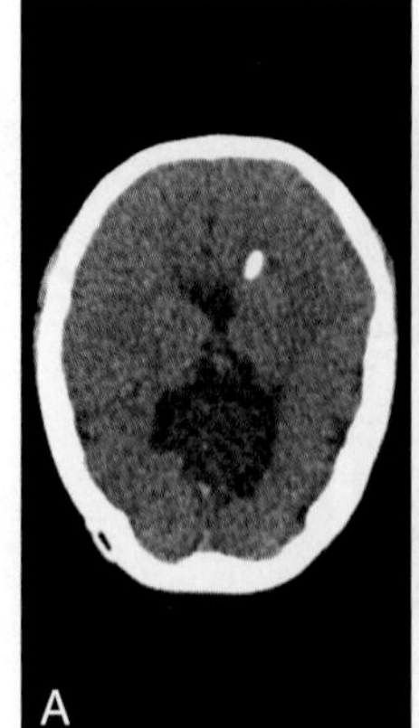

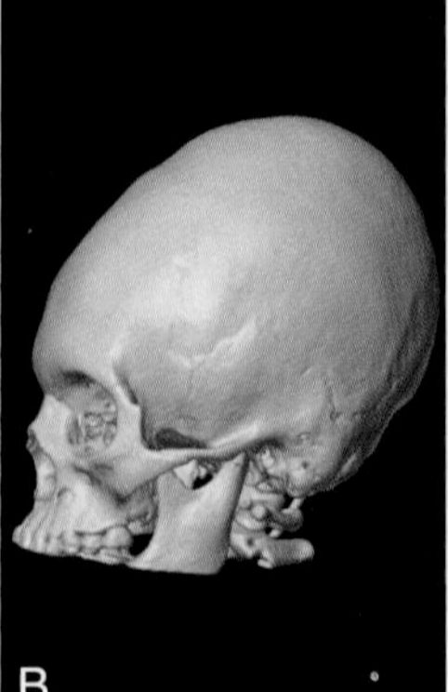

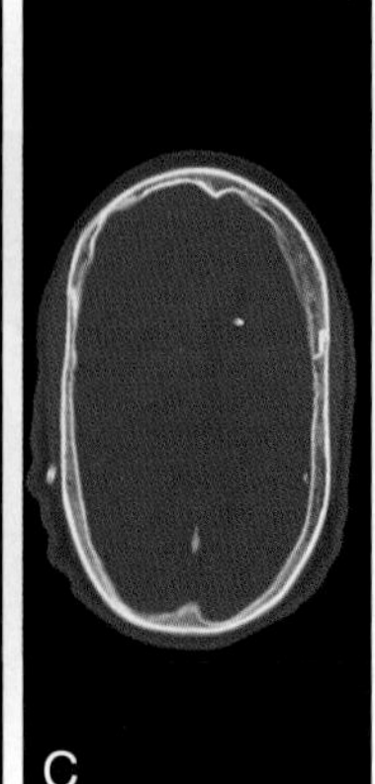

Fig. 11.22 Skull Thickening and Abnormal Calvarial Shape. (A and B) Axial CT and 3D reformat CT demonstrate calvarial thickening, microcephaly, and flattening of the frontal bones due to chronic shunting in a 12-year-old patient with prematurity-related hydrocephalus. (C) Axial head CT in a 13-year-old with shunted hydrocephalus demonstrates scaphocephaly due to chronic shunting.

Key Points

Background

- Shunt malfunction occurs in 30% to 40% of children within 1 year and in approximately 50% of children within 2 years of surgery. Lifetime risk for shunt malfunction is 80%.
- Some studies have shown myelomeningocele, intraventricular hemorrhage, tumor, and postmeningitis hydrocephalus associated with higher shunt failure, while a large prospective study did not find these associations.
- Young patients experience higher rates of shunt failure as well as those with cardiac comorbidities.
- Causes of shunt malfunction:
  - Catheter obstruction with tissue or cells accounts for 50% of shunt failures.
  - Valve obstruction or malfunction accounts for 4% to 6% of shunt failures.
  - Shunt tubing fracture accounts for 3% to 21% of failures and is usually a delayed problem.
  - Shunt tubing disconnection typically is an early problem.
  - Shunt migration can occur as the child grows and is more common with ventriculoatrial catheters.
  - Shunt infections account for 3% to 20% of failures; 90% of shunt infections occur in the first 6 months after shunt placement. Infections are most commonly due to coagulase-negative *Staphylococcus* (60%) and *Staphylococcus aureus* (20%). Risk factors include young age, prior shunt revision or neurosurgical procedure, and gastrostomy tube.
- Symptoms: Infants present with feeding difficulty, nausea/vomiting, irritability, and bulging fontanelle. Older children present with headache, nausea/vomiting, somnolence, cognitive difficulty, and papilledema.
- Slit ventricle syndrome (SVS) refers to patients with symptoms of shunt malfunction who have slit-like ventricles on imaging. Although approximately 50% of patients have slit-like ventricles on imaging, only 11% have SVS. SVS usually is a late presentation, occurring approximately 6.5 after shunt placement. Etiology is due to either overdrainage of CSF or decreased ventricular compliance. Four SVS subtypes have been described: (1) postural headache due to CSF overdrainage; (2) on-off again symptom complex due to reduced ventricle compliance to mild variations in CSF volume, which manifests with elevated CSF pressure in extracranial regions such as a spinal syrinx; (3) recurrent proximal catheter obstructions due to collapse of the ventricle around the shunt and an enlarged contralateral ventricle; (4) subdural fluid collections due to overdrainage.

Imaging

- Typical imaging evaluation is a series of shunt radiographs that visualize of the entire shunt system and either head ultrasound (if neonatal age), CT, or MRI. Shunt radiographs are performed to assess catheter continuity, kinks, and valve setting. Ultrasound, CT, or MRI is needed for visualization of the ventricles.
- Most common appearance of shunt malfunction is an interval enlargement of the ventricles from baseline. Other findings include fluid along the shunt catheter in the brain parenchyma, transependymal edema, change in catheter position, catheter tubing disconnection, fracture, or kinking.
- Ventricular enlargement may not occur in as much as 15% of shunt malfunctions. Therefore, unchanged ventricular size does not exclude a shunt malfunction. Distal shunt failure is more common in patients without ventricular enlargement during shunt malfunction.
- Overdrainage can result in extraaxial fluid collections and/or subdural hematomas. Extraaxial collections are more common following shunting of severe ventriculomegaly.
- Slit ventricles and post-shunt baseline ventriculomegaly are risk factors for shunt failure.
- Catheter removal can result in intraventricular hemorrhage due to avulsion from bound choroid plexus.
- Trapped fourth ventricle is seen as a dilated fourth ventricle after shunting the lateral ventricle and most commonly occurs in the setting of prior infection or hemorrhage and as a result of adhesions obstructing the fourth ventricular outflow sites.
- A peritoneal pseudocyst can occur in the setting of a low-grade VP shunt infection as a result of inflammatory thickening of a peritoneal membrane.
- New imaging advancements: Ultrafast MRI using MRI sequences such as T2 HASTE acquire T2W imaging in shorter time than conventional T2W sequences and are a useful tool to reduce radiation from CT. Ultrafast MRI can be performed without sedation and reliably demonstrates the ventricular size and catheter position.

REFERENCES

1. Sellin JN, Cherian J, Barry JM, et al. Utility of computed tomography or magnetic resonance imaging evaluation of ventricular morphology in suspected cerebrospinal fluid shunt malfunction. *J Neurosurg Pediatr.* 2014 Aug;14(2):160–166.
2. Hanak B, Bonow RH, Harris CA, et al. Cerebrospinal fluid shunting complications in children. *Pediatr Neurosurg.* 2017;52(6):381–400.
3. Riva-Cambrin J, Kestle JRW, Holubkov R, et al. Risk factors for shunt malfunction in pediatric hydrocephalus: a multi-center prospective cohort study. *J Neurosurg Pediatr.* 2016;17:382–390.
4. Orman Gm Bosemani T, Tekes A, et al. Scout view in pediatric CT neuroradiological evaluation: do not underestimate!. *Childs Nerv Syst.* 2014 Feb;30(2):307–311.
5. Sivaganesan A, Krishnamurthy R, Sahni D, et al. Neuroimaging of ventriculoperitoneal shunt complications in children. *Pediatr Radiol.* 2012 Sep;42:1029–1046.

IDIOPATHIC INTRACRANIAL HYPERTENSION

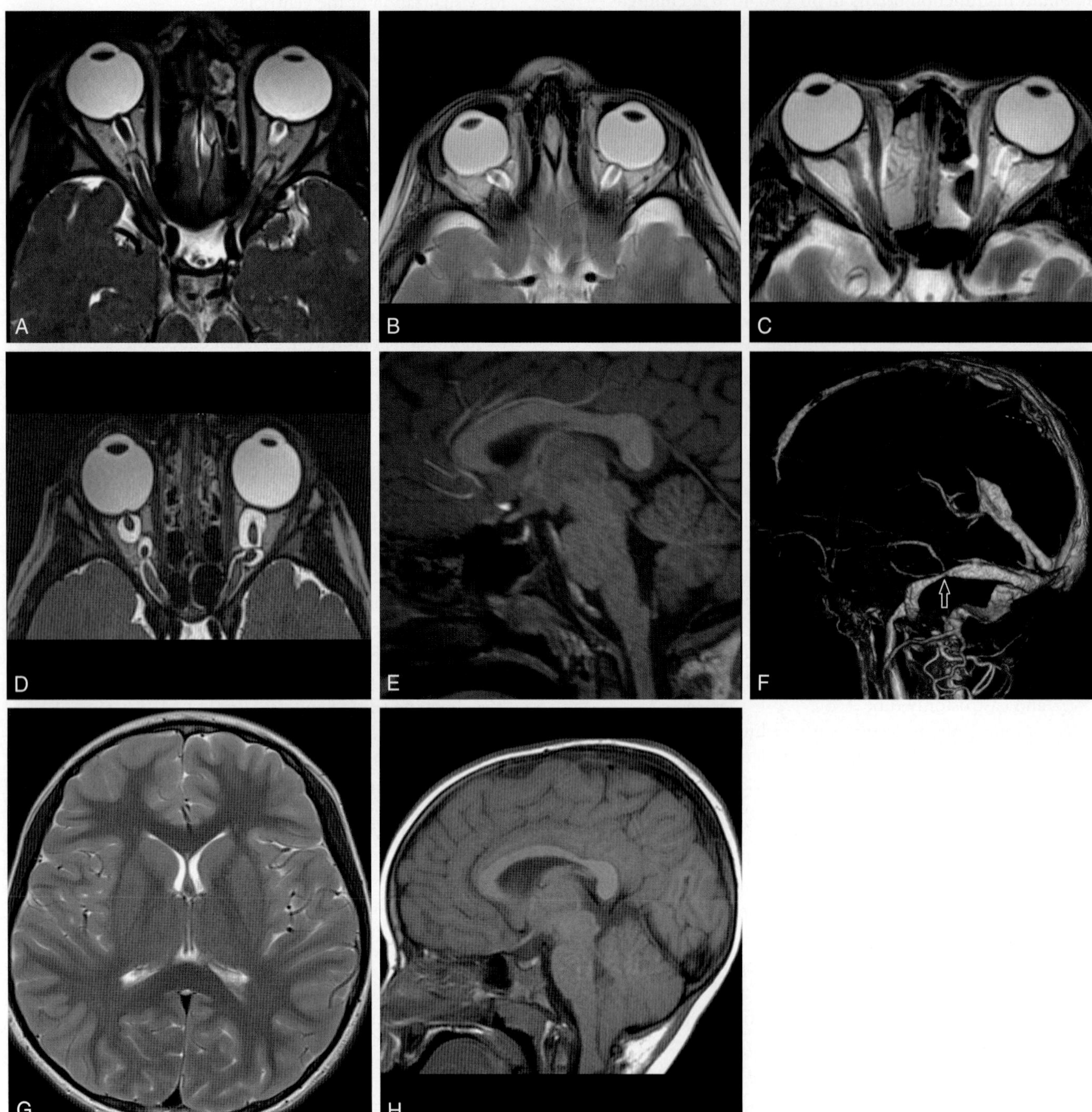

Fig. 11.23 Idiopathic Intracranial Hypertension. (A) Axial 3D T2W image with bulging of the optic discs indicative of papilledema. (B) Axial T2W image demonstrating optic nerve sheath dilatation. (C) Axial T2W image demonstrating posterior globe flattening. (D) Axial 3D T2W image demonstrating optic nerve tortuosity. (E) Sagittal T1W image with partially empty sella indicative of elevated intracranial pressure. (F) CT venogram volume rendered image demonstrating focal stenosis of the transvere sinus. (G) Axial T2W image demonstrating slit-like ventricles. (H) Sagittal T1W image demonstrating low cerebellar tonsils.

Key Points

Background

- Also known as pseudotumor cerebri
- Primary symptoms include headache (57–87%), papilledema (80–90%), vision loss (33%), cranial nerve 6 palsy (10–17%), nausea and vomiting (13–52%), transient vision obscurations (42%), pulsatile tinnitus (10%), and hearing loss
- Etiology unknown but possibly from abnormal CSF physiology (impaired outflow from venous stenosis, abnormal CSF production), or metabolic basis (affecting the rennin-angiotensin-aldosterone pathway)

- Secondary Intracranial Hypertension: refers to elevated intracranial pressure due to an identifiable cause such as venous thrombosis, corticosteroid withdrawal, tetracycline antibiotics, growth hormone administration, Addison's disease, and Aldosteronism
- Diagnostic Criteria
  A. Papilledema
  B. Normal neurologic examination except cranial nerve abnormalities
  C. Neuroimaging demonstrating normal parenchyma (no mass, hydrocephalus, structural lesion, or abnormal meningeal enhancement) for typical patients (female and obese), and normal MR venography for other patients
  D. Normal CSF composition
  E. CSF opening pressure > 25 cm H2O
  F. If papilledema is absent, diagnosis can be made with abducens palsy and criteria B–E
  G. If papilledema and abducens palsy are not present, then idiopathic intracranial hypertension (IIH) diagnosis can be made with criteria B–E and three of the following: empty sella, flattening of the posterior globe, distended perioptic subarachnoid space with or without optic nerve tortuosity, transverse sinus stenosis. Three or more of the MRI findings have a sensitivity of 62% and specificity of 95% for diagnosis of idiopathic intracranial hypertension
- Risk factors include postpuberty obesity (i.e., weight does not seem to be a risk factor in children <12 years), recent weight gain, polycystic ovarian syndrome, postpuberty female gender (i.e., equal male:female prevalence in young children), family history.
  ~30% of young children are asymptomatic.
- Treatment includes weight loss, acetazolamide, and surgical interventions (optic nerve sheath fenestration, CSF shunting, venous sinus stenting) depending on vision loss.

Imaging

- Role of imaging is to first exclude a mass, hydrocephalus, or sinus thrombosis.
- Identify MRI finding supportive of IIH (sensitivity/specificity in pediatric patients):
  - Optic disc bulging (32–40%, 100%)
  - Optic nerve sheath dilatation (46–97%, 67–100%)
  - Optic nerve tortuosity (30–68%, 83–95%)
  - Posterior globe flattening (56–97%, 90–100%)
  - Empty sella (43–64%, 64–100%)
  - Slit-like ventricles (3%, 100%)
  - Low cerebellar tonsils (7%, 100%)
  - Transverse sinus narrowing (96%, 83%)

REFERENCE

1. Friedman DI, Liu GT, Digre KB. Revised diagnostic criteria for the pseudotumor cerebri syndrome in adult and children. *Neurology.* 2013 Sept 24;81(13).

INTRACRANIAL HYPOTENSION

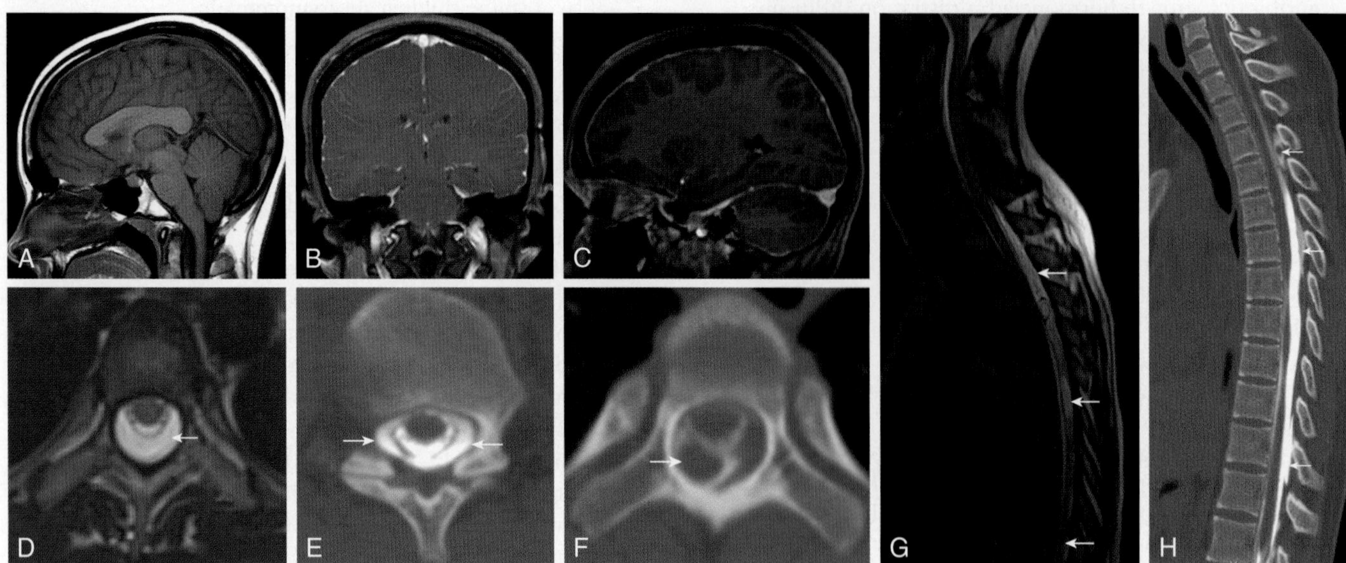

Fig. 11.24 Intracranial Hypotension. A 10-year-old with orthostatic headache. (A) Sagittal T1W image with low position of cerebellar tonsils, and enlarged pituitary gland. (B) Coronal T1W+C image and (C) Sagittal T1W+C with smooth dural thickening and enhancement along the cerebral hemispheres as well as distended transverse sinus indicated by the convex inferior margin of the transverse sinus (C). (D and G) Axial and sagittal 3D T2W image demonstrates a large epidural fluid collection in the thoracic spine *(arrow)* displacing the dural lining. (E, F, and H) Axial and sagittal CT myelogram images demonstrate epidural contrast indicative of active CSF leak. A focal area surrounded by contrast *(small arrow)* was found at surgery to be a pseudomeningocele and a source of the CSF leak. The patient was ultimately found to have Ehlers-Danlos.

Key Points

Background

- Intracranial hypotension is caused by low CSF pressure/volume.
- CSF hypotension can be secondary to fractures through the skull base (most commonly the anterior cranial fossa, resulting in rhinorrhea), overshunting, or surgical loss of CSF during brain or spine surgery, and can also occur spontaneously (most commonly from CSF leak cause by a perineural cyst, disc protrusion, or CSF-venous fistula).
- In the setting of trauma, a CT cisternogram allows for depiction of both the fracture site and confirmation of a CSF leak.
- Spontaneous intracranial hypotension (SIH) is uncommon in children and can be secondary to connective tissue disorders, causing weakness in the dura and/or nerve sheaths as well as CSF-venous fistulas reported with Gorham disease.
- Multiple symptoms can occur including but not limited to orthostatic headache and tinnitus.

Imaging

- Brain findings:
  - Low position of the cerebellar tonsils
  - Smooth diffuse dural thickening and enhancement
  - Enlarged dural sinuses (rounded/convex margins of the transverse sinus on sagittal images compared to normal flat or concave appearance)
  - Enlarged pituitary gland
  - Subdural effusion or hematoma
  - Narrowing of the mamillopontine distance
- Spine findings:
  - Extradural fluid collection caused by the CSF leak
  - Extravasation of intrathecal contrast into the epidural space on CT or MR myelography
  - Rare complication of CSF loss during surgery is a remote hemorrhage in the midcerebellar hemisphere. Etiology for this hemorrhage is unknown
  - Myelographic contrast uptake into a paraspinal vein from a fistula

REFERENCE

1. Schievink WI, Maya MM, Louy C, et al. Spontaneous intracranial hypotension in childhood and adolescence. *J Pediatr*. 2013 Aug;163(2):504–510.

BENIGN ENLARGEMENT OF SUBARACHNOID SPACES

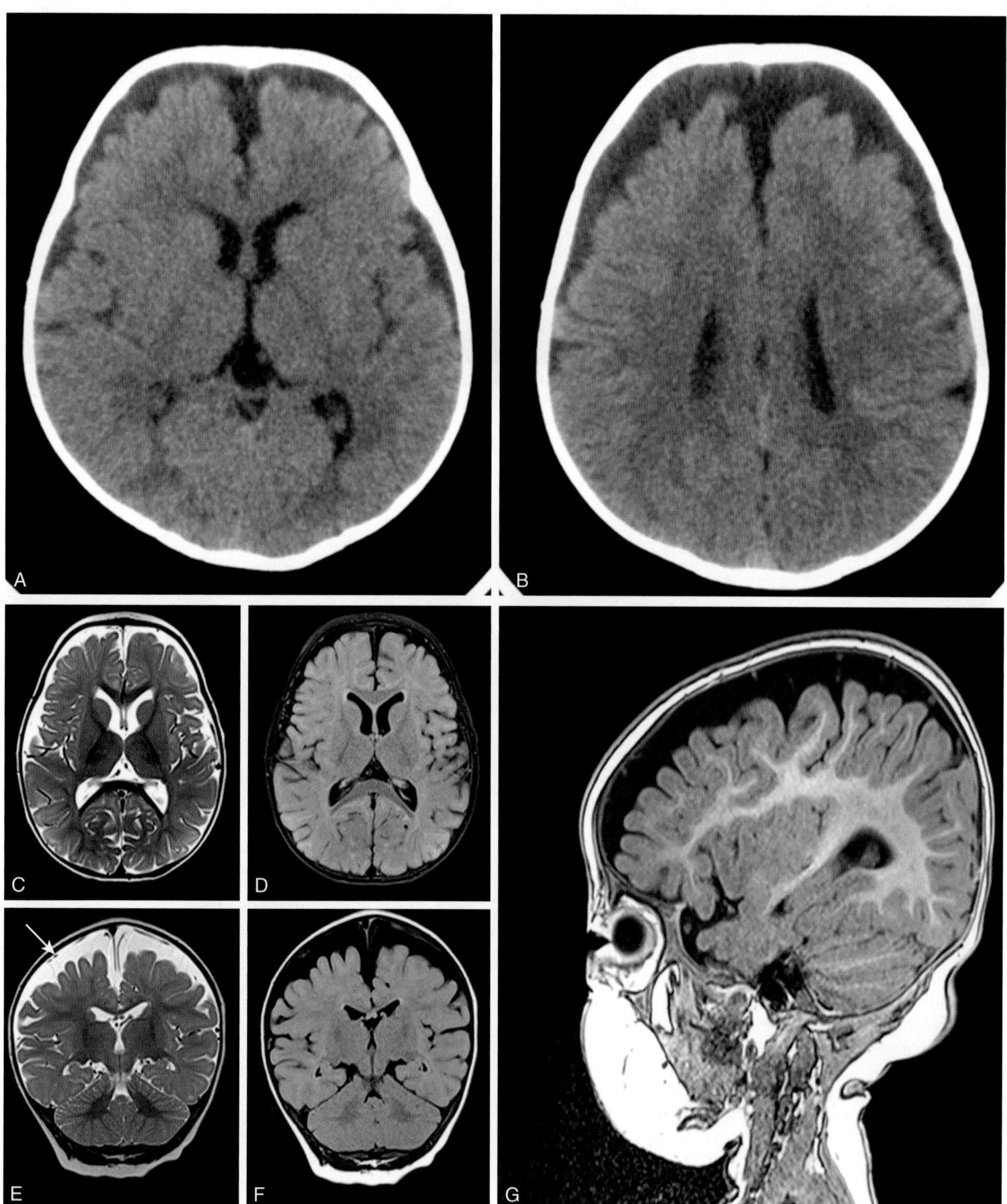

Fig. 11.25 Benign Enlargement of Subarachnoid Spaces. (A and B) Axial head CT images with enlarged extraaxial spaces. (C and E) Axial and coronal T2W, (D and F) axial and coronal FLAIR, and (G) sagittal T1W images with enlarged subarachnoid spaces as indicated by the cortical vessels closely opposed to the inner table of the calvarium. FLAIR images are useful in this setting for increasing sensitivity for detection of a subdural fluid collection.

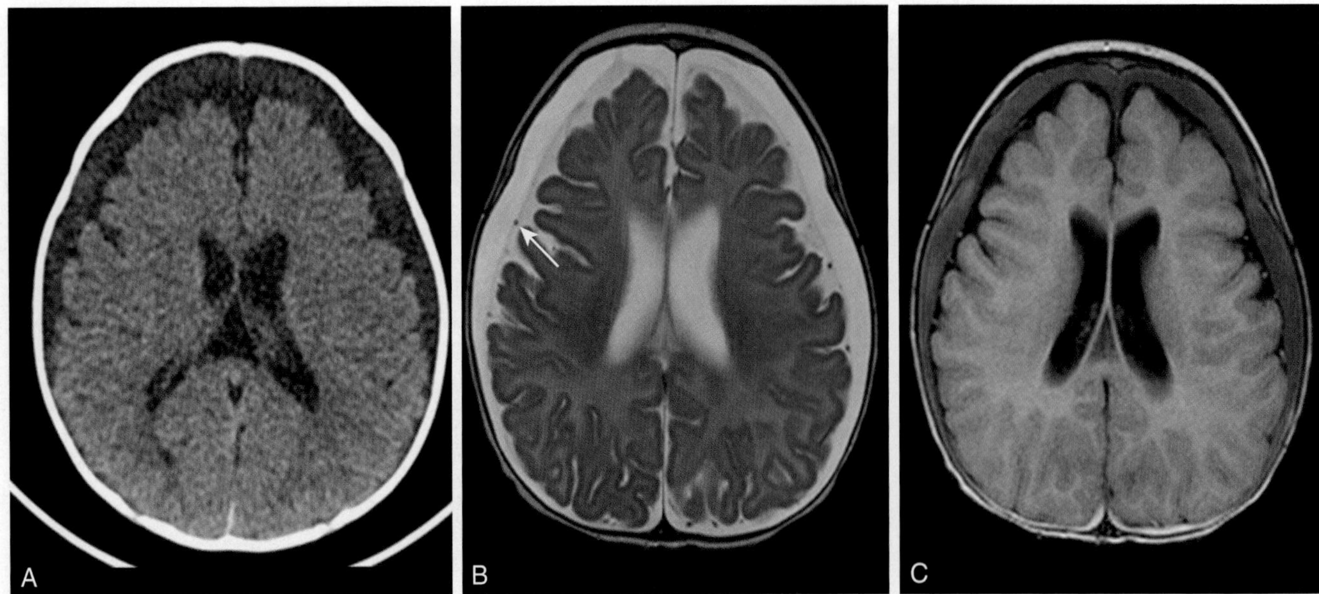

Fig. 11.26 Pitfall in Diagnosis of Benign Enlargement of Subarachnoidal Spaces in Infancy (BESSI): Subdural Fluid Collections. (A) Axial head CT with enlargement of the extraaxial spaces along the frontal lobes, which are proven to be bilateral subdural fluid collections using MRI with (B) axial T2W, and (C) axial FLAIR images that demonstrate the cortical vessels displaced inward, visible dural lining of the subdural collection, and the subdural fluid has higher signal intensity than normal CSF on FLAIR image. These finding should raise concern for potential abusive head trauma.

Key Points

Background

- Benign enlargement of the subarachnoid spaces in infancy (BESSI) refers to a transient prominence of the subarachnoid spaces in neonates and infants (2 to 8 months of age, mean 3.4 months).
- The children may become apparent because of frontal bossing, macrocephaly, or rapidly increasing head circumference but have no neurologic symptoms.
- BESSI is usually self-limiting. Half of patients end up with head circumference at or above the 97.5 percentile.
- The etiology of BESSI is unclear, but a transient immaturity of the arachnoid granulations is believed to be causative.

Imaging

- BESSI is characterized by a symmetric mild to moderate widening of the frontal subarachnoid spaces (>4 mm), including the anterior interhemispheric space. The sylvian fissures may also be prominent, and the anterior horn of the lateral ventricles are often at the upper limits of normal in size. Findings normalize after 12–18 months of age.
- Differentiation of enlarged subarachnoid spaces in BESSI from subdural effusions can be accomplished by identifying vessels extending from the brain surface to the inner table of the calvarium.
- In subdural effusions, the vessels are pushed away from the inner table of the calvarium. In addition, subdural effusions are compartmentalized in between split layers of the dura and do not intermix with the subarachnoid cerebrospinal fluid resulting in increased proteinaceous content and resultant increased signal intensity on FLAIR MR imaging.
- Controversy exists regarding whether BESSI predisposes children to subdural hemorrhage. In this setting, workup for nonaccidental trauma should be performed.

REFERENCES

1. Zahl SM, Egge A, Helseth E, et al. Clinical, radiological, and demographic details of benign external hydrocephalus: a population based study. *Pediatr Neurol.* 2019 Jul;96:53–57.
2. Fingarson AK, Ryan ME, McLone SG, et al. Enlarged subarachnoid spaces and intracranial hemorrhage in children with accidental head trauma. *J Neurosurg Pediatr.* 2017 Feb;19(2):254–258.
3. Tucker J, Choudhary A, Piatt J. Macrocephaly in infancy: benign enlargement of the subarachnoid spaces and subdural collections. *J Neurosurg Pediatr.* 2016 Jul;18(1):16–20.
4. McNeely PD, Atkinson JD, Saigal G, et al. Subdural hematomas in infants with benign enlargement of the subarachnoid spaces are not pathognomonic for child abuse. *AJNR Am J Neuroradiol.* 2006 Sep;27(8):1725–1728.

12 Orbital and Craniofacial Malformations

INTRODUCTION

Background

- Craniofacial malformations have characteristic osseous and soft tissue features, which lead to visible deformity. In addition, these anomalies can lead to loss of normal function of hearing, swallowing, and vision.
- These malformations frequently involve combinations of craniofacial locations.
- Several craniofacial malformations have known genetic causes. The most common genetic abnormality involves the fibroblast growth factor.

Imaging

- CT imaging with 3D reconstruction is the modality of choice. Although currently limited to research investigations, black bone MRI using an ultrashort TE sequence is a potential future alternative to CT.
- Because craniofacial malformations frequently involve multiple anatomic sites, an evaluation of craniofacial malformations requires a systematic assessment of the calvarium, orbits, nose, palate, maxilla, mandible, temporal bone, and spine.
- Once the combination of anomalies or a characteristic anomaly is identified, a diagnosis is often achieved.
- This section illustrates the congenital and acquired orbital and craniofacial malformations and clues to the diagnosis.

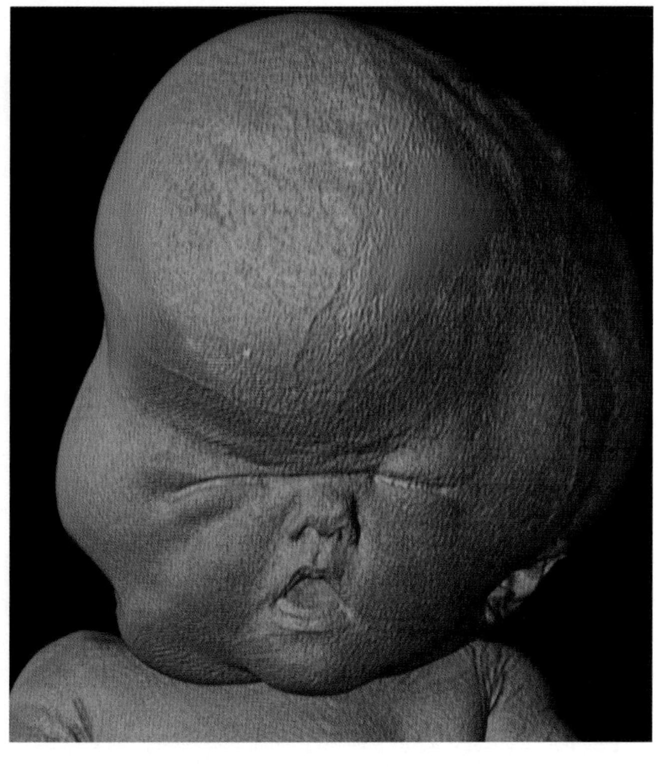

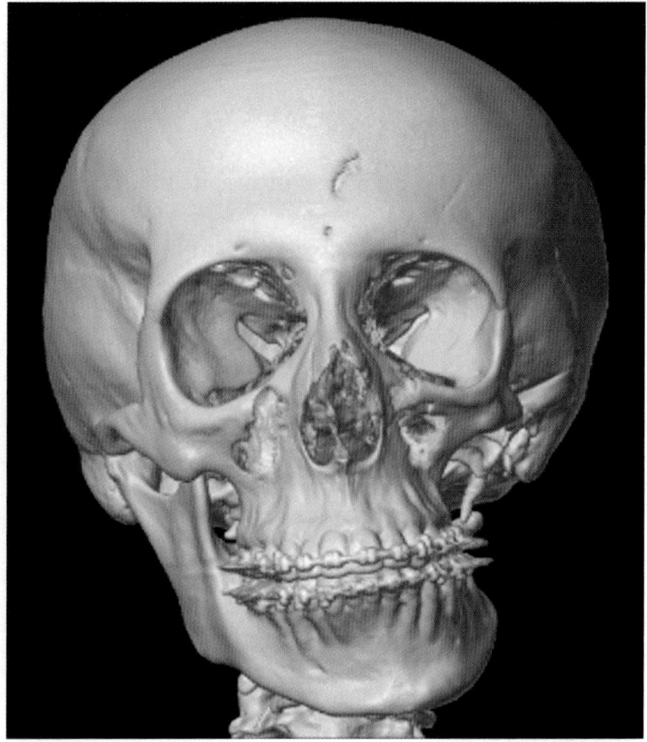

CRANIOSYNOSTOSIS: OVERVIEW

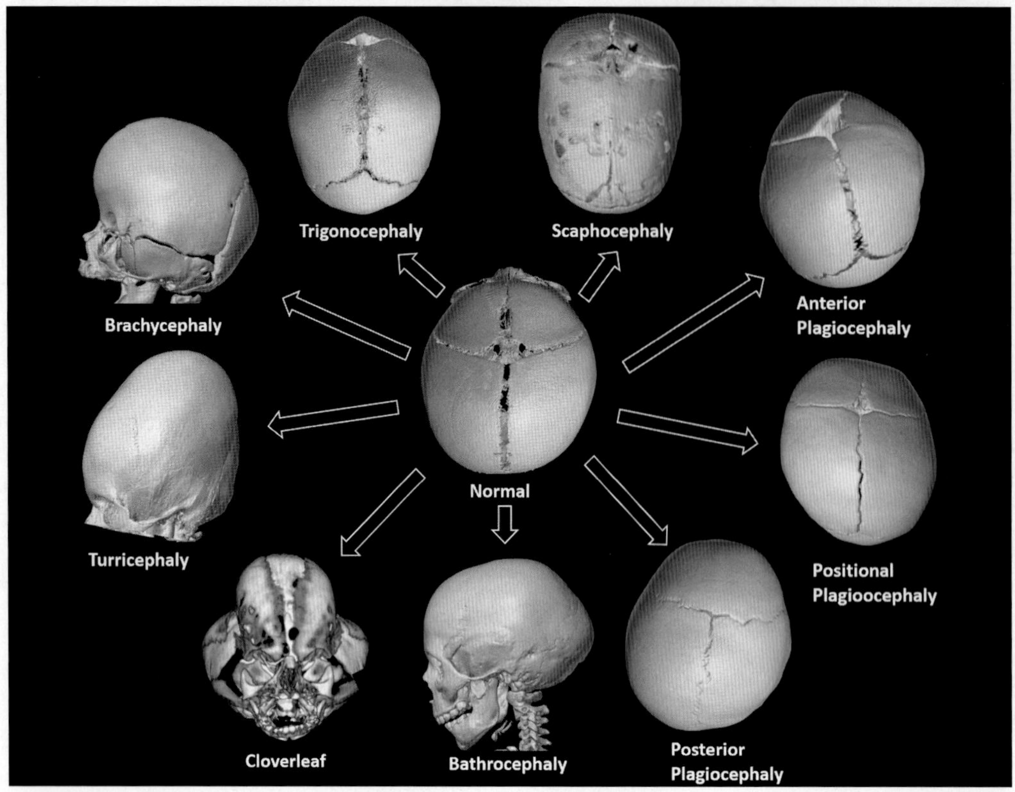

Fig. 12.1 Craniosynostosis: Overview skull shapes in caused by craniosynostosis with exception of positional plagiocephaly.

Key Points

Background

- Craniosynostosis is the premature fusion of the cranial sutures.
- Craniosynostosis is categorized as single or multiple and syndromic or nonsyndromic. Syndromic craniosynostosis is associated with other anomalies of the face, trunk and/or extremities.
- There is an association between craniosynostosis and intracranial hypertension, particularly in complex or syndromic craniosynostosis. However, no correlation between craniosynostosis and hydrocephalus has been established.
- Craniosynostosis has been shown to be associated with altered brain morphology but not overall brain volume. These alteration may account for observed problems with language, attention, information processing, and visual spatial skills.
- Etiology unknown; 15% are syndromic causes, most commonly due to FGFR, TWIST1, or MSX2 gene mutations
- Secondary causes can include brain malformations and shunting, which lead to altered pressure exerted on the calvarium

Imaging

- CT imaging with 3D reconstruction is the modality of choice.
- Ultrasound has been suggested as an alternative modality but is operator dependent and requires user expertise.
- Black Bone MRI may emerge in the future as an alternative to CT.
- Syndromic craniosynostosis is often associated with jugular foramen stenosis, tonsillar herniation, altered venous drainage, and accessory transosseous venous drainage, which may impact surgical approach.
- Plagiocephaly which refers to flattening of the skull is often imaged to assess for craniosynostosis but is most commonly due to positional flattening that occurs in infants from laying asymmetrically on one side of the posterior calvarium rather than fusion of a suture.

REFERENCES

1. Attaya H, Thomas J, Alleman A. Imaging of Craniosynostosis from Diagnosis through Reconstruction. *Neurographics.* 2011;01:121–128.
2. Eley KA, Watt-Smith SR, Sheerin F, et al. Black Bone" MRI: a potential alternative to CT with three-dimensional reconstruction of the craniofacial skeleton in the diagnosis of craniosynostosis. *Eur Radiol.* 2014;24(10):2417–2426.
3. Garza RM, Khosla RK. Nonsyndromic craniosynostosis. *Semin Plast Surg.* 2012;26(2):53–63.

METOPIC CRANIOSYNOSTOSIS

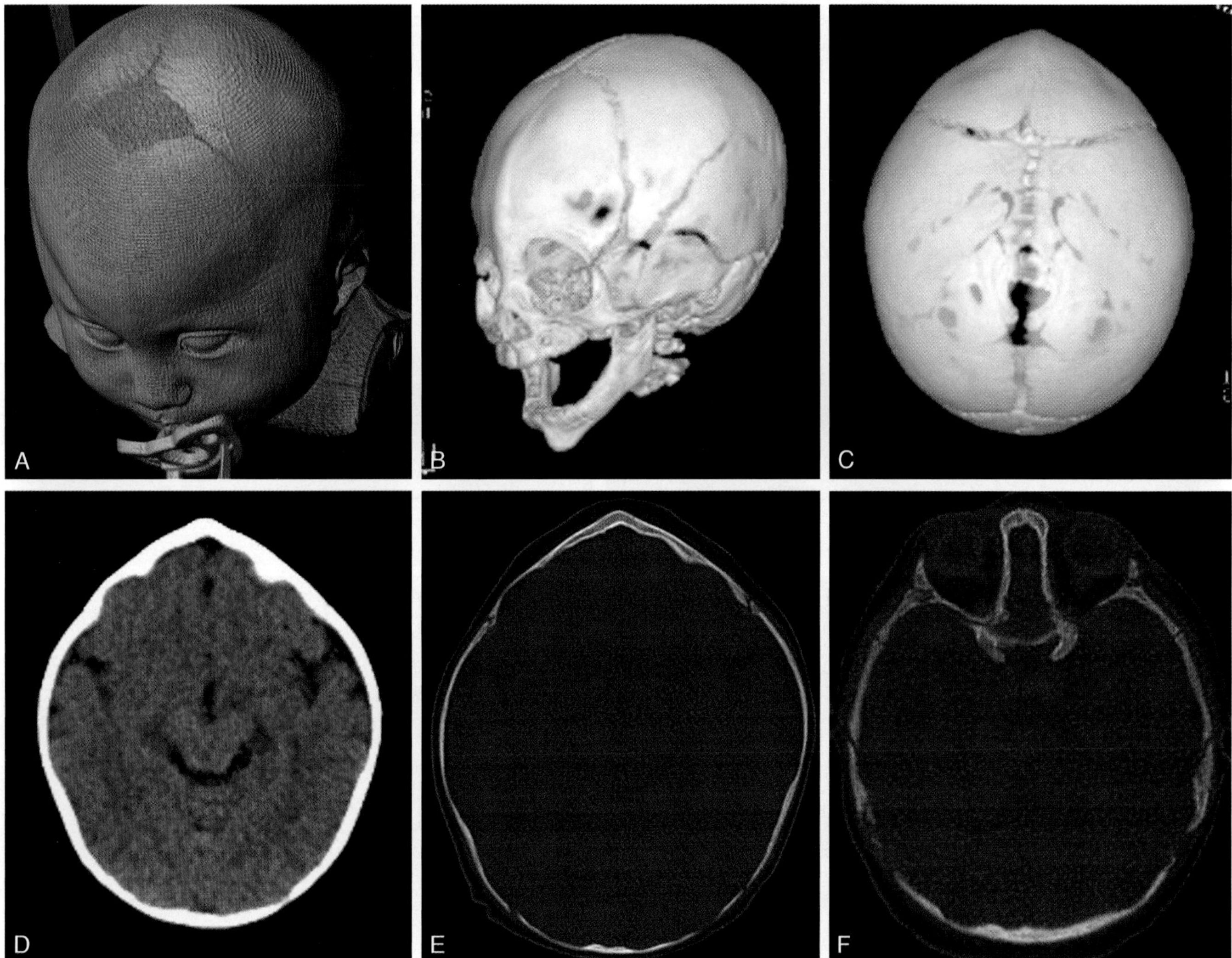

Fig. 12.2 Metopic Craniosynostosis. (A to F) 3D volumetric CT and axial CT images demonstrating metopic craniosynostosis characterized by early closure of the metopic suture and trigonocephaly of the frontal bone as well as potential for crowding of the frontal lobes and hypotelorism.

Key Points

- Normal fusion of the metopic suture occurs at 6 to 9 months
- Premature fusion results in trigonocephaly +/– hypotelorism
- ~25% of metopic craniosynostosis is nonsyndromic

REFERENCES

1. Attaya H, Thomas J, Alleman A. Imaging of Craniosynostosis from Diagnosis through Reconstruction. *Neurographics.* 2011;01:121–128.
2. Garza RM, Khosla RK. Nonsyndromic craniosynostosis. *Semin Plast Surg.* 2012;26(2):53–63.

SAGITTAL CRANIOSYNOSTOSIS

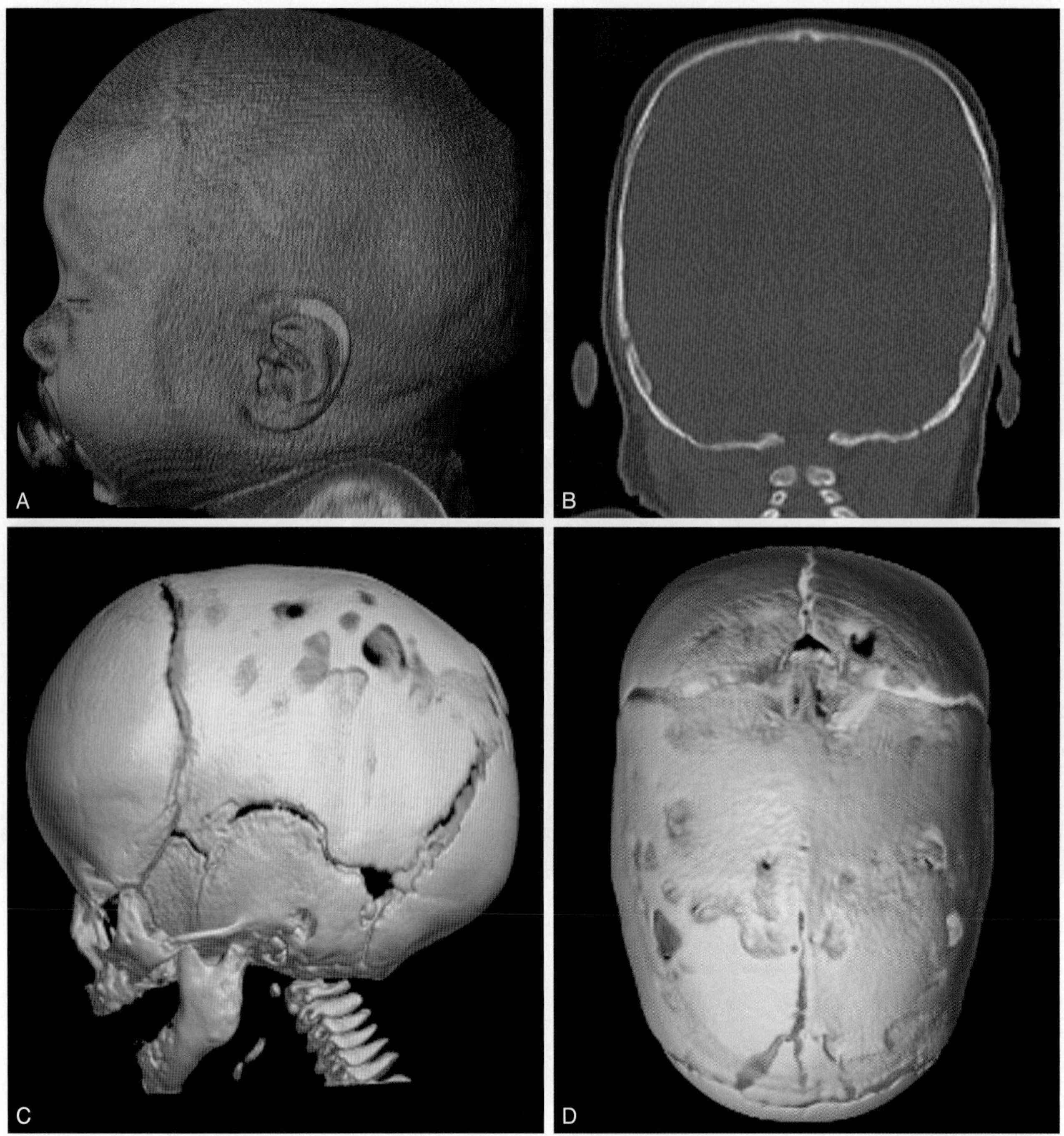

Fig. 12.3 Sagittal Craniosynostosis. (A to D) 3D volumetric CT images and coronal CT images demonstrating sagittal craniosynostosis with associated elongation of the calvarium called scaphocephaly.

Key Points

- Normal fusion of the sagittal suture occurs at ~22 years
- Most common craniosynostosis (40% to 60% of craniosynostosis); 45% of nonsyndromic craniosynostosis; 20% of syndromic craniosynostosis
- Results in scaphocephaly which is AP elongation and narrowed biparietal distance of the calvarium

REFERENCE

1. Attaya H, Thomas J, Alleman A. Imaging of Craniosynostosis from Diagnosis through Reconstruction. *Neurographics*. 2011;01:121–128.

CORONAL CRANIOSYNOSTOSIS

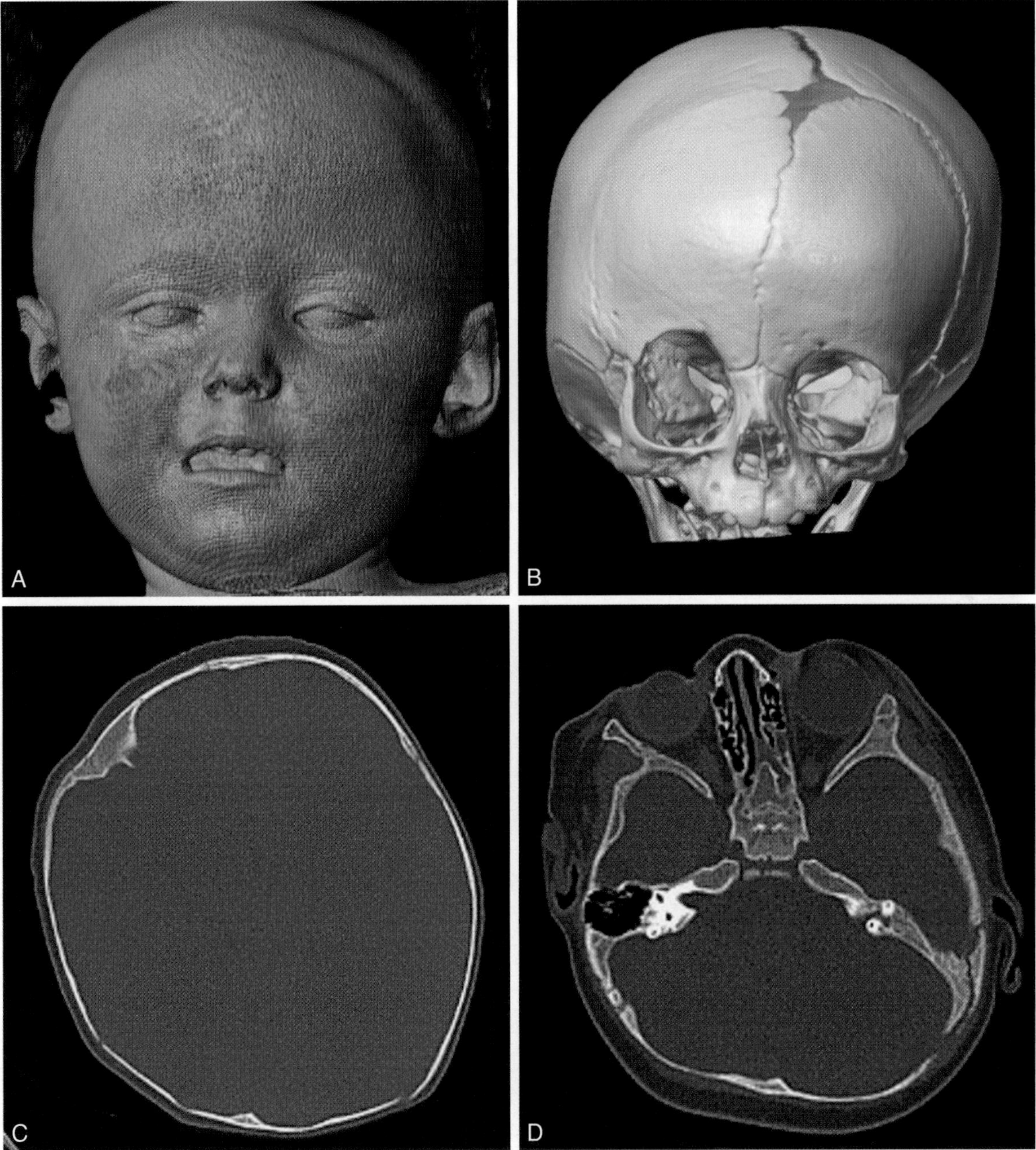

Fig. 12.4 Coronal Craniosynostosis. (A to D) 3D volumetric and axial CT images demonstrating unilateral right coronal craniosynostosis and associated flattening of the calvarium, also known as plagiocephaly. Note the characteristic facial twist and contralateral bulging of the frontoparietal skull.

Key Points

- The coronal suture normally fuses at ~24 years of age
- Unilateral fusion: 25% of nonsyndromic craniosynostosis; results in anterior plagiocephaly, uplifted superolateral corner of the orbit (harlequin eye deformity), contralateral bulging of the frontoparietal skull, "facial twist", and proptosis
- Bilateral fusion: Usually syndromic (i.e., Apert, Crouzon); results in brachycephaly which is a shortening of the skull in AP dimension.

REFERENCES

1. Attaya H, Thomas J, Alleman A. Imaging of Craniosynostosis from Diagnosis through Reconstruction. *Neurographics*. 2011;01:121–128.
2. Garza RM, Khosla RK. Nonsyndromic craniosynostosis. *Semin Plast Surg*. 2012;26(2):53–63.

LAMBDOID CRANIOSYNOSTOSIS

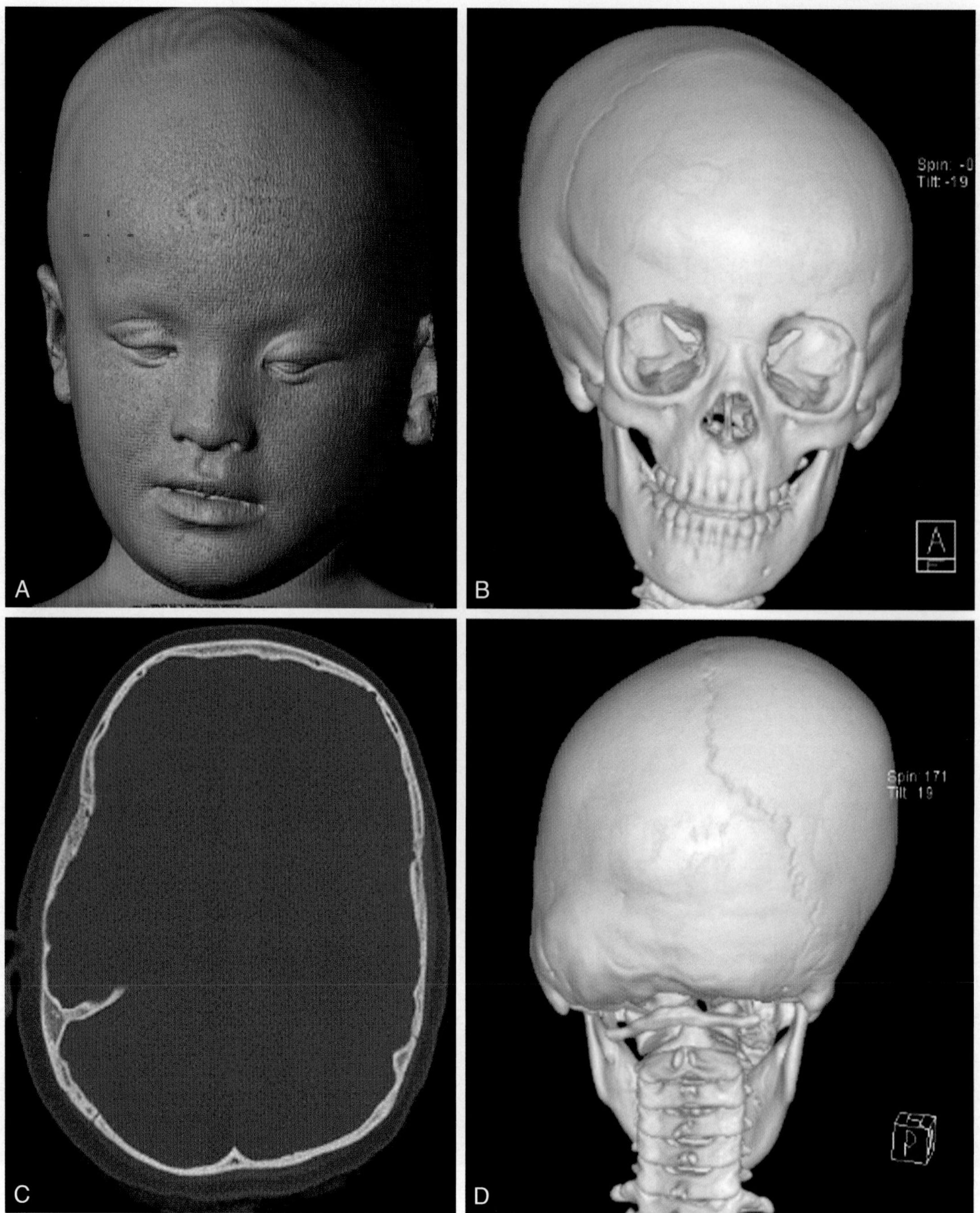

Fig. 12.5 Lambdoid Craniosynostosis. (A to D) 3D volumetric and axial CT images demonstrating left lambdoid craniosynostosis, with associated posterior plagiocephaly. Note the findings of ipsilateral mastoid bulge, contralateral parietal bulge, and inferior position of the ipsilateral ear.

Key Points

- Unilateral fusion results in posterior plagiocephaly; bilateral fusion results in brachycephaly
- Unilateral fusion results in an ipsilateral mastoid bulge, contralateral parietal bulge, thickened ridge along the suture, and inferior displacement of the external auditory canal (EAC) which is a useful clinical finding to differentiate from positional plagiocephaly.
- Less common than metopic, coronal, and sagittal suture craniosynostosis
- Lambdoid suture normally fuses at ~26 years of age

REFERENCE

1. Attaya H, Thomas J, Alleman A. Imaging of Craniosynostosis from Diagnosis through Reconstruction. *Neurographics*. 2011;01:121–128.

CLOVERLEAF SKULL

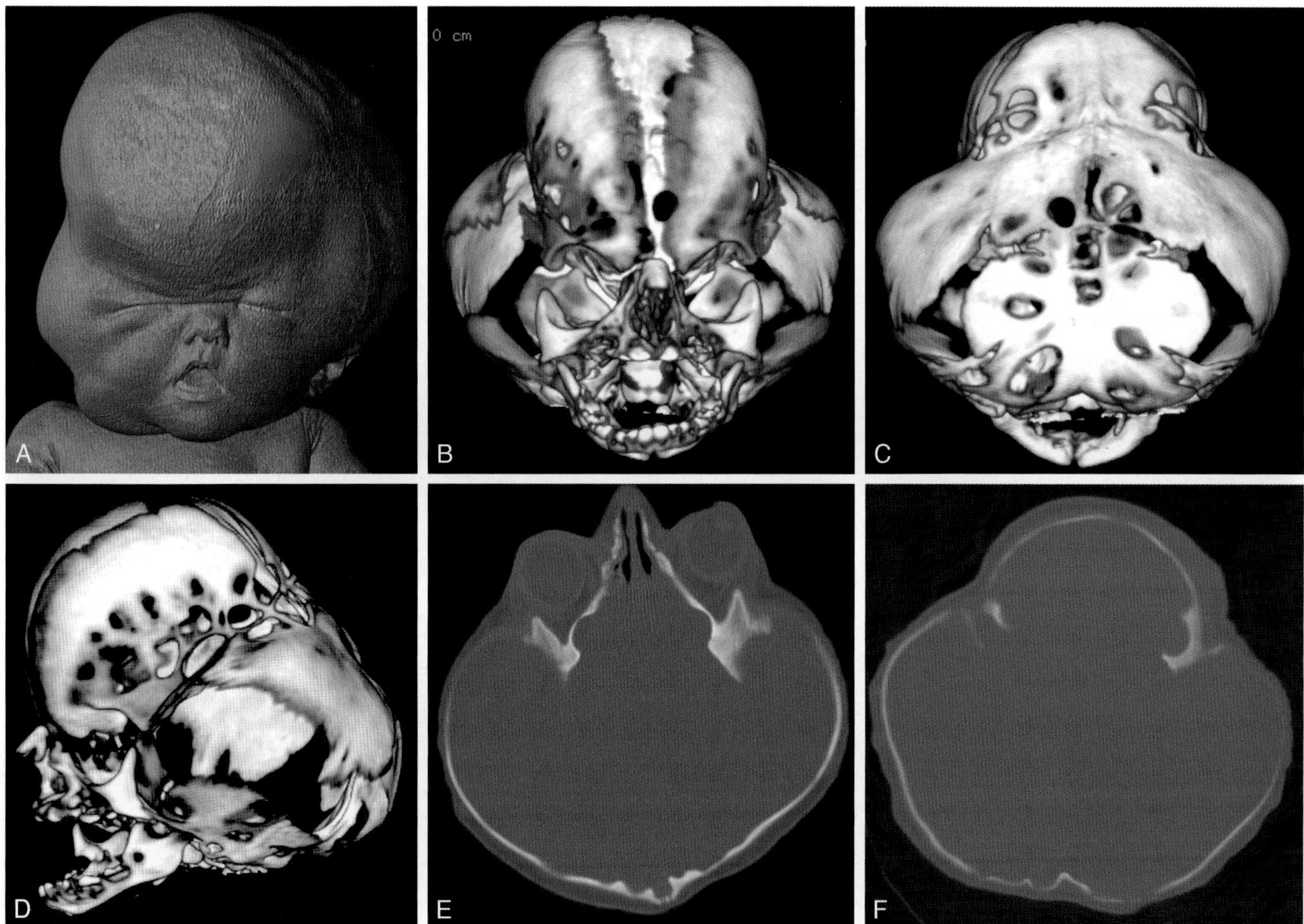

Fig. 12.6 Cloverleaf Skull. (A to F) 3D volumetric and axial CT images demonstrating multisuture craniosynostosis resulting in a cloverleaf pattern.

Key Points

- Also known as Kleeblattschadel deformity
- Multisuture craniosynostosis (sagittal, coronal, and lambdoid), resulting in a trilobed or cloverleaf pattern
- Associated with Apert, Crouzon, and Pfeiffer syndrome

REFERENCE

1. Attaya H, Thomas J, Alleman A. Imaging of Craniosynostosis from Diagnosis through Reconstruction. *Neurographics.* 2011;01:121–128.

APERT SYNDROME

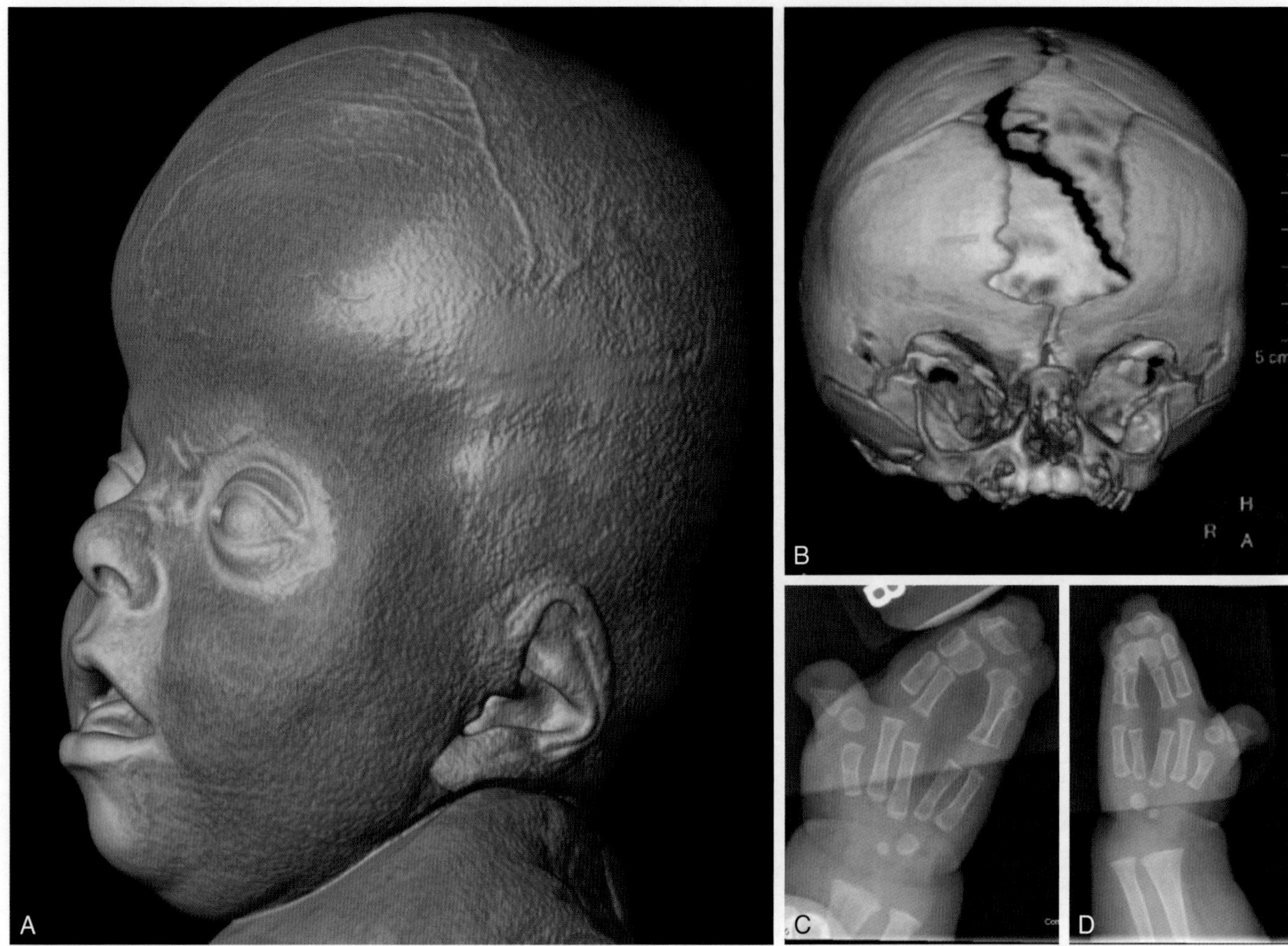

Fig. 12.7 Apert Syndrome. (A and B) 3D volumetric CT images demonstrate bilateral coronal craniosynostosis and brachycephaly. (C and D) AP hand radiographs demonstrate bilateral syndactyly.

Key Points

Background

- Autosomal dominant; FGFR2 mutation
- Varying degrees of developmental delay, mild to moderate intellectual disability

Imaging

- Skull: *Bicoronal craniosynostosis* resulting in brachycephaly; may have widened metopic suture; harlequin eye deformity
- Face: Midface hypoplasia, choanal stenosis, pyriform aperture stenosis, and cleft palate
- Intracranial malformations: Callosal agenesis/dysgenesis, ventriculomegaly/hydrocephalus, temporal lobe dysgyria, Chiari I, and venous outflow stenosis
- *Symmetric syndactyly* (fusion) of the hands and feet
- Other anomalies: Cervical segmentation anomalies, cardiovascular, respiratory, GI, and GU anomalies

REFERENCES

1. Rossi A. Pediatric Neuroradiology 1st edition. Springer-Verlag Berlin Heidelberg.
2. Lowe LH, Booth TN, Joglar JM, et al. Midface anomalies in children. *Radiographics*. 2000;20(4):907–922.

APERT SYNDROME

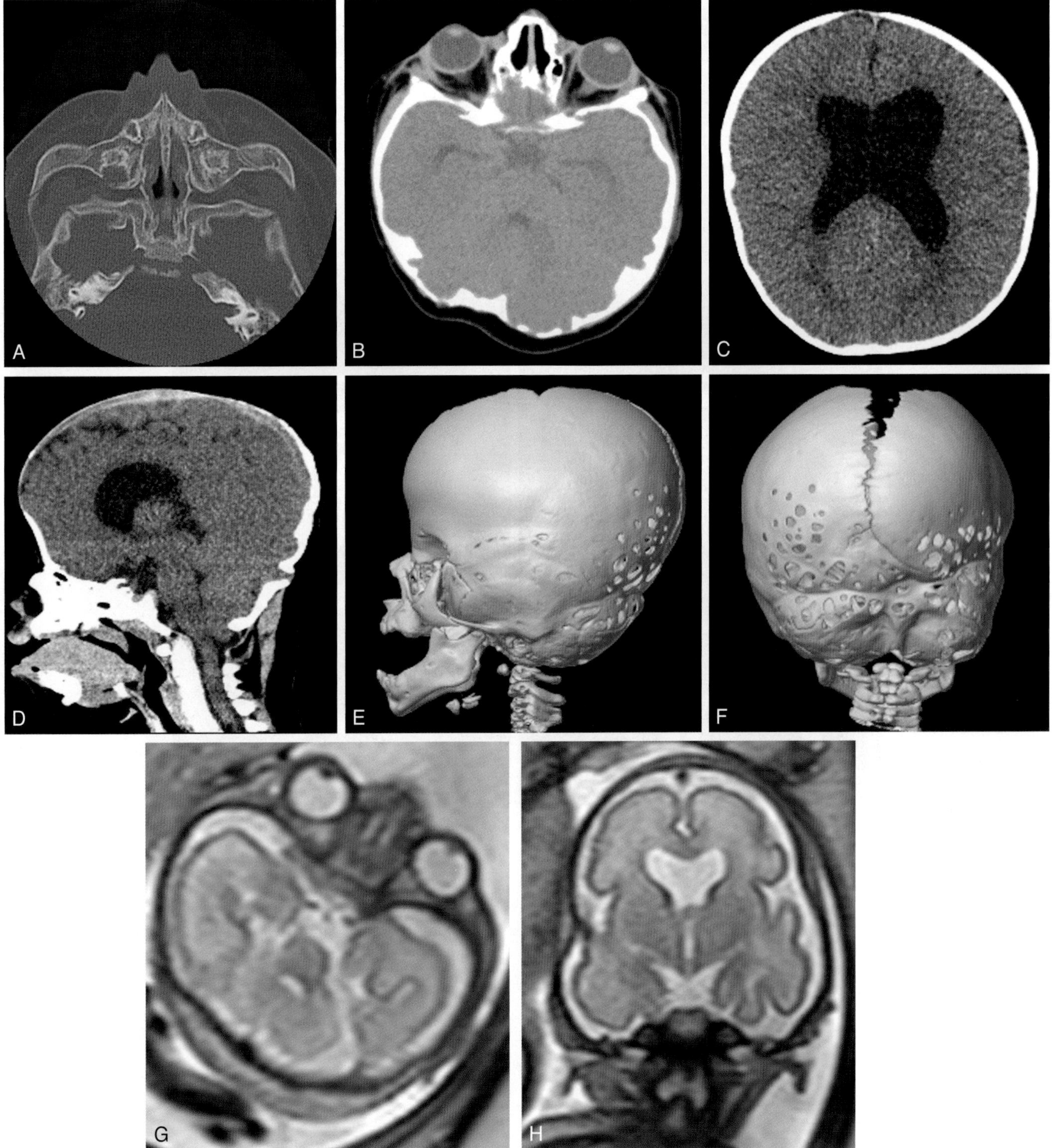

Fig. 12.8 Apert Syndrome. (A to F) Multiplanar CT images and 3D volumetric CT images demonstrating bilateral coronal craniosynostosis, brachycephaly, hypertelorism, pyriform aperture stenosis, ventriculomegaly, and Chiari I malformation. (G and H) Axial and coronal T2W fetal MR images demonstrate bilateral temporal lobe dysgyria, ventriculomegaly, and absent septum pellucidum.

CROUZON SYNDROME

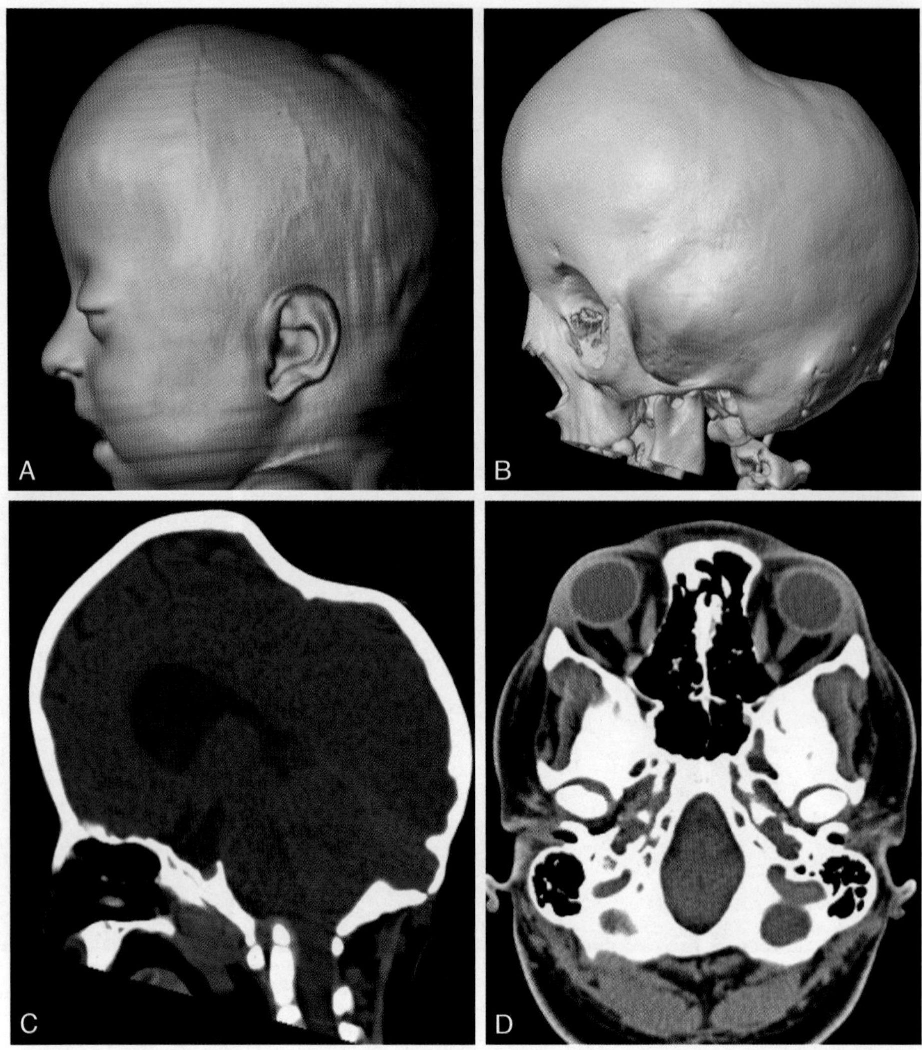

Fig. 12.9 Crouzon Syndrome. (A to D) 3D volumetric CT images and multiplanar CT images hypertelorism, craniosynostosis of the metopic and coronal sutures, basilar invagination, Chiari I malformation, and nasopharynx.

Key Points

Background

- Also known as craniofacial dysostosis
- Autosomal dominant. *FGRF2* gene mutation; normal intelligence

Imaging

- Skull: *Multiple craniosynostosis* combinations can be seen resulting in turricephaly, trigonocephaly, brachycephaly, scaphocephaly, and cloverleaf skull
- Face: Hypertelorism, shallow orbits, proptosis, maxillary hypoplasia, prognathia, basilar kyphosis, AP narrowing of the nasopharynx, stenosis or atresia of EAC, and cleft palate
- Intracranial malformations: midline anomalies including callosal agenesis/dysgenesis, Chiari I, hydrocephalus, venous outflow stenosis/anomalous drainage
- Additional anomalies: Cervical segmentation anomalies, stylohyoid ligament calcification, musculoskeletal deformities, and skin lesions
- Normal hands and feet

REFERENCES

1. Rossi A. Pediatric Neuroradiology 1st edition. Springer-Verlag Berlin Heidelberg.
2. Lowe LH, Booth TN, Joglar JM, et al. Midface anomalies in children. *Radiographics*. 2000;20(4):907–922.

UNCOMMON CRANIOSYNOSTOSES

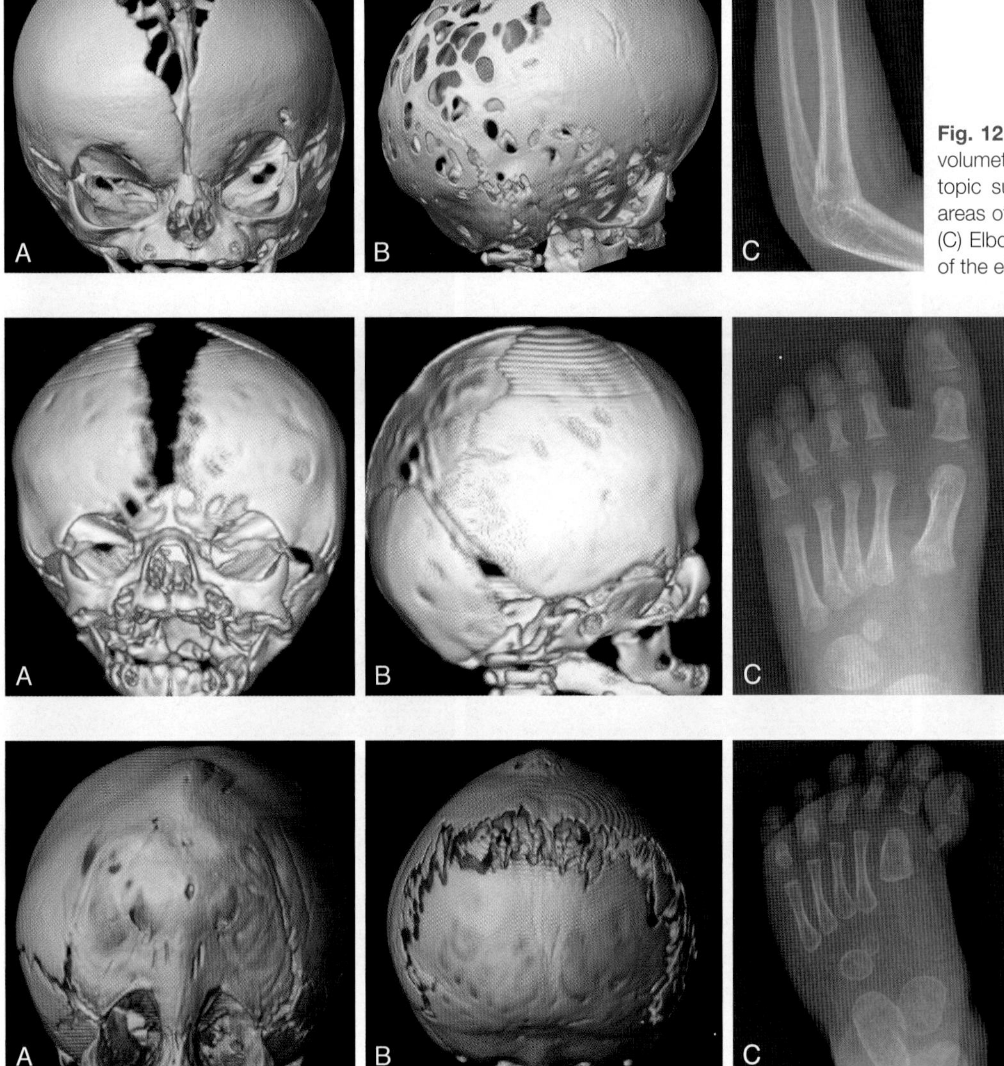

Fig. 12.10 Pfeiffer Syndrome. (A and B) 3D volumetric CT images demonstrate wide metopic suture, bicoronal craniosynostosis, and areas of osseous thinning of the parietal bone. (C) Elbow radiograph demonstrating ankylosis of the elbow joint.

Fig. 12.11 Saethre Chotzen Syndrome. (A and B) 3D volumetric CT images demonstrate wide metopic suture, wide gap between the parietal bones, and bicoronal craniosynostosis. (C) Foot radiograph demonstrating cutaneous syndactyly between the second and third toes.

Fig. 12.12 Carpenter Syndrome. (A and B) 3D volumetric CT images demonstrate metopic, sagittal, and bicoronal craniosynostosis, ridging along the midline of the skull, downsloping orbits, and multiple intrasutural ossification centers in the arc-like lambdoid suture. (C) Foot radiograph demonstrating polydactyly.

Key Points

- Pfeiffer: Autosomal dominant; *FGFR1* or *FGFR2* gene; multiple suture craniosynostosis, midface hypoplasia, broad and radially deviated thumbs, ankylosed elbows, brachydactyly, and syndactyly; usually normal intelligence
- Saethre Chotzen: Autosomal dominant; *TWIST1* gene; coronal synostosis (unilateral or bilateral), syndactyly, brachydactyly, ptosis, hypertelorism, and beaked nose; usually normal intelligence
- Carpenter syndrome: Autosomal recessive; *RAB23* or *MEGF8* gene; multiple suture synostosis, down-slanting palpebral fissures, mandibular and/or maxillary hypoplasia, brachydactyly, polydactyly, cutaneous syndactyly, cryptorchidism and cardiac anomalies; mild to moderate intellectual disability is common
- Muenke syndrome: Autosomal dominant; *FGRF3* gene; coronal synostosis (unilateral or bilateral), broad toes, brachydactyly, and down-slanting palpebral fissures; usually normal intelligence

REFERENCE

1. Lattanzi W, Barba M, Di Pietro L, et al. Genetic advances in craniosynostosis. *Am J Med Genet A*. 2017 May;173(5):1406–1429.

BATHROCEPHALY

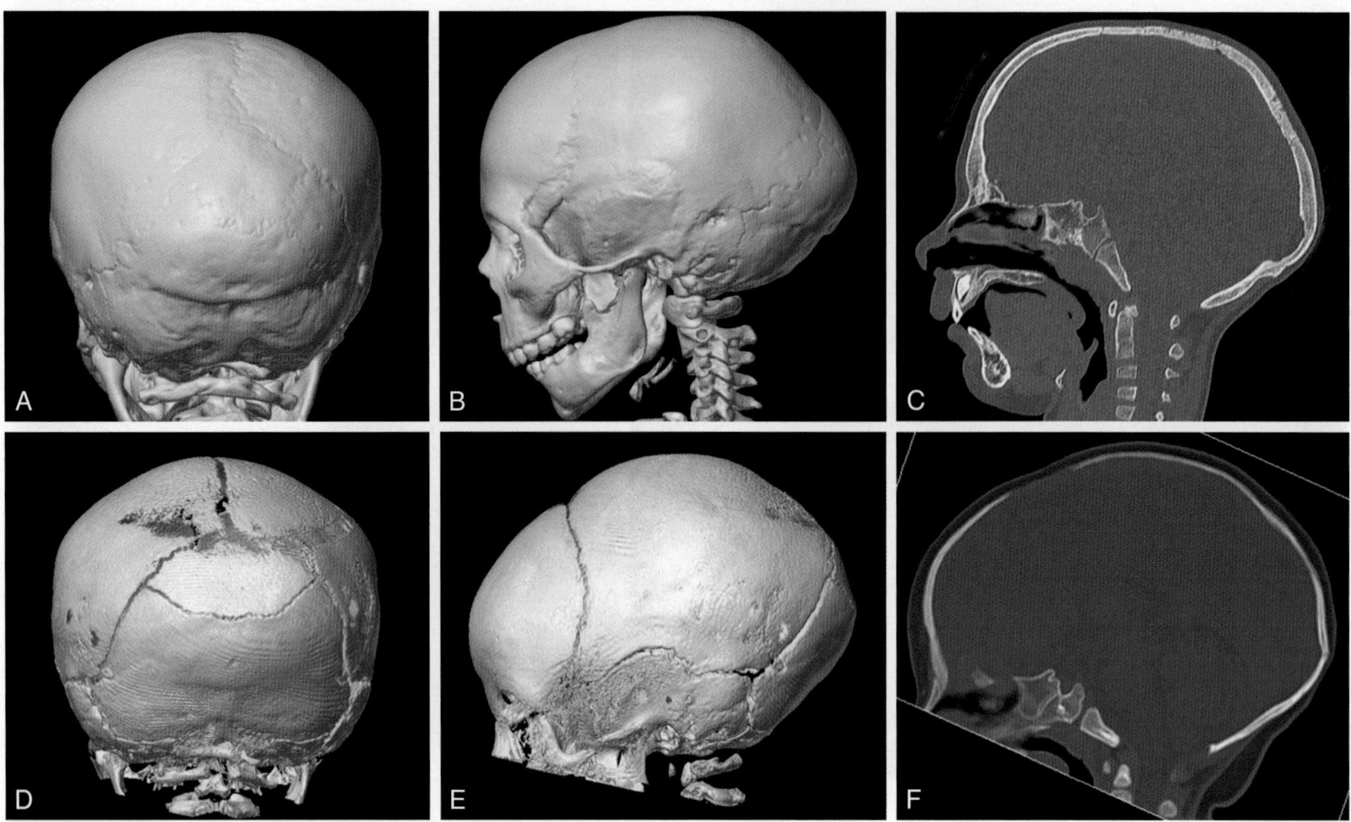

Fig. 12.13 Bathrocephaly. (A to B, D to E) 3D volumetric CT images and (C, F) sagittal reformat CT in two separate patients demonstrating dorsal symmetric midline protuberance of the occipital calvarium with a persistent mendosal suture.

Key Points

- Midline symmetric dorsal protuberance of the occipital calvarium
- May be associated with persistence of the mendosal suture
- No intervention is warranted

REFERENCE

1. Gallagher ER, Evans KN, Hing AV, et al. Bathrocephaly: a head shape associated with a persistent mendosal suture. *Cleft Palate Craniofac J*. 2013 Jan;50(1):104–108.

PIERRE ROBIN SEQUENCE

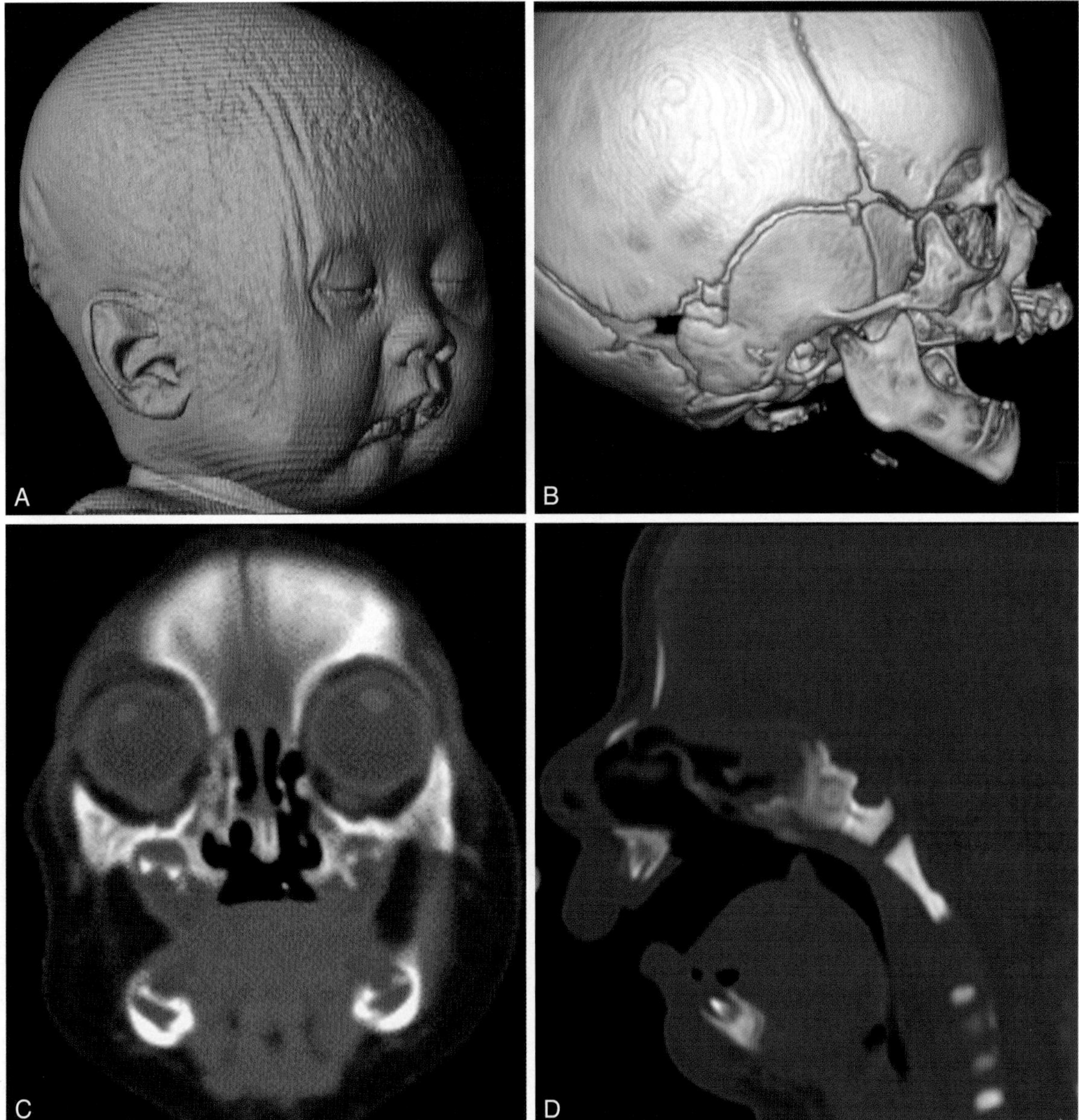

Fig. 12.14 Pierre-Robin. (A to D) 3D volumetric CT images and coronal and sagittal CT images demonstrate micrognathia, retrognathia, glossoptosis, and cleft palate. Low-set ears are also present.

Key Points

Background

- Pierre Robin sequence (PRS) can occur by itself (isolated PRS) or part of a multiple anomaly disorder ("syndromic PRS"). Isolated PRS is often associated with mutation in the SOX9 gene. Syndromic PRS can be caused by collagen gene mutations (Stickler syndrome), 22q11.2 microdeletion (velocradiofacial syndrome), and Treacher Collins syndrome. Stickler syndrome has PRS plus abnormalities of the eyes (retinal detachment, myopia), ears (hearing loss; ossicular malformation), skeleton and joints. Velocardiofacial syndrome has Pierre Robin plus cardiac anomalies, immune system disorders, endocrine disorders, hearing loss, GI and renal abnormalities, and skeletal abnormalities.
- Varying degrees of airway obstruction
- Mandibular distraction is used to treat airway obstruction

Imaging

- Triad of micrognathia, glossoptosis and U-shaped cleft palate

REFERENCE

1. Meyers AB, Zei MG, Denny AD. Imaging neonates and children with Pierre Robin sequence before and after mandibular distraction osteogenesis: what the craniofacial surgeon wants to know. *Pediatr Radiol.* 2015 Aug;45(9):1340–1392.

MICROGNATHIA

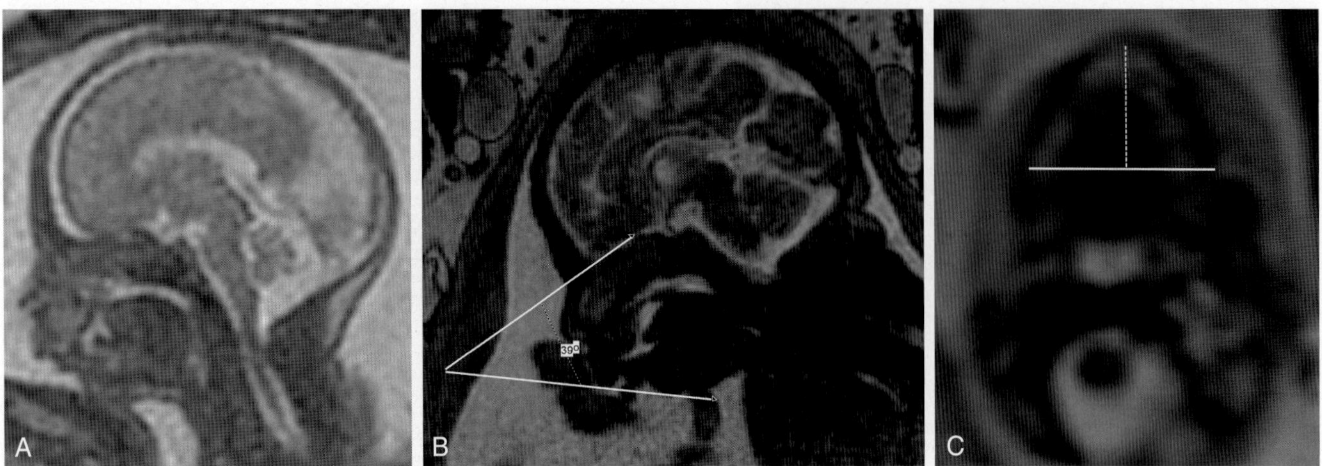

Fig. 12.15 Micrognathia. (A) Sagittal T2W image of micrognathia, retrognathia, and glossoptosis in a patient with Pierre-Robin sequence. (B) Sagittal T2W fetal image in a different patient demonstrating the inferior facial angle is abnormally low measuring 39°. (C) Axial T2W fetal image demonstrating the AP diameter (dashed line) of the mandible in a patient with micrognathia.

Key Points

Background

- The formation of the mandible begins after the 6th week of gestation, requires interactions between the ectoderm of the branchial arches and neural crest cells from the dorsal neural tube, and is susceptible to disruption by genetic and environmental causes.
- Micrognathia occurs in 1:1000 births, is thought to be due to hypoplasia of neural crest cells, and may be isolated or occur in conjunction with other abnormalities. Micrognathia usually occurs simultaneously with retrognathia which is the abnormal posterior position of the mandible with respect to the maxilla.
- Micrognathia is found in over 300 chromosomal and non-chromosomal conditions, some of which include Pierre Robin sequence, Trisomy 13 and 18, DiGeorge Syndrome, Treacher Collins syndrome, Meckel-Gruber syndrome, and Smith-Lemli-Opitz syndrome
- Micrognathia can lead to neonatal respiratory distress, feeding difficulty, and developmental delay

Imaging

- In utero diagnosis is usually made with ultrasound and less commonly with MRI
- Fetal measurements used to diagnose micrognathia and retrognathia include:
  - Inferior facial angle (IFA): In midsagittal view of the face, the IFA is the angle formed by a line is drawn perpendicular to the vertical part of the forehead at the nasal root with line joining the mentum and anterior margin of the upper lip. The normal angle measures 65° +/- 16° and an angle less than 49° is diagnostic of retrognathia with 100% sensitivity and 99% specificity.
  - Anterior-posterior diameter (APD): On axial image through the mandible the APD is the distance of a line drawn posteriorly from the mandibular symphysis intersecting a line drawn between both mandibular angles (usually found by locating the masseter insertion). The mean APD is 19 +/- 2.3 mm.
  - Jaw Index: the Jaw Index = (mandibular APD)/(cerebral biparietal diameter) × 100. A jaw < 23 mm demonstrated 100% sensitivity and 98% specificity for diagnosis of micrognathia.
  - Mandible width/maxilla width: A ratio obtained in axial plane 10 mm posterior to the anterior cortex of the mandible and at the level of the maxillary alveolus. This ratio measures 1.02 +/- 0.12 and is constant in the 2nd trimester. A ratio < 0.78 is used to diagnose micrognathia.

REFERENCES

1. Nemec U, Nemec SF, Brugger PC, et al. Normal mandibular growth and diagnosis of micrognathia at prenatal MRI. *Prenat Diagn*. 2015 Feb;35(2):108–116.
2. Rotten D, Levaillant JM, Martinez H, Ducou le Pointe H, Vicaut E. The fetal mandible: a 2D and 3D sonographic approach to the diagnosis of retrognathia and micrognathia. *Ultrasound Obstet Gynecol.* 2002 Feb;19(2):122–130.
3. Paladini D, Morra T, Teodoro A, Lamberti A, Tremolaterra F, Martinelli P. Objective diagnosis of micrognathia in the fetus: the jaw index. *Obstet Gynecol.* 1999 Mar;93(3):382–386.

HEMIFACIAL MICROSOMIA

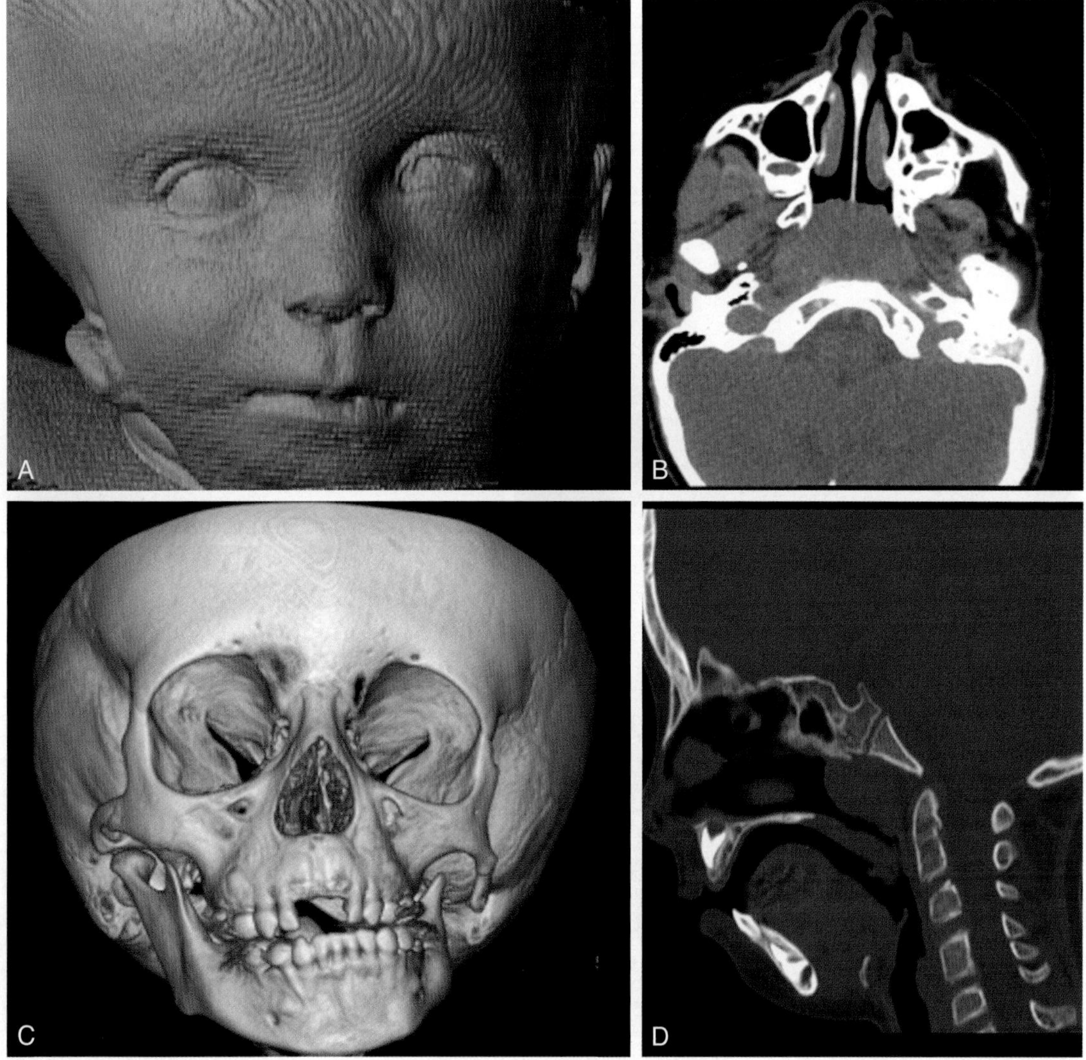

Fig. 12.16 Hemifacial Microsomia. (A to D) 3D volumetric CT images and axial and sagittal CT images demonstrate left mandibular hypoplasia, leftward jaw angulation, left external auditory canal atresia, hypoplastic left muscles of mastication, and segmentation anomalies of the C2-C3 and C5-C6 vertebrae.

Key Points

Background

- Also known as Goldenhar and oculoauriculovertebral syndrome
- Asymmetric malformation affecting the first and second pharyngeal arches
- Second most common craniofacial abnormality after cleft lip and palate
- Etiology unknown but associated with genetic and environmental causes. Potentially due to embryonic hemorrhage at the anastomosis that precedes the formation of the stapedial artery. Damage to the Meckel cartilage that forms the mandible and middle ear may account for the skeletal abnormalities

Imaging

- Unilateral mandibular hypoplasia (ramus, condyle, and coronoid process), small glenoid fossa, hypoplastic zygomatic arch, EAC atresia or stenosis
- Cleft palate +/− cleft lip
- Vertebral anomalies
- Hypoplasia of the muscles of mastication and the parotid gland

REFERENCE

1. Kabak SL, Savrasova NA, Zatochnaya VV, et al. Hemifacial macrosomia: skeletal abnormalities evaluation using CBCT (case report). *J Radiol Case Rep*. 2019 Nov;13(11):1–9.

TREACHER COLLINS

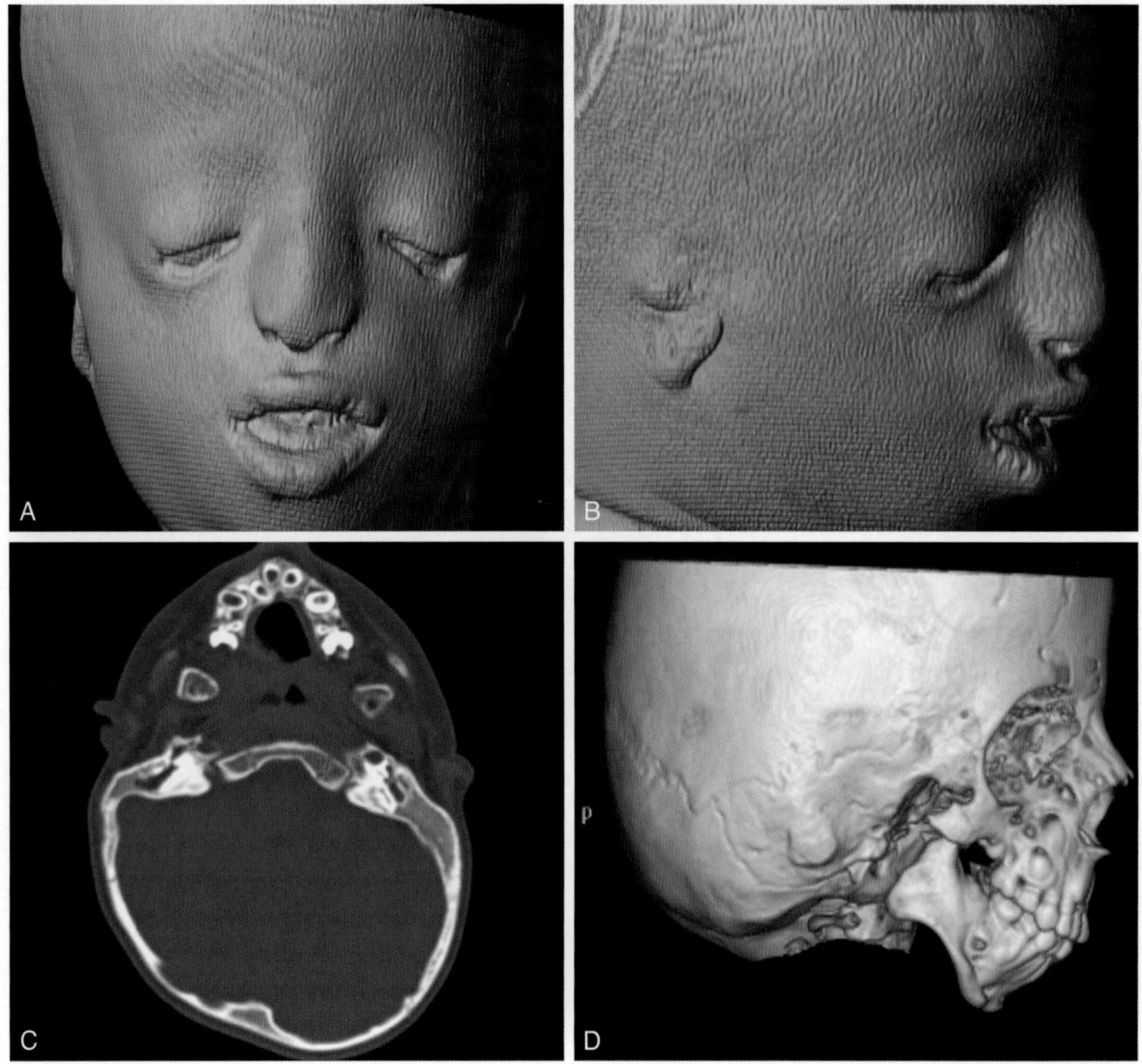

Fig. 12.17 Treacher Collins. (A to D) 3D volumetric CT images and axial CT image demonstrate bilateral mandibular and maxillary hypoplasia, retrognathia, and bilateral external auditory canal atresia.

Key Points

Background

- Also known as mandibulofacial dysostosis
- Caused by mutations in TCOF1 gene (80% of patients) or POLR1B, POLR1C, or POLR1D genes. TCOF1 and POLR1B cause autosomal dominant inheritance; intelligence is usually normal

Imaging

- Face: Cleft lip and palate, micrognathia, and glossoptosis which are features of Pierre Robin sequence as well as maxillary hypoplasia
- Eye: Coloboma
- Ear: Microtia, EAC atresia, ossicle malformations, and inner ear anomalies
- Often bilateral and symmetric anomalies. No limb anomalies

REFERENCE

1. Lowe LH, Booth TN, Joglar JM, et al. Midface anomalies in children. *Radiographics*. 2000;20(4):907–922.

CLEIDOCRANIAL DYSPLASIA

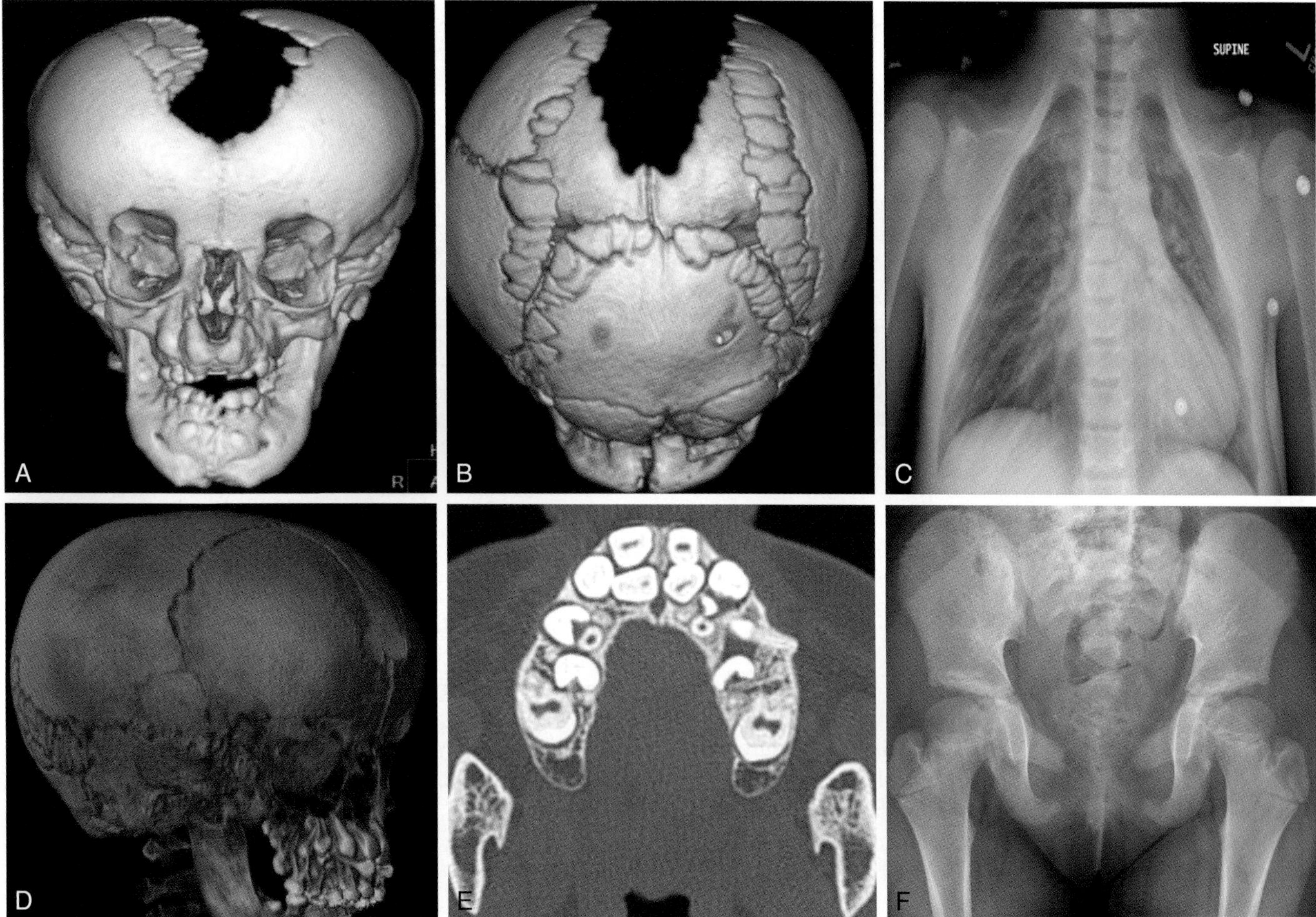

Fig. 12.18 Cleidocranial Dysplasia. (A and B) 3D volumetric CT images demonstrate wide metopic and sagittal sutures, inverted pear-shaped calvarium, and multiple intrasutural ossicles (also known as wormian bones). (C) AP chest radiograph demonstrates absent clavicles. (D and E) 3D volumetric CT and axial CT image demonstrate delayed eruption of primary teeth and impacted supernumerary teeth. (F) AP pelvis radiograph demonstrates wide pubic symphysis.

Key Points

Background

- Developmental anomaly of the bones and teeth
- *RUNX2* gene mutation detected in 65% of patients. *RUNX2* is involved with osteoblast differentiation and skeletal development

Imaging

- Skull: Wormian bones, wide sutures, inverted pear-shaped calvarium, late closure of the fontanelle
- Face: Midface retrusion, prognathia, delayed eruption of primary teeth, and impacted supernumerary teeth
- Ear: EAC atresia or stenosis, ossicular anomalies
- Orbits: Hypertelorism
- Other: partial or complete aplasia of the *clavicles.* Short stature. Delayed ossification of the pelvic bones. Widened pubic symphysis.

REFERENCE

1. Farrow E, Nicot R, Wiss A, et al. Cleidocranial dysplasia: a review of clinical, radiological, genetic implications and a guidelines proposal. *J Craniofac Surg*. 2018 mar;29(2):382–389.

MORNING GLORY DISC ANOMALY

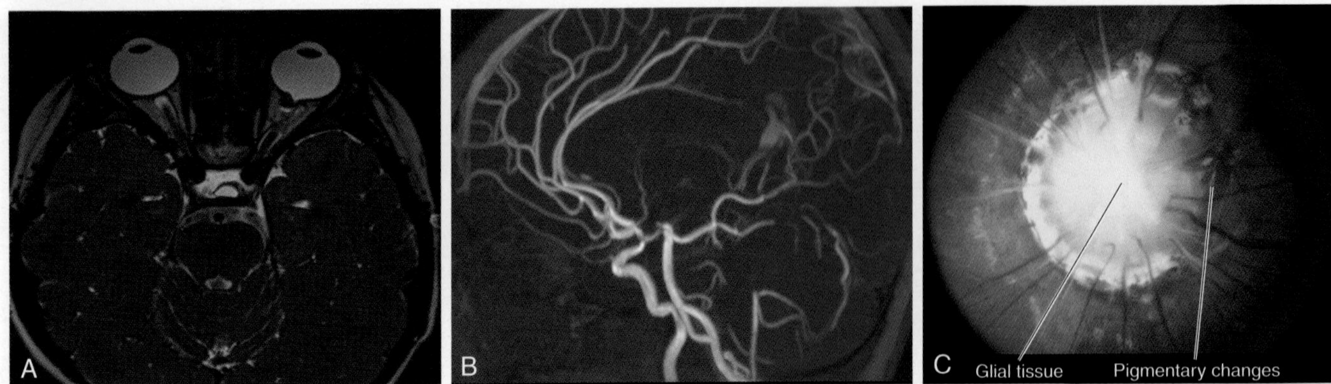

Fig. 12.19 Morning Glory Disc Anomaly. (A) Axial T2W image demonstrating abnormal left optic disc with funnel shape disc, elevation of the adjacent retinal surface, and effaced distal optic nerve sheath. (B) Sagittal volumetric MR angiography image demonstrating left supraclinoid internal carotid artery stenosis. (C) Morning glory syndrome demonstrating the characteristic appearance with central white glial tissue, surrounding pigmentary changes, and straightened spoke-like vessels radiating from the disc. (C from Kaiser PK, Friedman NJ, Pineda R II. *The Massachusetts Eye and Ear Infirmary Illustrated Manual of Ophthalmology.* 5th ed. Elsevier; 2021.)

Key Points

Background

- Rare congenital malformation of the optic nerve
- Etiology unknown but possibly from failure of closure of the fetal fissure or primary mesenchymal anomaly
- Enlarged, funnel-shaped excavation in the optic disc; an annulus of chorioretinal pigmentary changes that surrounds the optic disc excavation; and a central glial tuft overlying the optic disc

Imaging

- Funnel-shaped morphology of the optic disc, adjacent elevation of the retinal surface, and abnormal tissue associated with the distal intraorbital segment of the optic nerve effacing the subarachnoid space at that level, and discontinuity of uveal scleral coat at the optic nerve insertion
- Associated anomalies: Midline craniofacial and skull base defects (basal encephalocele), vascular abnormalities (carotid stenosis, moyamoya), agenesis of corpus callosum, and PHACES syndrome

REFERENCES

1. Vachha BA, Robson CD. Imaging of Pediatric Orbital Disease. *Neuroimaging Clin N Am.* 2015 Aug;25(3):477–501.
2. Ellika S, Robson CD, Heidary G, et al. Morning glory disc anomaly, characteristic MR imaging findings. *AJNR Am J Neuroradiol.* 2013;35(5):525–528.

PERSISTENT FETAL VASCULATURE

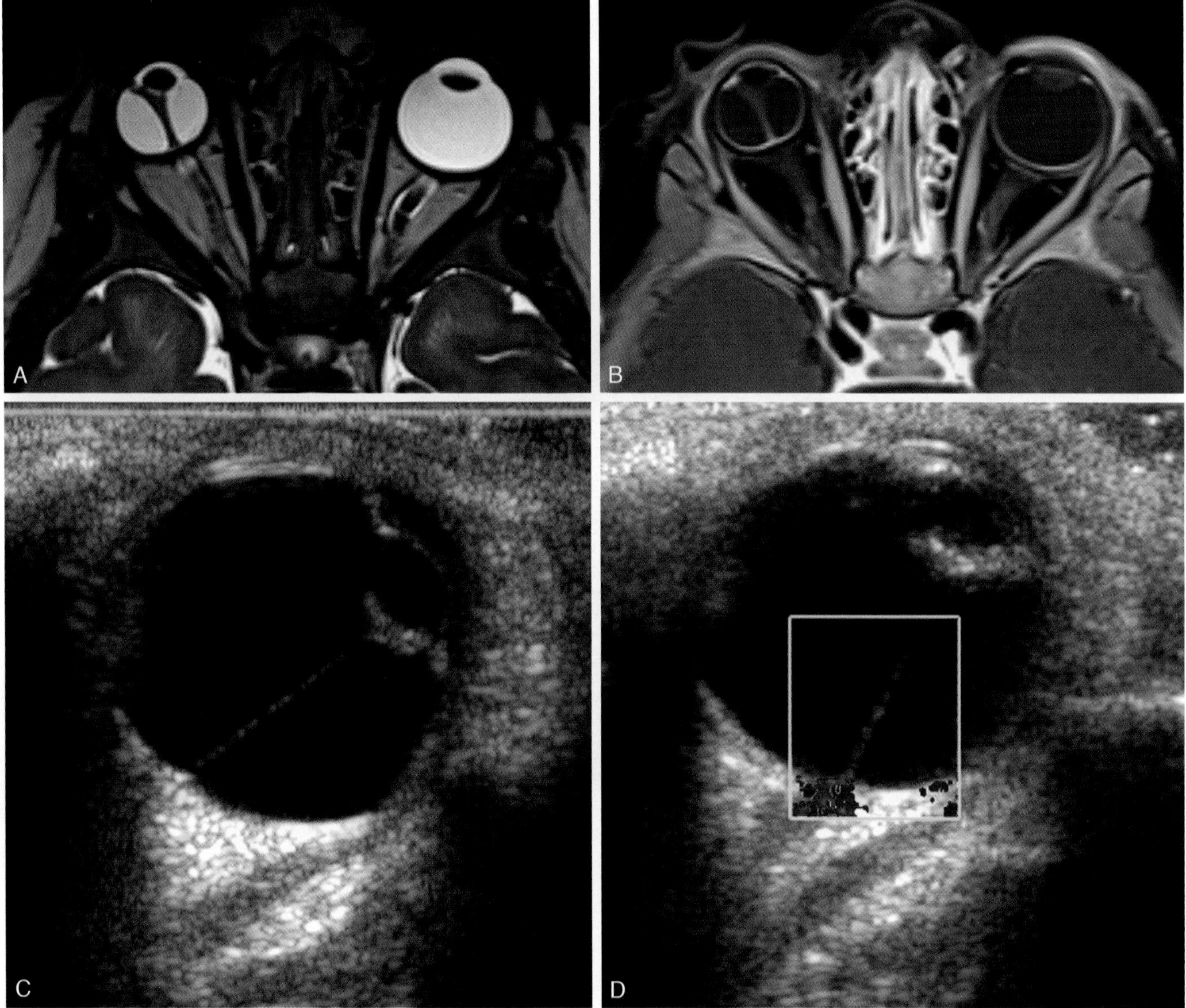

Fig. 12.20 Persistent Hyperplastic Primary Vitreous. (A) Axial T2W and (B) axial T1W+C images demonstrate small right globe with abnormal intraocular triangular and linear tissue ("martini sign"). (C and D) Ultrasound images of the globe without and with color Doppler demonstrate the persistent fetal vasculature of PHPV.

Key Points

Background

- Also known as persistent hyperplastic primary vitreous (PHPV)
- Primary vitreous is the embryonic vasculature to the eye, predominantly supplied by the hyaloid artery. Cloquet's canal contains the hyaloid artery and extends from optic nerve to posterior aspect of lens. Normal regression occurs at 20 weeks' gestational age. PHPV results from failure of normal regression
- Clinical: Unilateral process; leukocoria; limited treatment options

Imaging

- Small globe
- Triangular retrolental mass (martini glass sign) demonstrating T1 and T2 hypointense signal and enhancement
- Anterior displaced lens
- Retinal or posterior hyaloid detachment
- Hemorrhage and debris
- No calcification

REFERENCE

1. Vachha BA, Robson CD. Imaging of Pediatric Orbital Disease. *Neuroimaging Clin N Am*. 2015 Aug;25(3):477–501.

MICROPHTHALMIA

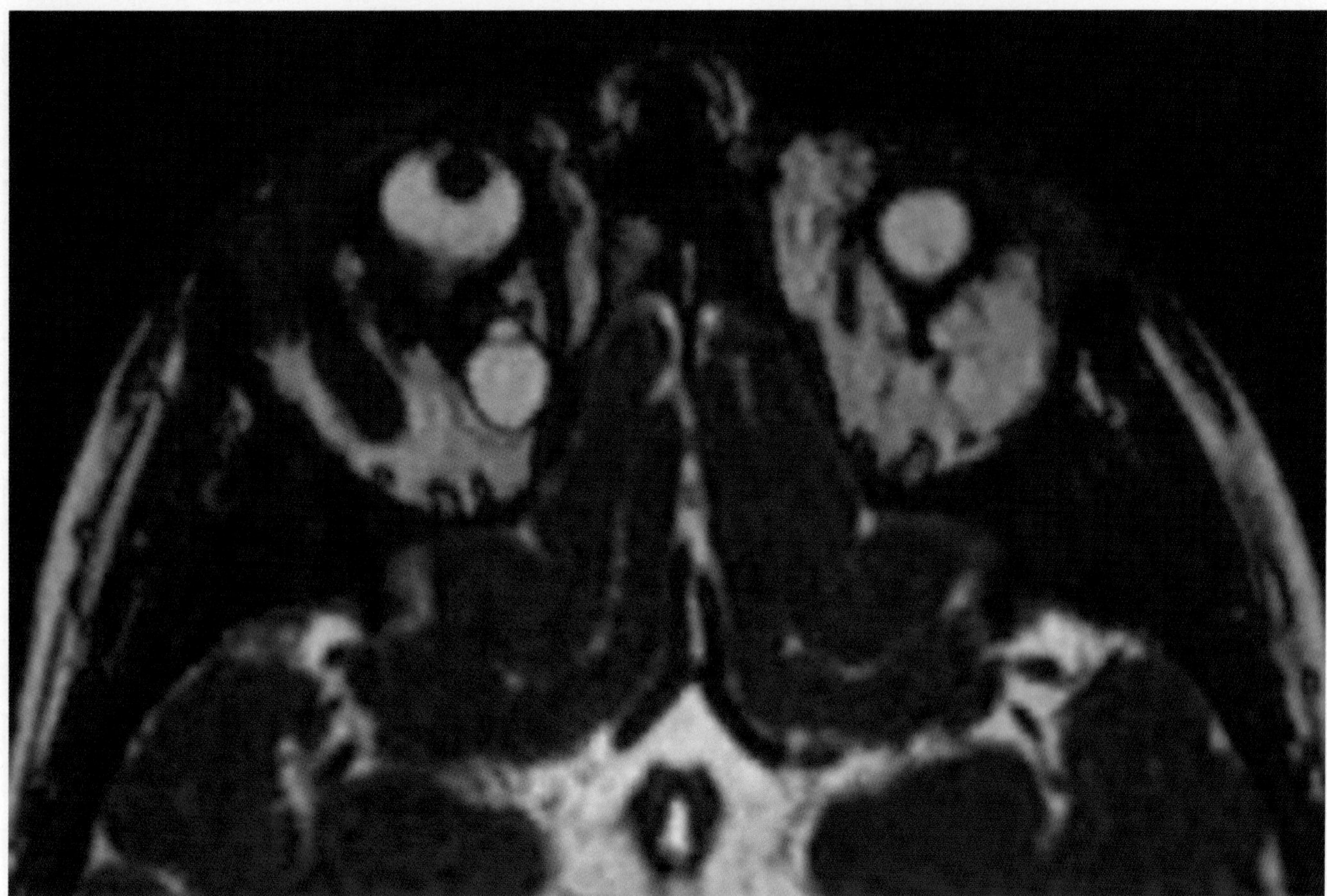

Fig. 12.21 Microphthalmia. A T2W image demonstrating small right and left globes with colobomatous cyst in the right orbit.

Key Points

Background

- Can be inherited due to genetic abnormality or acquired (e.g., infection, retinopathy of prematurity, trauma) and can be associated with brain malformations, including agenesis of the corpus callosum, basal encephalocele, and microcephaly
- Simple microphthalmia refers to an intact globe with mildly decreased length
- Complex microphthalmia includes anterior or posterior segment globe dysgenesis

Imaging

- The globe size is measured using the axial ocular length, which is distance from the anterior cornea to the optic nerve insertion
- Microphthalmia measures less than 2 standard deviations from the mean, which is <19 mm in a 1-year-old or <21 mm in an adult
- Severe microphthalmia refers to axial length <10 mm at birth or <12 mm after 1 year of age

REFERENCE

1. Vachha BA, Robson CD. Imaging of Pediatric Orbital Disease. *Neuroimaging Clin N Am*. 2015 Aug;25(3):477–501.

RETINOPATHY OF PREMATURITY

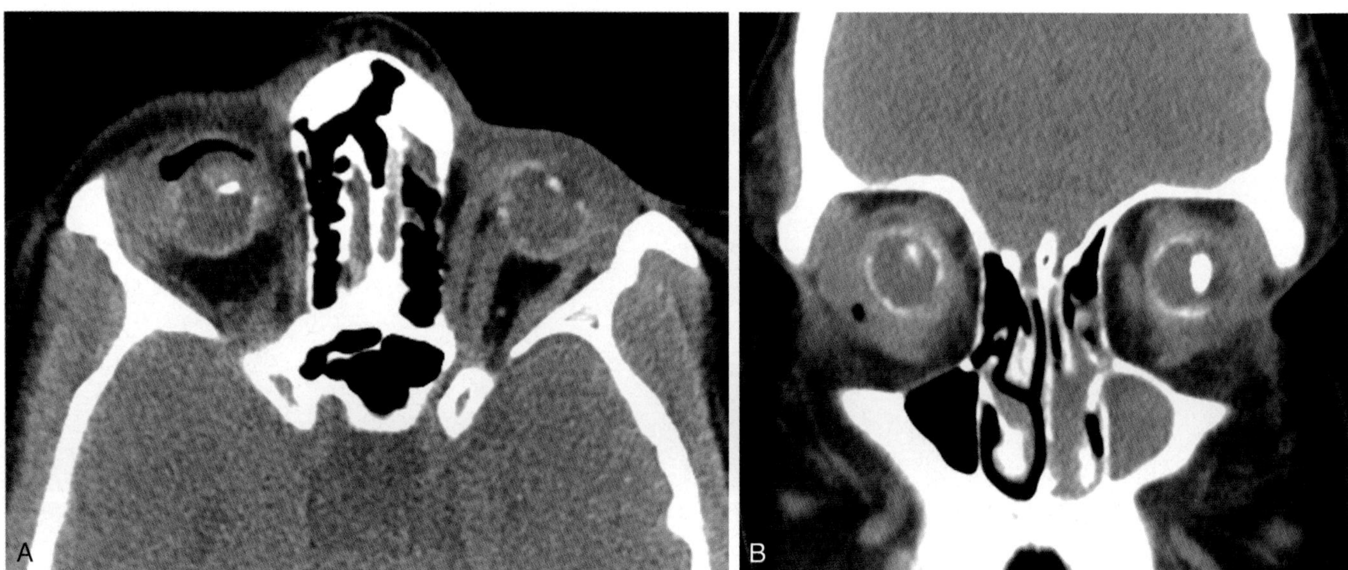

Fig. 12.22 Retinopathy of Prematurity. (A and B) Axial and coronal CT images demonstrate small right and left globes with dystrophic calcifications and abnormal lenses. Calcification is not a prominent feature of ROP but can be seen.

Key Points

Background

- A vasculoproliferative disorder occurring in premature newborns with very low birth weight
- Presumed etiology from hyperoxygenation. Greater duration of oxygen exposure associated with severity of disease

Imaging

- Usually bilateral small globes
- Chronic stage demonstrates retrolental hyperdense mass +/− retinal detachment
- Calcification occasionally present but not a dominant feature

REFERENCE

1. Rossi A. Pediatric Neuroradiology 1st edition. Springer-Verlag Berlin Heidelberg.

UNCOMMON OCULAR ANOMALIES

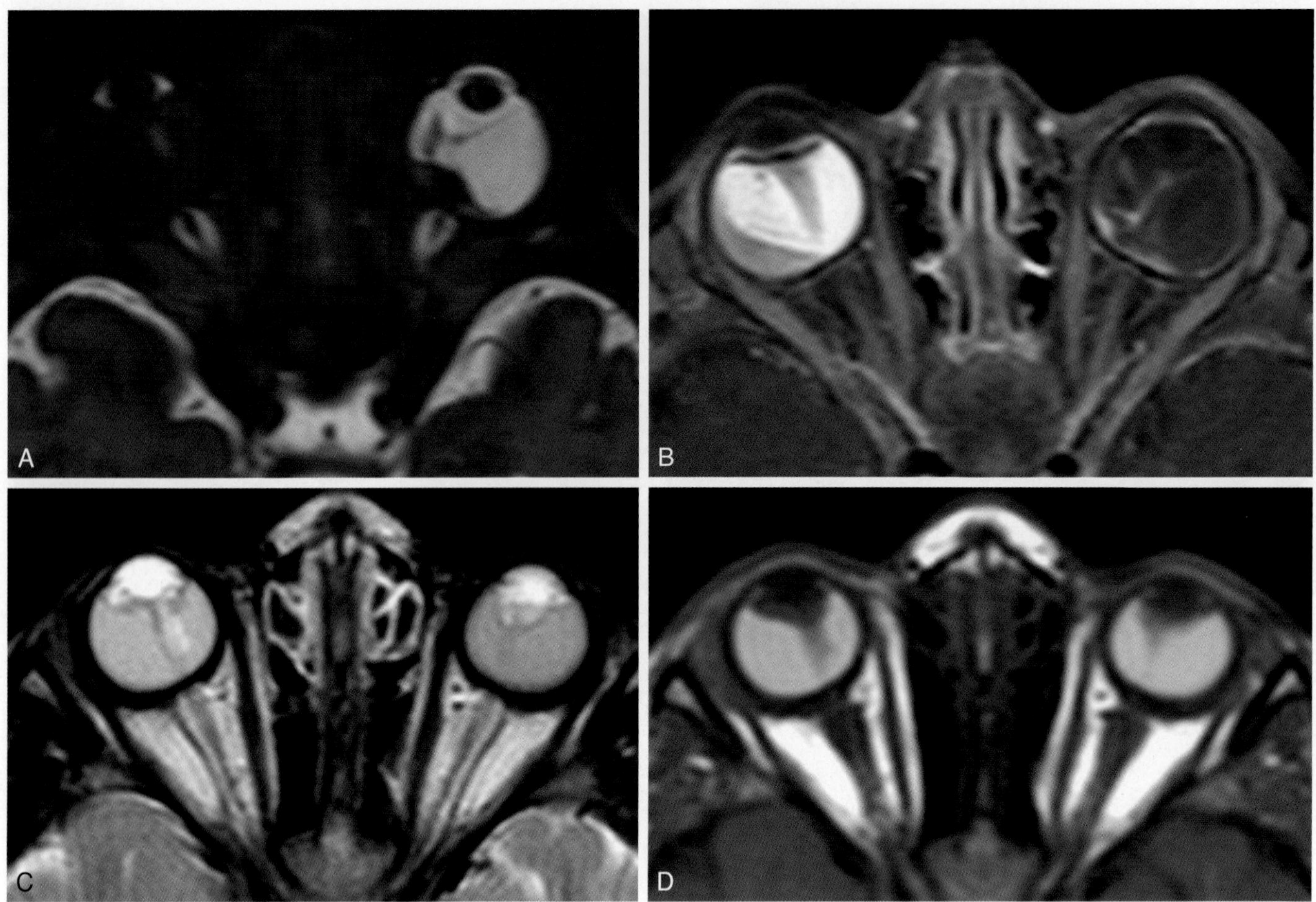

Fig. 12.23 Norrie Disease. (A) Axial T2W and (B) axial T1W+C images demonstrate bilateral PHPV as well as retinal detachments, and subretinal hemorrhagic effusions. (C) Axial T2W and (D) axial T1W images demonstrate bilateral PHPV with retinal detachments, and subretinal proteinaceous effusions.

Key Points

- Norrie disease: X-linked disorder caused by mutation in the Norrie disease protein *(NDP)* gene. Presents with leukocoria, vision loss, and progressive hearing loss. Imaging on CT demonstrate hyperdense vitreous without calcification. MRI demonstrates bilateral PHPV, retinal detachment, and subretinal hemorrhagic effusion.
- Coats disease: Rare exudative retinopathy with retinal telangiectasias leading to subretinal exudates and retinal detachment. Usually isolated but can also occur with Norrie disease. Presents with leukocoria and vision loss. Imaging demonstrates retinal detachment, subretinal effusion with T1W hyperintensity on MRI from proteinaceous, hemorrhagic, and cholesterol crystals; 90% unilateral; hyperdense fluid on CT but no calcification. Treated with laser photocoagulation and cryotherapy.

REFERENCE

1. Payabvash S, Anderson JS, Nascene DR. Bilateral persistent fetal vasculature due to a mutation in the Norrie disease protein gene. *Neuroradiol J*. 2015 Dec;28(6):623–627.

RADIOTHERAPY-RELATED HEMIFACIAL ATROPHY

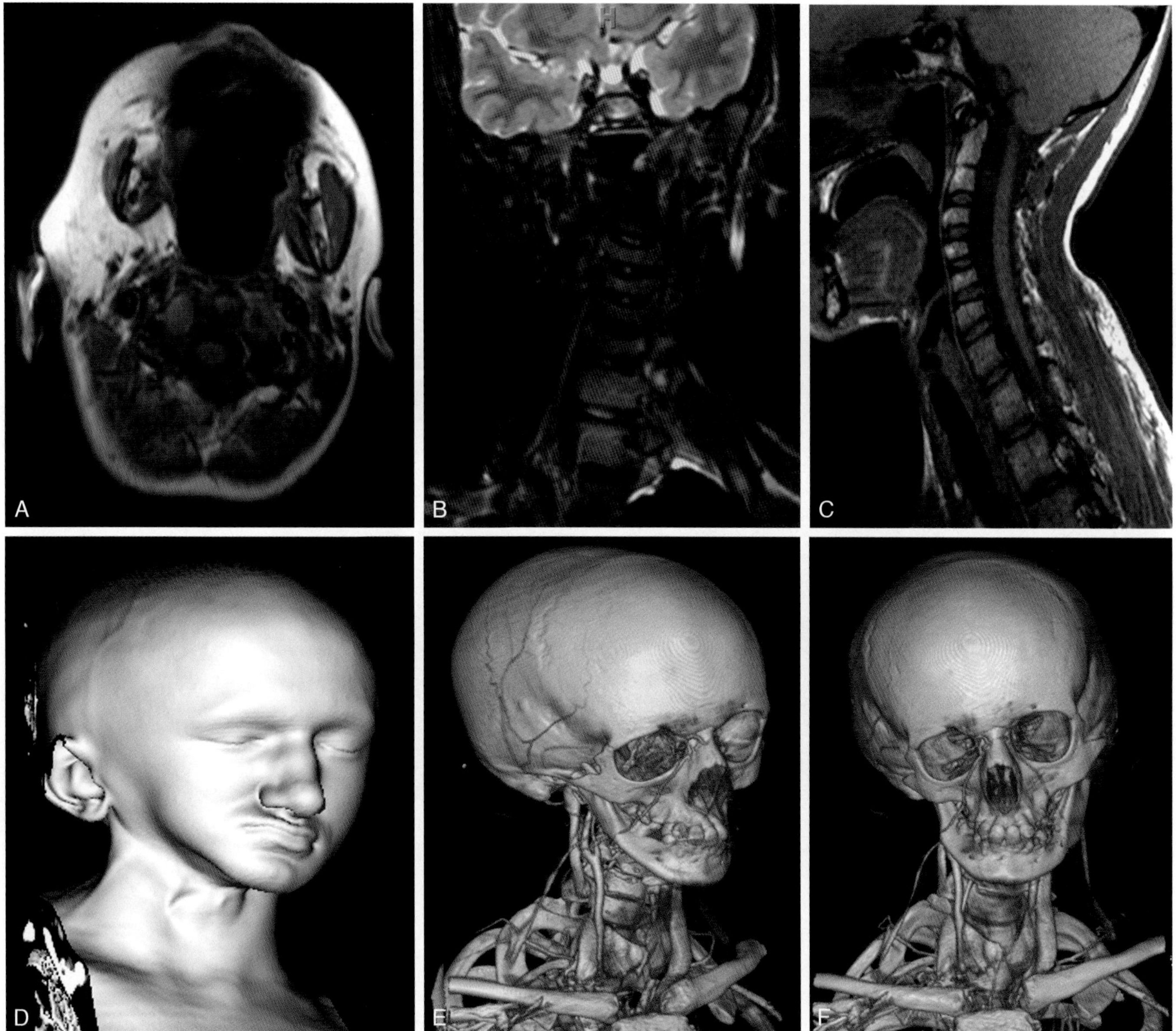

Fig. 12.24 Radiotherapy-Related Atrophy. (A) Axial T1W, (B) coronal T2W fat saturation, and (C) sagittal T1W images demonstrate right masseter and medial pterygoid muscle atrophy, reduced height, and fatty marrow in the C3-C6 vertebral bodies and basilar invagination. (D to F) 3D volumetric CT images demonstrate the right facial atrophy and right head tilt.

Key Points

- Following head and neck radiotherapy, soft tissue atrophy of the muscles, subcutaneous fat, and salivary glands can occur and result in facial asymmetry.
- The age at which the facial tissue is least at risk for atrophy and the duration from time of radiotherapy to tissue atrophy has yet to be researched.

CHOANAL ATRESIA

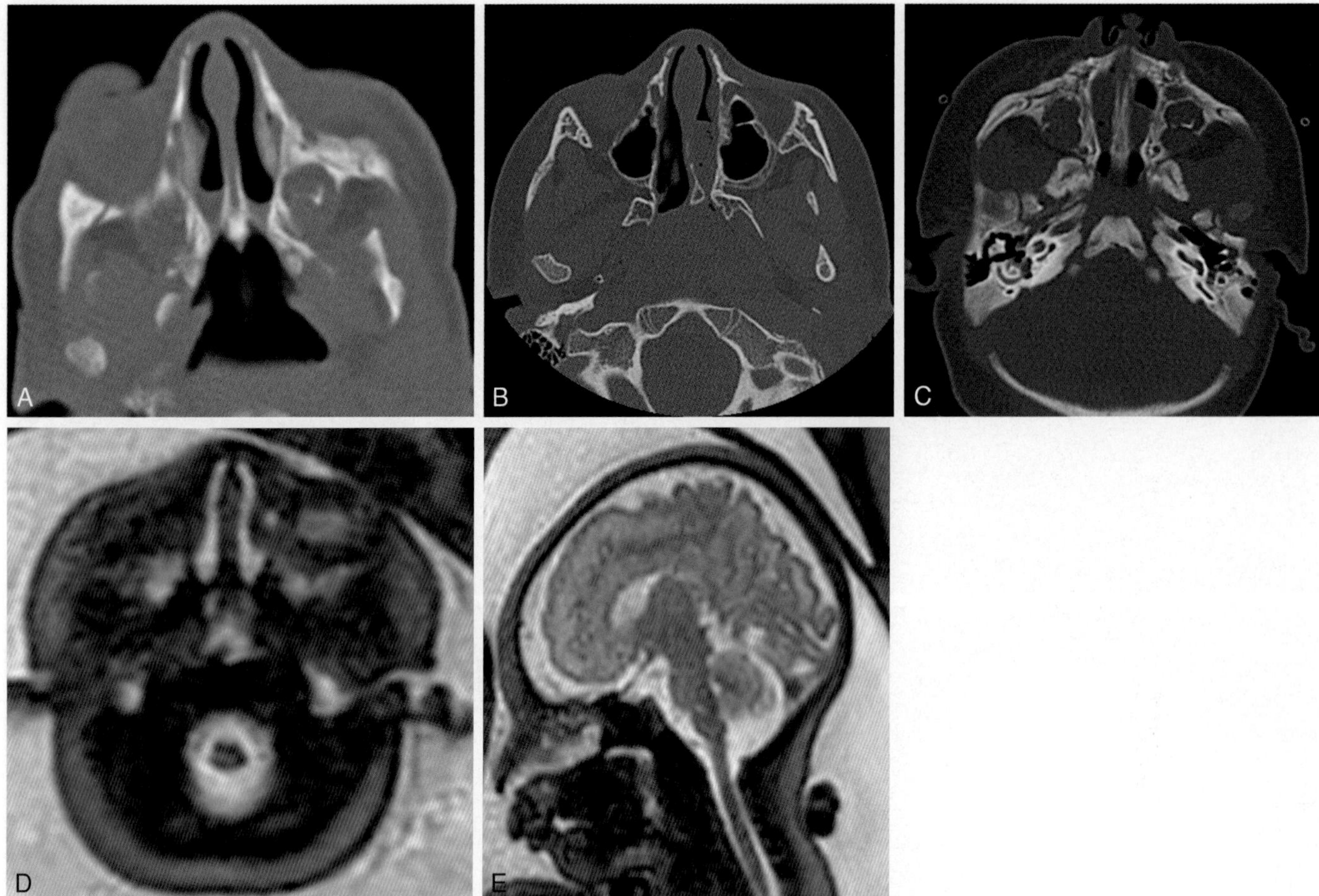

Fig. 12.25 Choanal Atresia. (A) Axial CT image demonstrates narrow bilateral choana with membranous occlusions. (B) Axial CT image demonstrating left choana osseous narrowing and membranous occlusion. (C) Axial CT image demonstrating bilateral osseous choanal narrowing with membranous occlusion. (D and E) Axial and sagittal T2W fetal images demonstrate bilateral choanal atresia seen as dark signal interrupting the T2 hyperintense fluid signal in the posterior nasal cavity.

Key Points

Background

- Most common cause of neonatal nasal obstruction (1 per 5000 to 8000 neonates). Common cause of inability to pass nasogastric tube
- 66% unilateral (present late or are asymptomatic); 33% bilateral (neonates with respiratory distress). Bilateral requires securing an airway in the neonate
- Associated with numerous conditions e.g., CHARGE, Apert syndrome, Treacher Collins syndrome, cleft palate, congenital heart disease, and craniosynostosis
- Choanal atresia can present on fetal imaging with polyhydramnios.

Imaging

- Obstruction or narrowing (<3.4 mm) of choanal opening
- Posterior nasal cavity obstruction/narrowing, medial bowing of posterior nasal cavity, thickening of posterior vomer (>3.4 mm); mixed bony and membranous atresia in 70%, pure bony atresia in 30%

REFERENCES

1. Lowe LH, Booth TN, Joglar JM, et al. Midface anomalies in children. *Radiographics*. 2000;20(4):907–922.
2. Slovis TL, Renfro B, Watts FB, et al. Choanal atresia: precise CT evaluation. *Radiology*. 1985;155(2):345–348.

CHARGE SYNDROME

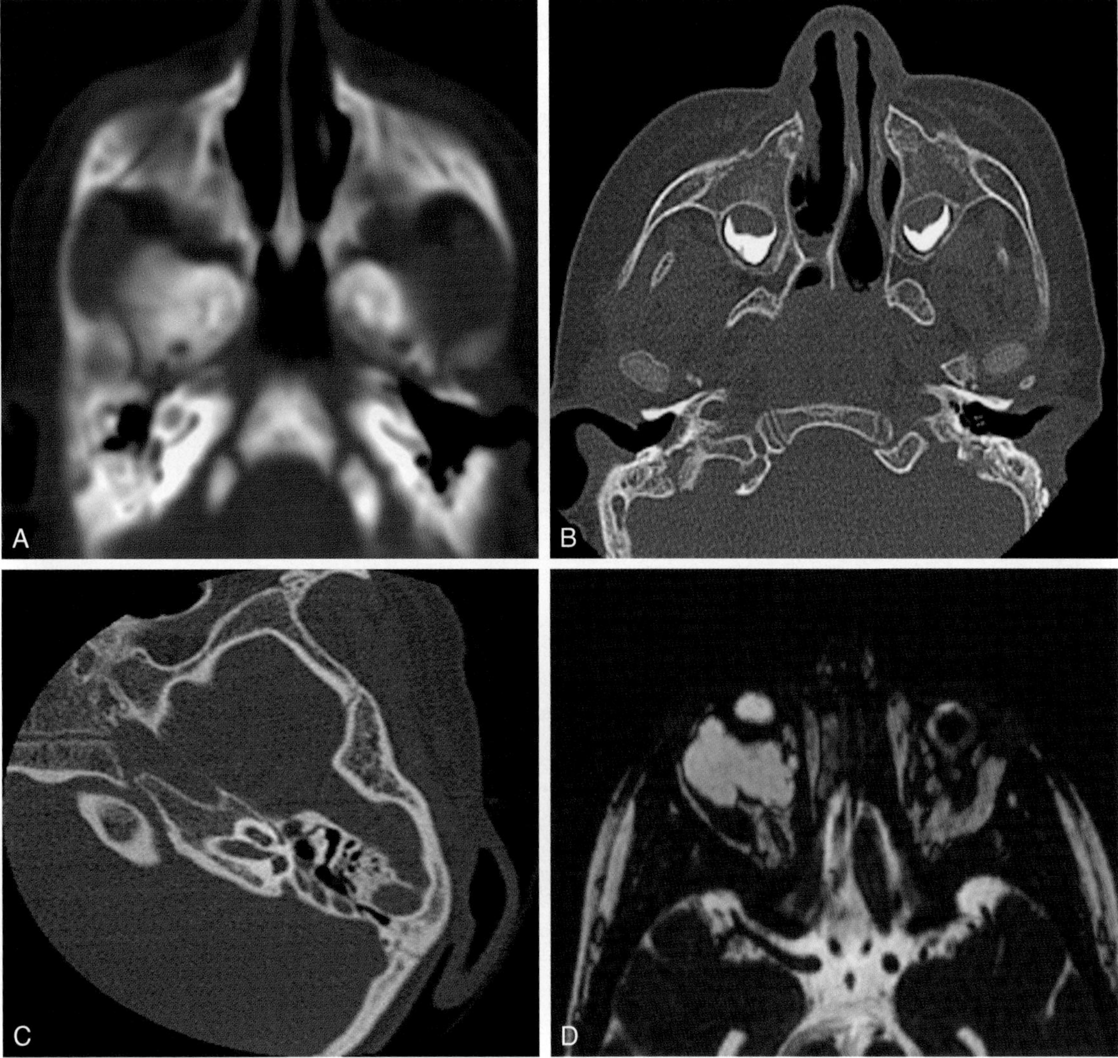

Fig. 12.26 CHARGE Syndrome. (A) Axial CT image demonstrates bilateral choanal atresia with osseous and membranous occlusion. (B) Axial CT image demonstrating right choanal atresia. (C) Axial CT image demonstrating left cochlear aperture stenosis and large vestibular aqueduct. (D) Axial T2 W image demonstrating bilateral microphthalmia and large right coloboma.

Key Points

Background

- CHARGE:
  Coloboma of the eye[a]
  Heart defects
  Atresia of the choana[a]
  Retardation of growth and/or development,
  Genital and/or urinary abnormalities
  Ear abnormalities, and deafness[a]
- Most cases are sporadic with *CHD7* gene mutation as the cause (in 2/3)

([a] Major criteria)

Imaging

- Face: Choanal atresia, cleft palate, coloboma, parotid dysplasia, prominent emissary veins
- Temporal bone: Dysplasia of the vestibule, semicircular canals, IAC, cochlea; cochlear nerve hypoplasia; absent cochlear aperture; large vestibular aqueduct
- Skull: Hypoplasia, J-shaped sella, dorsally angulated clivus
- Olfactory nerve hypoplasia, groove and sulcus dysplasia
- CNS brainstem hypoplasia, vermian hypoplasia, ventriculomegaly

REFERENCE

1. Hoch MJ, Patel SH, Jethanamest D, et al. Head and neck MRI findings in CHARGE syndrome. *AJNR Am J Neuroradiol.* December 2017;38:2357–2363.

PYRIFORM APERTURE STENOSIS

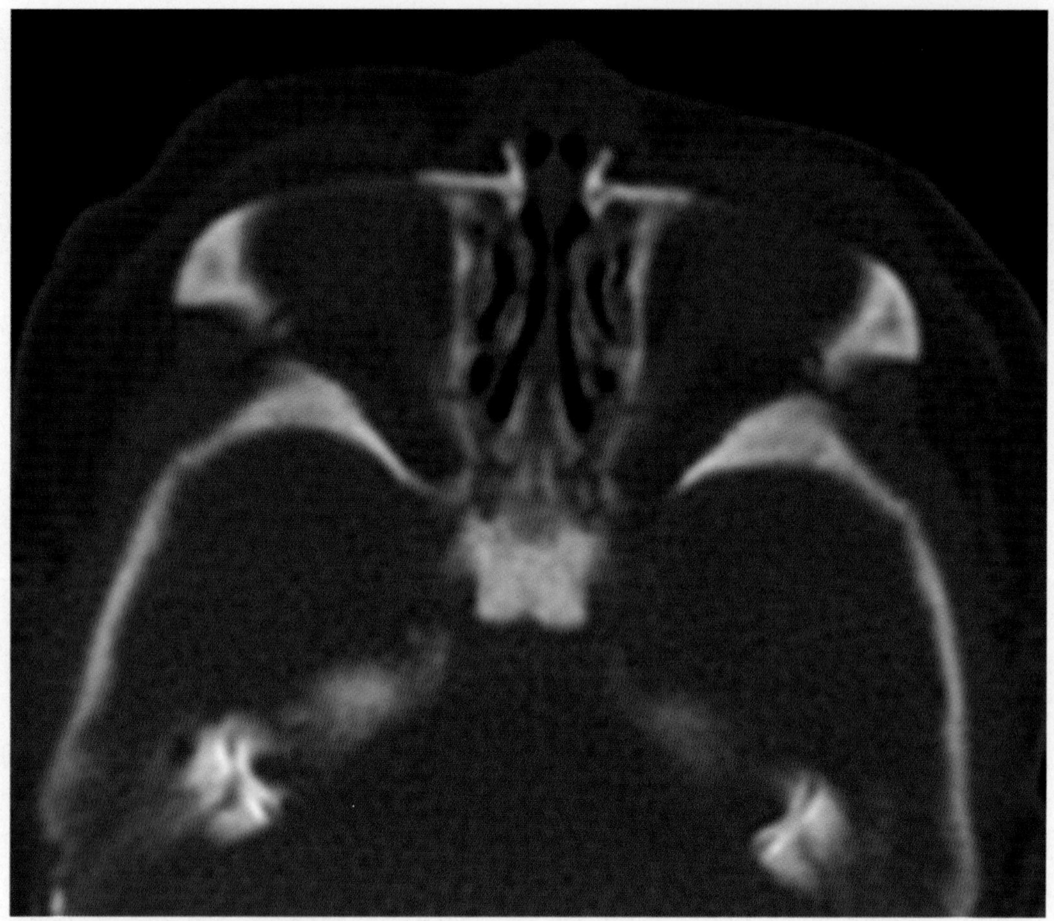

Fig. 12.27 Pyriform Aperture Stenosis. Axial CT image demonstrates narrow bilateral pyriform apertures.

Key Points

Background

- Rare cause of airway obstruction in the neonate caused by hypertrophy and fusion of the medial nasal processes

Imaging

- Narrowing of the pyriform aperture <11 mm; inward bowing and thickening of the nasal process of the maxilla
- Associated anomalies: central maxillary incisor, hemangioma, holoprosencephaly, hypopituitarism

REFERENCE

1. Lowe LH, Booth TN, Joglar JM, et al. Midface anomalies in children. *Radiographics*. 2000;20(4):907–922.

13 Temporal Bone Malformations

INTRODUCTION

Background

- Within a space of less than a few centimeters, the temporal bone contains highly specialized small anatomic structures that allow for hearing and balance.
- The temporal bone is composed of five parts (petrous, tympanic, squamosal, mastoid, and zygomatic) and is subdivided as the inner ear, middle ear, and external ear.
- The inner ear converts mechanical pressure into electrical signal to provide hearing and balance function. The inner ear contains the cochlea, vestibule, semicircular canals, cochlear aqueduct, vestibular aqueduct, oval window, and round window. The cochlea has 2½ turns, and the cochlear nerve enters the cochlea through the cochlear aperture to terminate on an osseous structure called the modiolus. The modiolus is attached to an osseous structure called the spiral lamina, forming a structure similar to a threaded screw. The spiral lamina has two membranes that separate each turn of the cochlea into three compartments. From lateral to medial the layers are the scala vestibuli → vestibular membrane (also known as Reissner membrane) → scala media (also known as cochlear duct) → basilar membrane → scala tympani. The scala vestibule terminates at the oval window, and the scala tympani terminates at the round window. The scala media contains the organ of Corti, which has the sensory receptors of the cochlear nerve and contains endolymph, whereas the scala tympani and scala vestibuli contain perilymph. The vestibule contains the utricle and saccule and with the three semicircular canals (lateral, superior, and posterior) provides balance information.
- The middle ear is subdivided into the epitympanum, mesotympanum, and hypotympanum and contains the ossicles (malleus, incus, and stapes) (Figure 13.2). The first branchial apparatus gives rise to the malleus, incus, and tensor tympani, while the second branchial apparatus gives rise to the stapes and facial nerve. The epitympanum communicates with the mastoid through the aditus ad antrum and the nasopharynx through the eustachian tube.
- The external ear includes the auricle and external auditory canal and arises from the first branchial apparatus.
- The facial nerve in the temporal bone consists of the canalicular, labyrinthine, genu, tympanic, and mastoid segments and exits the temporal bone at the stylomastoid foramen.

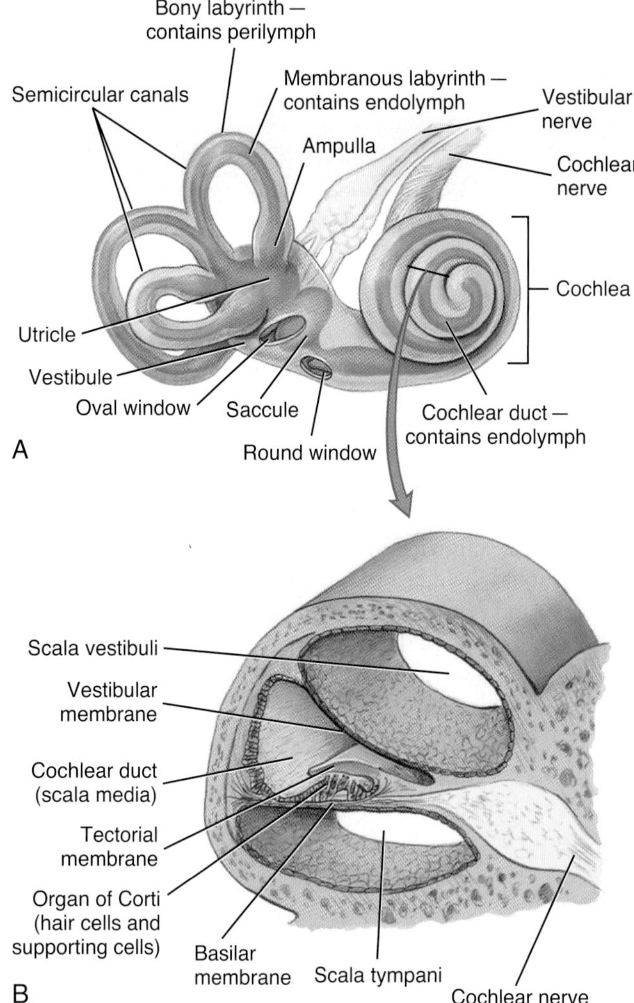

Fig. 13.1 The Inner Ear. (A) The bony labyrinth (tan) is the hard outer wall of the entire inner ear and includes the semicircular canals, vestibule, and cochlea. Within the bony labyrinth is the membranous labyrinth (purple), which is surrounded by perilymph and filled with endolymph. Each ampulla in the vestibule contains a crista ampullaris that detects changes in head position and sends sensory impulses through the vestibular nerve to the brain. (B) Section of the membranous cochlea. Hair cells in the organ of Corti detect sound and send the information through the cochlear nerve. The vestibular and cochlear nerves join to form the eighth cranial nerve. (From Applegate E: The anatomy and physiology learning system, 4th ed, St Louis, 2010, Saunders. In Rogers JL, Brashers VL: McCance & Huether's pathophysiology: the biologic basis for disease in adults and children, 9th ed, St. Louis, 2023, Elsevier.)

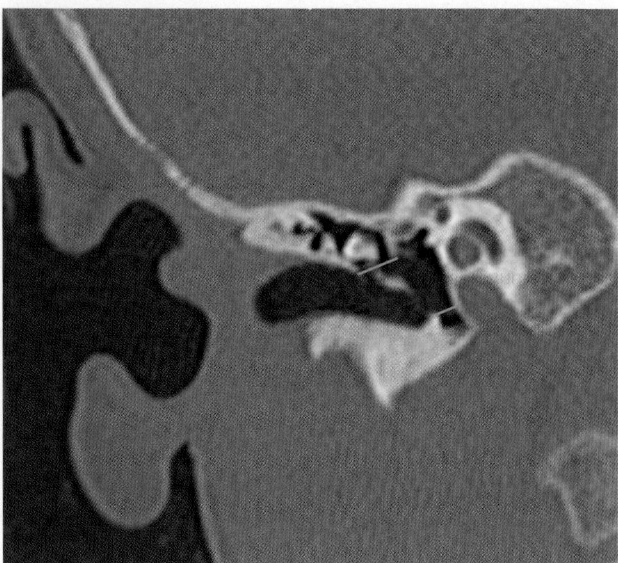

Fig. 13.2 Compartments of the middle ear.

- Malformations of the temporal bone can result in sensorineural and/or conductive hearing depending on the anatomic structure involved.

Imaging

- An imaging approach to malformations of the temporal bone should include a systematic assessment of the inner, middle, and external ear. Conductive hearing loss is typically a problem of the external or middle ear, while sensorineural hearing loss is a problem of the inner ear.
- MRI should be performed with 3D T2W sequences with 1-mm slice thickness. The advantage of MRI over CT is that MRI allows for visualization of the cochlear nerve, whereas CT may only infer the small size of the cochlear nerve based on a small internal auditory canal or cochlear aperture.
- CT allows for thin section imaging with fast acquisition, which may eliminate need for sedation in some patients. CT imaging of the temporal bone should be acquired with bone algorithm using 1 mm or less axial slice thickness and reformatted into coronal plane. Sagittal and oblique reformatted images can be helpful for evaluating ossicular erosions or malformations and for evaluating dehiscence of semicircular canals. Soft tissue algorithms should be reviewed for intracranial or periauricular abnormalities.
- MRI of the temporal bone should include thin-section 3D T2W sequences with 1 mm or less slice thickness and precontrast thin section (3 mm or less) T1W imaging. Precontrast T1W imaging is useful for evaluation of T1W hyperintense signal in the inner ear, which signifies proteinaceous or hemorrhagic fluid from a labyrinthitis, as well as for masses such as lipomas or dermoid cysts which have lipid. Thin-section postcontrast T1W imaging can be added if there is need for assessing for inner ear enhancement from labyrinthitis and for a vestibular schwannoma. The advantage of MRI over CT is that MRI allows for visualization of the cochlear nerve, whereas CT may only infer small size of the cochlear nerve based on a small internal auditory canal or cochlear aperture.
- The following cases illustrate common and uncommon malformations in children affecting the inner, middle, and external ear.

INNER EAR MALFORMATIONS

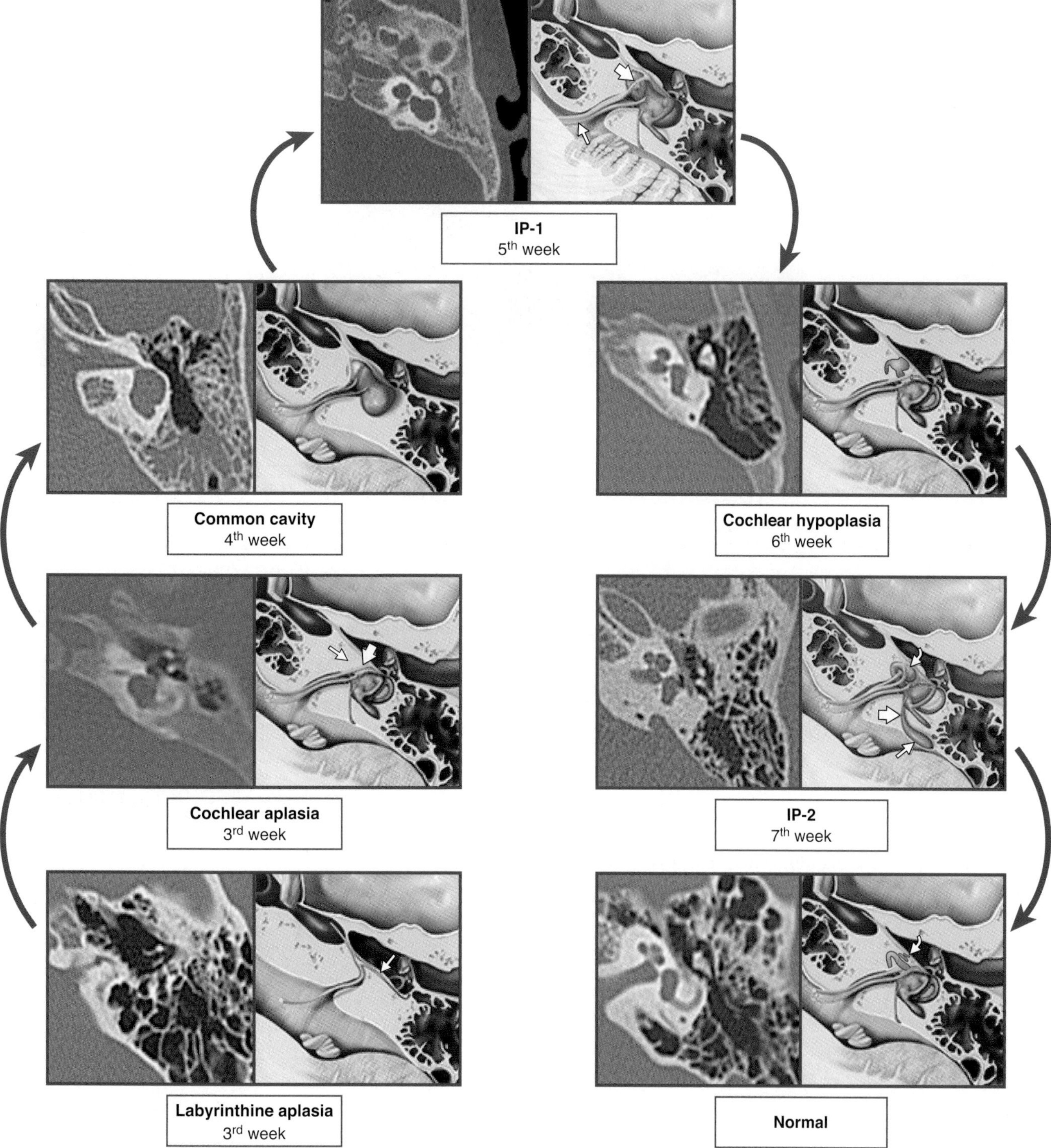

Fig. 13.3 The spectrum of inner ear malformation imaging findings reflects the timing of insult during gestation. Earlier insults lead to less formation of inner ear structures. (Illustrations from StatDX, Copyright © 2022 Elsevier.)

INCOMPLETE PARTITION ANOMALY TYPE 1 (IP-1)

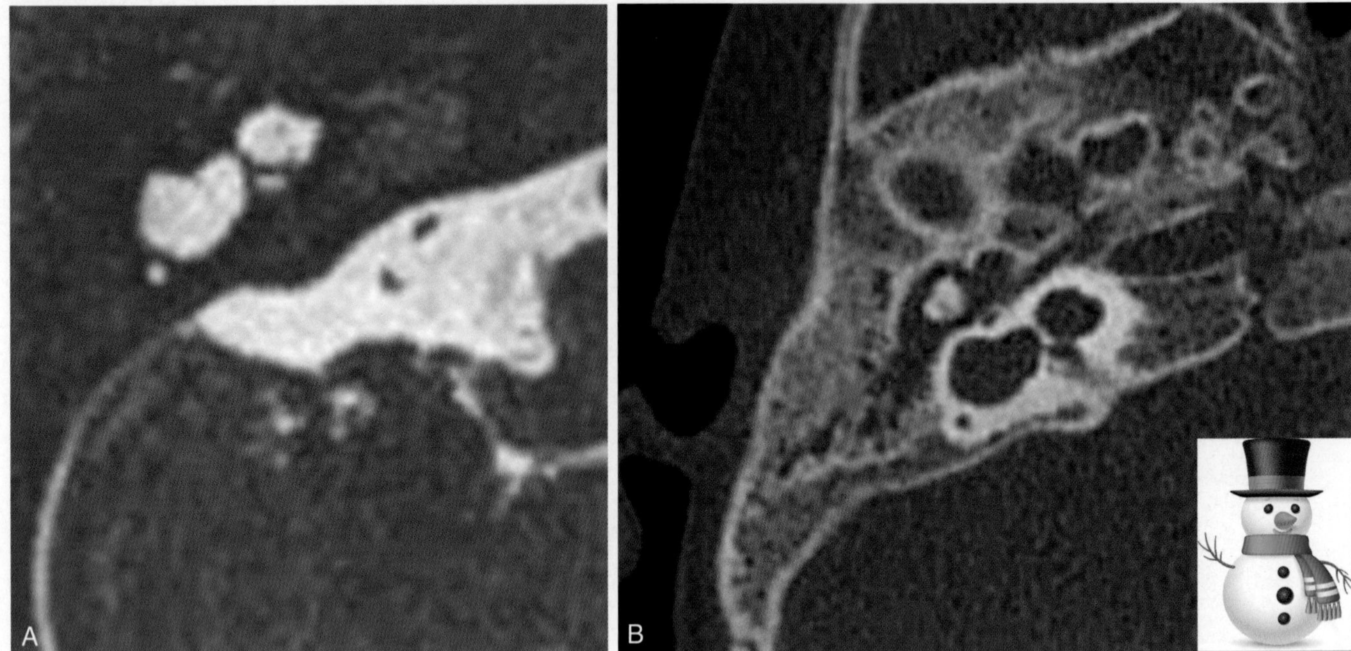

Fig. 13.4 Incomplete Partition Anomaly Type 1. (A) Axial T2W and (B) axial CT images demonstrate a cystic cochleovestibular anomaly with a "snowman" or "figure-8" morphology, absent interscalar septum, and absent modiolus. (B, inset image of snowman © istock.com/Vectorcreator.)

Key Points

Background

- Cystic cochleovestibular anomaly
- Developmental arrest in the fifth gestational week

Imaging

- Snowman shape/figure of 8 shape to the cochlea and vestibule
- Cystic cochlear malformation, which is separate from the vestibule
- Absent interscalar septum
- Absent modiolus
- Wide internal auditory canal (IAC)
- Vestibular aqueduct rarely large
- Cochlear nerve often hypoplastic

REFERENCE

1. Joshi VM, Navlekar SK, Kishore GR, et al. CT and MR imaging of the inner ear and brain in children with congenital hearing loss. *Radiographics*. 2012 May-Jun;32(3):683–698.

INCOMPLETE PARTITION ANOMALY TYPE 2

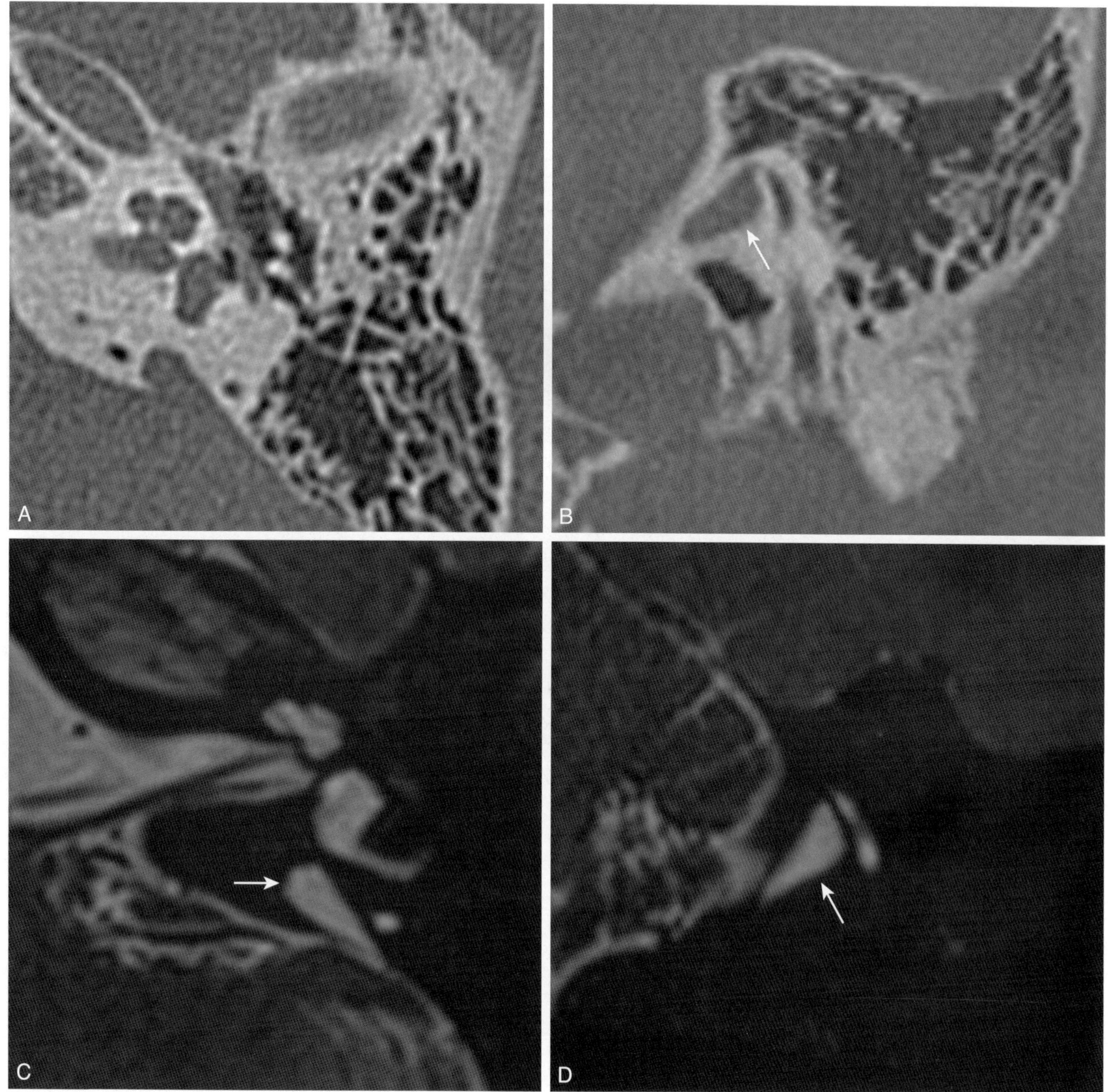

Fig. 13.5 Incomplete Partition Anomaly Type 2. (A and B) Axial and coronal 3DT2W CT and (C and D) axial images demonstrate malformation of the apical and middle turns of the cochlea and an enlarged vestibular aqueduct (*arrows*). A normal cochlear nerve is visible.

Key Points

Background

- Developmental arrest in the seventh week of gestation. More common than IP-1

Imaging

- Malformation of the apical and middle turns of the cochlea, and normal basal turn
- Absent interscalar septum between apical and middle turn
- Large vestibular aqueduct
- May have absent or deficient modiolus
- Cochlear nerve and semicircular canals usually normal. Greater success with cochlear implant

REFERENCE

1. Joshi VM, Navlekar SK, Kishore GR, et al. CT and MR imaging of the inner ear and brain in children with congenital hearing loss. *Radiographics*. 2012 May-Jun;32(3):683–698.

LATERAL SEMICIRCULAR CANAL DYSPLASIA

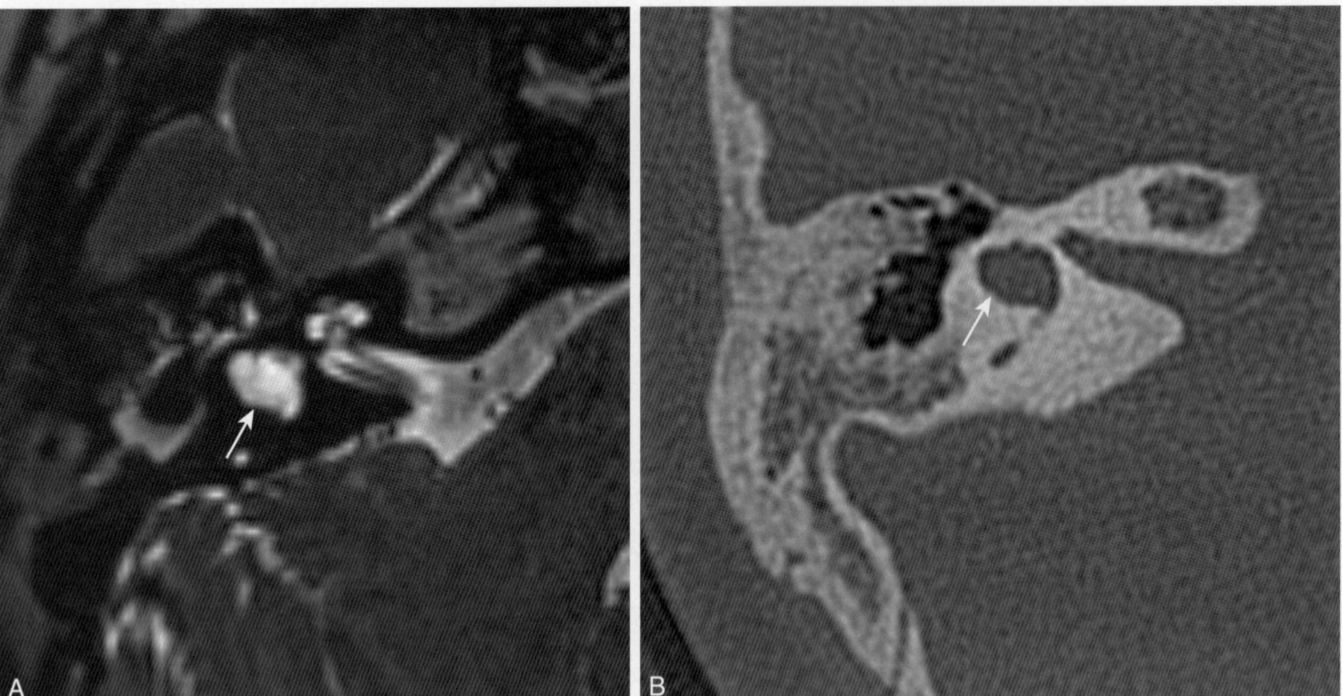

Fig. 13.6 Lateral Semicircular Canal Dysplasia. (A) Axial T2W and (B) axial CT images demonstrate malformation of the lateral semicircular canal (*arrow*) seen as lack of separation of the canal from the vestibule.

Key Points

Background

- Semicircular canals begin development between the sixth and eighth week of gestation and are complete at the 19th to 22nd weeks.
- Superior canal develops first, then the posterior canal, then the lateral canal.
- Earlier gestational insults will involve more of the semicircular canals. Consequently, the lateral semicircular canal is the most common canal to be malformed as well as malformed in isolation.

Imaging

- Lateral semicircular canal appears as a short and wide canal, often unseparated from the vestibule.
- Cochlea can be normal in appearance or malformed.

REFERENCE

1. Joshi VM, Navlekar SK, Kishore GR, et al. CT and MR imaging of the inner ear and brain in children with congenital hearing loss. *Radiographics*. 2012 May-Jun;32(3):683–698.

TIMELINE OF INNER EAR MALFORMATIONS

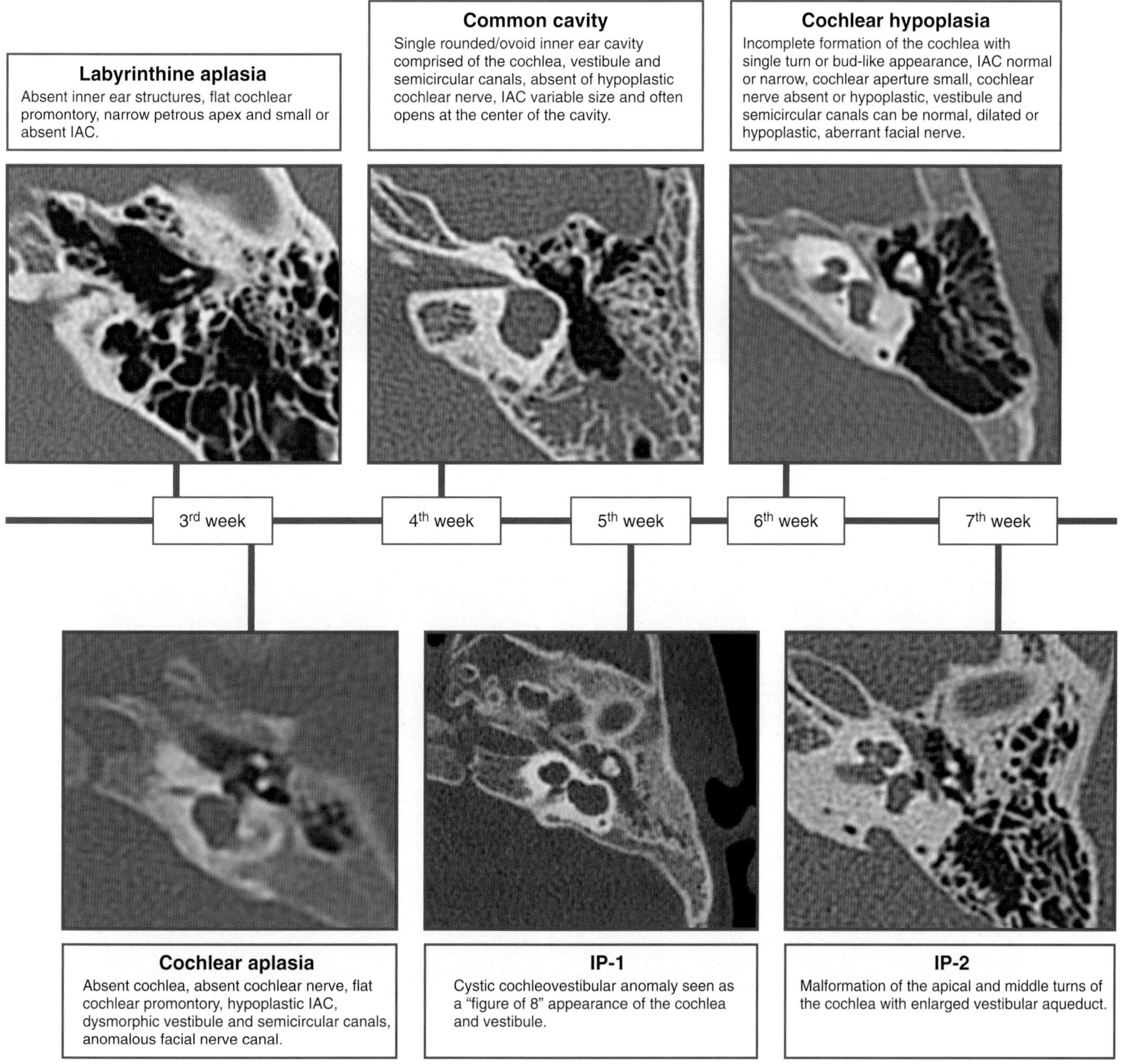

Fig. 13.7 Timeline of Inner Ear Malformations. The severity of the inner ear malformation reflects the timing of insult during gestation.

COCHLEAR NERVE HYPOPLASIA

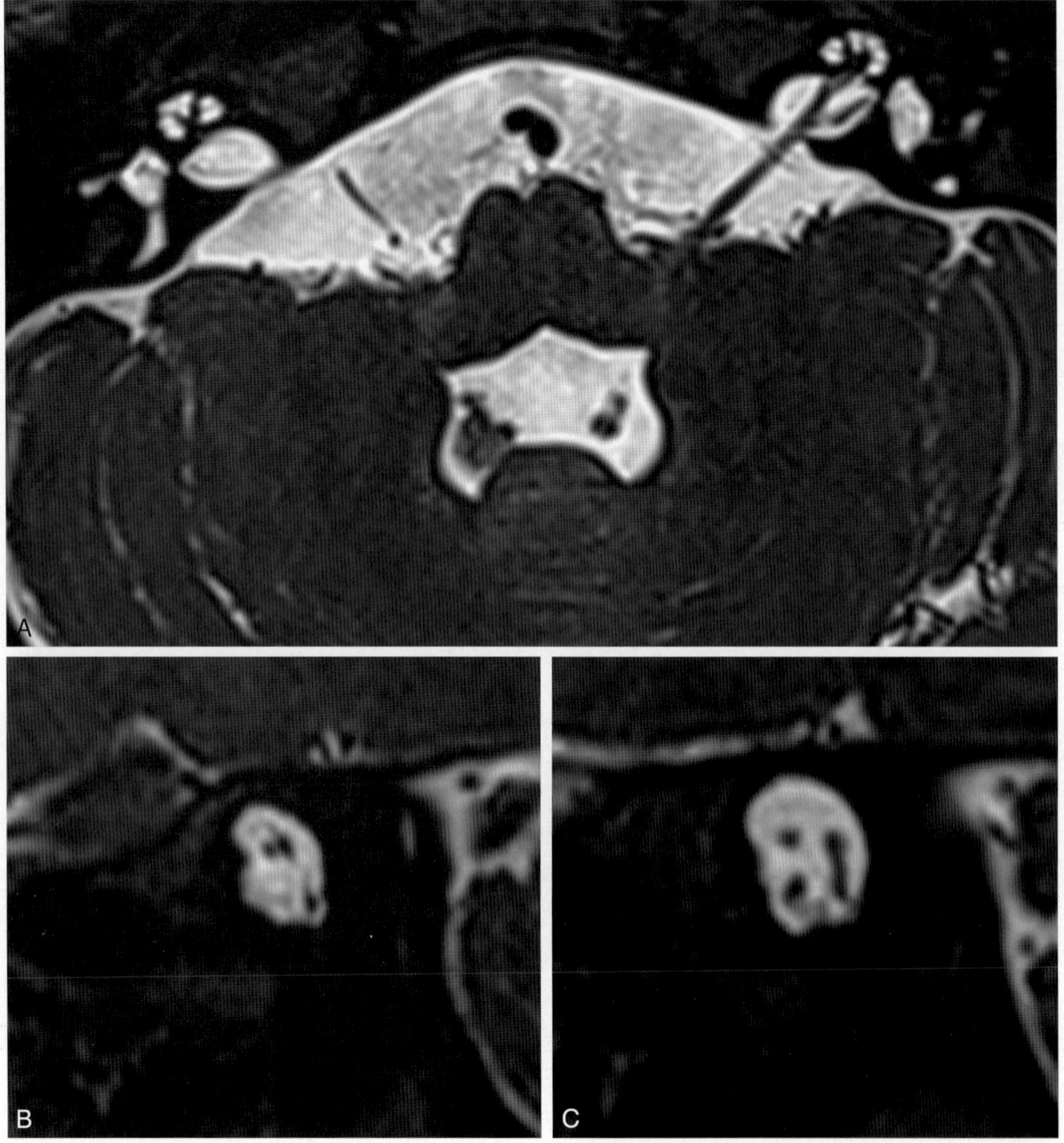

Fig. 13.8 Cochlear Nerve Hypoplasia. (A) Axial T2W, (B) right sagittal oblique T2W, and (C) left sagittal oblique T2W images demonstrate the lack of a right cochlear nerve beneath the facial nerve. Popular mnemonic "7 up, Coke down" refers to the normal appearance, which is cranial nerve 7 above and cranial nerve 8 below in the anterior aspect of the internal auditory canal.

Key Points

Background

- Diagnosed in 12% to 18% of pediatric sensorineural hearing loss (SNHL)
- The labyrinth starts development at 3 weeks' gestation with formation of the otic placode, which will become the otic vesicle. At 7 weeks' gestation the spiral organ of Corti develops from the cochlear duct and fibers from the spiral ganglia form the cochlear nerve

Imaging

- Lack of visible cochlear nerve.
- IAC may be small, but a normal sized IAC and normal inner ear structures do not exclude a nerve deficiency.
- Cochlear aperture often small.
- May or may not have associated inner ear anomalies.

REFERENCE

1. Joshi VM, Navlekar SK, Kishore GR, et al. CT and MR imaging of the inner ear and brain in children with congenital hearing loss. *Radiographics*. 2012 May-Jun;32(3):683–698.

BRANCHIO-OTO-RENAL SYNDROME

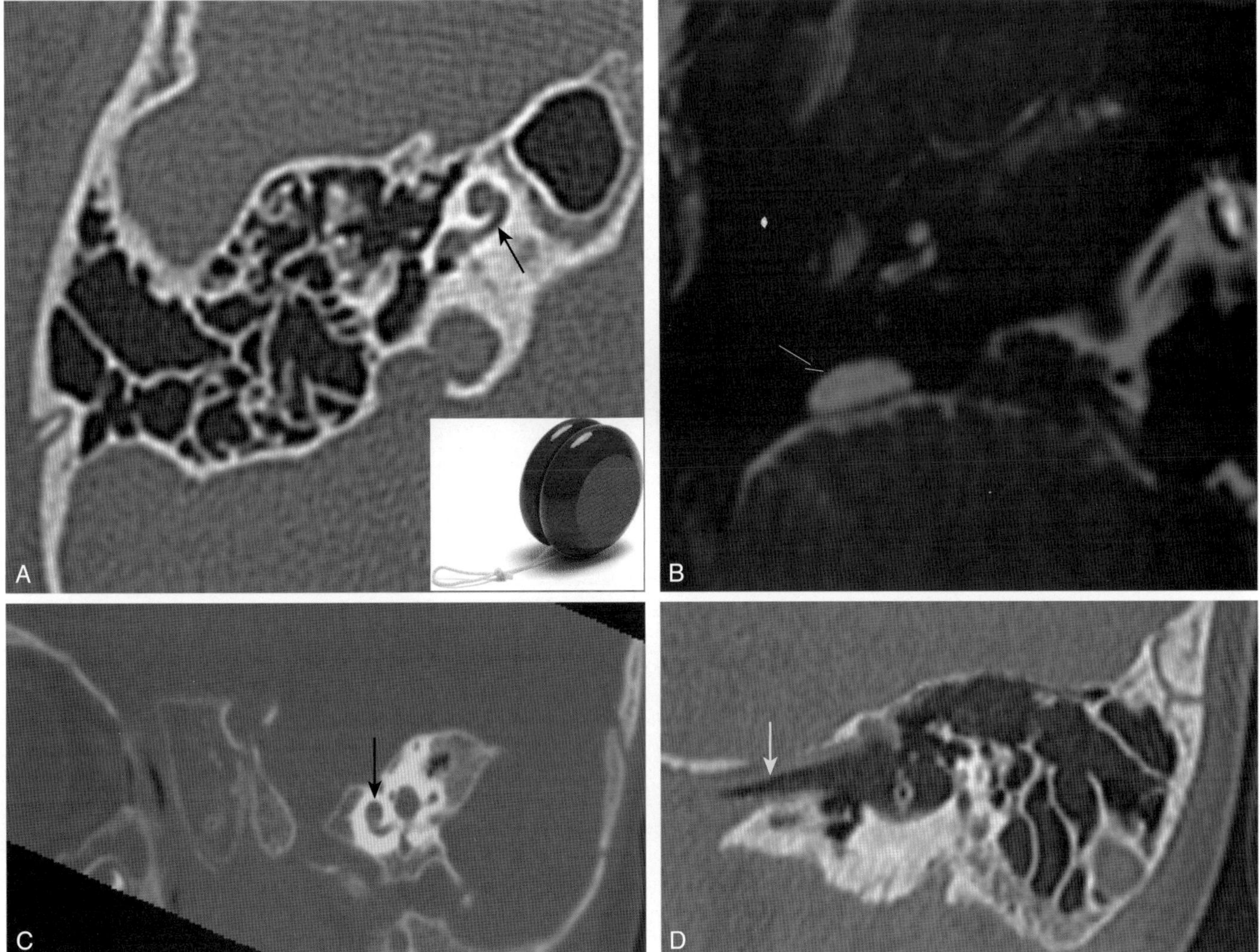

Fig. 13.9 Branchio-oto-renal Syndrome. (A, C, D) Multiplanar CT images and (B) axial T2W images demonstrate characteristic unwound cochlea (*blue arrow*), enlarged vestibular aqueduct (*red arrow*), and prominent eustachian tube (*yellow arrow*). (A, inset image of yo-yo © istock.com/Michael Burrell.)

Key Points

Background

- Autosomal dominant; mutation in *EYA1 (BOR1, BOR2), SIX5 (BOR2)* and *SIX1 (BOR3, BOS3)* genes
- Ear anomalies: Hearing loss (mild to profound). Preauricular pits or tags, malformed middle and inner ear
- *Renal* anomalies: Spectrum including malformed, collecting system duplication, and renal agenesis
- *Branchial* anomalies: Fistulas or cysts

Imaging

- *Unwound cochlea*; widened cochlear aperture; enlarged vestibular aqueduct; patulous IAC; prominent eustachian tube

REFERENCES

1. Talenti G, Manara R, Brotto D, et al. High-resolution 3T magnetic resonance findings in cochlear hypoplasias and incomplete partition anomalies: a pictorial essay. *Br J Radiol.* 2018;91(1089):20180120.
2. Hsu A, Desai N, Paldino MJ. The unwound cochlea: A specific imaging marker for branchio-oto-renal syndrome. *AJNR Am J Neuroradiol.* 2018 Dec; 39(12):2345–2349.

X-LINKED DEAFNESS

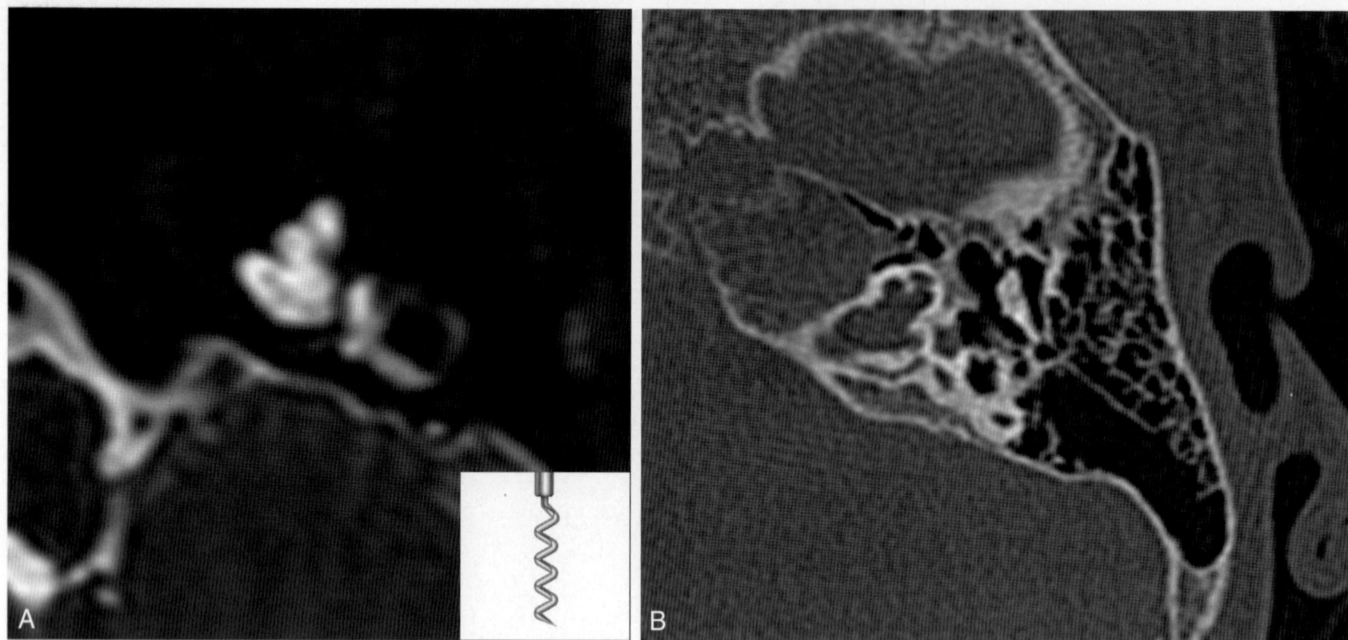

Fig. 13.10 X-Linked Deafness. (A) Axial T2W and (B) axial CT images demonstrate corkscrew malformation of the cochlea and absent modiolus. (A, inset image of corkscrew © istock.com/UASUMY)

Key Points

Background

- Also known as stapes gusher, or incomplete partition anomaly type 3
- X-linked cause of mixed hearing loss caused by POU3F4 gene mutation

Imaging

- Absent modiolus, and absent lamina cribrosa (bony partition between basal turn of cochlea and IAC)
- Cochlear hypoplasia with corkscrew appearance to the cochlea
- Enlarged IAC
- Aberrant and/or widening of the canal for the labyrinthine segment of the facial nerve
- Variable enlargement of vestibular aqueduct
- "Stapes gusher": Because there is abnormal communication between the perilymph and CSF, there is potential for leakage if stapes is removed
- Hypothalamic hamartoma is associated with the POU3F4 gene mutation

REFERENCE

1. Talenti G, Manara R, Brotto D, et al. High-resolution 3T magnetic resonance findings in cochlear hypoplasias and incomplete partition anomalies: a pictorial essay. *Br J Radiol.* 2018;91(1089):20180120.

OVAL WINDOW ATRESIA

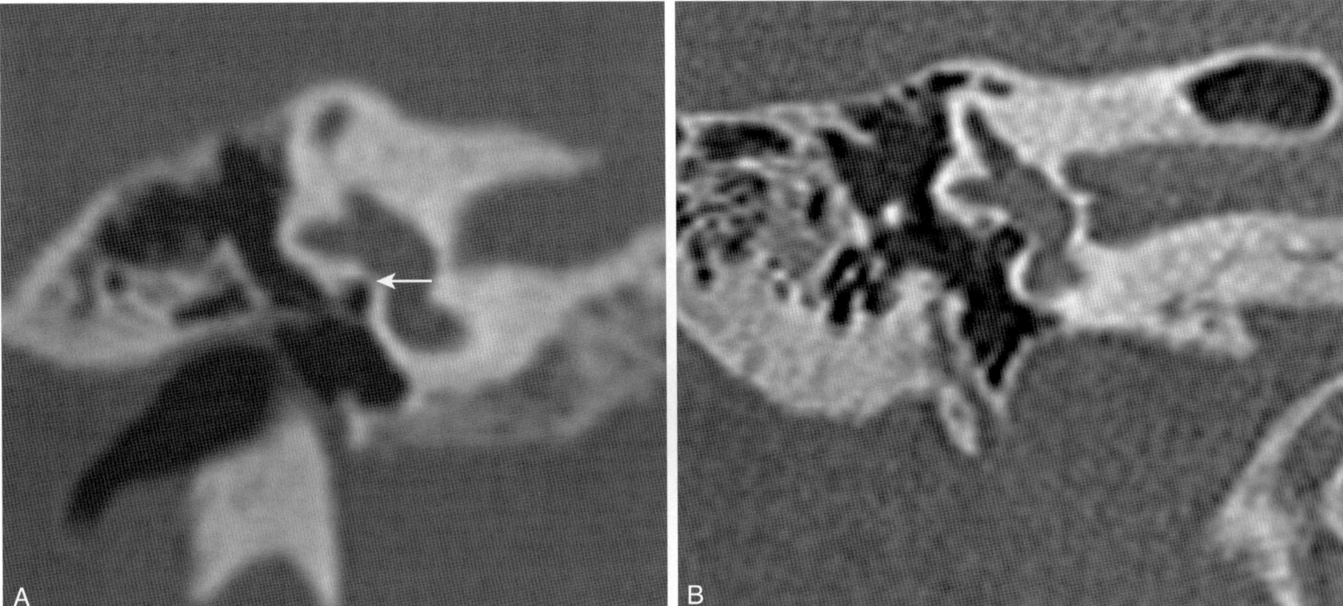

Fig. 13.11 Oval Window Atresia. (A) Coronal reformat CT demonstrating thickened oval window/absence of normal thinning of the bone at the oval window (*arrow*) as seen on a normal patient coronal CT image. In addition, the tympanic segment of the facial nerve is not seen below the lateral semicircular canal as is seen on this (B) coronal reformat CT from a normal patient.

Key Points

Background

- Malformation of the oval window defined by absence of the oval window and presence of a bony plate between the middle ear and vestibule
- Incidence and etiology are unknown. Possible etiologies include abnormal displacement of the facial nerve during the fifth and sixth weeks of gestation, preventing normal contact between the stapes and the otic capsule. Alternatively, during the seventh week of gestation the primitive stapes fails to fuse with the primitive vestibule
- Often seen in associated with other anomalies and syndromes such as external auditory canal (EAC) atresia and CHARGE syndrome
- Results in moderate to severe mixed or conductive hearing loss

Imaging

- Coronal CT images best demonstrate thickening of the bone at the oval window and potential aberrant tympanic segment of the facial nerve.
- Associated findings include malformed or absent lenticular process of the incus, absent or posteriorly directed stapes, and aberrant tympanic segment of the facial nerve located at the atretic oval window.
- Axial CT images are useful for assessing the incus and stapes.

REFERENCES

1. Hughes A, Danehy A, Adil E. Case 226: Oval window atresia. *Radiology*. 2016 Feb;278(2):626–631.
2. Booth TN, Vezina LG, Karcher G, et al. Imaging and clinical evaluation of isolated atresia of the oval window. *AJNR Am J Neuroradiol.* 2000 Jan;21(1):171–174.
3. Zeifer B, Sabini P, Sonne J. Congenital absence of the oval window: radiologic diagnosis and associated anomalies. *AJNR Am J Neuroradiol.* 2000 Feb;21(1):322–327.

OSSICULAR ANOMALIES

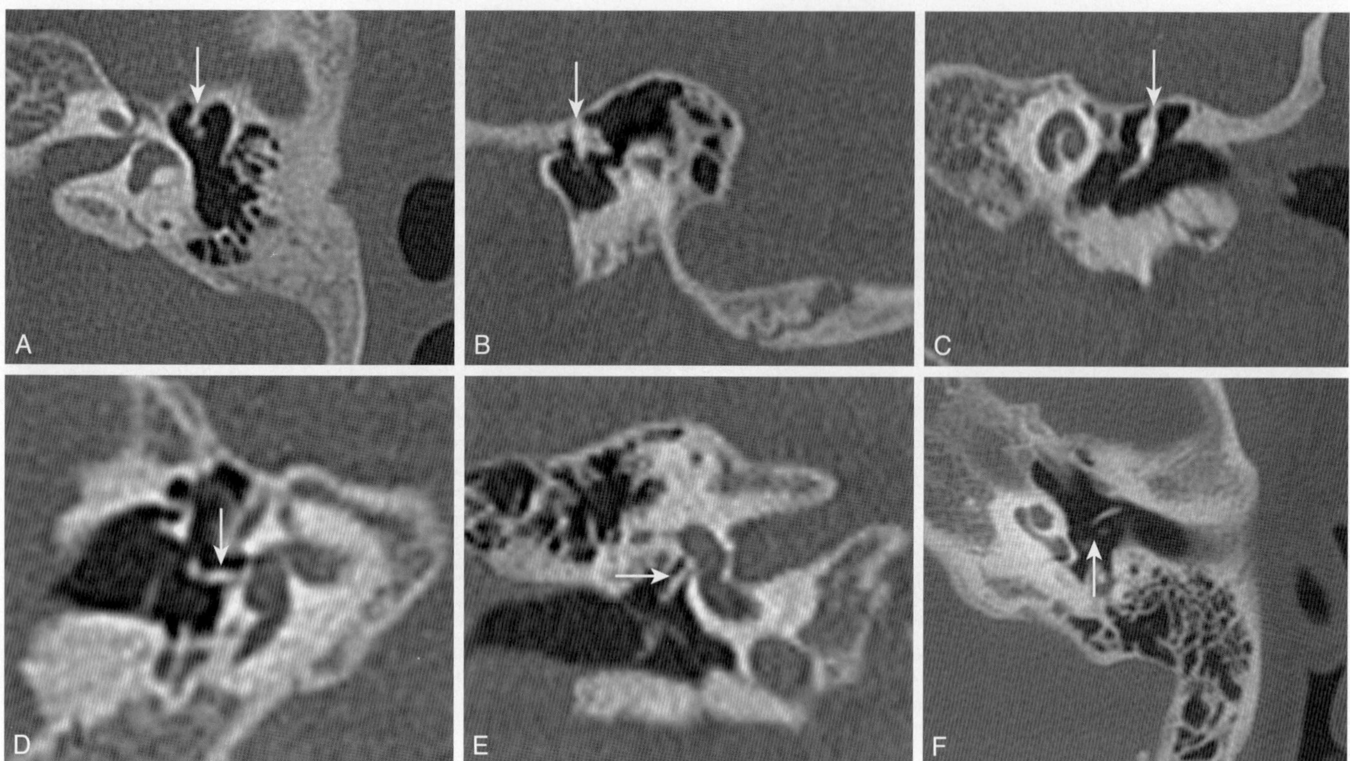

Fig. 13.12 Ossicular Anomalies. Malleus fixation: (A to C) Multiplanar CT images demonstrate an osseous bar fixating the head of the malleus (*arrows*). Monopod stapes: (D and E) Multiplanar CT images demonstrate a single thickened crus of the stapes (*arrows*). Incudo-stapedial dislocation: (F) Axial CT image demonstrates a gap between the incus and stapes (*arrow*).

Key Points

- Embryology: The malleus, incus, and stapes crus develop from the first and second branchial arches, while the stapes footplate and annular ligament develop from the otic capsule.
- Uncommon cause of conductive hearing loss.
- The ossicles as well as portions of the ossicles can be congenitally absent, dysplastic, ankylosed, and/or fixed to the tympanic cavity. Stapes malformation is the most common ossicular anomaly. Stapes tendon can be ossified.
- EAC atresia is commonly associated with ossicular malformations.
- Uncommonly, trauma can result in an acquired ossicular anomaly, most commonly ossicular dislocation.
- Middle ear cavity inflammation from tympanosclerosis, cholesteatoma, and cholesterol granuloma can result in ossicular fixation.

REFERENCES

1. Mukherji SS, Parmar HA, Ibrahim M, et al. Congenital malformations of the temporal bone. *Neuroimaging Clin N Am.* 2011 Aug;21(3):603–619.
2. Martin C, Timoshenko AP, Dumollard JM, et al. Malleus head fixation: histopathology revisited. *Acta Otolaryngol.* 2006 Apr;126(4):353–357.
3. Gentric JC, Rousset J, Garetier M, et al. High-resolution computed tomography of isolated congenital anomalies of the stapes: A pictorial review using oblique multiplanar reformation in the "axial stapes" plane. *J Neuroradiol.* 2012 Mar;39(1):57–63.
4. Park K, Choung YH. Isolated congenital ossicular anomalies. *Acta Otolaryngol.* 2009 Apr;129(4):419–422.

ABERRANT INTERNAL CAROTID ARTERY

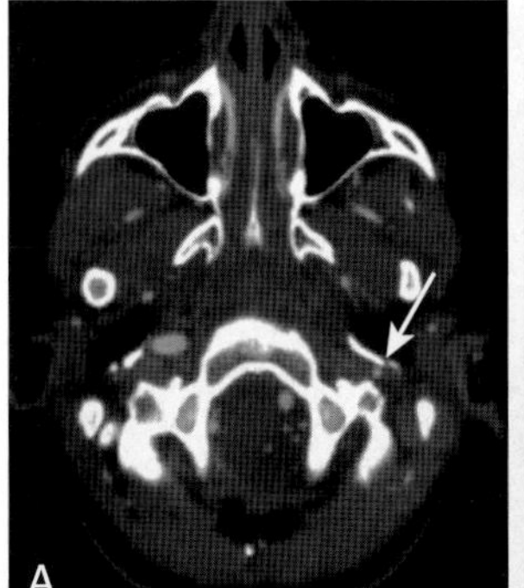

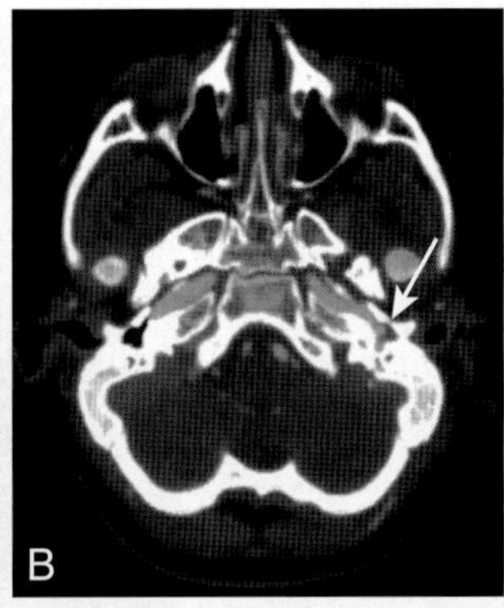

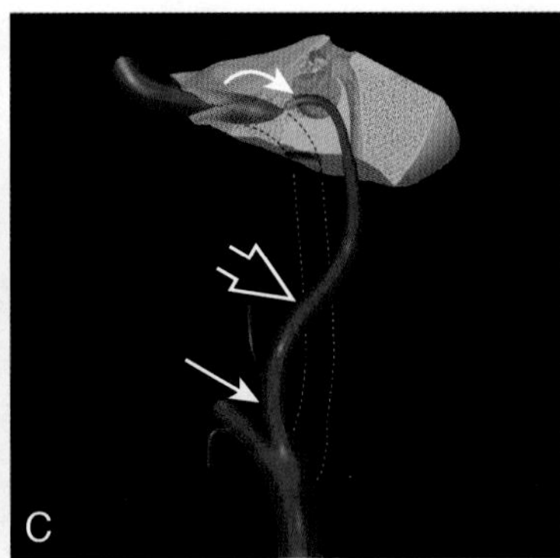

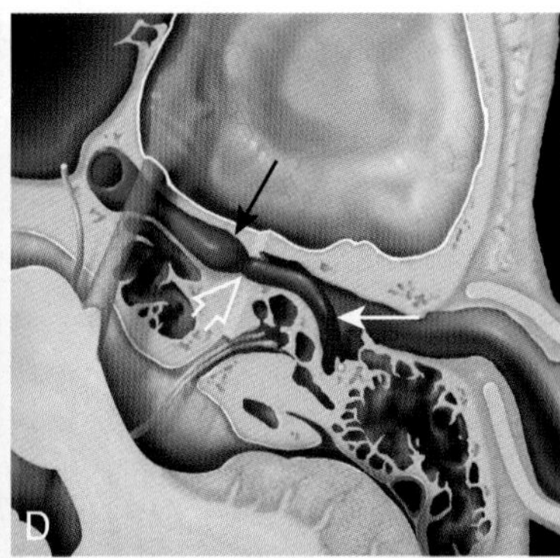

Fig. 13.13 Aberrant Internal Carotid Artery. (A and B) Axial CT angiogram images demonstrate a small inferior tympanic artery (*arrows*), which traverses through the middle ear cavity to join the horizontal petrous segment of the internal carotid artery (ICA). (C) Illustration depicts the failure of the cervical ICA to develop (*dotted lines*) with the ascending pharyngeal (*white solid arrow*), inferior tympanic (*white open arrow*), and caroticotympanic (*white curved arrow*) arteries providing an alternative collateral arterial channel, resulting in an aberrant ICA. (D) Axial illustration of the left temporal bone illustrates a classic aberrant internal carotid artery (*white solid arrow*) rising along the posterior cochlear promontory and crossing along the medial middle ear wall to rejoin the horizontal petrous ICA (*black solid arrow*). At the point of reconnection to the horizontal petrous ICA, stenosis (*white open arrow*) is often present. (C and D illustrations from StatDX, Copyright © 2022 Elsevier.)

Key Points

Background

- Involution of the cervical internal carotid artery (ICA) and secondary enlargement of the inferior tympanic artery (typically arising as a branch of the ascending pharyngeal artery and enters through the inferior tympanic canaliculus) and the caroticotympanic artery (a branch of the petrous portion of the internal carotid artery), which join at the horizontal segment of the petrous ICA. The aberrant ICA courses across the inferior cochlear promontory.
- May present with retrotympanic mass and pulsatile tinnitus.

Imaging

- Typical imaging findings include absence of the cervical ICA, a small artery in the neck that is the inferior tympanic artery that enters the inferior tympanic canaliculus in the temporal bone and extends through the middle ear cavity across the cochlear promontory to connect to the petrous ICA and a persistent stapedial artery.
- A lateralized petrous ICA, which is distinct from an aberrant ICA, has a preserved cervical ICA, does not enlarge the inferior tympanic canaliculus, and protrudes into the anterior mesotympanum.

REFERENCES

1. Swartz JD, Loevner LA. Imaging of the Temporal Bone. 4th edition. Thieme Medical Pub.
2. Glastonbury CM, Harnsberger HR, Hudgins PA, et al. Lateralized petrous internal carotid artery: imaging features and distinction from the aberrant internal carotid artery. *Neuroradiology.* 2012;54(9):1007–1013.

PERSISTENT STAPEDIAL ARTERY

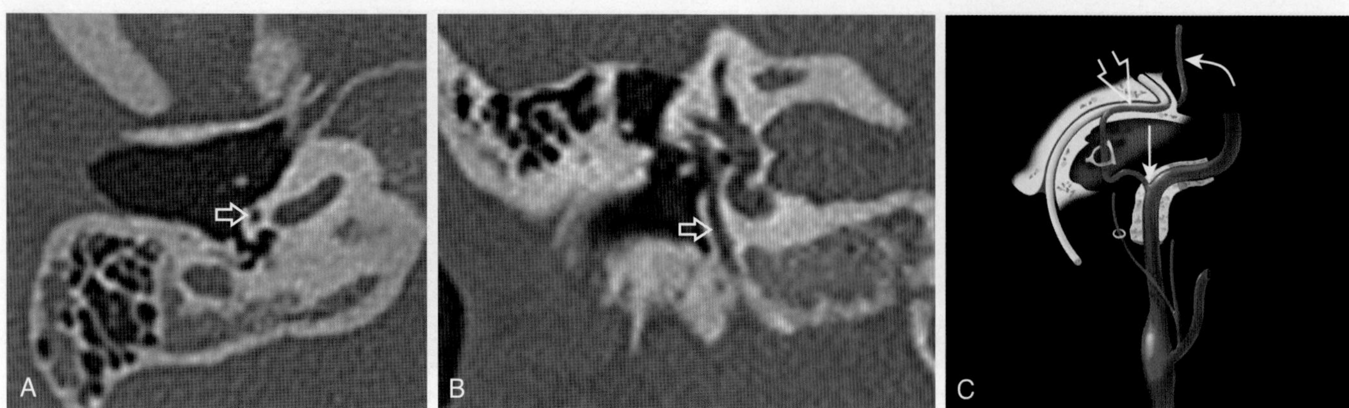

Fig. 13.14 Persistent Stapedial Artery. (A and B) Axial and coronal reformat CT images demonstrate linear density traversing the cochlear promontory consistent with a persistent stapedial artery (*arrows*). (C) Illustration shows the persistent stapedial artery (PSA) arising from the vertical segment of the petrous internal carotid artery (*white solid arrow*), passing through the stapes, and traveling along the tympanic segment of the facial nerve (*white open arrow*) to become the middle meningeal artery (*white curved arrow*). (C Illustration from StatDX, Copyright © 2022 Elsevier.)

Key Points

Background

- Rare vascular anomaly that may present as a reddish pulsatile mass on otoscopic examination or incidental finding.
- The stapedial artery arises from the hyoid artery at week 4 to 5 and passes through the obturator foramen of the stapes. The stapedial artery normally regresses at week 10. Middle meningeal artery arises from the persistent stapedial and the foramen spinosum is absent.
- Preoperative identification is important to prevent injury during surgery.
- May be isolated or associated with an aberrant ICA, which is formed from anastomosis between the inferior tympanic artery with the caroticotympanic artery.

Imaging

- Linear soft tissue density crossing the cochlear promontory
- Hypoplastic or absent foramen spinosum

REFERENCE

1. Yilmaz T, Bilgen C, Savas R, et al. Persistent stapedial artery: MR angiographic and CT findings. *AJNR Am J Neuroradiol.* 2003;24(6):1133–1135.

EXTERNAL AUDITORY CANAL ATRESIA

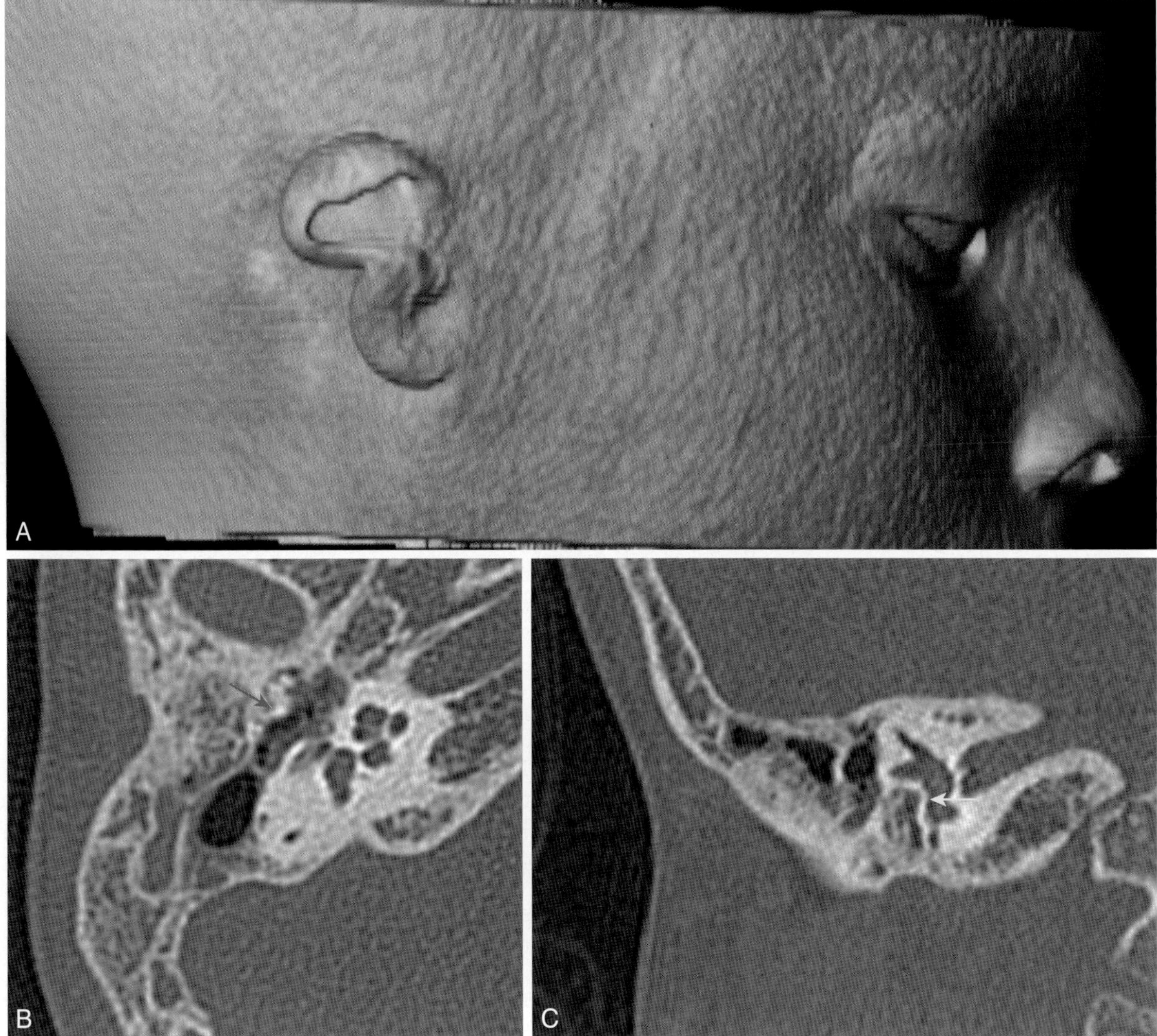

Fig. 13.15 External Auditory Canal Atresia. (A) A 3D volumetric CT image demonstrating malformation of the auricle. (B) Axial CT and (C) coronal reformat CT images demonstrate absent external auditory canal, atretic middle ear cavity, dysplastic incus (*red arrow*), absent stapes, and oval window atresia (*yellow arrow*).

Key Points

Background

- External auditory canal (EAC) develops from the first branchial cleft at 6 weeks' gestation.
- At 26th week of gestation the bony EAC canalizes from medial to lateral to fuse with the cartilaginous EAC. Failure to canalizes leads to EAC atresia.
- Anomalies of the middle ear are frequently associated with EAC atresia.

Imaging

- Jahrsdoerfer grading system (10-point scale) used to determine surgical candidacy with greater success with higher score. Includes the following:
- Stapes present (2 points)
- Oval window patent (2 mm vertically) (1 point)
- Middle ear space size and aeration with size measured from the promontory to the atretic bone laterally with <3 mm being inadequate (1 point)
- Facial nerve course normal (1 point)
- Malleus-incus complex normal (1 point)
- Incus-stapes complex normal (1 point)
- Mastoid pneumatization whether aerated, opacified, or bony (1 point)
- Round window greater than 1 mm (1 point)
- Appearance of the external ear (1 point)

REFERENCE

1. Nguyen VT, Paek G, Hu J, et al. Presurgical CT Evaluation of Congenital Aural Atresia. *Neurographics*. 2015 Sept-Oct;5(5):231–237.

COCHLEAR CLEFT

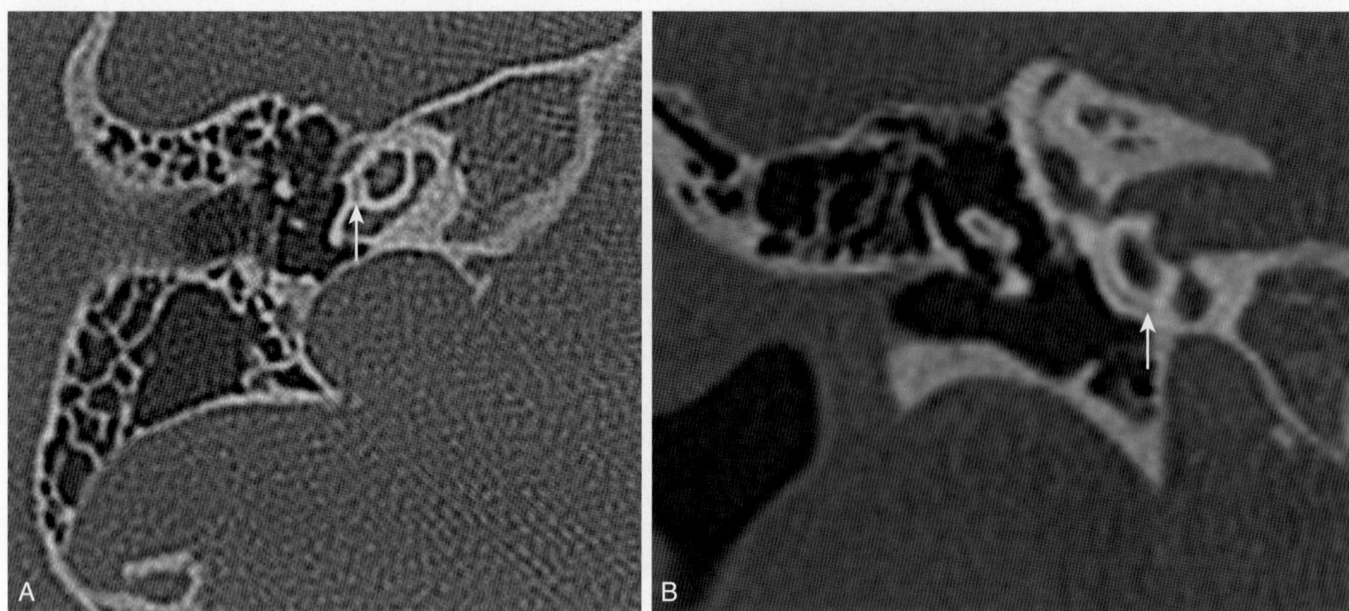

FIG. 13.16 Cochlear Cleft. (A) Axial CT and (B) coronal reformat CT images demonstrate the characteristic linear hypodensity lateral to the cochlear compatible with a cochlear cleft (*arrows*).

Key Points

Background

- A normal CT finding of a thin linear lucency within the otic capsule corresponding to fatty marrow from incomplete ossification of the otic capsule. The cochlear cleft is separate from the fissula ante fenestram.

Imaging

- Cochlear clefts are visible in approximately 34% of children on temporal bone CT.
- The prevalence of visible cochlear clefts decreases with increasing age of children.
- Should not be confused with otosclerosis, which does not have the same linear contiguous appearance and is also rare in children.

REFERENCES

1. Chadwell JB, Halsted MJ, Choo DI, et al. The cochlear cleft. *AJNR Am J Neuroradiol.* 2004 Jan 25(1):21–24.
2. Pucetaite M, Quesnel AM, Juliano A, et al. The cochlear cleft: CT correlation with histopathology. *Oto Neurotol.* 2020 Jul; 41(6):745–749.

14 Neck, Face, Orbit, and Temporal Bone Masses

APPROACH TO NECK MASSES

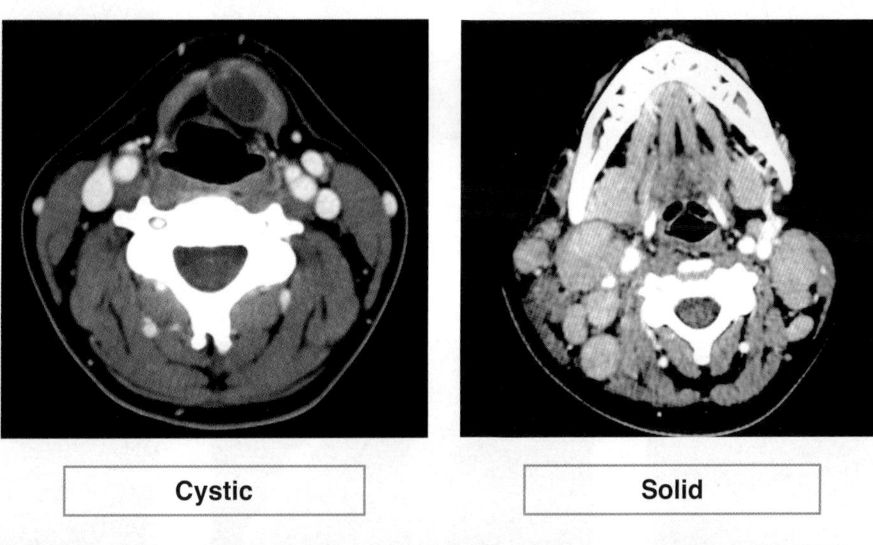

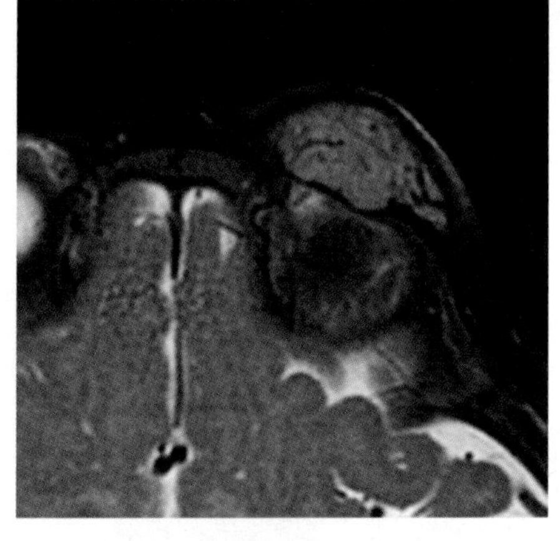

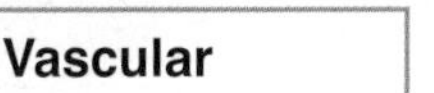

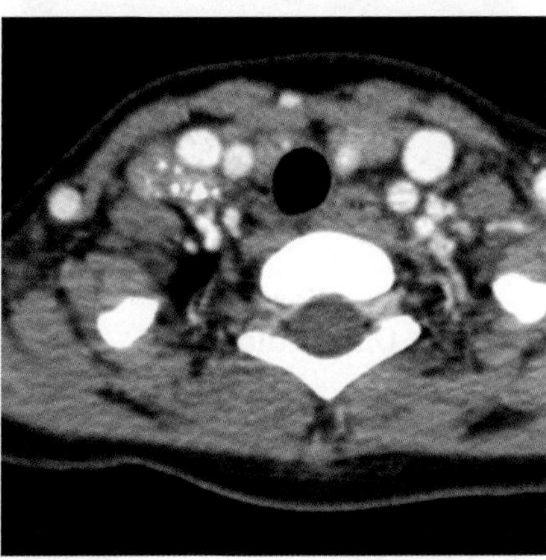

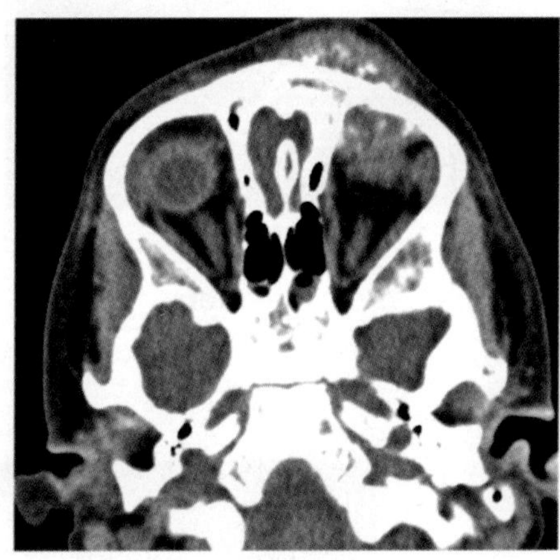

BACKGROUND AND APPROACH TO NECK MASSES

- Neck masses are commonly encountered in children, and a wide range of etiologies is possible such that familiarity with anatomic locations and a diagnostic approach is necessary in order to arrive at a specific diagnosis or to narrow the differential diagnosis.
- A particularly helpful approach is to determine whether the mass best falls within categories of a cystic, solid, vascular, calcified, or bone-associated mass. Each of these main categories will contain several possible lesions, many of which have helpful clues.
- This chapter will illustrate the many common and uncommon etiologies for neck masses in children.

DIFFERENTIAL DIAGNOSIS OF A CYSTIC NECK MASS

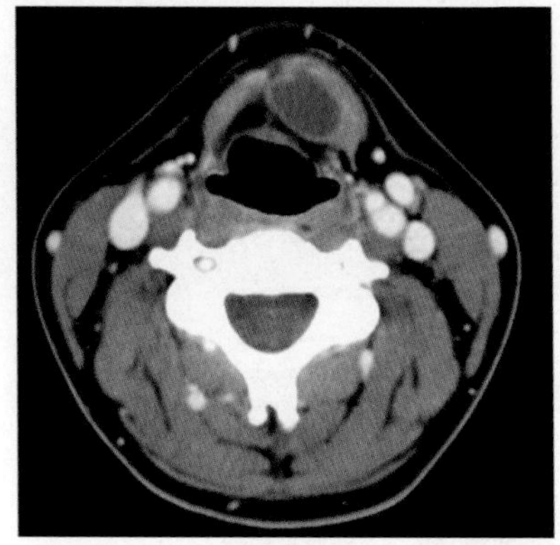

Thyroglossal Duct Cyst

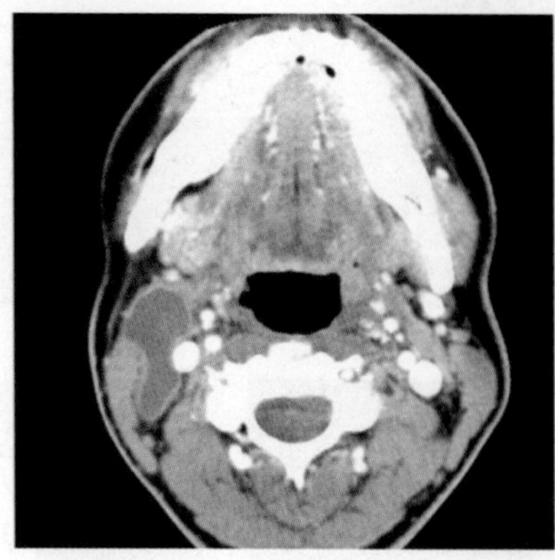

Branchial Cleft Cyst

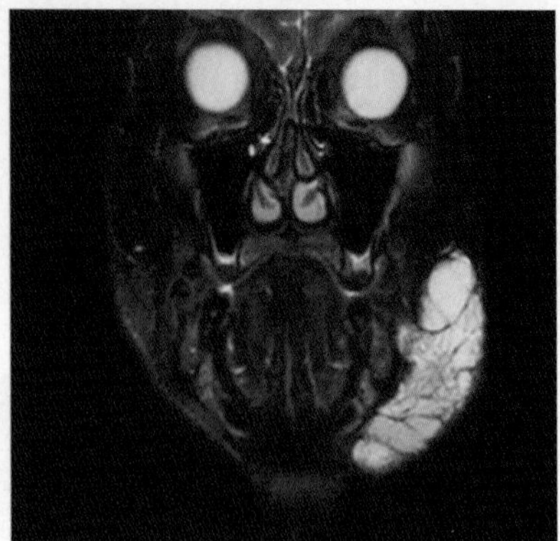

Lymphatic Malformation

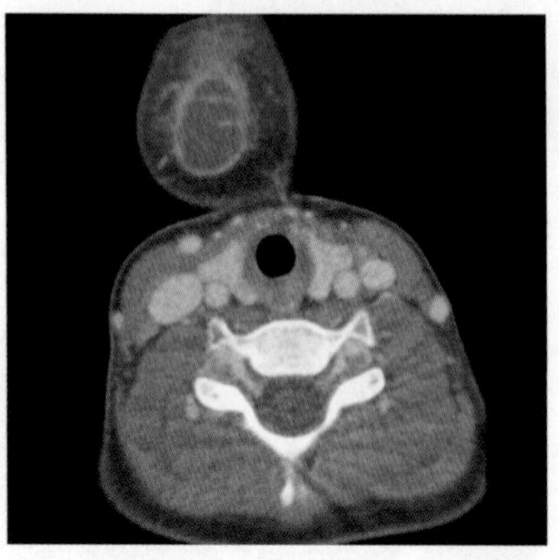

Infection

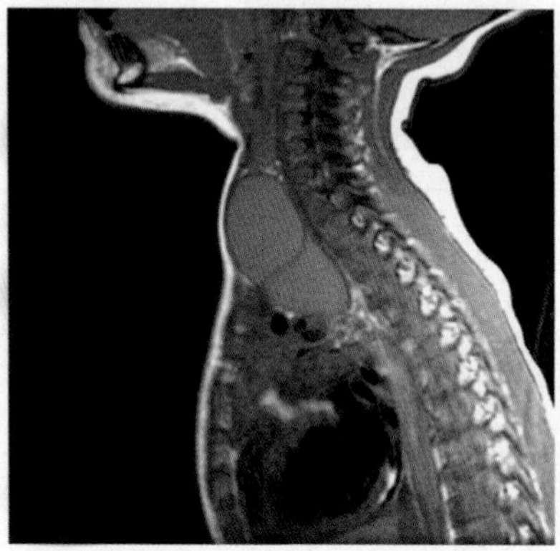

Foregut Duplication Cyst

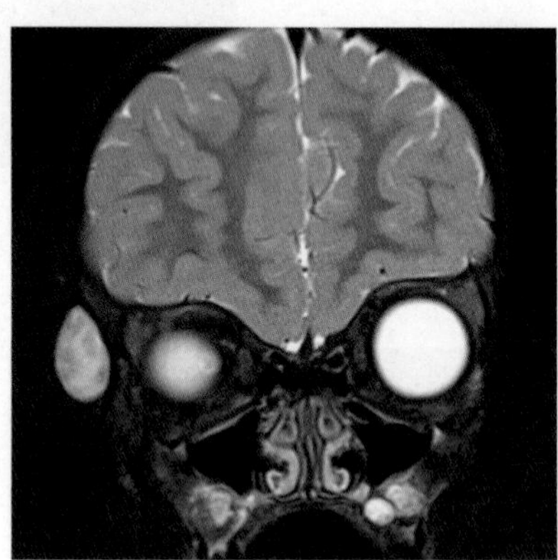

Epidermoid Cyst

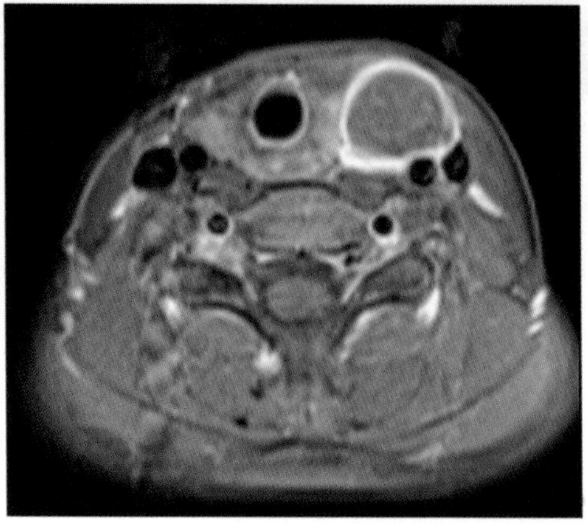

Thymic Cyst

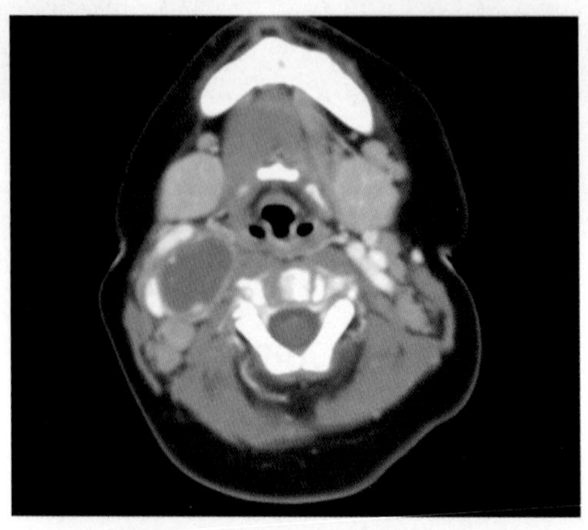

Neoplasm

THYROGLOSSAL DUCT CYST

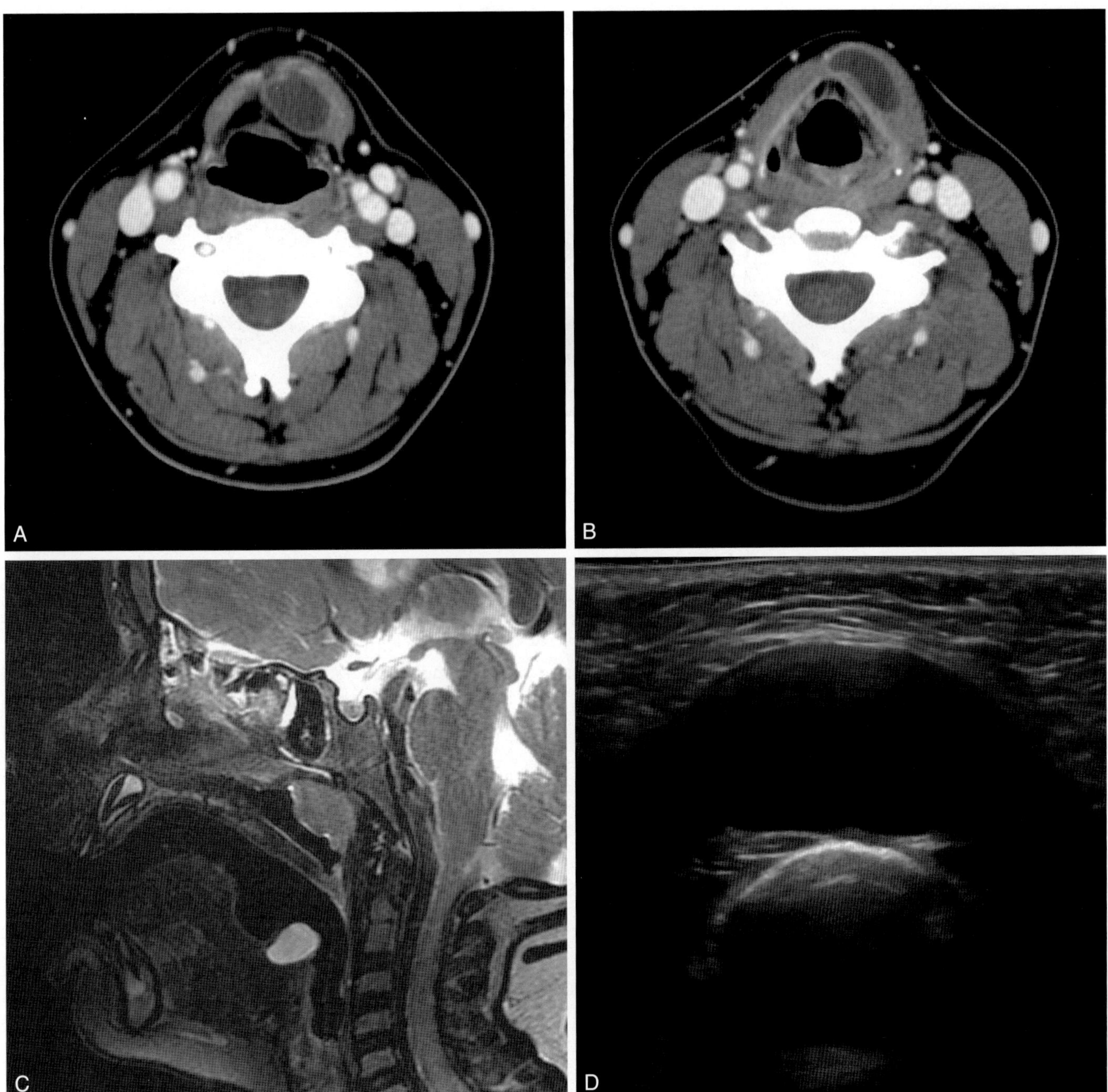

Fig. 14.1 Thyroglossal Duct Cyst: Typical Imaging Appearances. (A and B) Axial contrast-enhanced CT (CECT) images demonstrate an ovoid non-enhancing fluid density mass in the left anterior neck associated with the strap muscle. (C) Sagittal T2W fat saturation image demonstrates a fluid intensity cyst at the base of the tongue. (D) Transverse ultrasound image demonstrates an anechoic cyst in the anterior neck.

THYROGLOSSAL DUCT CYST

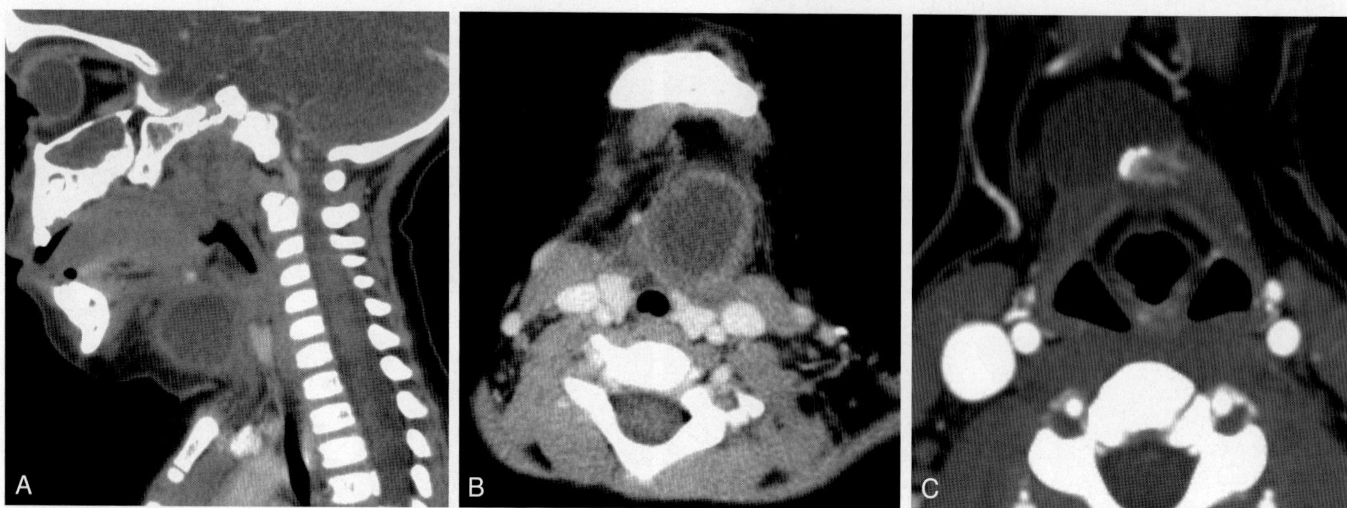

Fig. 14.2 Thyroglossal Duct Cyst: Uncommon Imaging Appearances. (A and B) Sagittal and axial CECT images demonstrate a peripherally enhancing fluid density lesion with thick walls and surrounding inflammation consistent with and infected thyroglossal duct cyst. (C) Axial CECT demonstrates a fluid density cyst with posterior nodular calcification consistent with papillary thyroid cancer arising in a thyroglossal duct cyst.

Key Points

Background

- Most common congenital malformation in the neck, accounting for 70% of congenital neck malformations
- Found from the foramen cecum to the thyroid gland; *midline/paramedian location in the neck*

Imaging

- Ultrasound: anechoic
- CT: Thin wall; uniform fluid density; no solid component
- MRI: Thin wall; nonenhancing; no solid component; T2W hyperintensity; ADC hyperintense
- Suprahyoid thyroglossal duct cyst: Comprise 20% of TGDCs; midline location.
- Hyoid/infrahyoid TGDC: Comprise 80% of TGDCs; located within 2 cm of midline; associated with strap muscles.
- May present with superinfection and demonstrate thickening of the cyst wall surrounding inflammation on imaging as well as secondary skin fistula.
- Rarely (<1%) may develop thyroid neoplasm (most commonly papillary thyroid cancer). The presence of Ca^{2+} can indicate neoplasm.
- Differential Diagnosis: Dermoid/epidermoid cyst.

REFERENCE

1. Glastonbury CM, Davidson HC, Haller JR, et al. The CT and MR imaging features of carcinoma arising in thyroglossal duct remnants. *AJNR Am J Neuroradiol.* 2000 Apr;21(4):770–774.

BRANCHIAL CLEFT ANOMALIES

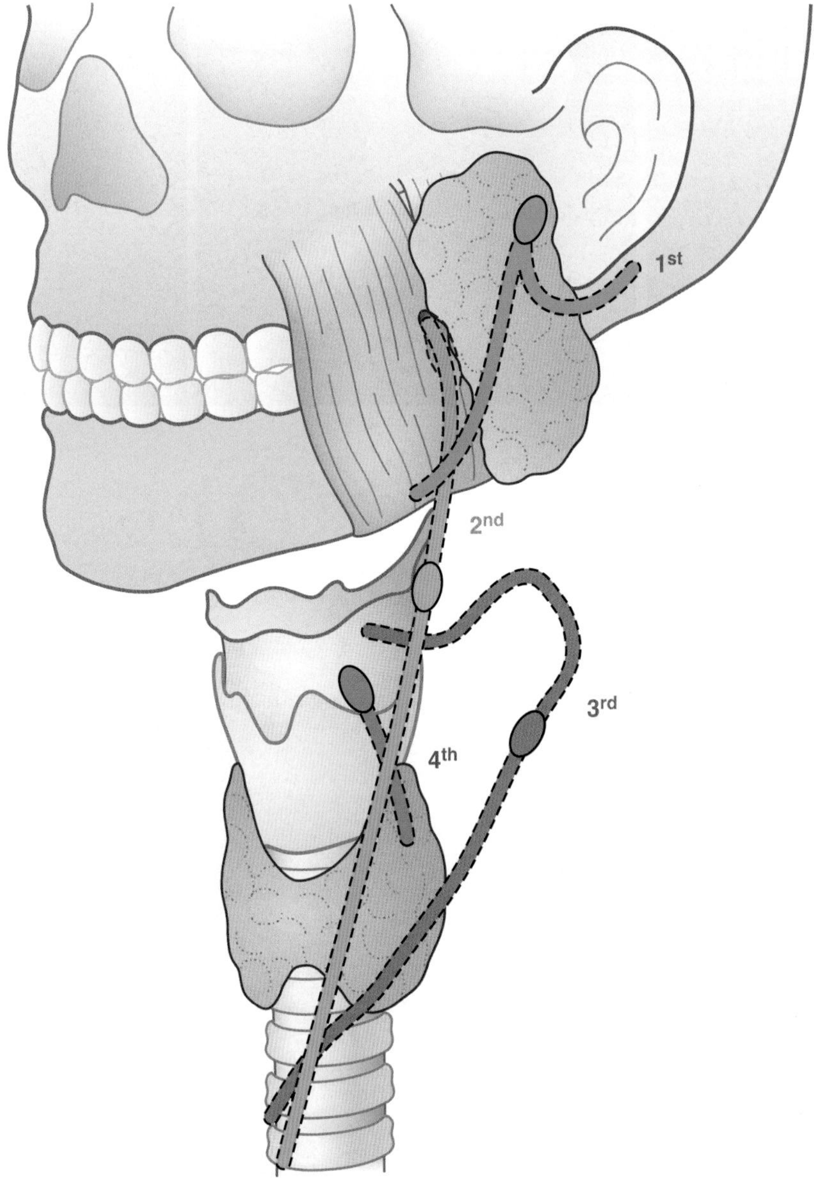

Fig. 14.3 Branchial Cleft Anomalies. The first branchial cleft anomaly (blue) can be found along a path from the external auditory canal to the peri-auricular space or through the periparotid space to the angle of the mandible. The second branchial cleft anomaly (green) is found along a path from superomedial to inferolateral from the palatine tonsil, extending laterally between the external and internal carotid arteries, anterolateral to the common carotid artery and medial to the sternocleidomastoid muscle before exiting the skin anterior to the junction of the middle and lower thirds of the sternocleidomastoid muscle at the level of the thyroid gland to the sternocleidomastoid muscle. The third branchial cleft anomaly (red) is found along a path from the upper pyriform sinus extending laterally to posterior to the carotid artery and sternocleidomastoid muscle and exiting the skin anterior to the lower third of the SCM to the anterolateral neck. The fourth branchial cleft anomaly (purple) is found along a path from the lower pyriform sinus extending inferiorly in the tracheoesophageal groove into the thyroid gland where most anomalies are clinically found, as shown here. The path continues (not shown) inferiorly to loop around the aorta in a posterior to anterior direction on the left side and subclavian artery on the right side and ascends posterior to the common carotid artery and exits the skin anterior to the sternocleidomastoid muscle.

Key Points

Background

- Branchial cleft anomalies commonly result in cystic neck masses but can also result in sinus tracts and fistula.
- Each anomaly has a specific course in the neck in which a cyst can be found.
- From most common to least common are the second, first, fourth, and third branchial cleft anomalies.

FIRST BRANCHIAL CLEFT ANOMALY

Cystic

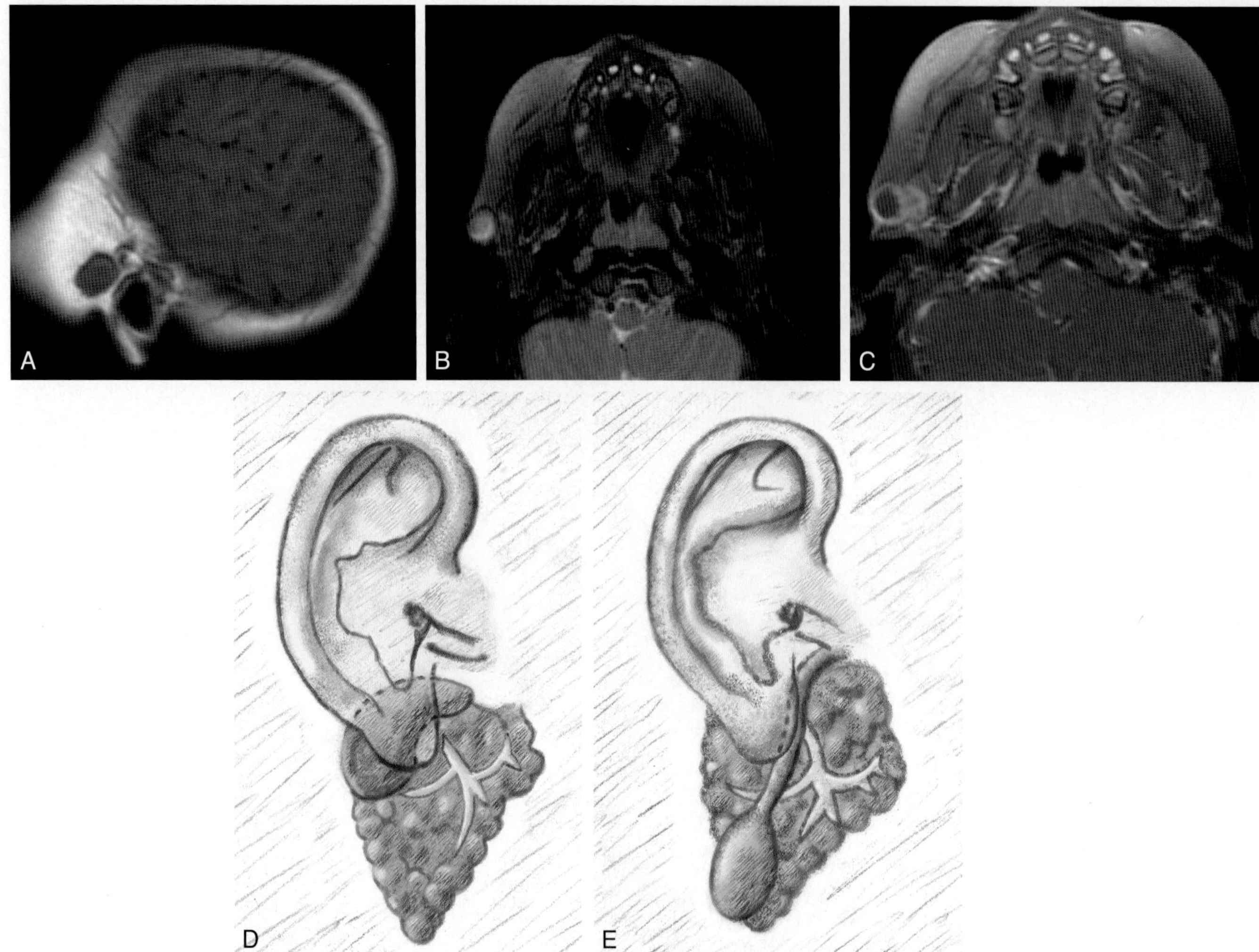

Fig. 14.4 First Branchial Cleft Cyst. (A) Sagittal T1W, (B) axial T2W fat saturation, and (C) axial T1W+C fat saturation images demonstrate a peripherally enhancing fluid intensity lesion in the right preauricular space. (D and E) Illustrations of the course of type 1 and type 2 first branchial cleft cysts.

Key Points

Background

- 8% of branchial cleft remnants
- May become superinfected or lead to otitis externa. Recurrent otitis externa should raise suspicion for a first branchial cleft anomaly.

Imaging

- Subdivided into:
  - Type 1: Periauricular
  - Type 2: Periparotid/extending from the external auditory canal (EAC) to angle of mandible
- Thin walled fluid filled cyst. Less common to have sinus tract or fistula
- Differential Diagnosis: Parotid tumor or necrotic lymph node

REFERENCE

1. Friedman ER, John SD. Imaging of pediatric neck masses. *Radiol Clin North Am.* 2011 Jul;49(4):617–632.

FIRST BRANCHIAL CLEFT ANOMALY

Cystic

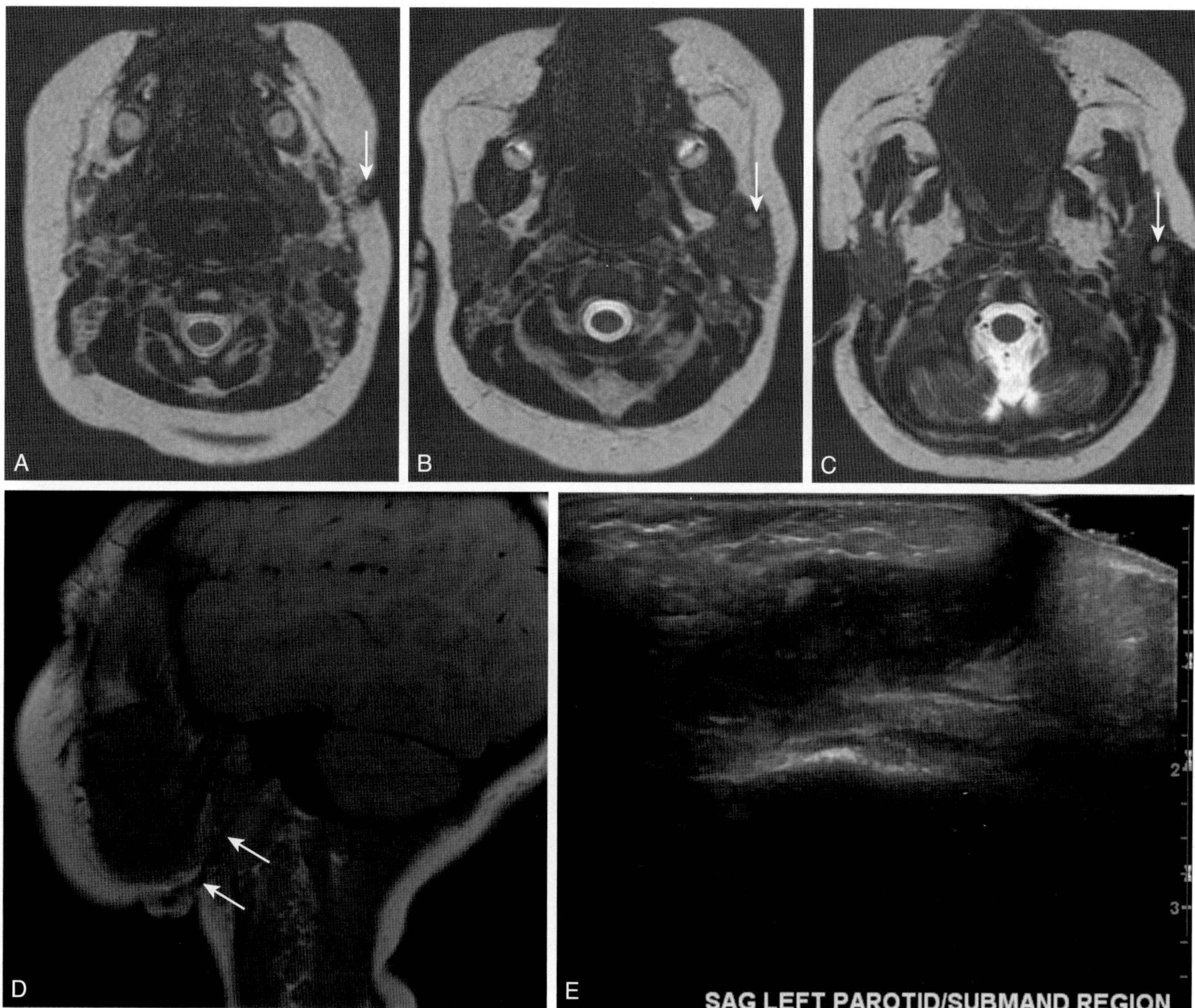

Fig. 14.5 First Branchial Cleft Fistula. (A to C) Axial T2W and (D) sagittal T1W images demonstrate a fluid-filled tract from the left external auditory canal to the left side of the face consistent with a first branchial cleft fistula. (E) Ultrasound image demonstrates a typical hypoechoic appearance of the tract.

SECOND BRANCHIAL CLEFT ANOMALY

Cystic

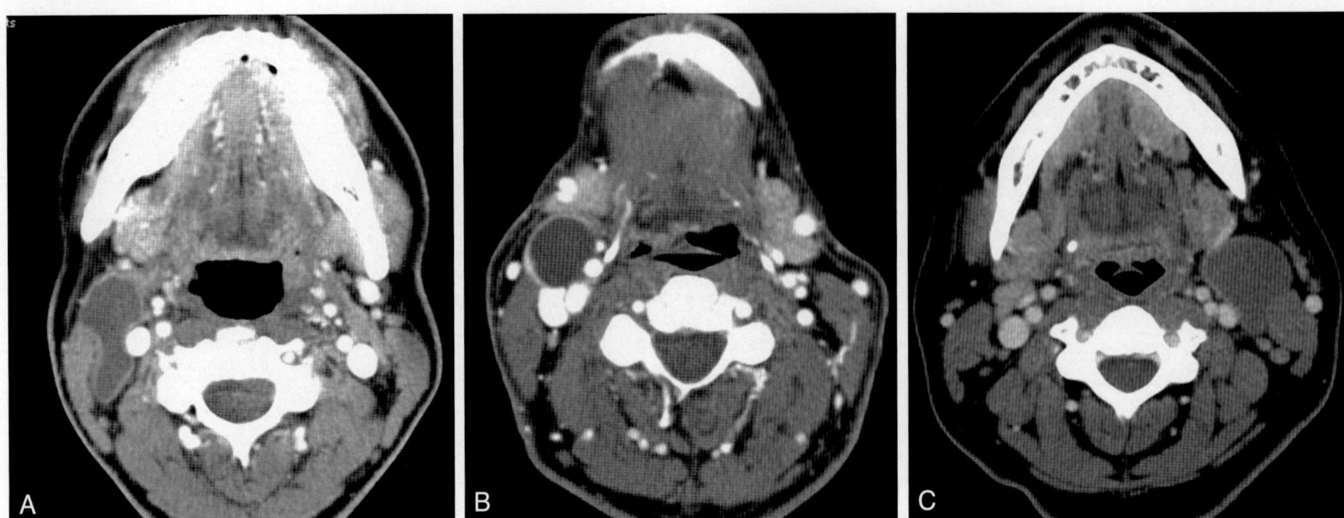

Fig. 14.6 Second Branchial Cleft Cyst: Typical Appearance. (A to C) Axial CECT images of different second branchial clefts cysts found in typical location posterolateral to the submandibular gland, lateral to the carotid space, and anteromedial to the sternocleidomastoid muscle.

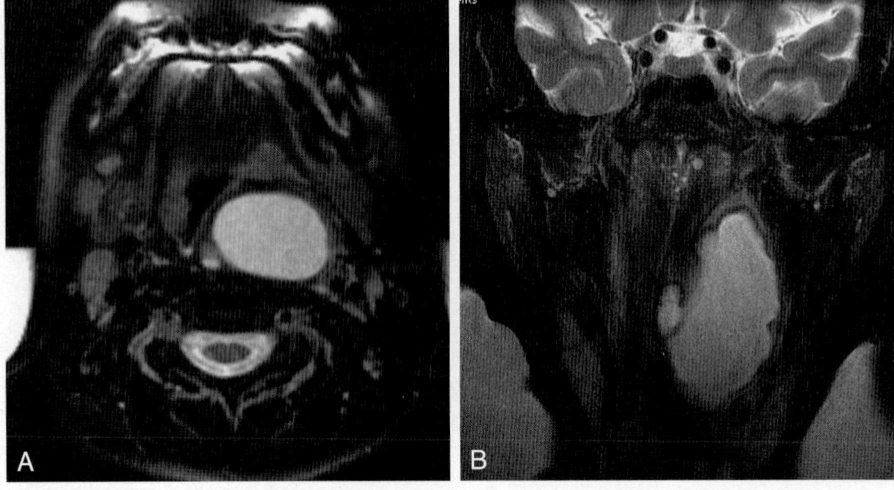

Fig. 14.7 Second Branchial Cleft Cyst: Atypical Appearance. (A and B) Axial and coronal T2W fat saturation images demonstrate an irregular walled cyst posterior to the palatine tonsil. Pathology was a second branchial cleft cyst.

Key Points

Background

- Most common branchial cleft anomaly (children 66%–75% vs adults >90%)
- Occurs along a tract that courses from *palatine tonsil* → anterior and lateral to the carotid space and posterior to the submandibular gland → lateral neck anterior and medial to sternocleidomastoid muscle (SCM) → existing the skin at the level of the thyroid gland anterior to the junction of the middle and inferior thirds of the SCM

Imaging

- Most commonly a cyst but can also occur as a sinus tract or fistula.
- Most common location: Lateral neck located posterolateral to submandibular gland, lateral to carotid space, and anteromedial to SCM
- Uncommon locations: Inferior along the infrahyoid carotid space; superior into the parapharyngeal or carotid space; lateral pharyngeal wall
- Fistula opening usually located at the junction of the middle and lower third of the SCM
- Differential Diagnosis: Suppurative/necrotic node, or lymphatic malformation

REFERENCE

1. Friedman ER, John SD. Imaging of pediatric neck masses. *Radiol Clin North Am*. 2011 Jul;49(4):617–632.

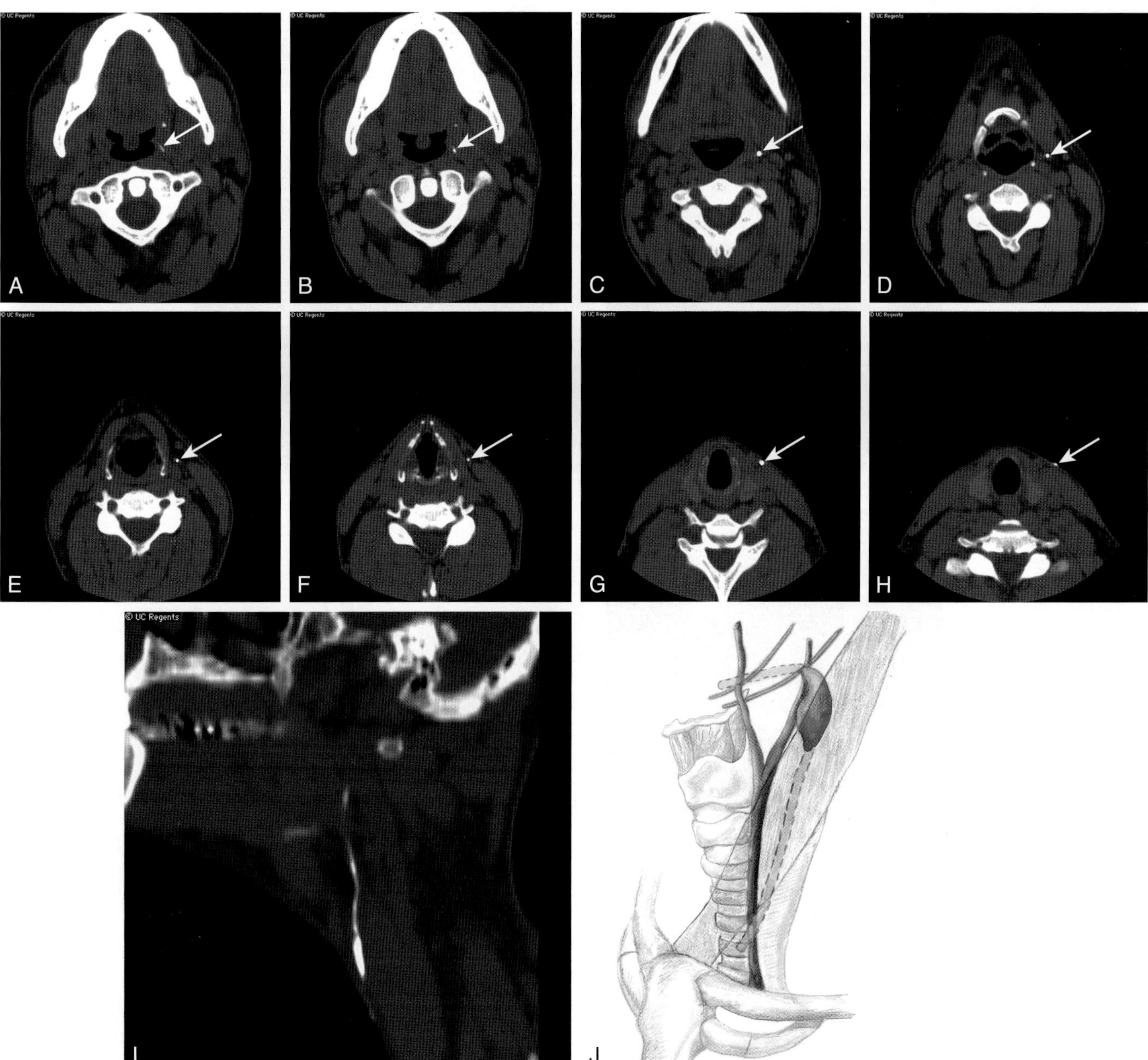

Fig. 14.8 Second Branchial Cleft Fistula. (A to H) Axial CT images following oral barium ingestion demonstrate the path of the second branchial cleft fistula from the left palatine tonsil, posterior to the submandibular gland, lateral neck anterior to the sternocleidomastoid muscle, and exiting the skin surface anterior to the sternocleidomastoid muscle at the level of the thyroid gland. (I) Sagittal reformat CT image demonstrating the fistula tract containing contrast material. (J) Illustration of the course of a second branchial cleft anomaly (blue) which can occur along a path from superior to inferior from the tonsillar fossa, extending laterally superficial to the glossopharyngeal and hypoglossal nerves (yellow structures), between the external and internal carotid arteries (red structures), and extending inferiorly along the lateral aspect of the common carotid artery (red structure) and medial to the sternocleidomastoid muscle before exiting the skin anterior to the junction of the middle and lower thirds of the sternocleidomastoid muscle at the level of the thyroid gland.

THIRD BRANCHIAL CLEFT ANOMALY

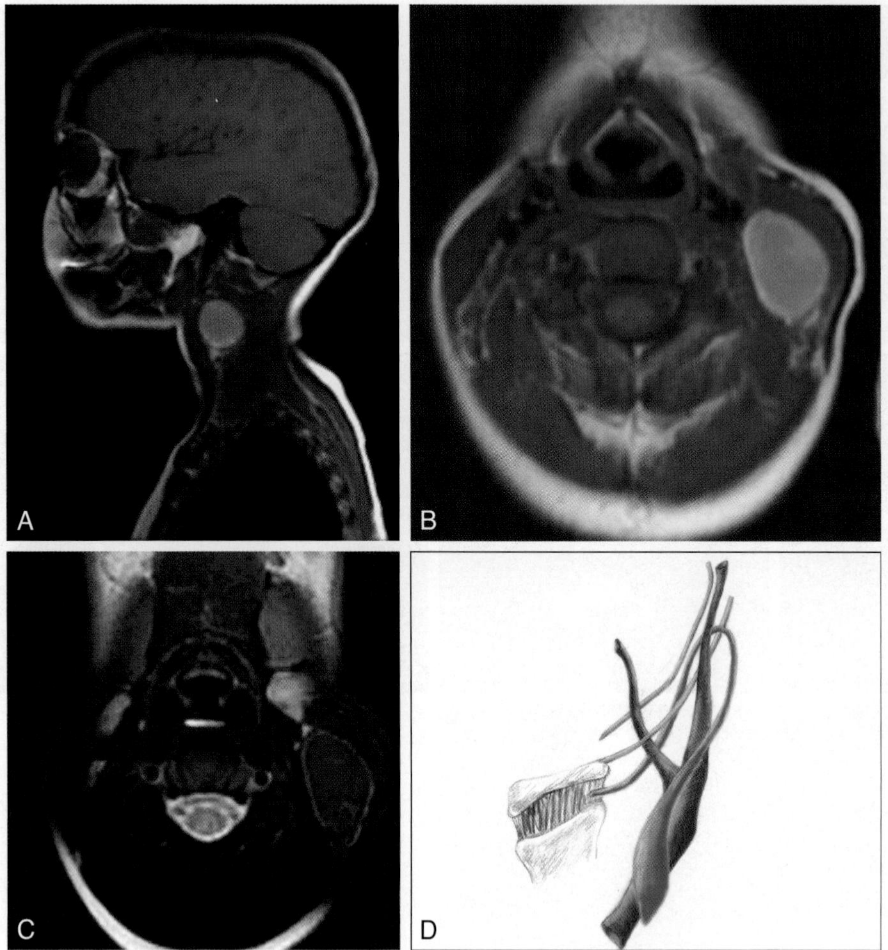

Fig. 14.9 Third Branchial Cleft Cyst. (A and B) Sagittal and axial T1W and (C) axial T2W images demonstrate a T1W hyperintense, T2W hypointense cyst in the posterior triangle of the left neck. The fluid signal is indicative of proteinaceous contents and is atypical. This lesion was biopsied and pathology confirmed a third branchial cleft cyst. The differential diagnosis would include a lymphatic malformation. (D) Illustration of the course of a third branchial cleft anomaly (blue) which extends from the pyriform sinus, above the superior laryngeal nerve (not shown) and between cranial 9 and 12 (yellow structures), posterior to the internal carotid artery (red) and sternocleidomastoid muscle and exiting the skin anterior to the lower third of the SCM.

Key Points

Background

- Includes cervical thymic cyst and third branchial cleft cyst

Imaging

- Third branchial cleft cyst: Rare; unilocular cystic mass.
- Location: most are found in the posterior triangle of the neck, lower anterior neck along anterior SCM or submandibular space.
- Third branchial cleft fistula courses from the upper *pyriform sinus* → above the superior laryngeal nerve and between the cranial nerve 9 and 12 → posterior to the carotid artery and posteromedial to the SCM → exiting through the skin along anterior border of lower one-third of the SCM.
- Differential Diagnosis: Lymphatic malformation.
- Note that a cervical thymic cyst is cyst from the third branchial pouch, which is different from the branchial cleft. See Thymic Cyst section for further details.

REFERENCE

1. Friedman ER, John SD. Imaging of pediatric neck masses. *Radiol Clin North Am*. 2011 Jul;49(4):617–632.

FOURTH BRANCHIAL CLEFT ANOMALY

Cystic

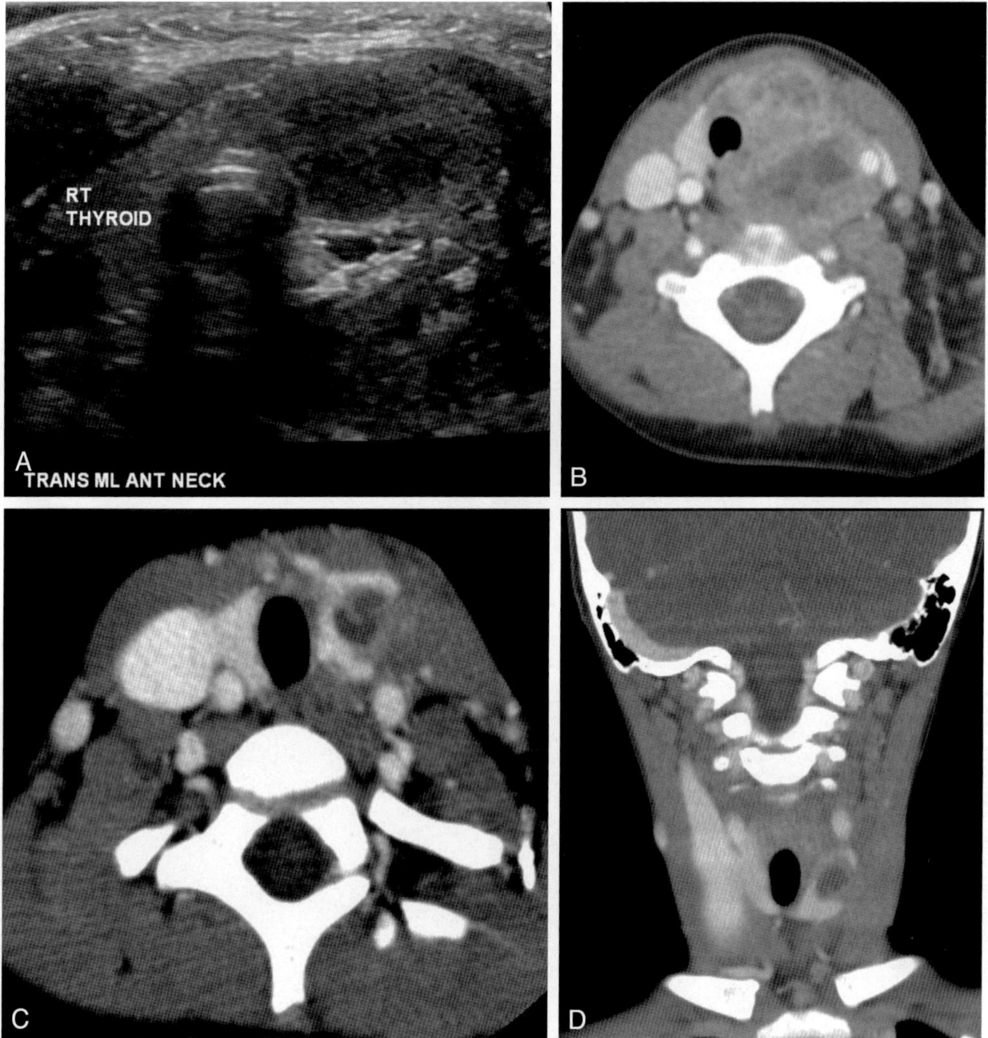

Fig. 14.10 Fourth Branchial Cleft Anomaly. (A) Transverse ultrasound image of the thyroid gland demonstrates abnormal enlargement and hypoechoic appearance of the left lobe. (B) Axial CECT image of the same patient demonstrates enlarged left thyroid lobe with areas of low density consistent with thyroid infection and abscess formation due to a fourth branchial cleft anomaly. A different patient presenting with left neck swelling and (C and D) axial and coronal CECT images demonstrate a fluid density lesion in the left lobe of the thyroid gland consistent with thyroid gland infection due to a fourth branchial cleft anomaly.

Key Points

Background

- Presents with thyroid gland infection (usually unilateral left thyroid lobe).
- Some combine third and fourth branchial cleft anomalies due to difficulty distinguishing the two. The location of the sinus tract with respect to the superior laryngeal nerve is key for differentiating the 3rd and 4th cleft anomalies.

Imaging

- Most commonly a sinus tract from the lower *piriform sinus* → below the superior laryngeal nerve → tacheoesophageal groove to the thyroid gland, usually the left lobe (80%). Although not clinically seen, the path follows the course of the recurrent laryngeal nerve and continues inferiorly to loop around the aorta in a posterior to anterior direction on the left side and subclavian artery on the right side and ascends posterior to the common carotid artery and exits the skin anterior to the sternocleidomastoid muscle.
- Thyroid gland infection typically seen on CT as an enlarged lobe, low-density areas in the lobe, organized fluid collections (abscess), and adjacent soft tissue inflammation and possible SCM myositis
- Barium swallow study followed by CT scan can demonstrate the sinus tract

REFERENCE

1. Friedman ER, John SD. Imaging of pediatric neck masses. *Radiol Clin North Am*. 2011 Jul;49(4):617–632.

FOURTH BRANCHIAL CLEFT ANOMALY

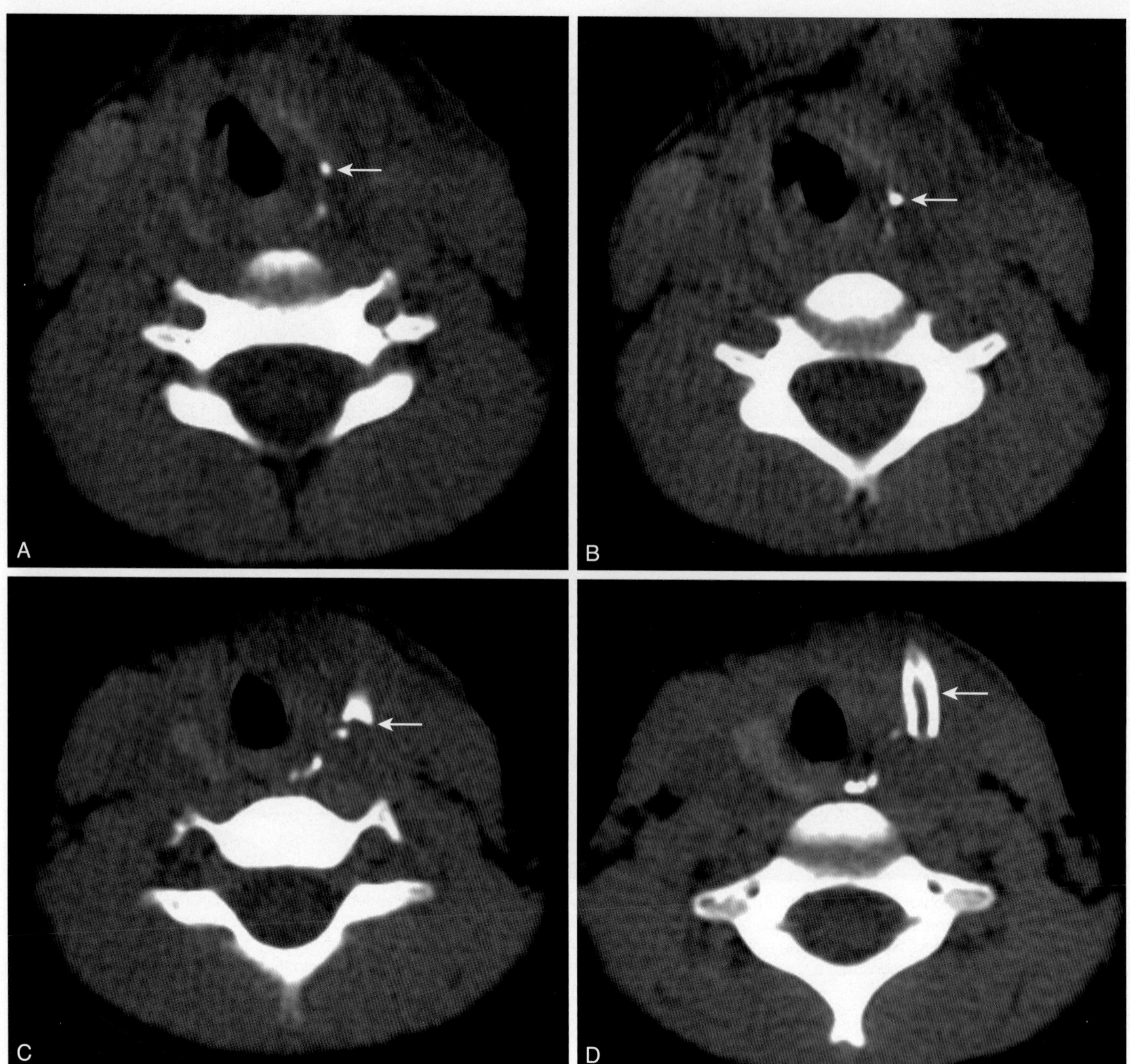

Fig. 14.11 Fourth Branchial Cleft Sinus Tract. (A to D) Axial CT images following ingestion of contrast material demonstrates extension of contrast from the left pyriform sinus into the medial left neck and terminating in the left lobe of the thyroid gland consistent with a fourth branchial cleft sinus tract.

SUMMARY: BRANCHIAL CLEFT ANOMALIES

Cystic

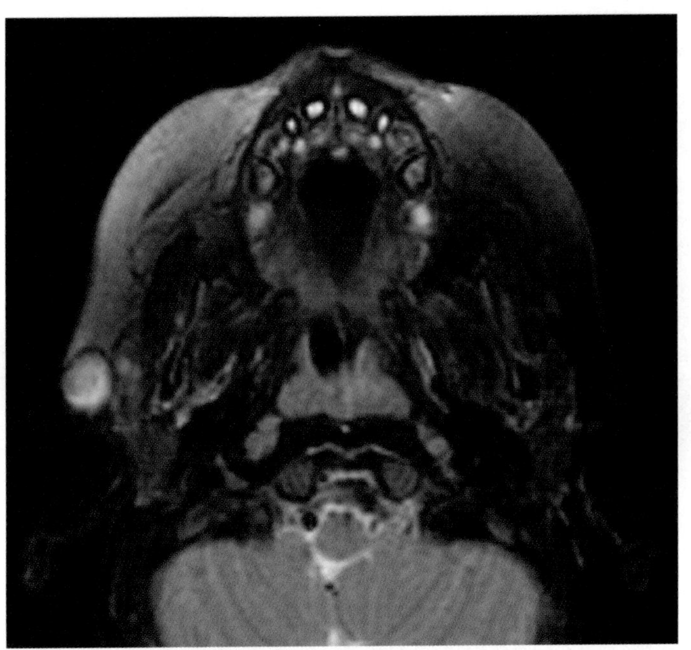

First Branchial Cleft Cyst

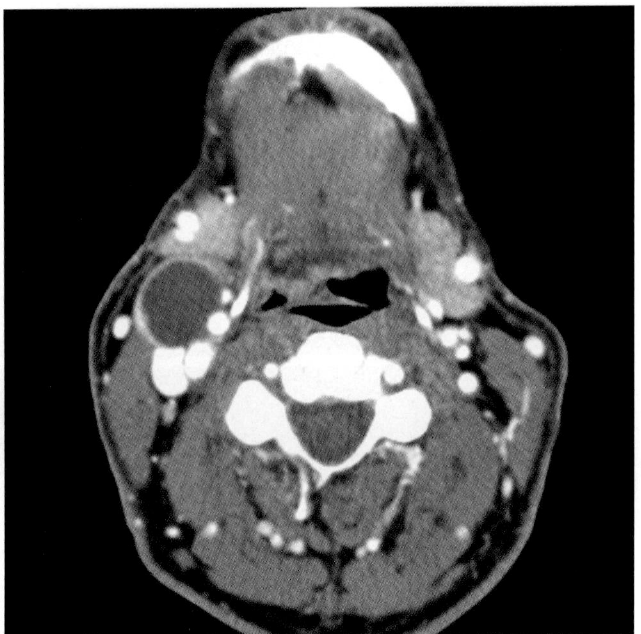

Second Branchial Cleft Cyst

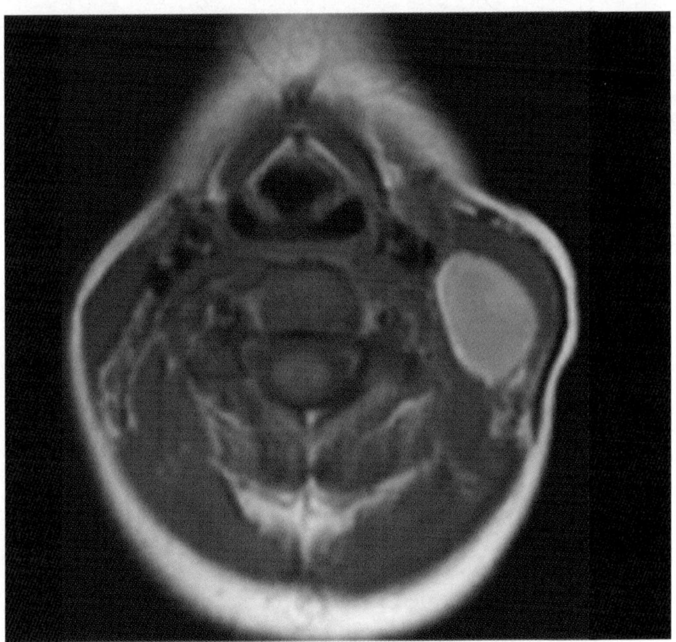

Third Branchial Cleft Cyst

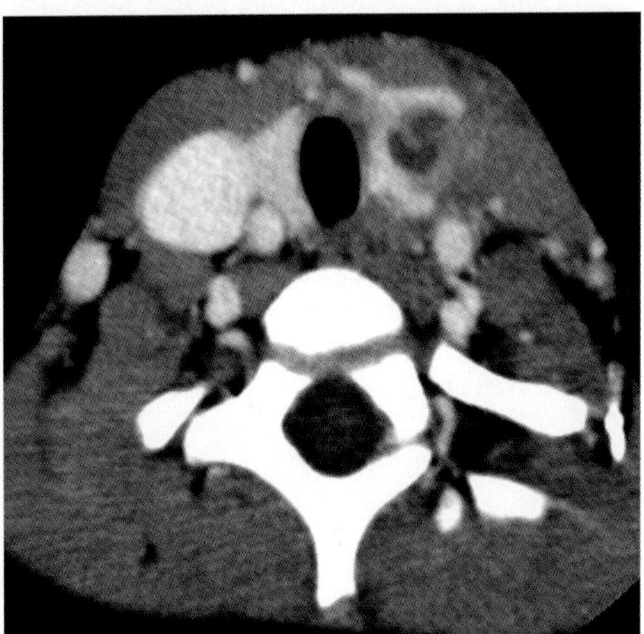

Fourth Branchial Sinus Cyst

LYMPHATIC MALFORMATION

Cystic

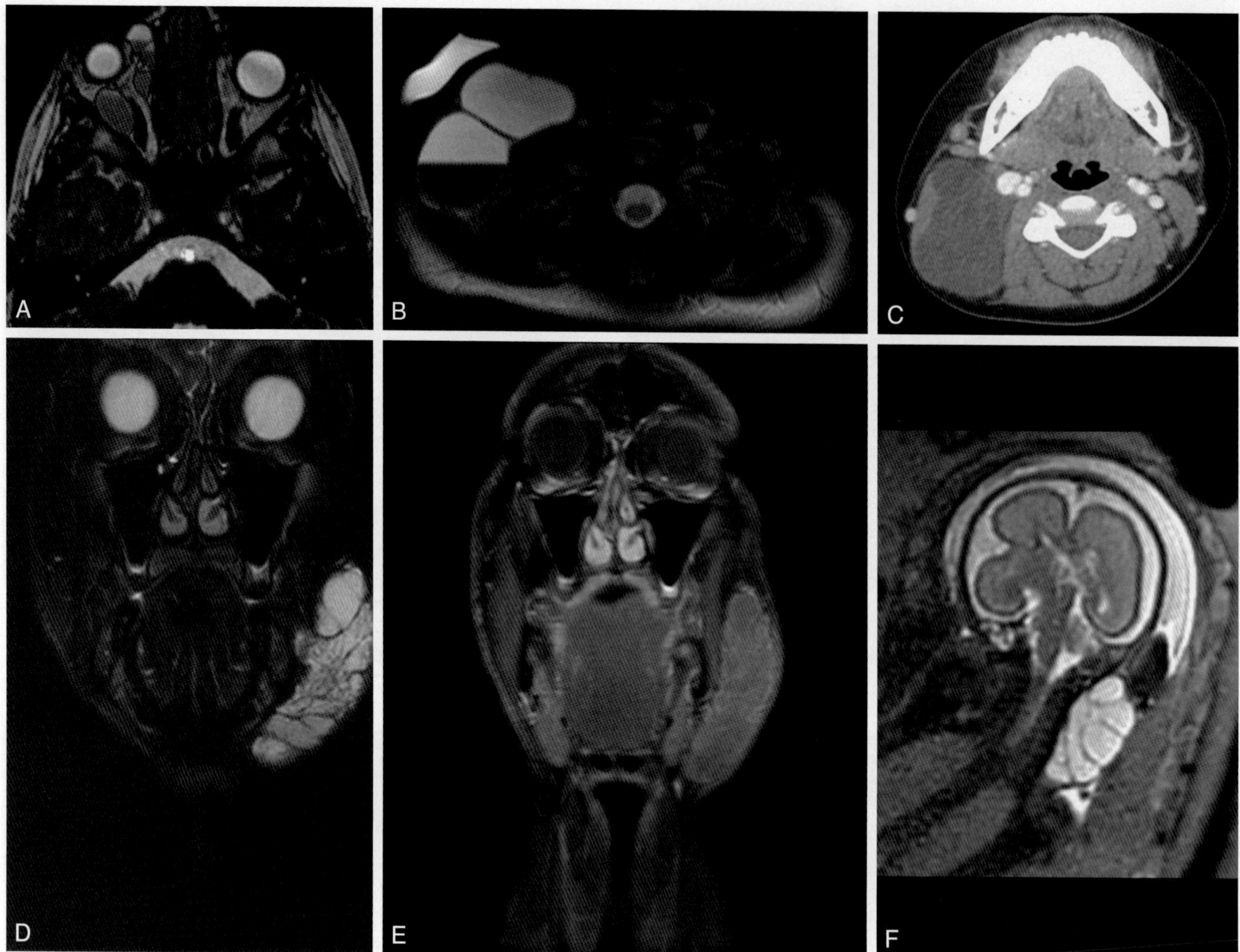

Fig. 14.12 Lymphatic Malformation: Imaging appearances in multiple patients. (A) Axial T2W image of the orbits demonstrates a multilocular right preseptal and postseptal fluid intensity lesion with fluid-fluid levels. (B) Axial T2W fat saturation image demonstrates a macrocystic cyst in the right lateral neck and supraclavicular fossa with internal layering fluid-fluid level. (C) Axial CECT image demonstrates a macrocystic fluid density cyst in the posterior triangle of the right neck with mass effect on the sternocleidomastoid muscle. (D) Coronal T2W fat saturation and (E) coronal T1W+C fat saturation images demonstrate a T2W hyperintense nonenhancing macrocystic lymphatic malformation. (F) Coronal T2W fetal MR image demonstrates a macrocystic lymphatic malformation in the lateral neck.

Key Points

Background

- Previously referred to as cystic hygroma or lymphangioma.
- Cystic mass composed of chyle-filled endothelial lined channels.
- Categorized as a slow or no-flow malformation.
- 90% present by 2 years of age. 75% occur in the neck.
- May present with rapid proptosis or acute neck mass if internal hemorrhage occurs or when a viral infection stimulates fluid production.

Imaging

- Transpatial/multispatial cystic mass in the face and neck.
- Macrocystic: Low density, hypoechoic; lobular, cystic areas with fluid-fluid levels; no-flow voids; nonenhancing except for septations or if venous component is present.
- Microcystic (<2 mm cyst size) may appear hyperechoic and may simulate an enhancing mass due to the close proximity of the septations.

REFERENCE

1. Friedman ER, John SD. Imaging of pediatric neck masses. *Radiol Clin North Am.* 2011 Jul;49(4):617–632.

THYMIC CYST

Cystic

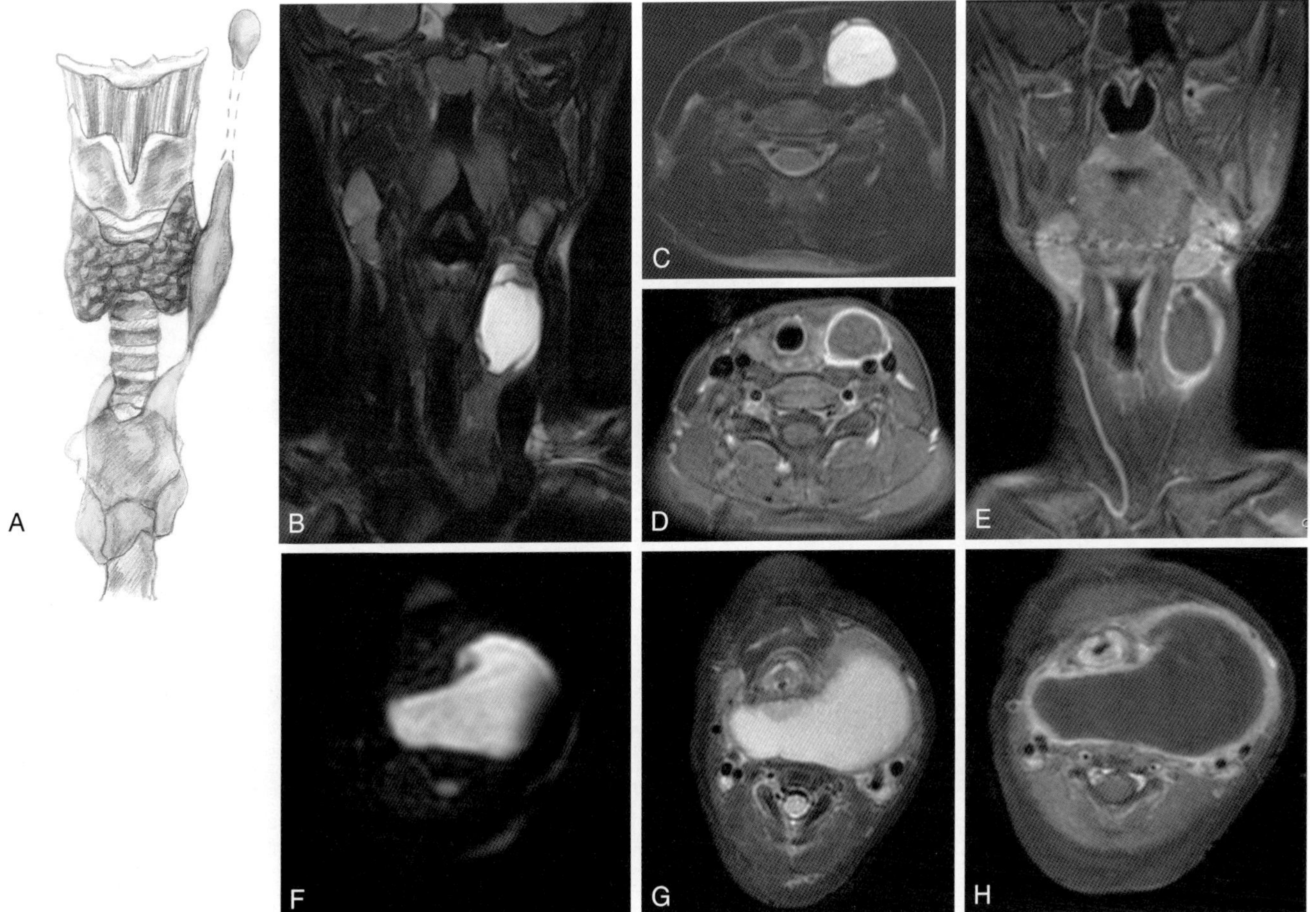

Fig. 14.13 Thymic Cyst. (A) Illustration of the tract of the thymus and possible ectopic thymus or thymic cyst in the neck. (B and C) Coronal and axial T2W fat saturation and (D and E) axial and coronal T1W+C fat saturation images demonstrate a fluid intensity cyst with thin peripheral enhancement in the left anterolateral neck along the course of the thymopharyngeal duct. Neonate with neck swelling: (F) axial DWI, (G) axial T2 fat saturation, and (H) axial T1W+C fat saturation images demonstrate a diffusion restricting fluid collection in the left lateral neck and retropharyngeal space. Biopsy performed during drainage confirmed an ectopic thymic cyst with *Escherichia coli* superinfection.

Key Points

Background

- Cystic remnant of the thymopharyngeal duct, which is a derivative of the third branchial *pouch* (as opposed to branchial cleft)
- Course of the thymopharyngeal pouch is from the piriform sinus → anterolateral neck along the parotid sheath → midline mediastinum
- A rapidly enlarging neck mass in a neonate can occur from superinfection of a thymic cyst due to communication between the aerodigestive tract and the cyst. Treated with drainage and surgical resection

Imaging

- Unilocular cyst in the lateral neck; typically fluid signal
- Superinfection can result in diffusion restriction from purulent material.
- Extends into the retropharyngeal space when large
- 50% are continuous with the mediastinal thymus.

REFERENCE

1. Billings KR, Rollins NR, Timmons C, et al. Infected neonatal cervical thymic cyst. *Ototaryngol Head Neck Surg*. 2000;123:651–654.

FOREGUT DUPLICATION CYST

Cystic

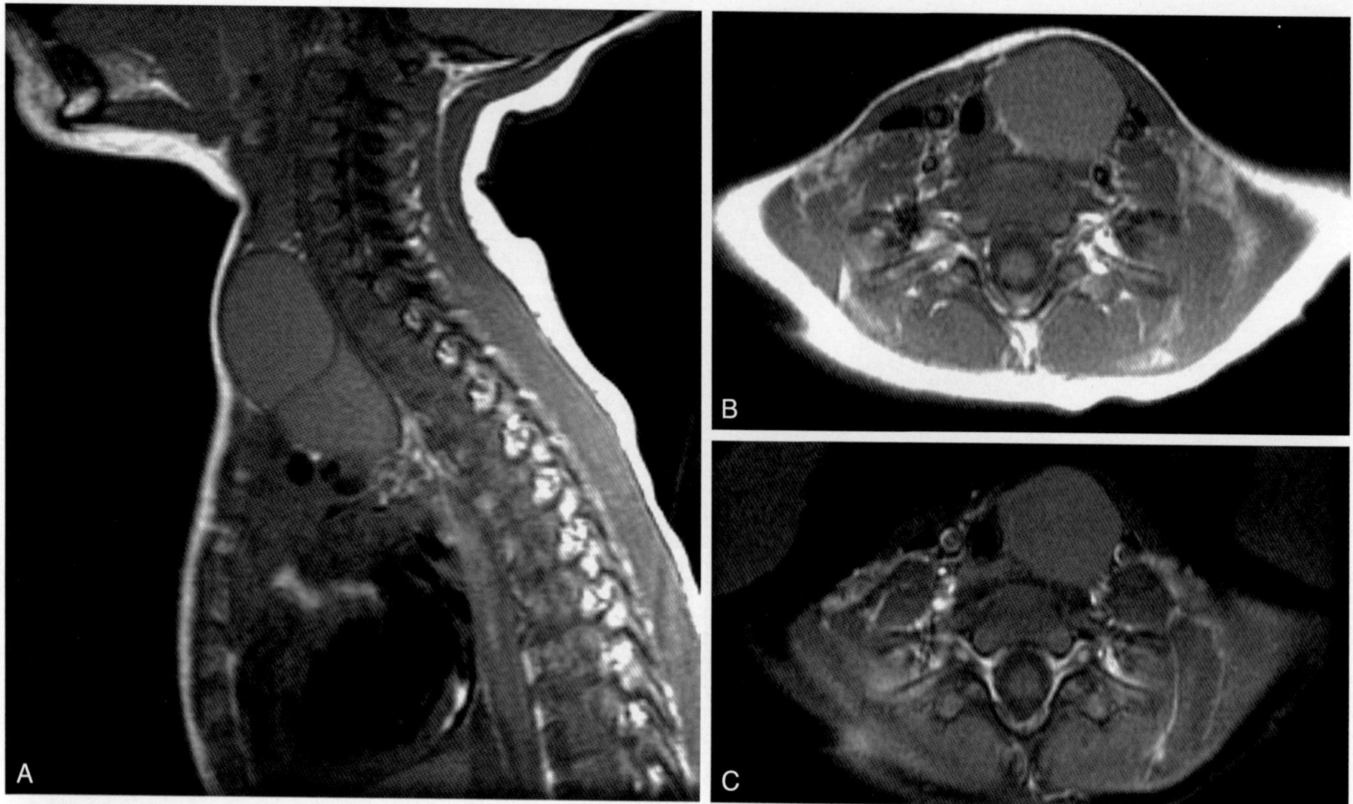

Fig. 14.14 Foregut Duplication Cyst. (A and B) Sagittal and axial T1W and (C) axial T1W+C fat saturation images demonstrate a nonenhancing proteinaceous cyst with T1W hyperintense signal in the central neck displacing the trachea and esophagus to the right side.

Key Points

Background

- Three types: Bronchogenic, esophageal, and neurogenic.
- Duplication cysts can be found from the mouth to the anus. Foregut anlage gives rise to the pharynx, respiratory tract, esophagus, stomach, and first and second parts of the duodenum.

Imaging

- Foregut duplication cysts are usually *midline*, often infrahyoid, floor of mouth, or posterior mediastinal.
- Often discovered incidentally.
- Differential Diagnosis: Thymic cyst.

REFERENCES

1. Eaton D, Billings K, Timmons C, et al. Congenital foregut duplication cysts of the anterior tongue. *Arch Otolaryngol Head Neck Surg.* 2001;127(12):1484–1487.
2. Balakrishnan K, Fonacier F, Sood S, et al. Foregut duplication cysts in children. *JSLS.* 2017 Apr–Jun;21(2):e2017.

DERMOID CYST

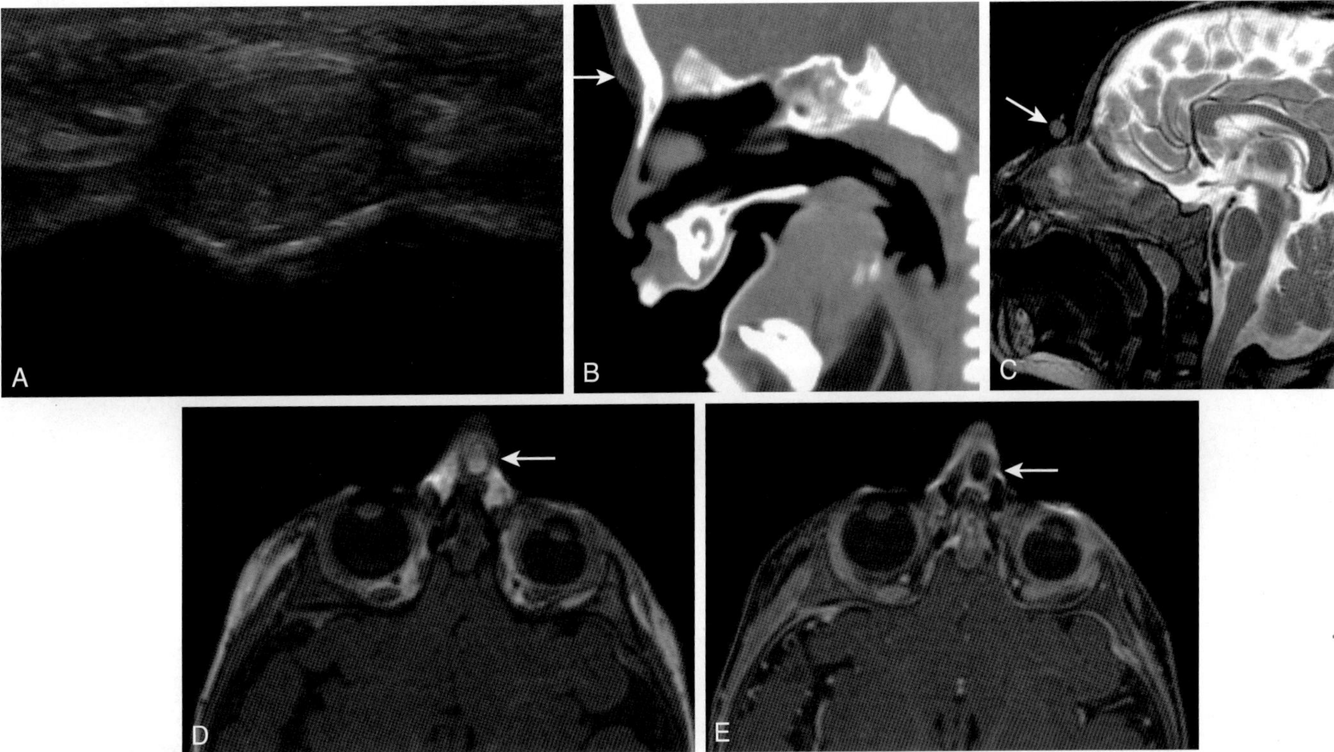

Fig. 14.15 Dermoid Cyst. (A) Ultrasound image demonstrating an isoechoic nodule located at the nasal bridge. (B) Sagittal reformat CT image demonstrates a fat density nodule at the nasal bridge. (C) Sagittal T2W image demonstrates mild T2W hyperintense nodule at the nasal bridge. (D and E) Axial T1W and T1W+C fat saturation images demonstrate a nodule at the nasal bridge with T1W hyperintense signal that loses signal with fat saturation and demonstrates thin peripheral enhancement.

Key Points

Background

- Congenital malformation due to skin elements pulled into the prenasal space along with the regressing dural diverticulum.
- Occur from the tip of the nose to the crista galli. More common than epidermoid cysts. CNS connection in ~50%. Sinus tract opening, dimple or tuft of hair at the skin surface is present in 84%.
- Surgical removal to prevent intracranial infection.

Imaging

- CT: Wide foramen cecum; bifid crista galli; fat density
- MRI: Nonenhancing; T1 hyperintensity
- Differential Diagnosis: Encephalocele, and nasal glioma/hamartoma

REFERENCES

1. Lowe LH, Booth TN, Jogler JM, et al. Midface anomalies in children. *Radiographics*. 2000 Jul–Aug;20(4):907–922.
2. Huisman TA, Schneider JF, Kellenberger CJ, Martin-Fiori E, Willi UV, Holzmann D. Developmental nasal midline masses in children: neuroradiological evaluation. *Eur Radiol*. 2004 Feb;14(2):243–249.

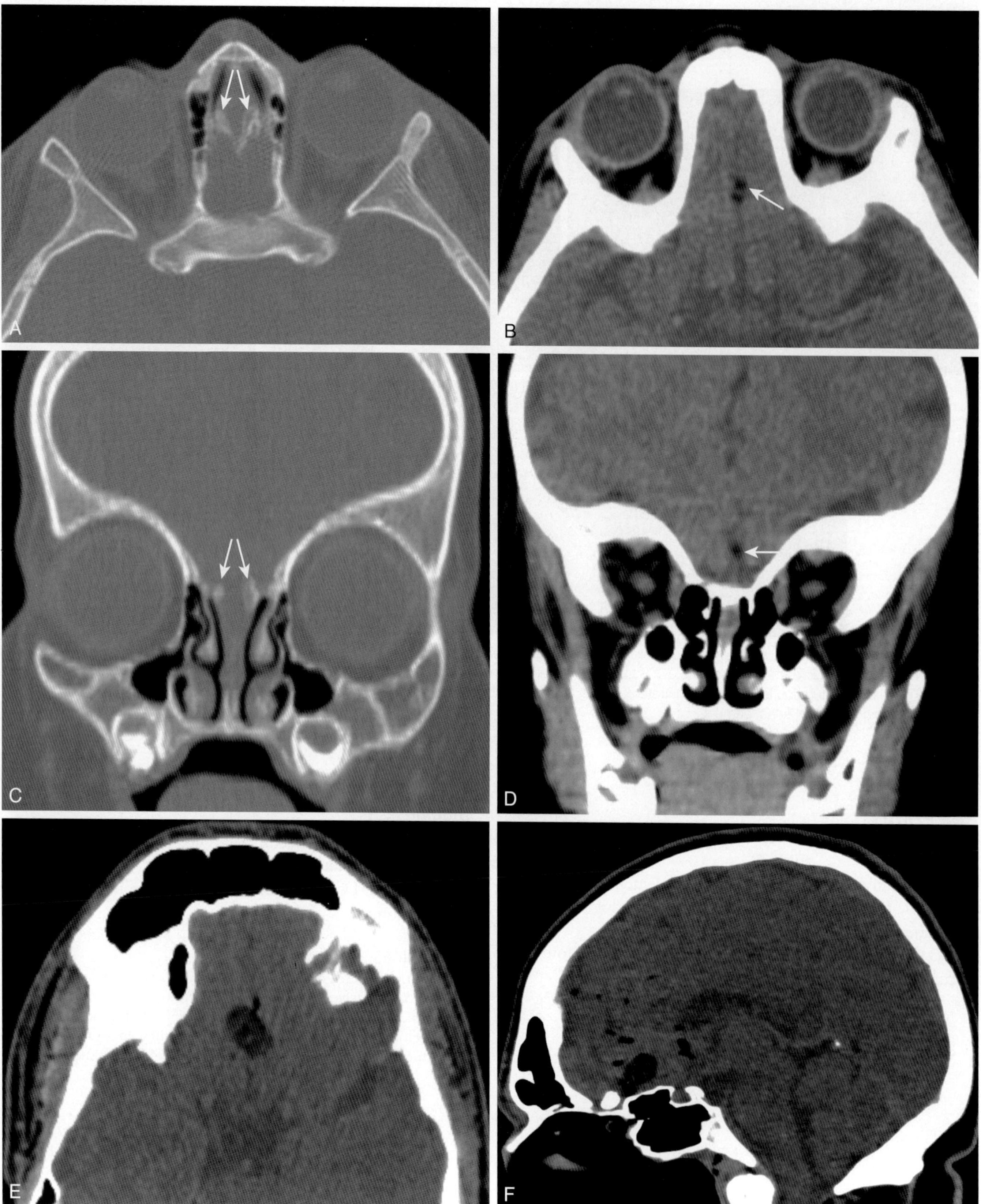

Fig. 14.16 Nasal Dermoid Cyst. (A to D) Axial and coronal CT images at 11 months of age demonstrate bifid crista galli and focal fat density in the midline above the crista galli. (E and F) Axial and coronal CT images at 17 years of age demonstrate interval enlargement of the dermoid cyst and rupture of the cyst into the subarachnoid spaces.

EPIDERMOID CYST

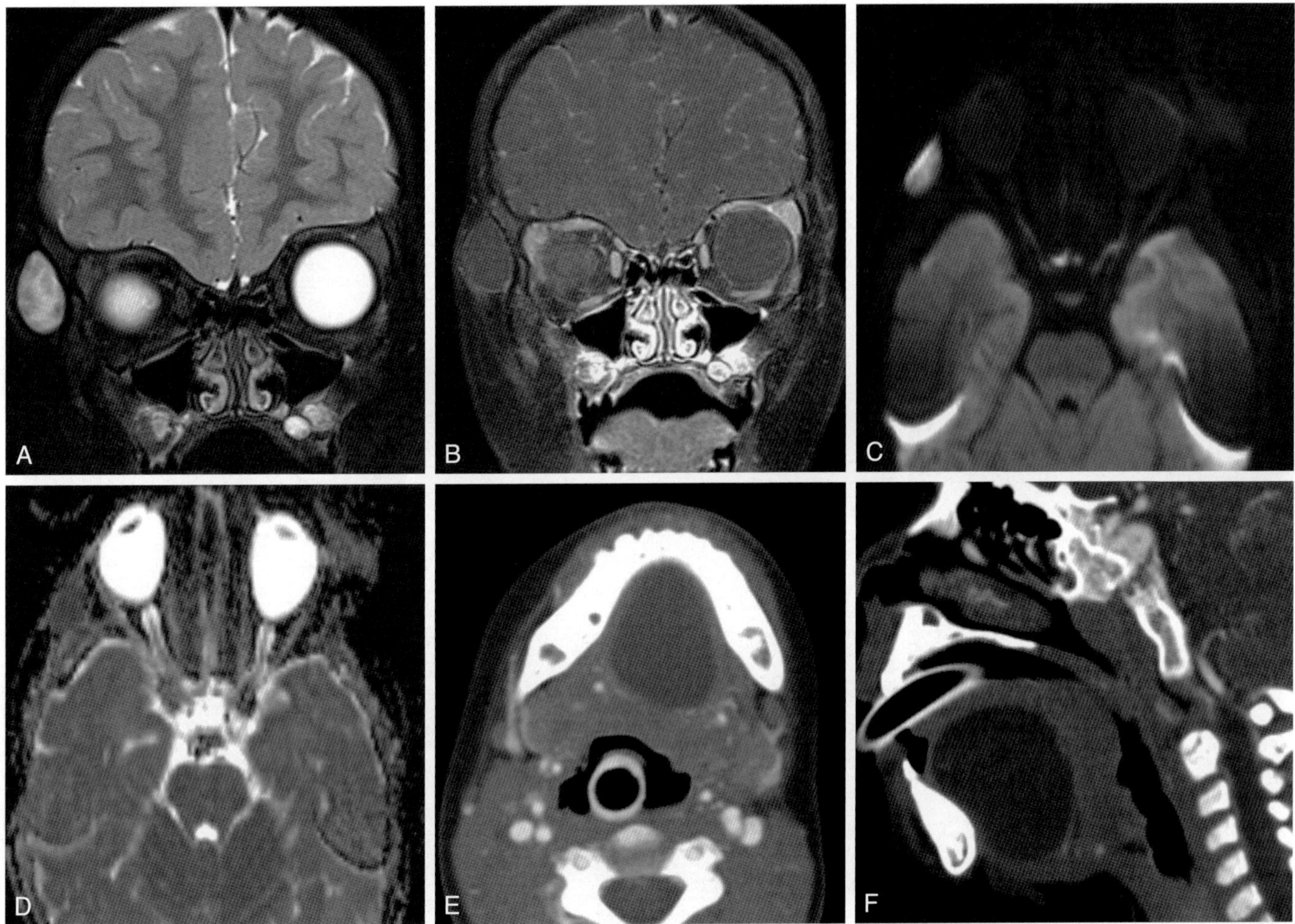

Fig. 14.17 Epidermoid Cyst. (A) Coronal T2W fat saturation, (B) coronal T1W+C fat saturation, (C) axial DWI, and (D) axial ADC images demonstrate a nonenhancing T2W hyperintense cyst with diffusion restriction in the right lateral orbit adjacent to the frontozygomatic suture. Different patient with a dermoid cyst: (E and F) Axial and sagittal CECT images demonstrate a floor of mouth epidermoid cyst with fluid density and no areas of enhancement.

Key Points

Background

- Benign cyst arising from an epidermal rest

Imaging

- Common locations: Lateral orbit and floor of mouth
- Midline or paramedian in location
- Fluid density/intensity; T2 hyperintensity; diffusion restriction
- Can become superinfected if a coexistent dermal sinus tract from the skin is present

REFERENCE

1. Vachha BA, Robson CD. Imaging of pediatric orbital disease. *Neuroimaging Clin N Am*. 2015 Aug;25(3):477–501.

RANULA

Cystic

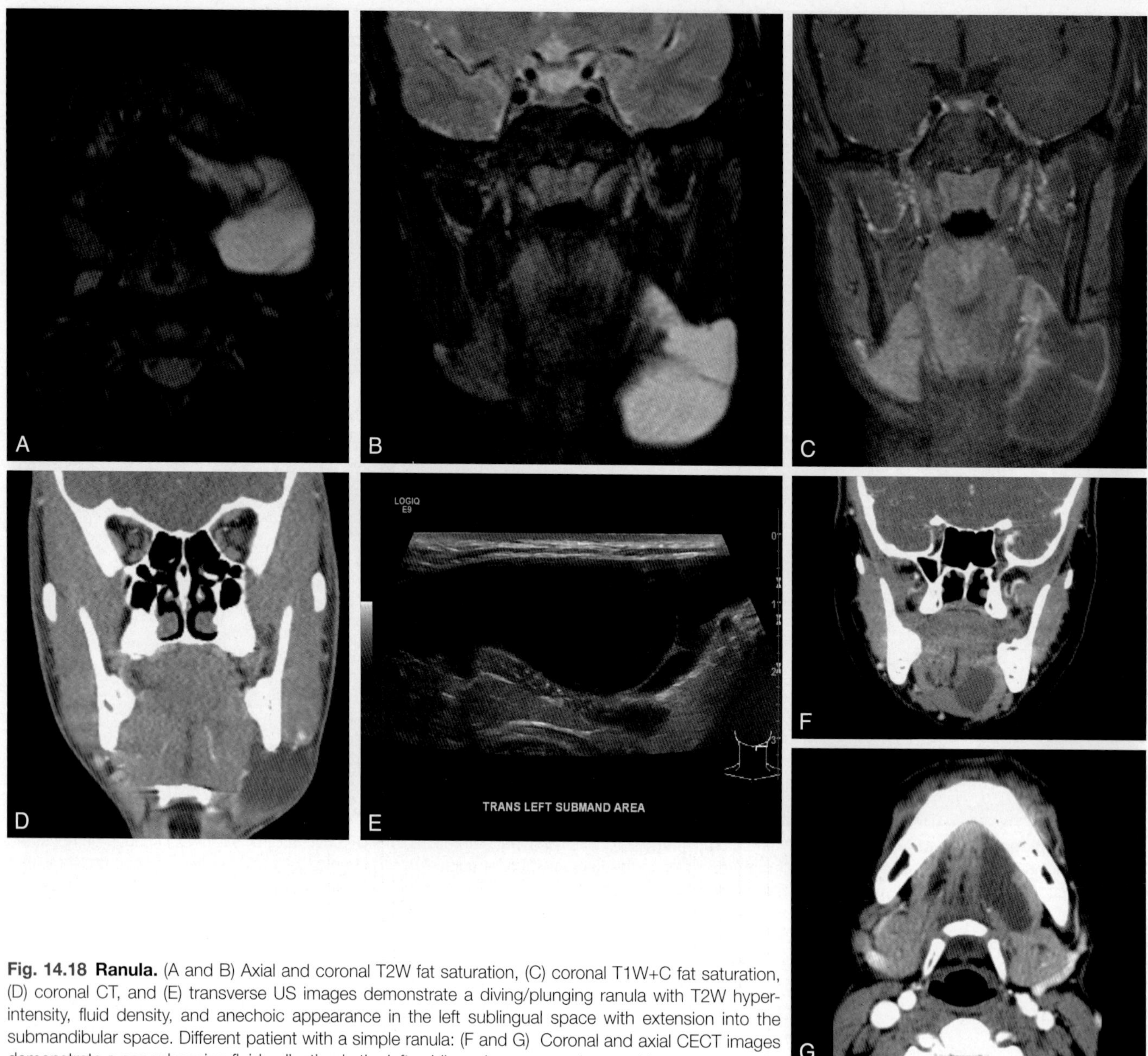

Fig. 14.18 Ranula. (A and B) Axial and coronal T2W fat saturation, (C) coronal T1W+C fat saturation, (D) coronal CT, and (E) transverse US images demonstrate a diving/plunging ranula with T2W hyperintensity, fluid density, and anechoic appearance in the left sublingual space with extension into the submandibular space. Different patient with a simple ranula: (F and G) Coronal and axial CECT images demonstrate a nonenhancing fluid collection in the left sublingual space consistent with a simple ranula.

Key Points

Background

- Retention cyst of the sublingual gland or minor salivary glands resulting from trauma or inflammation

Imaging

- Unilocular fluid density/intensity; thin wall.
- Simple ranula is confined to the sublingual space.
- Diving ranula extends into the submandibular space with a pointed/tail toward the sublingual space.

REFERENCE

1. Som PM, Curtin HD. *Head and Neck Imaging*. 5th ed. St. Louis: Mosby Elsevier; 2011.

PAPILLARY THYROID CANCER

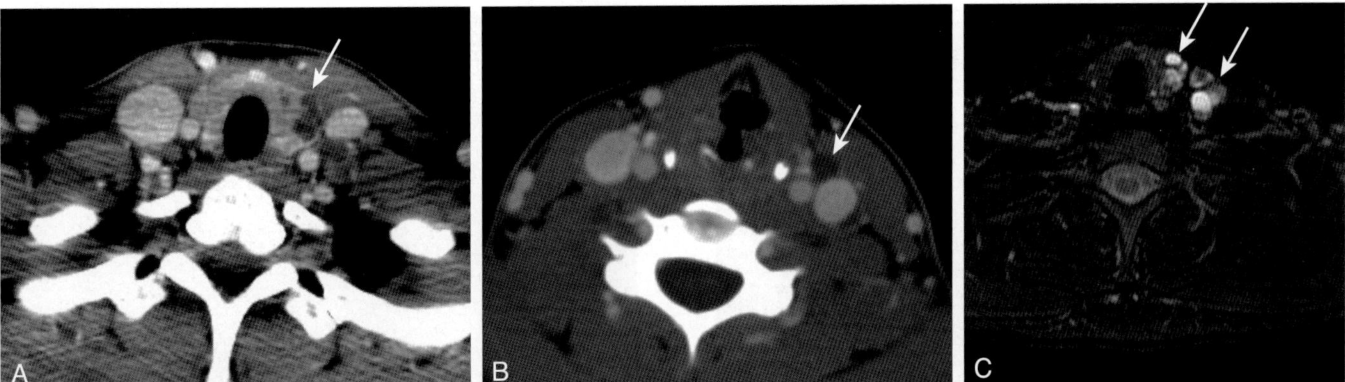

Fig. 14.19 Papillary Thyroid Cancer. (A) Axial CECT demonstrates a low-density mass in the left lobe of the thyroid gland and low density nodal metastasis to the left level 4 location. (C) Axial T2W fat saturation image demonstrates the left thyroid lobe T2W hyperintense mass and the cystic nodal metastases in the left level 4 location.

Key Points

Background

- The annual incidence of thyroid cancer is low in children younger than 15 years (2 per million), although prepubertal children tend to have a more aggressive presentation. The incidence is higher in children aged 15 to 19 years (17.6 per million).

Imaging

- CT: Hypodense nodule/mass compared to thyroid gland and muscles. Often, the mass contains dystrophic calcification. Metastatic thyroid carcinoma can have solid or cystic nodes and may have calcifications.
- MRI: Metastatic lymph nodes may have T2W hyperintensity from cystic degeneration and/or intrinsic high T1W signal due to thyroglobulin and/or hemorrhage.
- Important to assess for extrathyroidal extension, lymph node involvement, and lung metastasis.

REFERENCE

1. Harness JK, Sahar DE, et al. Childhood thyroid carcinoma. In: Clark O, Duh Q-Y, Kebebew E, eds. *Textbook of Endocrine Surgery*. 2nd ed. Philadelphia, PA: Elsevier Saunders Company; 2005:93–101.

DIFFERENTIAL DIAGNOSIS OF A VASCULAR NECK MASS

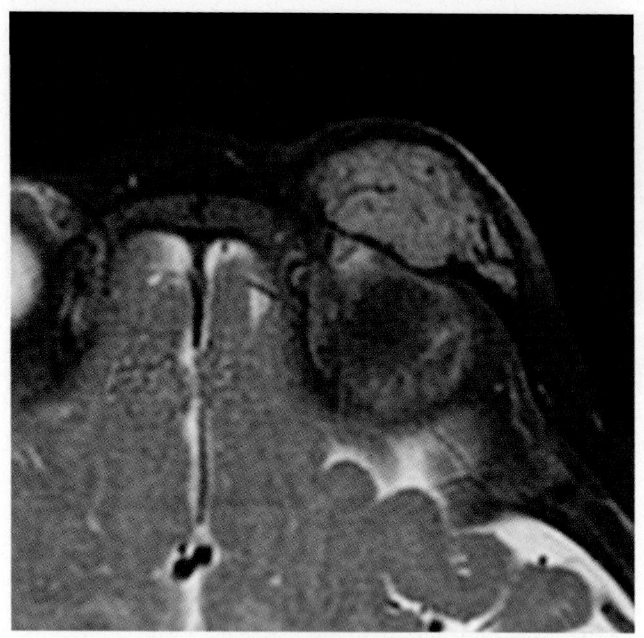

Infantile Hemangioma

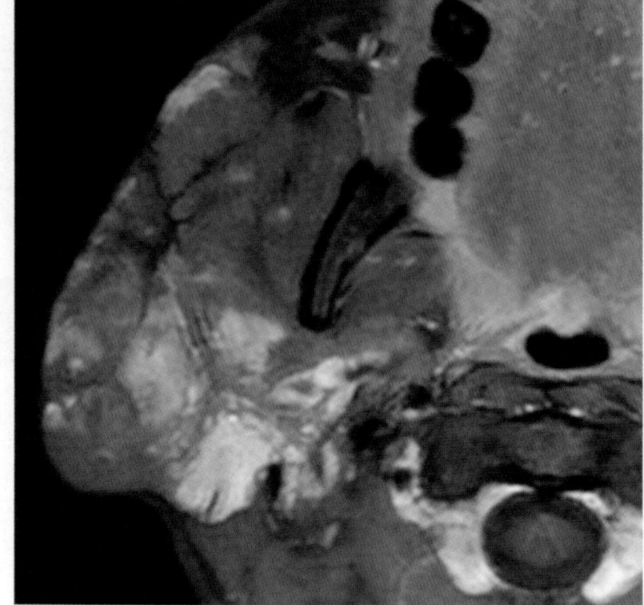

Venolymphatic Malformation

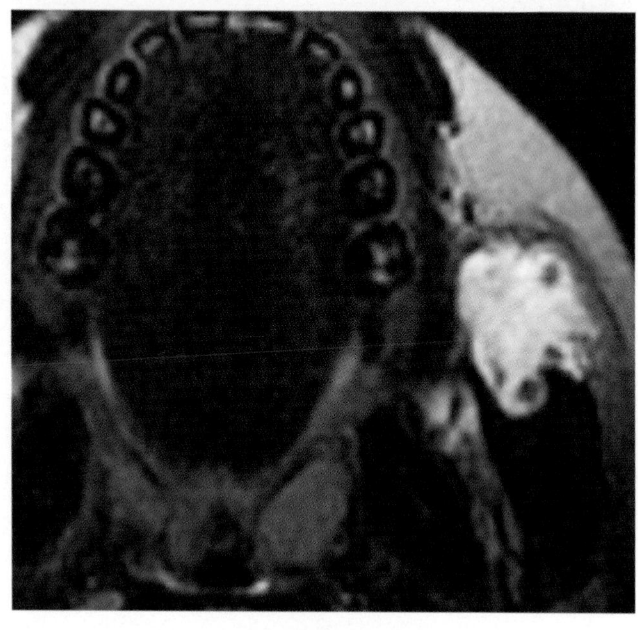

Venous Malformation

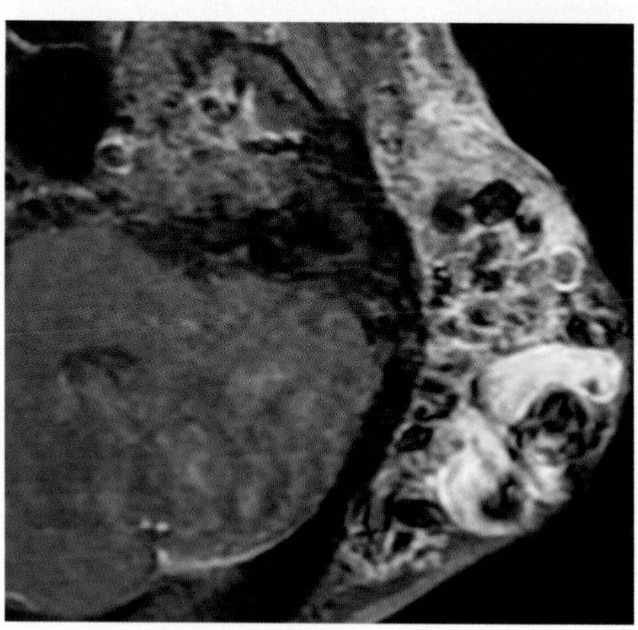

AVM

INFANTILE HEMANGIOMA

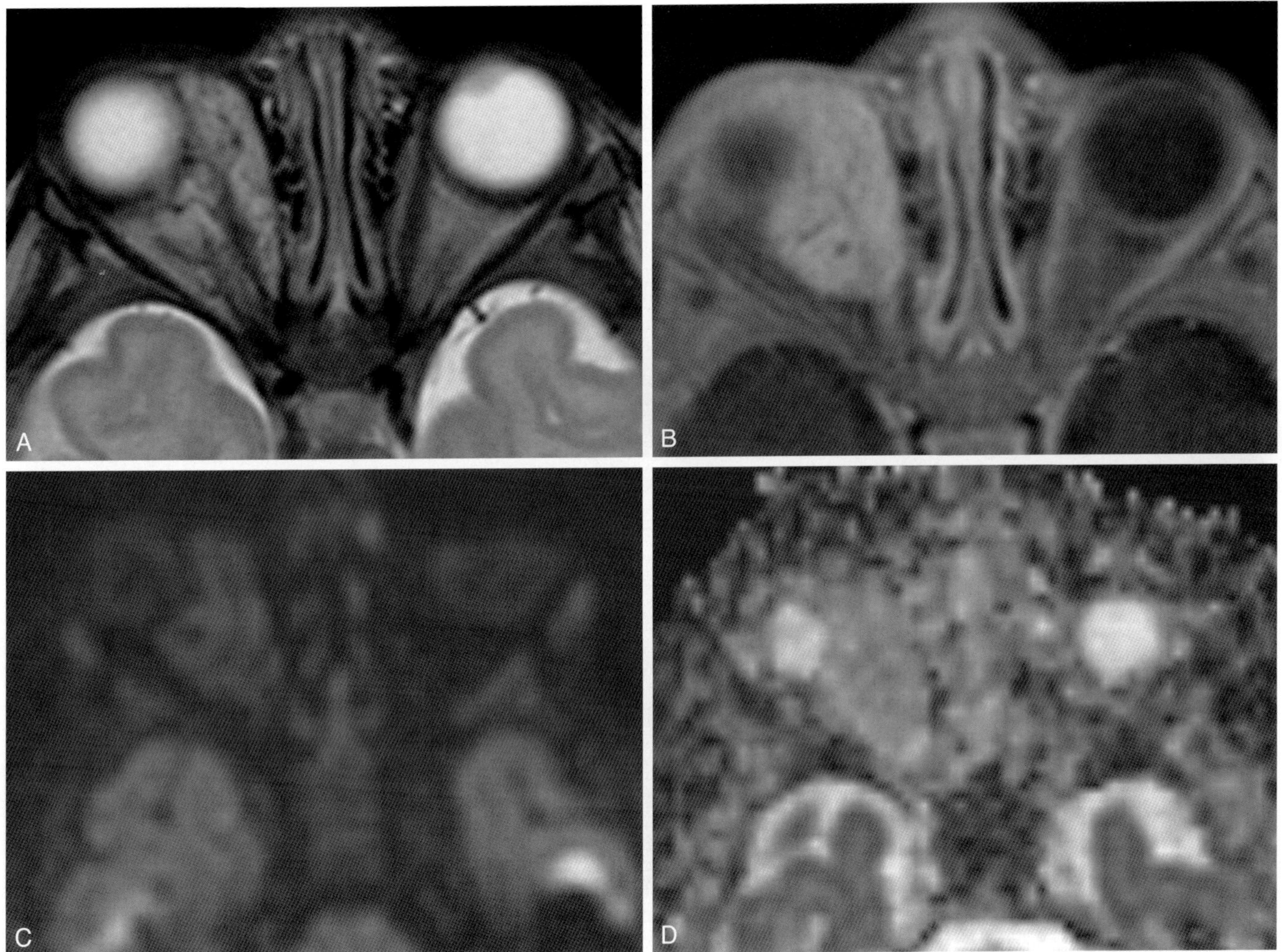

Fig. 14.20 Infantile Hemangioma. (A) Axial T2W, (B) axial T1W+C fat saturation, (C) axial DWI, and (D) axial ADC images demonstrate a mildly T2W hyperintense mass with thin linear T2W hypointense flow voids, homogeneous avid enhancement and facilitated diffusion in the post septal right orbit displacing the right globe.

Key Points

Background

- The most common benign tumor of infancy. 95% present before 6 months of age. Often involute spontaneously.
- Predilection for superior orbit, eyelid, and supranasal periorbita (can be intraconal and extend to superior orbital fissure).
- Associated with PHACES syndrome:
  - **P**osterior fossa malformation
  - **H**emangioma
  - **A**rterial anomaly
  - **C**oarctation of the aorta
  - **E**ye abnormality
  - **S**ternal defect and supraumbilical raphe.
- Treatment options include propranolol steroids, interferon, laser therapy, and surgical excision.

Imaging

- Circumscribed or infiltrative
- US: Variable echogenicity with high flow velocity
- CT: Solid tissue density; homogenous enhancement; no gross Ca^{2+}
- MRI: Mild T2W hyperintensity; flow voids; intense enhancement; ADC hyperintense, which helps distinguish from orbital rhabdomyosarcoma

REFERENCES

1. Baer AH, Parmar HA, McKnight CD, et al. Head and neck vascular anomalies in the pediatric population. *Neurographics*. 2014 March(4):2–19.
2. Kralik SF, Haider KM, Lobo RR, et al. Orbital infantile hemangioma and rhabdomyosarcoma in children: differentiation using diffusion-weighted magnetic resonance imaging. *JAAPOS*. 2018 Feb;22(1):27–31.

CONGENITAL HEMANGIOMA

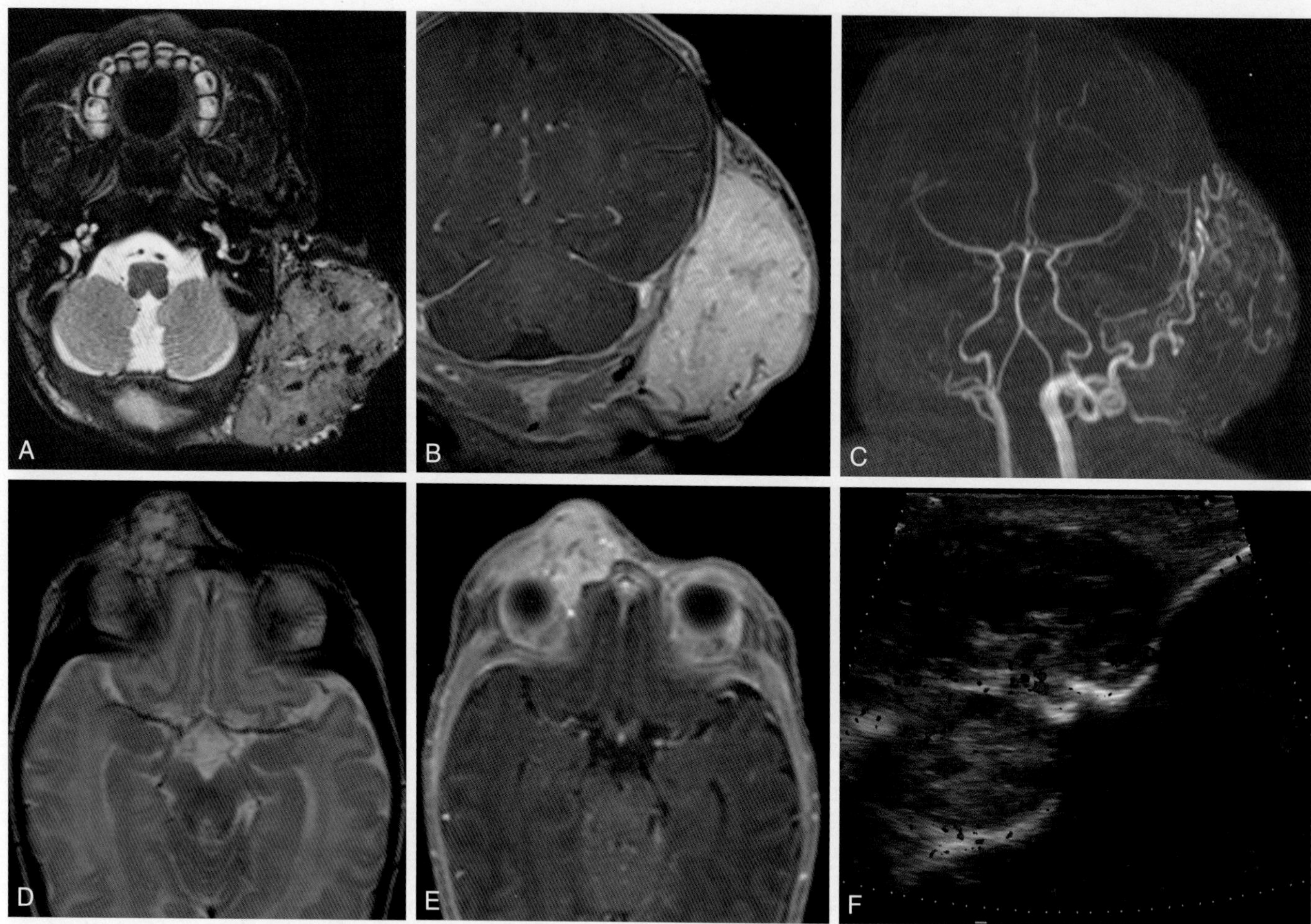

Fig. 14.21 Congenital Hemangioma. (A) Axial T2W fat saturation, (B) axial T1W+C fat saturation, and (C) 3D volumetric MR angiography images demonstrate a mildly T2W hyperintense mass with linear T2 hypointense flow voids, homogeneous avid enhancement, and arterial supply from the external carotid artery. (D) Axial T2W fat saturation, (E) axial T1W+C fat saturation, and (F) ultrasound images demonstrate a mildly T2W hyperintense mass with linear T2W hypointense flow voids, homogeneous avid enhancement, and significant vascularity on color Doppler ultrasound.

Key Points

Background

- Benign vascular tumor present at birth.
- Rapidly involuting congenital hemangioma (RICH) and non-involuting congenital hemangioma (NICH).
- RICH usually regress by 14 months, while NICH proportionally grows with the child without regression.
- Neither expresses GLUT-1 transporter, which differs from infantile hemangiomas; may result in vascular shunting or thrombocytopenia when large; does not respond to treatment with propranolol.

Imaging

- Avidly enhancing mass with flow voids and enlarged arterial feeding vessels; may contain calcification and visible vessels on US to greater degree than infantile hemangiomas

REFERENCES

1. Gorincour G, Kokta V, Rypens F, et al. Imaging characteristics of two subtypes of congenital hemangiomas: rapidly involuting congenital hemangioma and non-involuting congenital hemangiomas. *Pediatr. Radiol.* 2005;35:1178–1185.
2. Baer AH, Parmar HA, McKnight CD, et al. Head and neck vascular anomalies in the pediatric population. *Neurographics.* 2014 March(4):2–19.

KAPOSIFORM HEMANGIOENDOTHELIOMA

Vascular

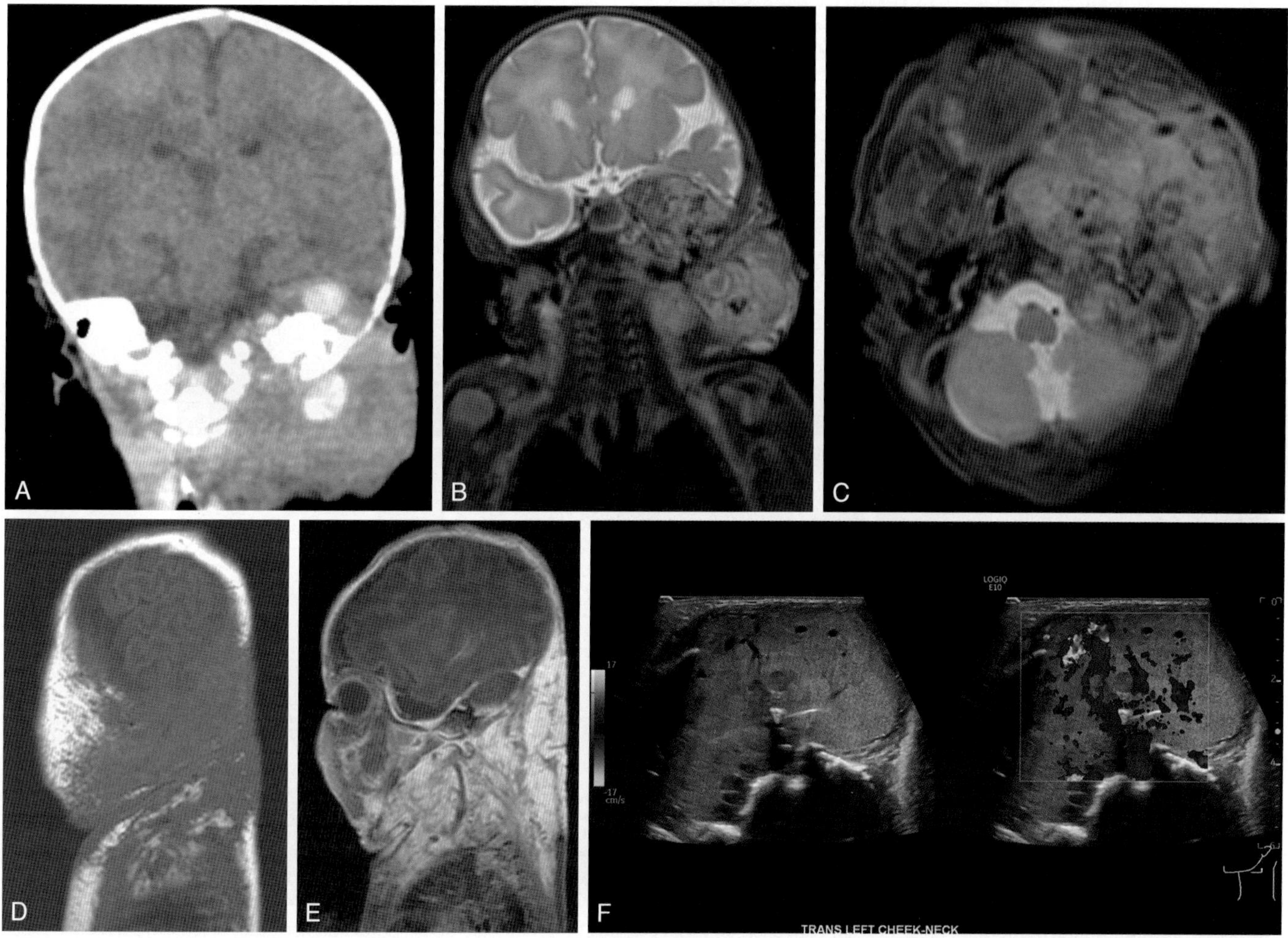

Fig. 14.22 Kaposiform Hemangioendothelioma. (A) Coronal CT image demonstrates an aggressive soft tissue mass with bone destruction of the left temporal bone and internal hemorrhage. (B and C) Coronal and axial T2W fat saturation images demonstrates a T2W hyperintense mass with internal flow voids centered in the left temporal bone with intracranial extension. (D) Sagittal T1W, (E) sagittal T1W+C, and (F) ultrasound image demonstrate and infiltrative soft tissue mass in the lateral neck with homogeneous enhancement and significant vascularity.

Key Points

Background

- Rare congenital vascular tumor, with a prevalence rate of 1 per 100,000
- Aggressively infiltrates the normal tissues with epithelial cells, lymphatic channels, and vascular spaces
- May result in thrombocytopenia (Kasabach Merritt)
- Treated with surgical resection and medical therapy (corticosteroids and other medications)

Imaging

- MRI: Solitary or diffuse infiltrative solid mass with aggressive appearance, flow voids related to feeding and draining vessels, and hemorrhage; T2W hyperintense relative to muscle; may have scattered areas of hemorrhage and diffusion restriction
- May mimic an infantile hemangioma because of the flow voids
- US: Solid mass with hypervascular appearance

REFERENCE

1. Hu PA, Zhou ZR. Clinical and imaging features of kaposiform hemangioendothelioma. *Br J Radiol.* 2018 Jun;91(1086):20170798.

VENOUS MALFORMATION

Vascular

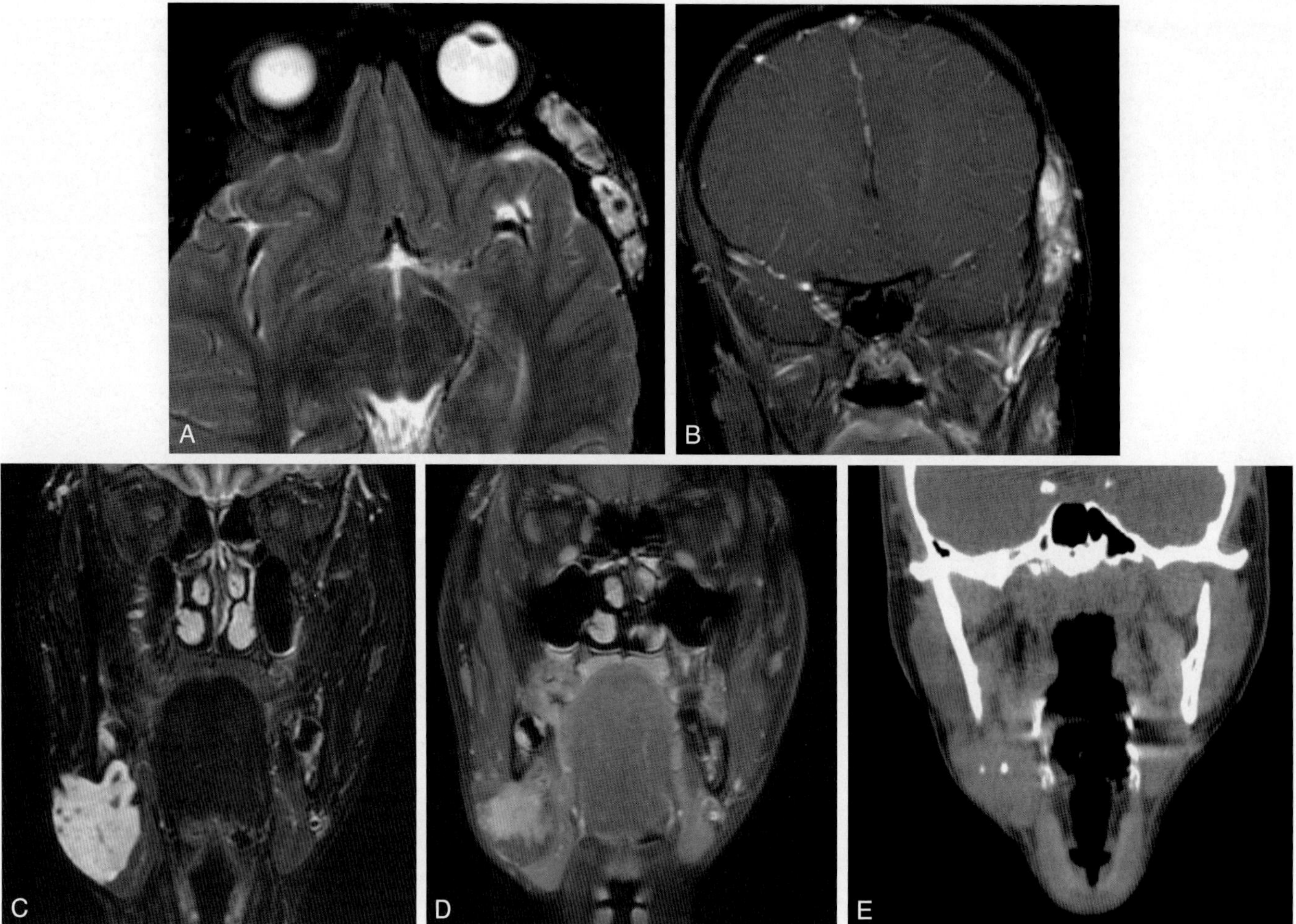

Fig. 14.23 Venous Malformation. (A) Axial T2W fat saturation and (B) coronal T1W+C fat saturation images demonstrate a T2W hyperintense mass with rounded T2W hypointense phleboliths and incomplete enhancement. (C) Coronal T2W fat saturation and (D) coronal T1W+C fat saturation images demonstrate a T2W hyperintense mass with rounded T2W hypointense phleboliths and incomplete enhancement, while (E) coronal CT demonstrates an isodense mass with rounded calcifications (phleboliths).

Key Points

Background

- Also known as cavernous hemangioma, cavernous malformation, stork bite, port wine stain, or port wine hemangioma
- Slow-flow vascular malformation; present at birth; soft, compressible, bluish mass; most common vascular malformation of head and neck
- Associated syndromes: Klippel-Trenauney, Proteus, Maffuci, Gorham-Stout, blue-rubber bleb nevus, and Bockenheimer.

Imaging

- US: Hypoechoic, and shadowing phleboliths.
- CT: Isodense to hypodense to muscle on noncontrast CT; coarse Ca^{2+} represent phleboliths
- MRI: T2W hyperintense; progressively enhances; dynamic contrast-enhanced MRA may be very helpful in revealing the specific contrast enhancement pattern, facilitating differentiation from other similar appearing lesions.

REFERENCES

1. Nasseri F, Munjal K, Ginsberg LE, et al. Imaging review of craniofacial masses in children. *Neurographics*. 2015 Sept/Oct;5(5):217–230.
2. Baer AH, Parmar HA, McKnight CD, et al. head and neck vascular anomalies in the pediatric population. *Neurographics*. 2014 March(4):2–19.

VENOUS MALFORMATION

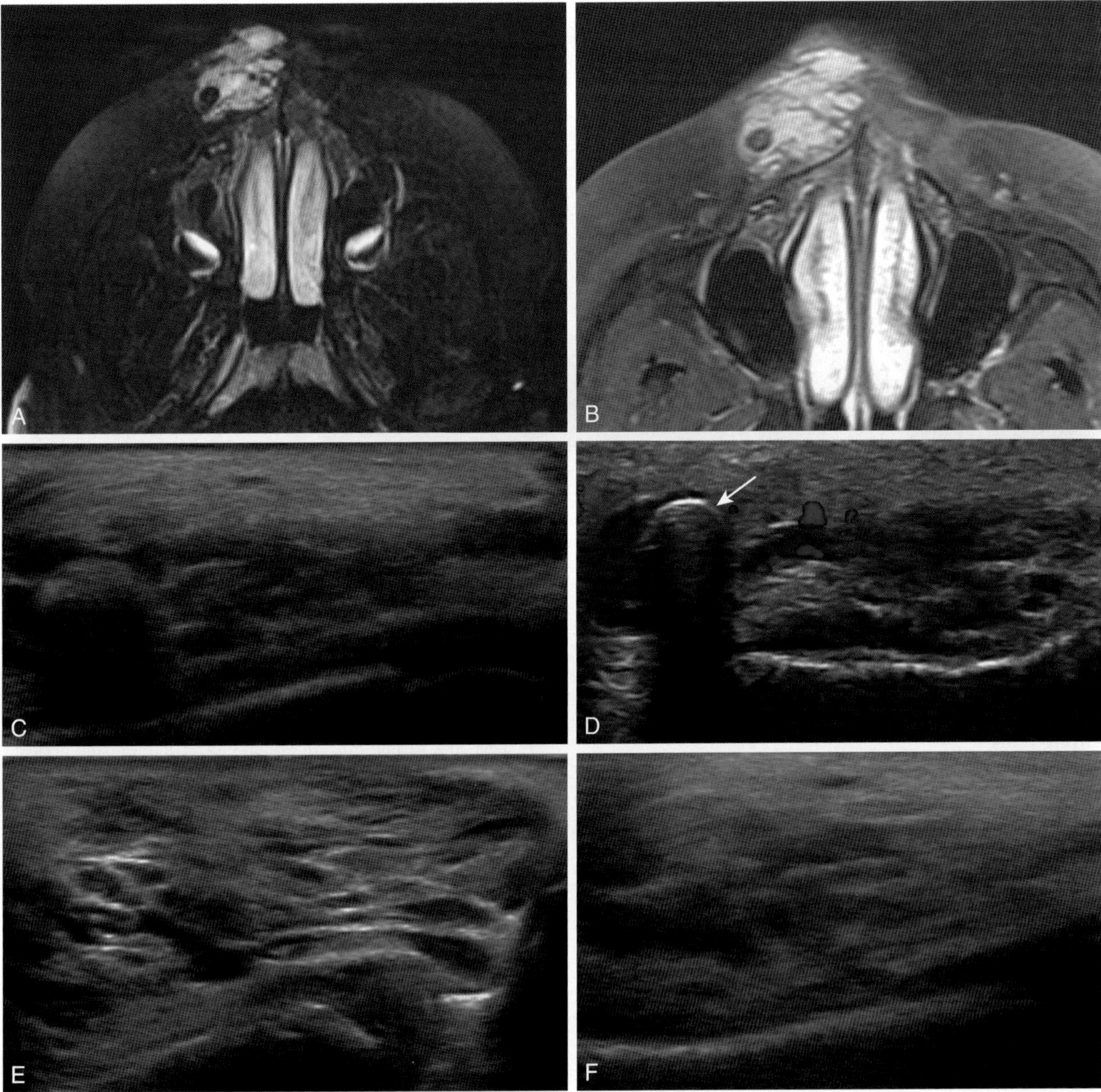

Fig. 14.24 Venous Malformation. (A) Axial T2W fat saturation and (B) axial T1W+C fat saturation images demonstrate a T2W hyperintense mass with rounded T2W hypointense phleboliths and diffuse enhancement. (C to F) Multiple ultrasound images demonstrate the venous malformation with mixed hypoechoic and isoechoic areas, mild vascularity, and a rounded phlebolith with posterior acoustic shadowing.

ARTERIOVENOUS MALFORMATION

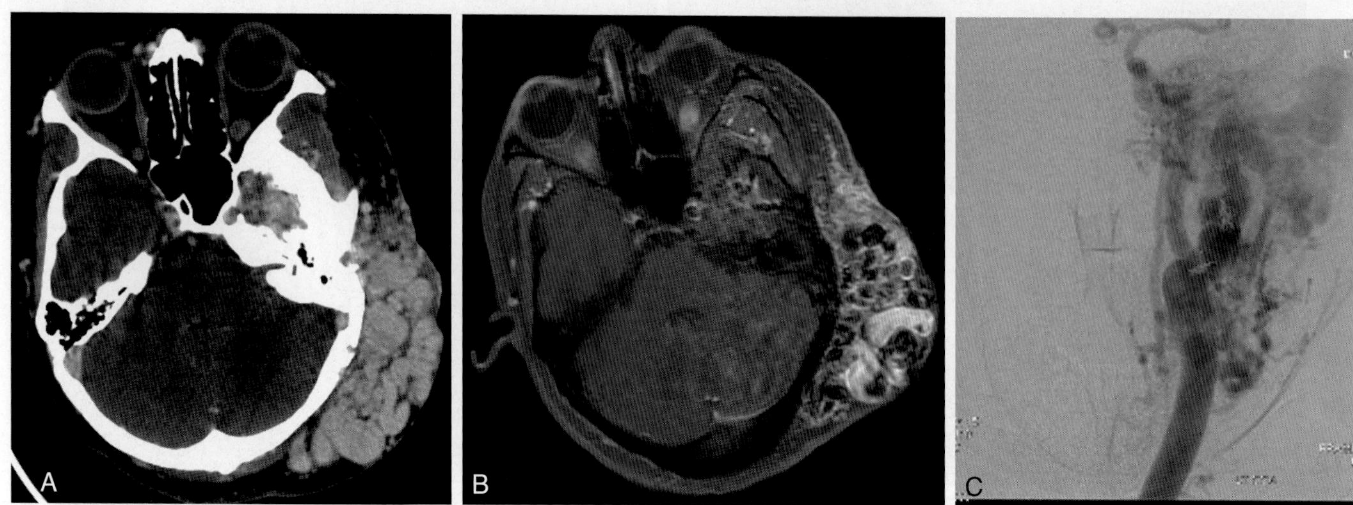

Fig. 14.25 Arteriovenous Malformation. (A) Axial CECT image demonstrates a large tangle of enhancing vessels in the left temporal and occipital scalp. (B) Axial T1W+C fat saturation image demonstrates the tangle of enhancing and nonenhancing vessels due to arterial and venous flowing blood. (C) Catheter angiography following left common carotid artery injection demonstrates typical appearance of the arteriovenous malformation with early draining vein.

Key Points

Background

- High-flow *malformation* between feeding arteries and draining veins
- Associated syndromes: Osler-Weber-Rendu, Parkes-Weber, and Cobb syndrome

Imaging

- Tangle of arteries and veins; no solid parenchyma

REFERENCE

1. Baer AH, Parmar HA, McKnight CD, et al. Head and neck vascular anomalies in the pediatric population. *Neurographics.* 2014 March(4):2–19.

DIFFERENTIAL DIAGNOSIS OF A COMMON SOLID NECK MASS

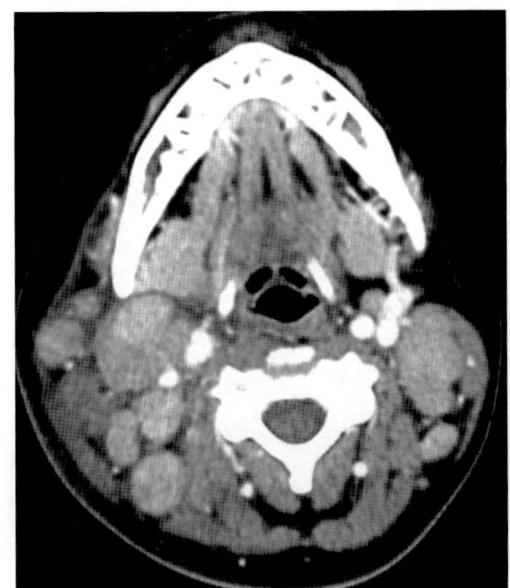

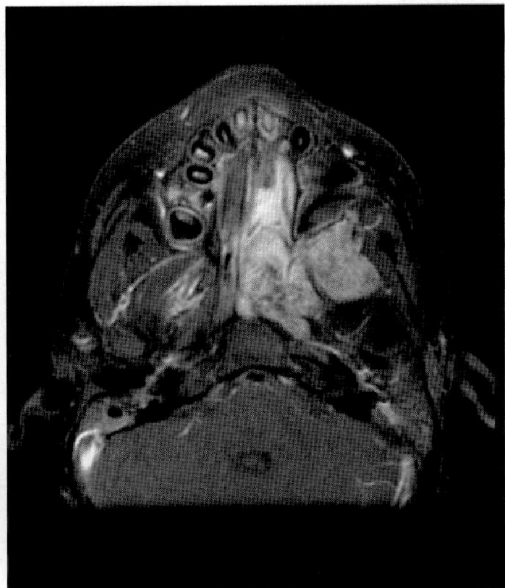

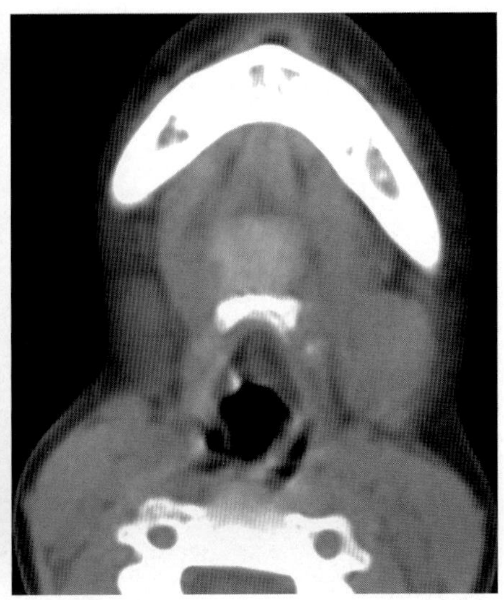

Nodal:
- Reactive lymphadenopathy and Lymphadenitis
- Lymphoma
- Nasopharyngeal carcinoma
- Neuroblastoma
- Rosai-Dorfman

Nonnodal:
- Rhabdomyosarcoma
- Juvenile angiofibroma
- Nerve sheath tumor
- Mucoepidermoid carcinoma
- Pilomatrixoma
- Fibrosarcoma
- Myofibromatosis
- Fibromatosis coli

Congenital:
- Ectopic thyroid
- Ectopic thymus
- Teratoma
- Nasal glial hamartoma

ECTOPIC THYROID GLAND

Solid

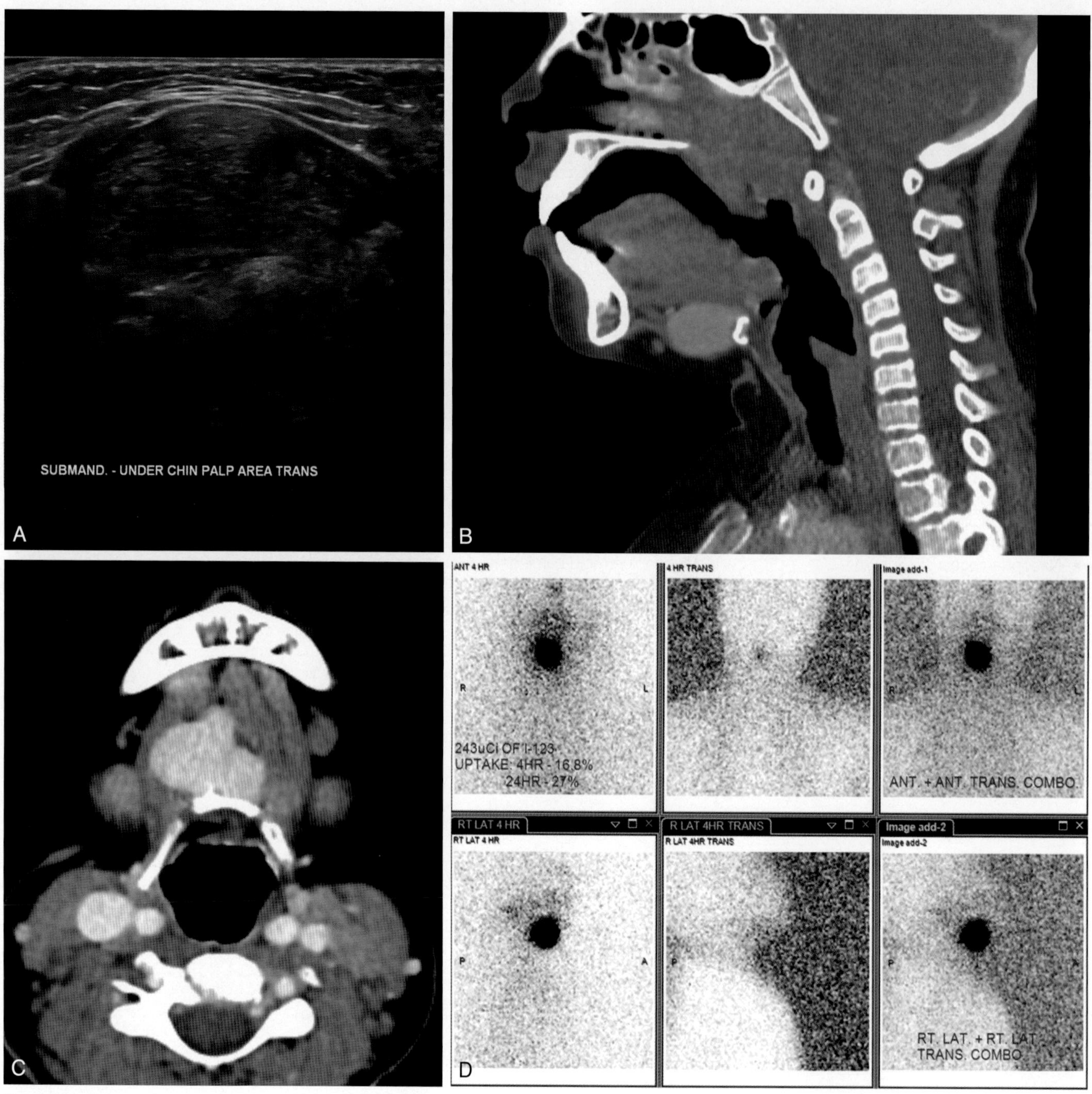

Fig. 14.26 Ectopic Thyroid Gland. (A) Transverse ultrasound image demonstrates an isoechoic mass and (B and C) sagittal and axial CECT images demonstrate a hyperdense mass inferior to the tongue and anterior to the hyoid bone. (D) Multiplanar I-123 nuclear medicine images demonstrate uptake in the submental space consistent with a ectopic thyroid gland.

Key Points

Background

- Also known as lingual thyroid gland
- Midline or paramedian along the course of the thyroglossal duct; usually located at the base of the tongue
- In 75% of patients, no cervical thyroid gland is present
- May expand during puberty

Imaging

- Ultrasound: isoechoic or hyperechoic
- CT: Hyperdense soft tissue similar to normal thyroid gland
- MRI: Isointense to mild hyperintense on T1W, and mild hyperintense on T2W relative to the tongue

REFERENCE

1. Friedman ER, John SD. Imaging of pediatric neck masses. *Radiol Clin North Am*. 2011 Jul;49(4):617–632.

NASAL GLIAL HETEROTOPIA

Solid

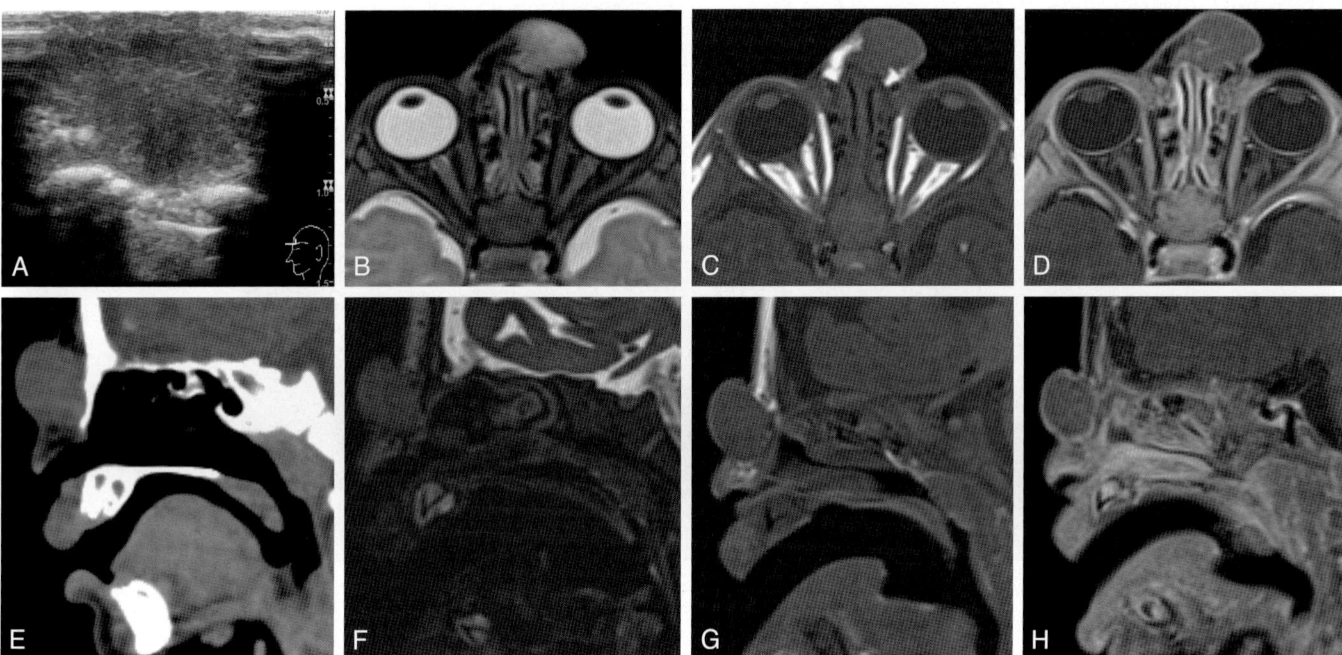

Fig. 14.27 Nasal Glial Heterotopia. (A) Focussed ultrasound over the nasal bridge demonstrates an isoechoic nodule. (B and F) Axial and sagittal T2W, (C and G) axial and sagittal T1W, (D and H) axial and sagittal T1W+C fat saturation, and (E) sagittal CT images demonstrate a soft tissue density and T2W hyperintense mass without enhancement and without diffusion restriction (DWI/ADC not shown).

Key Points

Background

- Nasal glioma is a heterotopia/dysplastic neural glial and fibrovascular tissue separated from the brain.
- Occurs along the tract of the foramen cecum or frontonasal suture.
- 10% to 30% are attached to the brain by a fibrous stalk through a defect in the cribriform plate.
- May become superinfected and result in meningitis. Treated with surgical resection.

Imaging

- Solid, circumscribed, nonenhancing, no diffusion restriction, and no macroscopic fat; midline; no CSF connection intracranially
- Locations: Extranasal (60%) located along the nasal dorsum, glabella, medial canthus, nasopharynx, mouth or pterygopalatine fossa; intranasal (30%) located in the nasal cavity; mixed extranasal-intranasal (10%) communicate through a bone defect in the nasal bone, or rarely the orbital plate, frontal bone, or sinus

REFERENCE

1. Lowe LH, Booth TN, Joglar JM, et al. Midface anomalies in children. *Radiographics*. 2000;20(4):907–922.

ECTOPIC THYMUS

Solid

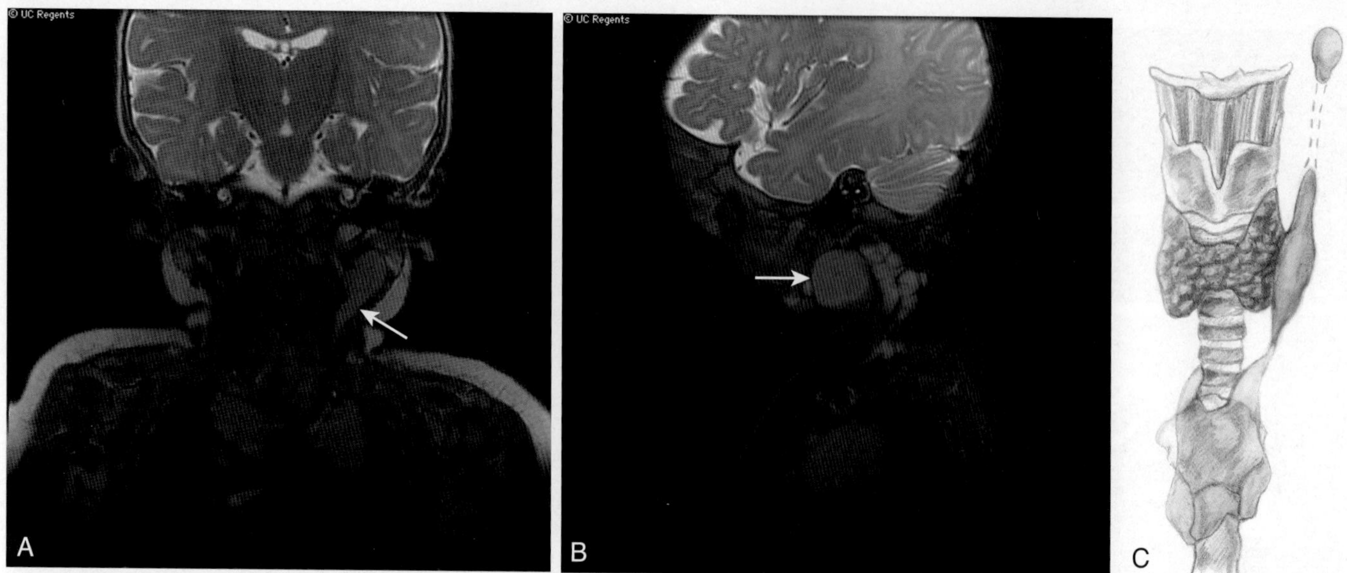

Fig. 14.28 Ectopic Thymus. (A and B) Coronal and sagittal T2W images demonstrate a left lateral neck mild T2W hyperintense mass that follows a similar signal pattern as normal thymus tissue. (C) Illustration of the course of the thymopharyngeal duct and potential location of ectopic thymus (blue structure).

Key Points

Background

- 80% to 90% are asymptomatic; rarely present with stridor, dyspnea, and/or dysphagia due to compression of the trachea and/or esophagus.
- *Usually shrinks by age of 5 years and no treatment is necessary.* If symptomatic, surgical removal is the treatment of choice.

Imaging

- Solid homogeneous neck mass similar in appearance to mediastinal thymic tissue along the course of normal thymic descent, from the angle of the mandible to the superior mediastinum (thymopharyngeal duct).
- 60% to 70% on the left side; 20% to 30% on the right side; remaining 5% to 7% in the midline.
- US can be diagnostic via demonstration of "starry" parenchyma.
- Approximately 50% of all cervical thymic masses may be continuous with the mediastinal thymus by direct extension or by connection to a vestigial remnant or a solid cord.

REFERENCE

1. Wang J, Fu H, Yang H, et al. Clinical management of cervical ectopic thymus in children. *J Pediatr Surg*. 2011 Aug;46(8):e33–e36.

LYMPHOMA

Solid

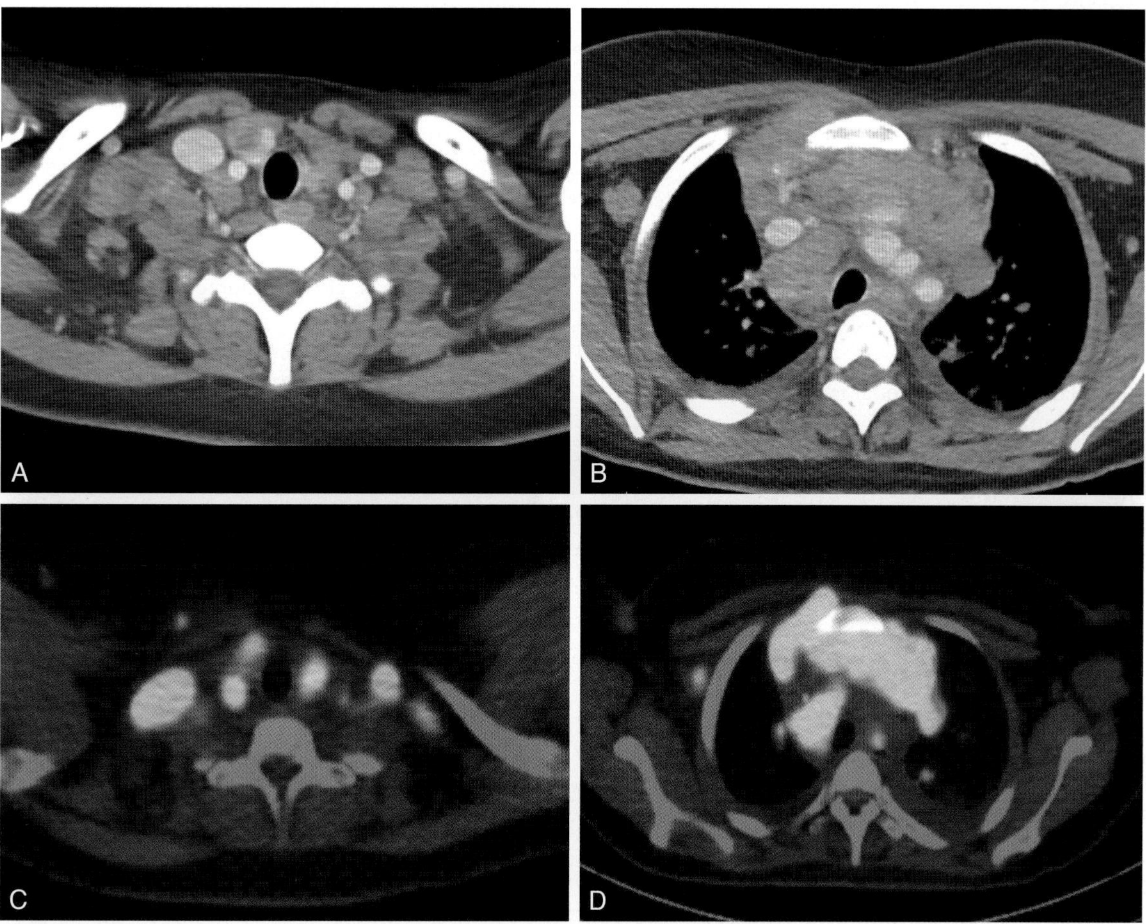

Fig. 14.29 **Hodgkin Lymphoma.** (A and B) Axial CECT and (C and D) corresponding FDG PET-CT images demonstrate multiple FDG avid enlarged lymph nodes in the central infrahyoid neck, bilateral supraclavicular fossa, right axilla, and mediastinum.

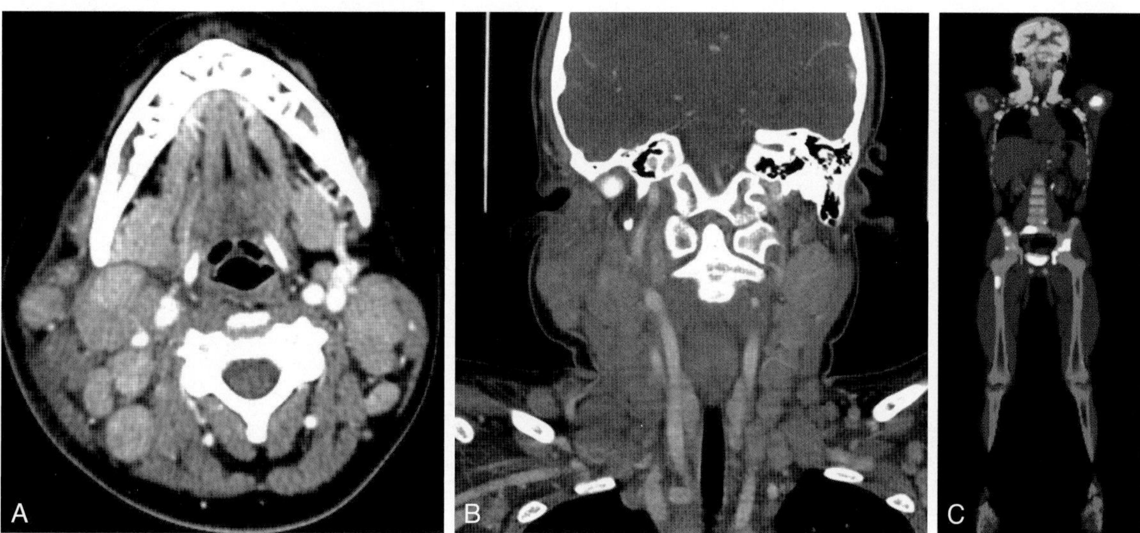

Fig. 14.30 **Non-Hodgkin Lymphoma.** (A and B) Axial and coronal CECT images demonstrate multiple pathologically enlarged lymph nodes in the right and left neck and left axilla. (C) Coronal FDG PET-CT image demonstrates multiple FDG avid enlarged lymph nodes in the bilateral neck and multifocal tumor in the ribs, pelvis, sacrum, and femur.

Key Points

- Lymphoma is caused by the malignant transformation of lymphoid cells.
- Third most common malignancy in children behind leukemia and CNS tumors.
- Most common pediatric H&N malignancy.

Hodgkin Lymphoma

- Named after Thomas Hodgkin, who, in 1832, reported "peculiar enlargement" of cervical and other lymph nodes associated with splenic enlargement
- Most common form of lymphoma
- Epstein-Barr virus (EBV) positivity in 70% to 80%
- Teenagers
- Primarily nodal disease; extranodal is uncommon
- Overall 5-year survival is 91%

Non-Hodgkin Lymphoma

- Age 2 to 12.
- Extranodal more common including Waldeyer ring, and parotid gland in the neck.
- Four main subtypes in children: Burkitt lymphoma (40%), lymphoblastic lymphoma (30%), diffuse large B-cell lymphoma (20%), and anaplastic large cell lymphoma (10%).
- Burkitt lymphoma: associated with a history of EBV infection. African form often in the maxilla and mandible.
- Overall 5-year survival is 76% for ages <10 years and 70% for ages 10 to 19 years.

Background

- Hodgkin lymphoma presents with painless cervical lymphadenopathy and constitutional symptoms, i.e., fatigue, anorexia, fever, and night sweats (B-symptoms).
- Non-Hodgkin lymphoma presentation varies depending on the areas involved.
- Nonbenign lymphadenopathy should be suspected in the setting of age >10 years, lymphadenopathy duration >6 weeks, lymph node >2.5 cm, supraclavicular lymph nodes (particularly left sided), matted lymph nodes, and/or more than one noncontiguous lymph node location involved.
- Chemotherapy is the primary treatment of lymphoma.

Imaging

CT

- CT of the neck, chest, abdomen, and pelvis is performed for staging.
- Hodgkin lymphoma: enlarged soft tissue density lymph nodes that most commonly involve the lower cervical nodes, supraclavicular nodes, mediastinal nodes (present in two-thirds of patients), and axillary nodes. 35% have splenic involvement seen as focal nodules or splenomegaly. Involvement of the lung, cortical bone, or kidneys is uncommon.
- Non-Hodgkin lymphoma: involves the lymph nodes, Waldeyer ring, bone marrow, CNS, mediastinum, lungs, GI tract, liver, spleen, kidneys, and skin depending on the subtype.

PET-CT

- Used to assess response to treatment; tumors demonstrate avid FDG uptake.

REFERENCES

1. Nasseri F, Munjal K, Ginsberg LE, et al. Imaging review of craniofacial masses in children. *Neurographics*. 2015 Sept/Oct;5(5):217–230.
2. Abramson SJ, Price AP. Imaging of pediatric lymphomas. *Radiol Clin North Am*. 2008 Mar;46(2):313–338.

RHABDOMYOSARCOMA

Solid

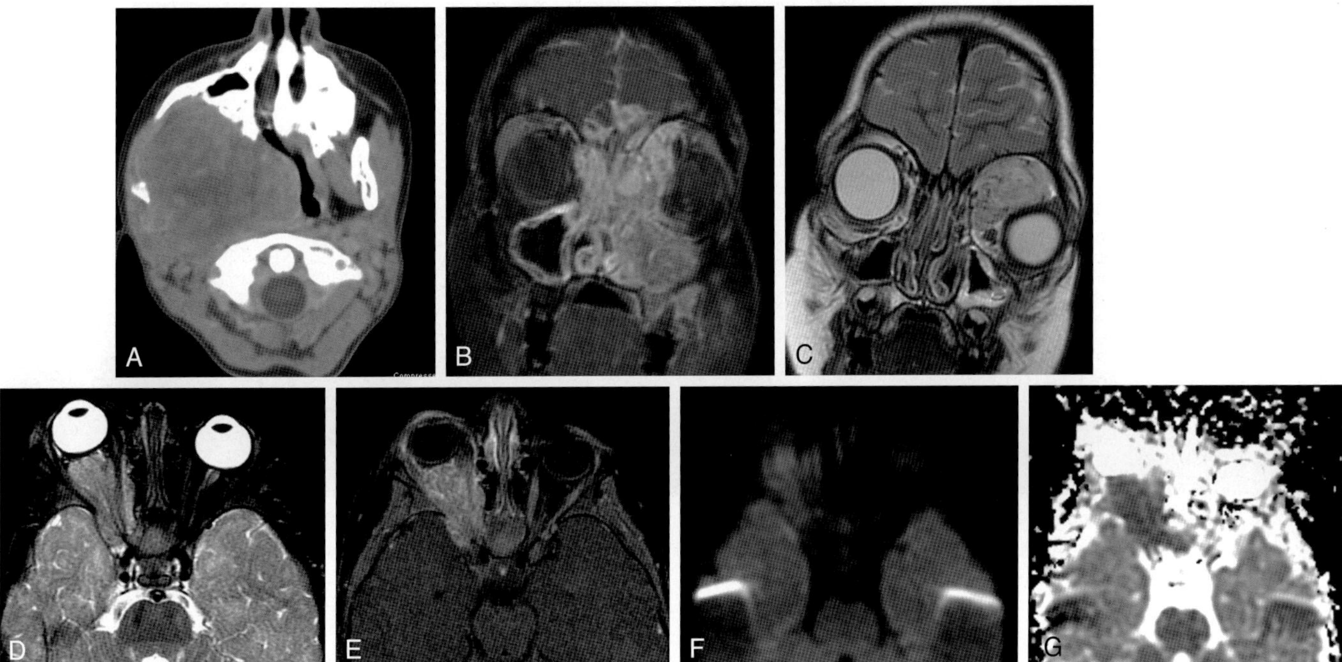

Fig. 14.31 Rhabdomyosarcoma. (A) Axial CT demonstrating a large soft tissue mass centered in the right masticator space extending to the nasopharynx. (B) Coronal T1W+C fat saturation image demonstrating a parameningeal rhabdomyosarcoma as an enhancing mass in the ethmoid sinuses, left maxillary sinus, left medial orbit, and intracranial extension. (C) Coronal T2W image demonstrates a left orbital rhabdomyosarcoma with mild T2W hyperintensity and linear flow voids mimicking an infantile hemangioma. (D) Axial T2W fat saturation, (E) axial T1W+C fat saturation, (F) axial DWI, and (G) axial ADC images demonstrate a mild T2W hyperintensity with linear flow voids right post septal orbital mass extending in to the superior orbital fissure with homogenous enhancement mimicking an infantile hemangioma; however, ADC hypointensity indicates a hypercellular neoplasm. Infantile hemangiomas would demonstrate ADC hyperintense signal.

Key Points

Background

- The most common soft tissue sarcoma in children. Second most common malignant tumor in the H&N in children.
- Mean age 5 to 6 years, 75% are younger than 10 years.
- Three pathological types: embryonal (75%), alveolar (15%), and pleomorphic/undifferentiated (15%). Embryonal types usually occur in younger children and have a good prognosis. Alveolar types typically occur in older children and have worse prognosis. Pleomorphic type is usually seen in adults and typically involves the extremities.

Imaging

- Three locations:
  - Orbital (25%)
  - Parameningeal (50%): nasopharynx, nasal cavity, parapharygeal, paranasal sinus, middle ear, mastoid, infratemporal, and pterygopalatine
  - Nonparameningeal (25%)
- CT: Soft tissue density mass; parameningeal and nonparameningeal locations typically have aggressive features including bone destruction and necrosis. Orbital masses may have more benign features.
- MRI: Modality of choice for detecting perineural extension, skull base and orbit extension. Restricted diffusion on DWI is a useful tool to differentiate rhabdomyosarcoma from hemangioma or venolymphatic malformation.
- Neck imaging should also be performed for cervical lymphadenopathy which can be found in 10% to 20%.

REFERENCE

1. Nasseri F, Munjal K, Ginsberg LE, et al. Imaging review of craniofacial masses in children. *Neurographics*. 2015 Sept/Oct;5(5):217–230.

RHABDOMYOSARCOMA

Solid

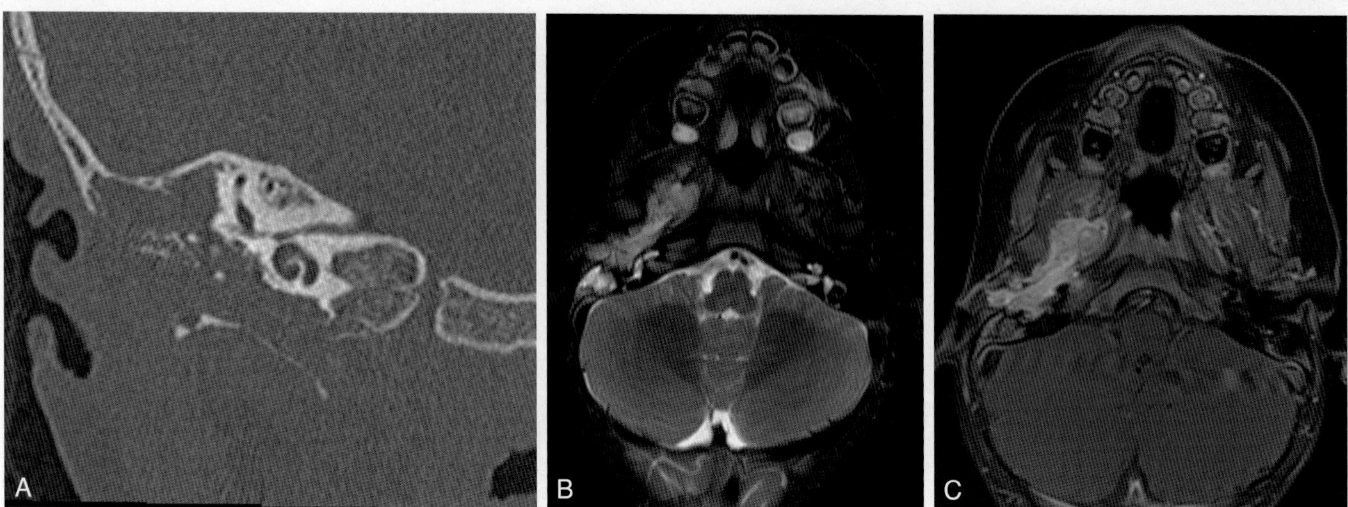

Fig. 14.32 Rhabdomyosarcoma: Temporal Bone. (A) Coronal CT demonstrating aggressive lytic destruction of the right mastoid and external auditory canal. (B) Axial T2W fat saturation and (C) Axial T1W+C fat saturation images demonstrate a T2W hyperintense enhancing soft tissue mass in the right middle ear cavity, eustachian tube, and lateral pterygoid muscle.

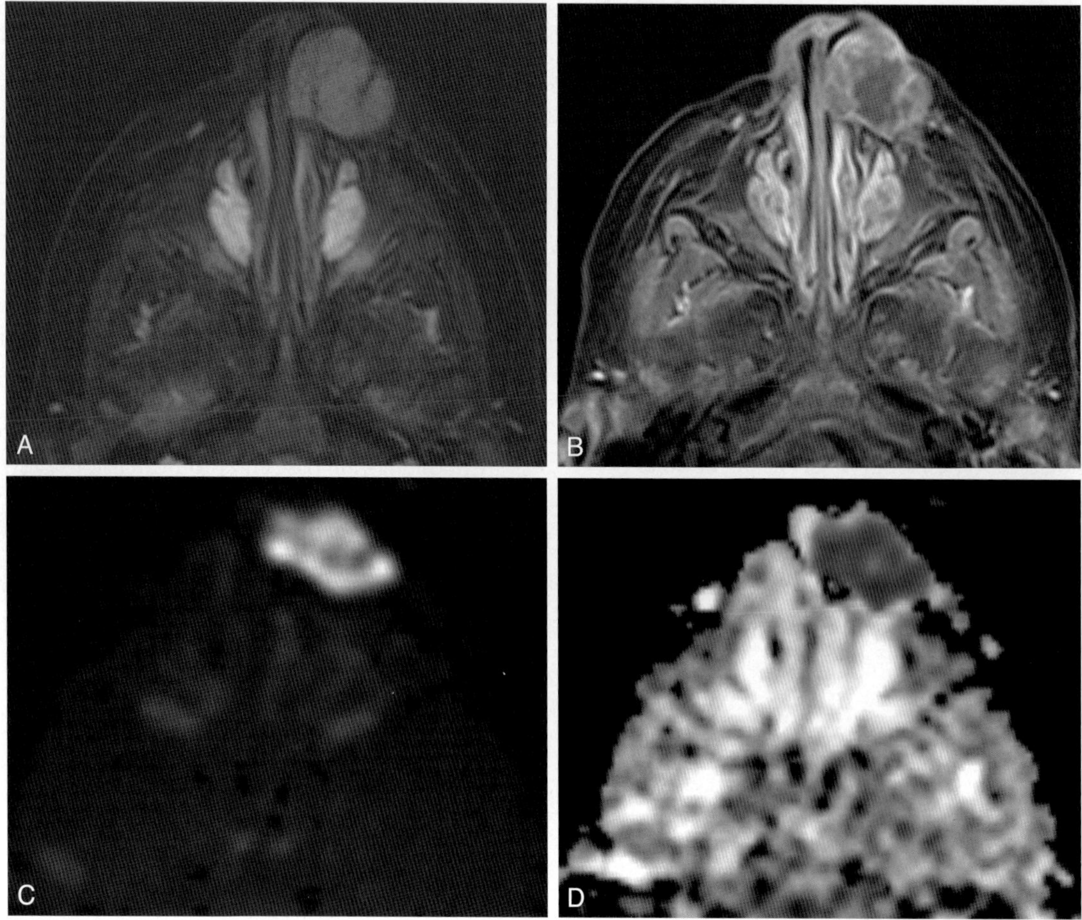

Fig. 14.33 Rhabdomyosarcoma. (A) Axial T2W fat saturation, (B) axial T1W+C fat saturation, (C) axial DWI, and (D) axial ADC images demonstrate a mild homogeneous T2W hyperintense mass with heterogeneous enhancement and diffusion restriction involving the left side of the nose and nasolabial fold.

RHABDOMYOSARCOMA

Solid

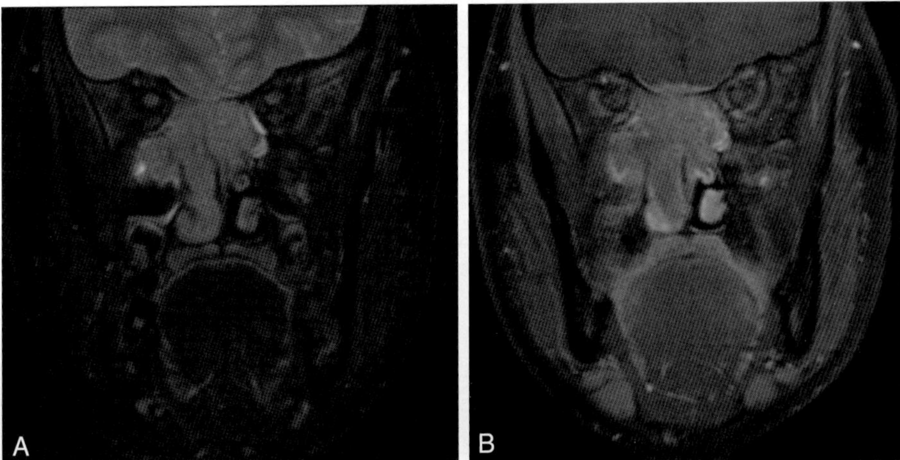

Fig. 14.34 Rhabdomyosarcoma. (A) Coronal T2W fat saturation and (B) coronal T1W+C fat saturation images demonstrate a mild homogeneous T2W hyperintense mass with mild enhancement involving the bilateral nasal cavities, ethmoid sinuses, right maxillary sinus, and intracranial extension into the dura of the anterior cranial fossa.

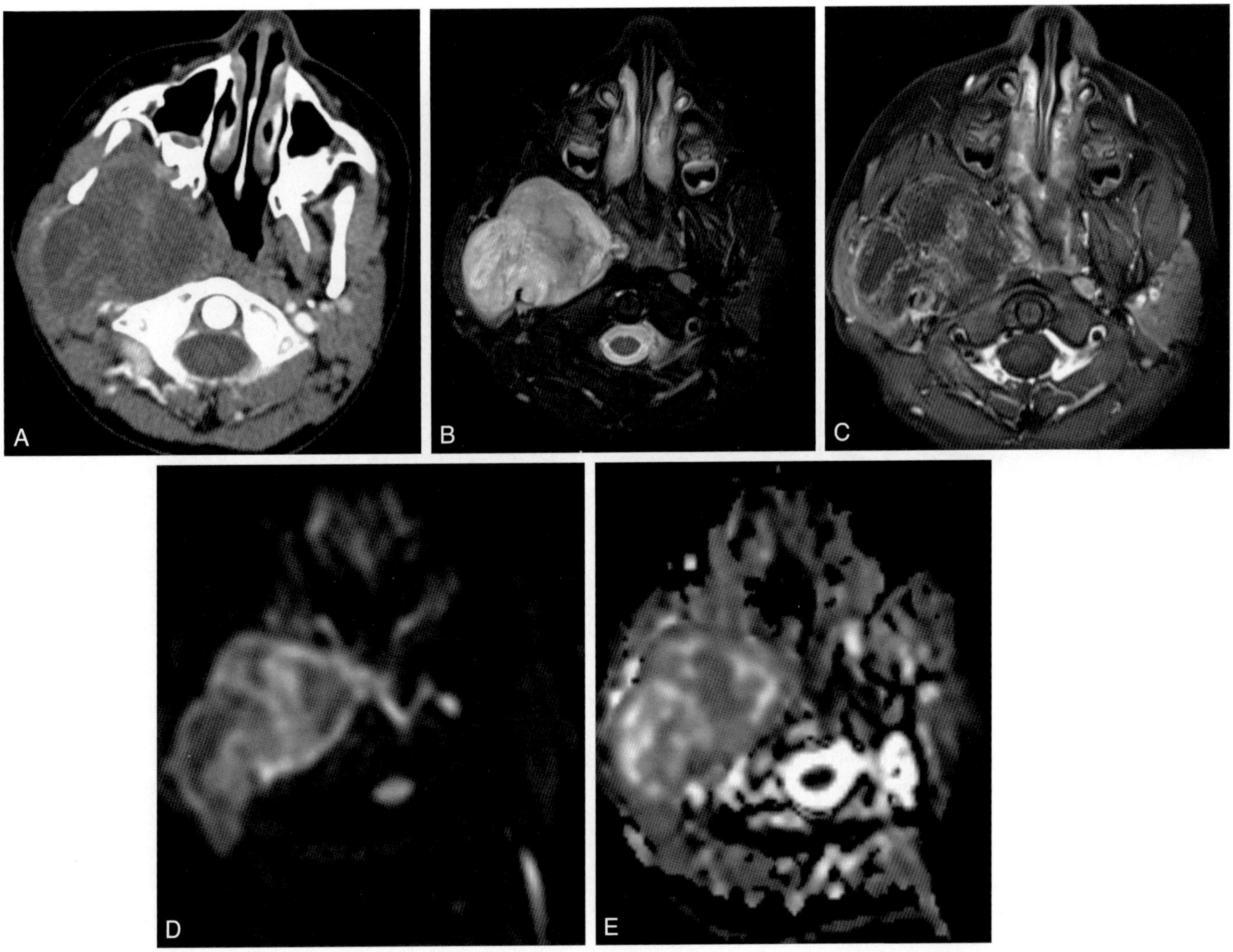

Fig. 14.35 Rhabdomyosarcoma. (A) Axial CECT, (B) axial T2W fat saturation, (C) axial T1W+C fat saturation, (D) axial DWI, and (E) axial ADC images demonstrate heterogeneous density soft tissue mass in the right parapharyngeal space with homogeneous T2W hyperintensity, heterogeneous enhancement, and areas of diffusion restriction.

JUVENILE ANGIOFIBROMA

Solid
Vascular

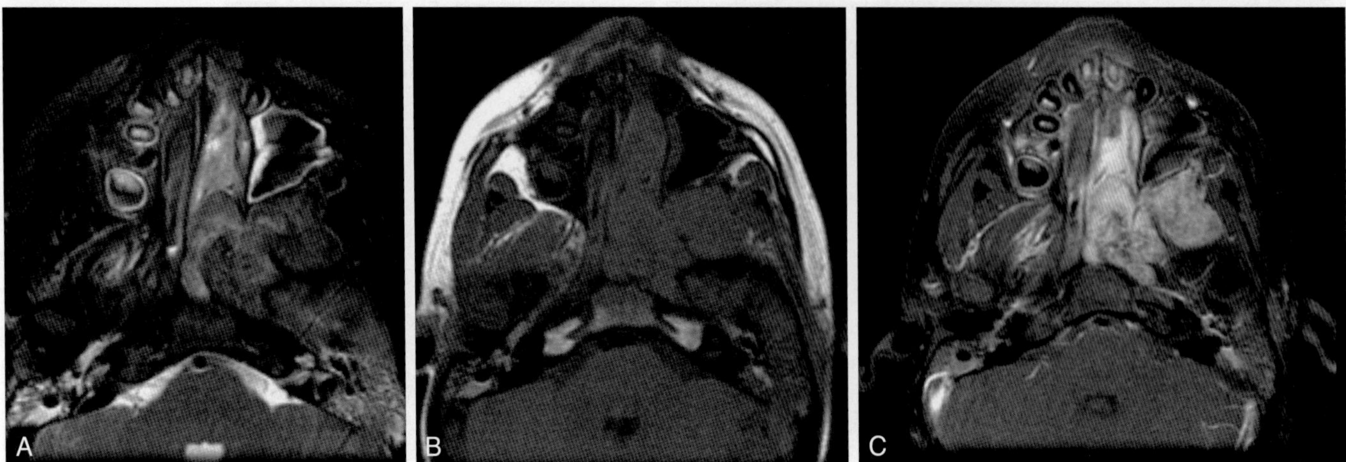

Fig. 14.36 Juvenile Angiofibroma. (A) Axial T2W fat saturation and (B and C) axial T1W and T1W+C fat saturation images demonstrate heterogeneous T2W homogenously enhancing mass in the left pterygopalatine fossa, left retromaxillary space, nasopharynx, and nasal cavity.

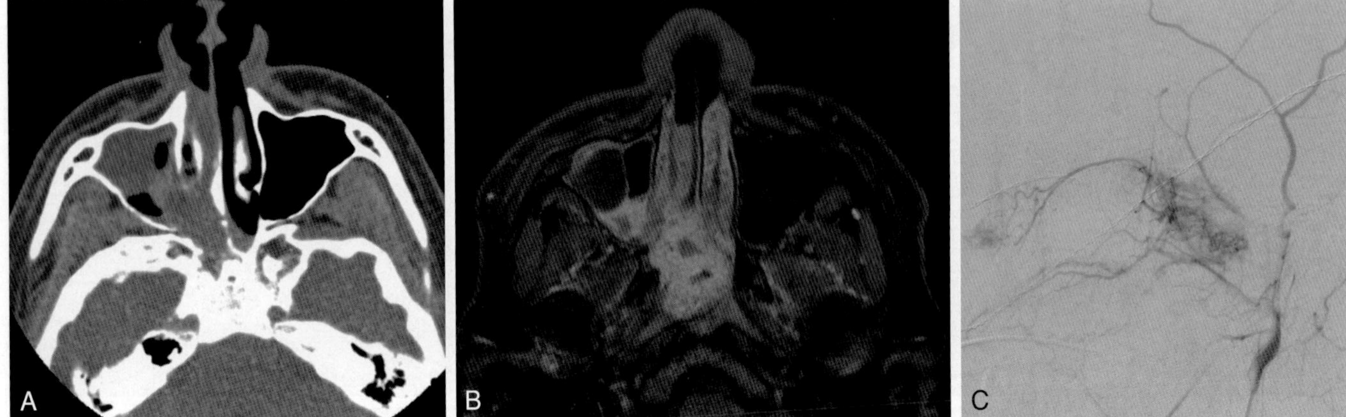

Fig. 14.37 Juvenile Angiofibroma. (A) Axial CT and (B) axial T1W+C fat saturation images demonstrate a soft tissue mass in the left nasal cavity, maxillary sinus and nasopharynx with heterogeneous enhancement. (C) Catheter angiography demonstrates a hypervascular mass.

Key Points

Background

- Benign locally aggressive vascular tumor
- Male:female ratio 9:1; age 8 to 25
- Presents with nasal obstruction, rhinorrhea, and epistaxis
- Treated with embolization followed by surgical resection

Imaging

- Hypervascular mass centered in the sphenopalatine foramen; extends into the nasal cavity, nasopharynx, infratemporal fossa, sphenoid and ethmoid sinus, central skull base, and cavernous sinus; usually smooth remodeling of the orbit
- MRI: Heterogeneous; strongly enhancing; flow voids

REFERENCE

1. Nasseri F, Munjal K, Ginsberg LE, et al. Imaging review of craniofacial masses in children. *Neurographics*. 2015 Sept/Oct;5(5):217–230.

NASOPHARYNGEAL CARCINOMA

Solid

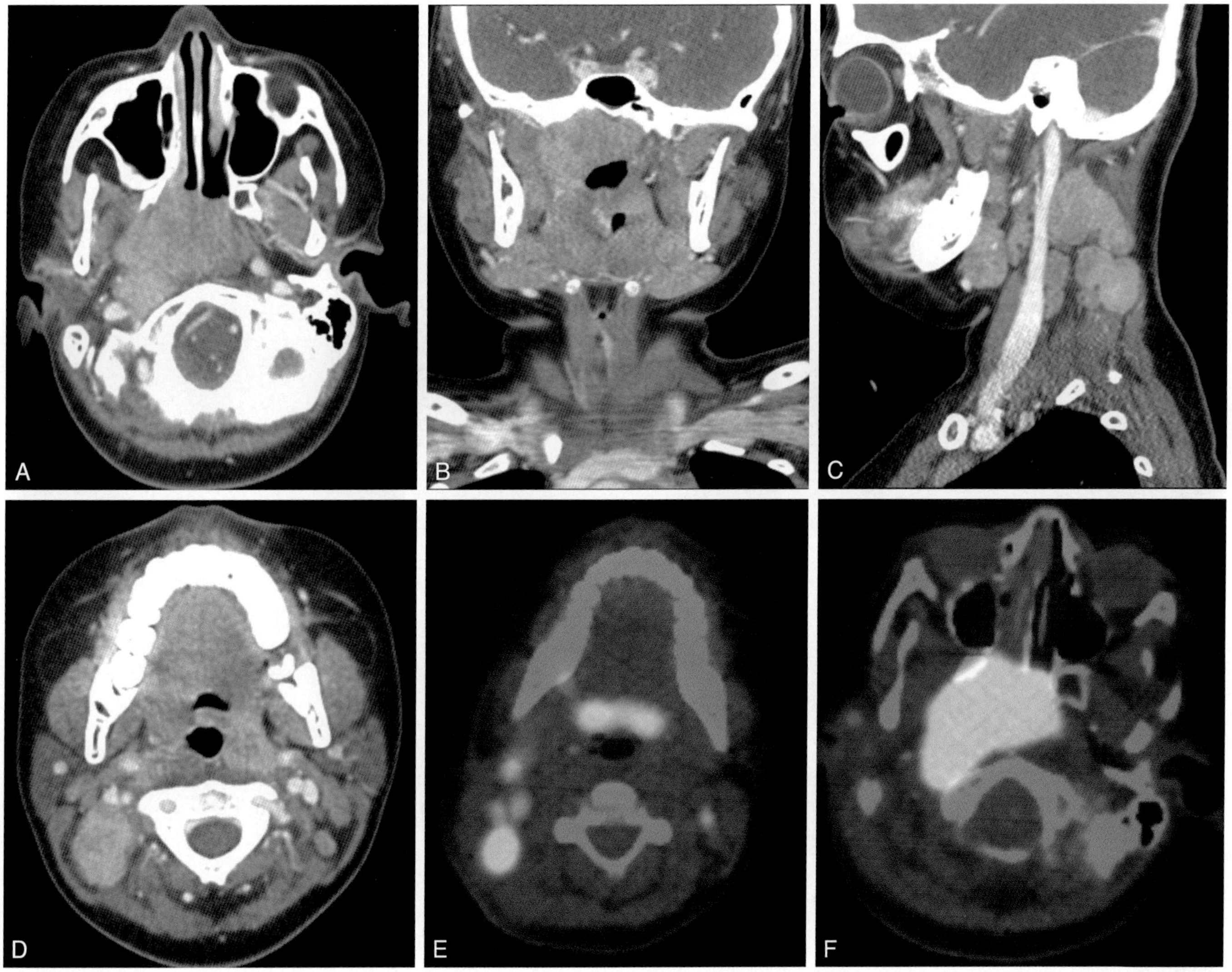

Fig. 14.38 Nasopharyngeal Carcinoma. (A to D) Axial and coronal CECT and (E and F) FDG PET-CT images demonstrate a homogeneously enhancing soft tissue mass in the nasopharynx with FDG uptake and enlarged right retropharyngeal and lateral neck lymph nodes with FDG uptake.

Key Points

Background

- More common in Asia and Africa
- Elevated EBV titers

Imaging

- Soft tissue density mass centered in the nasopharynx with variable extension into central skull base, cavernous sinuses, skull base foramen, and parapharyngeal spaces.
- Most have concurrent cervical lymphadenopathy (80%–90%).
- PET-CT demonstrates FDG primary tumor and metastatic nodes.

REFERENCE

1. Friedman ER, John SD. Imaging of pediatric neck masses. *Radiol Clin North Am*. 2011 Jul;49(4):617–632.

NEUROFIBROMA

Solid

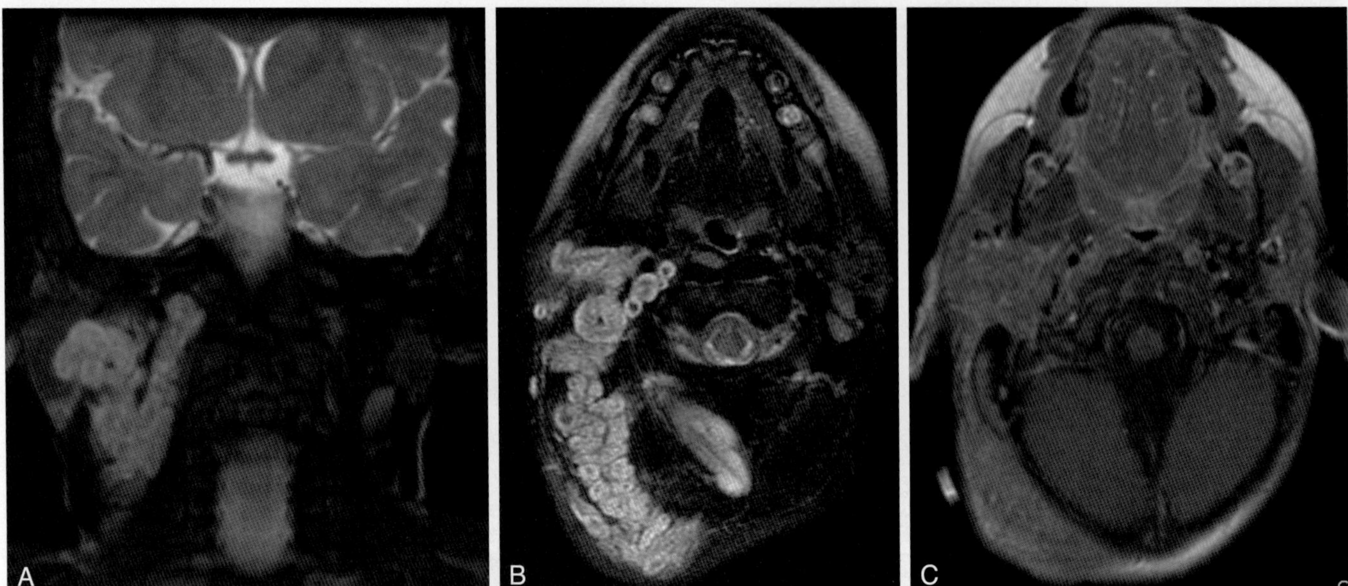

Fig. 14.39 Neurofibroma. (A and B) Coronal and axial T2W fat saturation and (C) axial T1W+C fat saturation images demonstrate a T2W hyperintense homogeneously enhancing multispatial soft tissue mass with "target sign" (peripheral T2W hyperintense, central T2W hypointense) involving the right lateral neck, parapharyngeal space, carotid space, and paraspinal space.

Key Points

Background

- Benign tumor of the peripheral nerve containing Schwann cells, fibroblasts intermixed tumor, and nerve fascicles
- Nearly all will have NF-1

Imaging

- Transpatial/multispatial
- "Target sign": Relatively characteristic with peripheral T2W hyperintensity and central low T2W intensity.
- Enhancement usually mild and homogeneous.
- Transformation to malignant peripheral nerve sheath tumor in 5% to 10%. Malignant peripheral nerve sheath tumor demonstrate rapid growth, FDG uptake, diffusion restriction, and necrosis.

REFERENCE

1. Nasseri F, Munjal K, Ginsberg LE, et al. Imaging review of craniofacial masses in children. *Neurographics.* 2015 Sept/Oct;5(5):217–230.

MALIGNANT PERIPHERAL NERVE SHEATH TUMOR

Solid

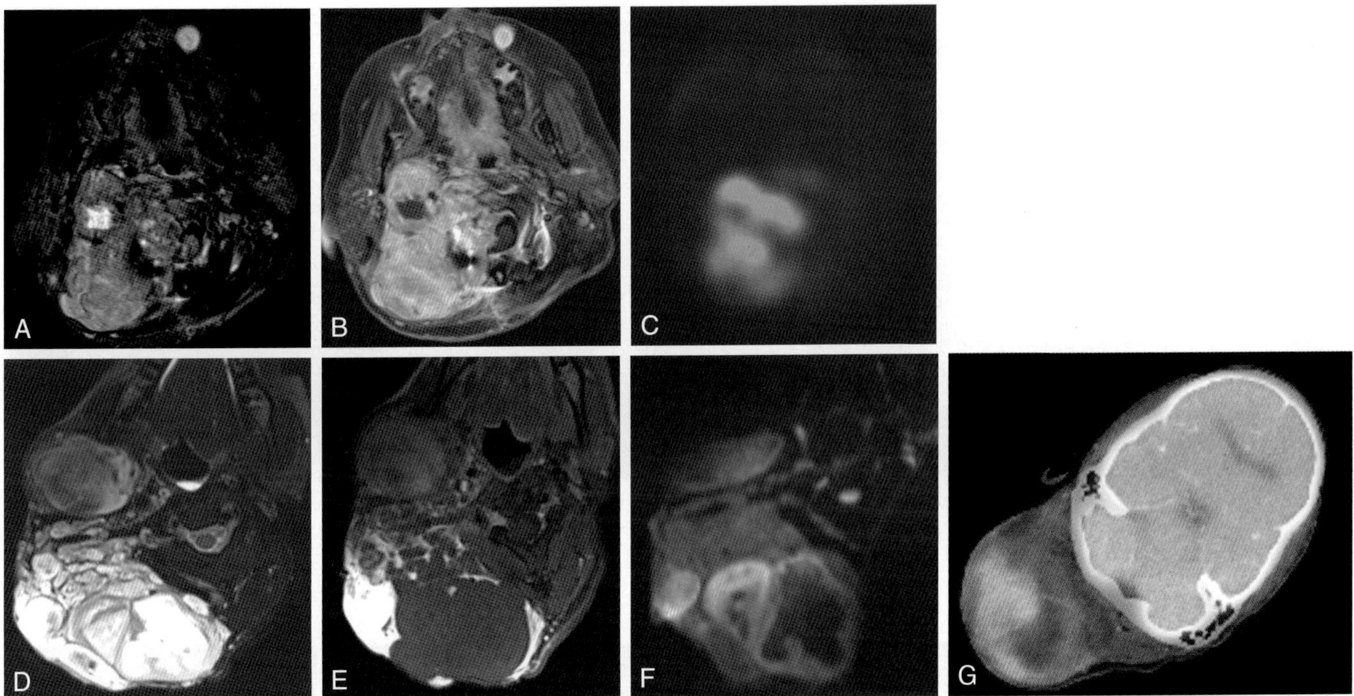

Fig. 14.40 Malignant Peripheral Nerve Sheath Tumor: Malignant Transformation of a Plexiform Neurofibroma. (A to C) Axial T2W fat saturation, axial T1W+C fat saturation, and axial DWI and (D to G) axial T2W fat saturation, axial T1W+C fat saturation, axial DWI, and axial FDG PET CT images demonstrate a multispatial soft tissue mass with areas of necrosis, diffusion restriction, and FDG uptake in the right lateral neck, parapharyngeal space, carotid space, and paraspinal space.

Key Points

Background

- Accounts for 3% to 10% of soft tissue sarcomas
- Symptoms: New or increased pain. Rapid growth of a known plexiform neurofibroma

Imaging

- MRI: Rapid growth, loss of target sign on T2, diffusion restriction and necrosis.
- PET CT: FDG avid, whereas benign neurofibromas are not FDG avid.

REFERENCE

1. Nasseri F, Munjal K, Ginsberg LE, et al. Imaging review of craniofacial masses in children. *Neurographics*. 2015 Sept/Oct;5(5):217–230.

TERATOMA

Solid
Cystic

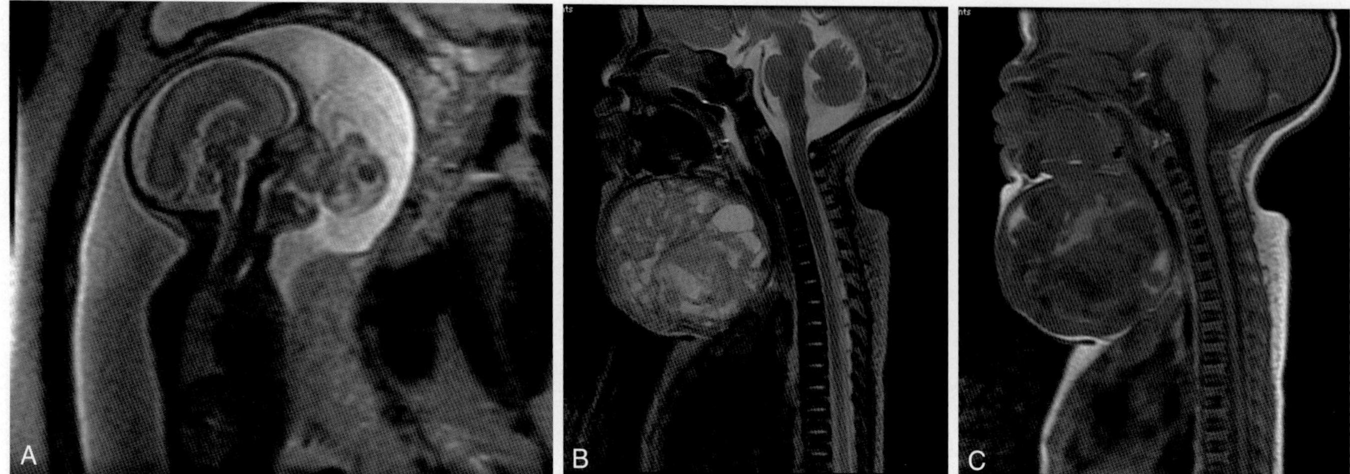

Fig. 14.41 Teratoma. (A) Sagittal T2W fetal MR image demonstrating a solid and cystic soft tissue mass arising from the maxilla consistent with epignathis. Different patient with (B) sagittal T2W and (C) sagittal T1W images demonstrate a circumscribed round anterior neck mass with internal T1W hyperintensity from fat and proteinaceous fluid compressing the trachea.

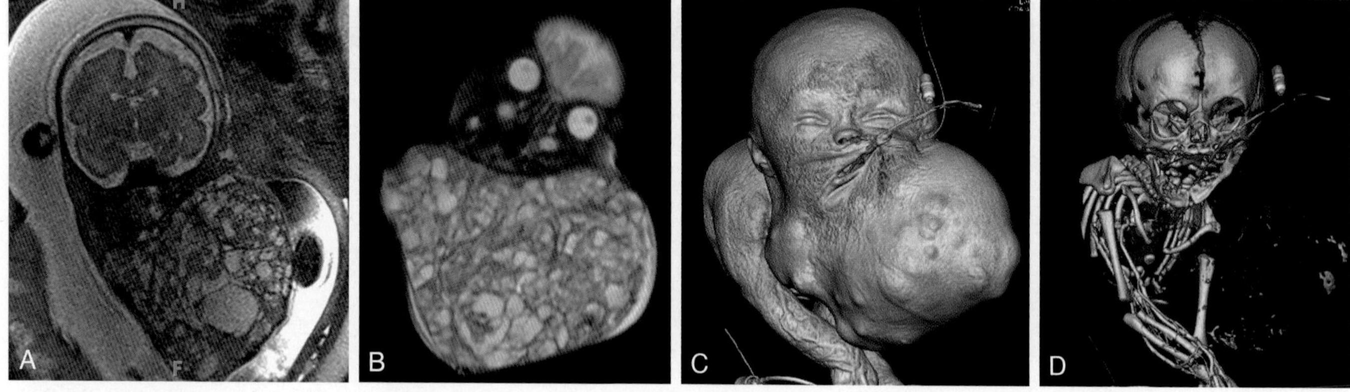

Fig. 14.42 Teratoma. (A) Coronal T2W fetal MR image, and postnatal (B) coronal T2W, and (C and D) 3D volumetric CT images demonstrate a solid and cystic midline anterior neck mass causing hypoplasia and deformity of the left side of the face and chest.

Key Points

Background

- Composed of elements of all three germ cell layers.
- Classified as mature, immature, or malignant. Most are benign teratomas.
- Most common head and neck congenital tumor.
- Treatment: Surgery; airway protection. Ex utero intrapartum treatment (EXIT) procedure used if diagnosed intrauterine. Polyhydramnios may coexist, requiring amnioreduction to prevent preterm labor.

Imaging

- Multilocular, usually midline, circumscribed, cystic, and solid; calcification in 50%; macroscopic fat variably present but useful for definitive diagnosis when present.
- Large neck teratomas can affect swallowing and result in polyhydramnios and pulmonary hypoplasia.
- Fetal MRI provides the best visualization of the cervical teratoma for determining need for EXIT procedure with the goal of securing the fetal airway. This includes determining the size and etiology of the neck mass, whether the airway is distorted, and whether the mass involves critical structures.

REFERENCE

1. Friedman ER, John SD. Imaging of pediatric neck masses. *Radiol Clin North Am.* 2011 Jul;49(4):617–632.

TERATOMA

Solid
Cystic

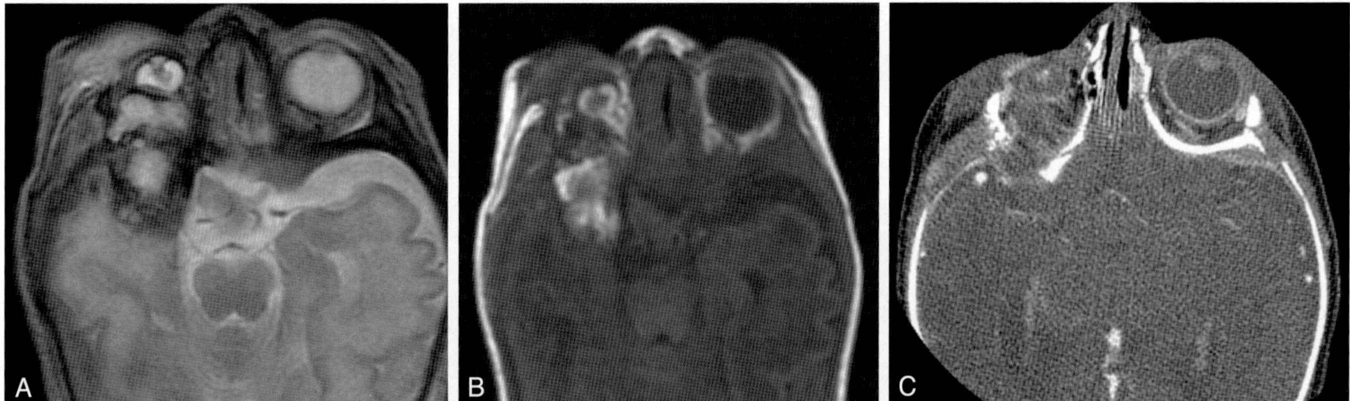

Fig. 14.43 Teratoma: Uncommon Appearance. (A) Axial T2W, (B) axial T1W, and (C) axial CECT images demonstrate a right orbital mass extending into the middle cranial fossa with areas of T2W hyperintensity, T1W hyperintensity, and associated microphthalmia of the right globe.

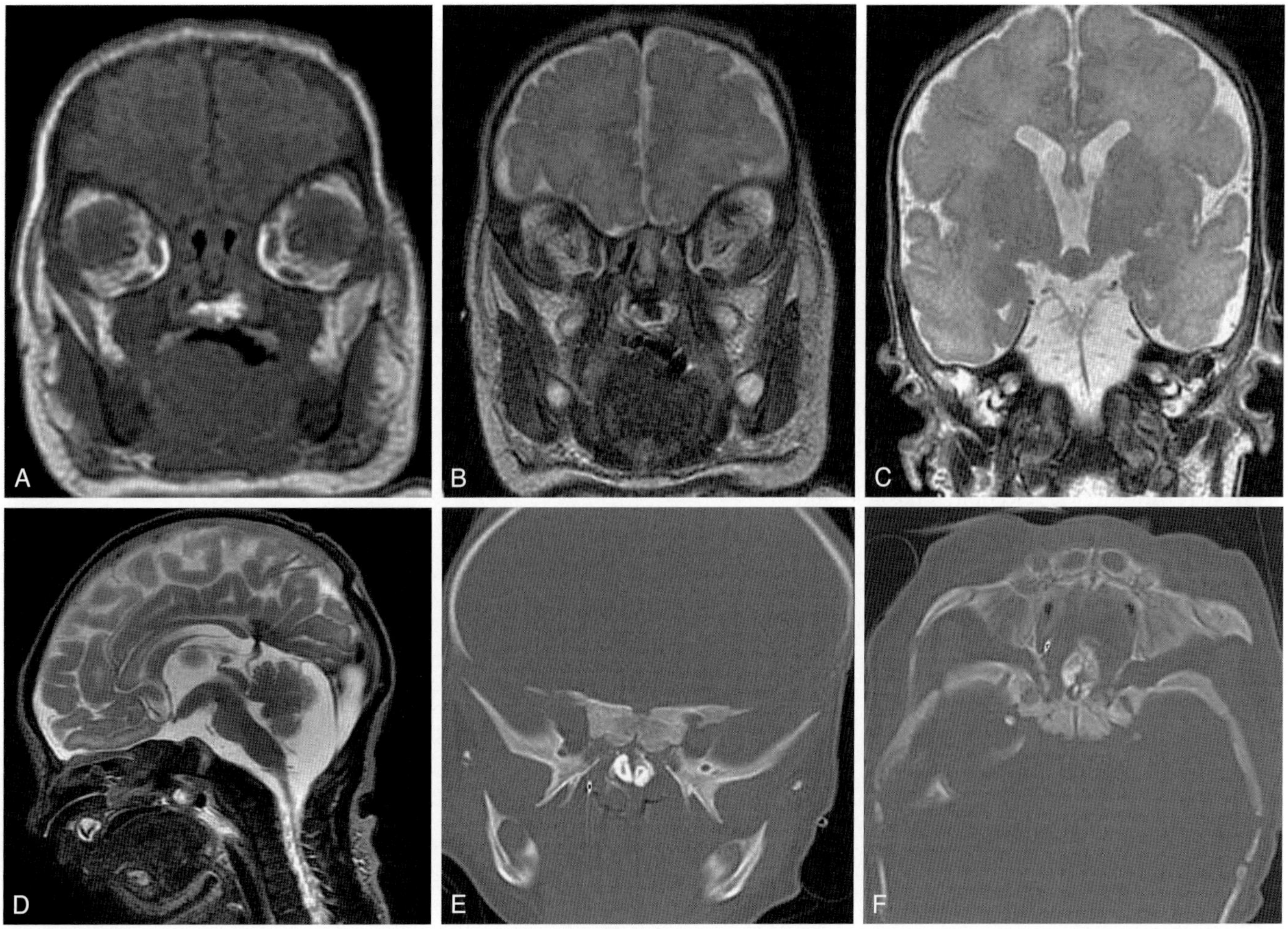

Fig. 14.44 Teratoma. (A) Coronal T1W, (B to D) coronal and sagittal T2W, and (E and F) coronal and axial CT images demonstrate a T1W hyperintense, mixed T2W hypointense, and hyperintense mass in the nasopharynx with hyperdense CT appearance due to tooth formation. Intracranial malformations including absent septum pellucidum and brainstem malformation are present, including a duplicated pituitary gland and thickened floor of the third ventricle due to fusion of the mammillary bodies.

INFANTILE MYOFIBROMATOSIS

Solid
Cystic

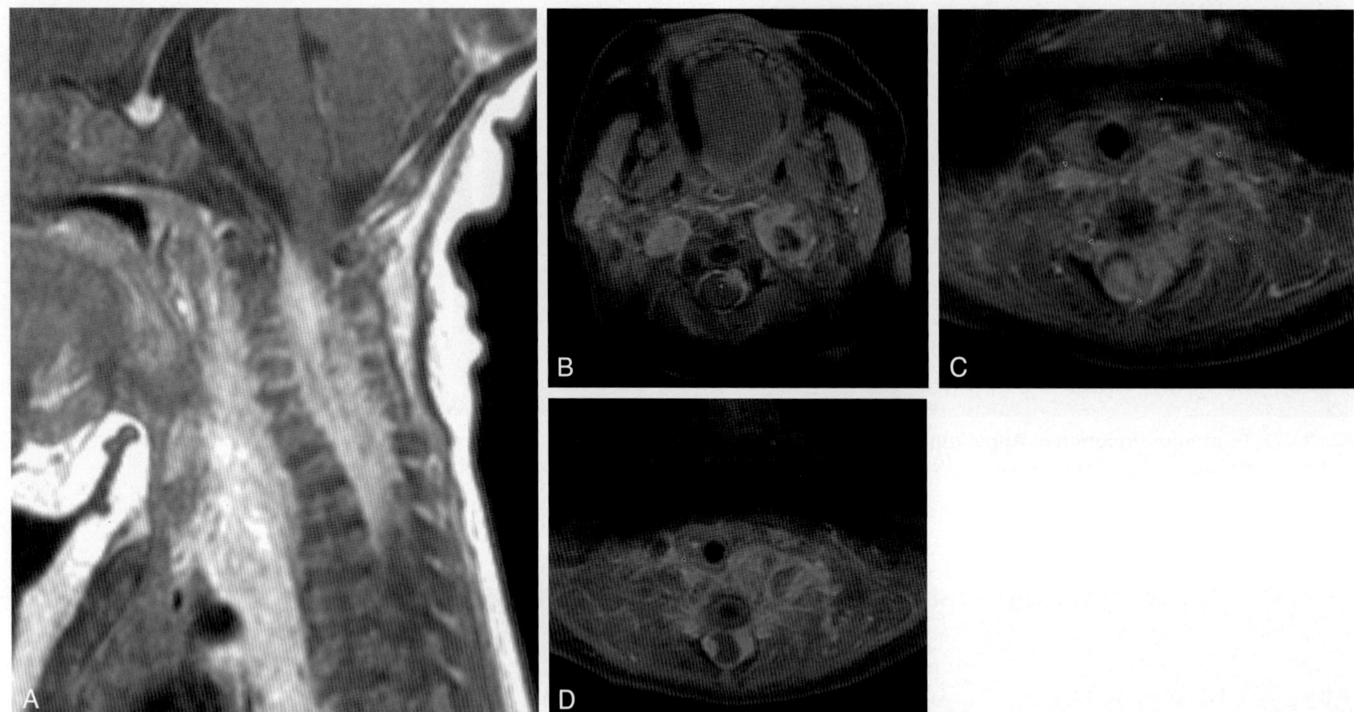

Fig. 14.45 Infantile Myofibromatosis. (A to D) Sagittal and axial T1W+C fat saturation images demonstrate infiltrative homogeneously enhancing soft tissue mass in the prevertebral space, mediastinum, epidural space, paraspinal spaces, and left supraclavicular fossa with intradural extension causing spinal cord compression.

Key Points

Background

- Solitary or multicentric myofibroblastic neoplasm.
- Despite the benign clinical behavior, histopathology demonstrates vascularity, necrosis, local invasion, and increased cellularity.
- Treated with surgical resection, if possible, and chemotherapy.

Imaging

- MRI: Infiltrative solid avidly enhancing mass with high cellularity (low ADC) that may mimic neuroblastoma.

REFERENCE

1. Beck JC, Devaney KO, Weatherly RA, et al. Pediatric myofibromatosis of the head and neck. *Arch Otolaryngol Head Neck Surg.* 1999;125(1):39–44.

INFANTILE FIBROSARCOMA

Solid

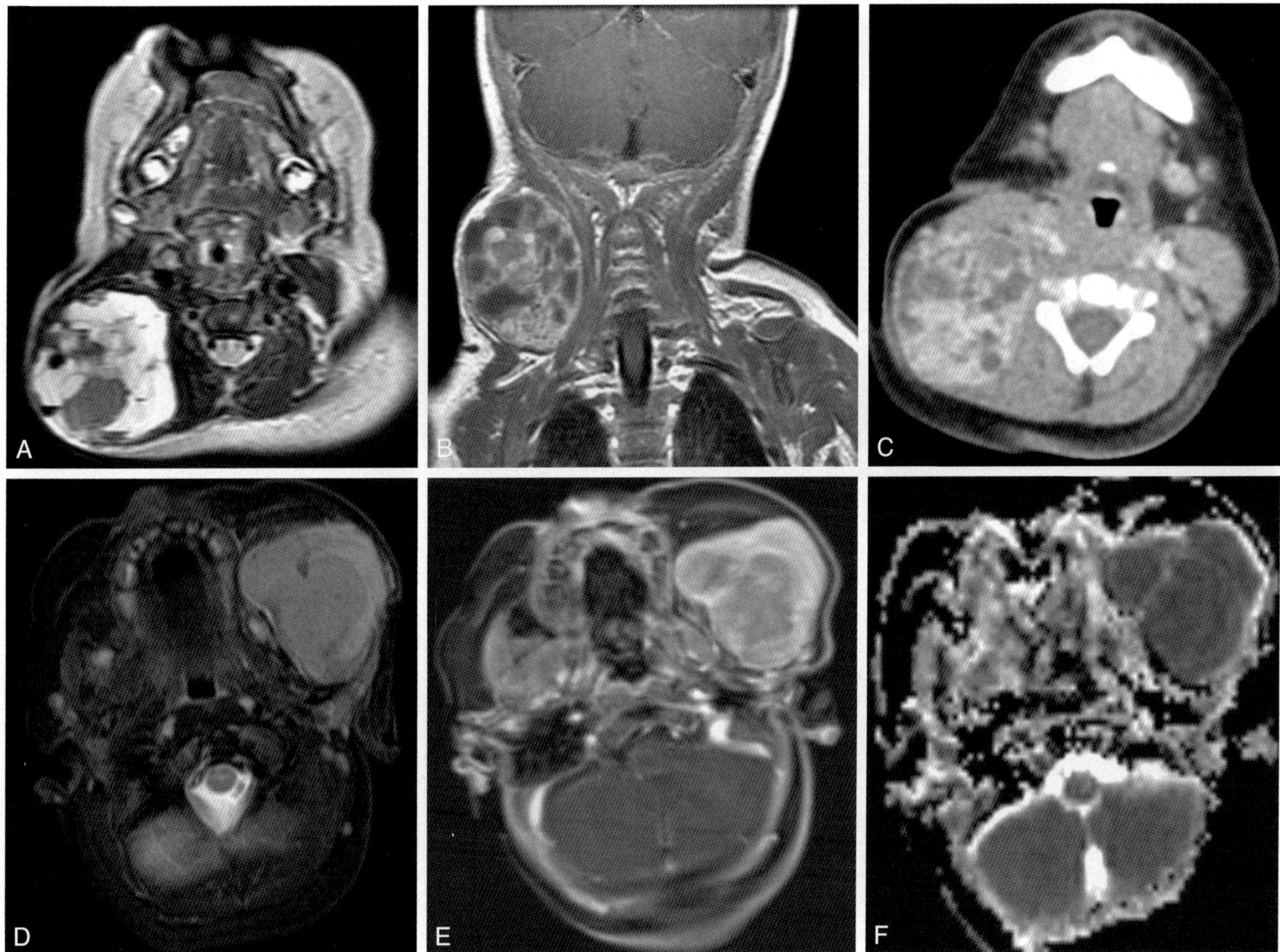

Fig. 14.46 Infantile Fibrosarcoma. (A) Coronal T2W, (B) coronal T1W+C, and (C) axial CECT images demonstrate an heterogeneously enhancing solid and cystic right lateral neck mass with internal fluid levels. (D) Axial T2W fat saturation, (E) axial T1W+C fat saturation, and (F) axial ADC images demonstrate a homogeneous T2W hyperintense enhancing mass with diffusion restriction.

Key Points

Background

- Solid and cystic mass that may mimic a teratoma or venolymphatic malformation.
- A rare mesenchymal tumor occurring at a rate of 5 per million.
- Most commonly occurs in the distal extremities.
- Metastatic disease in 5% to 8%.
- Treatment includes surgical excision and chemotherapy for residual or metastatic tumor. Survival rate is 85% to 95%.

Imaging

- Nonspecific but aggressive appearing soft tissue mass; areas of necrosis

REFERENCES

1. Hu Z, Chou PM, Jennings LJ, et al. Infantile fibrosarcoma—a clinical and histologic mimicker of vascular malformations: case report and review of the literature. *Pediatr Dev Pathol.* 2013 Sep–Oct;16(5):357–363.
2. Jain D, Kohli K. Congenital infantile fibrosarcoma: a clinical mimicker of hemangioma. *Cutis.* 2012 Feb;89(2):61–64.

MELANOTIC NEUROECTODERMAL TUMOR OF INFANCY

Solid

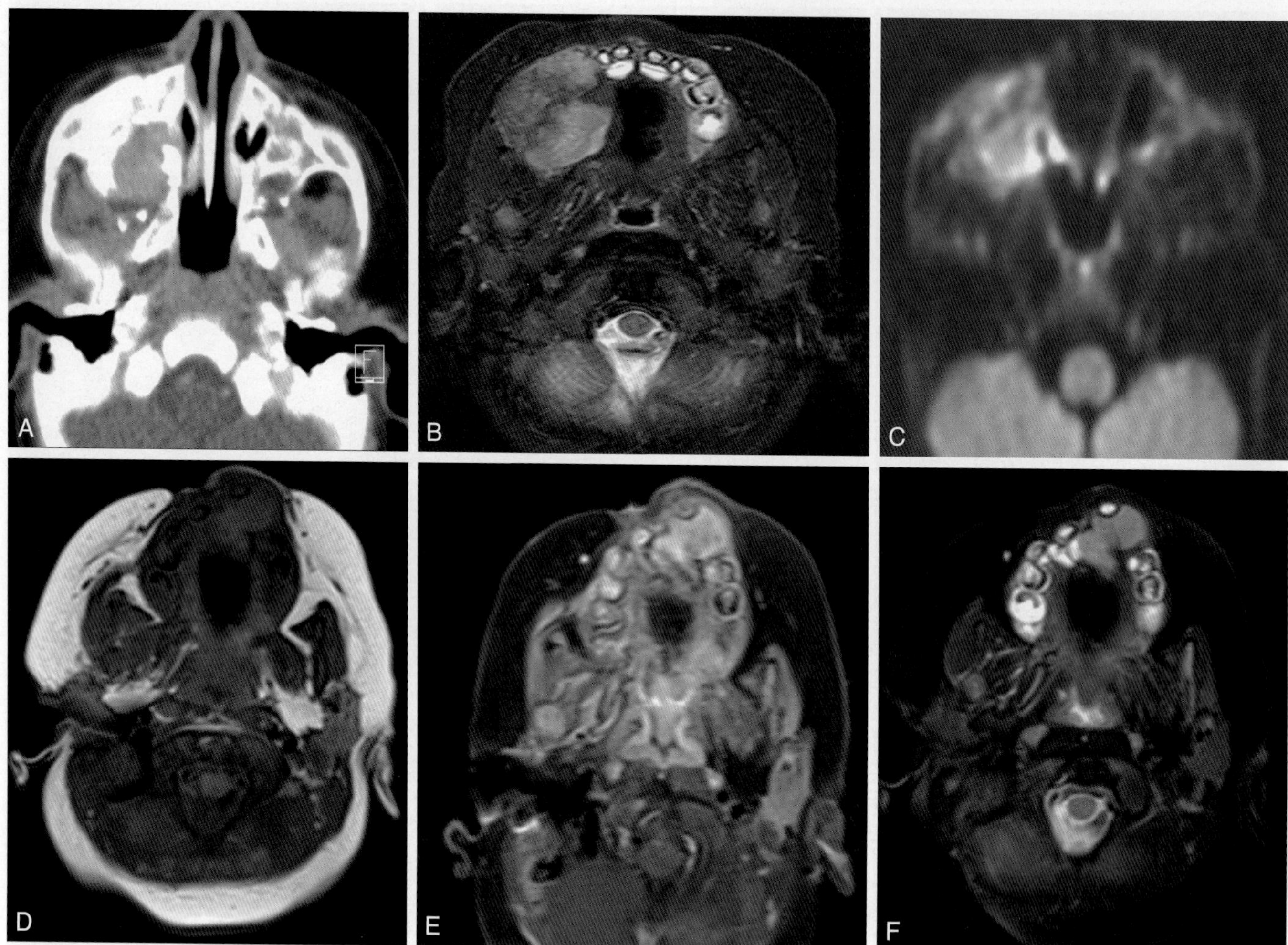

Fig. 14.47 Melanotic Neuroectodermal Tumor of Infancy. (A) Axial CT image demonstrates a hyperdense mass in the right maxilla. (B) Axial T2W fat saturation and (C) axial DWI images demonstrate and T2W mild hyperintense mass with diffusion restriction. (D) Axial T1W, (E) axial T1W+C fat saturation, and (F) axial T2W fat saturation images demonstrate a left anterior maxilla T2W hyperintense mass with homogeneous enhancement.

Key Points

Background

- Rare benign tumor of infancy.
- Predilection for the *anterior maxilla and occipital bone.* May also occur in the mandible.
- Rapidly growing tumor.
- Treated with surgical excision. Chemotherapy can be included for incompletely resected tumors.

Imaging

- MRI: Solid enhancing mass with high cellularity (*DWI restriction*)
- CT: *Aggressive* bone destruction, spiculations, lytic destruction, calcifications, and adjacent hyperostosis

REFERENCE

1. Agarwal P, Saxena S, Kumar S, et al. Melanotic neuroectodermal tumor of infancy: Presentation of a case affecting the maxilla. *J Oral Maxillofac Pathol.* 2010;14(1):29–32.

FIBROMATOSIS COLLI

Solid

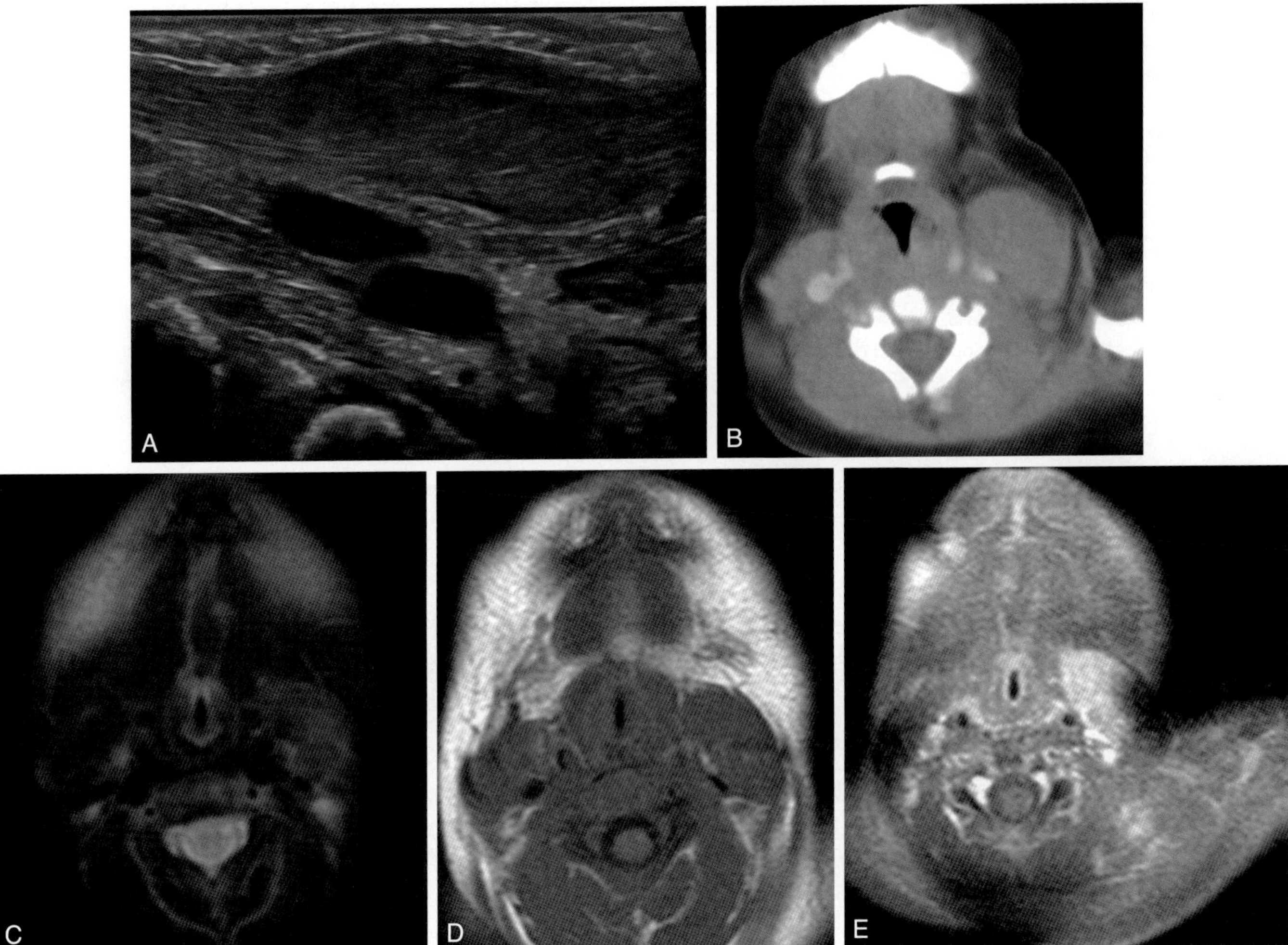

Fig. 14.48 Fibromatosis Colli. (A) Longitudinal ultrasound image demonstrates thickening of the sternocleidomastoid muscle. (B) Axial CT image demonstrates homogeneous soft tissue enlargement of the left sternocleidomastoid muscle. (C) Axial T2W fat saturation, (D) axial T1W, and (E) axial T1W+C fat saturation images demonstrate left sternocleidomastoid muscle enlargement, mild T2W hyperintensity, and enhancement. Although CT and MRI are not commonly performed for this indication, the appearance should not be misinterpreted as a neoplasm such as a rhabdomyosarcoma.

Key Points

Background

- Benign self-limited enlargement of the SCM
- Believed to be secondary to injury to the SCM with breech and difficulty deliveries
- May present as a neck mass, torticollis at 10 to 14 days postpartum. May enlarge for 2 to 4 months and then regress by 4 to 8 months
- Treated with physical therapy

Imaging

- Imaging not required, but if necessary, US is the modality of choice. CT and MRI are typically not necessary.
- 75% are right sided.
- US demonstrates fusiform enlargement of the SCM with intact muscle fiber architecture.
- CT demonstrates soft tissue density expansion of the SCM.
- MRI demonstrates T2W hyperintensity and contrast enhancement in the expanded SCM.

REFERENCE

1. Friedman ER, John SD. Imaging of pediatric neck masses. *Radiol Clin North Am*. 2011 Jul;49(4):617–632.

MUCOEPIDERMOID CARCINOMA

Solid

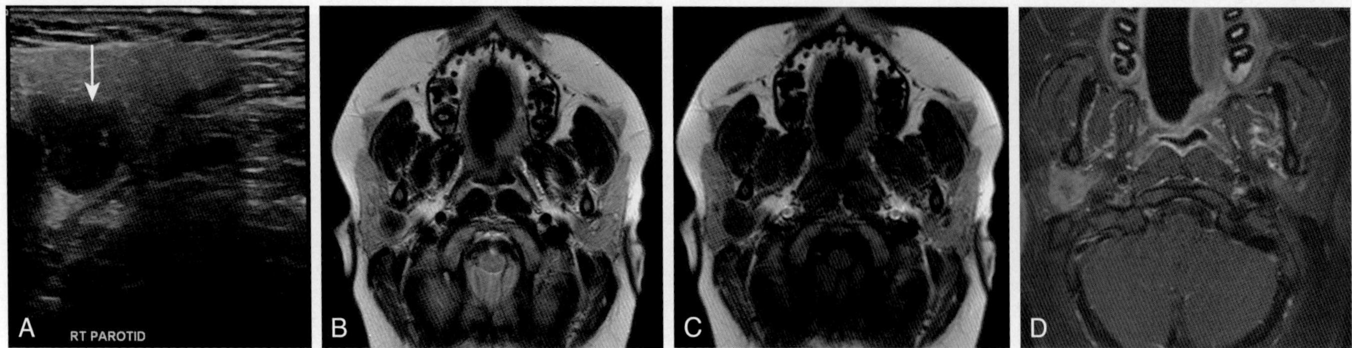

Fig. 14.49 Mucoepidermoid Carcinoma. (A) Focused ultrasound image demonstrates a hypoechoic mass in the parotid gland. (B) Axial T2W and (C and D) axial T1W and axial T1W+C fat saturation images demonstrate a round T2W hypointense nodule with thick enhancement in the right parotid gland.

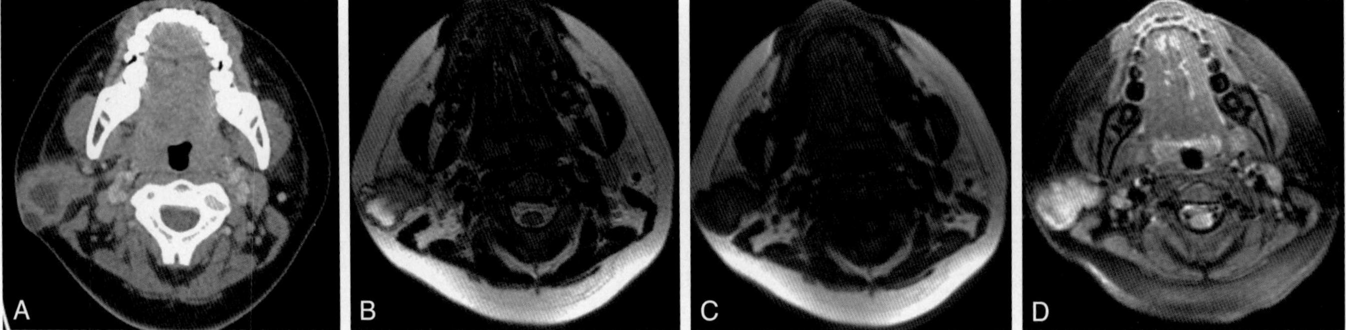

Fig. 14.50 Mucoepidermoid Carcinoma. (A) Axial CECT demonstrates a solid and cystic mass in the right parotid gland. (B) Axial T2W and (C and D) axial T1W and axial T1W+C fat saturation images demonstrate a solid and cystic mass with nearly homogeneous enhancement in the right parotid gland.

Key Points

Background

- Parotid tumors are rare in children.
- Most often occur in children older than 10 years.
- The most common parotid neoplasms in children are mucoepidermoid and acinic cell tumors.
- Complete excision with preservation of the facial nerve is the treatment of choice. Neck dissection is performed for regional metastases.

Imaging

- Mostly well defined but with some irregular margins; enhances but often areas of cystic degeneration; usually T2W hypointense and isointense signal

REFERENCE

1. Rahbar R, Grimmer JF, Vargas SO, et al. Mucoepidermoid carcinoma of the parotid gland in children: a 10-year experience. *Arch Otolaryngol Head Surg*. 2006 Apr;132(4):375–380.

RETINOBLASTOMA

Solid

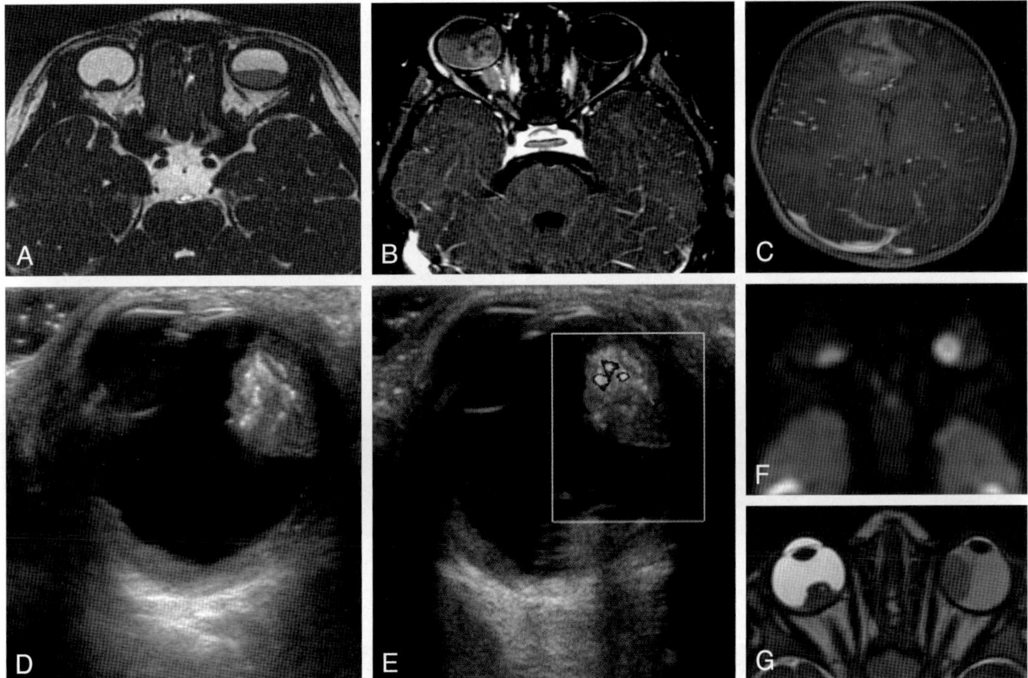

Fig. 14.51 Retinoblastoma: Common Patterns. (A) Axial T2W image demonstrates isointense nodules in the posterior right and left globes. (B) Axial T1W+C image demonstrates abnormal enhancing nodule in the posterior right globe, hyperintense vitreous, and enhancing optic nerve indicative of invasion. (C) Axial T1W+C image demonstrates abnormal leptomeningeal mass-like enhancement due to intracranial metastases. (D and E) Ultrasound images of the globe without and with color Doppler demonstrate an isoechoic nodule with internal hyperechoic foci from calcification and mild vascularity. (F and G) Axial DWI and axial T2W images demonstrate diffusion restriction of bilateral intraocular masses and left globe vitreous proteinaceous fluid.

Key Points

Background

- Most common primary ocular malignancy of childhood affecting ~300 children/year in the USA.
- Cancer develops from a two-hit model in which two events are necessary for the retinal cells to develop tumors. The first hit can be an inherited mutation and would be present in all cells of the body, and the second hit results in loss of function in the normal allele causing dysregulation of the cell cycle.
- Mean age at diagnosis is 18 months. 95% present before 5 years of age.
- Leukocoria is most common presenting sign. Strabismus is the next most common sign.
- Unilateral disease: sporadic form; 70% to 80% of patients; present at ~30 months of age.
- Bilateral/multilateral disease: inherited form; constitute 20% to 30% of patients; presents at younger age (14–16 months).
- Diagnosis based on ophthalmology examination and assisted with US, CT, and/or MRI.
- Risk factors for tumor dissemination include optic nerve invasion, extrascleral extension, and massive choroidal invasion.
- Multiple treatment options include chemotherapy, laser photocoagulation, chemotherapy, and enucleation depending on extent of disease. External beam radiotherapy is no longer recommended due to the high risk of a secondary cancer.

Imaging

- US: Provides high-resolution imaging of the intraocular mass
- CT: Hyperdense mass with characteristic Ca^{2+}; performed less commonly as MRI techniques have improved
- MRI: Used to evaluate extraocular spread, optic nerve extension, and brain involvement. Retinoblastomas demonstrate enhancement and diffusion restriction in a normal globe size. 3D T2W imaging helps to visualize small lesions. Retinal and/or vitreous hemorrhage is often present
- DDx: Coat disease (no Ca^{2+}); persistent hyperplastic primary vitreous (PHPV) (small globe); Toxocara endophthalmitis (rare)

REFERENCES

1. Kralik SF, Kersten R, Glastonbury CM, et al. Evaluation of orbital disorders and cranial nerve innervation of the extraocular muscles. *Magn Reson Imaging Clin N Am.* 2012 Aug;20(3):413–434.
2. Vachha BA, Robson CD. Imaging of pediatric orbital disease. *Neuroimaging Clin N Am.* 2015 Aug;25(3):477–501.
3. Chintagumpala M, Chevez-Barrios P, Paysse EA, et al. Retinoblastoma: a review of current management. *Oncologist.* 2007 Oct;12(1):1237–1246.

RETINOBLASTOMA: UNCOMMON PATTERNS

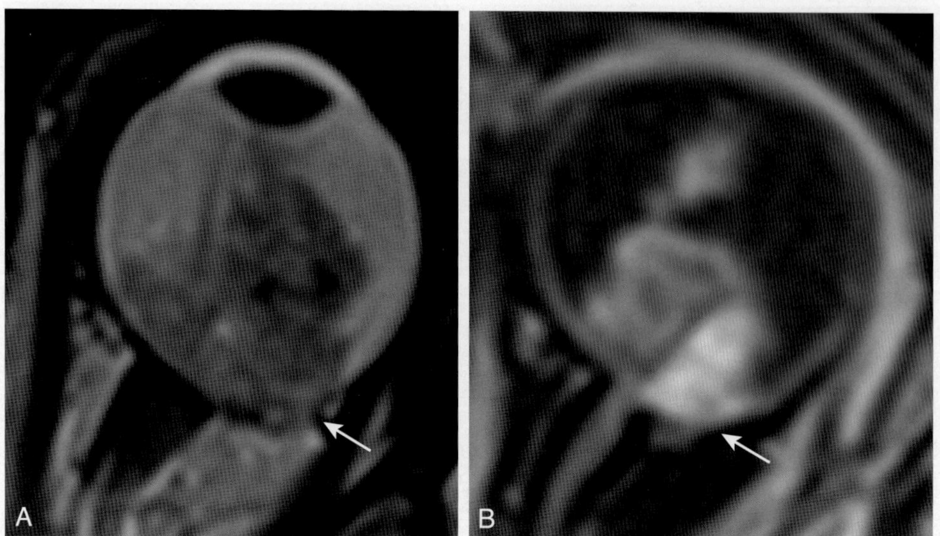

Fig. 14.52 Scleral Invasion. (A) Axial T2W and (B) axial T1W+C fat saturation images demonstrate a retinoblastoma with invasion through the sclera seen as discontinuity of the globe lining.

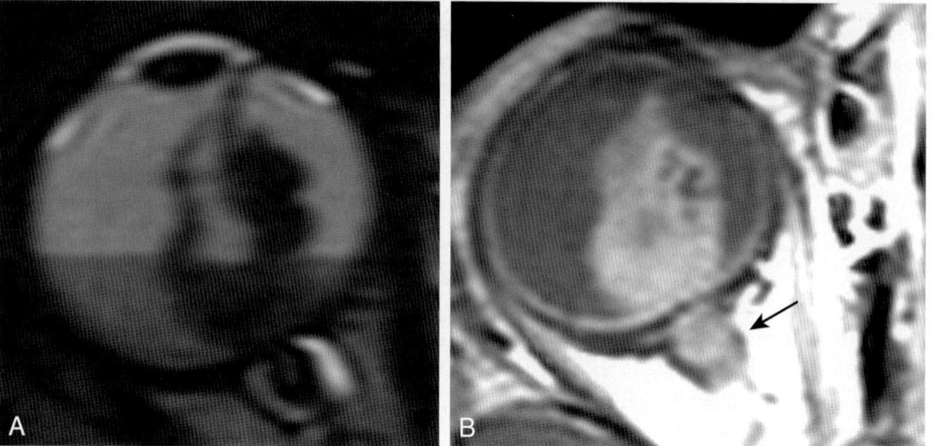

Fig. 14.53 Optic Nerve Invasion. (A) Axial T2W and (B) axial T1W+C images demonstrate a retinoblastoma with enhancement in the anterior optic nerve indicative of nerve invasion.

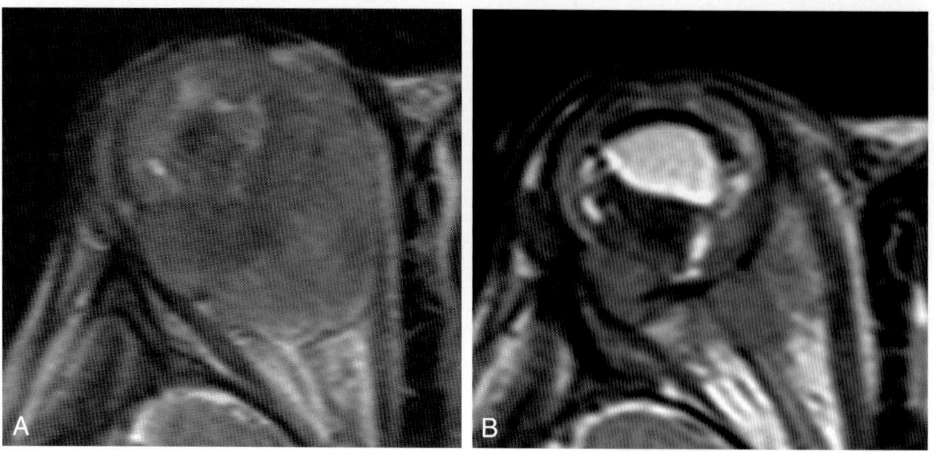

Fig. 14.54 Extraocular Invasion. (A and B) Axial T2W images demonstrate extensive extraocular invasion beyond the sclera and into the periorbital and retrobulbar spaces and optic nerve.

RETINOBLASTOMA: UNCOMMON PATTERNS

Solid

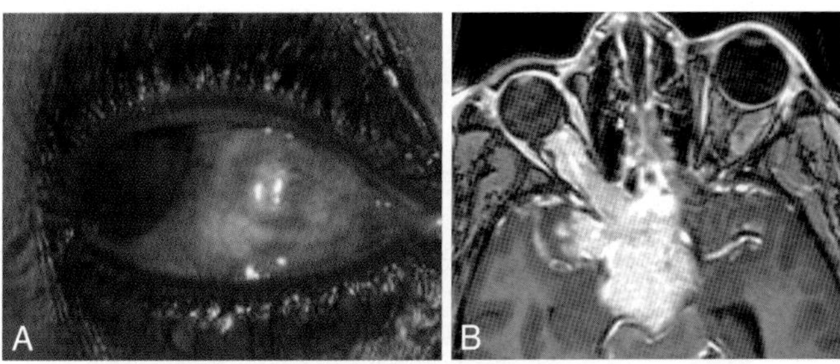

Fig. 14.55 Intracranial Extension. (A) Clinical image of the globe demonstrating erythematous conjunctiva and focal nodular tumor bulge. (B) Axial T1W+C image demonstrates a large enhancing intracranial mass in continuity with the right optic nerve.

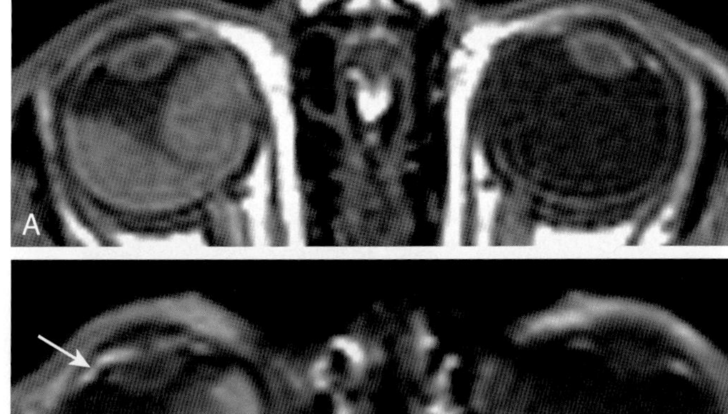

Fig. 14.56 Rubeosis Iridis. (A) Axial T1W and (B) axial T1W+C images demonstrate abnormal anterior chamber enhancement due to neovascularization as well as retinal detachment and enhancing mass in the right globe.

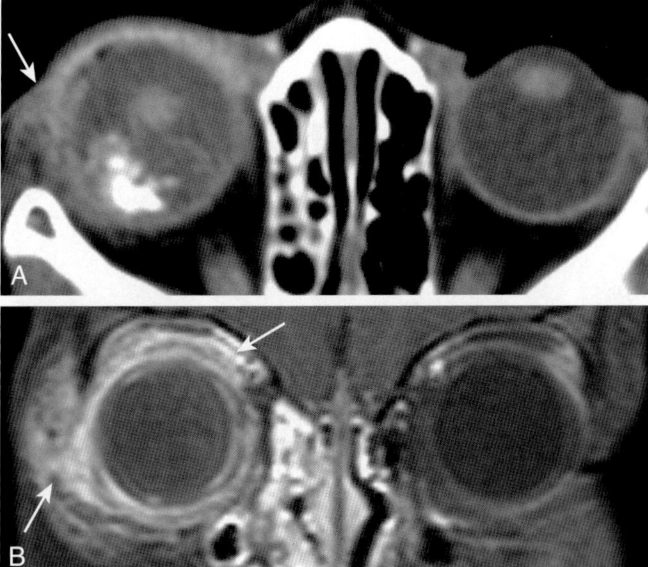

Fig. 14.57 Periorbital Inflammation. (A) Axial CT image demonstrates a partially calcified intraocular right globe mass. (B) Coronal T1W+C image demonstrates right periorbital inflammatory changes.

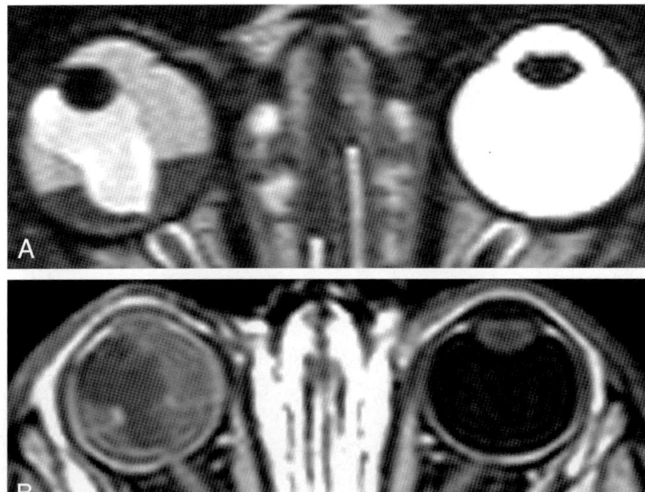

Fig. 14.58 Lens Dislocation. (A) Axial T2W and (B) axial T1W+C fat saturation images demonstrate lens dislocation, neovascularization of the iris, invasion of the ciliary body, and layering vitreous hemorrhage.

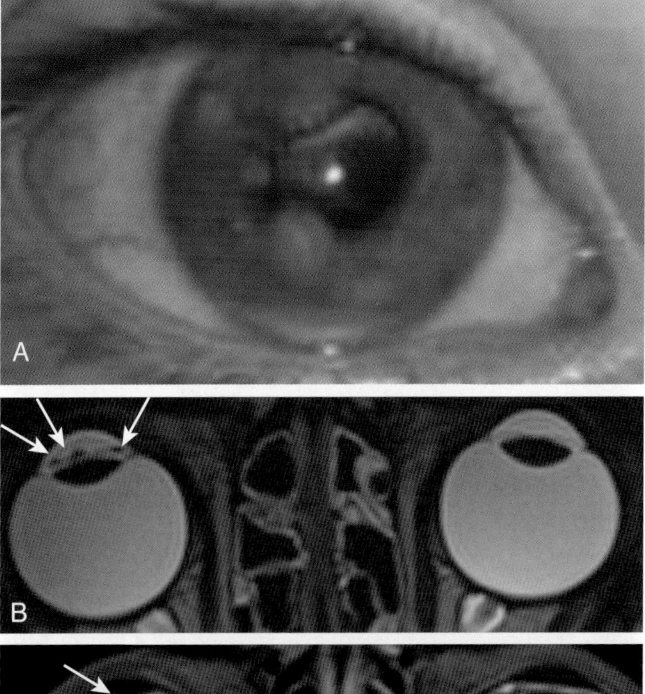

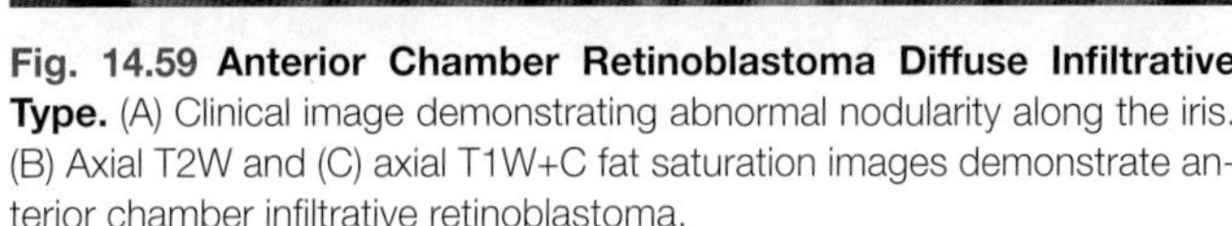

Fig. 14.59 Anterior Chamber Retinoblastoma Diffuse Infiltrative Type. (A) Clinical image demonstrating abnormal nodularity along the iris. (B) Axial T2W and (C) axial T1W+C fat saturation images demonstrate anterior chamber infiltrative retinoblastoma.

RETINOBLASTOMA: COMPLICATIONS

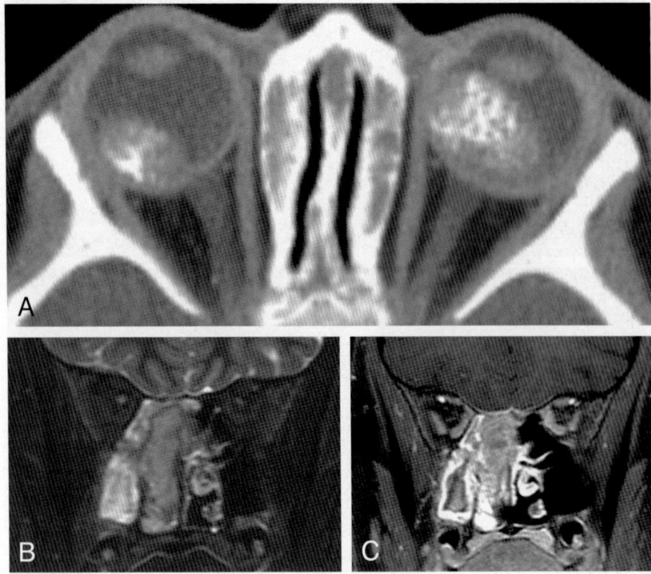

Fig. 14.60 Associated Malignancy. (A) Axial CT image demonstrating bilateral calcified intraocular masses, which were treated subsequently treated with enucleation and chemotherapy. Seven years later, the patient presented with epistaxis and was found to have a right-sided nasal cavity mass seen as a mild T2W hyperintense enhancing mass on (B) coronal T2W and (C) coronal T1W+C fat saturation images. Pathology was an esthesioneuroblastoma indicating a secondary malignancy due to germline Rb gene mutation.

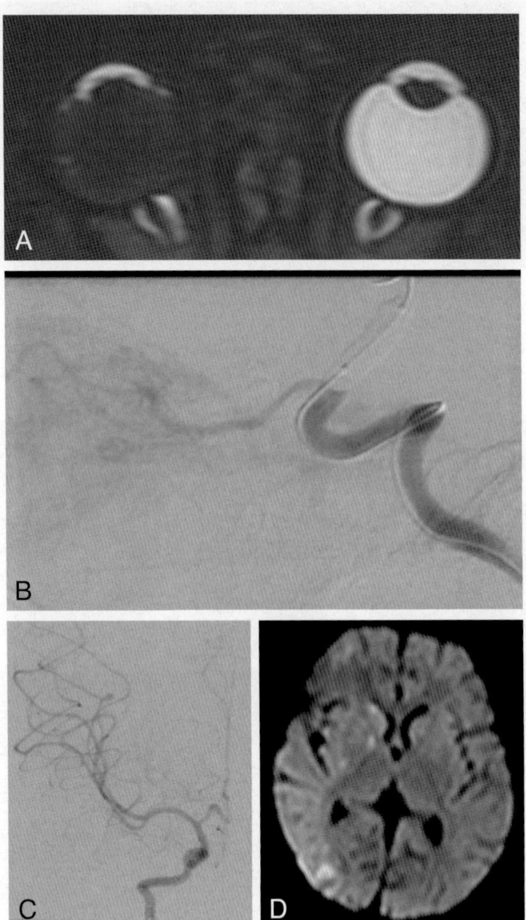

Fig. 14.61 Infarcts Following Chemotherapy. (A) Axial T2W image demonstrates a right intraocular mass. (B and C) Catheter angiography for ophthalmic artery intraarterial chemotherapy following supraclinoid ICA balloon occlusion and postprocedural right ICA angiogram are normal; however, (D) axial DWI demonstrated several small infarcts in the right cerebral hemisphere.

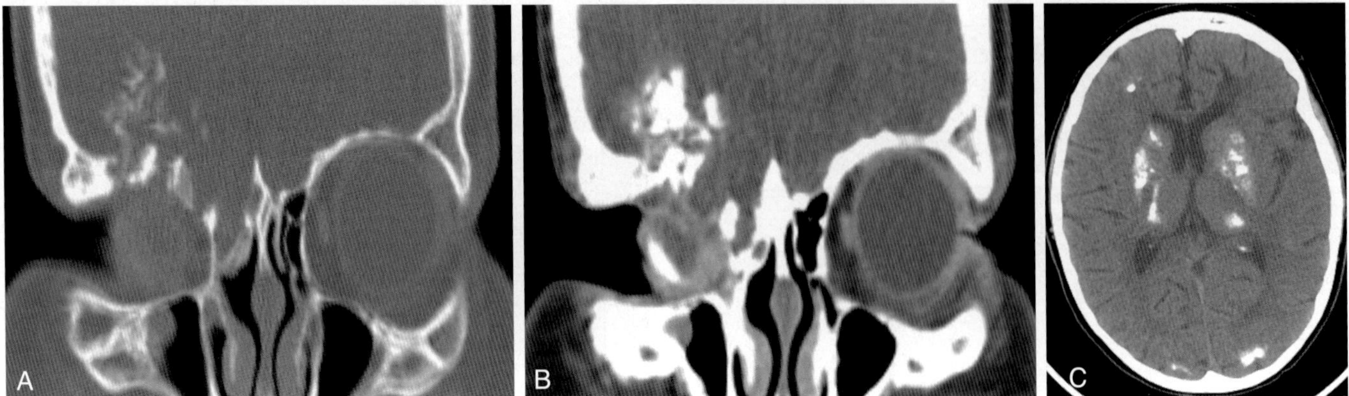

Fig. 14.62 Orbital Roof Osteonecrosis and Parenchymal Calcifications. Right globe retinoblastoma treated with enucleation, chemotherapy, and radiotherapy in 1989. (A to C) Coronal and axial CT images demonstrate right facial deformity, right orbital roof and frontal bone osteonecrosis, and intracranial parenchymal calcification.

PILOMATRIXOMA

Solid

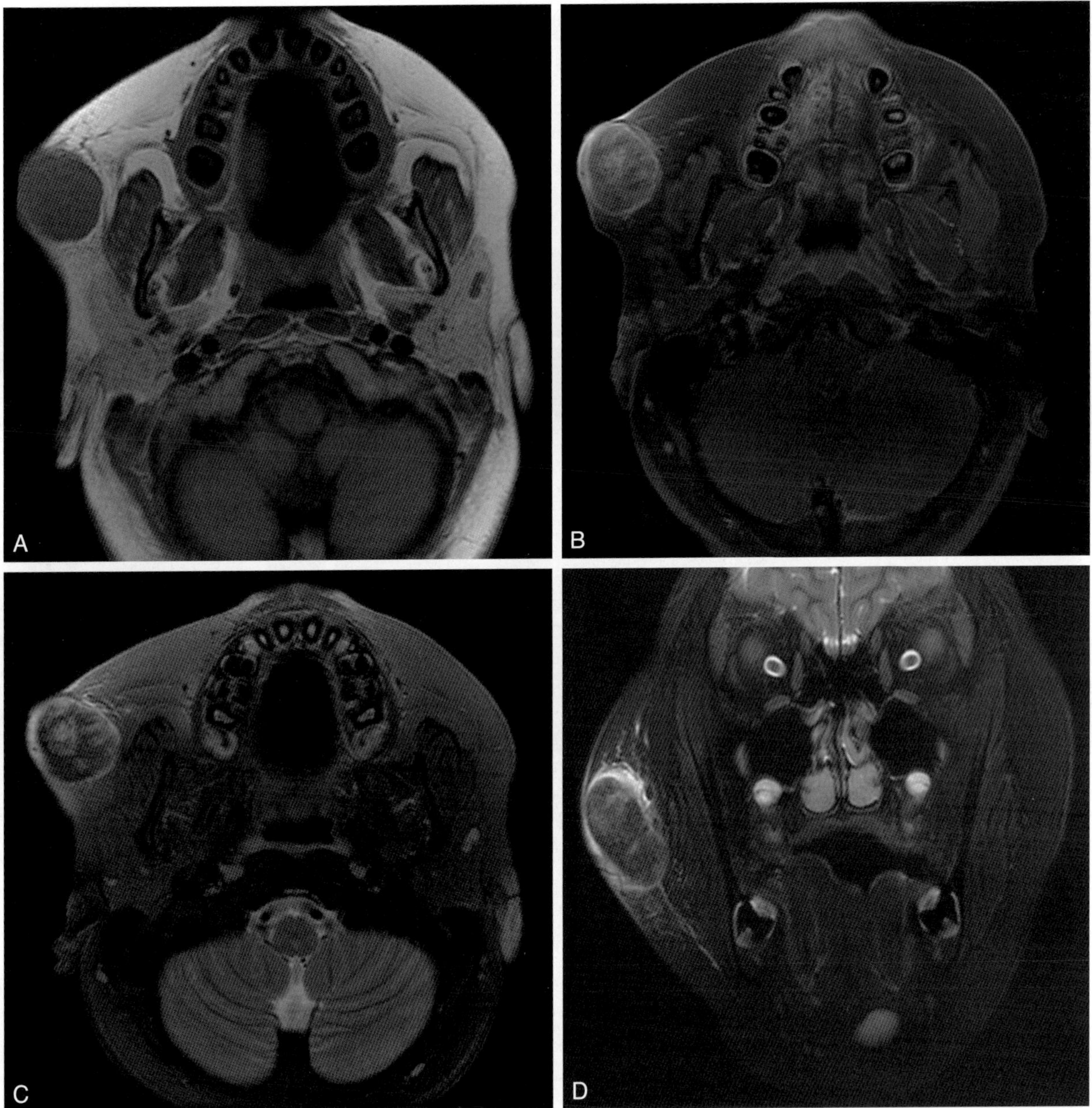

Fig. 14.63 Pilomatrixoma. (A) Axial T1W, (B) axial T1W+C fat saturation, and (C and D) axial and coronal T2W fat saturation images demonstrate heterogeneous T2W signal and enhancement in a right buccal space subcutaneous mass.

Key Points

Background

- Rare benign tumor of hair follicle origin
- Commonly in the first two decades of life

Imaging

- Heterogeneous *cutaneous/subcutaneous* mass; often contain calcifications
- 78% located in the head and neck; often the buccal space
- Differential Diagnosis: Sebaceous cyst, and hemangioma

REFERENCE

1. Guinot-Moya R, Valmaseda-Castellon E, Berini-Aytes L, et al. Pilomatrixoma. Review of 205 cases. *Med Oral Patol Oral Cir Bucal.* 2011 Jul 1;16(4):e552–e555.

ROSAI DORFMAN

Solid

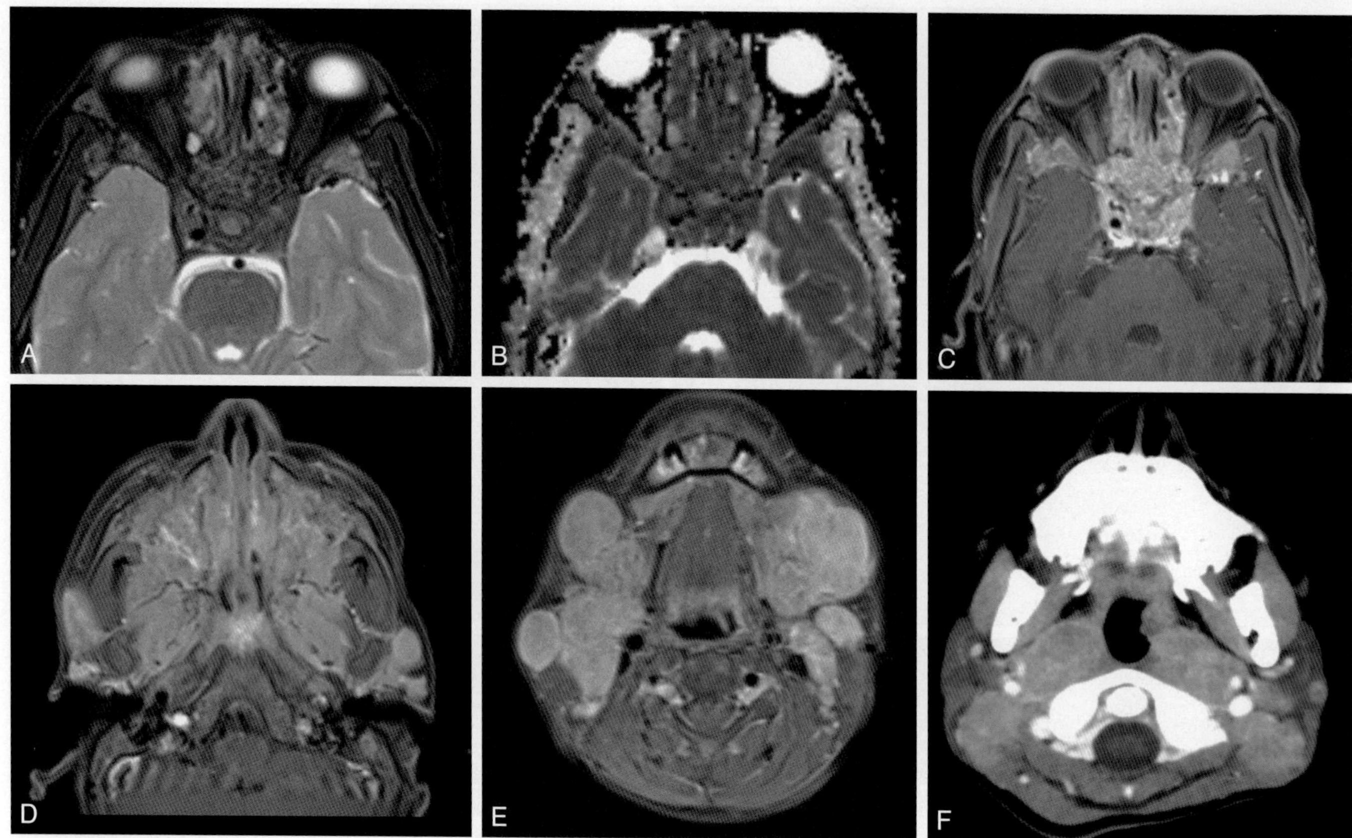

Fig. 14.64 Rosai Dorfman. (A) Axial T2W fat saturation, (B) axial ADC, (C to E) axial T1W+C fat saturation, and (F) axial CECT images demonstrate homogeneous enhancing soft tissue in the ethmoid and maxillary sinuses, greater wings of the sphenoid bones, pterygoid muscles, retromaxillary spaces, and bulky lymphadenopathy with hyperenhancement in the submandibular spaces, lateral retropharyngeal spaces, and the jugular chain lymph nodes. Paranasal sinus masses demonstrate low ADC signal indicative of hypercellularity.

Key Points

Background

- Rare, idiopathic, non-Langerhans cell histiocytic proliferative disease.
- Massive, painless, cervical lymphadenopathy in 90% of patients. 75% have extranodal disease involving the nasal cavity, parotid glands, skin, central nervous system (CNS), orbits, respiratory tract, and bones
- Accompanied by fever, weight loss, and hypergammaglobulinemia
- Intracranial Rosai Dorfman is rare and described in approximately 7% of cases. 83% have isolated CNS disease. CNS lesions most commonly occur as dural-based masses, most commonly involving the cavernous sinuses. Rarely involves the parenchyma
- Presence of S100 positive cells with an intact cell within the cytoplasm of another cell

Imaging

- Soft tissue density nonnecrotic masses; orbital and central skull base involvement of the dura and cavernous sinus involvement is common; homogenous enhancing and hypercellular on DWI (low ADC)

REFERENCE

1. Wang Y, Camelo-Piragua S, Abdullah A, et al. Neuroimaging features of CNS histiocytosis syndromes. *Clin Imaging*. 2020;60:131–140.

DIFFERENTIAL DIAGNOSIS OF A BONE-ASSOCIATED MASS

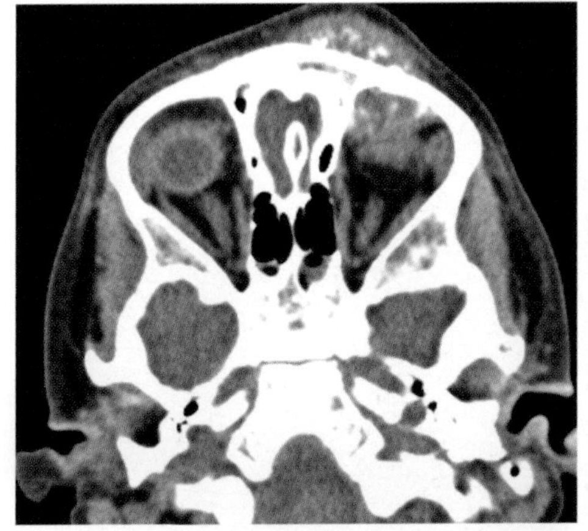

Neuroblastoma

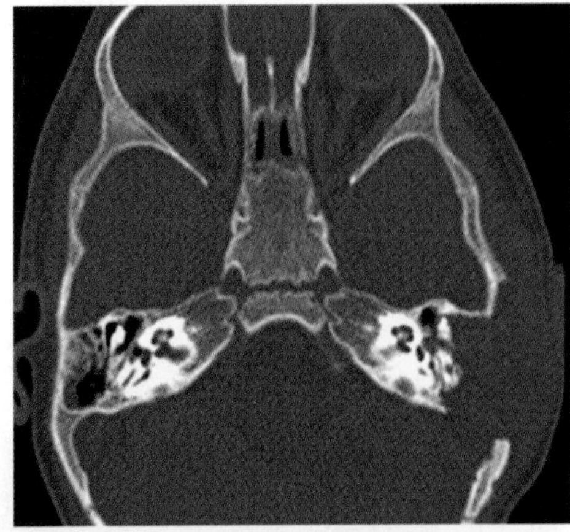

Langerhans Cell Histiocytosis

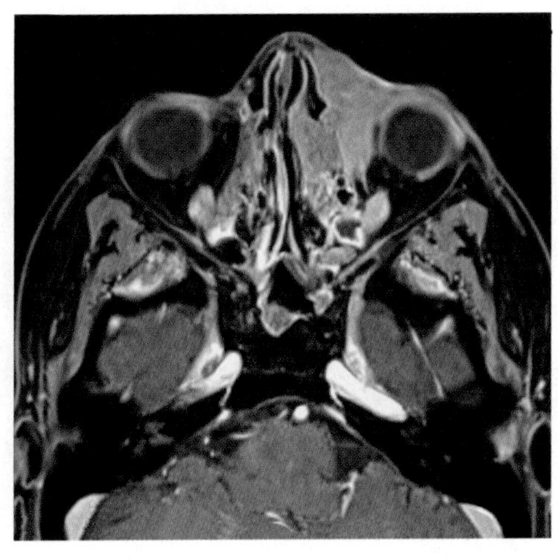

Leukemia

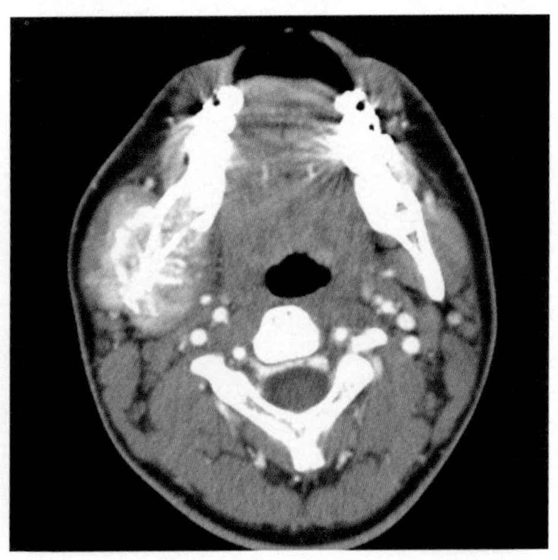

Ewing Sarcoma

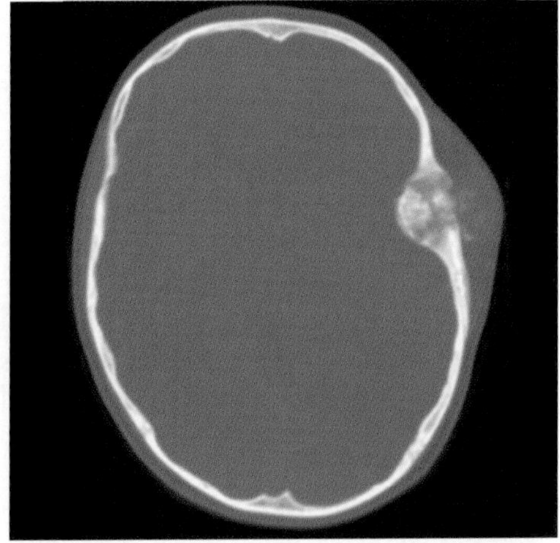

Osteosarcoma

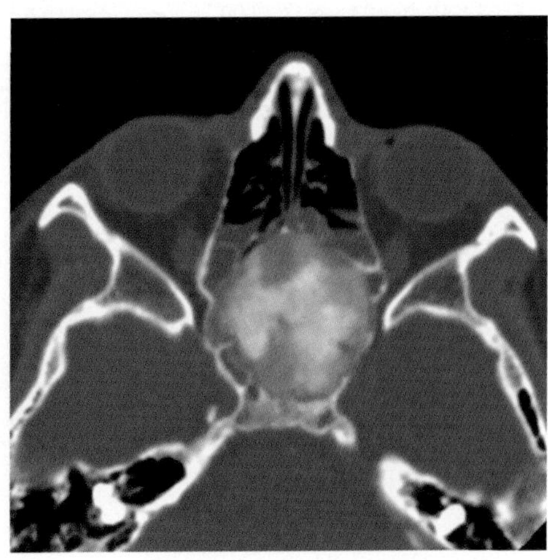

Fibroosseous Lesions

NEUROBLASTOMA

Bone-associated
Calcified
Cystic

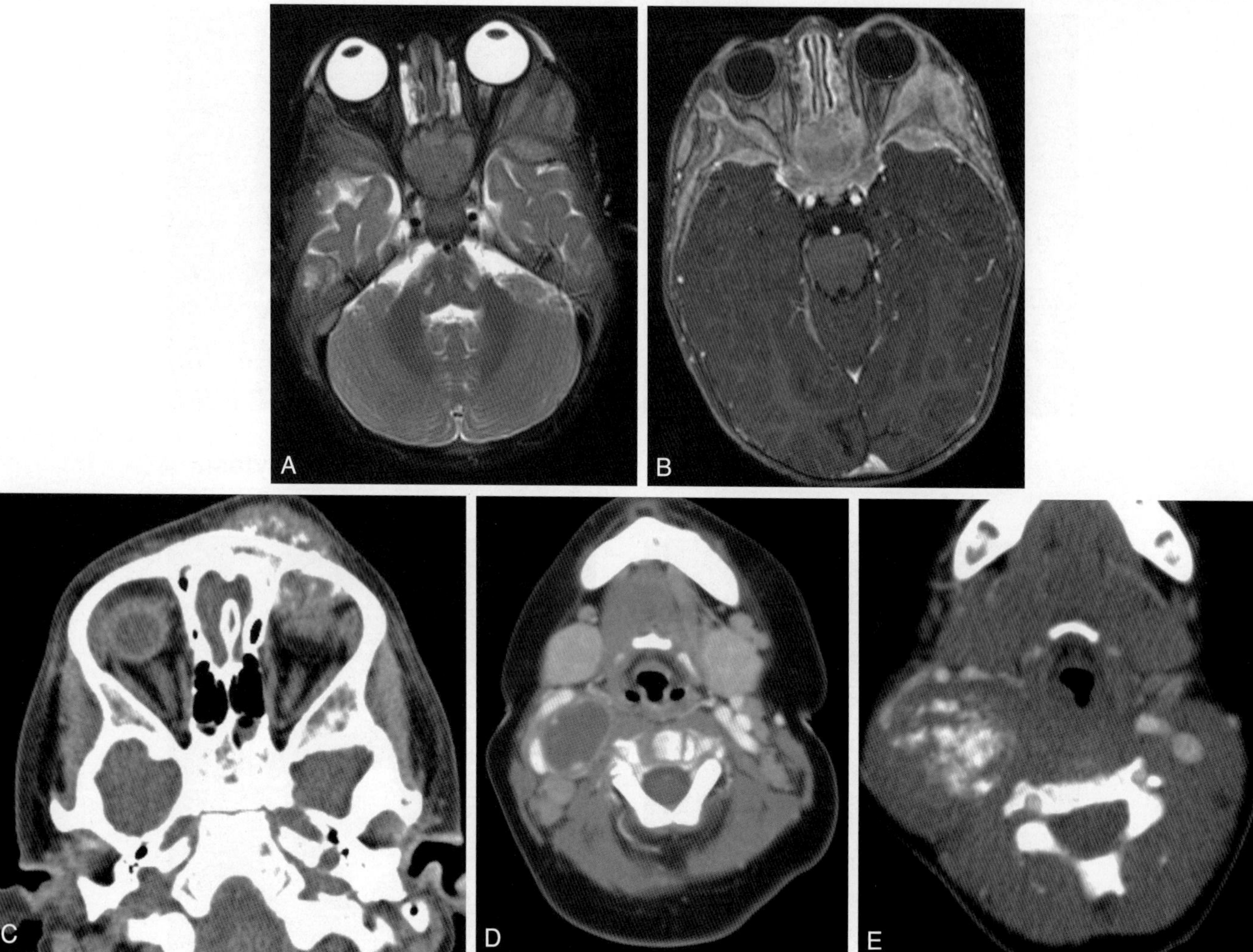

Fig. 14.65 Neuroblastoma: Imaging Patterns Seen in the Head and Neck. (A) Axial T2W fat saturation and (B) axial T1W+C fat saturation images demonstrate symmetric T2W mild hyperintense homogeneously enhancing masses in the lateral walls of the orbits with soft tissue extension. (C) Axial CECT image demonstrates a mass centered in the left paramedian aspect of the frontal bone with soft tissue extension and small foci of calcification. (D) Axial CECT demonstrates a cystic mass in the right lateral neck with peripheral nodular enhancement. (E) Axial CECT image demonstrates a large right lateral neck soft tissue mass with internal calcification.

Key Points

Background

- Malignant tumor of the sympathetic nervous system.
- Most common solid extracranial tumor in children <5 years of age
- Bone metastases is present in two-thirds of patients at diagnosis.
- Presentation: 20% to 55% with ophthalmic manifestations including proptosis and "raccoon eyes" (periorbital ecchymosis); Horner syndrome; opsoclonus myoclonus; ataxia

Imaging

- Tumors in the H&N region usually involve the calvarium and orbit, and most are from metastatic disease. The H&N region is the primary site of disease in 5% of patients.
- CT: Lytic, permeative, and "hair on end" periosteal reaction; often associated soft tissue mass; cystic/necrotic mass with calcification when involving the neck
- MRI: Variable enhancement; diffusion restriction
- Differential Diagnosis: LCH, leukemia, and Ewing sarcoma

REFERENCE

1. Vachha BA, Robson CD. Imaging of pediatric orbital disease. *Neuroimaging Clin N Am.* 2015 Aug;25(3):477–501.

LANGERHANS CELL HISTIOCYTOSIS

Bone-associated

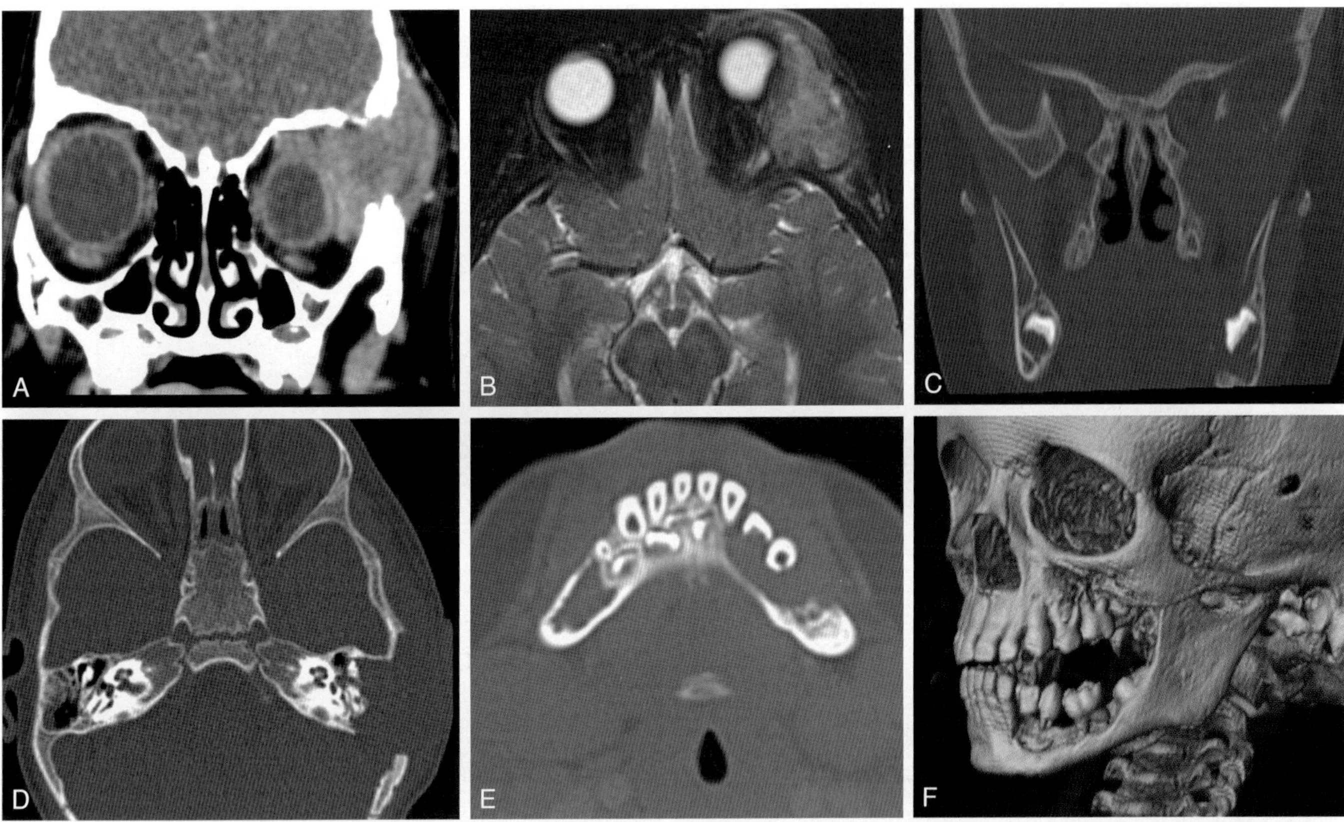

Fig. 14.66 Langerhans Cell Histiocytosis. (A) Coronal reformat CECT, (B) axial T2W fat saturation, and (C) coronal reformat CT images demonstrate a well-defined lytic bone lesion in the left lateral wall of the orbit with associated soft tissue mass. (D) Axial CT image demonstrates a well-defined lytic defect in the left temporal bone. (E and F) Axial and 3D volumetric CT images demonstrates well-defined lytic bone lesion in the left mandibular body resulting in "floating teeth" appearance.

Key Points

Background

- Infiltration by abnormal histiocytic cells.
- Average age of onset is 1 to 3 years.

Imaging

- H&N locations involve bones of the calvarium, orbit, maxilla, temporal bone, mandible, and central skull base.
- The calvarium is the most common bony site involved in the head and neck.
- Temporal bone involvement can mimic otitis media and mastoiditis.
- Orbital involvement can result in proptosis and swelling.
- Mandibular involvement can result in floating tooth and gingival bleeding.
- CT: Well-defined and sharply marginated lytic bone lesion; no periosteal reaction; frequently there is an associated enhancing soft tissue mass
- MRI: heterogeneous T2W; signal heterogeneous enhancement; uncommonly contain fluid-fluid levels

REFERENCES

1. Vachha BA, Robson CD. Imaging of pediatric orbital disease. *Neuroimaging Clin N Am*. 2015 Aug;25(3):477–501.
2. Nasseri F, Munjal K, Ginsberg LE, et al. Imaging review of craniofacial masses in children. *Neurographics*. 2015 Sept/Oct;5(5):217–230.

GRANULOCYTIC SARCOMA

Bone-associated

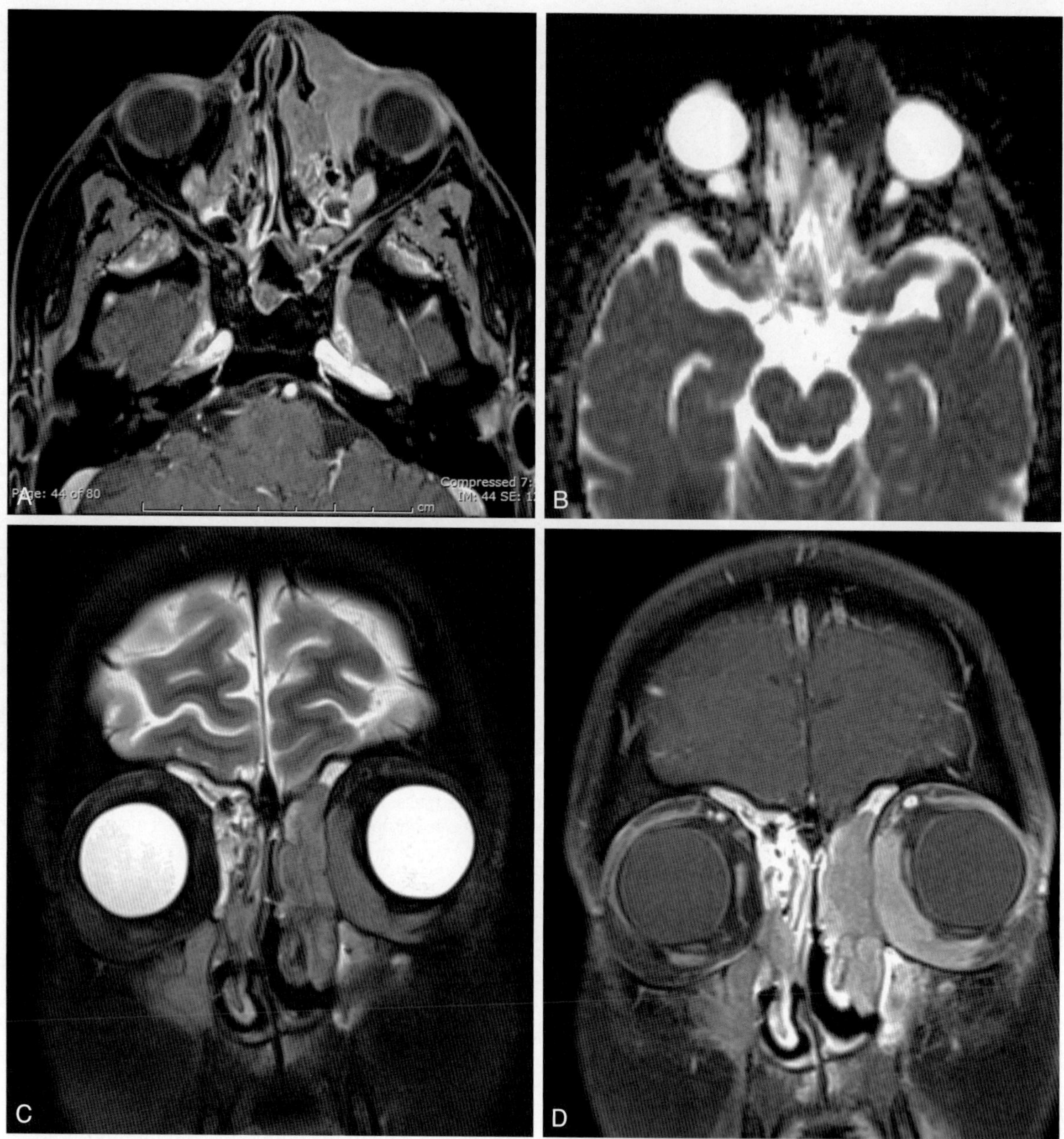

Fig. 14.67 Granulocytic Sarcoma. (A) Axial T1W+C fat saturation, (B) axial ADC, (C) coronal T2W fat saturation, and (D) coronal T1W+C fat saturation images demonstrate homogeneous enhancing mild T2W hyperintense soft tissue in the ethmoid and maxillary sinuses, nasal cavity, and left orbit with diffusion restriction indicative of hypercellularity.

Key Points

Background

- Also known as a chloroma
- Acute myelogenous leukemia involving the orbits, skull base, and paranasal sinuses

Imaging

- CT: Minimal bone destruction; permeative; lytic changes
- MRI: Diffusion restriction, infiltrative, homogenous enhancement
- Can infiltrate the optic nerve and globe and result in vision loss

REFERENCE

1. Vachha BA, Robson CD. Imaging of pediatric orbital disease. *Neuroimaging Clin N Am*. 2015 Aug;25(3):477–501.

EWING SARCOMA

Bone-associated

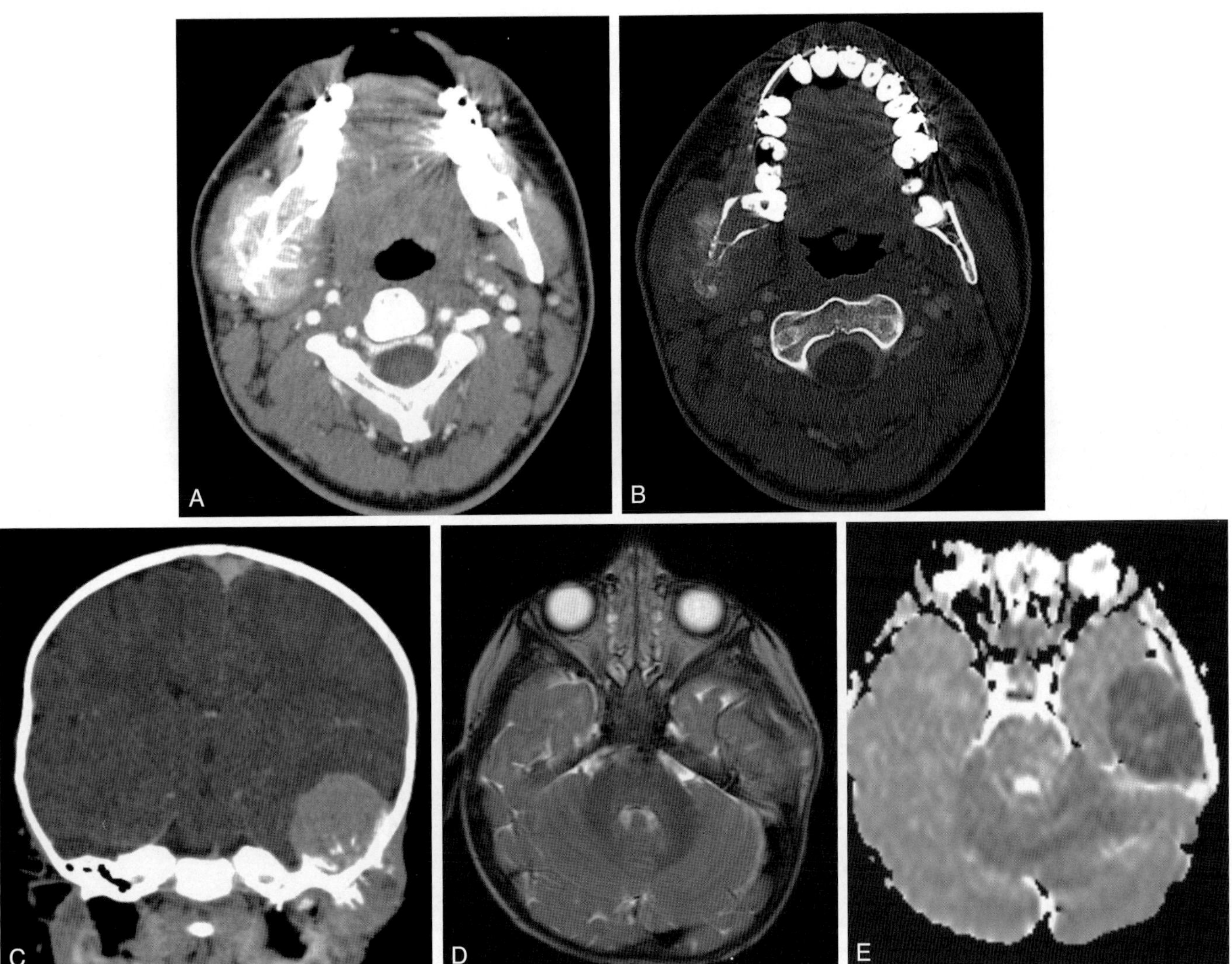

Fig. 14.68 Ewing Sarcoma. (A and B) Axial CECT images demonstrate an enhancing mass arising from the right mandible with aggressive speculated bone periosteal reaction. Different patient with Ewing Sarcoma: (C) Coronal CECT, (D) axial T2W, and (E) axial ADC images demonstrate an enhancing mass in the squamosal left temporal bone with soft tissue extension and low ADC signal indicative of hypercellularity.

Key Points

Background

- Malignant neuroectodermal bone tumor
- Second most common malignant bone tumor of childhood after osteosarcoma

Imaging

- The H&N region most commonly involves the mandible
- CT: Lytic, permeative, aggressive periosteal reaction (sunburst, spiculated, brushlike, Codman triangle), and homogeneously dense soft tissue component
- MRI: T2 heterogeneous, avid homogeneous enhancement, and hypercellular on DWI (low ADC)

REFERENCE

1. Nasseri F, Munjal K, Ginsberg LE, et al. Imaging review of craniofacial masses in children. *Neurographics*. 2015 Sept/Oct;5(5):217–230.

OSTEOSARCOMA

Bone-associated

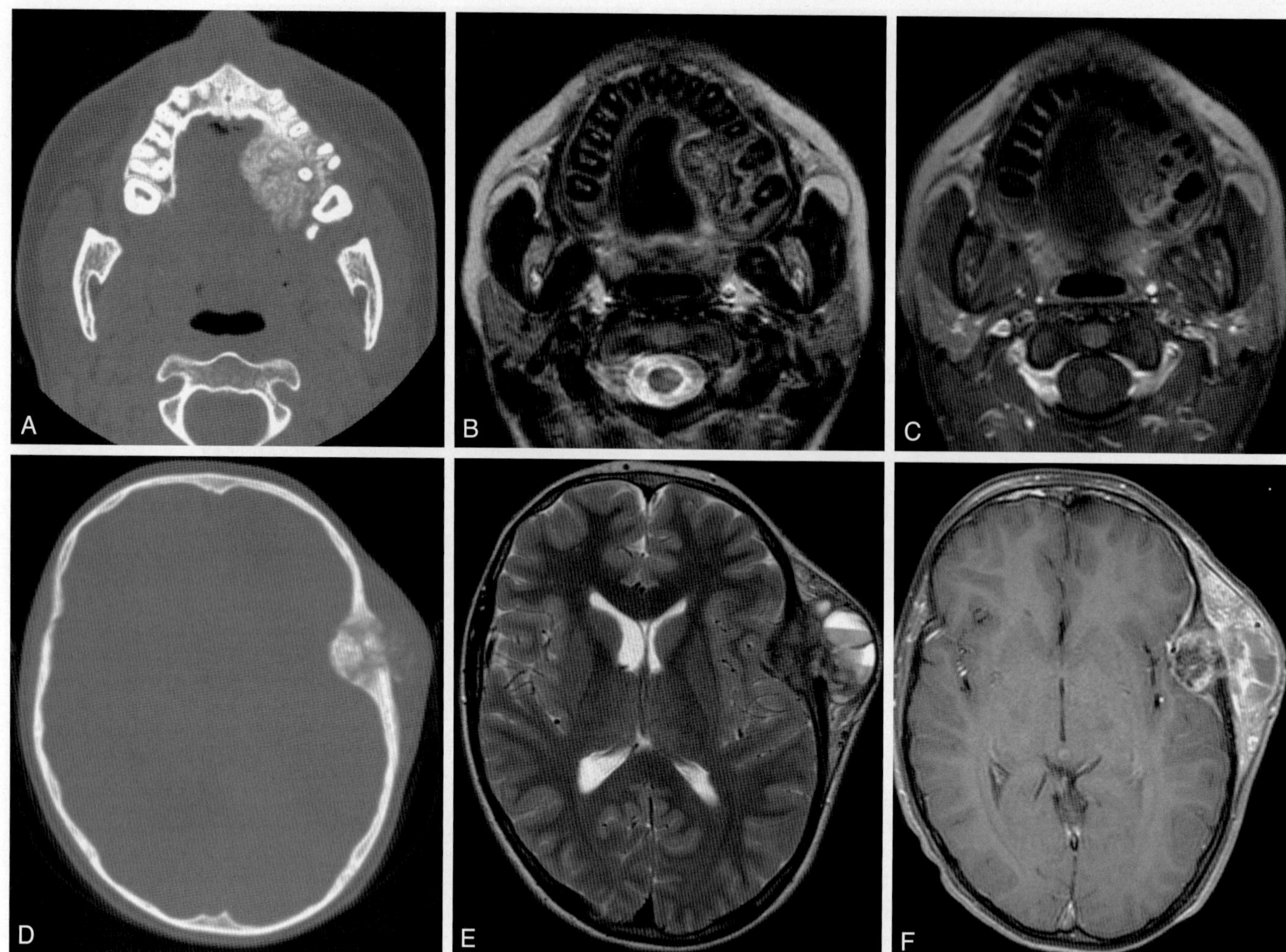

Fig. 14.69 Osteosarcoma. (A) Axial CT, (B) axial T2W, and (C) axial T1W+C fat saturation images demonstrate an ossified mass with mixed T2W signal and mild enhancement arising from the left maxilla. (D) Axial CT, (E) axial T2W, and (F) axial T1W+C images demonstrate an enhancing mass arising from the left side of the calvarium with ossification, heterogeneous enhancement, and internal fluid-fluid levels consistent with an osteosarcoma with secondary aneurysmal bone cyst formation.

Key Points

Background

- H&N location accounts for <10% of all osteosarcomas.
- Rare in children. More common in the third and fourth decades.
- Most commonly involves the mandible and maxilla.
- Radiotherapy-related osteosarcomas can occur in hereditary retinoblastoma survivors.

Imaging

- CT: Lytic bone lesion with mineralization, and aggressive periosteal reaction
- MRI: heterogeneous T1W, T2W, and T1W+C intensity

REFERENCE

1. Nasseri F, Munjal K, Ginsberg LE, et al. Imaging review of craniofacial masses in children. *Neurographics*. 2015 Sept/Oct;5(5):217–230.

FIBROOSSEOUS LESIONS

Bone-associated

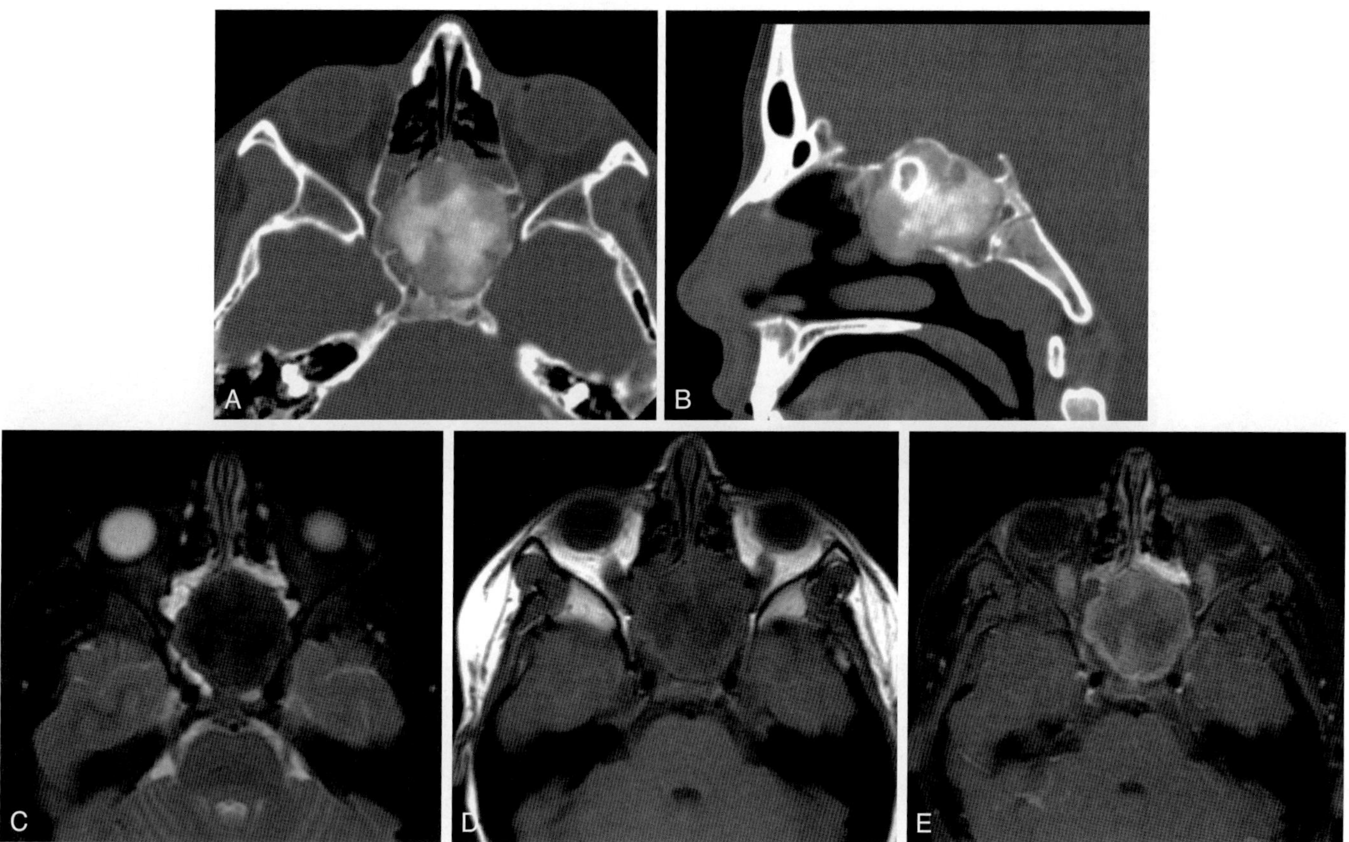

Fig. 14.70 Ossifying Fibroma. (A and B) Axial and sagittal CT images demonstrate an expansile mass arising from the ethmoid and sphenoid sinus with ossification and ground glass matrix. (C) Axial T2W fat saturation, (D) axial T1, and (E) axial T1W+C fat saturation images demonstrate a T2W hypointense mass with heterogeneous enhancement. The mass results in narrowing of the orbital foramen. This example demonstrates how MRI appearance can be misleading to a diagnosis of a malignancy while CT appearance leads to a diagnosis of a benign lesion.

Key Points

Background

- Fibroosseous lesions include fibrous dysplasia, ossifying fibroma, and nonossifying fibroma.
- Benign but locally aggressive bone neoplasm.
- 85% involve the facial bones; 12% involve the calvarium; 4% are extracranial.
- Majority of fibrous dysplasia are sporadic, while a minority occur with McCune-Albright syndrome which includes precocious puberty, café au lait spots, and polyostotic fibrous dysplasia and Mazabraud syndrome which include soft tissue myxomas.
- Treated with local excision. Recurrence up to 56%.

Imaging

- CT: Expansile, well defined with varying ossification and ground glass components; juvenile form more aggressive
- MRI: Usually low T1W and low or heterogeneous T2W signal; usually enhance; may contain fluid-fluid levels
- Differential Diagnosis: Fibrous dysplasia: less well defined

REFERENCE

1. Nasseri F, Munjal K, Ginsberg LE, et al. Imaging review of craniofacial masses in children. *Neurographics*. 2015 Sept/Oct;5(5):217–230.

FIBROOSSEOUS LESIONS

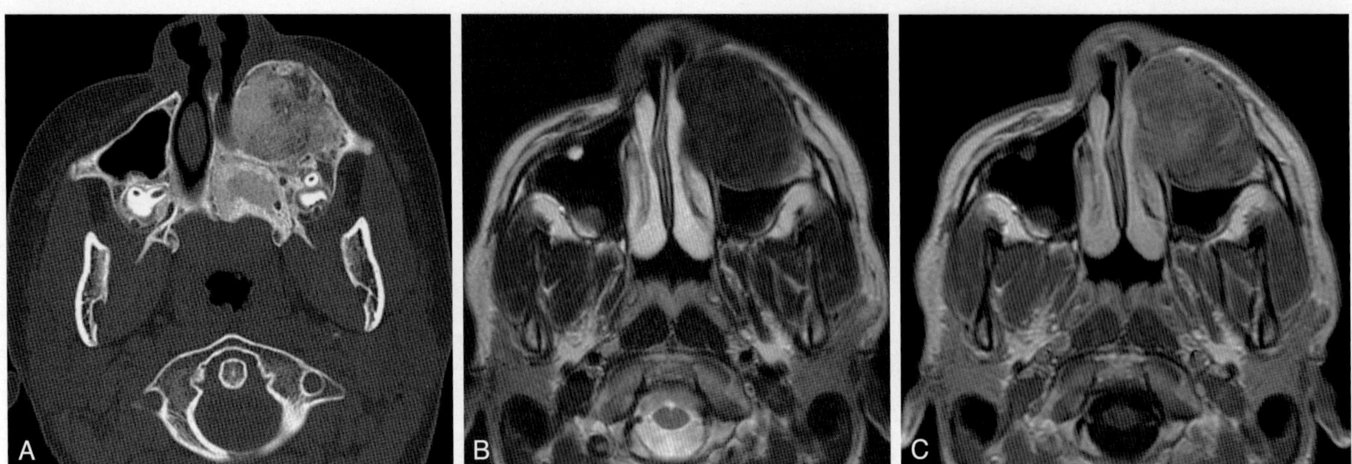

Fig. 14.71 Fibrous Dysplasia. A 10-year-old with fibrous dysplasia. (A) Axial CT demonstrates an expansile ground-glass mass in the left maxilla. (B) Axial T2W and (C) axial T1W+C images demonstrate T2 hypointensity and mild diffuse enhancement consistent with a fibrooseous lesion. Surgical resection confirmed the pathology of fibrous dysplasia.

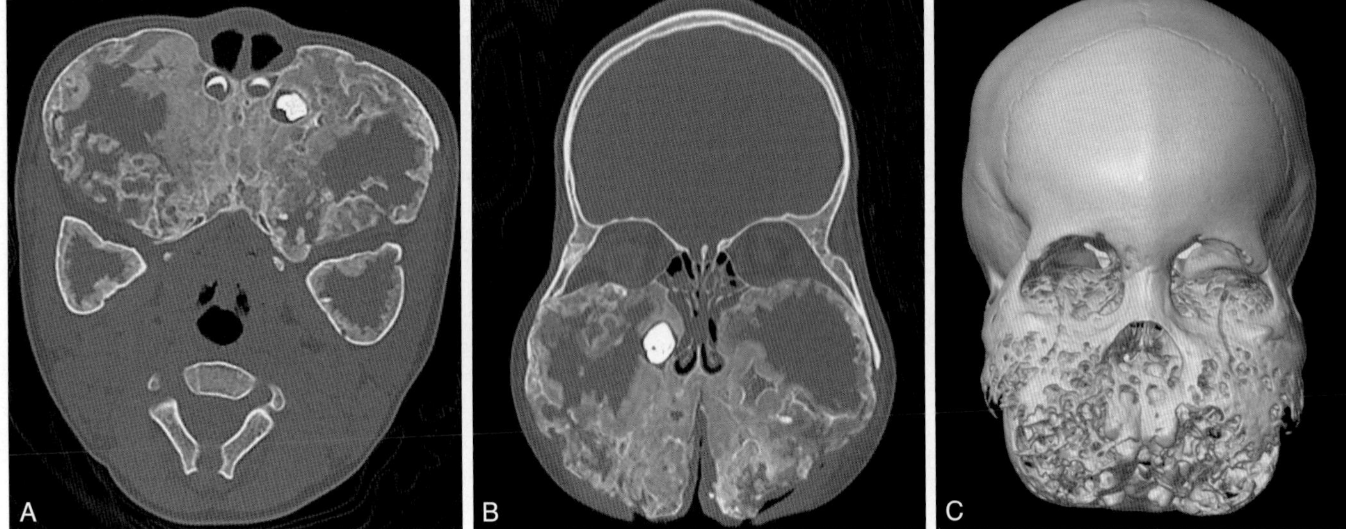

Fig. 14.72 Fibrous Dysplasia. A 4-year-old with fibrous dysplasia. (A and B) Coronal CT and volumetric CT images demonstrate severe expansion of the bilateral mandible and maxilla with combination of ground-glass and lucent areas consistent with fibrous dysplasia pattern also known as cherubism.

GIANT CELL GRANULOMA

Bone-associated

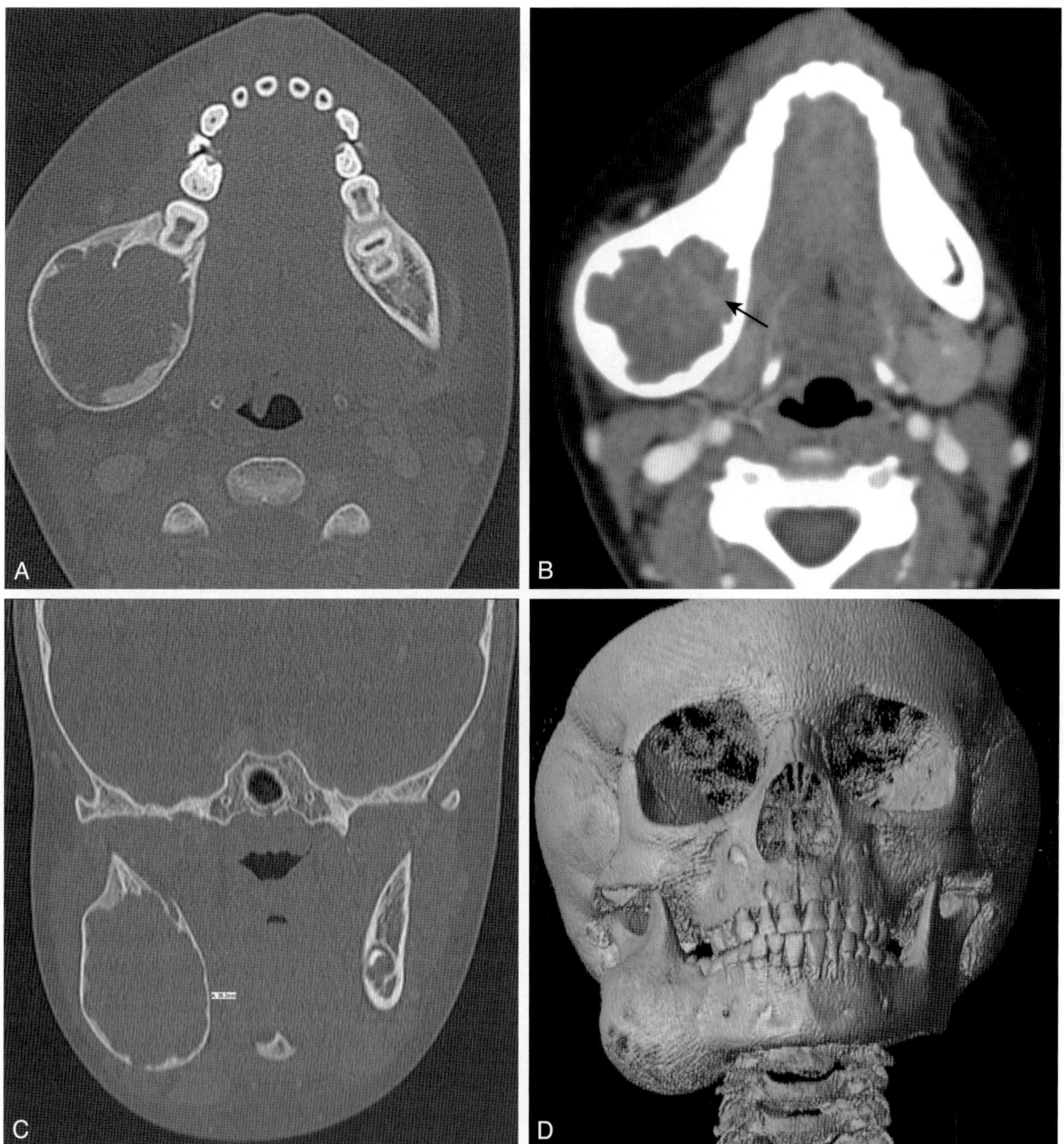

Fig. 14.73 Giant Cell Granuloma. (A to D) Axial, coronal, and 3D volumetric CT images demonstrate an expansile lytic bone lesion arising from the right mandible without a soft tissue mass. Internal areas of hyperdensity due to hemorrhage are present.

Key Points

Background

- Benign locally aggressive bone tumor.
- Etiology presumed due to reaction to intraosseous hemorrhage from trauma or inflammation.
- Majority occur in mandible and maxilla.

Imaging

- Well defined; expansile; lytic; unilocular or multilocular; with or without internal hemorrhage
- Differential Diagnosis: Aneurysmal bone cyst, odontogenic cyst, brown tumor, and ameloblastoma

REFERENCE

1. Nasseri F, Munjal K, Ginsberg LE, et al. Imaging review of craniofacial masses in children. *Neurographics*. 2015 Sept/Oct;5(5):217–230.

AMELOBLASTOMA

Bone-associated

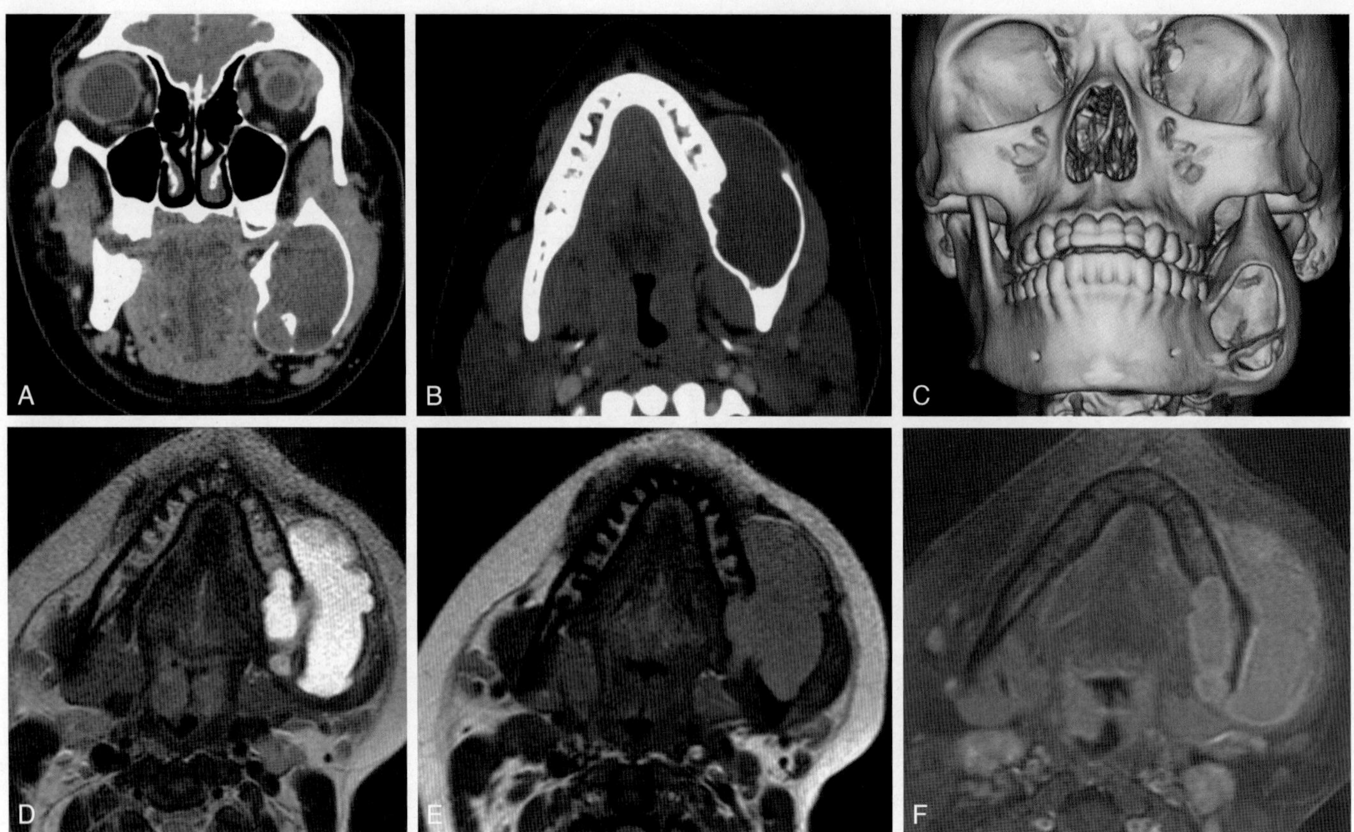

Fig. 14.74 Ameloblastoma. (A to C) Coronal, axial, and 3D volumetric CT images demonstrate an expansile lytic bone lesion arising from the left mandible without a soft tissue mass. (D) Axial T2W, (E) axial T1W, and (F) axial T1W+C fat saturation images demonstrate T1W and T2W hyperintensity from proteinaceous fluid thin peripheral enhancement.

Key Points

Background

- Benign, locally aggressive bone tumor of the mandible arising from odontogenic epithelial enamel-forming cells that fail to regress during embryonic development.
- More common in ages 20 to 40.
- 80% of cases involve the posterior mandible/third molar region.
- Treated with en bloc resection due to high recurrence with incomplete resection or curettage.

Imaging

- CT: Expansile; unilocular or multilocular; soap-bubble; cortical thinning/destruction; and erosion of roots of teeth.
- MRI demonstrates fluid signal; may be T1W hyperintense due to cholesterol crystals.

REFERENCE

1. Nasseri F, Munjal K, Ginsberg LE, et al. Imaging review of craniofacial masses in children. *Neurographics*. 2015 Sept/Oct;5(5):217–230.

UNCOMMON MAXILLARY AND MANDIBULAR LESIONS

Bone-associated

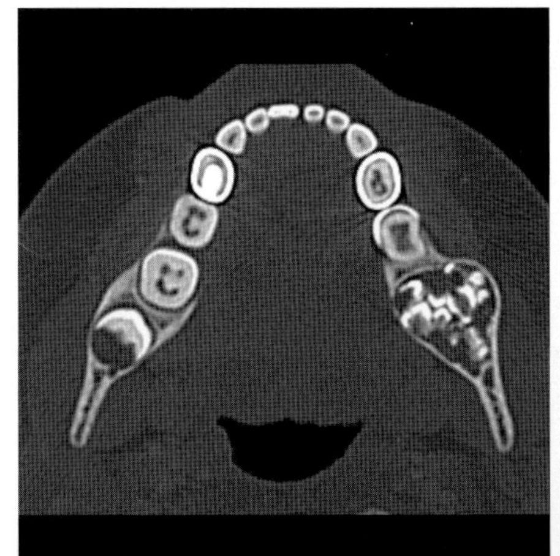
Compound odontoma

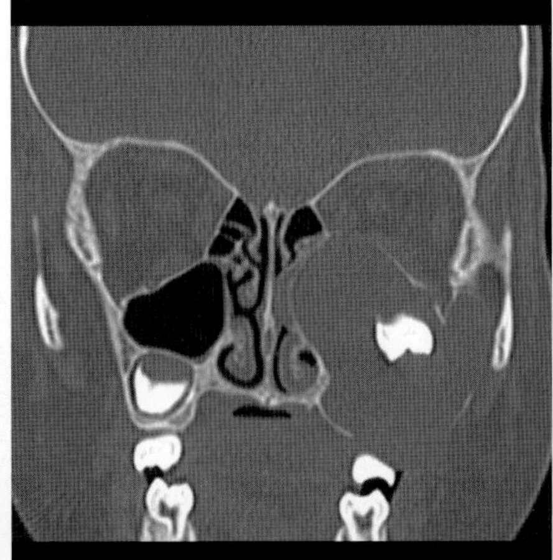
Dentigerous cyst

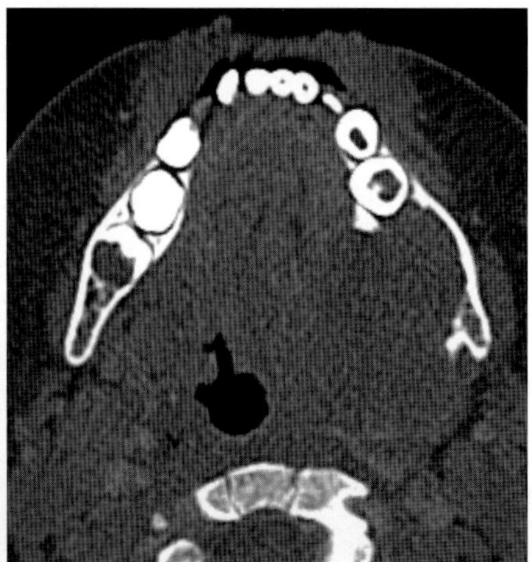
Desmoid fibroma

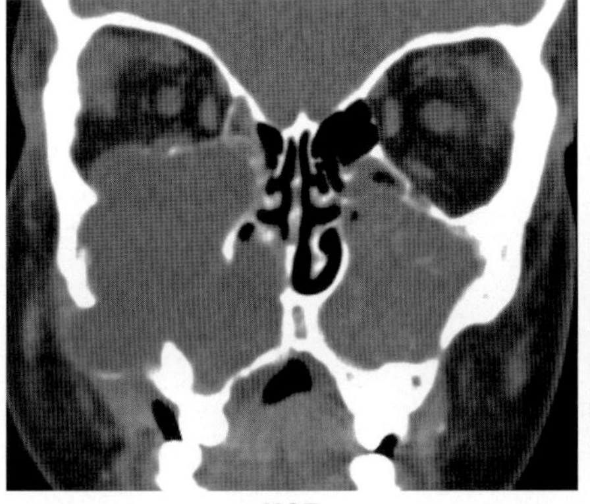
KOT

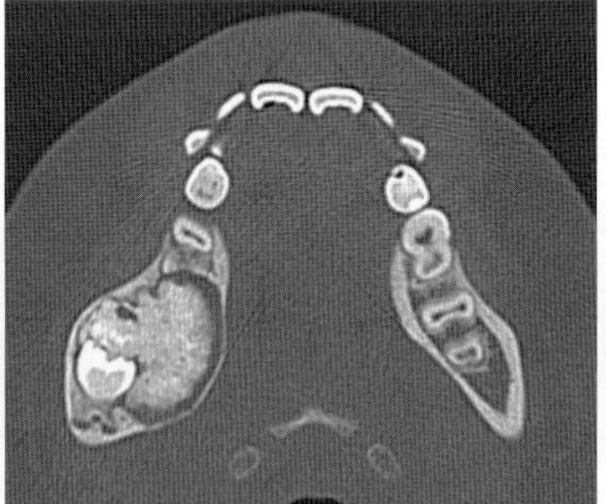
Ameloblastic fibroodontoma

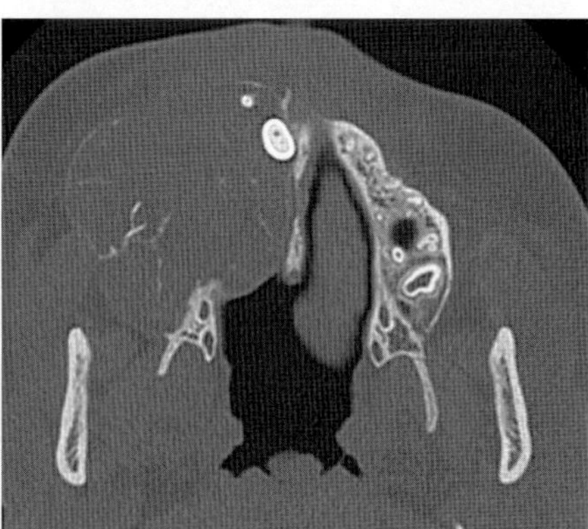
Odontogenic myxoma

Key Points

Compound Odontoma

An odontogenic hamartoma that is classified as simple, compound, and complex. Simple odontomas have the appearance of supranumerary teeth. Compound odontomas have the appearance of multiple small tooth-like structures. Complex odontomas have amorphous hyperdensity with peripheral lucent halo.

Dentigerous Cyst

A well-defined, expansile, unilocular lytic bone lesion associated with the crown of an unerupted tooth.

Desmoid Fibroma

A slow-growing, locally invasive soft tissue mass with well-defined or infiltrative appearance that can lead to lytic changes in the adjacent bone.

Keratocystic Odontogenic Tumor (KOT)

Well-defined, expansile, fluid-filled, unilocular lytic lesion usually centered between the roots of the teeth; associated with basal cell nevus syndrome.

Ameloblastic Fibroodontoma

A rare mixed odontogenic tumor seen in children. Associated with delayed tooth eruption and painless swelling. Imaging demonstrates an expansile sclerotic lesion with radiolucent margin. Treated with surgical resection.

Odontogenic Myxoma

Well-defined, lytic lesion with multiple trabeculae similar in appearance to ameloblastoma

REFERENCES

1. Kumar LKS, Manuel S, Khalem SA, et al. Ameloblastic fibro-odontoma. *Int J Surg Case Rep*. 2014;5(12):1142–1144.
2. Cure JK, Vattoth S, Shah R. Radiopaque jaw lesions: an approach to the differential diagnosis. *Radiographics*. 2012 Nov–Dec;32(7):1909–10925.
3. Kingston CA, Owens CM, Jeanes A, et al. Imaging of desmoid fibromatosis in pediatric patients. *AJR Am J Roentgenol*. 2002 Jan;178(1):191–199.

15 Infectious and Inflammatory Disorders of the Head and Neck

INTRODUCTION

Background

- Head and neck infections are extremely common in children.
- Locations of infections include the lymph nodes, salivary glands, aerodigestive tract, orbit, sinuses, and temporal bone. Consequently, an initial approach to head and neck infections and inflammatory conditions includes appropriate categorization of the anatomic site, followed by determination of extension into adjacent anatomic sites.
- Complications from spread from one anatomical site can cause significant morbidity and mortality. In particular, infections involving the orbits, sinuses, and temporal bones have the greatest potential for intracranial spread of infection.

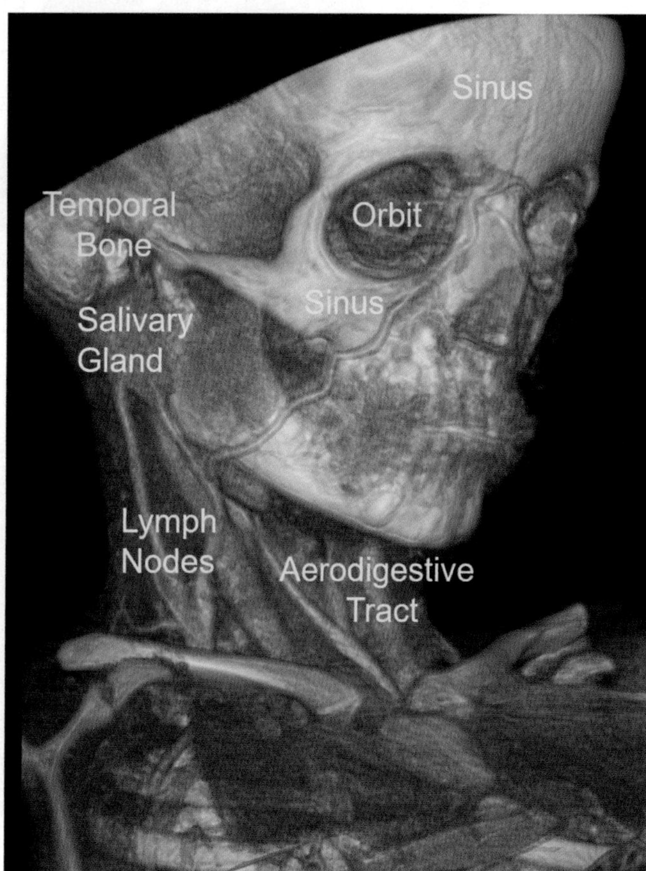

Imaging

- Imaging modalities to assess infections of the face and neck include radiographs, ultrasound, CT, and MRI. This chapter will demonstrate face and neck infection findings on these modalities.
- Radiographs have a limited role, with the exception for airway infections and foreign bodies.
- Ultrasound can be used for assessing for abscess and lymph nodes in the neck but has no role in evaluating infections of the sinuses and temporal bones.
- Contrast-enhanced CT (CECT) imaging is often performed for infections of the neck, temporal bone, orbits, and sinuses. This is due to the fast acquisition time, high spatial resolution, and capability of visualization of all anatomic sites. Consequently, the majority of neck infections are best visualized with CT and are demonstrated in this section.
- MRI is generally performed to assess complications of infections and intracranial spread of infection. MRI is also performed in the setting of specific infections such as invasive fungal sinusitis or inflammation such as juvenile idiopathic arthritis (JIA) or chronic recurrent multifocal osteomyelitis (CRMO).
- This chapter will use a location-based approach for demonstrating infections of the neck that are commonly imaged.

LYMPHADENITIS AND SUPPURATIVE LYMPH NODES

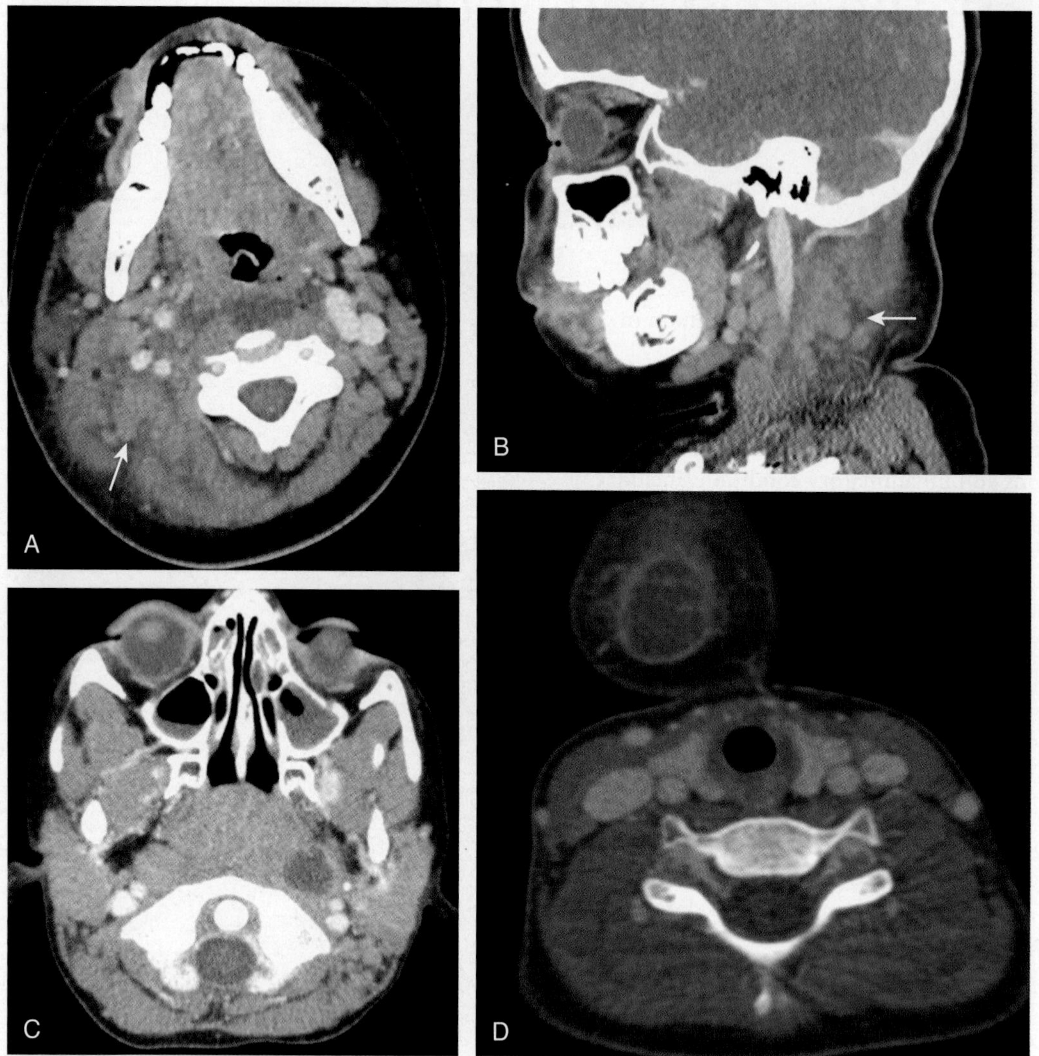

Fig. 15.1 Lymphadenitis and Suppurative Lymph Nodes. (A and B) Axial and sagittal CECT images demonstrate increased number and mild enlargement of right lateral neck lymph nodes (*arrows*) with surrounding inflammation, as well as a retropharyngeal effusion. (C) Axial CECT image demonstrates a peripherally enhancing low-density mass consistent with a suppurative left lateral retropharyngeal lymph node in addition to enlarged and enhancing nasopharyngeal mucosa from pharyngitis. (D) Axial CECT demonstrating a peripherally enhancing mass in the submental space consistent with a suppurative lymph node.

Key Points

Background

- Lymphadenitis refers to infectious enlargement and inflammation of the lymph nodes.
- Suppurative lymph nodes refer to necrosis/abscess formation within a lymph node.
- Viral and bacterial causes are most frequent.

Imaging

- CT: Soft tissue density enlargement of the lymph nodes. Suppurative lymph nodes demonstrate central low density/necrosis.
- Associated findings: *Perinodal inflammation*, compression, and/or occlusion of the internal jugular vein (IJV).
- Differential Diagnosis:
  - Lymphoma, and nasopharyngeal carcinoma: Consider these diagnoses for non-suppurative lymphadenopathy that does not resolve after appropriate treatment and consider biopsy to exclude malignancy

REFERENCE

1. Friedman ER, John SD. Imaging of pediatric neck masses. *Radiol Clin North Am.* 2011 Jul;49(4):617–632.

INFECTIOUS MONONUCLEOSIS

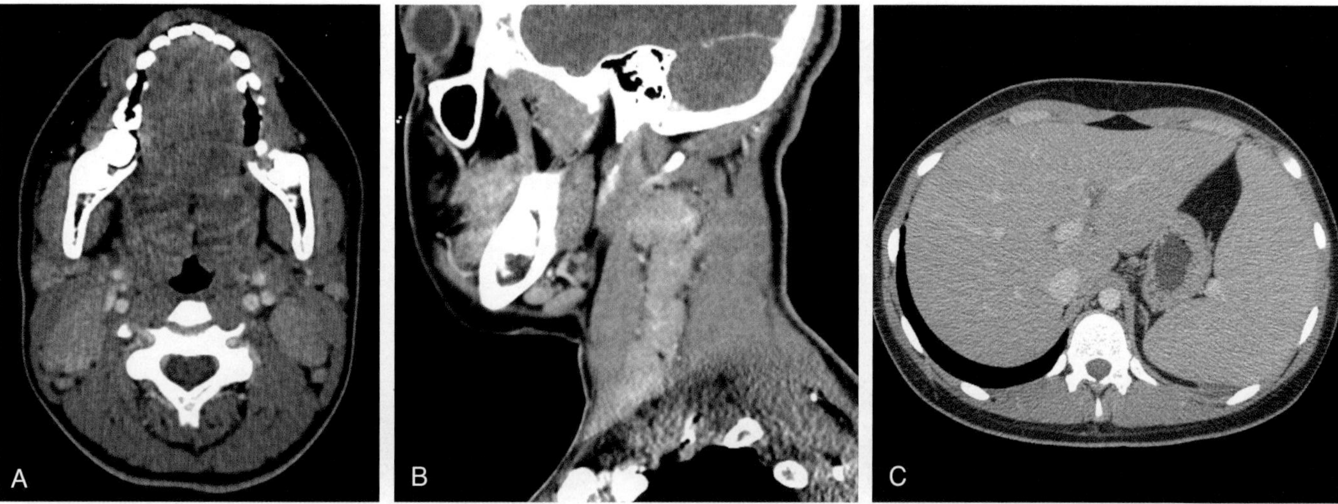

Fig. 15.2 Infectious Mononucleosis. A 14-year-old with fever, pharyngitis, and neck swelling. (A and B) Axial and sagittal CECT images demonstrates increased number and mild enlargement of bilateral jugular chain lymph nodes and enlarged and striated palatine tonsils consistent with lymphadenopathy and tonsillitis. (C) Axial CECT image of the abdomen demonstrates splenomegaly.

Key Points

Background

- Epstein-Barr virus (EBV) is the causative agent spread by human to human contact. 90% to 95% of adults are EBV seropositive. Most cases are subclinical. Peak incidence of infection is 15 to 24 years of age.
- *Clinical triad includes lymphadenopathy, fever, and pharyngitis.* Additional signs and symptoms include fatigue, rash, splenomegaly, atypical lymphocytosis, aseptic meningitis, Guillain-Barre syndrome, encephalomyelitis, transverse myelitis, and optic neuritis. Rare "Alice in Wonderland" syndrome can be triggered by EBV infection and results in distortion of visual perception, body image, and experience of time. Lymphadenopathy peaks in the first week and gradually decreases over the next 2 to 3 weeks. Fatigue may last for 6 months in a minority of patients.
- Diagnosis is made with heterophile antibody test in a patient with appropriate clinical presentation. False-negative heterophile antibody tests can occur in early infection and young children and may require EBV-specific antibody testing for diagnosis.
- Treatment with acetaminophen or nonsteroidal antiinflammatory medications.

Imaging

- Soft tissue density enlargement of jugular chain lymph nodes; enlarged, striated hyperenhancement of palatine tonsils; and splenomegaly are the most common imaging findings.

REFERENCE

1. Aronson MB, Auwaerter PG. Infectious mononucleosis. UpToDate. https://www.uptodate.com/contents/infectious-mononucleosis. Published March 19, 2021. Accessed September 23, 2022.

GRANULOMATOUS INFECTION

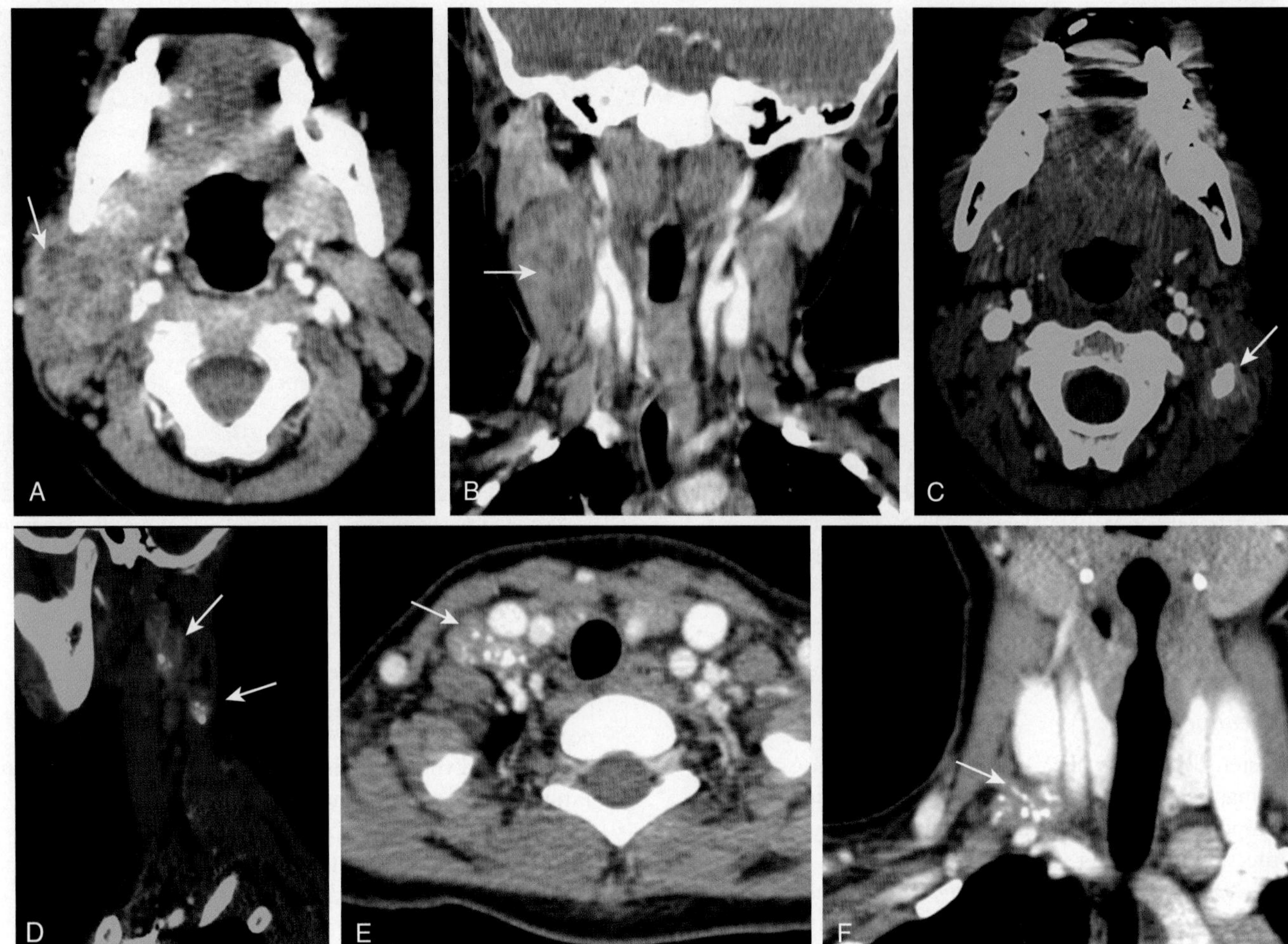

Fig. 15.3 Granulomatous Infection. (A and B) Axial and coronal CECT images demonstrate right lateral neck enlarged lymph nodes (*arrows*) with central low density. (C and D) Axial and coronal CECT images demonstrate enlarged enhancing and partial calcification of left lateral neck lymph nodes. (E and F) Axial and coronal CECT images demonstrate enlarged enhancing and partial calcification of right lateral neck lymph nodes (*arrows*).

Key Points

Background

- In children, most commonly due to non-tuberculous mycobacterium occurring in children aged 2 to 4 years. Associated violaceous skin discoloration. Frequently involves the parotid space and posterior triangle.
- Cat scratch disease is a chronic granulomatous infection due to *Bartonella henselae*. Typically involves the parotid gland, midcervical, and submandibular nodes. Cat scratch disease can also be seen in conjunction with enhancement of the optic nerve/globe junction due to an obliterative vasculitis.

Imaging

- Lymphadenopathy, and/or suppurative lymph nodes in 50% of patients
- *Sinus tract* formation in 10% of patients
- Chronic stage demonstrates multiple *calcified lymph nodes*

REFERENCES

1. Robson CD. Imaging of granulomatous lesions of the neck in children. *Radiol Clin North Am.* 2000 Sep;38(5):969–977.
2. Abedel Razek AAK, Castillo M. Imaging appearance of granulomatous lesions of the head and neck. *Eur J Radiol.* 2010;76:52–60.

KIKUCHI FUJIMOTO DISEASE

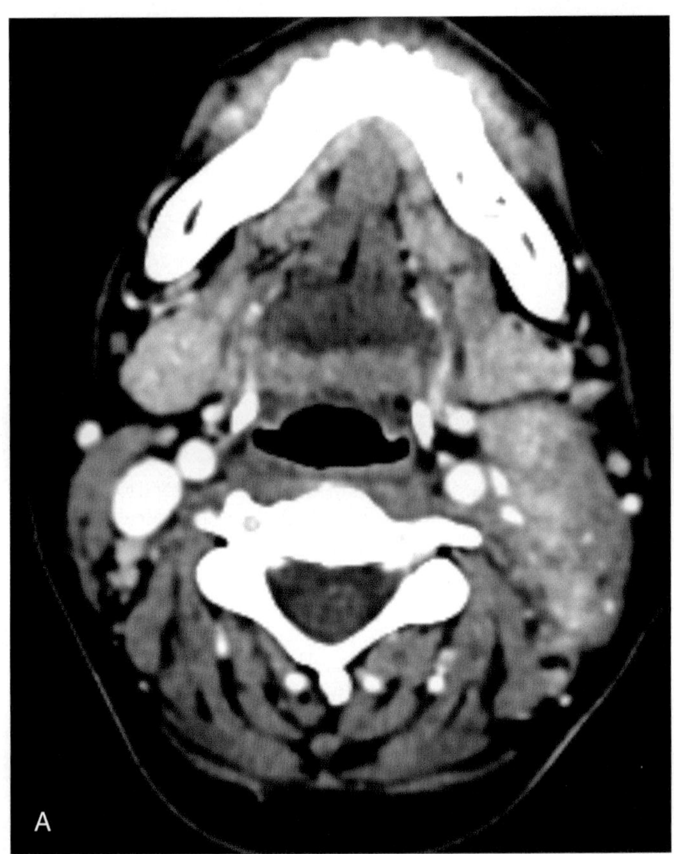

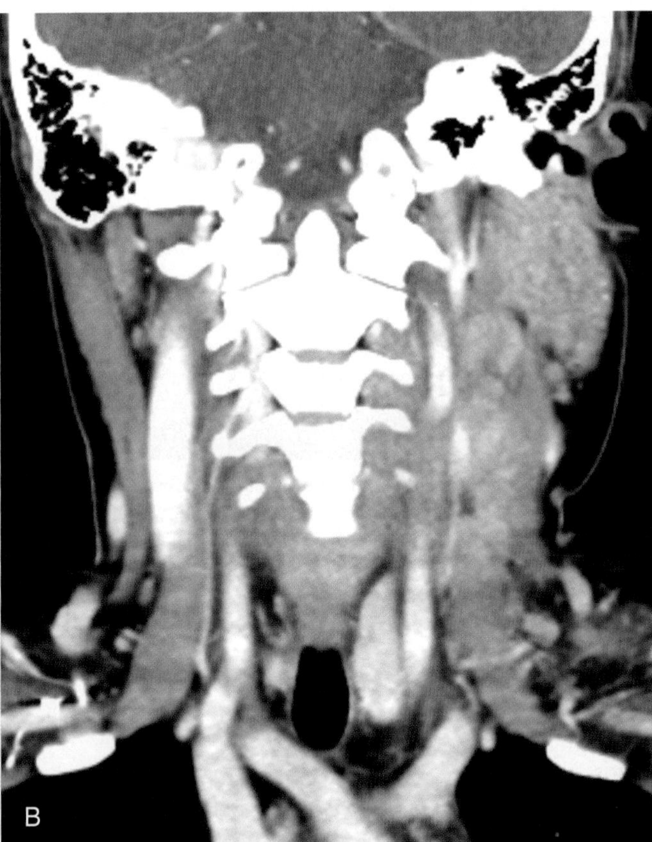

Fig. 15.4 Kikuchi Fujimoto Disease. (A and B) Axial and coronal CECT images demonstrate a conglomerate of mildly enlarged enhancing left lateral neck enlarged lymph nodes.

Key Points

Background

- A rare self-limiting histiocytic necrotizing lymphadenitis of unknown origin.
- Mean age is 24 years, with age range 12 to 40 years.
- Presents with *painful cervical lymphadenopathy* and *prolonged fever.*
- Diagnosis made through biopsy. No laboratory tests available for diagnosis.
- Cases of associated hemophagocytic lymphohistiocytosis have been reported.

Imaging

- *Unilateral* (60%–80%) lateral neck lymph nodes (levels 2–5) and less commonly remaining nodal locations of the body
- Appearance on contrast CT: Hyperenhancement of the lymph nodes relative to muscle density; *perinodal inflammation* in 93%; *homogeneous and necrotic lymph nodes*; small to *medium sized* nodal enlargement (mean node size 2.3 cm; range 1.8–3.1 cm)

REFERENCES

1. Han HJ, et al. Kikuchi's disease in children: clinical manifestations and imaging features. *J Korean Med Sci*. 2009 Dec;24(6):1105–1109.
2. Kwon SY, et al. CT findings in Kikuchi disease: analysis of 96 cases. *AJNR Am J Neurol*. 2004 Jun;25(6):1099–1102.

PHARYNGOTONSILLITIS AND PERITONSILLAR ABSCESS

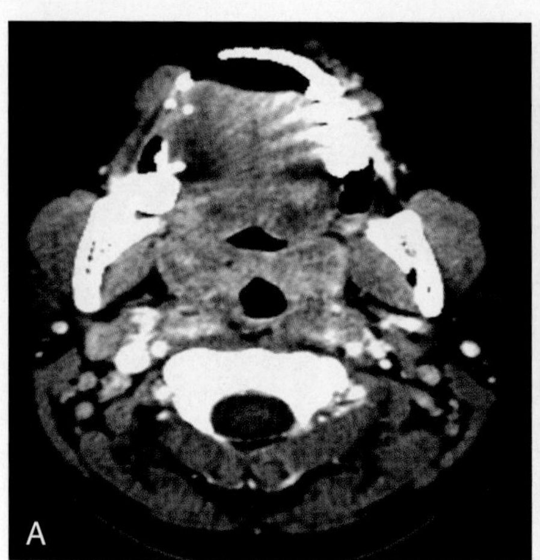

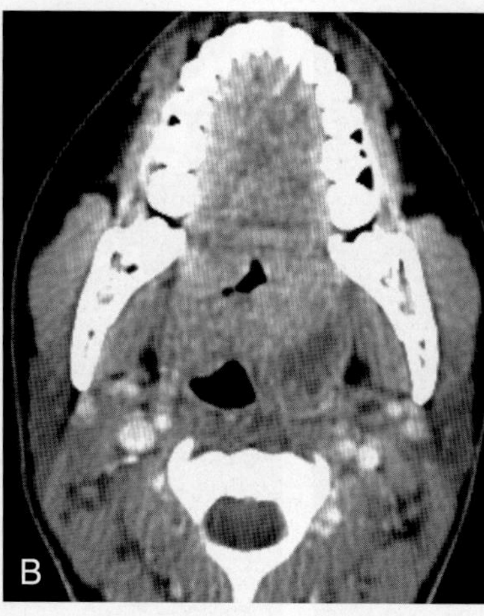

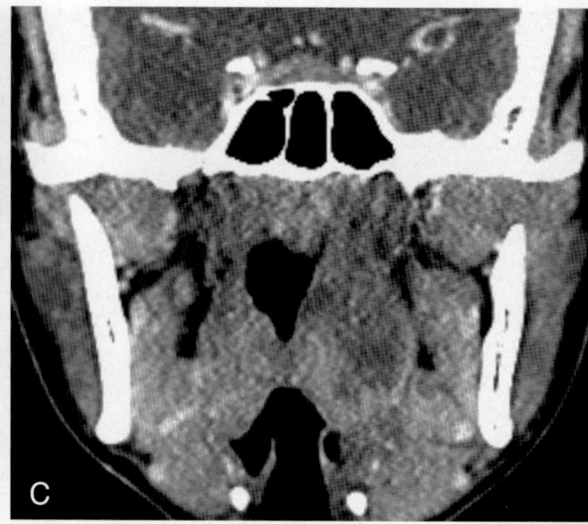

Fig. 15.5 Pharyngotonsillitis and Peritonsillar Abscess. (A) Axial CECT image demonstrates enlarged striated hyperenhancing palatine tonsils. (B and C) Axial and coronal CECT images demonstrate peripherally enhancing low-density collection in the left palatine tonsil, bilateral enlarged striated hyperenhancing palatine tonsils consistent with a pharyngotonsillitis and left peritonsillar abscess.

Key Points

Background

- Majority of cases of tonsillitis are viral infections and self-limiting.
- 30% of tonsillitis cases are bacterial and most commonly due to beta-hemolytic *Streptococcus*, *Streptococcus pneumoniae*, *Staphylococcus aureus*, and *Haemophilus influenzae.*
- Potential etiology of peritonsillar abscess is progression of acute exudative tonsillitis to abscess formation versus inflammation of Weber glands (minor salivary glands located in the soft palate superior to the tonsil, which are responsible for clearing tonsillar debris and digesting food particles).
- Symptoms: Fever, sore throat, stiff neck, dysphagia.
- Treatment: Drainage (typically abscesses >1 cm), antibiotics, supportive care, and possible steroids.

Imaging

- CT: Tonsillitis demonstrates enlarged, hyperenhancing striated palatine tonsils. Peritonsillar abscess is a peripherally enhancing fluid collection involving the palatine tonsil.
- Complications: Airway obstruction, aspiration pneumonia, deep neck cellulitis and/or mediastinitis, jugular thrombosis, and hemorrhage from carotid artery wall erosion.

REFERENCES

1. Hegde SV, et al. A space-based approach to pediatric face and neck infections. *Neurographics.* 2014;4:43–52.
2. Galioto NJ, et al. Peritonsillar abscess. *Am Fam Physician.* 2017;95(8):501–506.

LEMIERRE SYNDROME

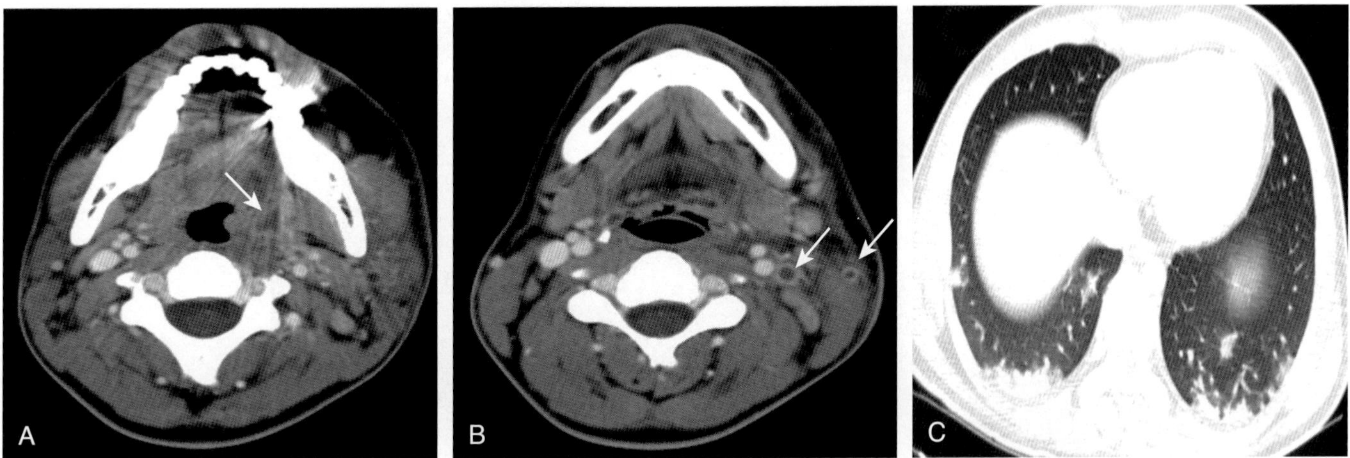

Fig. 15.6 Lemierre Syndrome. (A to C) Axial CECT images demonstrate a left peritonsillar abscess (*arrow*, image A), thrombosed left internal and external jugular veins (*arrows*, image B), and septic emboli in the lower lobes of the lungs.

Key Points

Background

- Rare complication of an oropharyngeal infection.
- Typically found in previously healthy teenagers.
- Results in septic dissemination with abscess formation in other parts of the body, most commonly the lungs, osteomyelitis, and arterial vasospasm or occlusion.
- Typically caused by *Fusobacterium* infection, which is an anaerobic Gram-negative bacterium found in normal oral flora.
- High morbidity/mortality associated if it is not treated in a timely manner.
- The infection spreads from the peritonsillar space to result in internal jugular vein (IJV) *thrombosis*.
- IJV involvement can be resultant *septic emboli to the lungs* or brain, thus causing an abscess. There may also be spread into the retropharyngeal space, resulting in osteomyelitis of the spine.
- Treatment is high-dose IV antibiotics. Anticoagulation is used in up to 27% of patients; however, the role of this treatment is not clear at this time.

Imaging

- Triad of pharyngitis, ipsilateral IJV thrombosis, and associated cavitary pulmonary nodules

REFERENCE

1. Hegde SV, et al. A space-based approach to pediatric face and neck infections. *Neurographics*. 2014;4:43–52.

RETROPHARYNGEAL ABSCESS

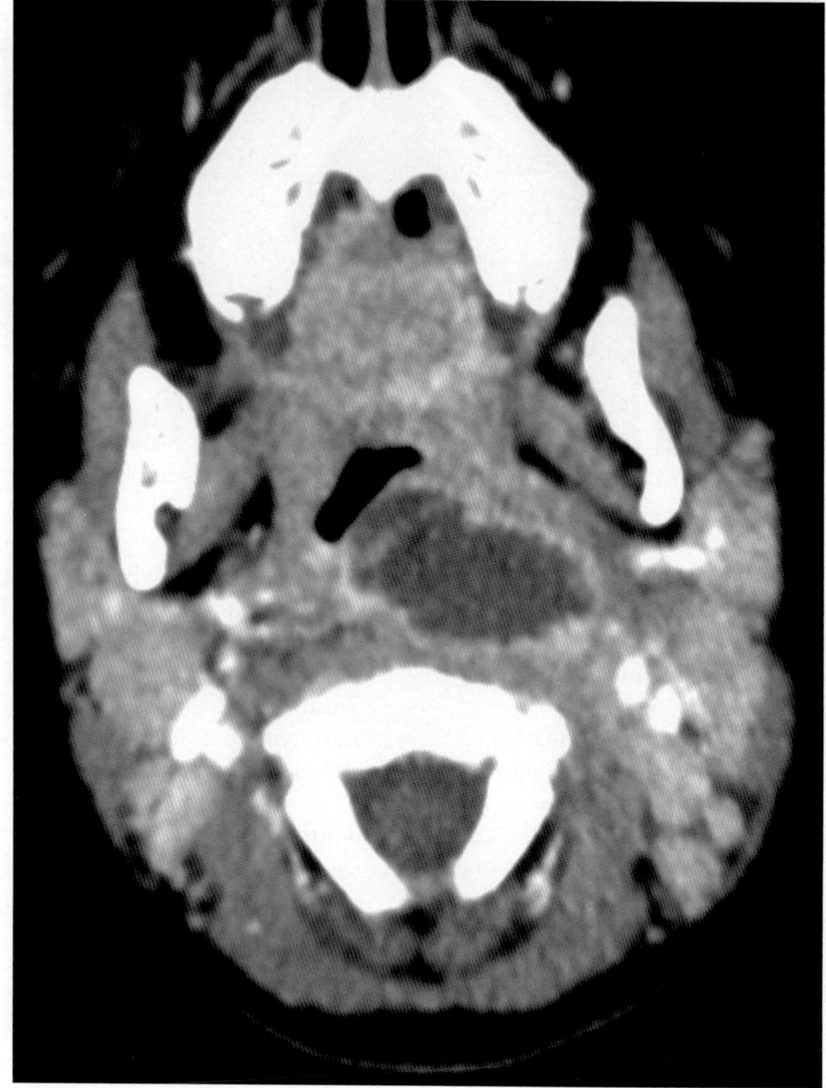

Fig. 15.7 Retropharyngeal Abscess. Axial CECT image demonstrates a peripherally enhancing left retropharyngeal fluid collection consistent with an abscess.

Key Points

Background

- The source of infection is often from rupture of a suppurative retropharyngeal lymph node.
- Potentially life threatening due to effect of airway.
- Surgical drainage often necessary.

Imaging

- Typical features of an abscess i.e. peripheral rim enhancement with central low density
- Usually associated with lymphadenopathy in the lateral neck
- Can extend into the mediastinum as well as cause IJV thrombophlebitis, or carotid pseudoaneurysm

REFERENCE

1. Hegde SV, et al. A space-based approach to pediatric face and neck infections. *Neurographics*. 2014;4:43–52.

LARYNGOTRACHEOBRONCHITIS (CROUP)

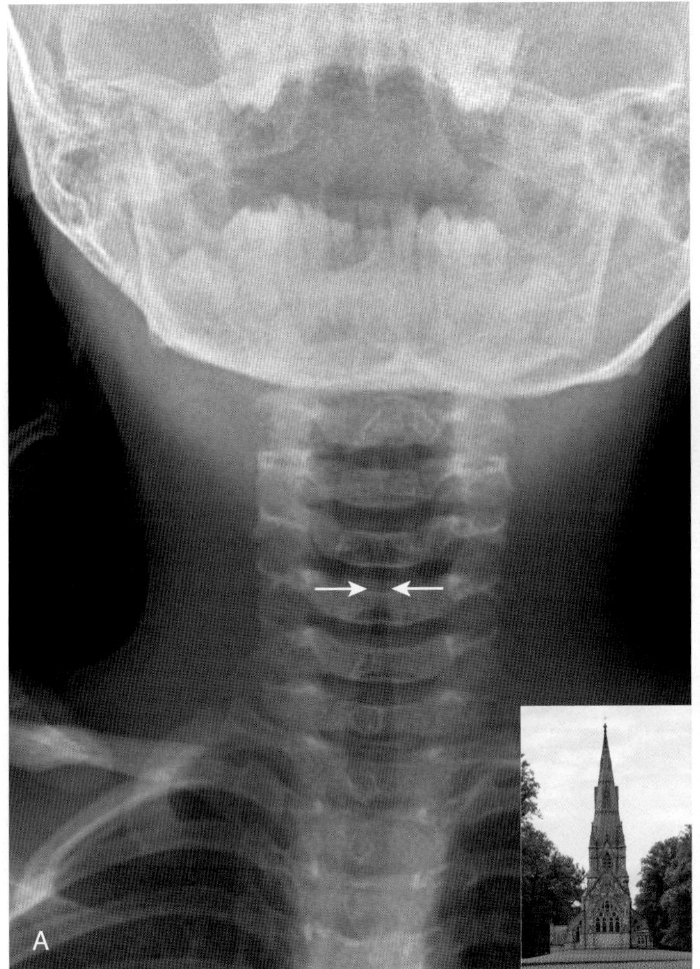

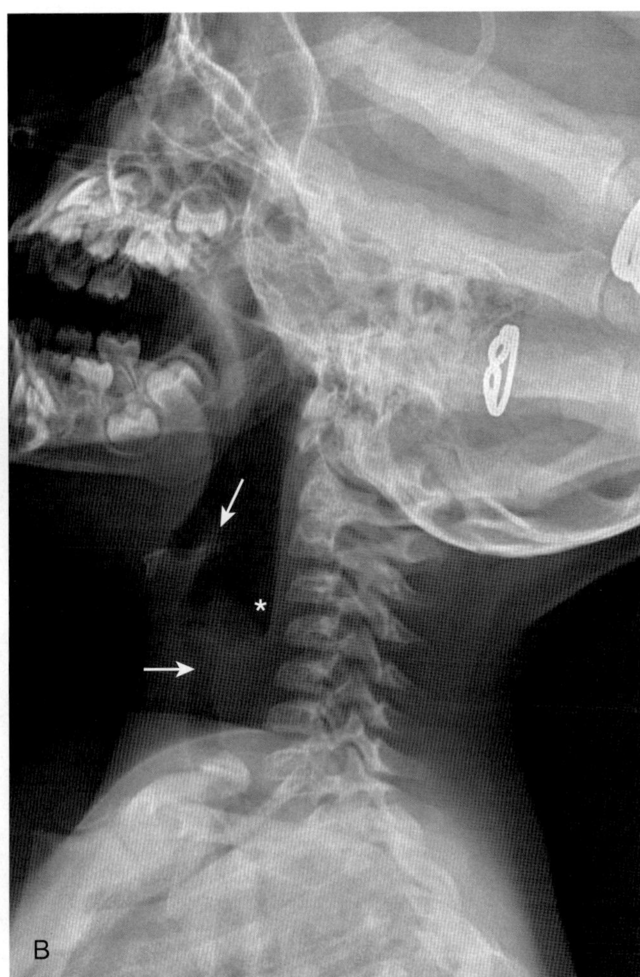

Fig. 15.8 Croup. A 2-month old with stridor. (A and B) AP and lateral radiographs of the soft tissue neck. The frontal radiograph demonstrates the characteristic shouldering of the subglottic trachea, also known as a steeple sign (*arrows*, image A), similar to a church steeple. The lateral radiograph demonstrates a normal epiglottis (upper *arrow*, image B). There is dilation of the hypopharyngeal region (*) and narrowing of the subglottic region (lower *arrow*, image B). (A, inset image of steeple © istock.com/daseaford.)

Key Points

Background

- Most common cause of upper airway obstruction in children aged 6 months to 3 years.
- The most common etiologic agents for viral croup are parainfluenza and influenza, which induce an inflammatory response resulting in subglottic edema and airway narrowing.
- Clinically, it is characterized by low-grade fever, inspiratory stridor, a characteristic barking cough, and hoarseness.

Imaging

- Typically a clinical diagnosis, but airway studies are often obtained for diagnostic confirmation and exclusion of other causes of acute-onset stridor, such as epiglottis.
- Characteristic "steeple" shape below the vocal cords on a frontal radiograph.
- Epiglottis, aryepiglottic folds, and prevertebral spaces are normal in croup.

EPIGLOTTITIS

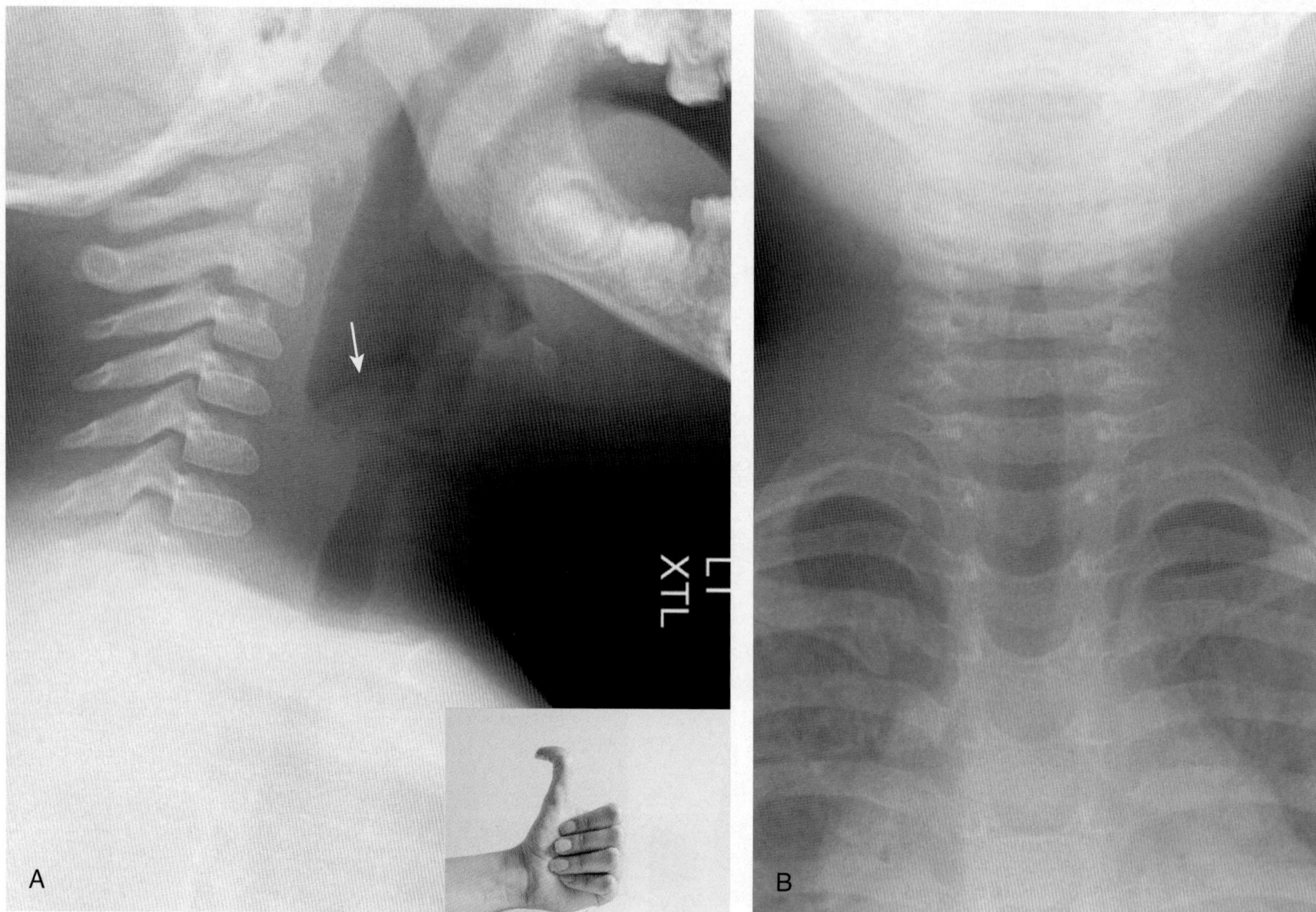

Fig. 15.9 Epiglottis. A 2-month old with stridor. (A and B) AP and lateral radiographs of the soft tissue neck. The lateral radiograph demonstrates marked thickening of the epiglottis (*arrow*) called the "thumb sign" similar to the photograph, as well as the aryepiglottic folds. The hypopharynx is dilated. The frontal radiograph does not demonstrate the shoulder of the subglottic larynx, as is found in croup. (A, insert image of thumb © istock.com/Anna Gorbacheva.)

Background

- Potential life-threatening cause of upper airway obstruction in children.
- Characterized by inflammation/swelling of the epiglottis and aryepiglottic folds but can also extend to involve the false cords and subglottic region.
- The agents that can result in epiglottis are *H. influenzae*, *Streptococcus* and *Staphylococcus*, *Morazella*, and *Pseudomonas*.
- With the increasing immunizations, the incidence of *H. influenzae* has dramatically decreased and so has epiglottitis.
- Typically occurs in children between 3 and 6 years of age.
- Patients typically appear toxic with acute stridor, dysphagia, fever, restlessness, drooling, and increased respiratory distress while lying down.

Imaging

- Typically diagnosed with radiography. Endoscopy is obtained for confirmation.
- Lateral radiograph demonstrates marked swelling/enlargement of the epiglottis ('thumb print' sign).

FOREIGN BODY INGESTION

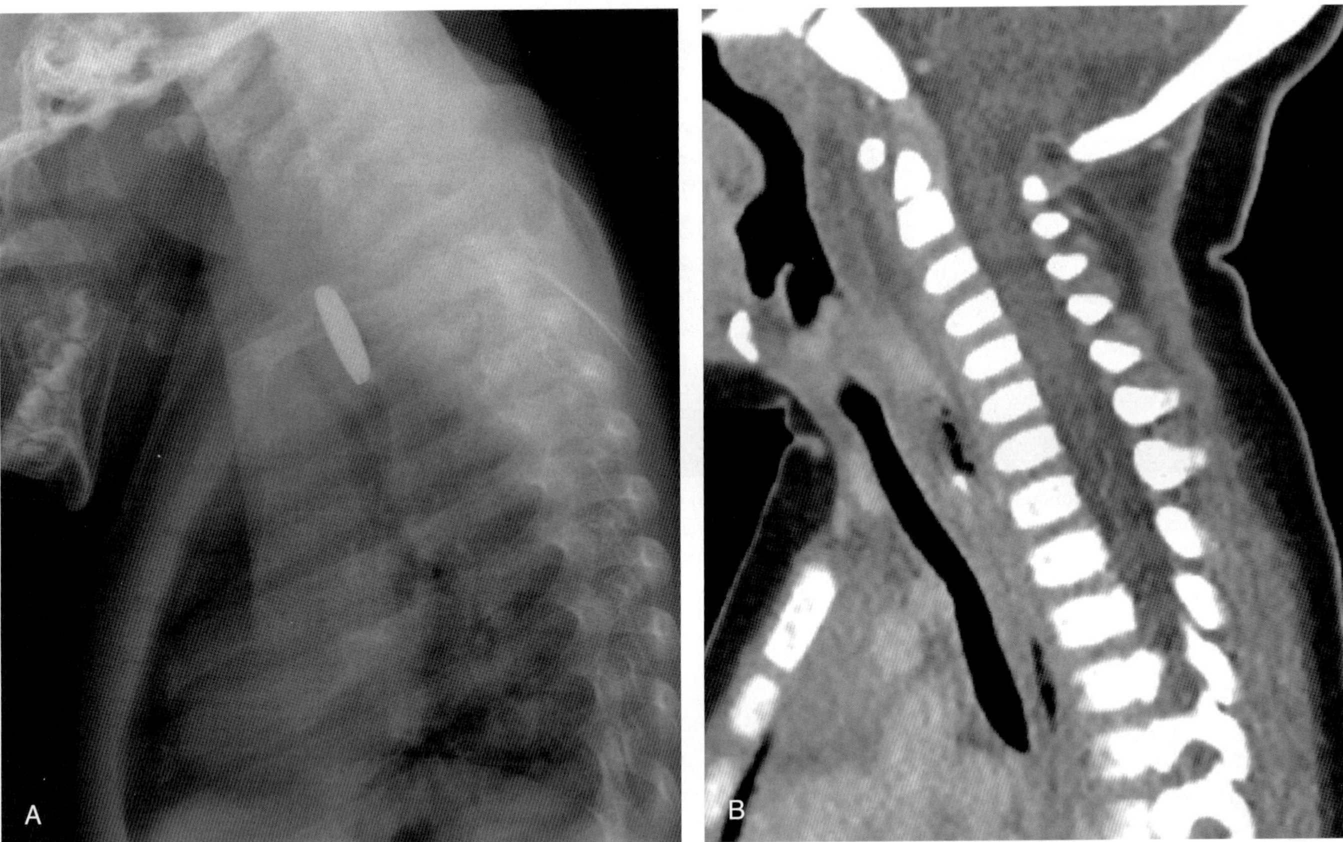

Fig. 15.10 Foreign Body Ingestion. (A) Lateral soft tissue radiograph demonstrates a metallic density from a battery in the esophagus. The step off on the edges of the battery differentiates this from a coin. (B) Sagittal reformat CECT image following endoscopic removal of the coin demonstrates a linear region of abnormal air in the posterior wall of the esophagus, mucosal edema, and retropharyngeal edema due to the perforation.

Key Points

- Foreign body ingestion is common in infants and young children.
- Button batteries can cause rapid-onset full thickness burns and esophageal perforation, occuring *within 2 hours of ingestion.*
- AP and lateral radiographs can confirm a battery rather than a coin by the double rim on AP projection and step off on the lateral projection.
- Batteries lodged in the esophagus should be removed as soon as possible. The majority of batteries found beyond the gastroesophageal junction will pass spontaneously unless swallowed with one or more magnets.
- Complications of battery ingestion include fistulas (aortoesophageal, trachea-esophageal), esophageal and tracheal stenosis, vocal cord paralysis, cellulitis, and discitis and osteomyelitis

REFERENCES

1. Semple T, et al. Button battery ingestion in children – a potentially catastrophic event of which all radiologists must be aware. *Br J Radiol.* 2018 Jan1081;91:20160781.
2. Young A, Tekes A, Huisman TAGM, et al. Spondylodiscitis associated with button battery ingestion" prompt evaluation with MRI. *Neuroradiol J.* 2015 Oct;28(5):504–507.

ODONTOGENIC INFECTION

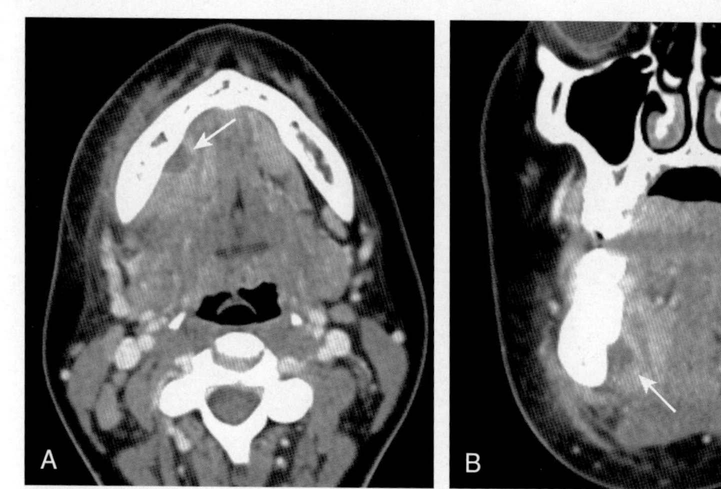

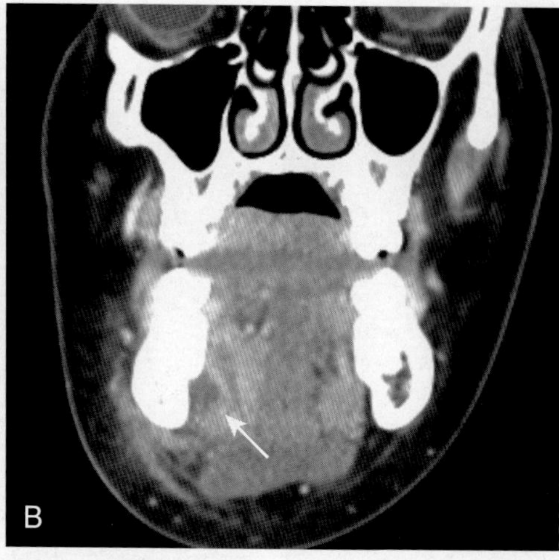

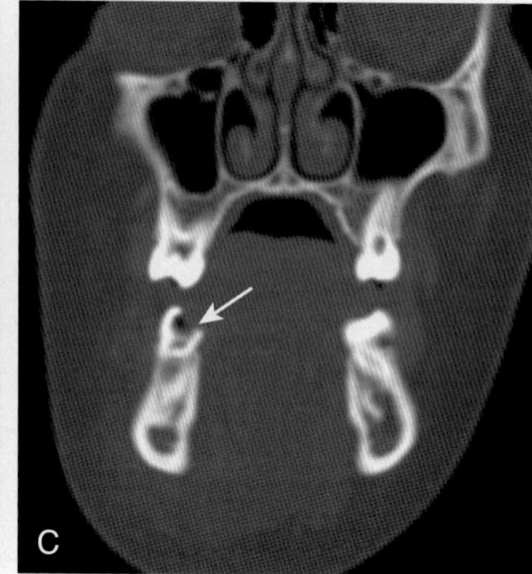

Fig. 15.11 Odontogenic Infection. (A to C) Axial and coronal CECT images demonstrate a peripherally enhancing fluid collection (*arrow*, image A and B) consistent with an abscess along the lingual cortical surface of the right mandible associated with edema in the right buccal and submandibular spaces. A large dental carie (*arrow*, image C) is present above the abscess, indicating the source of infection.

Key Points

Background

- Oral cavity infections are a common health care problem in children and are *most commonly from odontogenic origin*. Breakdown of tooth enamel allows for oropharyngeal bacteria to enter the tooth cavity, track into the root canal and into the mandible or maxilla, and lead to a periodontal infection. Subsequent acute infection leads to cellulitis, dentoalveolar abscess, fascia infection or necrotizing fasciitis, and potentially hematogenous spread. Chronic infection can lead to periapical cyst or granuloma, osteomyelitis, or fistula.
- Oral cavity infections are polymicrobial consisting of anaerobic and aerobic bacteria.
- Symptoms include odynophagia, facial pain, swelling, and erythema. Ludwig's angina is a rare, rapidly progressive gangrenous floor of mouth cellulitis and edema that can progress to airway obstruction.
- Early treatment is important to prevent systemic spread of infection. Treatment includes pain control, antibiotics, early tooth extraction, and incision and drainage of abscess when present.

Imaging

- CT with IV contrast is the modality of choice.
- Infections of the lower second and third molars tend to spread into the submandibular space because the root apices are below the mylohyoid muscle, while premolar infections tend to spread into the sublingual space because their roots are above the mylohyoid muscle.
- Findings include soft tissue edema and inflammation in the submental space, sublingual space, submandibular space, buccal space, masticator space, and/or infratemporal fossa with or without abscess formation and associated with dental caries, periapical dental lucency, and cortical bone breakthrough. Osteomyelitis is uncommon because of the rich vascular supply to the bones, but should be evaluated for.
- Ludwig's angina occurs when the cellulitis involves the bilateral submandibular, sublingual, and submental spaces. Retropharyngeal spread and oral airway compromise are rare.

REFERENCES

1. Lypka M, et al. Dentoalveolar infections. *Oral and Maxillofacial Surg Clin N Am*. 2011(23):415–424.
2. Johri A, et al. Should teeth be extracted immediately in the presence of acute infection? *Oral Maxillofacial Surg Clin N Am*. 2011(23):507–511.

PARANASAL SINUSITIS

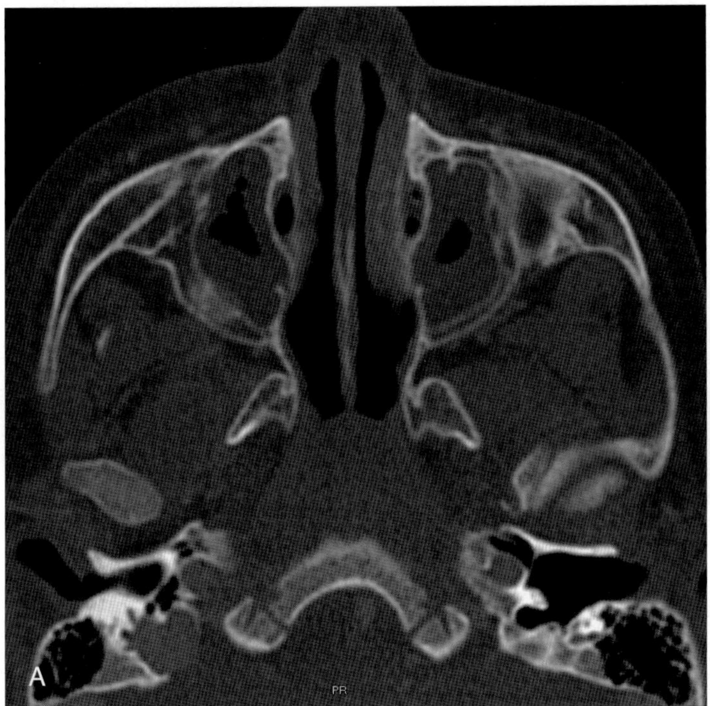

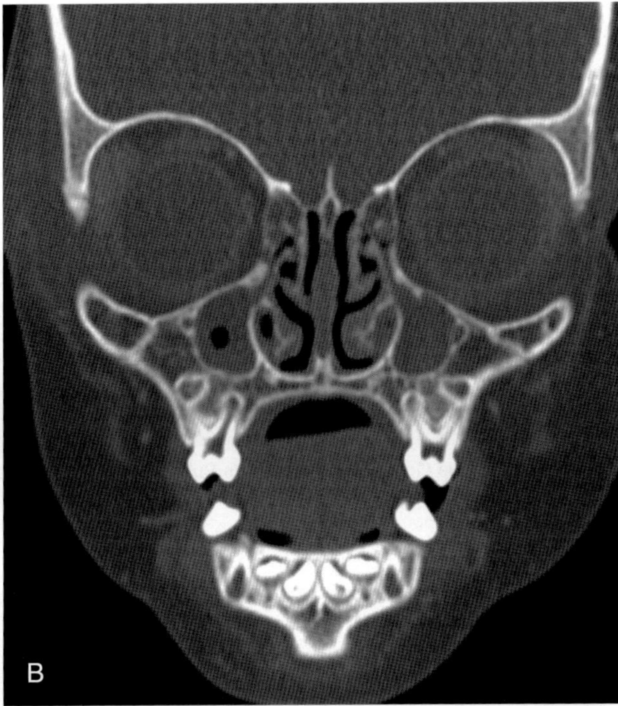

Fig. 15.12 Paranasal Sinusitis. (A) Axial and (B) coronal CT images demonstrate bilateral maxillary sinus air-fluid levels, mucosal thickening, and obstruction of the bilateral maxillary sinus ostium and infundibulum.

Key Points

Background

- Bacterial infection of the paranasal sinuses can develop when the nasal cavity or sinus mucosa becomes swollen/obstructs a sinus ostium resulting in decreased oxygen tension. The normal bacterial flora becomes altered, allowing overgrowth → acute bacterial sinusitis.

Imaging

- CT is the modality of choice for initial evaluation to assess extent and location, drainage pathways, bone changes (dehiscence, destruction, hyperostosis), and spread of infection beyond the sinuses.
- Acute sinusitis demonstrates air-fluid levels, sinus opacification, and drainage pathway obstruction.
- Chronic sinusitis demonstrates mucosal thickening, variable mucoperisoteal reaction, hyperdense sinus secretions, and potentially mucocele formation.
- MRI of the sinus is typically reserved for assessing complications of sinusitis, particularly intracranial and orbital extension and sinus thrombosis.

REFERENCE

1. Ludwig BJ, et al. Diagnostic imaging in nontraumatic pediatric head and neck emergencies. *Radiographics*. 2010 May;30(3):781–799.

SINUSITIS COMPLICATIONS

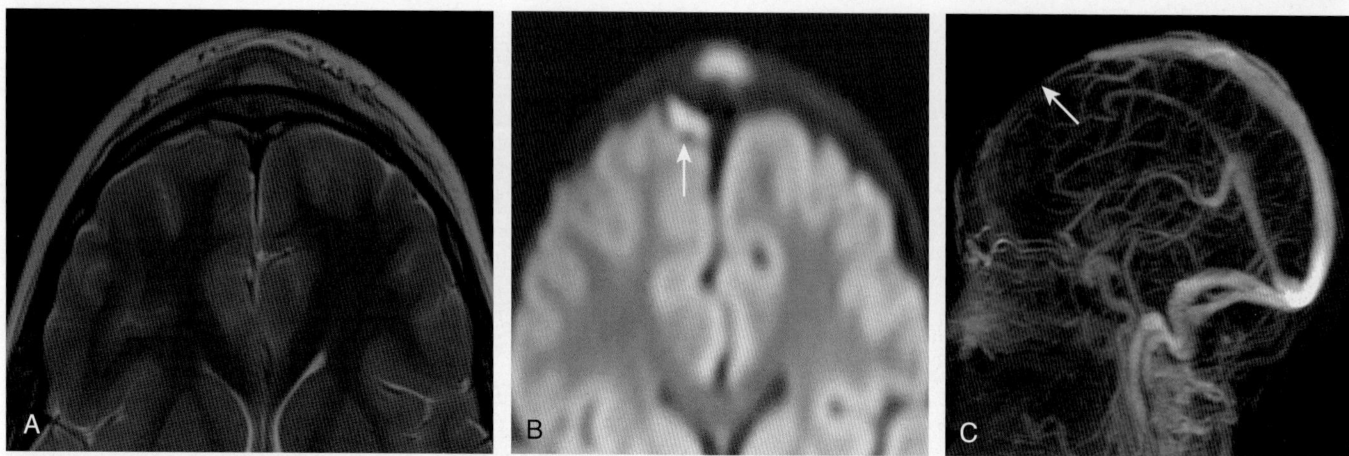

Fig. 15.13 Sinusitis Complications: Pott's Puffy Tumor, Empyema, and Sinus Thrombosis. (A) Axial T2W, (B) axial DWI, and (C) sagittal MR venogram volumetric images demonstrate subgaleal soft tissue thickening with diffusion restricting fluid collection consistent with an abscess (also called Pott's puffy tumor), right frontal extra axial diffusion restriction consistent with an empyema (*arrow*, image B), and thrombosis of the anterior superior sagittal sinus (*arrow*, image C).

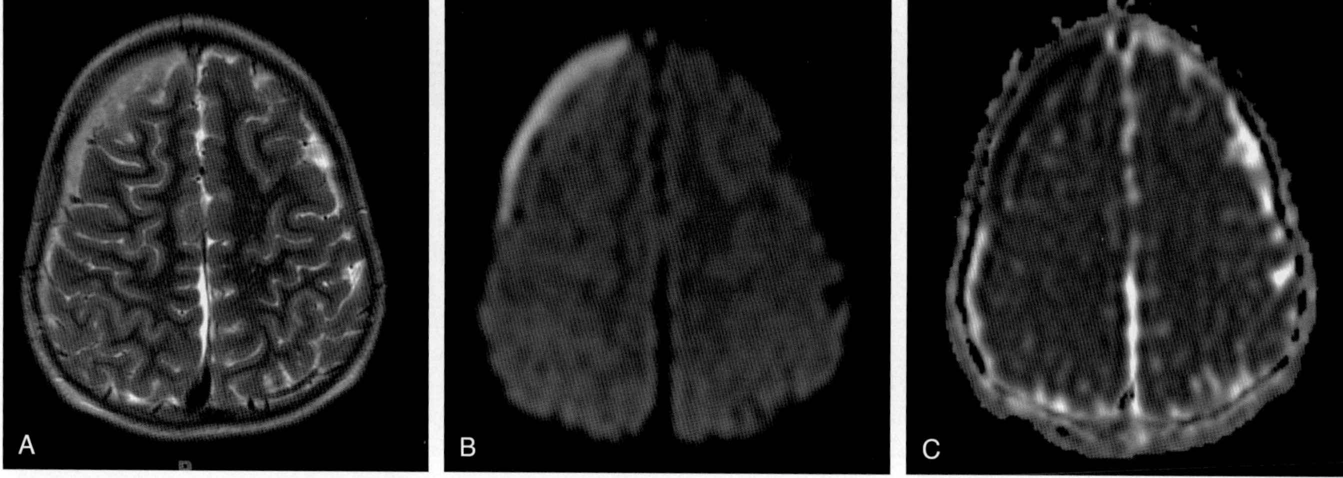

Fig. 15.14 Sinusitis Complications: Subdural Empyema. (A) Axial T2W, (B) axial DWI, and (C) axial ADC images demonstrate a T2 hyperintense diffusion restricting right frontal subdural fluid collection consistent with an empyema.

Key Points

- Infection from the sinuses can spread to the following sites and lead to:
  - *Orbit*: Cellulitis (preseptal, postseptal), abscess (periorbital, orbital, subperiosteal), thrombophlebitis. The Chandler classification organizes the severity of orbital complications secondary to rhinosinusitis as follows: stage 1, inflammatory edema (preseptal cellulitis); stage 2, orbital cellulitis; stage 3, subperiosteal abscess; stage 4, orbital abscess; stage 5, cavernous sinus thrombosis.
  - *Intracranial*: Empyema, cerebritis, cavernous sinus thrombosis, meningitis, abscess, sinus thrombosis. Subdural empyemas constitute a neurosurgical emergency as the infection can spread widely and via emissary veins result in infarcts, cerebral edema, sinus thrombosis, and elevated intracranial pressure. Epidural empyemas do not always require drainage as the dura can act as a mechanical barrier. Subdural empyemas are most often treated with a craniotomy, while epidural empyemas can be treated with burr hole drainage. Although at times imaging differentiating epidural from subdural empyema can be difficult, a subdural empyema will have acute neurologic symptoms, which can assist in the diagnosis.
  - *Scalp*: Cellulitis, abscess (Pott's puffy tumor).
  - *Bone*: Osteomyelitis.

REFERENCES

1. Orman G., et al. Imaging of paranasal sinus infections in children: a review. *J Neuroimaging*. 2020 Sep;30(5):572–586.
2. Gavriel H, et al. Dimension of subperiosteal orbital abscess as an indication for surgical management in children. *Otolaryngol Head Neck Surg*. 2011 Nov;145(5):823–827.
3. Lundy P, et al. Intracranial subdural empyemas and epidural abscesses in children. *J Neurosurg Pediatr*. 2019;24(1):14–21.

ALLERGIC FUNGAL SINUSITIS

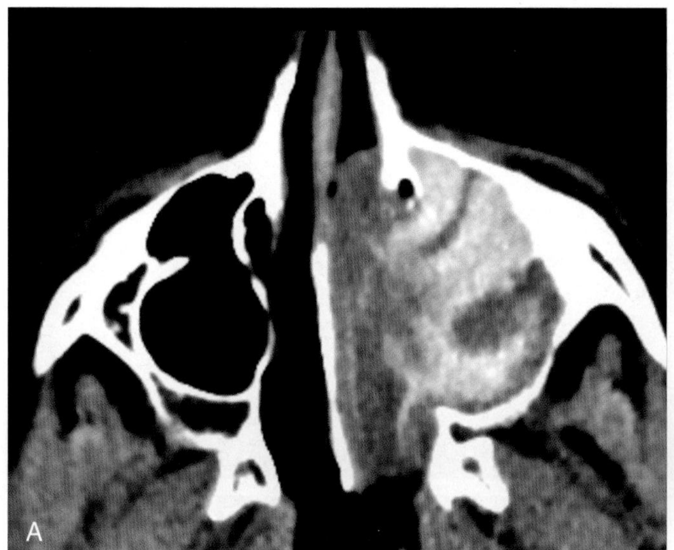

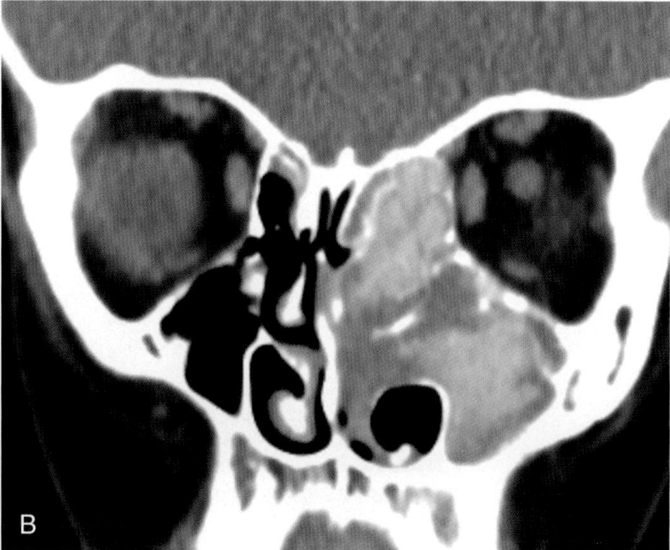

Fig. 15.15 (A and B) Axial and coronal noncontrast CT images demonstrate abnormal opacification of the left maxillary and ethmoid sinuses with centrally hyperdense, peripherally hypodense sinus secretions, sinus expansion, and sinus drainage pathway obstruction.

Key Points

Background

- An IgE-mediated hypersensitivity reaction to fungal antigens causing eosinophilic mucin and noninvasive fungus. The inflammatory response causes mucosal edema, sinus obstruction and stasis. The fungus proliferates and increases antigen exposure causing a self-perpetuating cycle.
- Most commonly occurs with Aspergillus but also occurs with other fungi including Alternaria, Bipolaris, Curvularia, Exserohilum and Phialophora
- Occurs in immunocompetent patients
- Symptoms of chronic rhinosinusitis including nasal congestion, rhinorrhea and nasal obstruction
- The sinus material has consistency similar to putty, grease, mud or crunchy peanut butter and a foul odor.
- Treated with topical steroids followed by surgical debridement and evacuation of obstructing material.

Imaging

- Unilateral (50%) or bilateral (50%)
- Most commonly affects the maxillary and ethmoid sinuses
- CT: *opacified and expanded sinuses with central hyperdense and peripheral hypodense sinus secretions;* possible areas of bone dehiscence due to the sinus expansion; can have associated sinonasal polyps
- MRI: not routinely performed for this diagnosis; sinus material can show T2W hypointensity and variable T1W signal but often T1W hyperintensity

REFERENCES

1. Aribandi M, McCoy VA, Bazan C 3rd. Imaging features of invasive and noninvasive fungal sinusitis: a review. *Radiographics*. 2007 Sep-Oct;27(5):1283–1296.
2. Schubert MS. Allergic fungal sinusitis: pathophysiology, diagnosis and management. *Med Mycol*. 2009;47 (Suppl 1):S324–330.
3. Thompson LD. Allergic fungal sinusitis. *Ear Nose Throat J*. 2011 Mar;90(3):106–107.

INVASIVE FUNGAL SINUSITIS

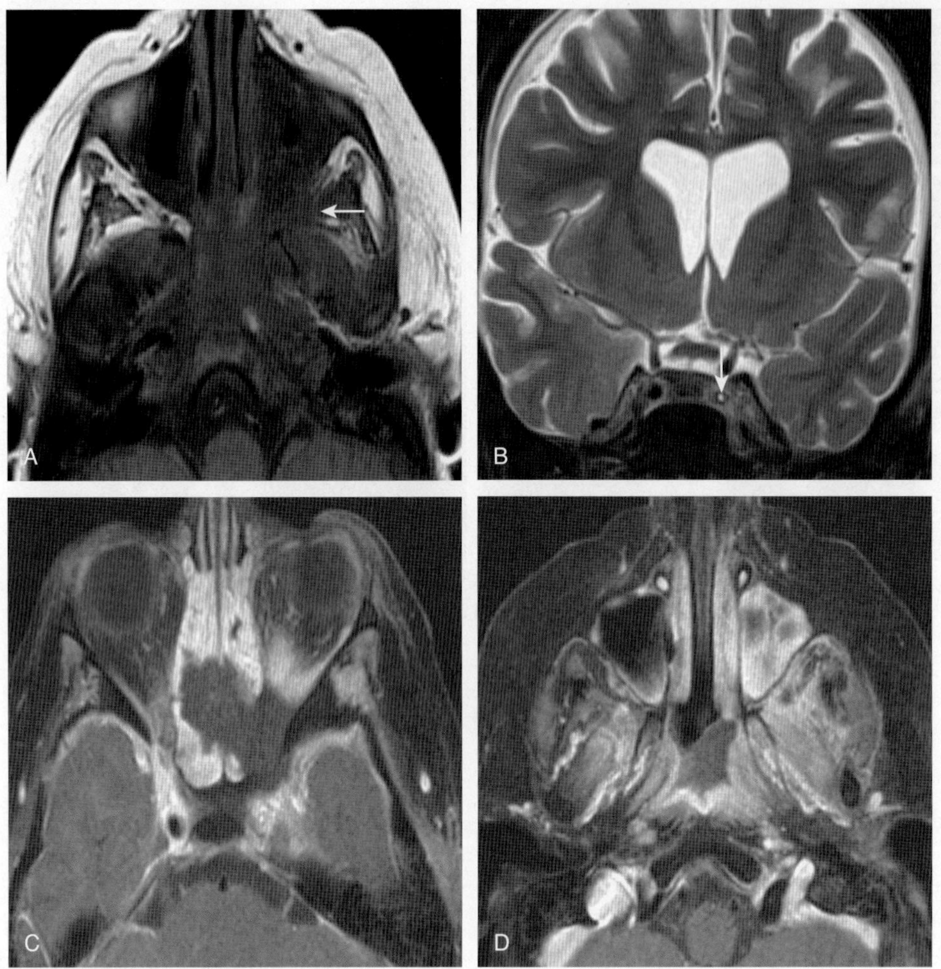

Fig. 15.16 Invasive Fungal Sinusitis. A 9-year-old with history of supratentorial PNET, immunosuppression, and neutropenia. (A) Axial T1W image demonstrates sinus mucosal thickening in the maxillary sinuses with abnormal left retromaxillary and pterygopalatine fossa T1 hypointense signal indicative of soft tissue extension of sinusitis. T1W imaging is very helpful for assessing loss of the normal T1 hyperintense fat surrounding the paranasal sinuses. (B) Coronal T2W shows the left cavernous sinus is enlarged and demonstrates loss of the flow void in the cavernous segment of the left internal carotid artery (ICA) indicative of cavernous sinus invasion and arterial thrombosis. (C and D) Axial T1W+C fat saturation images demonstrate a region of hypointense signal in the ethmoid and sphenoid sinuses and the left superior orbital fissure indicative of devascularization, adjacent enhancement of the left pterygoid muscles, and infratemporal fossa indicative of soft tissue extension of invasive fungal sinusitis.

Key Points

Background

- Rare aggressive infiltration by fungal organisms (typically mucormycosis or aspergillus) in the nasal cavity and paranasal sinuses.
- Usually immunocompromised patients secondary to chemotherapy, chronic immunosuppression drugs, poorly controlled diabetes, malnutrition, or corticosteroid treatment.
- Mortality ~ 50%.
- Rhinoscopy/endoscopy demonstrates pale grayish or black mucosa with bloody crusts.

Imaging

- CT: Bony destruction of paranasal sinus walls, inflammation of the soft tissues surrounding the sinuses (particularly important to assess the pterygopalatine fossa, retromaxillary space, premalar space, orbital apex and medial orbit fat for infiltration), cavernous sinus thrombosis, and carotid occlusion.
- MRI: More sensitive for extent of involvement, visualization of devascularized nonenhancing mucosa of the turbinates and sinuses, necrotic material visualization with diffusion restriction, cavernous sinus thrombosis, and intracranial extension that can result in empyema, cerebritis, abscess and ischemia.

REFERENCE

1. Orman G, et al. Imaging of paranasal sinus infections in children: a review. *J Neuroimaging*. 2020 Sep;30(5):572–586.

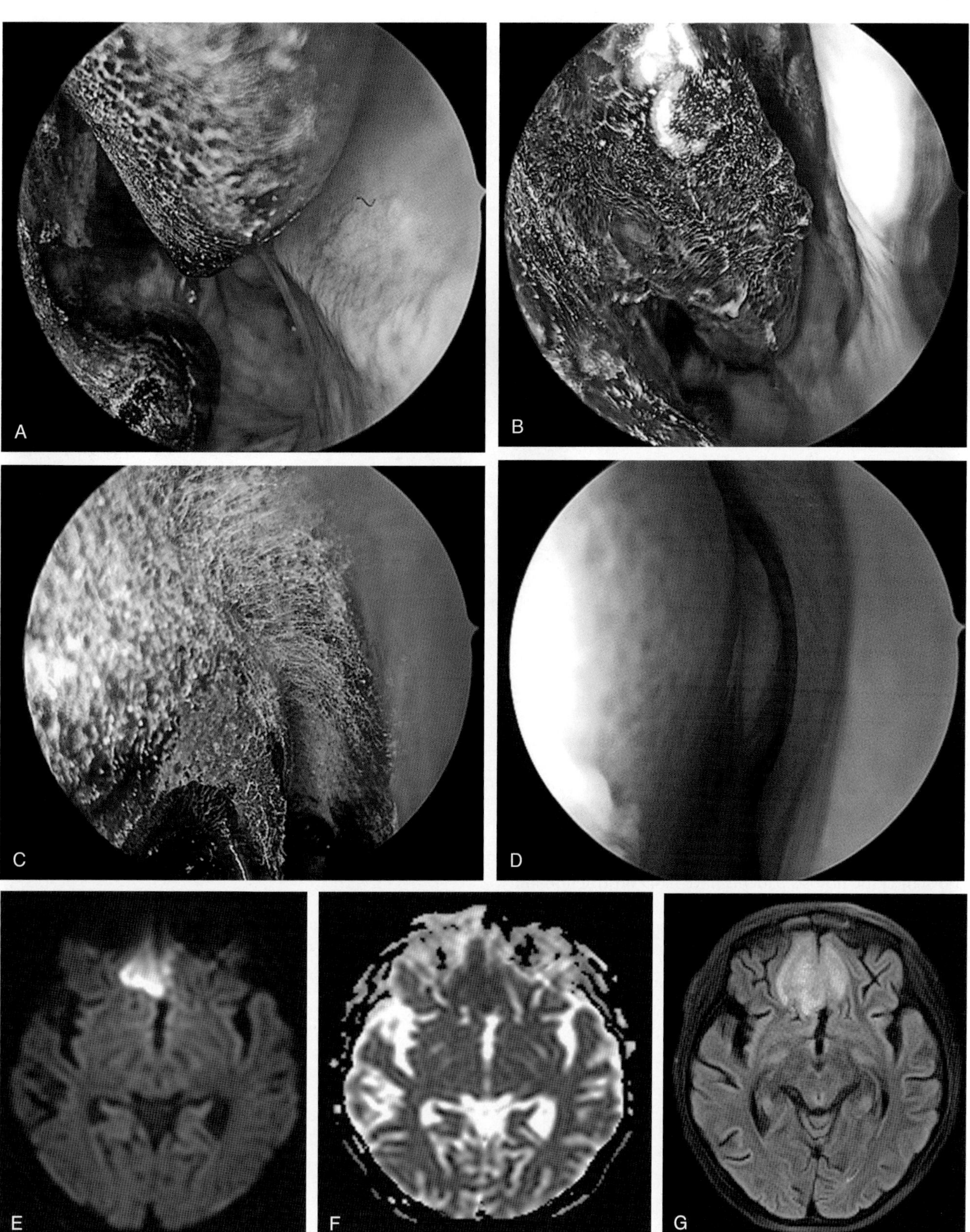

Fig. 15.17 Invasive Fungal Sinusitis. (A to D) Clinical images from nasal endoscope demonstrating dark mucosa in the nasal cavity and frond-like hyphae indicative of invasive fungal sinusitis compared to the normal mucosa seen in image D. (E) Axial DWI, (F) axial ADC, and (G) axial FLAIR images demonstrate intracranial diffusion restricting and FLAIR hyperintense extra-axial and parenchymal tissue consistent with empyema and cerebritis.

CYSTIC FIBROSIS

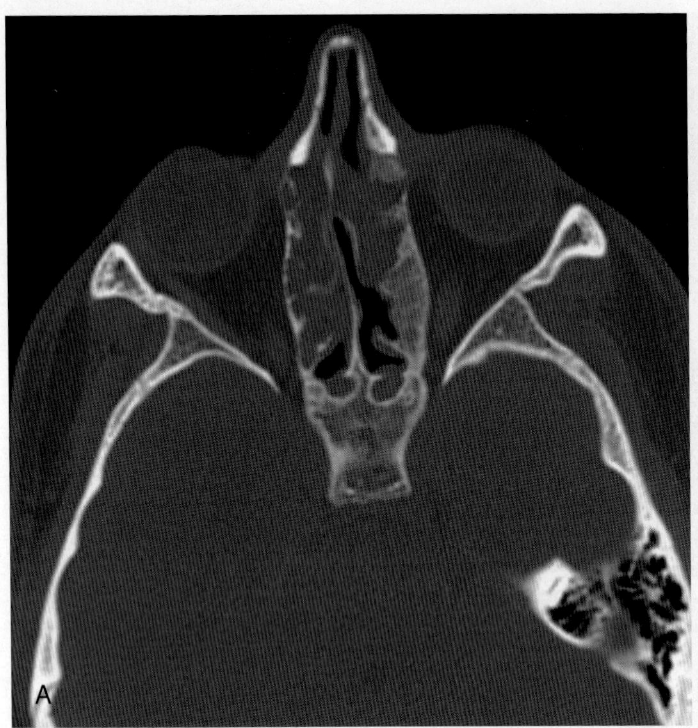

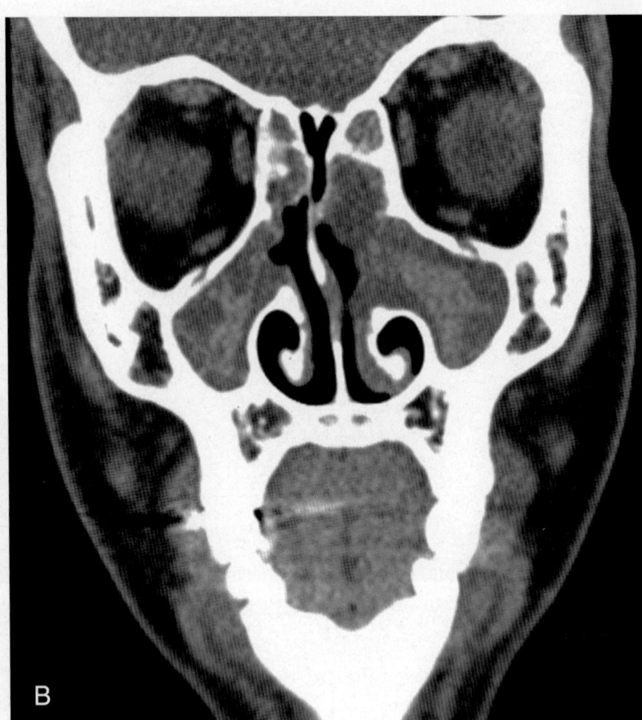

Fig. 15.18 Cystic Fibrosis. (A and B) Axial and coronal CT images demonstrate hypoplastic sphenoid sinuses, thickened and sclerotic ethmoid sinus walls, mucosal thickening in the sinuses and nasal cavities, and internal hyperdense material in the maxillary sinuses.

Key Points

Background

- Genetic defect involving chromosome 7. Regulates transmembrane passage of chlorine ion. High concentrations of chlorine, mucus thickness, and reduction of mucociliary clearance inflammation these children to inflammation and chronic infection of the respiratory tract.
- 100% of cystic fibrosis patients have nasal obstruction and chronic rhinosinusitis.

Imaging

- Similar to typical chronic sinusitis with sclerotic thickened bone (mucoperiosteal reaction/neoosteogenesis) due to the prolonged inflammation.
- *Hypoplasia of the sinuses, particularly the sphenoid sinuses.*
- *Hyperdense sinus secretions* on CT due to inspissated secretions.
- Intrasinus calcification and nasal polyps can also be seen.

REFERENCE

1. Eggesbo HB, et al. CT characterization of developmental variations of the paranasal sinuses in cystic fibrosis. *Acta Radiol.* 2001 Sep;42(5):482–493.

ORBITAL CELLULITIS

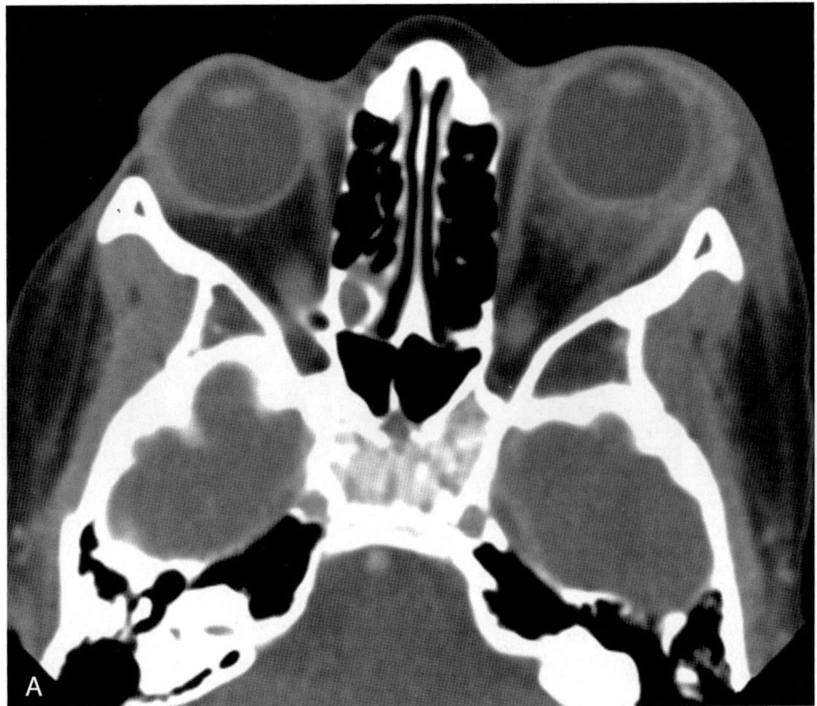

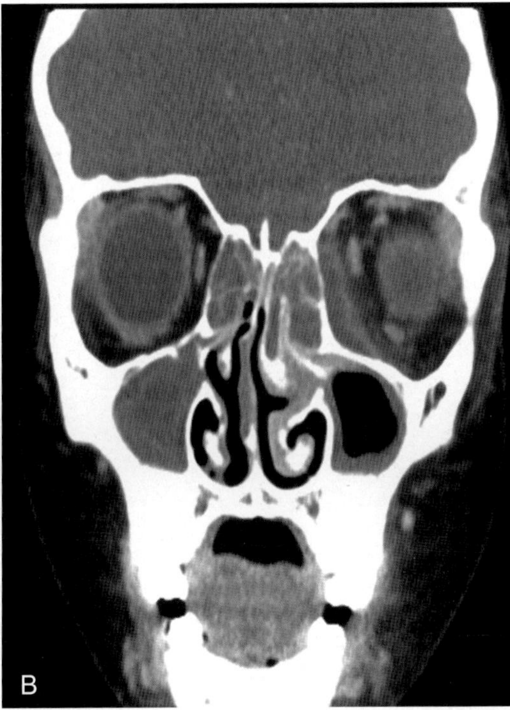

Fig. 15.19 Orbital Cellulitis. (A) Axial CECT image demonstrates left orbital preseptal and postseptal soft tissue thickening, edema, and inflammatory changes. (B) Coronal CT image in a different patient with a left medial and inferomedial peripherally enhancing fluid collection in the left orbit consistent with a subperiosteal abscess. The source of infection is likely an extension of the extensive ethmoid and maxillary acute sinusitis into the left orbit.

Key Points

Background

- The orbital septum is the anterior reflection of the periosteum of the orbital wall onto the tarsal plate of the eyelid, and divides the orbit into the preseptal and postseptal compartments.
- Preseptal cellulitis is typically treated with oral antibiotics.
- Postseptal cellulitis increases risk of abscess, blindness, venous thrombosis, intracranial extension, and death. Postseptal cellulitis typically treated with hospital admission for IV antibiotics with possible surgical management of the sinus infection and/or orbital infection.
- The most common cause of postseptal cellulitis is acute rhinosinusitis (60%–85%), and the most common cause of unilateral proptosis in a child is sinus-related orbital infection.
- The most common agents include *S. aureus*, *Staphylococcus epidermidis*, and *Streptococcus pyogenes* (~75%).
- Other causes: Stye, foreign body, dacryoadenitis/cystitis, dental abscess, and hematogeneous seeding (least common).
- Surgical drainage may be required in 12% of admitted patients.
- A subperiosteal abscess volume >0.5 mL, length >17 mm, and width >4.5 mm should be considered for drainage.
- Risk of vision loss reported to be 3% to 11%, and mortality ranging from 1% to 2.5%.

Imaging

- Soft tissue swelling, edema, and inflammatory changes in the preseptal and/or postseptal space.
- Assess for associated abscess, sinusitis, and/or complications seen with sinusitis.

REFERENCES

1. Kralik SF, et al. Evaluation of orbital disorders and cranial nerve innervation of the extraocular muscles. *Magn Reson Imaging Clin N Am.* 2012 Aug;20(3):413–434.
2. Ludwig BJ, et al. Diagnostic imaging in nontraumatic pediatric head and neck emergencies. *Radiographics.* 2010 May;30(3):781–799.
3. Tabarino F, et al. Subperiosteal orbital abscess: volumetric criteria for surgical drainage. *Int J Pediatr Otorhinolaryngol.* 2015 Feb;79(2):131–135.
4. Gavriel H, et al. Dimension of subperiosteal orbital abscess as an indication for surgical management in children. *Otolaryngol Head Neck Surg.* 2011 Nov;145(5):823–827.

DACRYOCYSTITIS

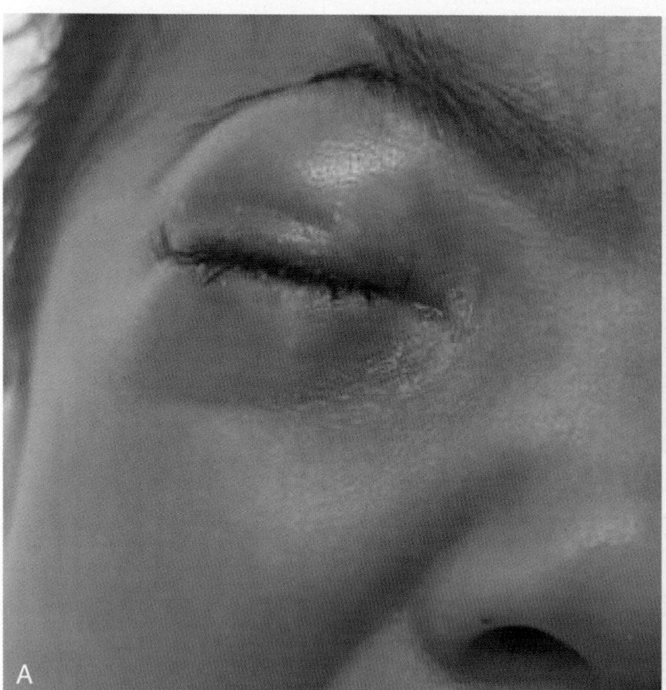

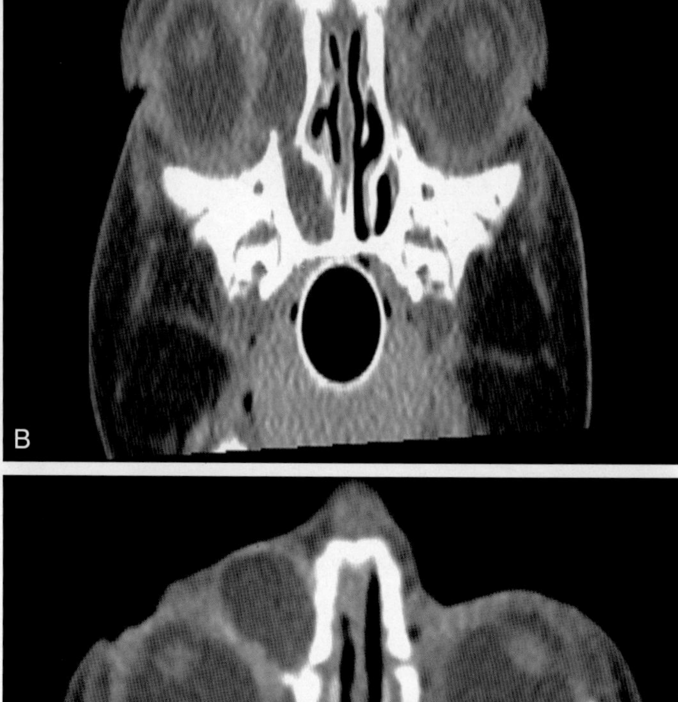

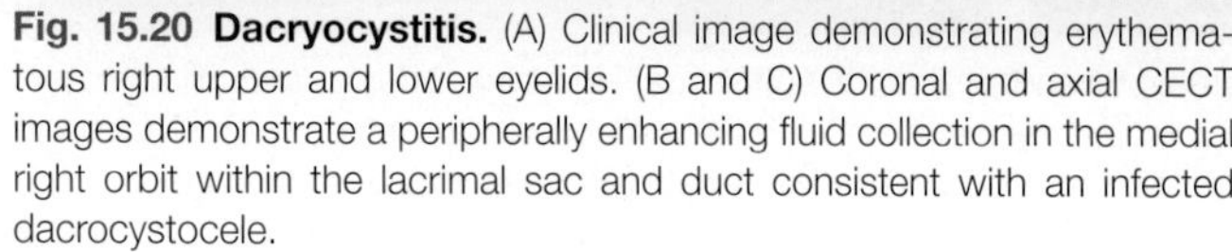

Fig. 15.20 Dacryocystitis. (A) Clinical image demonstrating erythematous right upper and lower eyelids. (B and C) Coronal and axial CECT images demonstrate a peripherally enhancing fluid collection in the medial right orbit within the lacrimal sac and duct consistent with an infected dacrocystocele.

Key Points

Background

- Infection and dilatation of the lacrimal sac secondary to impaired drainage along the nasolacrimal duct
- Clinical: Erythema and pain along the medial canthus with epiphora (overflow of tears onto the face)

Imaging

- Peripheral enhancement and dilatation of the lacrimal sac
- Preseptal inflammation and edema

REFERENCE

1. Ludwig BJ, et al. Diagnostic imaging in nontraumatic pediatric head and neck emergencies. *Radiographics*. 2010 May;30(3):781–799.

ORBITAL PSEUDOTUMOR

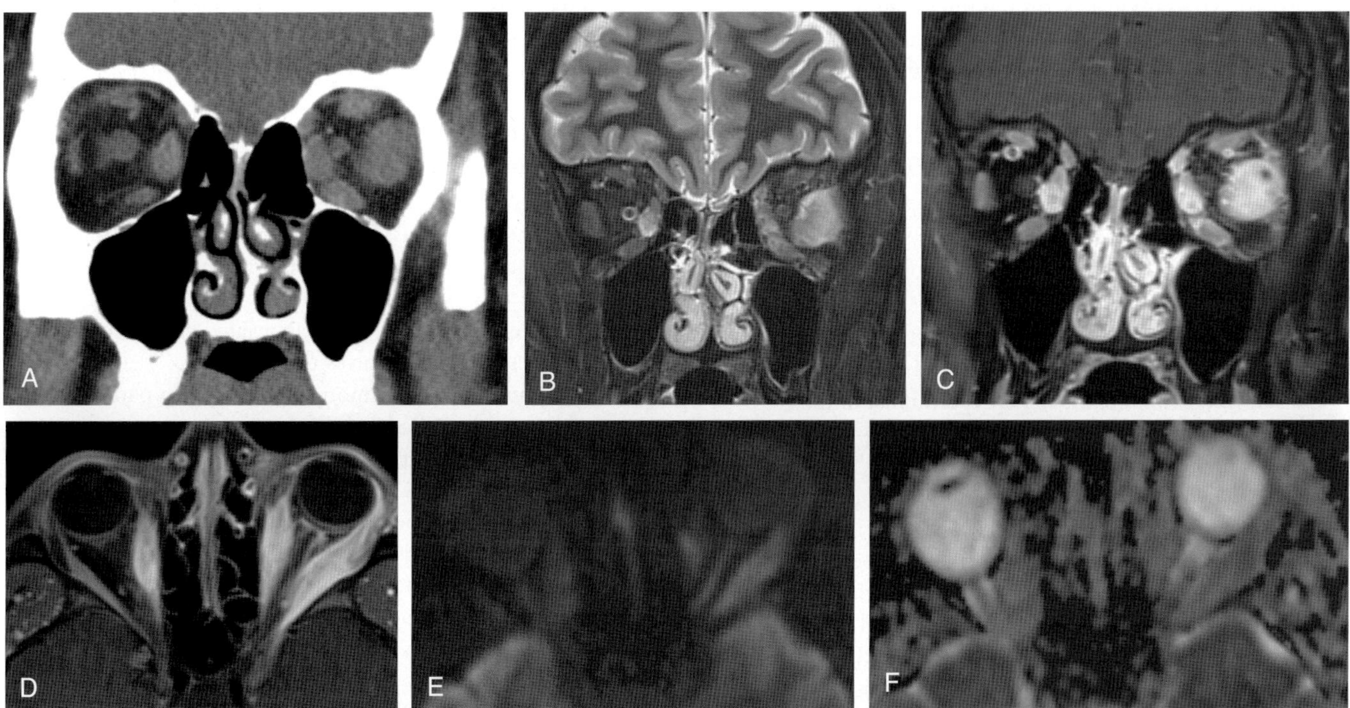

Fig. 15.21 Orbital Pseudotumor. (A) Coronal CT, (B) coronal T2W fat saturation, (C and D) coronal and axial T1W+C fat saturation, and (E and F) axial DWI and ADC images demonstrate enlarged, T2 hyperintense, homogeneously enhancing right medial rectus and left lateral rectus, medial rectus, inferior rectus, and superior oblique muscles with involved left lateral rectus myotendinous junction, and ADC isointense to mild hyperintense signal.

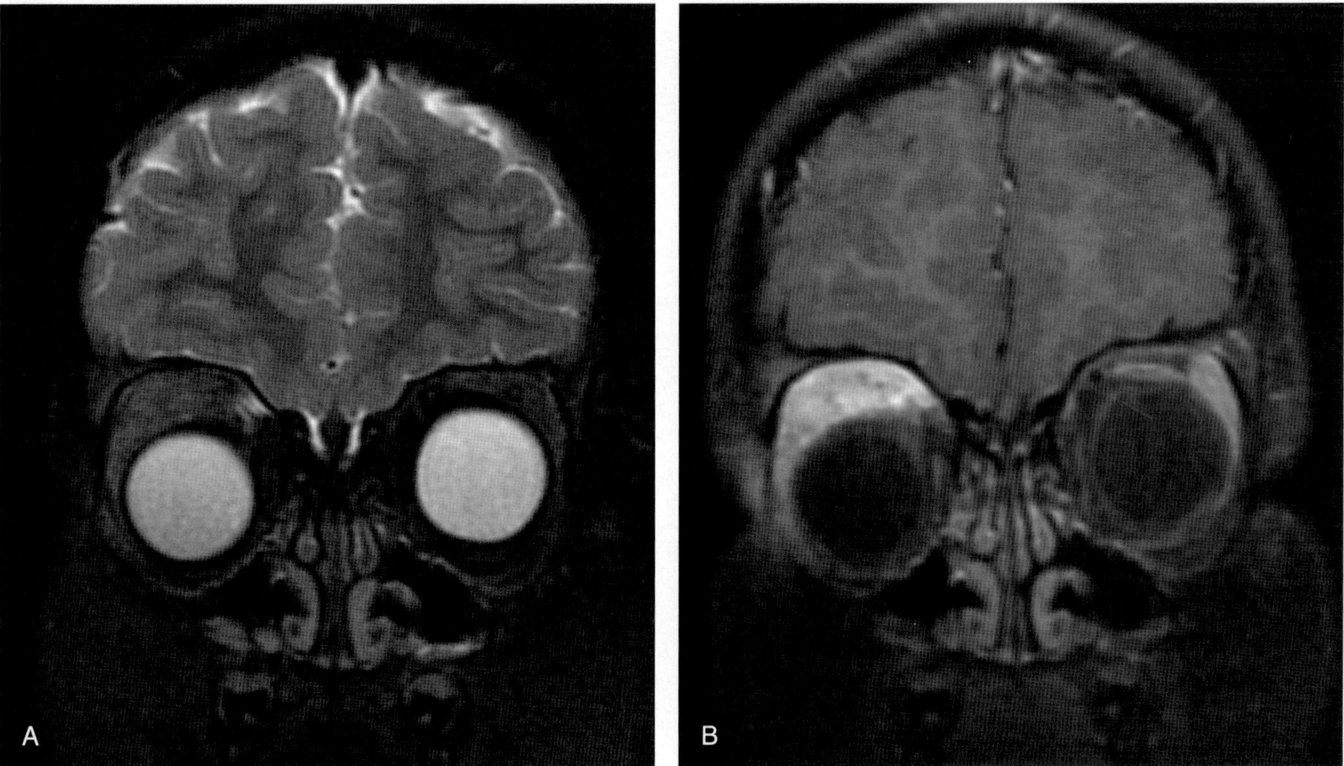

Fig. 15.22 Orbital Pseudotumor. (A) Coronal T2W and (B) coronal T1W+C fat saturation images demonstrate T2 isointense homogeneously enhancing mass in the postseptal superior right orbit that involves the superior rectus, lacrimal gland, and orbital fat.

Key Points

Background

- Also known as idiopathic orbital inflammation.
- Second most common cause of proptosis
- More commonly unilateral (except in children)
- Clinical
  - Acute: Pain, swelling, erythema, chemosis, optic neuropathy, and extraocular muscle dysmotility
  - Chronic: Diplopia and proptosis
- Responds to corticosteroid and immunosuppressive therapy

Imaging

- Multiple possible imaging patterns and appearances:
  - *Soft tissue inflammation*: T2 hyperintense and homogeneous enhancement of the preseptal and/or postseptal fat.
  - *Focal mass*: Usually a postseptal homogeneously enhancing mass with variable T2 signal. T2 signal can be hypointense due to fibrosis. ADC hyperintense signal compared to lymphoma, which demonstrates ADC hypointense signal. A small series showed that an ADC threshold of 1.0×10^{-3} mm^2/s reported 100% sensitivity and specificity for differentiation between pseudotumor and lymphoma.
  - *Extraocular muscle(s)*: Homogeneous enhancement of the muscles with involvement of the myotendinous junction.
  - *Lacrimal gland(s)*: Homogeneously enhancing and enlarged lacrimal glands.
  - *Optic nerve sheath* complex, sclera, uvea: Thin enhancement of the nerve sheath and globe.
  - *Cavernous sinus*: Homogeneous enhancement and enlargement of the cavernous sinus resulting in Tolosa Hunt, a syndrome consisting of painful ophthalmoplegia with neuropathy of cranial nerves 3 and 4, V1, and V2 in addition to orbital pain.
- Absence of additional cranial nerve, dural, or leptomeningeal enhancement. No regional or systemic lymphadenopathy.
- Differential Diagnosis: Imaging overlap with the following diagnoses leads to necessity for biopsy in many cases for diagnosis
  - IgG4-related disease: often associated cranial nerve involvement and involves the pancreas
  - Lymphoma: less common to present with pain, usually additional lymphadenopathy present
  - Sarcoidosis: frequently has pulmonary disease
  - Granulomatosis with polyangiitis: often chronic sinusitis findings are present
  - Graves orbitopathy: enlarged extraocular muscles, bilateral involvement of the muscles, and spares the myotendinous junction

REFERENCE

1. Kralik SF, et al. Evaluation of orbital disorders and cranial nerve innervation of the extraocular muscles. *Magn Reson Imaging Clin N Am*. 2012 Aug;20(3):413–434.

UVEITIS

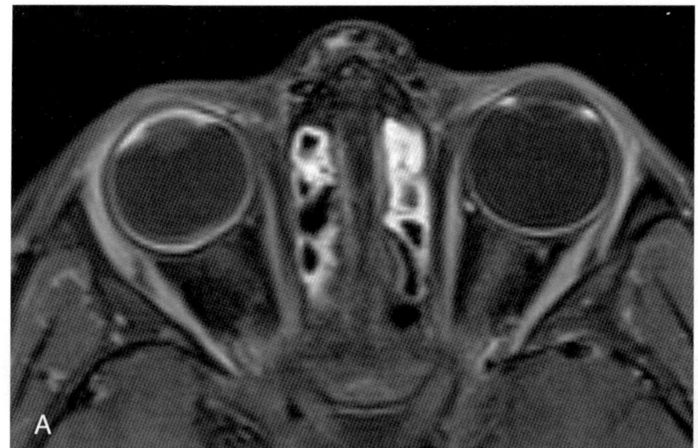

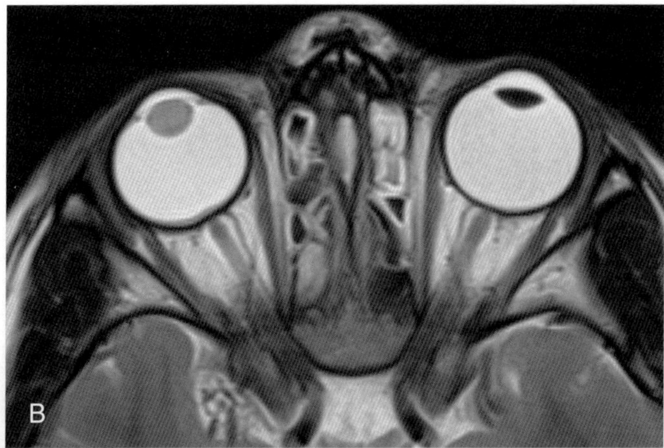

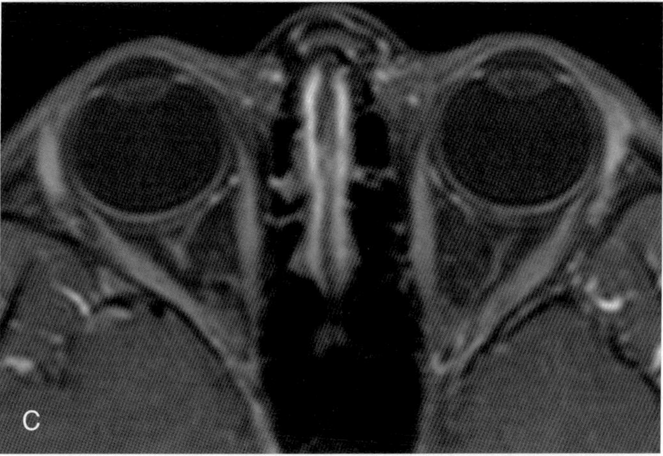

Fig. 15.23 Uveitis. (A) Axial T1W+C fat saturation image demonstrates abnormal enhancement of the right iris, ciliary bodies and posterior choroidal layer, and abnormal enhancement of the left ciliary bodies. (B) Axial T2W image demonstrates an enlarged and hyperintense right lens consistent with a cataract and a T2 hyperintense subretinal effusion. (C) Axial T1W+C fat saturation image of a normal globe for comparison.

Key Points

Background

- The uveal tract is a highly vascular middle layer of the ocular wall consisting of the choroid posteriorly and ciliary body and iris anteriorly. A uveitis is an inflammation of these structures.
- *Wide range of etiologies*. Noninfectious systemic inflammatory diseases including HLA-B27-related disease, rheumatoid arthritis, sarcoidosis, Behcet disease, relapsing polychondritis, and Vogt-Koyanagi-Harada syndrome. Infectious causes include toxoplasmosis, herpes simplex, varicella zoster, and tuberculosis. In many cases, an etiology is not discovered.
- Diagnosis is primarily clinical through history and physical examination.

Imaging

- Imaging not typically performed. MRI may be performed when the etiology is indeterminate, to assist in diagnosis such as assessment for involvement of other orbital structures (e.g., sarcoidosis), or unresponsive to treatment.
- MRI: hyperenhancing posterior choroidal layer, ciliary body, and iris. Abnormal vitreous signal (lack of fluid suppression on FLAIR). Subretinal effusion. Cataract formation.

REFERENCE

1. Li CQ, et al. Magnetic resonance imaging of uveitis. *Neuroradiology*. 2015;57:825–832.

ENDOPHALMITIS

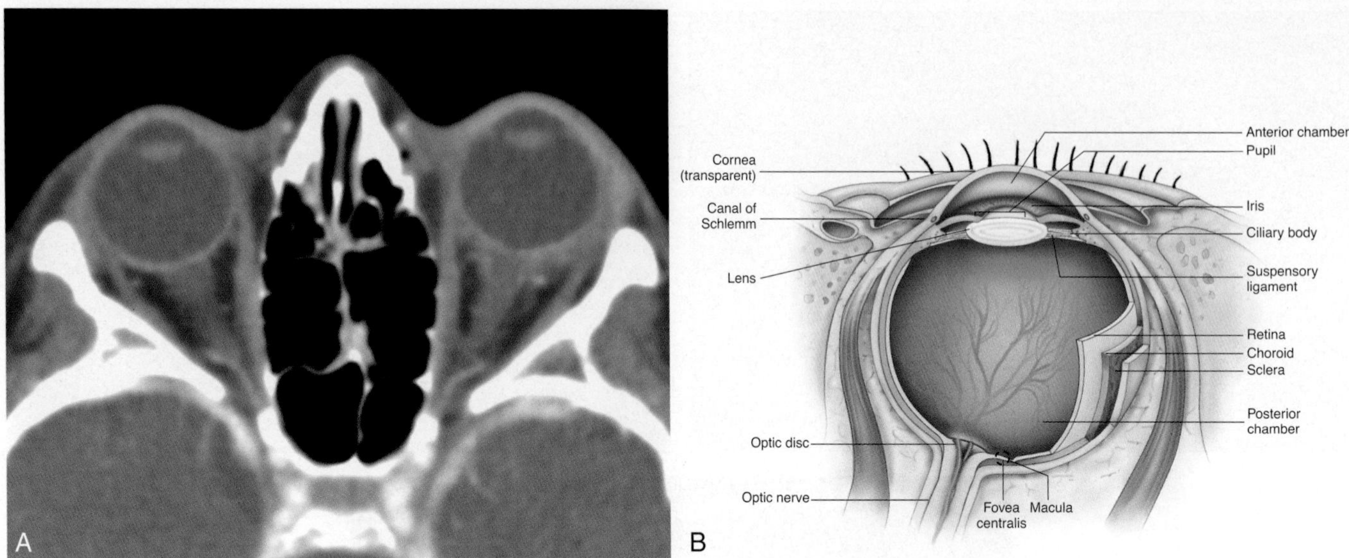

Fig. 15.24 Endophthalmitis. (A) Axial CECT image demonstrates thickening and ill-defined margins of the sclera of the left globe. (B) Illustration of the layers of the globe. (B from Lewis SL, Dirksen SR, Heitkemper MM, Bucher L, Harding MM. *Medical-Surgical Nursing: Assessment and Management of Clinical Problems*. 11th ed. St. Louis: Elsevier; 2020.)

Key Points

Background

- The three main layers of the globe are the sclera, choroid, and retina. The globe is surrounded by fascia called Tenon's capsule, which blends with the sclera at the corneoscleral junction and allows for a potential space between the fascia and the sclera.
- Bacteria, fungi, viruses, and parasites can cause endophthalmitis.
- Exogenous etiology includes surgery, trauma, or corneal ulcers. Endogenous etiologies cause infection through hematogenous spread.
- Presentation includes rapid-onset vision loss, eye pain, eyelid swelling, and conjunctival erythema.

Imaging

- CT and MRI can aid assessment of the extent of infection.
- Early findings include thick enhancement of the uvea and sclera progressing to abnormal vitreous.
- Advanced findings include thickening of the globe layers, retinal or choroidal detachment, exudate, globe deformity, and peribulbar inflammation.
- End-stage findings are of a calcified and shrunken globe (phthisis bulbi).

REFERENCE

1. Radhakrishnan R, et al. MR imaging findings of endophthalmitis. *Neuroradiol J*. 2016 Apr;29(2):122–129.

ACUTE PAROTITIS

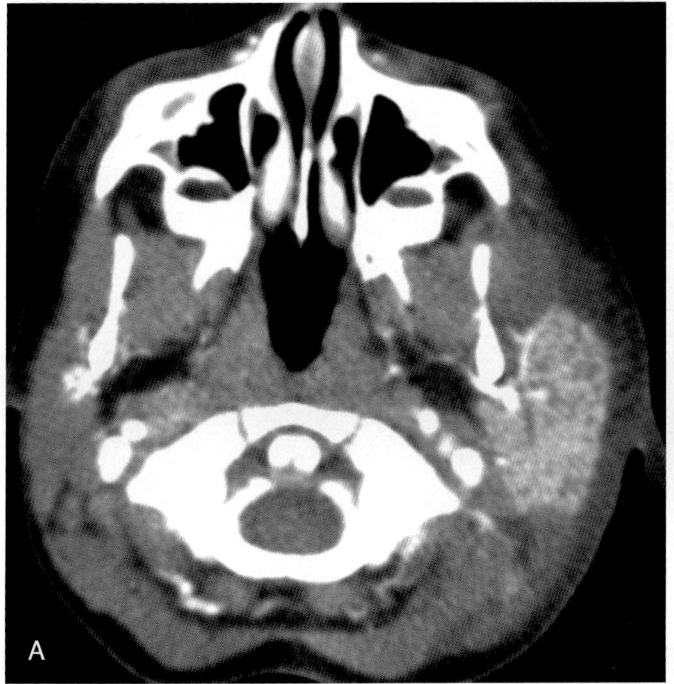

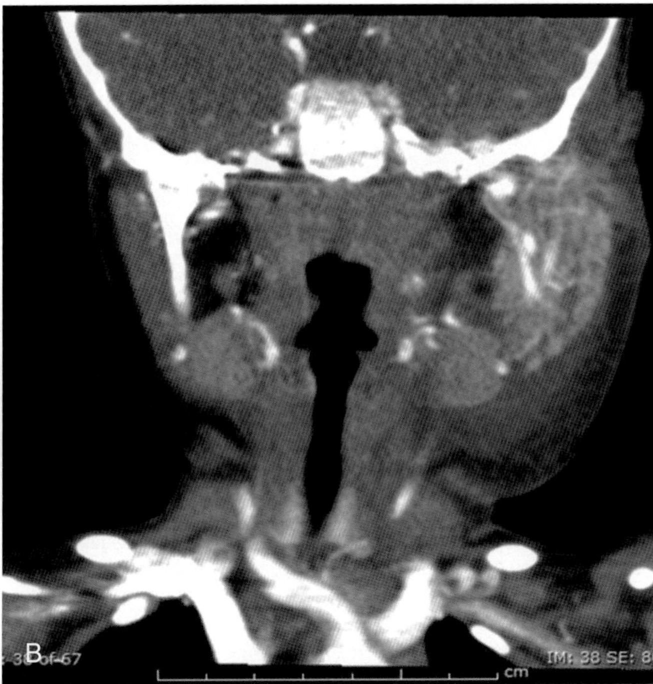

Fig. 15.25 Acute Parotitis. (A) Axial and (B) coronal CECT images demonstrate abnormal enlarged and homogeneously enhancing left parotid gland with surrounding soft tissue edema and inflammation in the periparotid space. No radiodense sialolith is visible.

Key Points

Background

- A common condition that most often affects the parotid and submandibular glands.
- Most commonly related to a viral infection that is usually diagnosed on clinical grounds.
- Mumps is by far the most common viral cause and typically affects both parotid glands.
- Presents as swelling and enlargement of the salivary glands.
- Acute (suppurative) bacterial sialoadenitis is uncommon in children, but recurrent parotitis is occasionally caused by *Streptococcus viridians*.
- Recurrent sialoadenitis can also occur due to sialoliths.
- *Juvenile recurrent parotitis* is the second most common cause of parotitis in children. It is a nonobstructive, nonsuppurative parotitis seen in children aged 3 to 6 years causing multiple episodes of parotid swelling, pain, fever, and malaise. Leads to glandular destruction and loss of 50% to 80% of function. Early diagnosis and treatment help reduce recurrence. Treated with antibiotics and sialography with iodinated oil.
- Recurrent sialoadenitis can also occur due to sialoliths. Sialoliths are most commonly found in the submandibular glands and in Wharton's ducts (85%).

Imaging

- Enlargement of the salivary gland ducts and calcified sialoliths on CT. Parenchymal atrophy occurs in chronic sialoadenitis.
- In children, ultrasound is most commonly the initial imaging study due to lack of radiation.

REFERENCES

1. Hegde SV, et al. A space-based approach to pediatric face and neck infections. *Neurographics*. 2014;4:43–52.
2. Katz P, et al. Treatment of juvenile recurrent parotitis. *Otolaryngol Clinics N Am*. 2009 Dec;42(6):1087–1091.

ACUTE OTITIS EXTERNA

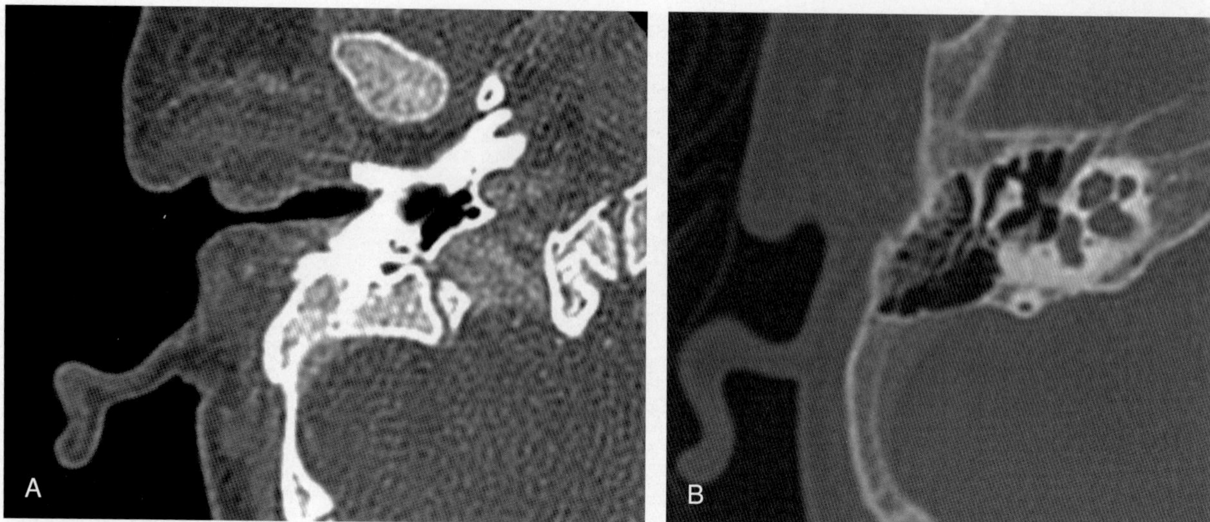

Fig. 15.26 Acute Otitis Externa. (A and B) Axial CECT images in soft tissue and bone algorithm demonstrates abnormal edema and inflammatory changes involving the right external auditory canal, preauricular and post auricular spaces with no abnormal fluid in the middle ear cavity or mastoid air cells.

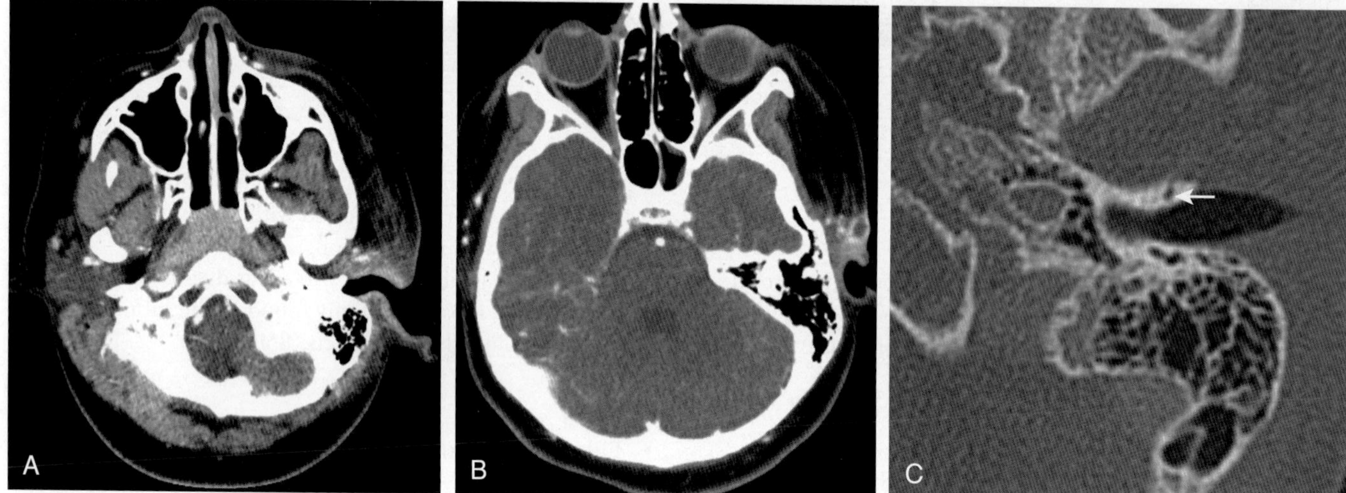

Fig. 15.27 Acute Otitis Externa Secondary to a First Branchial Cleft Fistula. (A) Axial CECT image demonstrates abnormal edema and inflammatory changes involving the left external auditory canal, preauricular, and postauricular spaces. (B and C) A 6-week follow-up CECT demonstrates left preauricular peripherally enhancing abscess and thin osseous tract through the anterior wall of the left external auditory canal seen on the high-resolution image C. A first branchial cleft fistula was confirmed on surgical resection.

Key Points

Background

- Acute otitis externa is a common acute infection of the external auditory canal caused by breakdown of the skin cerumen barrier.
- Risk factors include swimming, foreign body, and trauma.
- The most common pathogens causing otitis externa are *Pseudomonas aeruginosa*, *Staphylococcus epidermidis, S. aureus*, anaerobes, and fungus. Approximately one-third of infections are polymicrobial.
- Common signs and symptoms including otalgia, otorrhea, and hearing loss.

Imaging

- Imaging is typically not performed unless there is concern for abscess, skull base osteomyelitis, or recurrent otitis externa in which a first branchial cleft anomaly may be present.
- CT imaging findings include soft tissue edema, inflammatory changes involving the external auditory canal, auricle, preauricular, and/or post auricular spaces. Concurrent acute otitis media with or without acute mastoiditis is often present.

REFERENCE

1. Goguen LA. External otitis: Pathogenesis, clinical features, and diagnosis. UpToDate. https://www.uptodate.com/contents/external-otitis-pathogenesis-clinical-features-and-diagnosis. Published July 12, 2022. Accessed September 23, 2022.

ACUTE OTITIS MEDIA

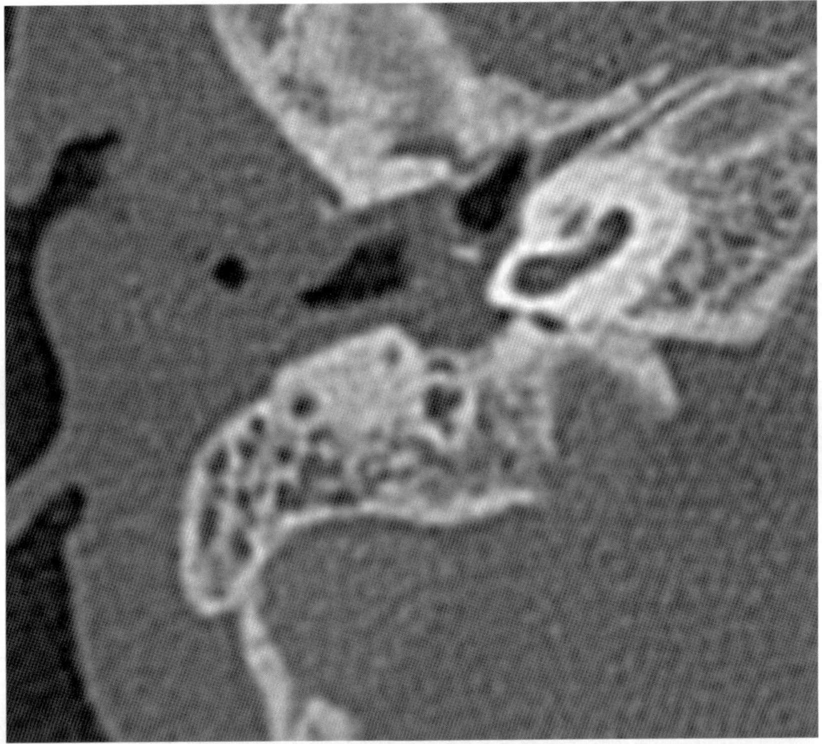

Fig. 15.28 Acute Otitis Media. Axial CT image demonstrates layering air-fluid level in the right middle ear cavity, fluid in the mastoid air cells, and narrowed external auditory canal due to edema.

Key Points

Background

- Acute otitis media is a common disorder in early childhood with rapid onset of middle ear cavity infection and inflammation.
- Common signs and symptoms include otalgia, otorrhea, fever, full or bulging tympanic membrane, and erythematous tympanic membrane.
- Often associated with a preceding upper respiratory tract infection that results in nasal and nasopharyngeal movement and functional Eustachian tube obstruction.
- Infections are due to bacteria and virus in 66%, bacteria only in 27%, and virus only in 4%. The most common pathogens are *S. pneumoniae*, nontypeable *H. influenzae*, and *Moraxella catarrhalis*.
- Treated with observation versus antibiotics depending on patient age, severity of symptoms, laterality, and presence of otorrhea. Tympanostomy tube placement performed for chronic middle ear effusion with hearing difficulty or recurrent acute otitis media.

Imaging

- Imaging is typically not performed unless there is concern for acute mastoiditis, deep neck cellulitis or abscess, meningitis, facial nerve palsy, petrous apicitis, and sepsis.
- CT imaging findings can include complete middle ear opacification or air fluid level in the middle ear cavity with mastoid opacification from effusion. No ossicular erosions.

REFERENCE

1. Rettig E, et al. Contemporary concepts in management of acute otitis media in children. *Otolaryngol Clin N Am*. 2014;47:651–672.

ACUTE MASTOIDITIS

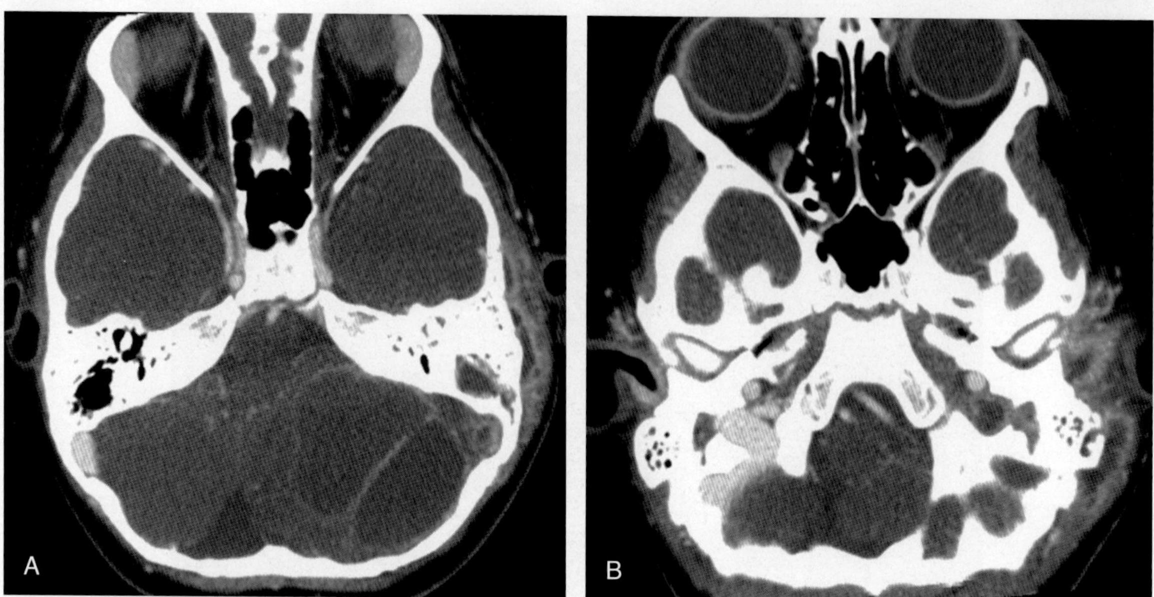

Fig. 15.29 Acute Mastoiditis With Intracranial Abscess and Sinus Thrombosis. (A and B) Axial CECT images demonstrate acute mastoiditis characterized by mastoid and middle ear cavity fluid, postauricular edema, inflammation and abscess formation, and complications including thrombosed left sigmoid sinus and intracranial abscess formation.

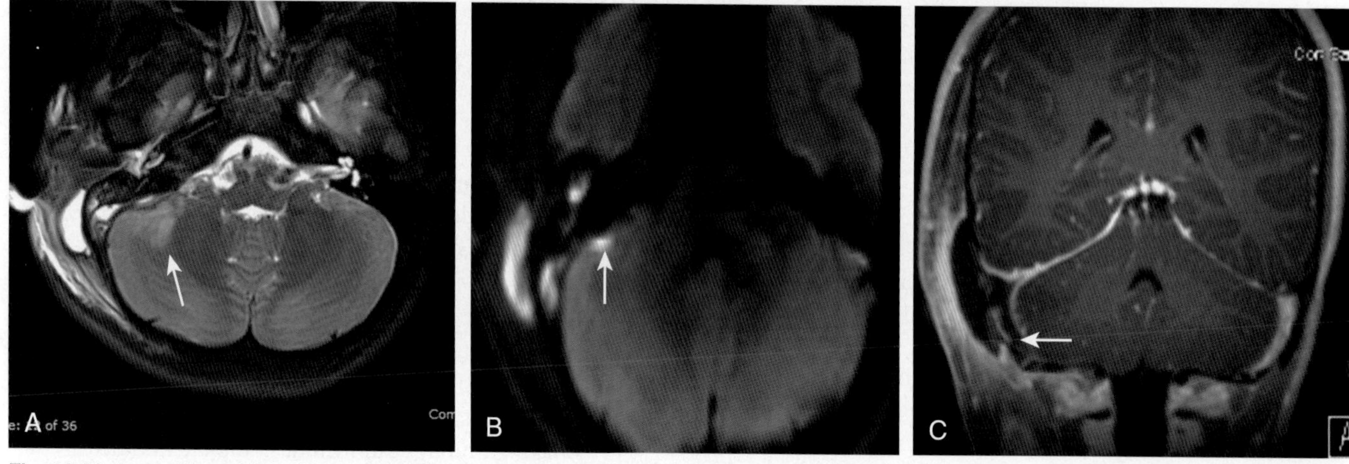

Fig. 15.30 Acute Mastoiditis With Intracranial Empyema, Cerebritis, Meningitis and Sinus Thrombosis. (A) Axial T2W, (B) axial DWI, and (C) coronal T1+C images demonstrate mastoid and middle ear cavity fluid, postauricular edema, inflammation and abscess formation (diffusion restriction), thrombosed right sigmoid sinus (*arrow*, image C), empyema (extra axial diffusion restriction; *arrow*, image B), leptomeningeal enhancement (meningitis), and right cerebellar edema (cerebritis, *arrow*, image A).

Key Points

Background

- Majority of infections from *S. pneumoniae* and *H. influenzae*
- Clinical presentation: Fever, periauricular erythema, swelling and tenderness

Imaging

- Imaging findings: Periauricular inflammation +/− abscess, middle ear cavity, and mastoid fluid
- Complications from intracranial spread: Dural sinus thrombosis, empyema, meningitis, and cerebritis
- CT with contrast is performed to identify mastoid fluid, erosions, periauricular inflammation, abscess, and sinus thrombosis.
- MRI with contrast is helpful to identify empyema, meningitis, cerebritis, and parenchymal abscess.

REFERENCE

1. Som PM, Curtin HD, Swartz JD, Hagiwana M. Inflammatory diseases of the temporal bone. In: Head and Neck Imaging. Vol I. 5th ed. St. Louis: Mosby Elsevier; 2011:1183–1230.

PETROUS APICITIS

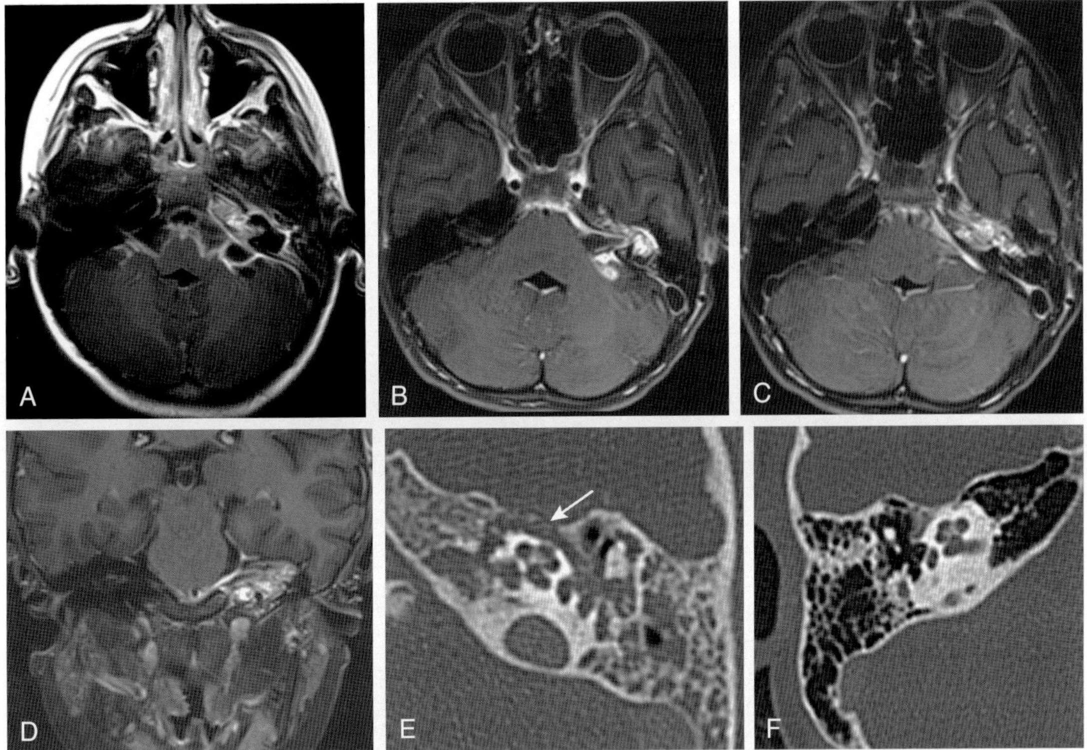

Fig. 15.31 8-Year-Old With Petrous Apicitis Secondary to Meningitis. (A) Axial T1W+C image demonstrates abnormal leptomeningeal enhancement along the brainstem and cranial nerves as well as abnormal enhancement of the left petrous apex. (B to D) Axial T1W+C images demonstrate petrous apex enhancement, adjacent dural thickening and enhancement, and left internal auditory canal (IAC) dural enhancement. (E) Axial CT image demonstrates abnormal fluid in the mastoid, middle ear, and petrous apex as well as abnormal osseous erosion (*arrow*) along the anterior wall of the petrous apex. (F) Axial CT image of a normal temporal bone for reference.

Key Points

Background

- Infection of the petrous apex, essentially an osteomyelitis, which occurs from spread of meningitis or acute mastoiditis through the pneumatized air cells of the petrous bone
- *Gradenigo syndrome*: Triad of otomastoiditis, facial pain (cranial nerve 5), and abducens palsy (cranial nerve 6)

Imaging

- CT: Demineralization and erosion of the petrous bone
- MRI: Homogeneous enhancement of the bone and adjacent dura and leptomeninges

REFERENCE

1. Som PM, Curtin HD, Swartz JD, Hagiwana M. Inflammatory diseases of the temporal bone. In: Head and Neck Imaging. Vol I. 5th ed. St. Louis: Mosby Elsevier; 2011:1183–1230.

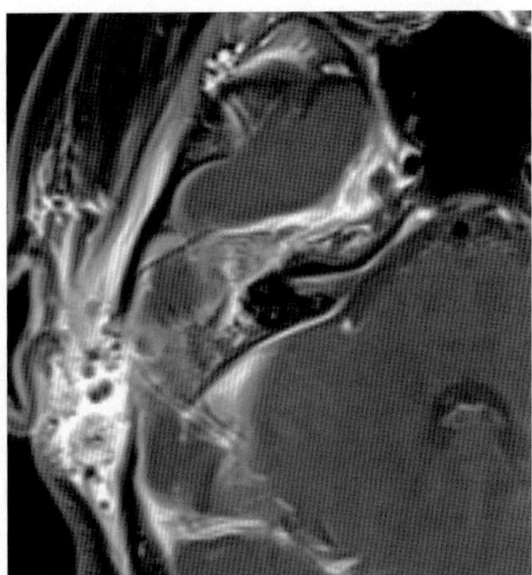

Fig. 15.32 14-Year-Old With Petrous Apicitis Secondary to Acute Otomastoiditis. Axial T1W+C image demonstrates abnormal petrous apex and adjacent dural enhancement secondary to extension of infection originating in the left middle ear and mastoid as indicated by the abnormal enhancement and periauricular enhancement.

CHRONIC OTITIS MEDIA

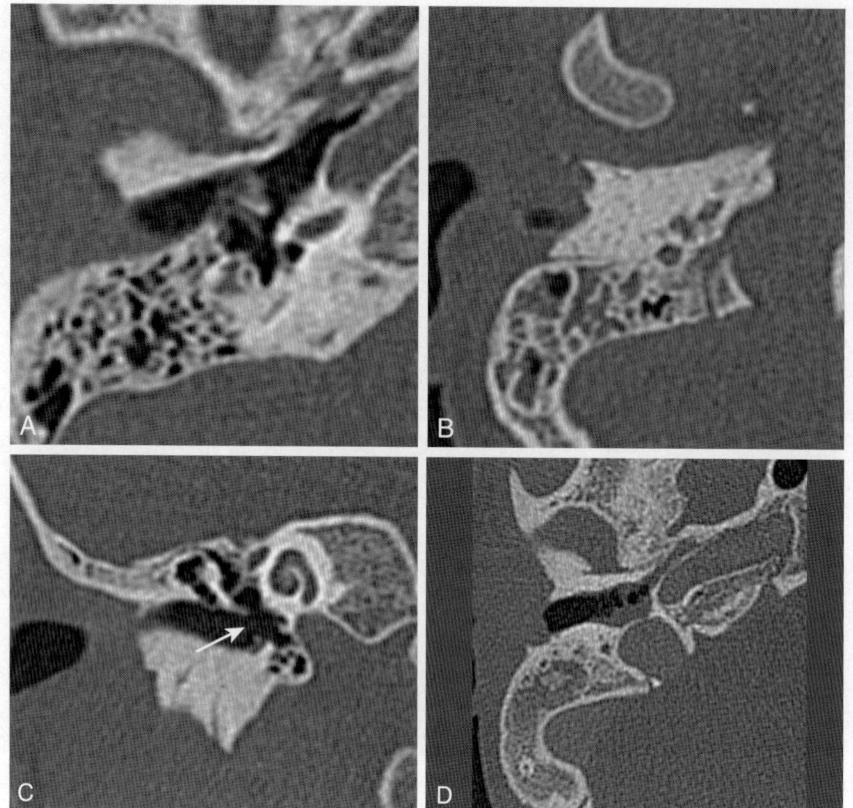

Fig. 15.33 Chronic Otitis Media. (A to C) Axial and coronal CT images demonstrate nondependent opacity in the middle ear cavity, mastoid effusion, and tympanic membrane perforation. (D) Axial CT image in a second patient with chronic otitis media demonstrates middle ear cavity fluid and mastoid sclerosis.

Key Points

Background

- Chronic otitis media is defined as otitis media persisting for >3 months from onset.
- Common signs and symptoms include persistent middle ear drainage, tympanic membrane perforation, and hearing loss (typically conductive loss).
- Pathogenesis presumed to be from bacterial pathogens including *Pseudomonas* and *Staphylococcus*, Eustachian tube dysfunction, and host immune response inflammation.
- Treated with aural antimicrobial medications and surgical options such as tympanoplasty and mastoidectomy.

Imaging

- Granulation tissue: Dependent and nondependent opacities in the middle ear that encase middle ear structures and enhances on T1+C MRI.
- Thickened and/or retracted and/or perforated tympanic membrane.
- Calcifications in the middle ear cavity or along the tympanic membrane indicative of tympanosclerosis.
- Complete or partial mastoid air cell opacification and mastoid sclerosis.
- Ossicular fixation and erosions are possible, particularly distal incus, but not a predominant feature compared to cholesteatoma.
- Associated cholesterol granuloma and acquired cholesteatoma formation.
- Differential Diagnosis: Cholesteatoma: middle ear soft tissue with bone erosions.
- Langerhans Cell Histiocytosis: imaging overlap with EAC cholesteatoma in early stages.
- Keratosis obturans: EAC soft tissue without erosion.

REFERENCES

1. Rettig E, et al. Contemporary concepts in management of acute otitis media in children. *Otolaryngol Clin N Am*. 2014;47:651–672.
2. Som PM, Curtin HD, Swartz JD, Hagiwana M. Inflammatory diseases of the temporal bone. In: Head and Neck Imaging. Vol I. 5th ed. St. Louis: Mosby Elsevier; 2011:1183–1230.

ACQUIRED CHOLESTEATOMA

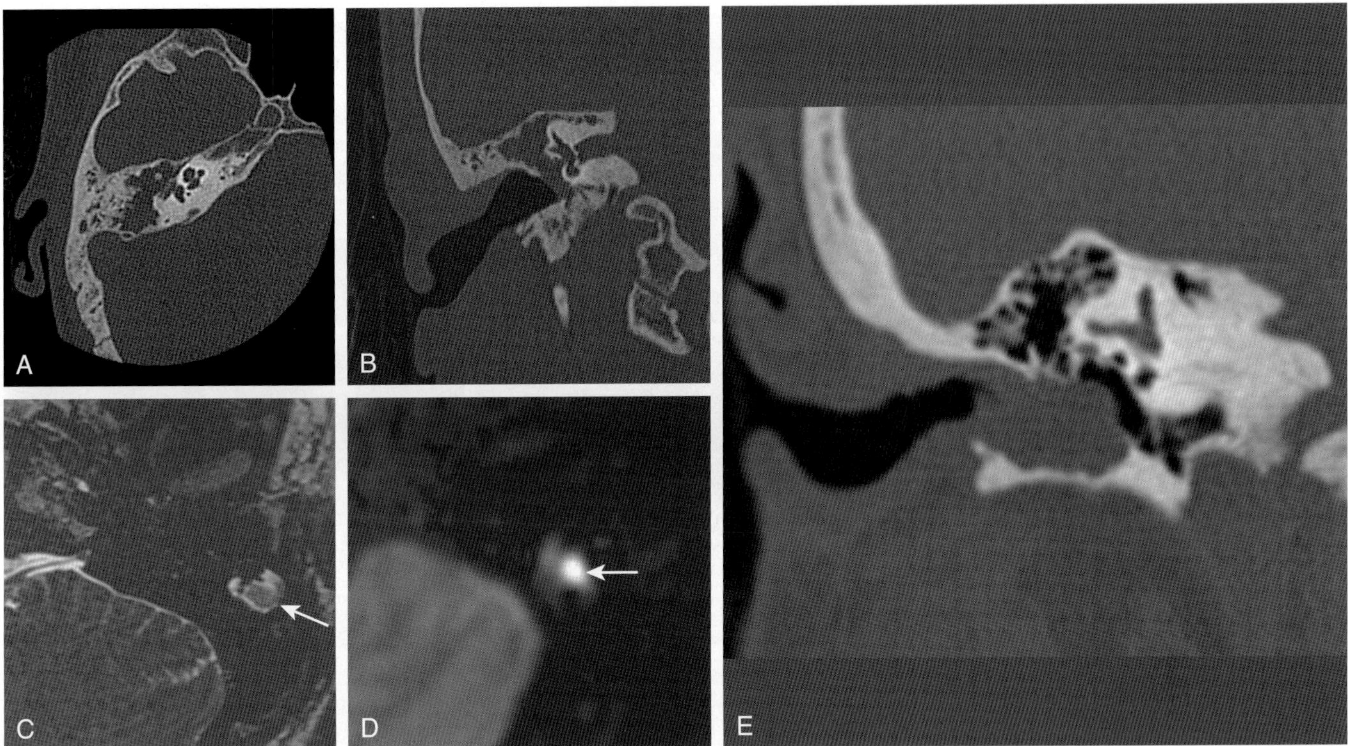

Fig. 15.34 Acquired Cholesteatoma. (A and B) Axial CT images demonstrate complete opacification of the middle ear cavity associated with erosion of the incus and majority of the malleus. Different patient: (C) Axial T2W and (D) axial DWI images demonstrate middle ear cavity fluid, T2 isointense nodule with diffusion restriction consistent with a cholesteatoma. Different patient: (E) Coronal CT image demonstrating soft tissue in the external auditory canal with erosions of the inferior wall of the external auditory canal consistent with an EAC cholesteatoma.

Key Points

Background

- Pathology: Squamous epithelium lined sac filled with keratin debris.
- Etiology presumed to be due to Eustachian tube dysfunction causing retraction pockets that disrupt normal migration of the skin on the external surface of the tympanic membrane and lead to accumulation of keratin debris.
- Acquired cholesteatomas arise from the pars flaccida or pars tensa. Can be subdivided as primary acquired cholesteatoma (when there is no prior history of otitis media) versus secondary cholesteatoma.
- Note: Congenital cholesteatomas are epidermoid cysts.

Imaging

- CT: Middle ear: Opacity involving the Prussak space and associated adjacent *erosion of ossicles* (most commonly long process of the incus), scutum, facial nerve canal, and tegmen tympani and less commonly the sigmoid plate. Lack of erosions does not exclude cholesteatoma.
- External auditory canal: EAC cholesteatoma demonstrates abnormal soft tissue thickening with *mild erosion of the osseous EAC.*
- LCH (imaging overlap), keratosis obturans (no erosion).
- MRI: Diffusion restriction, nonenhancing lesions. Recurrent cholesteatoma often imaged with MRI to differentiate granulation from cholesteatoma. Non echo-planar DWI demonstrates *diffusion restriction in recurrent cholesteatoma* (sensitivity 77%–100%, specificity 100%); detection limited to size >5 mm
- Differential Diagnosis: Chronic otitis media: no bone erosions; Langerhans Cell Histiocytosis: imaging overlap with EAC cholesteatoma in early stages; Keratosis obturans: EAC soft tissue without erosion.

REFERENCES

1. Shekdar KV, et al. Imaging of pediatric sensorineural hearing loss. *Neuroimag Clin N Am.* 2019;29:103–115.
2. Som PM, Curtin HD, Swartz JD, Hagiwana M. Inflammatory diseases of the temporal bone. In: Head and Neck Imaging. Vol I. 5th ed. St. Louis: Mosby Elsevier; 2011:1183–1230.

CHOLESTEROL GRANULOMA

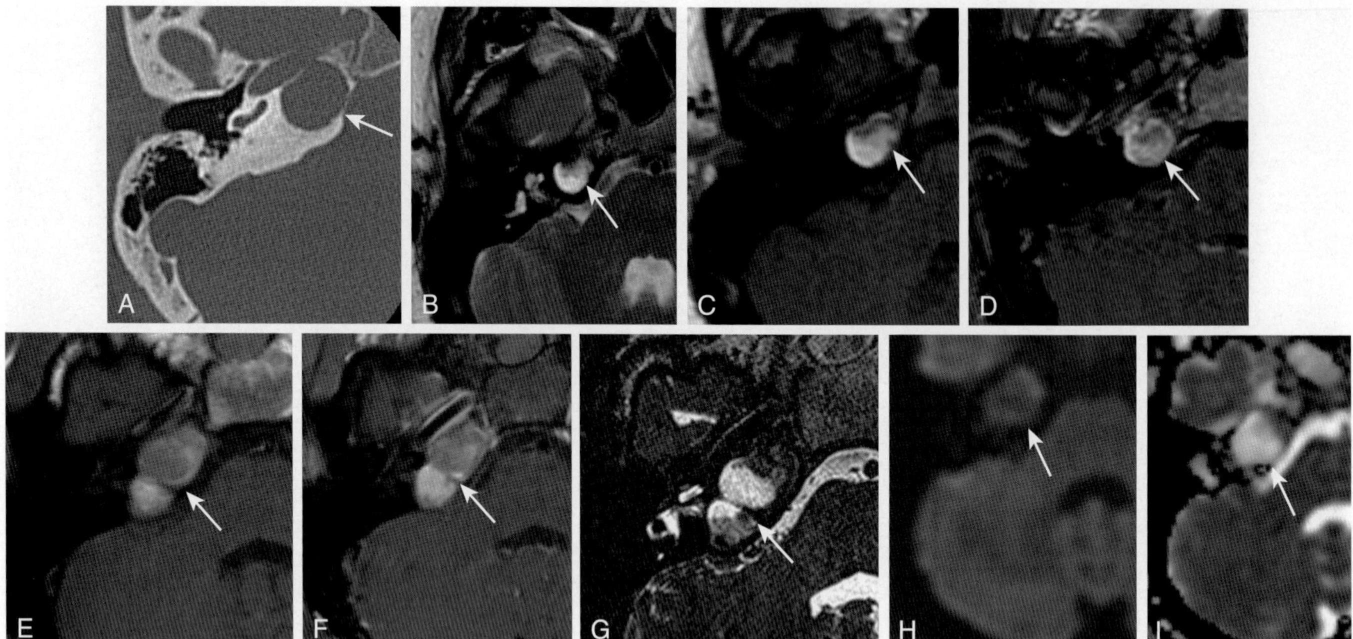

Fig. 15.35 Cholesterol Granuloma. (A to D) A 17-year-old with cholesterol granuloma. (A) Axial CT, (B) axial T2W, (C) axial T1W, and (D) axial T1W+C images demonstrate a circumscribed lytic lesion in the right petrous apex with T2 hyperintensity, T1 hyperintensity, and no enhancement consistent with a cholesterol granuloma. (E to I) A 15-year-old with cholesterol granuloma. (E) Axial T1W, (F) axial T1W+C, (G) axial T2W, (H) axial DWI, and (I) axial ADC map images demonstrate a T1 hyperintense, T2 heterogenous dumbbell-shaped lesion in the right petrous apex without enhancement and heterogeneous but nondiffusion restricting pattern consistent with a cholesterol granuloma.

Key Points

Background

- A foreign body reaction to cholesterol crystals. Poor ventilation, interference with drainage, and hemorrhage in a pneumatized space are predisposing factors to cyst formation. Negative pressure from air resorption leads to degradation of blood and cholesterol crystal formation.
- Can be found in the middle ear cavity and petrous apex.
- Typically arises from a pneumatized petrous apex (~10% of the population has a pneumatized petrous apex).
- Often asymptomatic and incidentally discovered by imaging. Can also present with hearing loss and headache. Surgical treatment depending on symptoms.

Imaging

- The combination of CT and MRI provides complementary diagnostic findings.
- CT: *Well-defined benign-appearing expansile lytic lesion in the petrous apex.*
- MRI: *T1 hyperintense*, T2 hyperintense and hypointense signal, *nonenhancing.*
- May expand and compromise the carotid canal, cavernous sinus, or cerebellopontine angle.
- Differential Diagnosis:
  - Chondrosarcoma: aggressive bone destruction
  - Petrous apicitis: nonexpansile enhancement
  - Mucocele: simple fluid signal (T1 hypointense, T2 hyperintense)
  - Petrous apex effusion: simple fluid, no expansion
  - Asymmetric pneumatization: fat signal on all sequences
  - Aneurysm: flow artifact
  - Metastasis: aggressive bone lucency or sclerosis

REFERENCE

1. Gore MR, et al. Cholesterol granuloma of the petrous apex. *Otolaryngol Clin N Am.* 2011;44:1043–1058.

LABYRINTHITIS OSSIFICANS

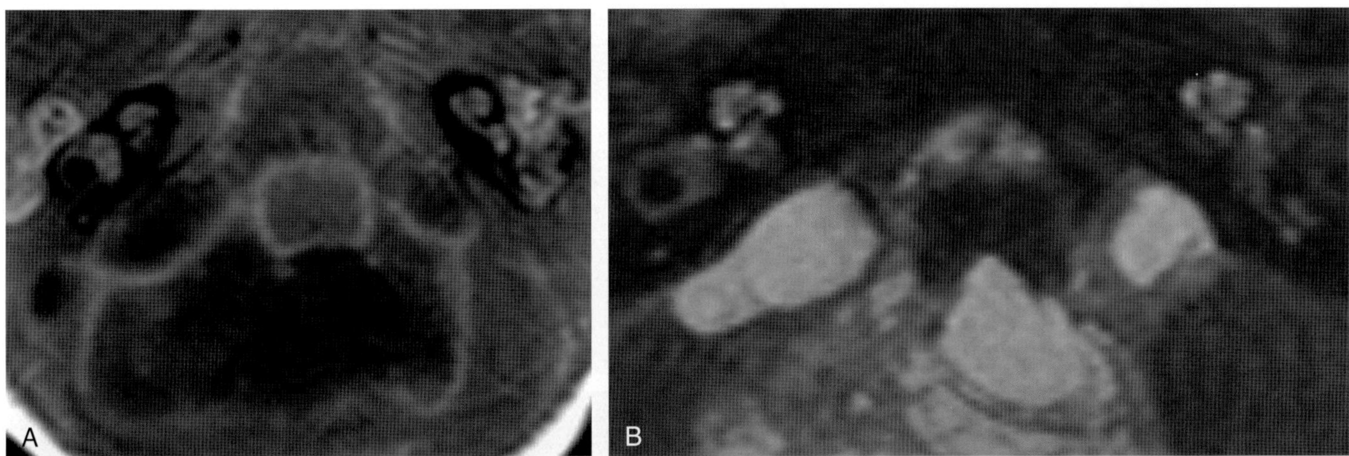

Fig. 15.36 **Labyrinthitis Ossificans.** (A and B) Axial T1W+C and (C) axial T2W images demonstrate abnormal enhancement and loss of normal T2 hyperintensity in the cochlea, vestibule, and semicircular canals consistent with acute labyrinthitis ossificans due to bacterial meningitis as indicated by abnormal leptomeningeal enhancement and arachnoid fluid loculations.

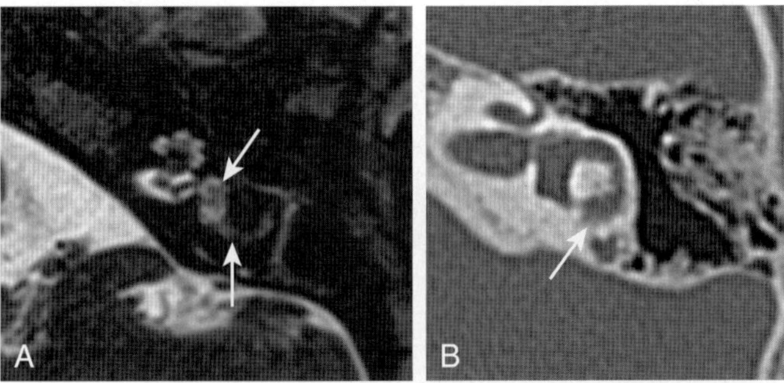

Fig. 15.37 **Labyrinthitis Ossificans.** (A) Axial T2W and (B) axial CT images demonstrate loss of fluid signal in the vestibule and semicircular canals (*arrows*) and abnormal ill-defined lucency along the margin of the lateral semicircular canal but without ossification (*arrow*).

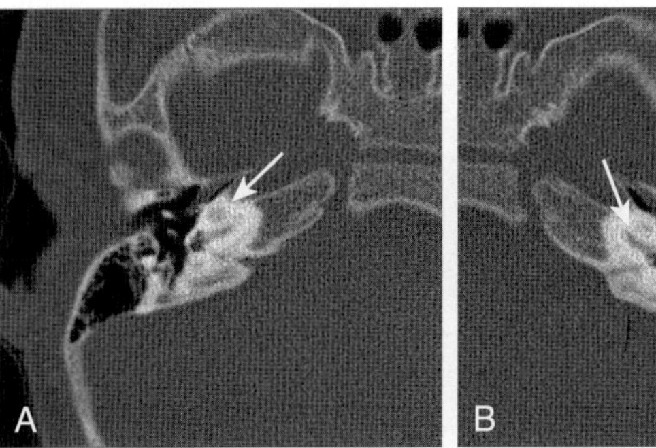

FIG. 15.38 **Labyrinthitis Ossificans.** (A and B) Axial CT images demonstrate ossification of the cochlea bilaterally (*arrows*).

Key Points

Background

- Hearing loss following meningitis is the most common cause of acquired bilateral sensorineural hearing loss (SNHL) in children.
- Most commonly the sequela of bacterial meningitis, most commonly *S. pneumoniae*. Bacteria enter the inner ear via the cochlear aqueduct.
- Cochlear implantation must be before ossification occurs and the implant can no longer pass through the ossification

Imaging

- Acute/subacute stage:
    - CT may be normal. Can also demonstrate lucency in the bone adjacent to the inner ear structures.
    - MRI demonstrates *inner ear enhancement.* MRI enhancement of inner ear structure demonstrates 61% sensitivity and 96% specificity for prediction of sensorineural hearing loss in infants with bacterial meningitis.
- Late stage:
    - CT demonstrates ossification of inner ear structures.
    - MRI demonstrates loss of fluid signal in the inner ear structures.

REFERENCES

1. Shekdar KV, et al. Imaging of pediatric sensorineural hearing loss. *Neuroimag Clin N Am.* 2019;29:103–115.
2. Orman G, et al. Accuracy of MR Imaging for detection of sensorineural hearing loss in infants with bacterial meningitis. *Am J Neuroradiol.* 2020 May.

CHRONIC RECURRENT MULTIFOCAL OSTEOMYELITIS

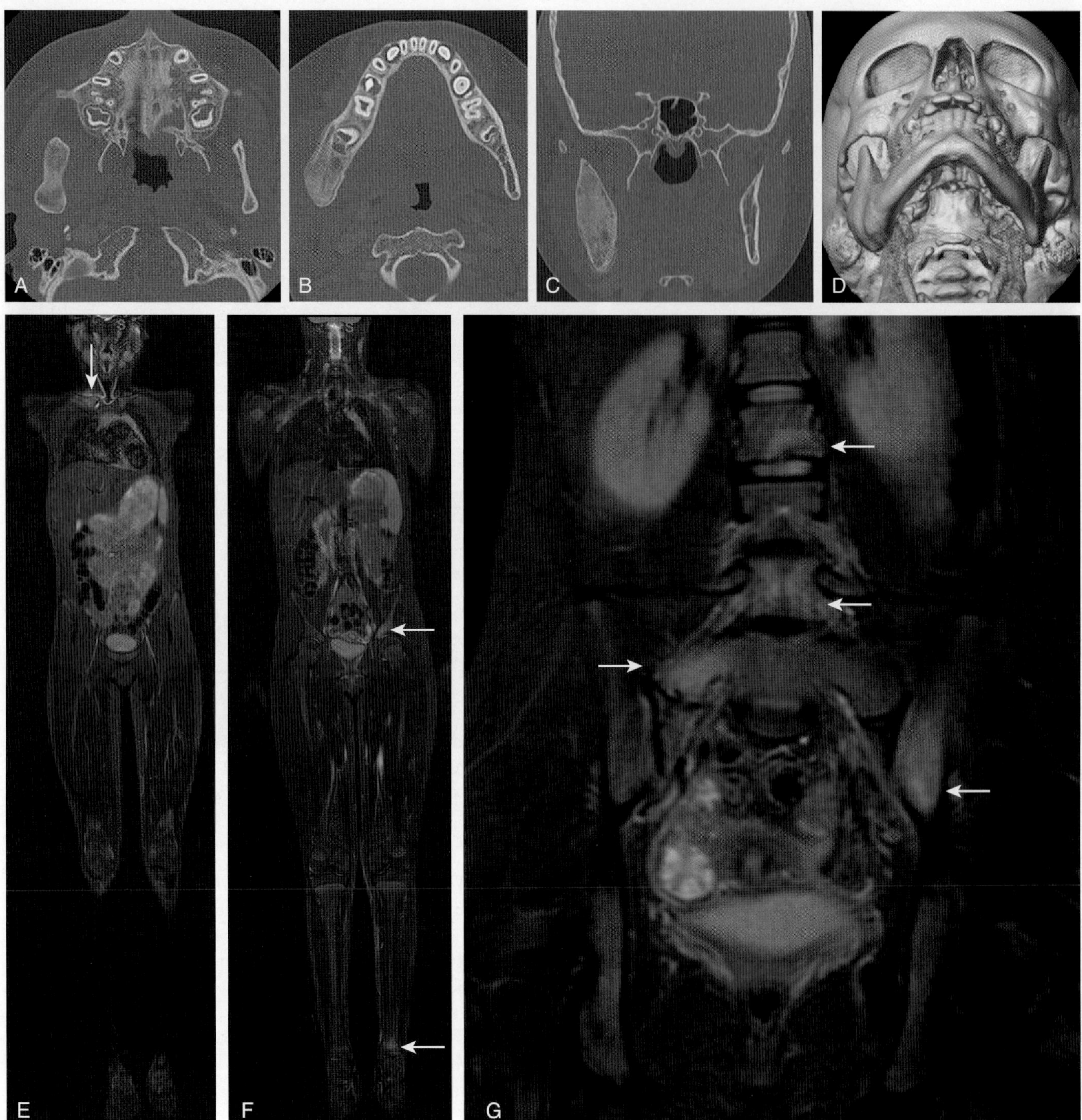

Fig. 15.39 CRMO. (A to D) Axial, coronal, and 3D volumetric CT images of the face demonstrate abnormal expansion and sclerosis in the right side of the mandible. (E to G) Whole-body STIR MR images demonstrate multifocal STIR hyperintensities in the bones including the right clavicle, left iliac, left distal tibia, right sacral ala, and L3 and L5 vertebral bodies (*arrows*).

Key Points

Background

- An idiopathic sterile inflammatory disorder with relapsing and remitting course.
- Clinical:
  - Average age of onset is 9 to 10 years. Female:male ratio 2:1.
  - Pain, swelling, reduced range of motion.
  - Most children appear well; systemic symptoms such fever, weight loss, and lethargy are less common.
  - Most commonly affects multiples bones (70%). Symmetric involvement in 60%.
  - Can result in vertebral fracture, deformity, and growth asymmetry.
  - Can recur at the initial site or develop at a remote site.
  - Elevated ESR, elevated CRP, and normal WBC count.
  - Coexisting inflammatory or autoimmune diseases in 25% can include dermatologic (e.g., psoriasis) and gastrointestinal (ulcerative colitis, Crohn disease) disorders.
- Biopsy required to exclude infection or malignancy. Biopsy specimens demonstrate inflammatory changes with granulocytic infiltration.
- Treatment: NSAIDs are used as first-line therapy. Methotrexate, TNF inhibitors, and bisphosphonates are second-line therapy.
- Disease monitored by pain symptoms, ESR and CRP levels, and imaging.
- Prognosis: 40% clinical remission after 1 to 5 years of follow-up. 50% recurrence rate. Risk factors for severe disease and poor outcome include male sex, multifocal disease, extra-rheumatologic disease, family history of associated disease, and CRP >1 mg/dL.

Imaging

- Most commonly involves the *metaphyses* of the long bones, *medial clavicles*, *mandible*, feet, pelvis, and spine
- *Whole-body MRI* used to assess all sites of disease
- MRI: Marrow edema, periosteal fluid, soft tissue inflammation
- CT: Range of appearance from lytic, to mixed lytic and sclerotic, to pure sclerosis and hyperostosis

REFERENCES

1. Zhao Y, et al. Chronic nonbacterial osteomyelitis and chronic recurrent multifocal osteomyelitis in children. *Pediatr Clin N Am.* 2018;65:783–800.
2. Khanna G, et al. Imaging of chronic recurrent multifocal osteomyelitis. *Radiographics.* 2009;29:1159–1177.

JUVENILE IDIOPATHIC ARTHRITIS

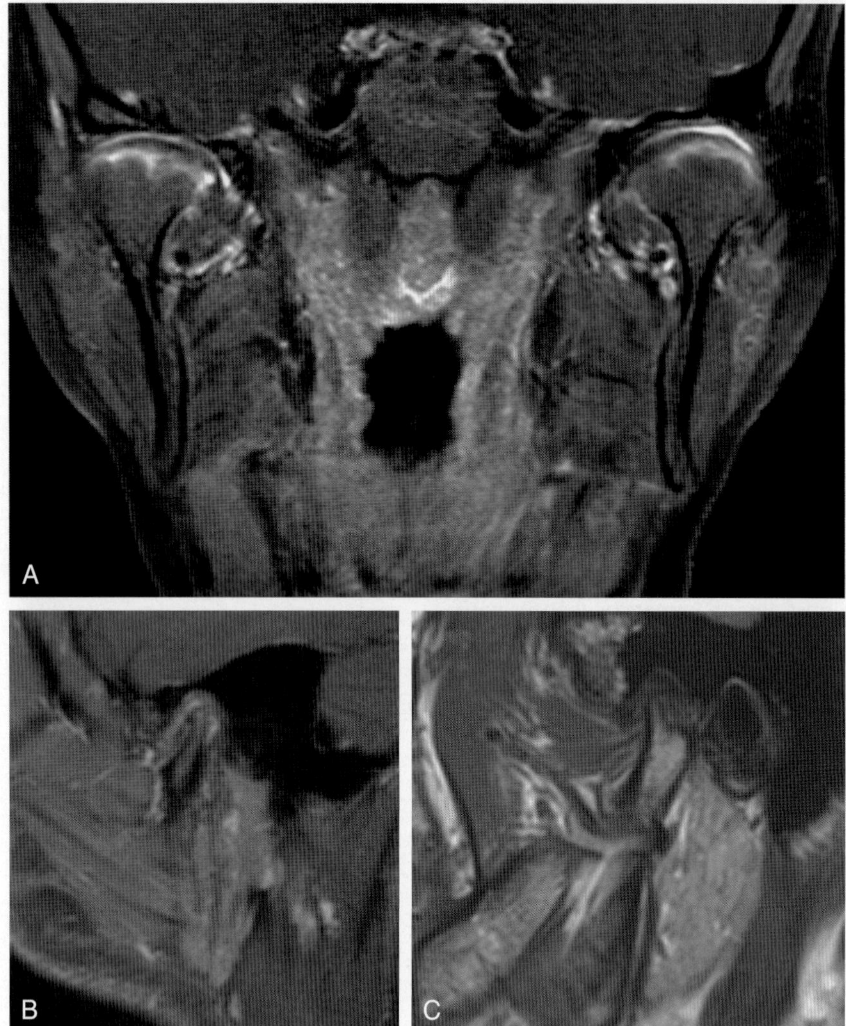

Fig. 15.40 Juvenile Idiopathic Arthritis. (A) Coronal T1W+C fat saturation, (B) sagittal T1W+C fat saturation, and (C) sagittal T1W images demonstrate abnormal synovial enhancement, condylar head bone marrow enhancement, and condylar head erosion.

Key Points

Background

- JIA is an immune-mediated inflammatory arthropathy.
- The temporomandibular joint (TMJ) is one of the most commonly involved joints in JIA, involved in 50% to 80% of children with JIA.
- Clinical symptoms include jaw pain, difficulty chewing, reduced range of motion, and morphologic changes to mandibular growth.
- Clinical symptoms and physical exam are limited for determining TMJ involvement. 71% of JIA patients with active TMJ synovitis were asymptomatic.
- TMJ JIA is often present at the beginning of JIA disease and may follow a clinical course that is independent from the other joints involved and systemic JIA treatment.

Imaging

- MRI is the modality of choice
- MRI protocols typically include coronal T1W, oblique sagittal proton density (open and closed mouth positions), T2W fat saturation or STIR, T1W, and T1W+C fat saturation images.
- MRI findings: *Synovial enhancement*, *condylar erosion* or deformity, condylar head bone marrow edema, secondary osteoarthritis, ramus shortening, *joint effusion*, and articular disc tear.
- CT findings: Less sensitive for findings of JIA; *condylar erosion* is the primary finding.

REFERENCE

1. Navallas M, et al. MR imaging of the temporomandibular joint in juvenile idiopathic arthritis: technique and findings. *Radiographics*. 2017 Mar–Apr;37(2):595–612.

16 Spine Malformations

SPINE MALFORMATION: EMBRYOLOGY AND APPROACH

Spine Embryology

The formation of the spine occurs from the second to sixth weeks of gestation through:

- Gastrulation (weeks 2–3): conversion of a bilaminar to trilaminar layer with the middle layer of the mesoderm.
- Primary neurulation (weeks 3–4): the notochord interacts with the overlying ectoderm to form the neural plate (Fig. 16.1A). The neural plate then bends to begin formation of the neural tube (Fig. 16.1B). Continued infolding of neural plate (Fig. 16.1C). Disjunction is the separation of the neural tube from the ectoderm (Fig. 16.1D).
- Secondary neurulation and retrogressive differentiation.
- Spinal dysraphisms occur when these processes are disrupted.

Classification of Spinal Dysraphisms and Imaging Approach

Spinal dysraphisms can be classified by embryologic anomaly (Box 16.1). This classification is important; however, an imaging algorithm as follows is more clinically useful (Fig. 16.2):

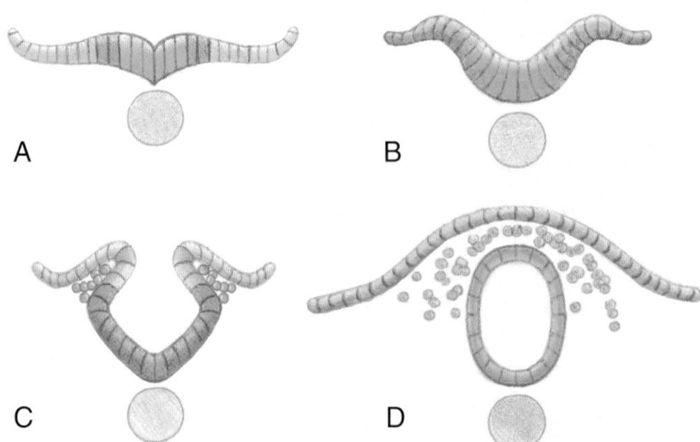

Fig. 16.1 Primary Neurulation (Weeks 3–4). The notochord interacts with the overlying ectoderm to form the neural plate (A). The neural plate then bends to begin formation of the neural tube (B). Continued infolding of neural plate (C). Disjunction is the separation of the neural tube from the ectoderm (D).

BOX 16.1
Embryologic Classification of Spinal Dysraphisms

Gastrulation Disorder

Midline notochord integration disorder:
- Dorsal enteric fistula
- Neurenteric cyst
- Diastematomyelia
- Dermal sinus tract

Notochord formation disorder:
- Caudal regression
- Segmental spinal dysgenesis

Primary Neurulation Disorder

Myelomeningocele
Myelocele
Lipomyelomeningocele
Lipomyelocele
Intradural lipoma
Nonterminal myelocystocele

Secondary Neurulation and Retrogressive Differentiation Disorder

Filar lipoma
Tight filum terminale
Terminal ventricle
Terminal myelocystocele

Unknown Origin

Meningocele

- Determine whether the malformation is exposed to the skin to determine whether the malformation is a closed or open defect.
- Determine whether there is a subcutaneous mass or not.
- Determine the necessary imaging features for final diagnosis.

This section will demonstrate the many types of spinal malformations, associated findings, and other genetic disorders that are associated with spinal malformations.

REFERENCE

1. Huisman TA, Rossi A, Tortori-Donati P. MR imaging of neonatal spinal dysraphia: what to consider?. *Magn Reson Imaging Clin N Am.* 2012 Feb;20(1):45–61.

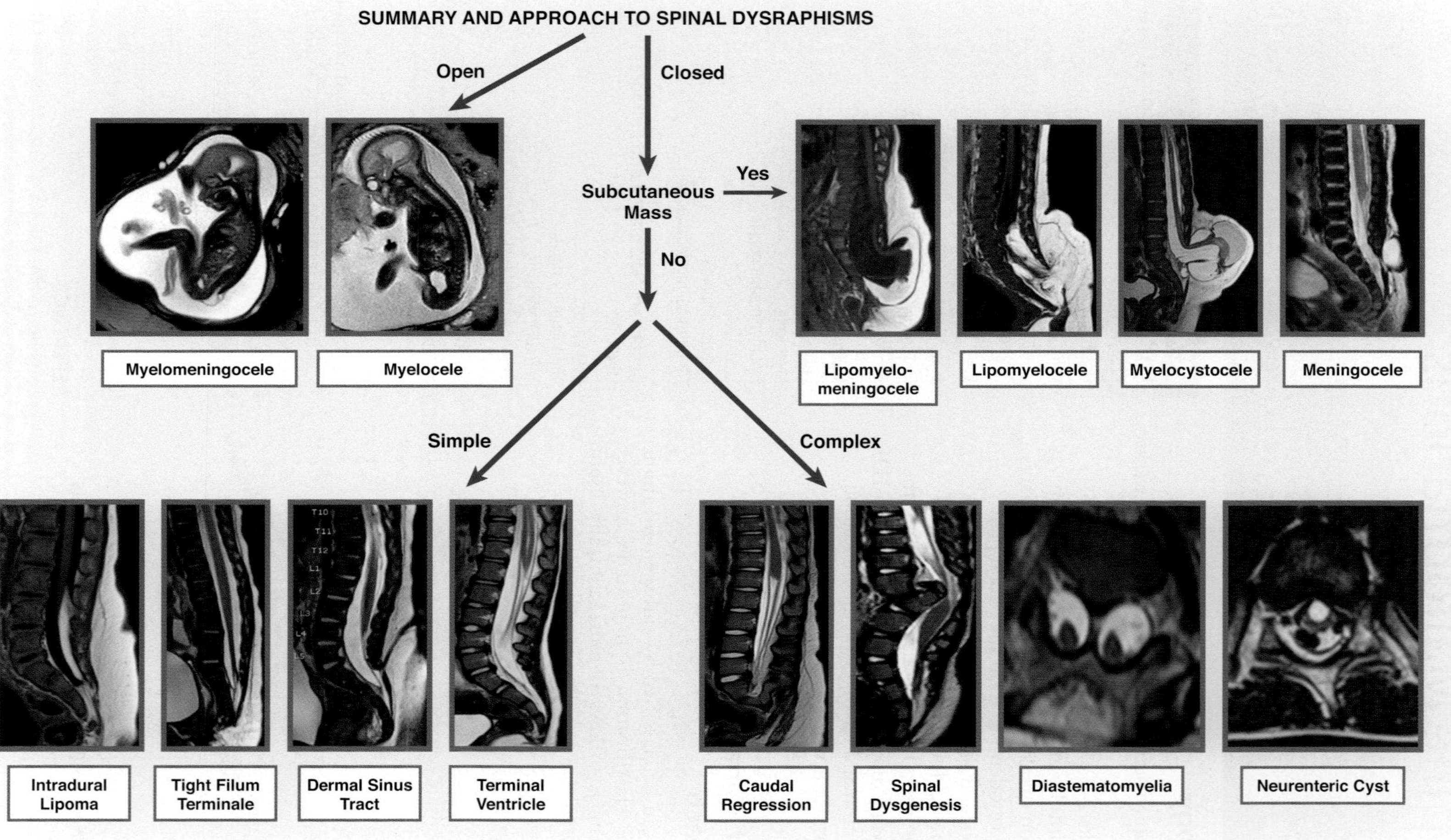

Fig. 16.2 Imaging Approach to Spinal Dysraphisms.

MYELOMENINGOCELE

OPEN Dysraphism

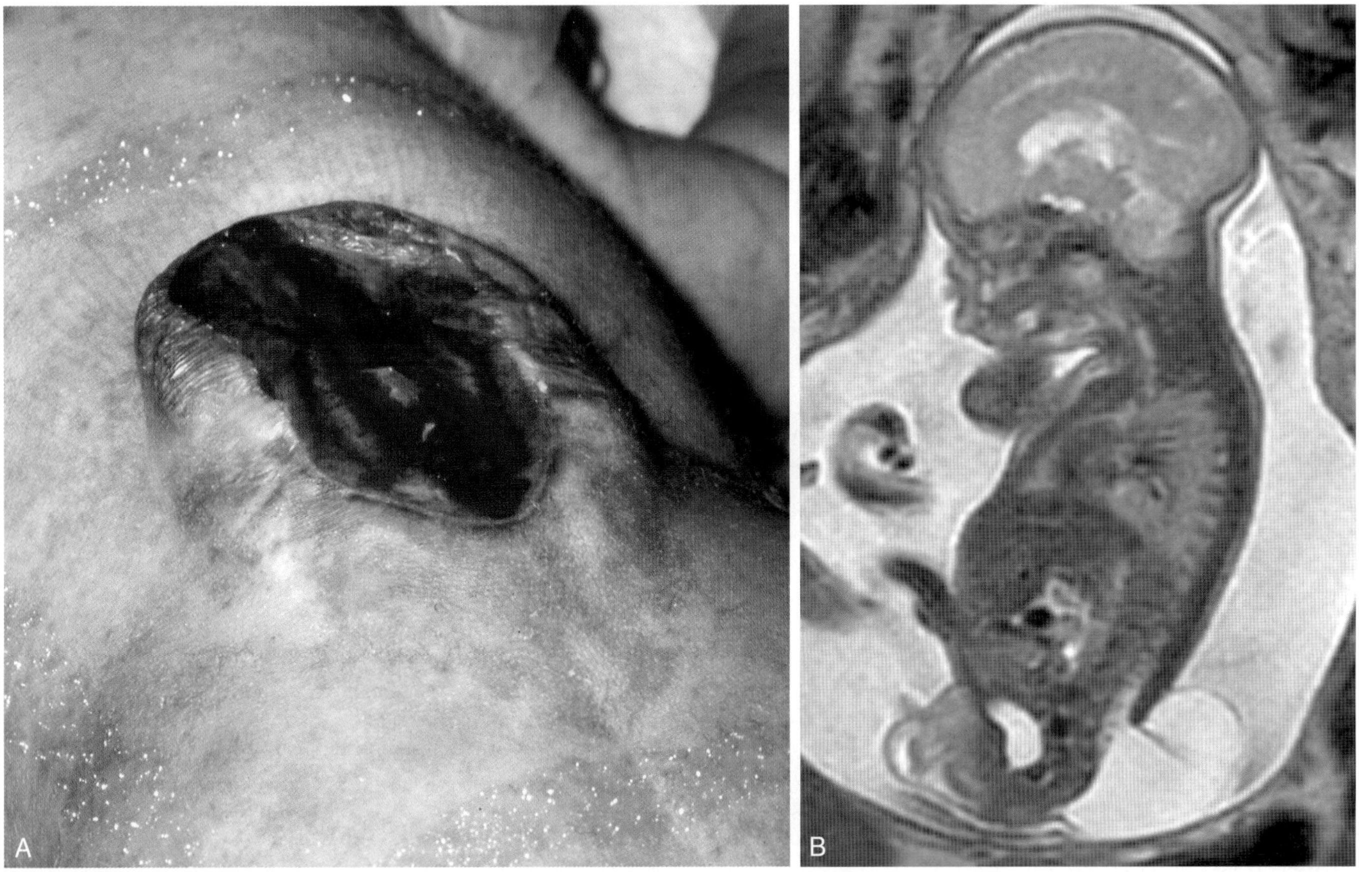

Fig. 16.3 **Myelomeningocele.** (A) Clinical photo of the open spinal dysraphism. (B) Sagittal T2W fetal MR image demonstrating the lumbosacral myelomeningocele sac, small posterior fossa, and ventriculomegaly. (A courtesy of Dr. William Whitehead.)

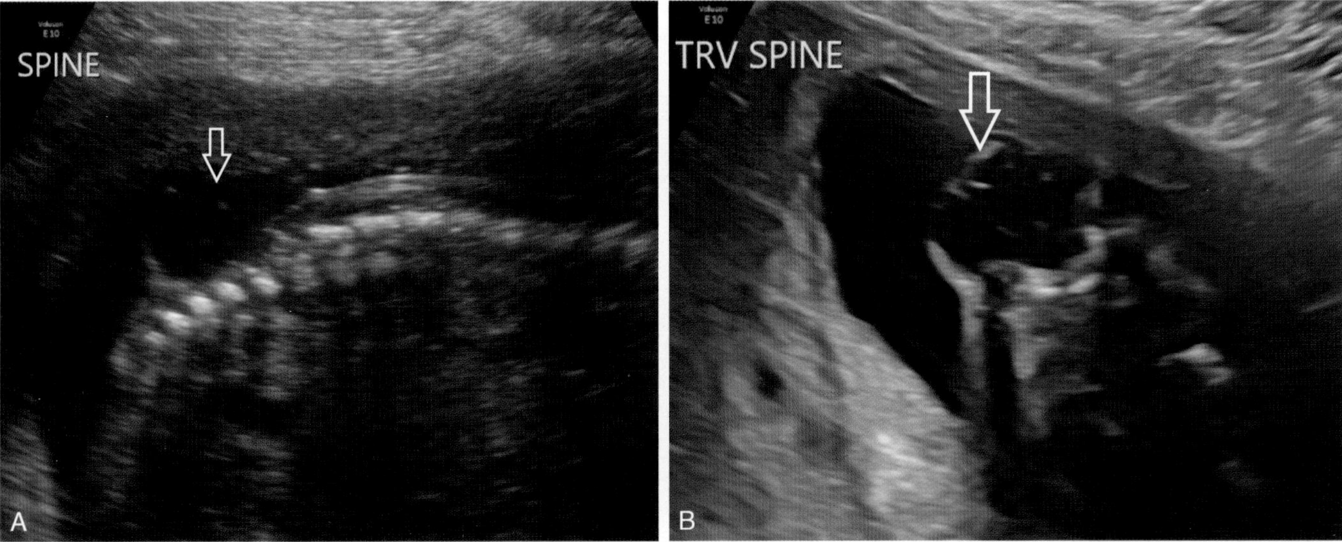

Fig. 16.4 **Myelomeningocele.** (A and B) Sagittal and axial fetal ultrasound images demonstrating the lumbosacral fluid-filled hypoechoic myelomeningocele sac.

MYELOCELE

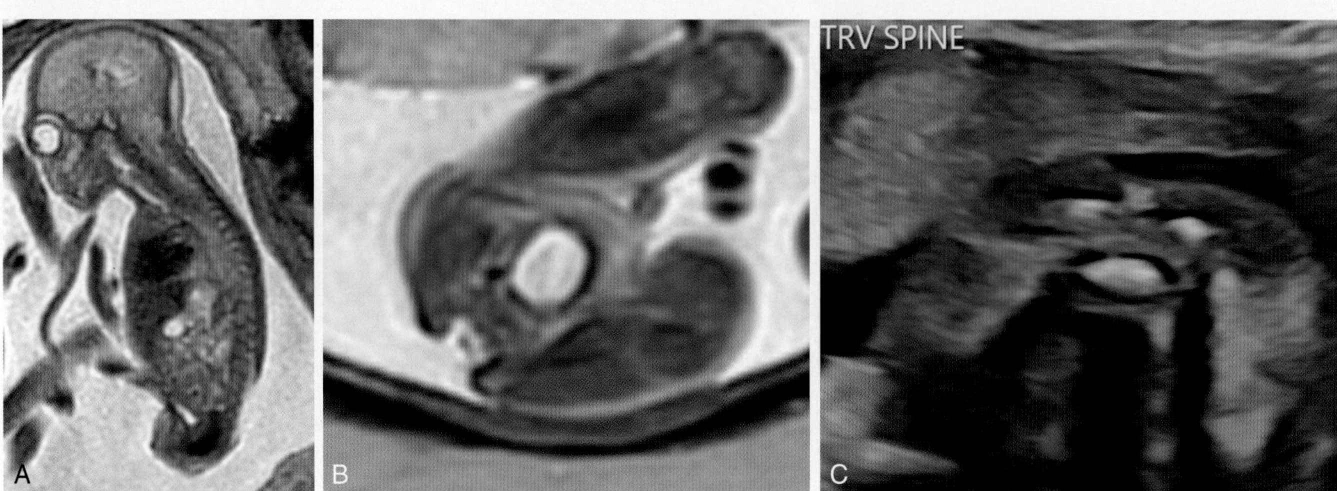

Fig. 16.5 Myelocele. (A and B) Sagittal T2W images demonstrate open spinal dysraphism in the lumbar and sacral spine without a sac. (C) Transverse ultrasound image demonstrates an open defect and hyperechoic neural placode at the skin surface without a sac.

Key Points

Background

- Also known as myeloschisis
- A myelocystocle is an open spinal dysraphism similar to myelomeningocele but differs from a myelomeningocele in that the exposed neural placode is flush with the skin and there is no herniating sac
- Myeloceles account for ~30% of open spinal dysraphisms
- Clinical implications of a myelocele as compared to a myelomeningocele have not been fully evaluated. One study has shown that myeloceles were more positively correlated with independent ambulation after prenatal repair compared to myelomeningocele.

Imaging

- Open neural tube defect with neural placode at the skin surface and no sac.
- On fetal MRI, myeloceles are associated with higher Chiari 2 grade (i.e effaced 4th ventricle and cisterna magna).

REFERENCE

1. Nagaraj UD, Bierbrauer KS, Stevenson CB, Peiro JL, Lim FY, Zhang B, Kline-Fath BM. Myelomeningocele versus myelocele on fetal MR images: are there differences in brain findings? *AJR Am J Roentgenol.* 2018 Dec;211(6):1376–1380.

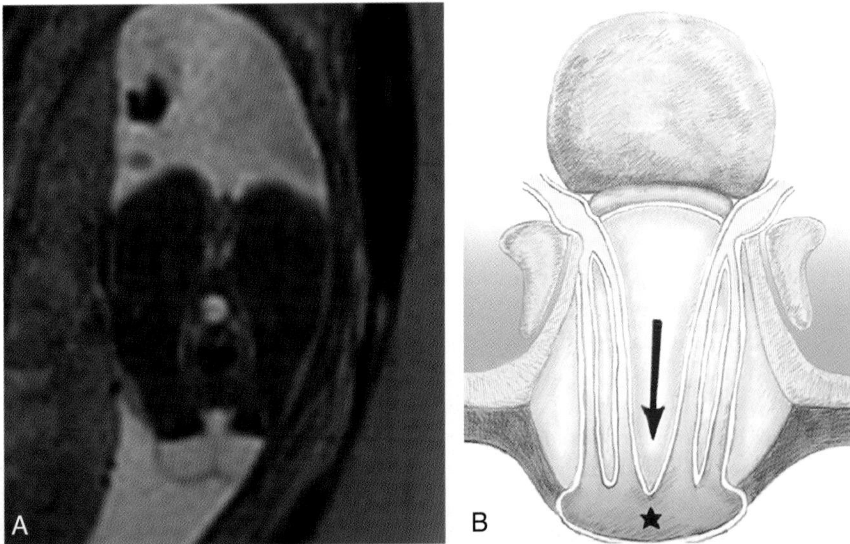

Fig. 16.6 Myelomeningocele. (A) Axial T2W fetal MRI of a lumbar MMC. (B) Illustration of an MMC seen as an open spinal dysraphism, herniated neural placode exposed at the skin surface.

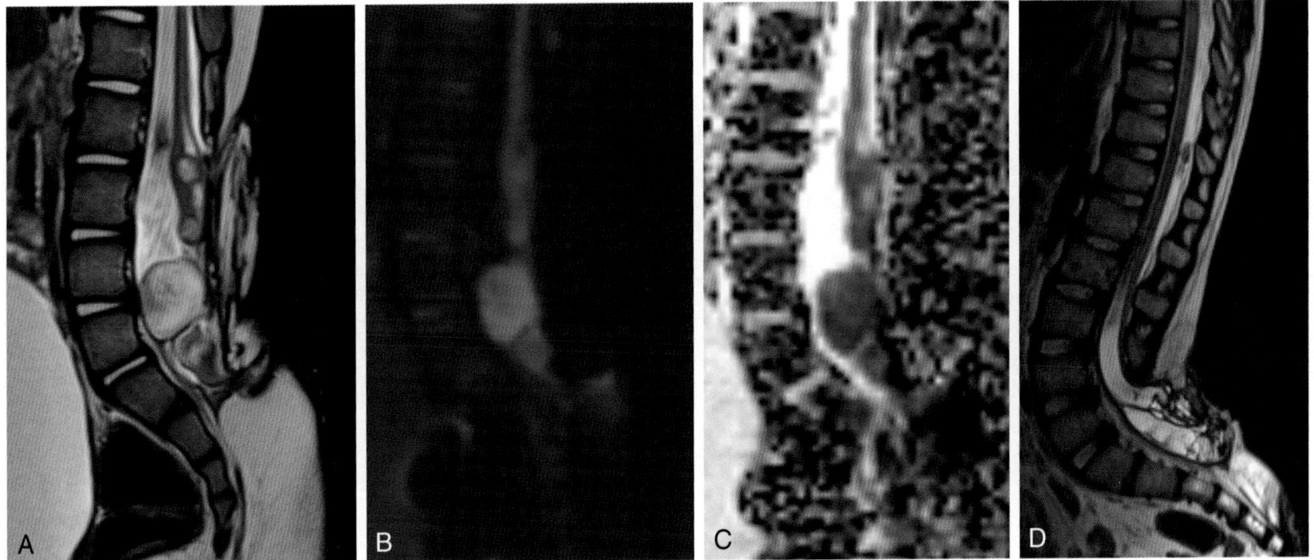

Fig. 16.7 Myelomeningocele: Post-surgical Findings. (A) Sagittal T2W, (B) sagittal DWI, and (C) sagittal ADC images in a 22-month-old patient with a surgically repaired lumbosacral myelomeningocele demonstrate rounded intradural masses with diffusion restriction indicative of epidermoid cysts which tether the spinal cord. (D) Sagittal 3D T2W image in a different patient with a previously repaired lumbosacral myelomeningocele with several intrathecal adhesions in the distal thecal sac. Adhesions, epidermoids, and syringohydromyelia are common findings in surgically repaired myelomeningoceles.

Key Points

Background

- *Open spinal dysraphism* and *primary neurulation* disorder due to failure of closure of the neural tube and nondisjunction.
- Neurological disabilities: paraplegia, incontinence, sexual dysfunction, skeletal deformities, pulmonary hypoplasia, breech position.
- The presumed etiology is multifactorial. Folate administration during pregnancy reduces incidence.
- Elevated amniotic fluid alpha-fetoprotein and acetylcholinesterase.
- Fetal/intrauterine surgery may limit neural placode injury, preventing/limiting the intrauterine "dual hit" injury of the exposed neural placode. Compared to postnatal repair, in utero repair is associated with decreased CSF shunting, less hindbrain herniation, and improved lower extremity motor function.

Imaging

- Accounts for ~70% of open spinal dysraphisms.
- An open/non-skin covered spinal dysraphism in which the neural placode and meninges herniate outside the spinal canal.
- Post-operative myelomeningoceles are associated with intrathecal adhesions, epidermoid cyst, and syrinx.
- Associated with *Chiari 2 malformation.*
- Differentiation of open spinal dysraphisms from closed spinal dysraphisms on fetal ultrasound and MRI can be challenging. The subcutaneous fat cannot always be differentiated from the neural placode on ultrasound and the expected T1W hyperintensity from fat in the defect is not reliably seen on MRI. Several reported imaging findings have been reported to help differentiate open vs closed spinal dysraphism as follows:
  - The wall thickness of the myelomeningocele sac was found to be thinner (0.7+/−0.6 mm) than with closed spinal dysraphisms (2.9+/−1.3 mm).
  - Continuity of the skin and subcutanoues tissues with the wall of the herniating sac or defect was seen in 94% of closed dysraphisms compared to 5% of open dysraphisms.
  - The lack of Chiari 2 malformation may also indicate a closed spinal dysraphism. Severe hindbrain herniation was seen in 6% of closed spinal dysraphisms compared to 82% with open spinal dysraphisms.
  - Ventriculomegaly was only present in 12.5% of closed spinal dysraphisms compared to 86% with open spinal dysraphisms.
  - Lastly, the clivus-supraoccipit angle was found to be larger (75 degrees +/−11 degrees) compared to open dysraphisms (53 degrees +/−10 degrees).
- Larger volumes of the myelomeningocele sac are associated with lower Chiari 2 grades (i.e. less effacement of the fourth ventricle and cisterna magna) but did not correlate with ventricular size or clubfoot. Larger areas of skin defect are associated with larger volumes of the lateral ventricles but did not correlate with the Chairi 2 grade or clubfoot.
- Myelomeningoceles repaired in utero demonstrate less hindbrain herniation on follow-up imaging. Intraventricular hemorrhage can be seen on both preoperative and post-operative fetal MRI.
- Hydrocephalus occurs in ~80%. Following in utero repair of a myelomeningocele the ventricles can increase in size on a follow up fetal MRI, however ultimately there is a postnatal decrease the incidence of hydrocephalus. Larger ventricular size on fetal MRI in open spinal dysraphisms has been shown to correlate with increased reuqirement of postnatal shunt placement.
- All myelomeningoceles are tethered by imaging, however the tethered cord syndrome occurs in 3–32% indicating the requirement of associated symptoms and urodynamic studies for evaluation. Tethering occurs as the spinal canal lengthens and due to adhesions. In utero repair is associated with equal or greater risk of tethered cord syndrome and greater risk of epidermoid cyst formation compared to postnatal repair. Retethering occurs at ~ 5–9 years of age which is the time of rapid growth of the spine. Patients with a conus position at or below S1 have poorer outcomes after detethering.

REFERENCES

1. Grimme JD, Castillo M. Congenital anomalies of the spine. *Neuro-imaging Clin N Am.* 2007 Feb;17(1):1–16.
2. Nagaraj UD, Bierbrauer KS, Peiro JL, Kline-Fath BM. Differentiating closed versus open spinal dysraphisms on fetal MRI. *AJR Am J Roentgenol.* 2016 Dec;207(6):1316–1323.
3. Woitek R, Dvorak A, Weber M, Seidl R, Bettelheim D, Schöpf V, Amann G, Brugger PC, Furtner J, Asenbaum U, Prayer D, Kasprian G. MR-based morphometry of the posterior fossa in fetuses with neural tube defects of the spine. *PLoS One.* 2014 Nov 13;9(11):e112585.

LIPOMYELOMENINGOCELE

CLOSED Dysraphism
Presence of a
Subcutaneous mass

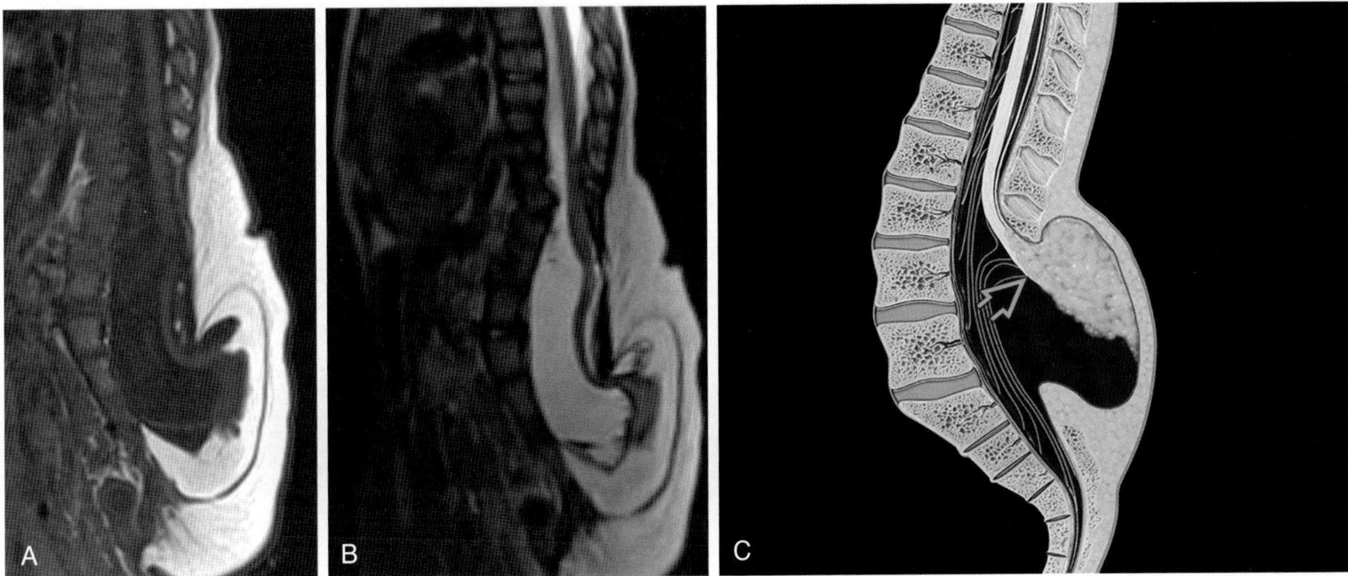

Fig. 16.8 Lipomyelomeningocele. (A) Sagittal T1W and (B) sagittal T2W images demonstrating a skin covered spinal dysraphism in the lumbosacral spine with herniation of the spinal cord and meninges outside the spinal canal that terminates on the enlarged subcutaneous fat. (C) Illustration of a lipomyelomeningocele demonstrating the herniation of spinal cord and meninges terminating on fat outside the spinal canal (*arrow*). (C from Ross JS, Moore KR. *Diagnostic Imaging: Spine*. Philadelphia: Elsevier; 2021.)

Key Points

Background

- Skin covered *closed spinal dysraphism* and *primary neurulation* disorder caused by premature disjunction of neural ectoderm from the cutaneous ectoderm while the overlying ectoderm closes, allowing mesodermal precursors to gain access to the central core of the open/nonclosed neural tube, enhancing the development of a coexisting lipoma
- The neural placode attaches outside the confines of the spinal canal onto fat which is in continuity with the enlarged subcutaneous fat.
- Clinical: Patients present with tethered cord signs and symptoms. Bladder dysfunction usually occurs first around 2 years of age followed by motor and sensory dysfunction by the teenage years. Progressive neurologic dysfunction occurs without detethering and there is limited recovery if detethering is performed after symptom progression.

Imaging

- Herniation of spinal cord and meninges *outside* the spinal canal and attached to the lipoma that is in continuity with the prominent or mass-like subcutaneous fat
- Associated with syrinx, diastematomyelia, spinal segmentation anomaly, caudal regression, and anorectal and genitourinary malformations

REFERENCES

1. Grimme JD, Castillo M. Congenital anomalies of the spine. *Neuroimaging Clin N Am.* 2007 Feb;17(1):1–16.
2. Huisman TA, Rossi A, Tortori-Donati P. MR imaging of neonatal spinal dysraphia: what to consider? *Magn Reson Imaging Clin N Am.* 2012 Feb;20(1):45–61.

LIPOMYELOMENINGOCELE

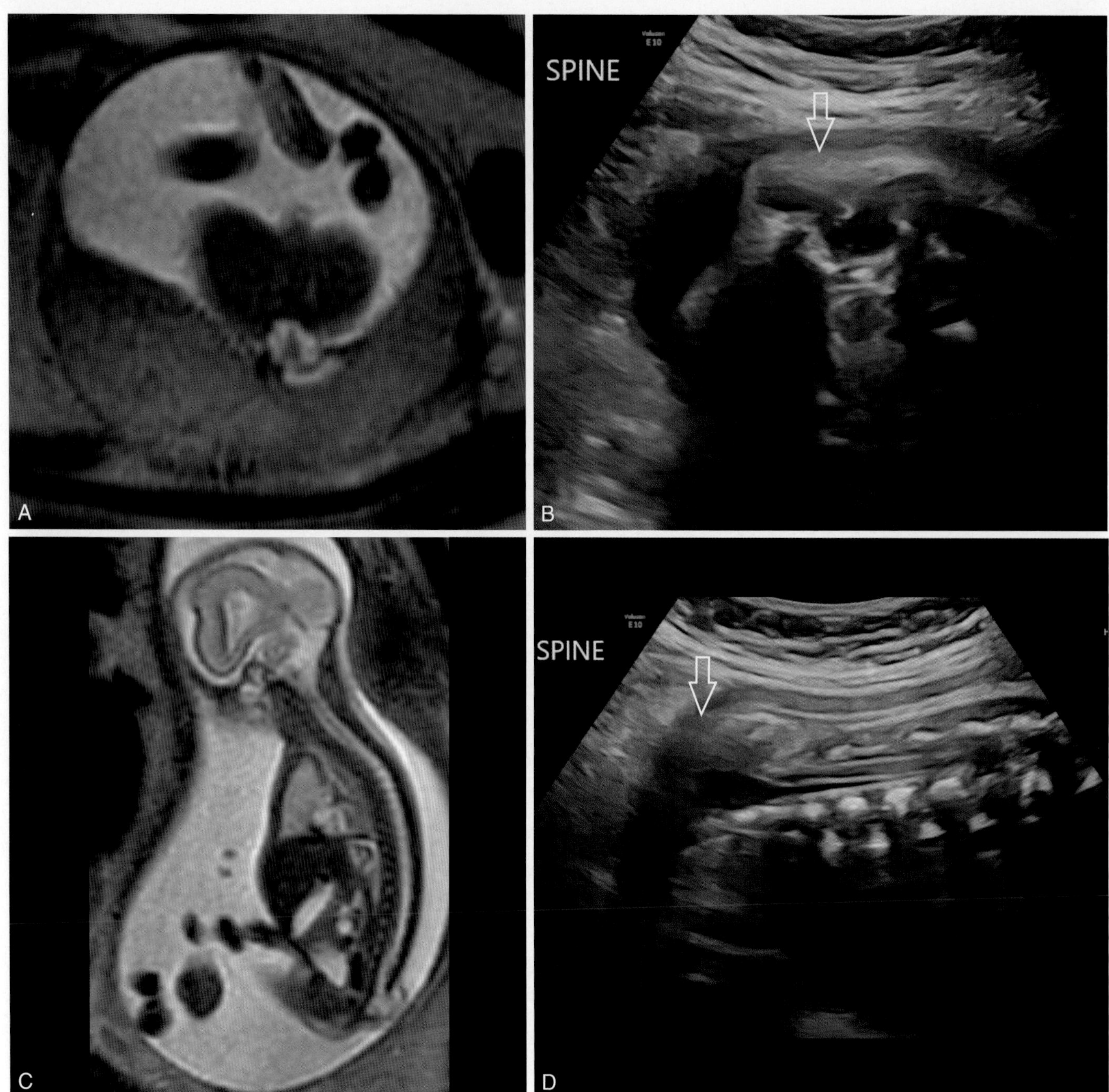

Fig. 16.9 Lipomyelomeningocele. (A and C) Axial and sagittal T2W fetal MR images and (B and D) transverse and sagittal ultrasound images demonstrating a skin covered spinal dysraphism in the lumbosacral spine with herniation of spinal cord and meninges outside the spinal canal that terminates on the hyperechoic subcutaneous fat (*arrows*). The diagnosis is more apparent on the ultrasound, indicating a complementary role of ultrasound and MRI.

LIPOMYELOCELE

CLOSED Dysraphism
Presence of a
Subcutaneous mass

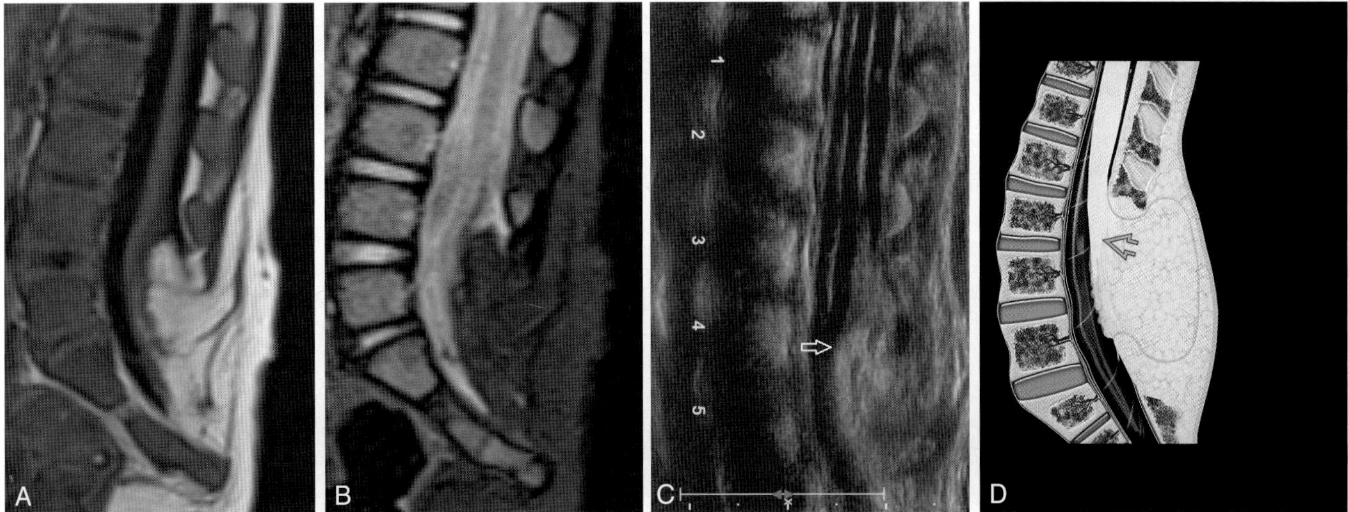

Fig. 16.10 Lipomyelocele. (A) Sagittal T1W, (B) sagittal STIR, and (C) sagittal ultrasound images demonstrate a skin covered lumbosacral dysraphism with low termination of the spinal cord onto fat within the spinal canal (*arrow*). The fat is in continuity with the subcutaneous fat through the posterior defect. (D) Illustration of a lipomyelocele showing the cord-fat junction within the confines of the spinal canal (*arrow*). (D from Ross JS, Moore KR. *Diagnostic Imaging: Spine.* Philadelphia: Elsevier; 2021.)

Key Points

Background

- *Closed spinal dysraphism with subcutaneous mass* and *primary neurulation* disorder caused by premature disjunction of neural ectoderm from the cutaneous ectoderm
- May present with lower extremity symptoms, back pain, and bowel/bladder dysfunction
- Early surgical intervention recommended to reduce neurological impairment

Imaging

- The spinal cord-lipoma attachment is inside the spinal canal and in continuity with prominence/mass-like subcutaneous fat. The lack of herniation of the cord and meninges differentiates a lipomyelocele from a lipomyelomeningocele.
- Associated with vertebral anomalies, terminal diastematomyelia, anorectal and genitourinary anomalies, epidermoid/dermoid, and dermal sinus tract

REFERENCES

1. Grimme JD, Castillo M. Congenital anomalies of the spine. *Neuroimaging Clin N Am.* 2007 Feb;17(1):1–16.
2. Barkovich AJ, Raybaud C: *Pediatric neuroimaging*, 6th ed., Philadelphia, 2019, Wolters Kluwer.

MENINGOCELE

CLOSED Dysraphism
Presence of a
Subcutaneous mass

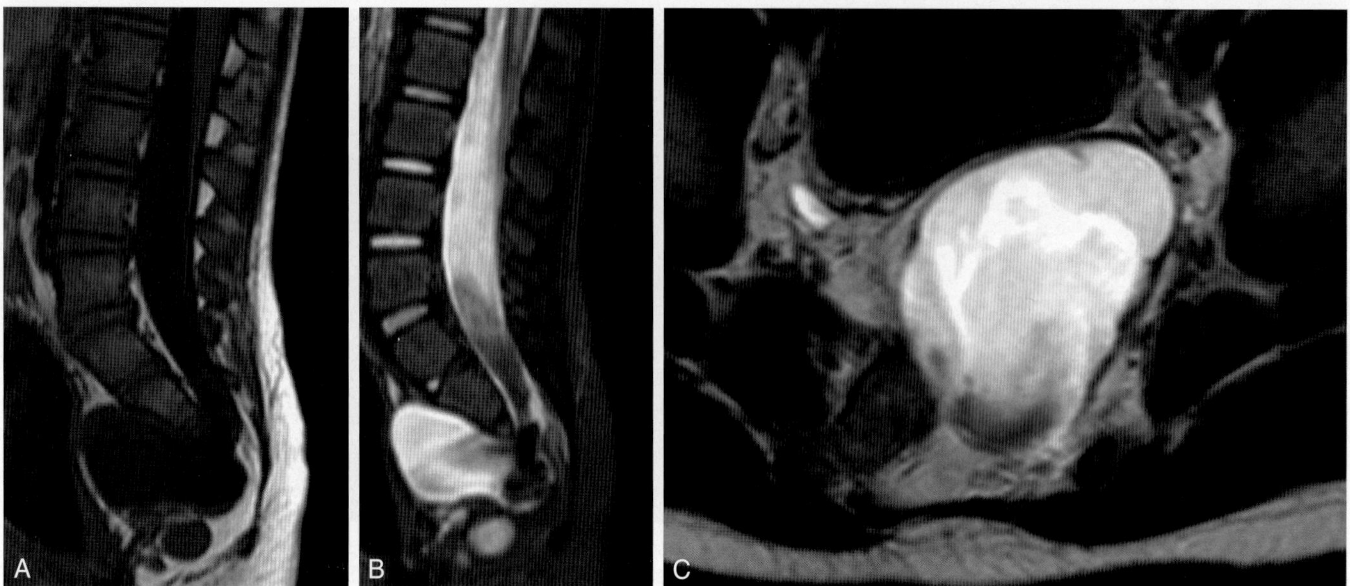

Fig. 16.11 Meningocele. (A) Sagittal T1W and (B and C) sagittal and axial T2W images demonstrate a presacral T2W hyperintense fluid collection in continuity with the CSF in the spinal canal through an anterior bone defect in the sacrum.

Key Points

Background

- *Closed spinal dysraphism* with unknown embryological etiology
- Herniation of fluid-filled meningocele sac through a defect in sacral or coccygeal vertebrae
- Symptoms secondary to result of pressure on the bowel, bladder, or nerve roots

Imaging

- *Fluid signal sac* with communication to the spinal canal.
- Associated with NF-1 and Marfan syndrome.

REFERENCE

1. Grimme JD, Castillo M. Congenital anomalies of the spine. *Neuroimaging Clin N Am*. 2007 Feb;17(1):1–16.

MYELOCYSTOCELE

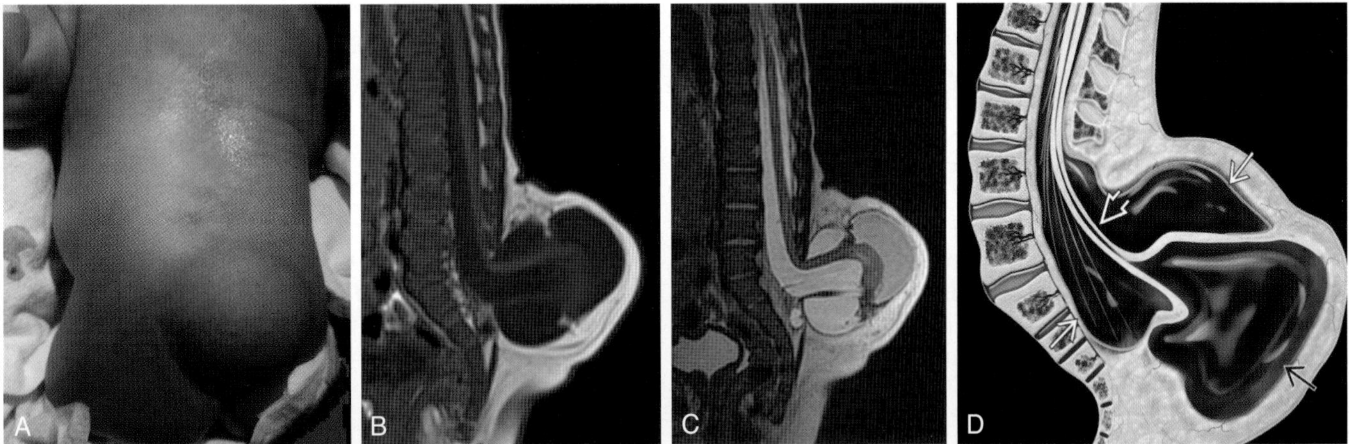

Fig. 16.12 Myelocystocele. (A) Clinical image of a neonate with a skin covered lumbosacral mass. (B) Sagittal T1W and (C) sagittal 3D T2W images demonstrate a closed lumbosacral spinal dysraphism with herniation of spinal cord and meninges and expanded central canal that herniates in the meningocele consistent with a terminal myelocystocele. (D) Illustration of a myelocystocele demonstrating a skin covered dysraphism with distal spinal cord fluid (*wide arrow*), expanded central canal (*black arrow*), and surrounding expanded subarachnoid space (*white arrow*). (D from Ross JS, Moore KR, *Diagnostic Imaging: Spine*. Philadelphia: Elsevier; 2021.)

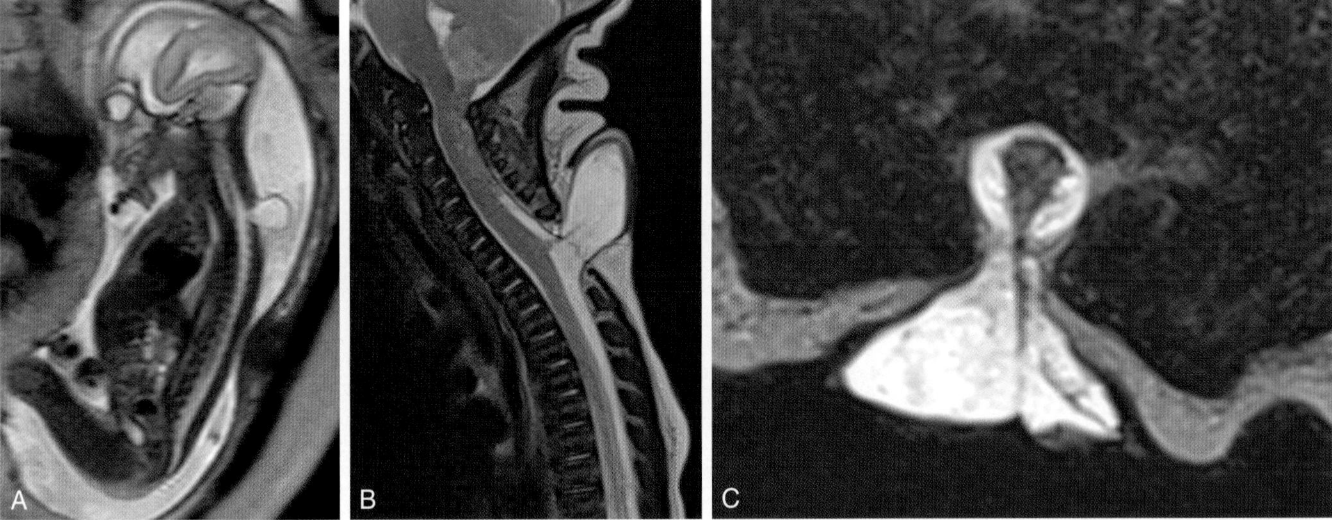

Fig. 16.13 Myelocystocele. (A) Sagittal T2W fetal MR image demonstrates a skin covered fluid filled sac at the cervicothoracic junction that appears to be a meningocele. (B and C) Postnatal sagittal and axial T2W images demonstrate the herniating sac consistent with a meningocele but also posterior tethering of the spinal cord by a bandlike structure consistent with a neurovascular stalk indicative of a nonterminal myelocystocele.

Key Points

Background

- *Closed spinal dysraphism.*
- A terminal myelocystocele consists of a skin-covered lumbosacral spinal dysraphism, an arachnoid-lined meningocele that is directly continuous with the spinal subarachnoid space, and a low-lying hydromyelic spinal cord that traverses the meningocele and then expands into a large terminal cyst which does not communicate with the subarachnoid space and is lined by ependyma and dysplastic glia. Terminal myelocystoceles are presumed to be a disorder of secondary neurulation caused by inability of CSF to exit the early neural tube causing the expansion and disrupting the overlying mesenchyme. Terminal myelocystoceles are associated with cloacal exstrophy, omphalocele, imperforate anus, ambiguous genitalia, caudal regression, and renal anomalies. Terminal myelocystoceles typically present with no bowel or bladder control and poor lower extremity function.
- A nonterminal myelocystocele consists of a skin-covered spinal dysraphism, a CSF filled cyst, a meningocele and variable amount of dorsal fat continuous with the subcutaneous fat. Type 1 consists of the meningocele sac

traversed by a fibroneurovascular stalk attached to the dome of the sac. Type 2 consists of focal hydromyelia that has displaced the posterior wall of the spinal cord into the meningocele sac. Nonterminal myelocystoceles are suspected to be disorders of primary neurulation with incomplete fusion of the dorsal neural folds/failure of the neural ectoderm to separate from the cutaneous ectoderm. Nonterminal myelocystoceles are associated with Chiari 2 malformations, hydrocephalus, ectopic cerebellar tissue, heterotopic renal tissue, and diastematomyelia. Nonterminal myelocystoceles often demonstrate no neurologic dysfunction at presentation.

- Etiology unknown. Possibly secondary to teratogens based on animal studies with retinoic acid.
- Early surgical repair maximizes neurological function

Imaging

- Divided into terminal and nonterminal myelocystoceles based on location.
- Hindbrain herniation can be seen in ~40% of patients with myelocystoceles.
- Skin covered spinal dysraphism/malformation with *herniated spinal cord and meninges*. The central canal is expanded and herniates into the meningocele.

REFERENCES

1. Grimme JD, Castillo M. Congenital anomalies of the spine. *Neuroimaging Clin N Am*. 2007 Feb;17(1):1–16.
2. Huisman TA, Rossi A, Tortori-Donati P. MR imaging of neonatal spinal dysraphia: what to consider? *Magn Reson Imaging Clin N Am*. 2012 Feb;20(1):45–61.
3. Rossi A, Piatelli G, Gandolfo C, Pavanello M, Hoffmann C, Van Goethem JW, Cama A, Tortori-Donati P. Spectrum of nonterminal myelocystoceles. *Neurosurgery*. 2006 Mar;58(3):509–15; discussion 509–515.

TERMINAL VENTRICLE

CLOSED Dysraphism
No Subcutaneous mass

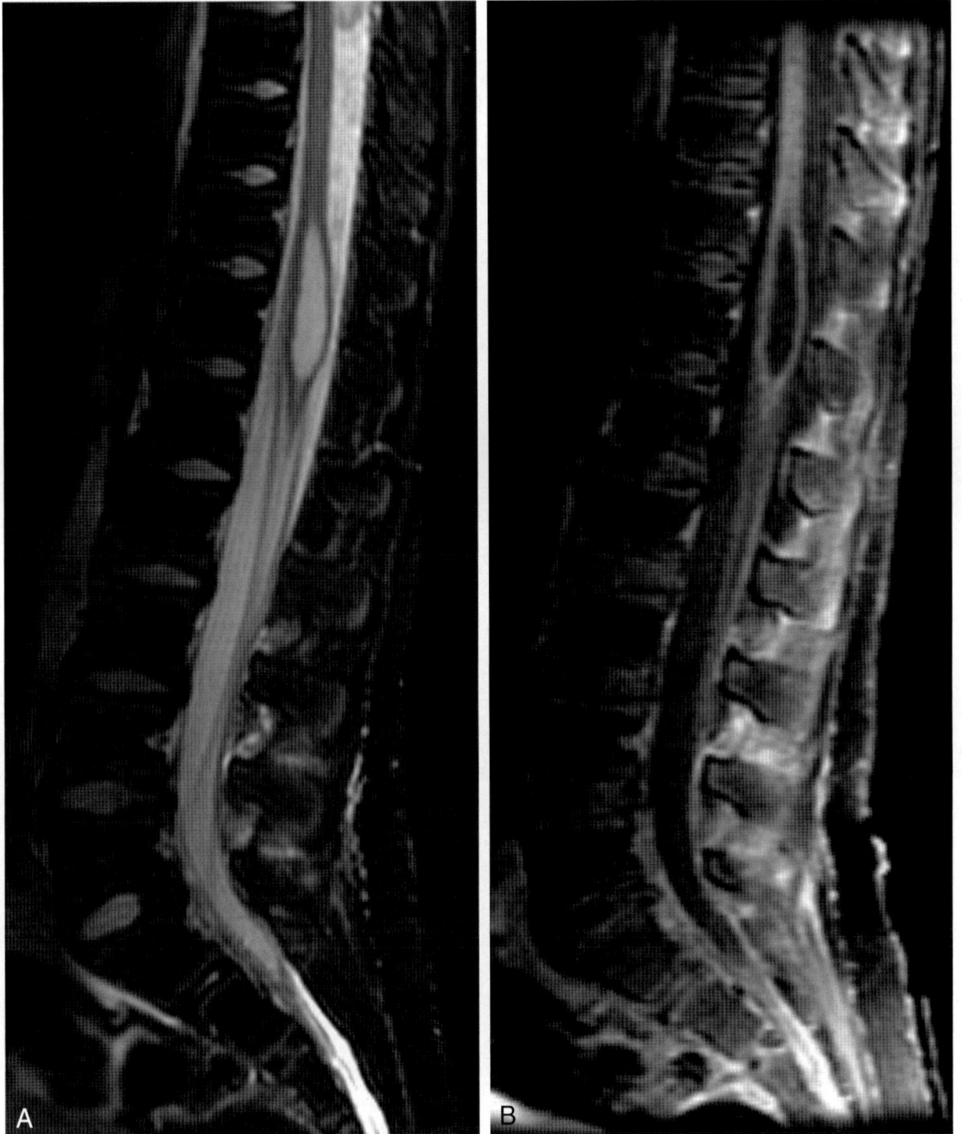

Fig. 16.14 Terminal Ventricle. (A) Sagittal T2W and (B) sagittal T1W+C images demonstrate T2W hyperintense expansion in the lower thoracic cord and conus without enhancement.

Key Points

Background

- *Closed spinal dysraphism* and *secondary neurulation* disorder
- Considered an incidental finding. It is uncommon for it to be associated with clinical deficits

Imaging

- Widening of the central canal in the conus
- Usually less than 10 mm in length and less than 2 to 4 mm in diameter

REFERENCE

1. Grimme JD, Castillo M. Congenital anomalies of the spine. *Neuroimaging Clin N Am.* 2007 Feb;17(1):1–16.

TETHERED SPINAL CORD, TIGHT FILUM TERMINALE, AND INTRADURAL LIPOMA

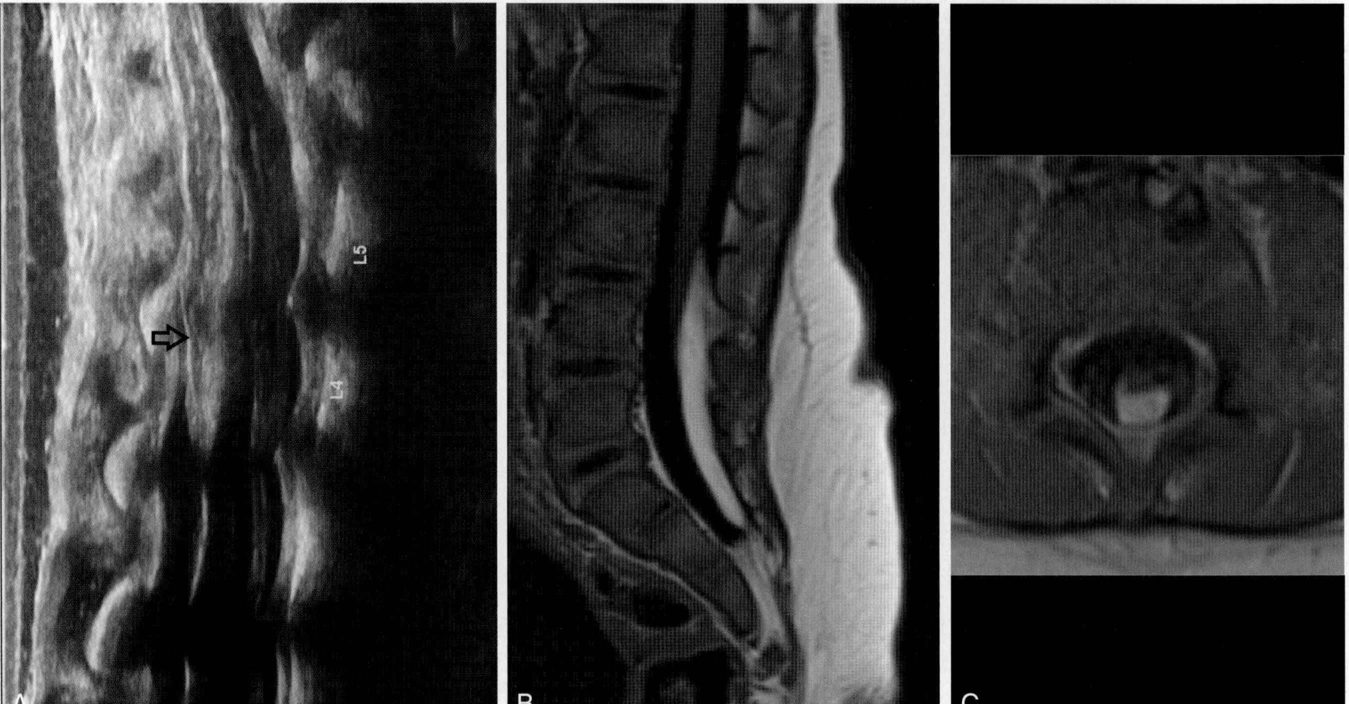

Fig. 16.15 Lipoma. (A) Sagittal ultrasound image demonstrates hyperechoic intrathecal mass. (B and C) Sagittal and axial T1W images demonstrate T1W hyperintense intrathecal mass consistent with a lipoma that tethers the spinal cord.

Key Points

Background

- A tight filum terminale is caused by a *secondary neurulation* disorder due to failure of regression of the caudal cell mass.
- Intradural lipomas occur as a result of *primary neurulation* disorder.
- The spinal cord can be tethered by a tight filum terminale as well as other spinal malformations and masses.
- The tethered cord syndrome occurs when there is tension on the spinal cord. The term is most often used to describe a clinical and radiological diagnosis with neurologic, orthopedic, and/or urologic symptoms in the presence of an abnormally low conus.
- The filum terminale in tethered cord syndrome patients demonstrates dense fibrous connective tissue compared to loose connective tissue in normal patients suggesting reduced elasticity. The reduced elasticity/increased tension on the spinal cord leads to decreased blood flow and oxidative metabolism. Improved blood flow to the conus has been shown to occur after detethering.
- Tethered cord syndrome occurs in 3–32% of myelomeningocele patients as the spine lengthens and due to adhesions.
- In the setting of caudal regression, the spinal cord is considered tethered if the conus terminates at or below the L1-2 interspace.
- Lipomyelomeningocele patients have bladder dysfuntion by age 2 and have progressive neurologic deterioration without detethering.
- The conus normally terminates at or above the inferior L2 vertebral body in 95% of children. The conus reaches an adult level by 3 months of age. A conus at the L2–3 disc space level can be normal in infants <3 months of age, but after 3 months of age, the L2–3 disc space and below is considered abnormal. The L3 level and below is considered abnormal in all children.
- Tethered cord syndrome most often presents between 4–8 years of age. Signs and symptoms in infants include cutaneous findings, lower extremity deformity, and anorectal malformation. Cutaneous findings are seen in ~80% of infants and findings that should lead to a high index of suspicion include a hairy patch, lipoma, hemangioma, atypical dimple, skin tag, nevus, and dermal sinus tract. A dimple superior to the gluteal cleft, outside the midline, and diameter greater than 5 mm warrant radiological investigation. Signs and symptoms in children include sensorimotor dysfunction, gait difficulty, scoliosis, foot deformity, back and lower extremity pain, and

incontinence. Signs and symptoms in teenagers include nondermatomal pain in the lumbosacral spine, perineum, and legs as well as incontinence.

- Tethered cord signs and symptoms include lower extremity sensorimotor abnormalities, abnormal reflexes, muscle atrophy, spastic gait, and foot deformity, as well as urinary incontinence, and scoliosis.
- Urodynamic studies are useful as findings can precede clinical symptoms. Detethering leads to improved or stable symptoms in 88% and improved urodynamics in 29–75%. Spinal column shortening leads to improvement in pain, weakness, and bowel/bladder dysfunction. Retethering occurs in ~5%, but higher incidence with complex etiologies such as lipomyelomeningocele and myelomeningocele (34%) compared to noncomplex etiologies (7%).

Imaging

- Tethered spinal cord from a tight filum terminale is seen on MRI as an abnormally low position of the conus with or without fibrofatty filum (<2 mm in diameter) or a filum lipoma (>2 mm in diameter). The conus may also be more posteriorly positioned in the spinal canal. Ultrasound can be used to determine the conus position and filum thickness in infants typically <4 months old but confirmation of abnormal findings with MRI is recommended.
- Lipomas can result in tethered spinal cord even when the conus terminates at a normal level.
- Lack of ventral shift in the conus with prone position can also be used to determine if there is a tethered spinal cord. Anterior-posterior movement greater than 10% of the spinal canal width when comparing prone to supine can exclude tethering (sensitivity 93%/Specificity 100%) but may be challenging to perform in sedated pediatric patients.
- Syrinx occurs in 25% and improves with detethering.
- The term occult tethered cord syndrome is used for symptomatic patients with a normal conus position. A randomized control study showed no benefit to support filum sectioning in these patients.
- There is varying surgical management chosen for an asymptomatic patient with a low conus +/– fatty filum. An asymptomatic patient with a normal conus position but fatty filum is seen on 1.5–5% of MRIs nad requires close clinical attention.

REFERENCE

1. Grimme JD, Castillo M. Congenital anomalies of the spine. *Neuroimaging Clin N Am.* 2007 Feb;17(1):1–16.

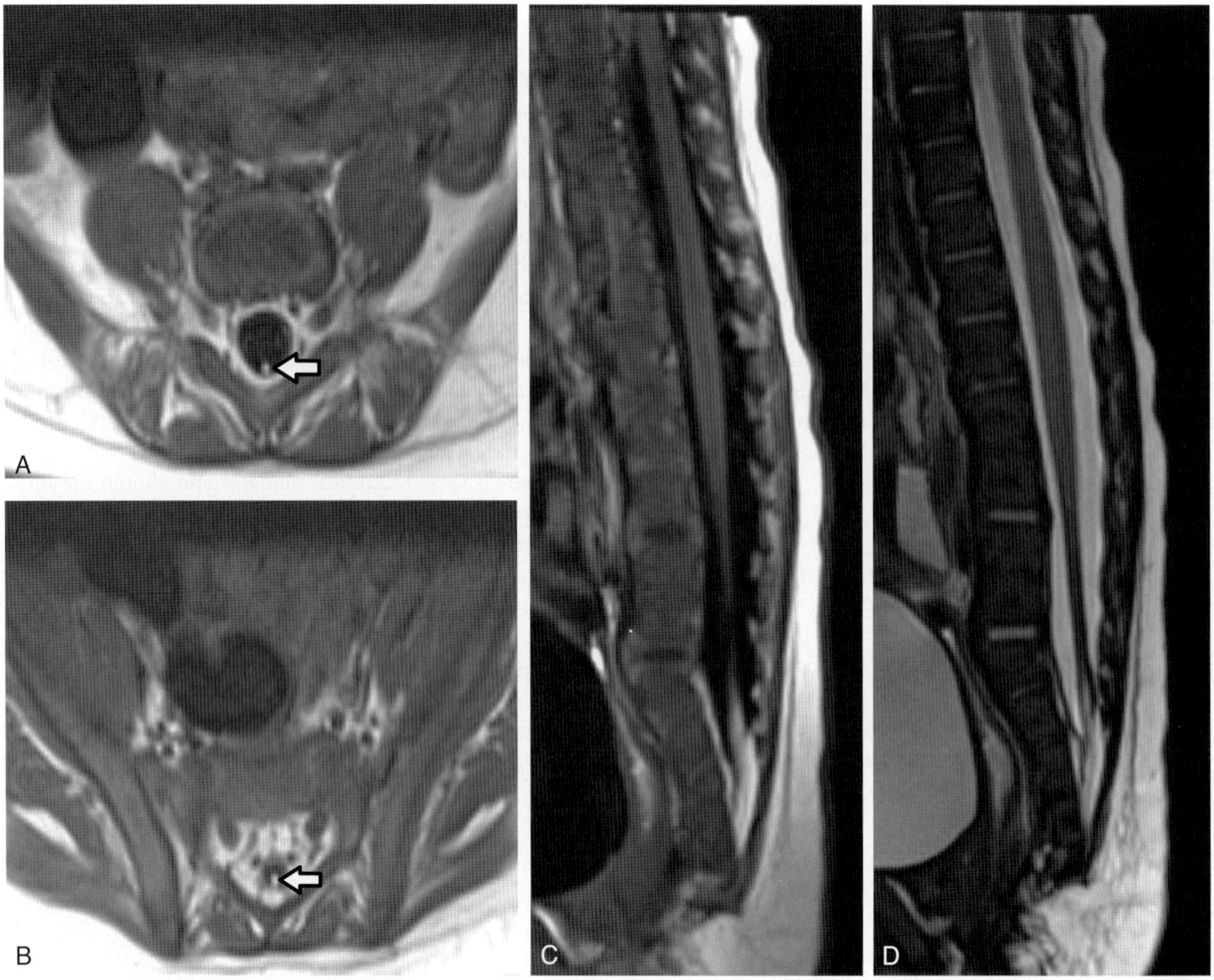

Fig. 16.16 Filar Lipoma and Tethered Spinal Cord. (A to C) Axial and sagittal T1W and (D) sagittal T2W images demonstrate T1W hyperintense signal from fat in the filum terminale and termination of the spinal cord at the L5-S1 level.

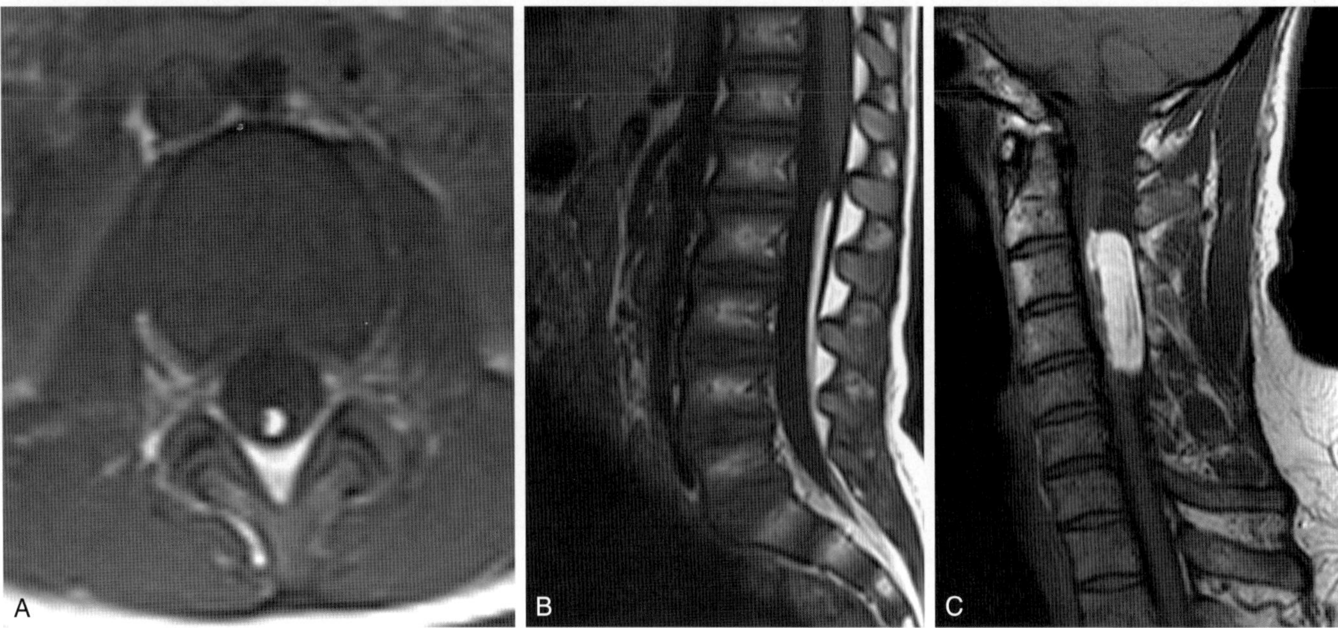

Fig. 16.17 Spinal Lipoma. (A and B) Axial and sagittal T1W images demonstrate T1W hyperintense signal from fat in the filum terminale and termination of the spinal cord at the lower L1 level. Cervical lipoma: (C) Sagittal T1W image demonstrates rare cervical lipoma.

DERMAL SINUS TRACT

CLOSED Dysraphism
No Subcutaneous mass

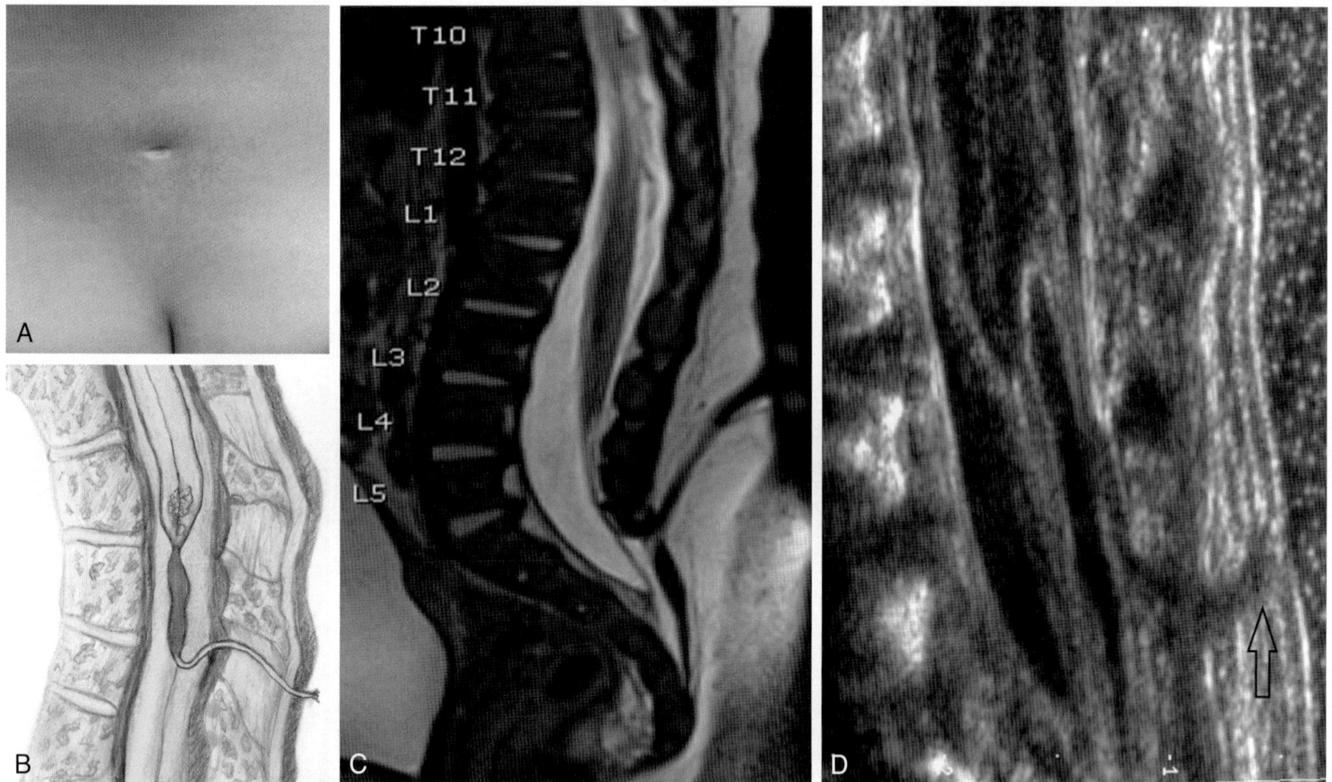

Fig. 16.18 Dermal Sinus Tract. (A) Clinical image of the skin surface pit of a dermal sinus tract. (B) Illustration of a dermal sinus tract that extends from the skin surface to the conus and a potential association with a dermoid or epidermoid cyst along the tract. (C) Sagittal T2W image demonstrates the linear T2 hypointense dermal sinus tract extending from skin surface to the dura. (D) Sagittal ultrasound image demonstrating the hypoechoic dermal sinus tract.

Key Points

Background

- Disorder of *gastrulation.*
- Epithelial tract extending inward from the skin surface.
- Midline or paramedian dimple/opening at the skin surface, which can have associated hyperpigmentation or hair patch.
- Communication from the skin surface with the brain or spinal canal can result in *meningitis or abscess.*

Imaging

- MRI: T1W and T2W hypointense tract extending from the skin surface to the spinal canal. Most commonly found in the lumbosacral and occipital regions, which are the last portions of the neural tube to close.
- Ultrasound: Hypoechoic linear tract.
- *May have an associated dermoid/epidermoid cyst.*
- Can result in spinal cord or nerve root tethering.
- The fistulous tract is best seen on T1W-weighted sequence *without* fat saturation.

REFERENCES

1. Grimme JD, Castillo M. Congenital anomalies of the spine. *Neuroimaging Clin N Am.* 2007 Feb;17(1):1–16.
2. Huisman TA, Rossi A, Tortori-Donati P. MR imaging of neonatal spinal dysraphia: what to consider? *Magn Reson Imaging Clin N Am.* 2012 Feb;20(1):45–61.

DERMAL SINUS TRACT COMPLICATION: SPINAL ABSCESS AND MENINGITIS

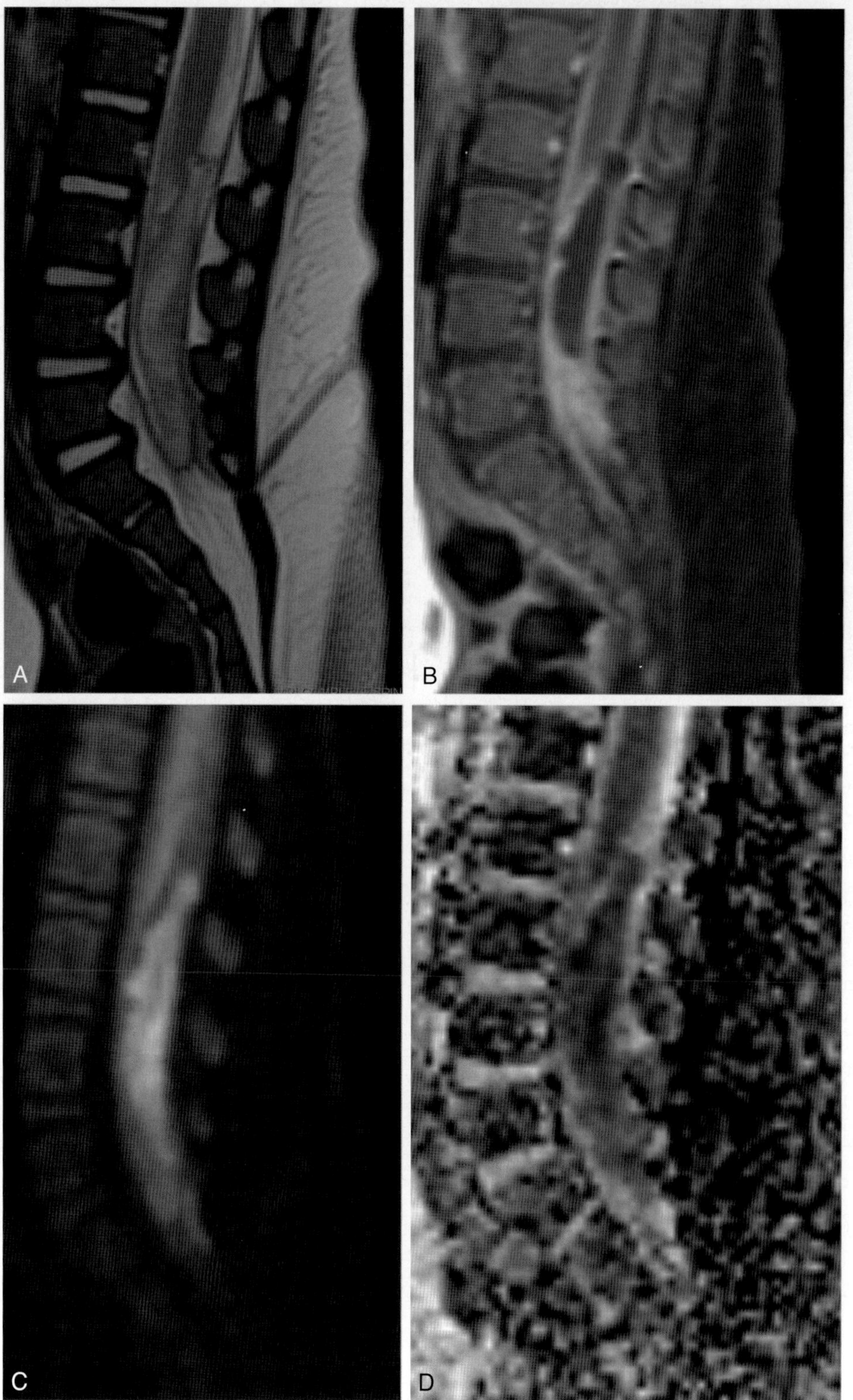

Fig. 16.19 Dermal Sinus Tract Complication: Spinal Abscess and Meningitis. A dermal sinus tract allows for communication from the skin surface to the spinal canal and a potential for infection to enter the spinal canal. (A) Sagittal T2W, (B) sagittal T1W+C, (C) sagittal DWI, and (D) sagittal ADC images demonstrate heterogenous T2W collection with peripheral enhancement and central diffusion restriction consistent with abscess. There is also abnormal spinal cord leptomeningeal enhancement consistent with meningitis.

EPIDERMOID CYST

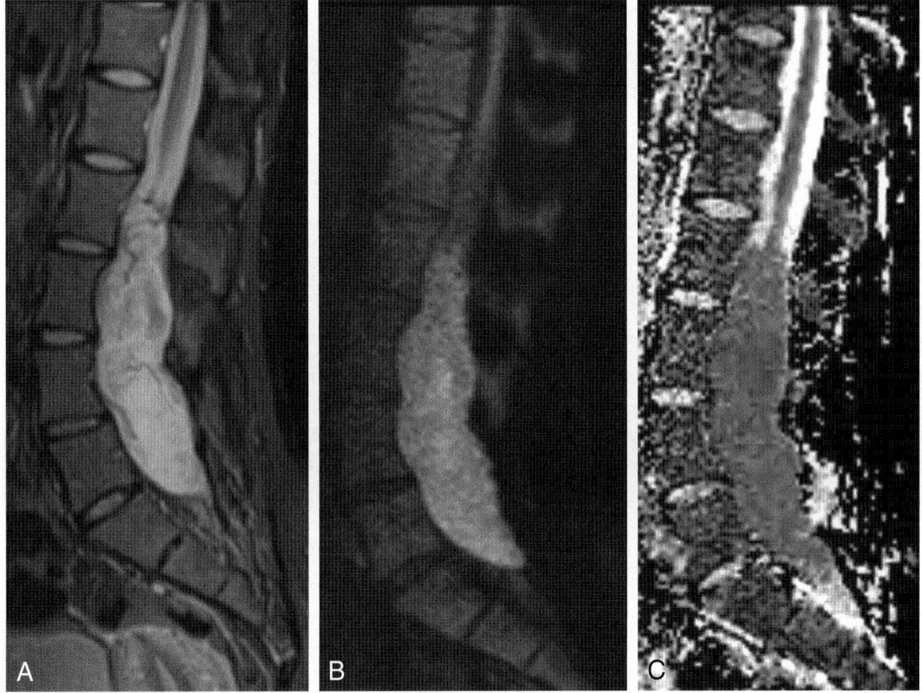

Fig. 16.20 Epidermoid Cyst. (A) Sagittal STIR, (B) sagittal DWI and (C) sagittal ADC demonstrate an intradural extramedullary mass with T2W hyperintensity, no enhancement (not shown), and diffusion restriction consistent with an epidermoid cyst.

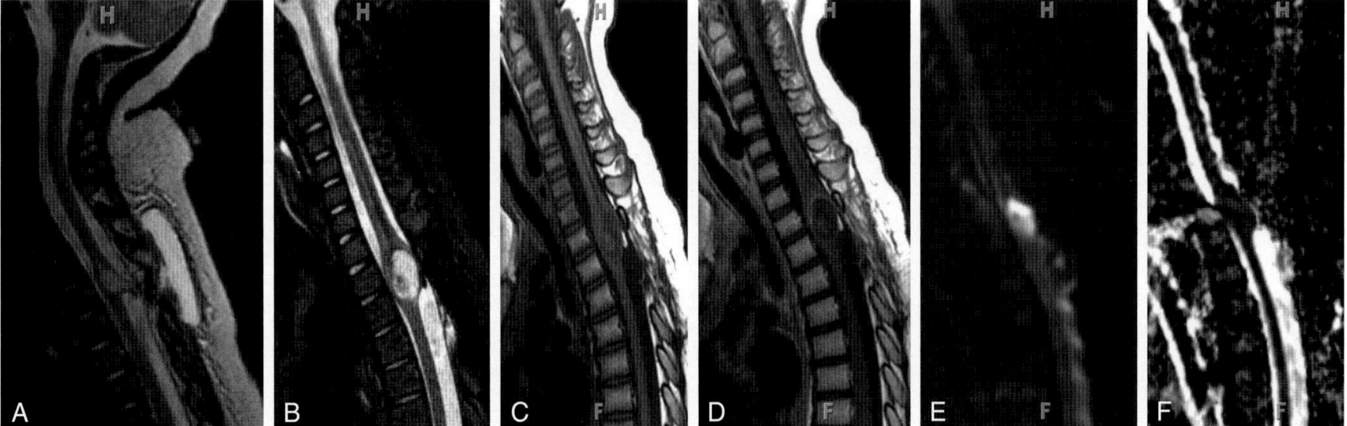

Fig. 16.21 Rare Intramedullary Epidermoid Cyst as a Complication From Spinal Surgery for Repair of a Skin Covered Meningocele. (A) Sagittal T2W demonstrates an upper thoracic meningocele. Following surgical resection, (B) sagittal T2W, (C and D) sagittal T1W and T1W+C, and (E and F) sagittal DWI and ADC images demonstrate an intradural T2W hyperintense mass with minimal peripheral enhancement and diffusion restriction consistent with an acquired epidermoid cyst.

Key Points

Background

- Most commonly associated with myelomeningocele repair or dermal sinus tract
- Often associated with dermal sinus tracts and vertebral abnormalities

Imaging

- Usually *extramedullary* T2W hyperintensity; no significant enhancement; *restricted diffusion*

REFERENCE

1. Rossi A, Gandolfo C, Morana F, et al. Tumors of the spine in children. *Neuroimaging Clin N Am.* 2007 Feb;17(1):17–35.

DIASTEMATOMYELIA

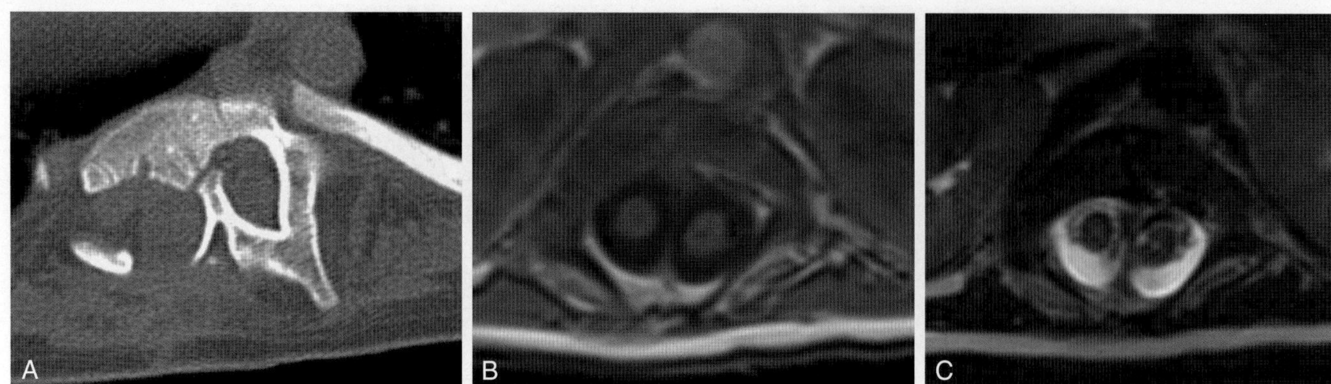

Fig. 16.22 Diastematomyelia. (A) Axial CT demonstrating a midline thoracic bone bar separating the spinal canal into two halves (type 1 diastematomyelia). (B and C) Axial T1W and T2W images demonstrate the two thecal sacs with hemicords separated in the midline by a bony bar (type 1 diastematomyelia).

Key Points

Background

- *Gastrulation* disorder
- Separation of the spinal cord into two symmetric or asymmetric hemicords, each containing a central canal, one dorsal horn (giving rise to a dorsal nerve root), and one ventral horn (giving rise to a ventral nerve root)
- Clinical manifestations: Cutaneous stigmata; clubfoot; scoliosis; tethered cord syndrome

Imaging

- Type I split cord malformation: 40% to 70%; separate dura surrounding each hemicord and typically a cartilage or osseous spur separating the sacs
- Type II: 30% to 60%; the two hemicords travel through a single subarachnoid space surrounded by a single dural sac
- Associated findings: Vertebral segmentation anomalies, hydromyelia, fibrofatty filum, dermal sinus tract, dermoid/epidermoid cyst, adhesions, myelocele, and myelomeningocele.

REFERENCES

1. Grimme JD, Castillo M. Congenital anomalies of the spine. *Neuroimaging Clin N Am*. 2007 Feb;17(1):1–16.
2. Orman G, Tijssen MPM, Seyfert D, Gassner I, Huisman TAGM. Ultrasound to evaluate neonatal spinal dysraphism: a first-line alternative to CT and MRI. *J Neuroimaging*. 2019 Sep;29(5):553–564.

DIASTEMATOMYELIA

CLOSED Dysraphism
No Subcutaneous mass

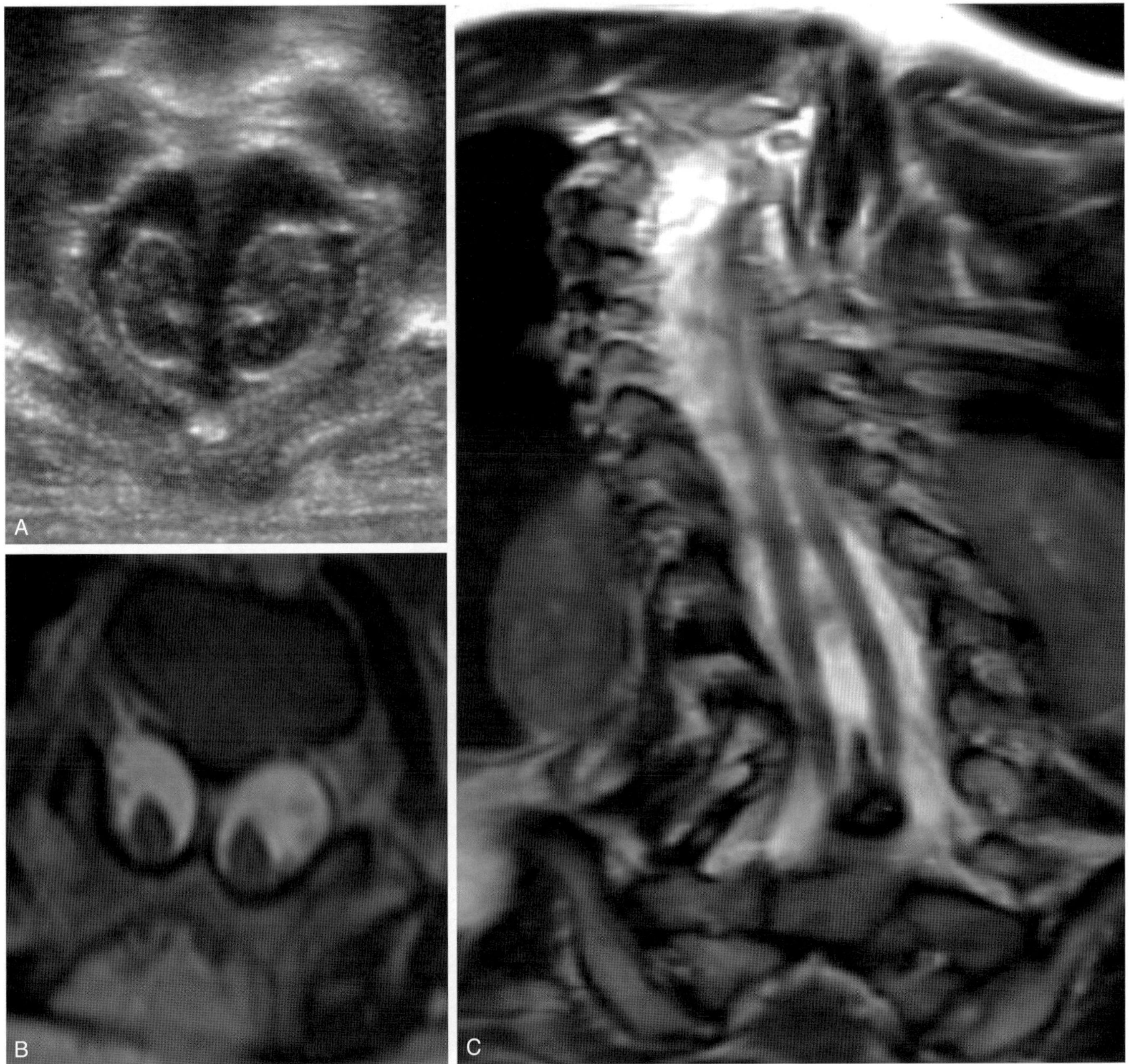

Fig. 16.23 Diastematomyelia. (A) Axial ultrasound appearance of diastematomyelia with two hemicords separated in the midline. (B and C) Axial and coronal T2W images from the same patient demonstrating a midline bone bar separating the spinal canal into two halves.

NEURENTERIC CYST

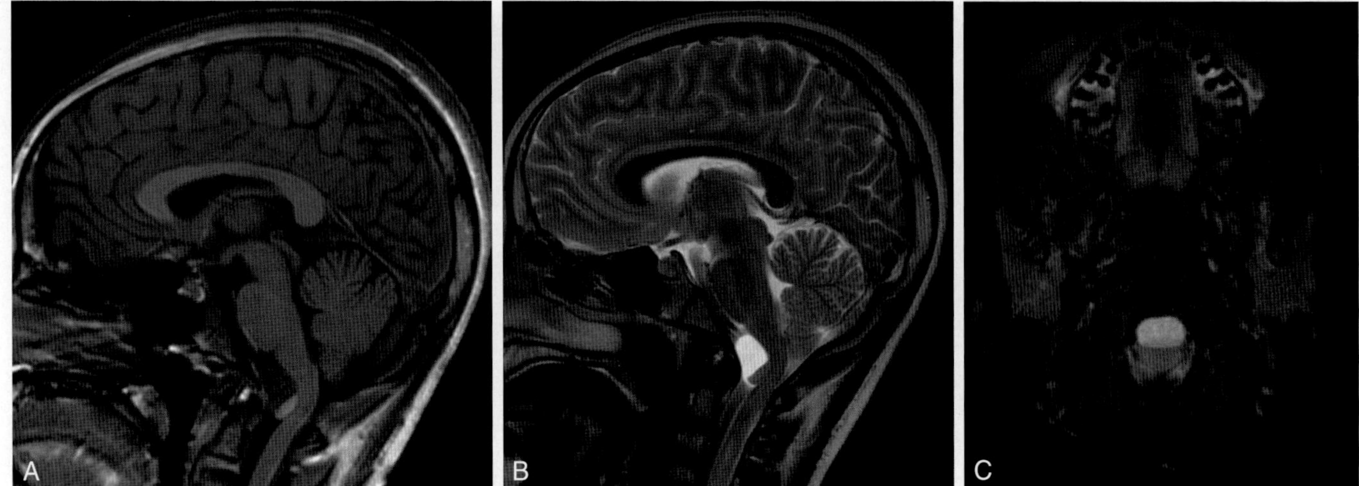

Fig. 16.24 Neurenteric Cyst. (A) Sagittal T1W, (B) sagittal T2W, and (C) axial FLAIR images demonstrate an intradural extramedullary lesion anterior to the medulla with posterior T1W hyperintense, T2W isointense signal likely from layering protein and anterior fluid that is T2W hyperintense but does not suppress on FLAIR. There is significant mass effect on the cord; however, no spinal cord edema is present indicating long-term presence of the lesion.

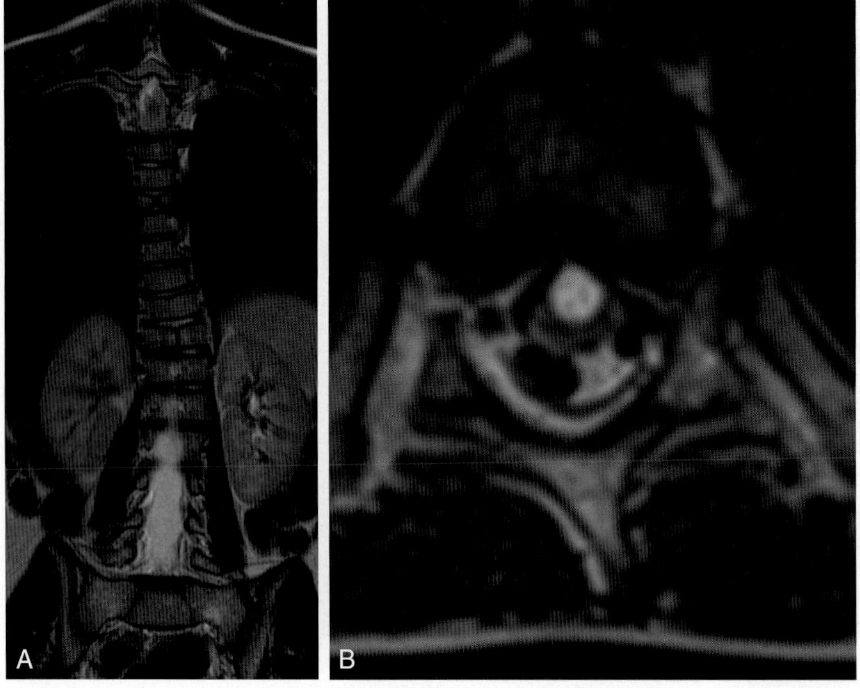

Fig. 16.25 Neurenteric Cyst. (A and B) Coronal and axial T2W images demonstrate thoracic vertebral segmentation anomalies and a T2W hyperintense intradural extramedullary lesion anterior to the spinal cord. There is mass effect on the cord; however, no spinal cord edema is present indicating long-term presence of the lesion.

Key Points

Background

- *Gastrulation* disorder
- Congenital cyst lined by epithelium

Imaging

- Location: Usually extradural and located prevertebral or paravertebral and *associated with vertebral segmentation anomaly*. Less commonly intradural or intramedullary
- MRI: Unilocular cyst with simple or proteinaceous fluid content resulting in T2W or T1W hyperintense internal signal. May have peripheral enhancement but no solid enhancement

REFERENCE

1. Rossi A, Gandolfo C, Morana G, et al. Tumors of the spine in children. *Neuroimaging Clin N Am*. 2007 Feb;17(1):17–35.

DORSAL ENTERIC FISTULA

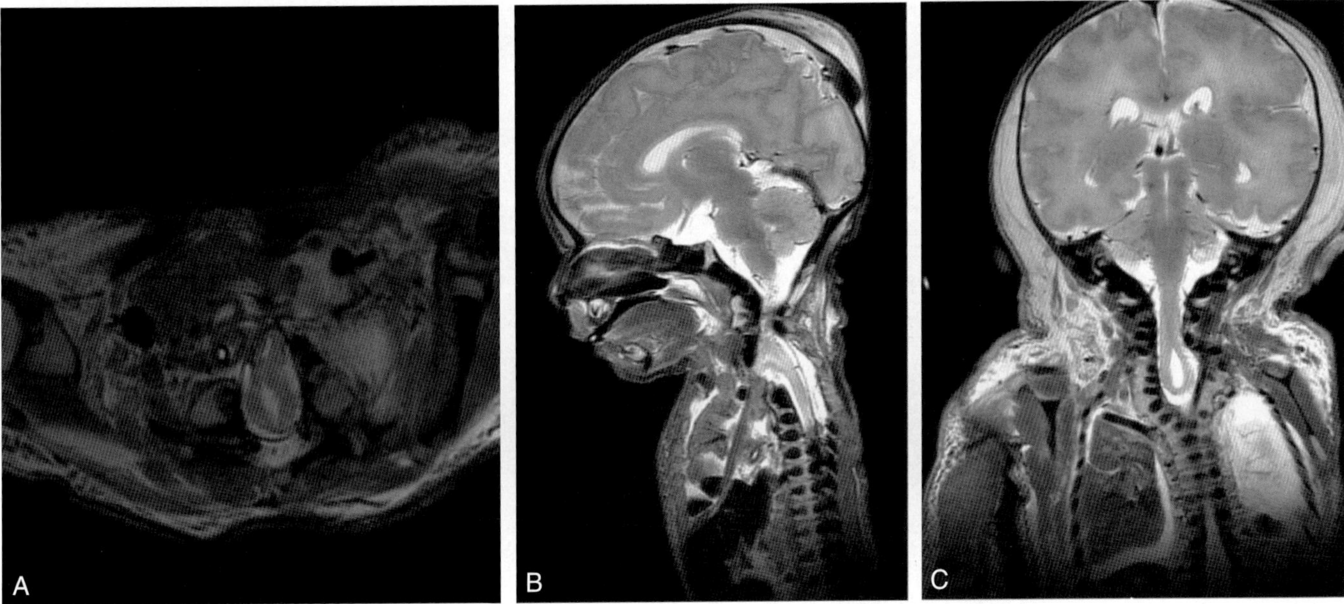

Fig. 16.26 Dorsal Enteric Fistula. A neonate with left sided-congenital diaphragmatic hernia. Postmortem MRI: (A to C) multiplanar T2W images demonstrate a fluid tract communicating between the aerodigestive tract and the spinal canal.

Key Points

Background

- *Gastrulation* disorder.
- Extremely rare malformation consisting of splitting of the notochord and communication between the ventral endoderm and dorsal ectoderm.
- Fistula connects the intestinal cavity to the midline dorsal skin traversing the vertebrae and spinal canal.
- Present in the neonatal period with a bowel ostium exposed mucus membrane that passes meconium.
- Enteric cysts and sinus tracts are included in the split notochord syndrome.

Imaging

- Visualization of a tract communicating from the intestinal tract through the spine to the posterior skin surface

REFERENCE

1. Barkovich AJ, Raybaud C: *Pediatric neuroimaging*, 6th ed., Philadelphia, 2019, Wolters Kluwer.

CAUDAL REGRESSION SYNDROME

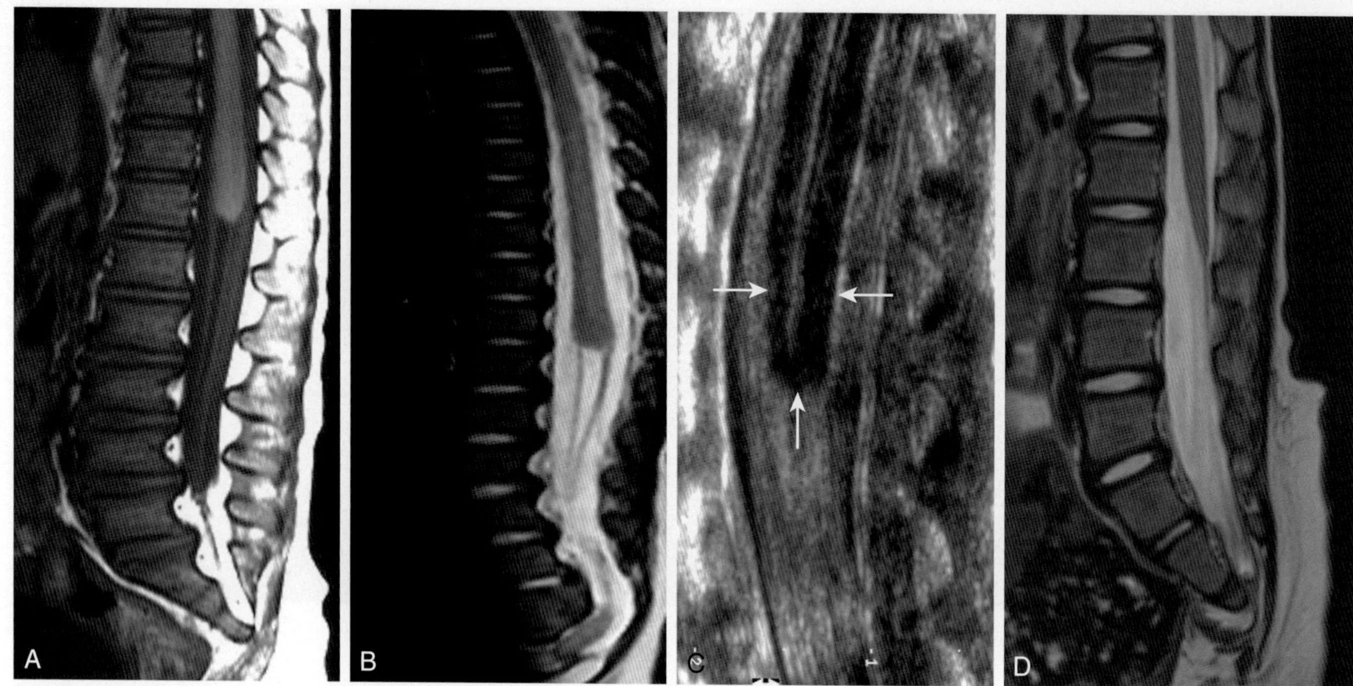

Fig. 16.27 Caudal Regression Syndrome. (A) Sagittal T1W, (B) sagittal T2W, and (C) sagittal ultrasound images demonstrate the absence of the coccyx and lower sacrum and the blunted/truncated appearance of the conus that terminates at the T12 level. (D) Sagittal T2W image in a different patient with a type 2 caudal regression demonstrating less vertebral body agenesis but abnormally low conus position.

Key Points

Background

- *Gastrulation* disorder.
- Agenesis or hypogenesis of the caudal spine associated with other cardiac, genitourinary, and gastrointenstinal anomalies.
- 30% are children of diabetic mothers.
- Secondary to congenital or acquired injury to the caudal cell mass with resultant deficient secondary neurulation. Often associated pelvic floor and genitourinary and pulmonary anomalies/hypoplasia. In addition, depending on the severity and cranial extension additional injury to the distal primary neural tube may have occurred.

Imaging

- Type 1: Blunted distal spinal cord that terminates at L1 or superior. Greater degree of vertebral agenesis.
- Type 2: Low-lying spinal cord that is tethered. Less severe degree of vertebral agenesis.

REFERENCE

1. Grimme JD, Castillo M. Congenital anomalies of the spine. *Neuroimaging Clin N Am.* 2007 Feb;17(1):1–16.

SEGMENTAL SPINAL DYSGENESIS

CLOSED Dysraphism
No Subcutaneous mass

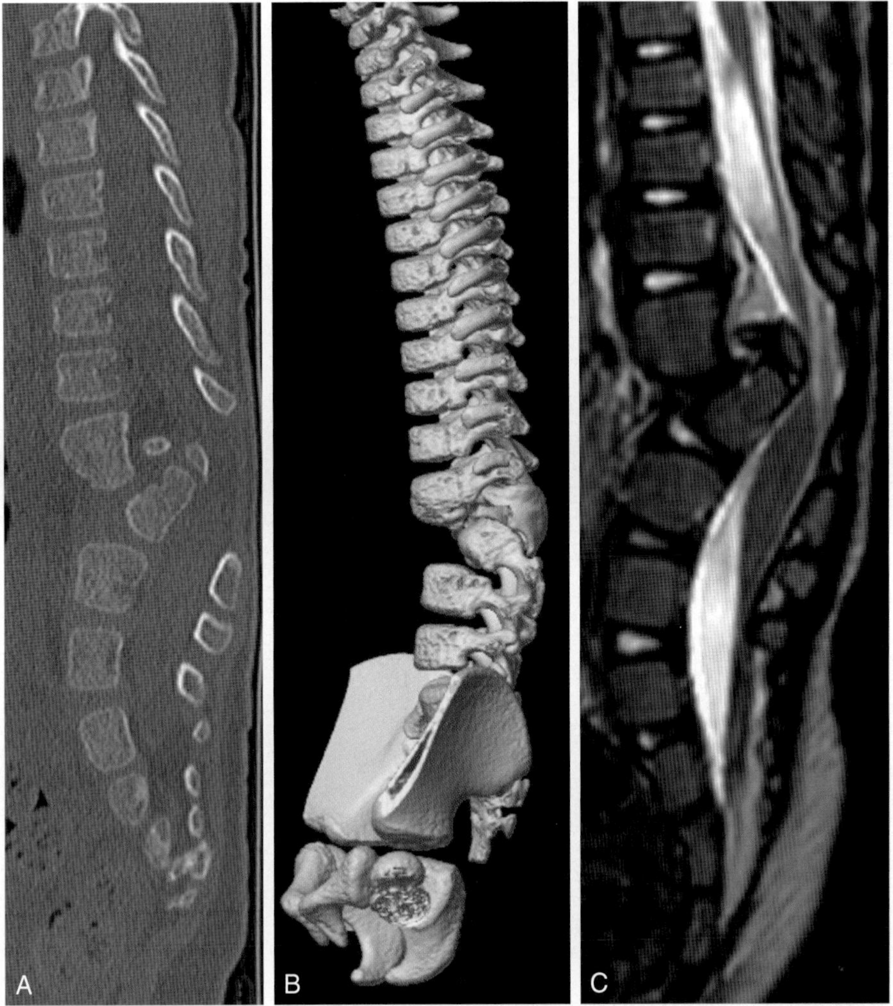

Fig. 16.28 Segmental Spinal Dysgenesis. (A) Sagittal reformat CT, (B) 3D volumetric CT, and (C) sagittal T2W images demonstrate a type 1 lumbar segmental spinal dysgenesis with hypoplastic vertebrae, a fibroconnective stalk, canal stenosis, kyphosis, and lower sacrum and coccygeal agenesis

Key Points

Background

- Etiology unknown. Possibly a disorder of *gastrulation*
- Abnormal segmental development of a vertebrae, and associated spinal cord and/or nerve roots. Results in scoliosis or kyphosis
- Includes paraplegia or paraparesis at birth and congenital deformity of the lower limbs
- Usually lower thoracic spine or lumbar spine
- Associated systemic anomalies of the heart, kidneys, and bladder

Imaging

- Type 1: Focal absence of spinal cord (or fibroneural/fibroconnective stalk) and one or more vertebral bodies, kyphosis, bone spur, canal stenosis between segments, low-lying cord often with bulky appearance, caudal agenesis, horseshow kidney, paraplegia, lower limb deformity (equinovarus)
- Type 2: Focal hypoplasia of the spinal cord and vertebrae without disconnection, focal canal stenosis, segmentation abnormality, +/– caudal agenesis, lower limb motor function present

REFERENCE

1. Chaturvedi A, Ayyamperumal B, Thirumaran R, et al. Segmental spinal dysgenesis – redefined. *Asian Spine J.* 2019 Apr;13(2):189–197.

ARACHNOID CYST

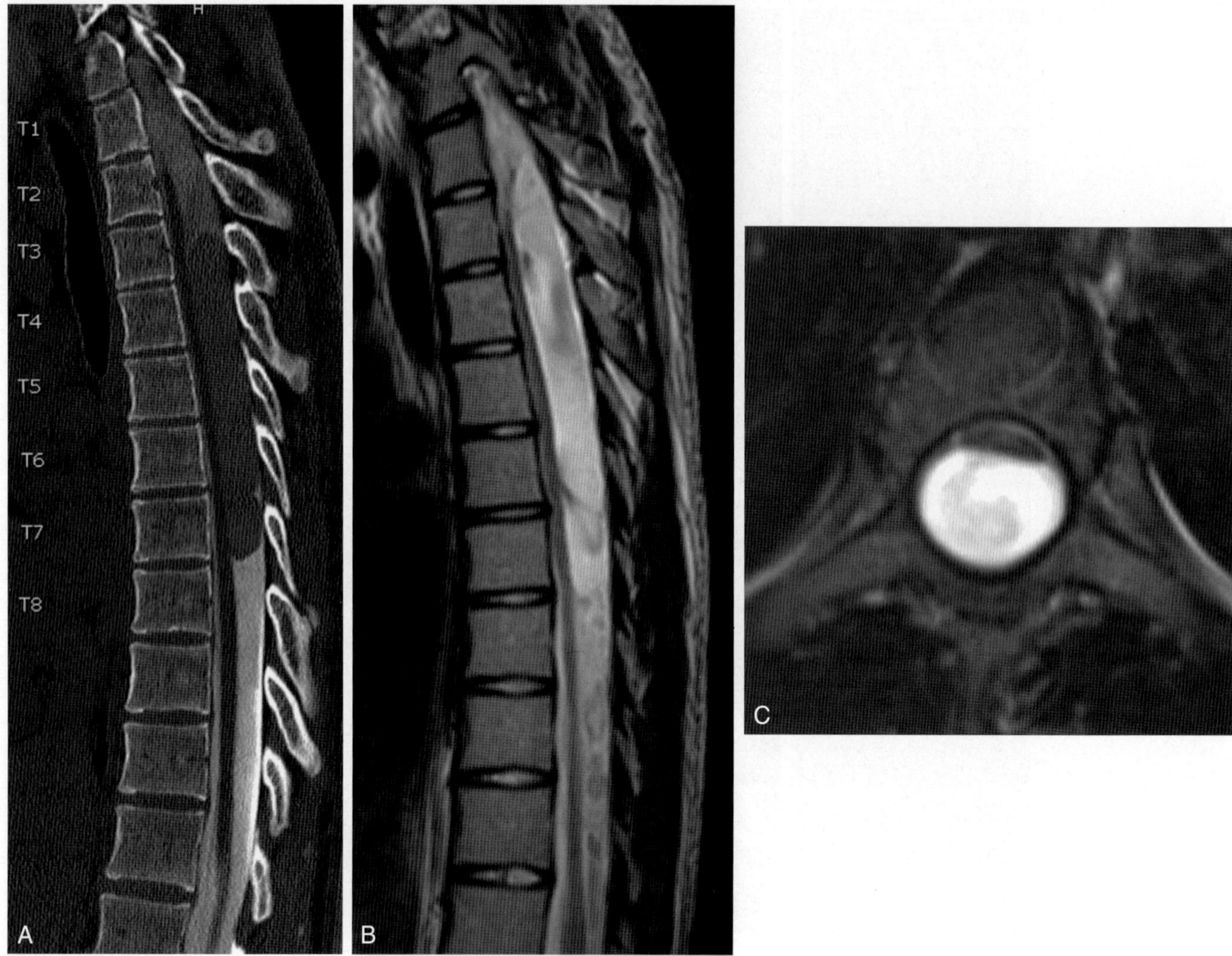

Fig. 16.29 Arachnoid Cyst. (A) Sagittal reformat CT myelogram image demonstrates an extramedullary mass that does not fill with intrathecal contrast in keeping with an arachnoid cyst. (B and C) Sagittal and axial T2W images demonstrate a T2W hyperintense fluid collection in the posterior thoracic thecal sac compressing the spinal cord.

Key Points

Background

- Congenital or secondary to prior infection, trauma, or surgery

Imaging

- Simple cyst located in the subdural or epidural space; may be anterior or posterior to the displaced or compressed spinal cord
- Usually has a mass effect on the spinal canal/cord
- *T2W hyperintense, nonenhancing, no diffusion restriction*

REFERENCE

1. Rossi A, Gandolfo C, Morana G, et al. Tumors of the spine in children. *Neuroimaging Clin N Am.* 2007 Feb;17(1):17–35.

SEGMENTATION/FORMATION ANOMALY

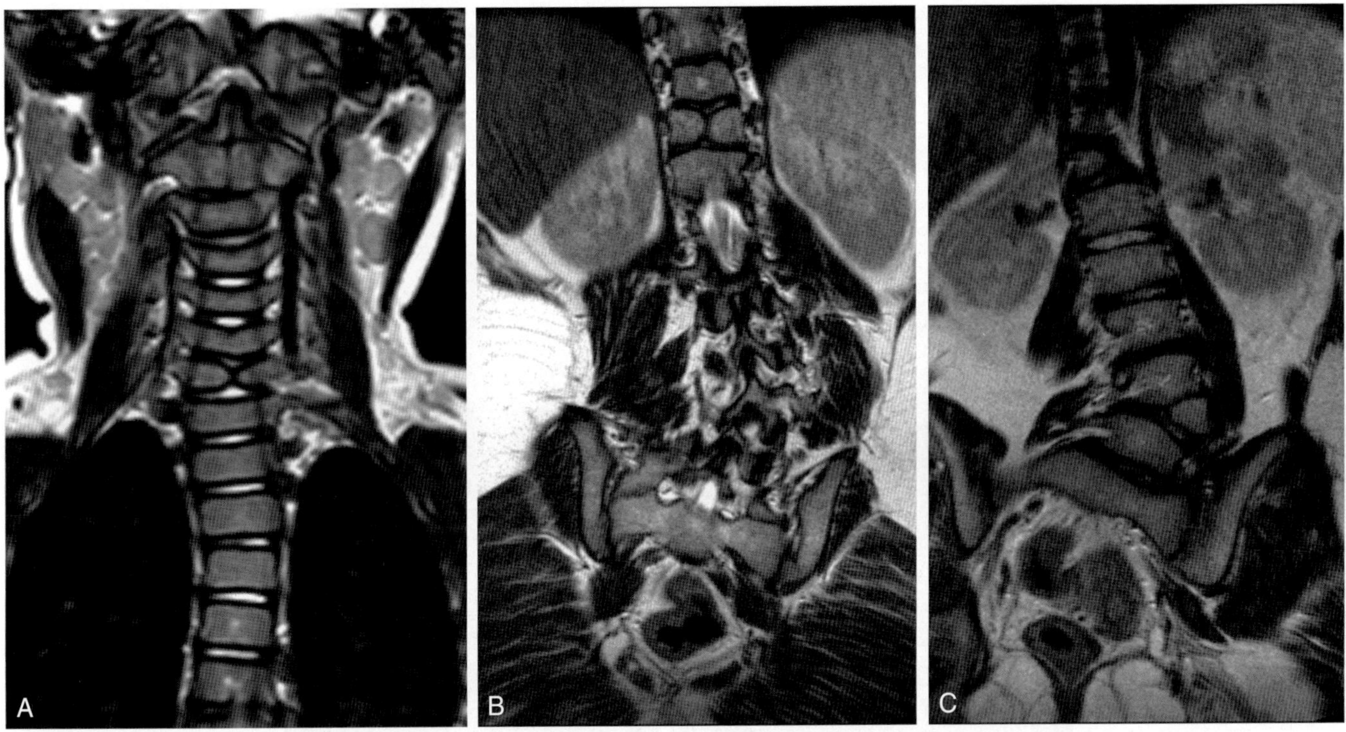

Fig. 16.30 Segmentation Anomaly. (A to C) Coronal T2W images demonstrate butterfly and hemivertebrae anomalies with associated scoliosis.

Key Points

Background

- Abnormal vertebrae formation
- Often results in scoliosis
- Associated with multiple spinal anomalies (diastematomyelia, tethered cord, etc.)

Imaging

- Spectrum includes hemivertebrae, butterfly vertebrae, small or absent intervertebral disc, fusion of vertebral body and/or posterior elements (transverse processes, lamina, facets, spinous processes), and AP narrowing of the vertebral bodies.

REFERENCE

1. Grimme JD, Castillo M. Congenital anomalies of the spine. *Neuroimaging Clin N Am*. 2007 Feb;17(1):1–16.

KLIPPEL FEIL

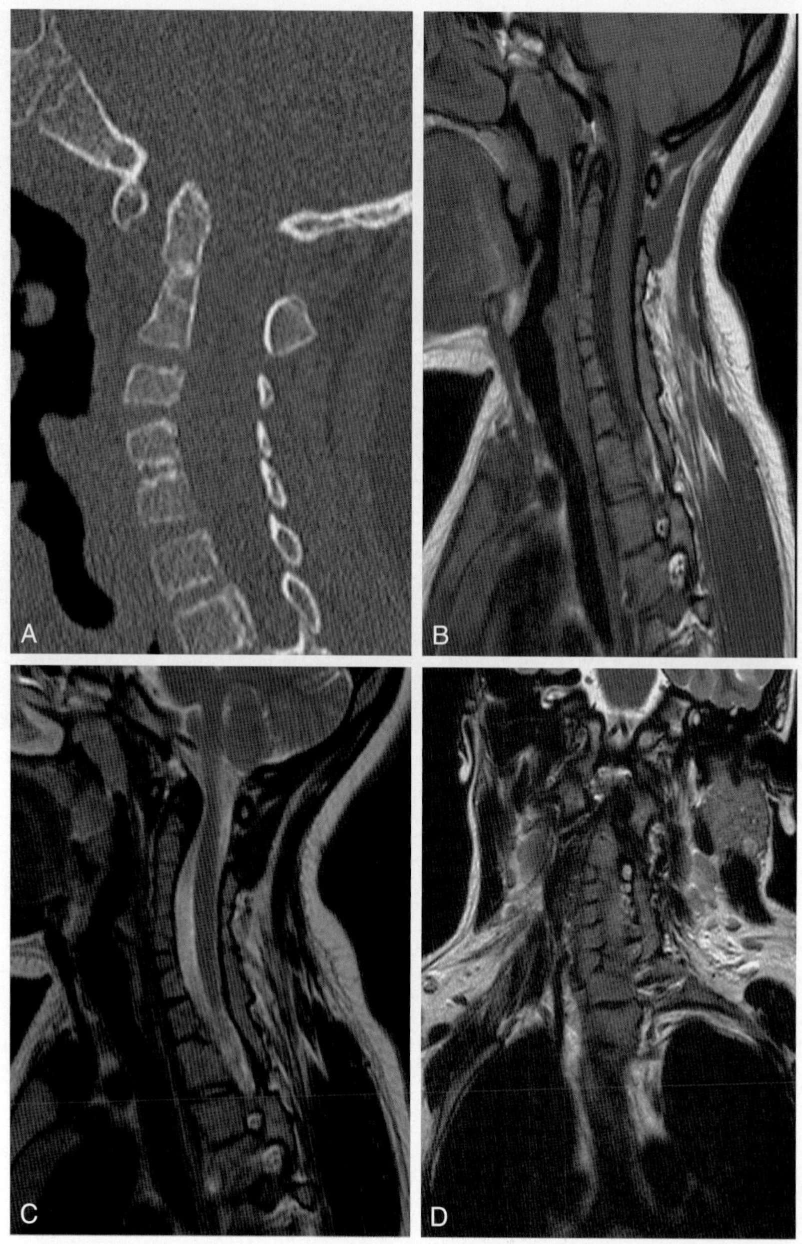

Fig. 16.31 Klippel-Feil syndrome. (A) Sagittal reformat CT demonstrates fused C2 and C3 vertebrae, C1 anterior arch assimilation with the clivus, and C5-6 rudimentary disc formation. Second patient: (B) sagittal T1W and (C and D) sagittal and coronal T2W images demonstrate numerous cervical segmentation anomalies and gracile appearance of the bones.

Key Points

Background

- Segmentation anomaly involving two or more cervical vertebrae; most commonly involves the C2–3 level.
- Coexisting petrous bone anomalies must be excluded in symptomatic patients.

Imaging

- Fusion of two or more cervical vertebrae
- Associations: Scoliosis, Sprengel deformity, temporal bone anomalies (microtia, external auditory canal (EAC) stenosis, inner ear anomalies, large vestibular aqueduct, internal auditory canal (IAC) malformation), cervical ribs, rib anomalies, genitourinary, and cardiac abnormalities

REFERENCE

1. Grimme JD, Castillo M. Congenital anomalies of the spine. *Neuroimaging Clin N Am*. 2007 Feb;17(1):1–16.

ACHONDROPLASIA

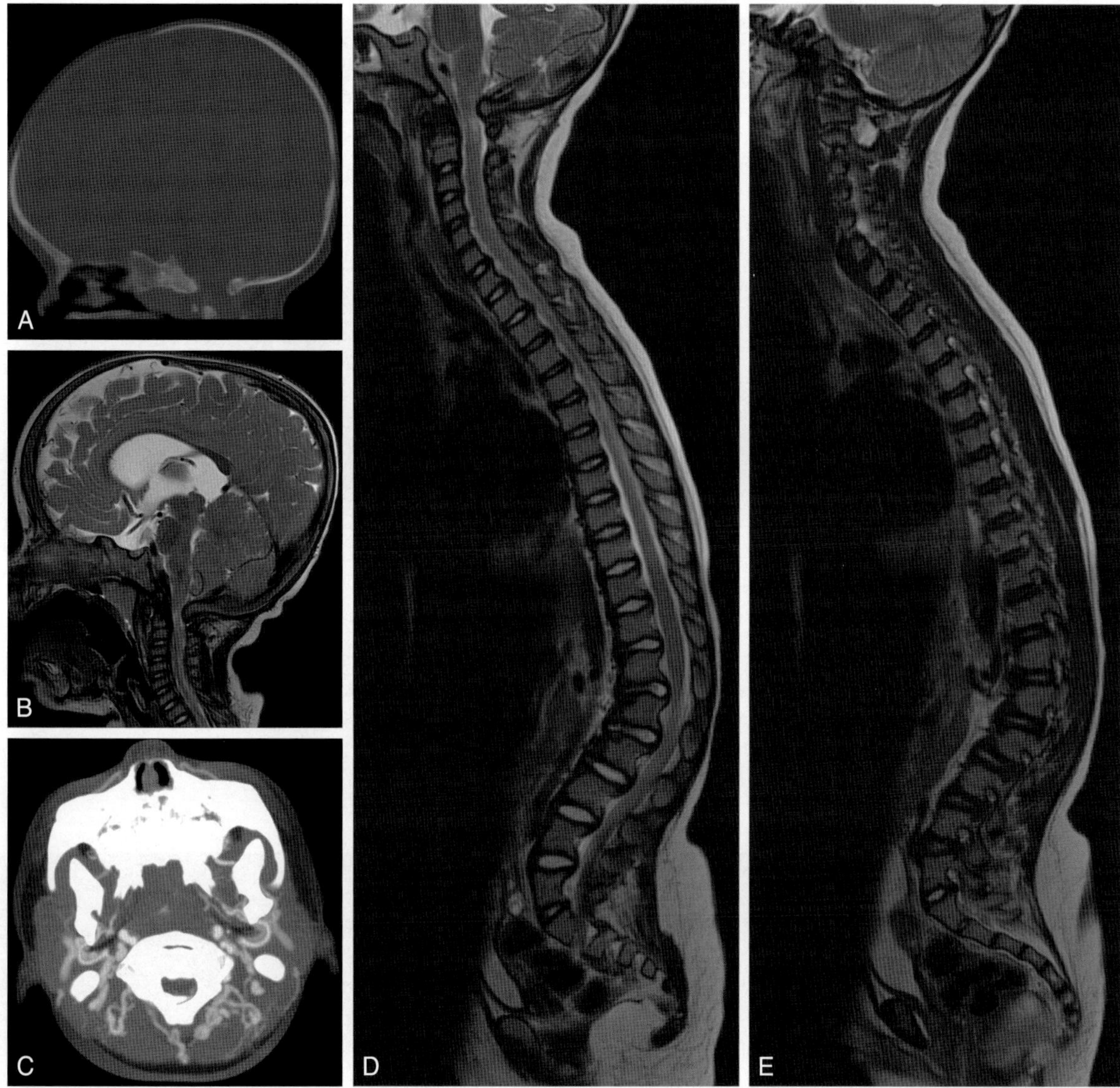

Fig. 16.32 Achondroplasia. (A) Sagittal reformat CT and (B) sagittal T2W images demonstrate fusion of the spheno-occipital synchondrosis, J-shaped sella, foramen magnum stenosis, upper spinal cord compression with abnormal T2W hyperintense cord signal from myelomalacia, and ventriculomegaly. (C) Axial CT venogram demonstrates an increased number of venous collaterals in the upper cervical spine due to jugular foramen stenosis and collateral formation. (D and E) Sagittal T2W images demonstrate foramen magnum stenosis, cord compression, cord myelomalacia, thoracolumbar junction kyphosis, short pedicles, and narrow spinal canal diameter.

Key Points

Background

- Autosomal dominant disorder caused by genetic mutation of the fibroblast growth factor receptor (FGFR3)
- Leads to abnormal enchondral bone formation
- Leads to dwarfism with greater involvement of proximal limbs

Imaging

- Early closure of spheno-occipital synchondrosis.
- Foramen magnum stenosis. Additional narrowing of the skull base foramina may exist.
- Large emissary veins and venous collateral formation at the skull base, possibly secondary to impaired normal venous drainage by the jugular veins due to a narrowing of the jugular foramina. Prominent veins may be seen overlying the cerebral hemispheres.
- Ventriculomegaly from venous hypertension.
- Short pedicles resulting in spinal stenosis, flattened vertebral bodies, thoracolumbar kyphosis, and scalloping of the dorsal contour of the vertebral bodies.

REFERENCE

1. Bosemani T, Orman G, Hergan B, et al. Achondroplasia in children: correlation of ventriculomegaly, size of foramen magnum, and jugular foramina, and emissary vein enlargement. *Childs Nerv Syst*. 2015 Jan;31(1):129–133.

OSTEOGENESIS IMPERFECTA

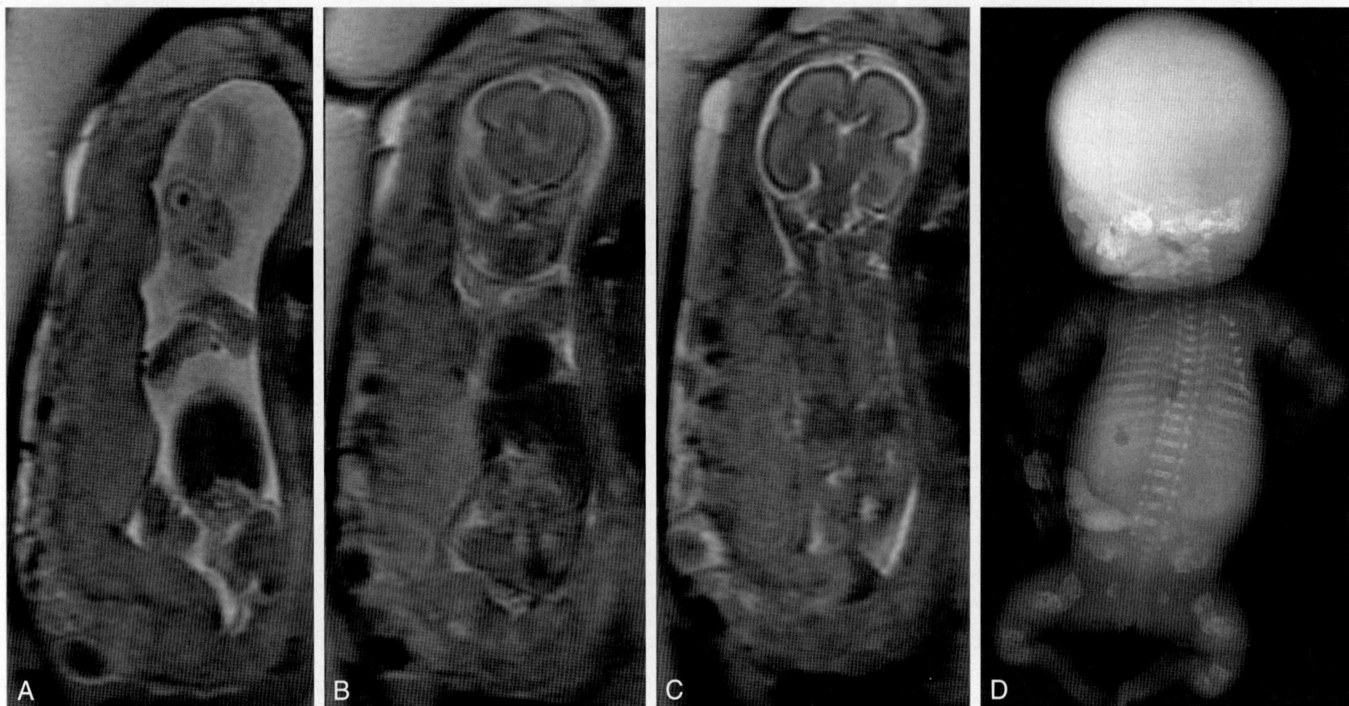

Fig. 16.33 Osteogenesis Imperfecta Type 2. (A to C) Coronal and sagittal T2W fetal MR images demonstrating small chest size and shortened limbs. (D) Postmortem AP radiograph demonstrating small chest, small vertebral bodies, and short limbs with fractures. Genetic testing confirmed type 2 osteogenesis imperfecta type 2.

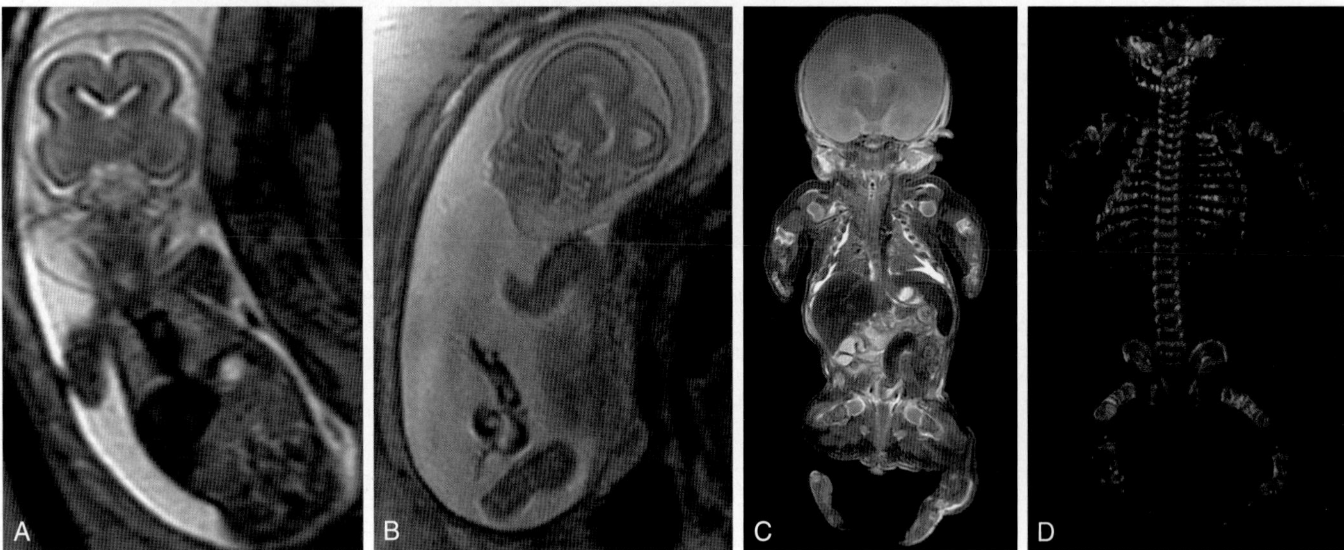

Fig. 16.34 Osteogenesis Imperfecta Type 2. (A and B) Coronal and sagittal T2W fetal MR images demonstrate a small chest, short limbs, and hydrops of the face and scalp. (C) Coronal postmortem T2W image and (D) postmortem volumetric CT image demonstrate similar findings of small chest size and shortened limbs with multiple rib and extremity fractures. Genetic testing confirmed type 2 osteogenesis imperfecta.

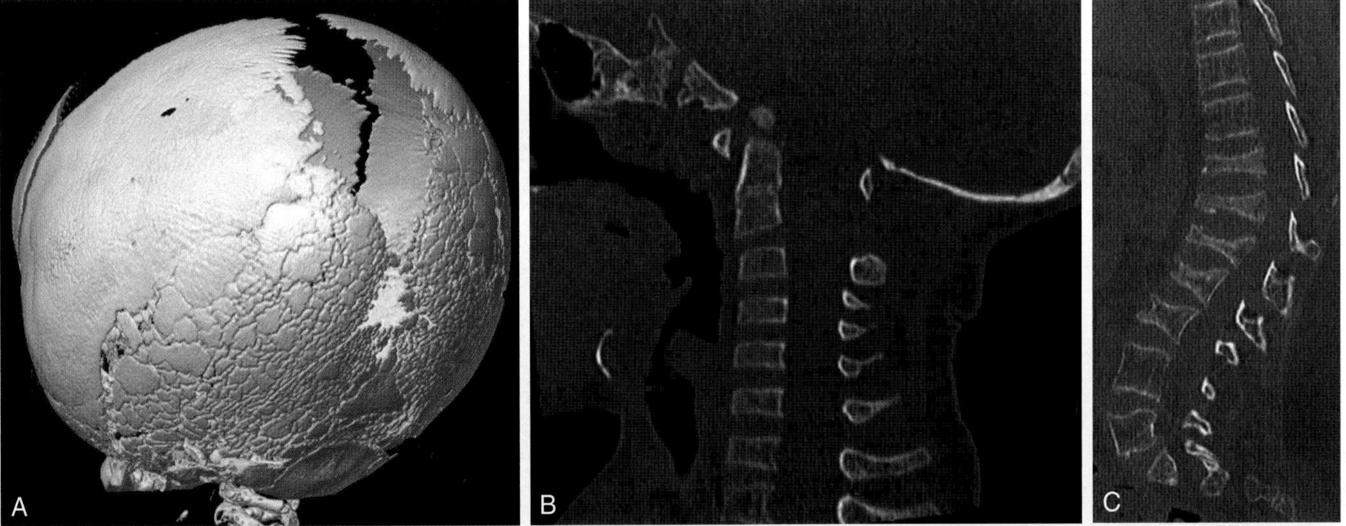

Fig. 16.35 Osteogenesis Imperfecta Type 3. (A) A 1-year-old with numerous wormian bones in the occipital bone seen on volumetric CT image. (B) A 7-year-old with platybasia and basilar invagination seen on sagittal CT reformat image. (C) A 13-year-old with multiple spinal compression fractures, demineralization of the bones, exaggerated lumbar lordosis, and mild scoliosis (not shown).

Key Points

Background

- Genetic disorder (most often affecting collagen COL1A1 or COL1A2 genes) affecting skin, teeth, sclera, ligaments, and bones.
- Clinical features include fragile bones/teeth, blue sclerae, hearing loss, and skeletal deformity.
- There are four main types of osteogensis imperfecta; however, there are now known to be 21 genetic mutations resulting in osteogenesis imperfecta.
  1. Type 1: Most common form (50%) and mildest form. Usually diagnosed in childhood with multiple bone fractures, often associated with minimal trauma. Patients have blue sclera and increasing incidence of hearing loss with age.
  2. Type 2: Most severe type causing shortened arms and legs, small chest causing under developed lungs, soft skull, multiple fractures or long bones with deformity, micrognathia, and usually lethal in utero or neonatally.
  3. Type 3: Presents in infants due to extremely fragile bones and large head size, and often results in short stature, scoliosis, exaggerated lordosis or kyphosis, basilar invagination, and platybasia. Hearing loss occurs in the first decade.
  4. Type 4: Moderate severity, which can resemble either type 1 or 3. Fractures most commonly occur before puberty. May lead to scoliosis and hearing loss.

Imaging

- Multiple spinal imaging findings due to skeletal dysplasia, including platybasia, basilar invagination, platyspondyly, codfish vertebrae (biconcave central depression), scoliosis, and osteopenia.
- Calvarium demonstrates multiple wormian bones, in particular within the occipital calvarium. Temporal bone malformations can have associated hearing loss.

REFERENCE

1. Barkovich AJ, Raybaud C: *Pediatric neuroimaging*, 6th ed., Philadelphia, 2019, Wolters Kluwer.

MUCOPOLYSACCHARIDOSIS

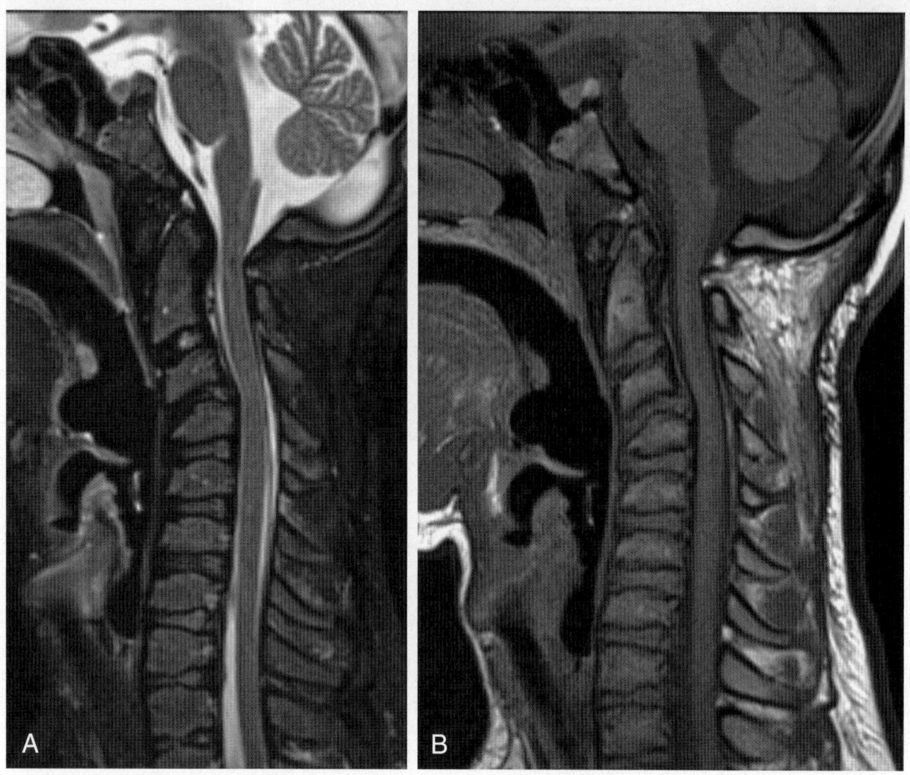

Fig. 16.36 Mucopolysaccharidoses. A 14-year-old with MPS-3 (Hunter syndrome). (A) Sagittal T2W and (B) sagittal T1W images demonstrate foramen magnum stenosis, shortened clivus, J-shaped sella, and inferior beaking of the vertebral bodies

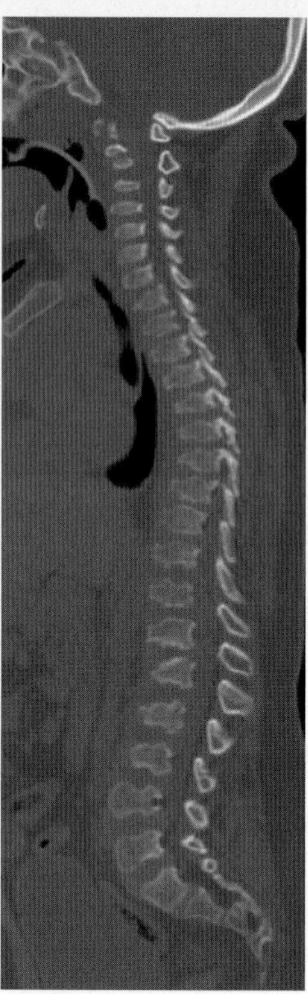

Fig. 16.37 Mucopolysaccharidoses. A 9-year-old with MPS-7 (Sly syndrome). Sagittal reformat CT image demonstrates foramen magnum stenosis, shortened clivus, and inferior beaking of the vertebral bodies.

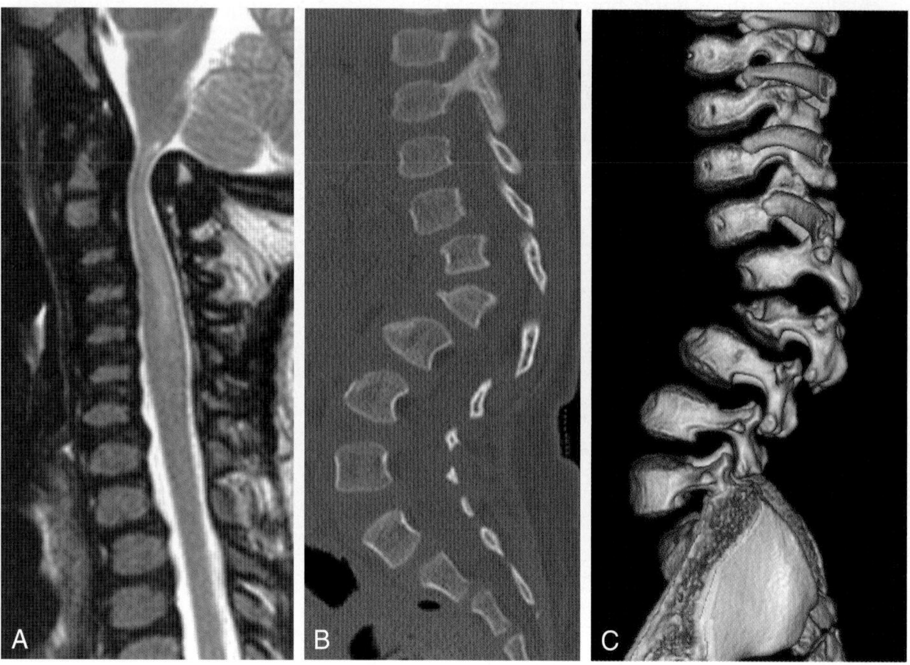

Fig. 16.38 Mucopolysaccharidoses. A 4-year-old with MPS-6 (Maroteaux-Lamy syndrome). (A) Sagittal T2W image demonstrates foramen magnum stenosis, cord compression and myelomalacia, and small cervical vertebral bodies. (B and C) Sagittal and 3D volumetric CT images demonstrate inferior beaking of the vertebral bodies and thoracolumbar junction kyphosis.

Key Points

Background

- A group of lysosomal storage disorders with enzyme deficiencies resulting in failure to degrade mucopolysaccharides (also known as glycosaminoglycans[GAGs]).
- Accumulation of GAGs around vessels and leptomeninges may result in the perivascular spaces and/or impaired resorption of CSF in the arachnoid granulations.
- Autosomal recessive except MPS-2 (Hunter), which is X-linked.

Classification:

- *Seven distinct types* that are further divided into subtypes according to enzyme deficiency and clinical severity. MPS-5 was reclassified as MPS-1S and MPS-8 were retracted.
- MPS-1: 1H (Hurler) subtype is the most severe, with cognitive and multisystemic involvement; 1H/S (Hunter/Scheie) subtype has intermediate severity; 1S (Scheie) subtype is the least affected and no cognitive decline; all due to alpha-L-iduronidase deficiency.
- MPS-2: Hunter syndrome due to iduronate-2-sulfatase deficiency; mild and severe subtypes depending on neurologic impairment.
- MPS 3: Sanfilippo syndrome A–D (subtypes) due to multiple enzyme deficiencies.
- MPS-4: Morquio syndrome A and B (subtypes) due to *N*-acetylgalactosamine-6-sulfatase and galactose 6-sulfatase deficiency.
- MPS-6: Maroteaux-Lamy syndrome due to *N*-acetylgalactosamine-4-sulfatase deficiency.
- MPS-7: Sly syndrome due to beta-glucoronidase deficiency.
- MPS-9: Natowicz syndrome due to hyaluronidase deficiency; rarest of the MPS.

Clinical:

- Urinary GAG testing done for screening and enzyme assay for confirmation.
- MPS 1–3 and 7 have cognitive impairment in the first year of life.
- MPS 4 and 6 usually do not have cognitive impairment but more frequent spinal stenosis.
- Multiple organ systems are involved, leading to hepatosplenomegaly, mental retardation, and skeletal anomalies (also known as dysostosis multiplex; MPS 1, 2, 4, 6, 7).
- Some MPS can be treated with intravenous enzyme replacement or stem cell transplantation.

Spine Imaging

- *Early closure of spheno-occipital synchondrosis*, thoracolumbar junction kyphosis, disc degeneration, hypoplastic dens, ligamentous thickening, craniocervical junction stenosis, and craniocervical junction instability.
- Vertebral body morphology due to failure of ossification of the peripheral secondary ossification centers due to the accumulation of the glycosaminoglycans.
- *Vertebral deformities* include platyspondyly, round or bullet-shaped vertebral bodies, wedge deformity, central vertebral body beaking (MPS-4) or anterior inferior beaking (other MPSs), and posterior scalloping of the vertebral body.
- Compressive myelopathy at the craniocervical junction and thoracolumbar junction.
- MPS-4 and 6 frequently have skeletal dysplasia, compressive myelopathy, and cervical instability.

REFERENCES

1. Nicolas-Jiwan M, Al Sayed M. Mucopolysaccharidoses: overview of neuroimaging manifestations. *Pediatr Radiol.* 2018;48:1503–1520.
2. Reichert R, Goncalves Campos L, Vairo F, et al. Neuroimaging findings in patients with mucopolysaccharidosis: what you really need to know. *Radiographics.* 2016 Sept–Oct;36(5):1448–1462.
3. Wagner MW, Poretti A, Benson JE, Huisman TA. Neuroimaging findings in pediatric genetic skeletal disorders: a review. *J Neuroimaging.* 2017 Mar;27(2):162–209.

SYRINGOHYDROMYELIA

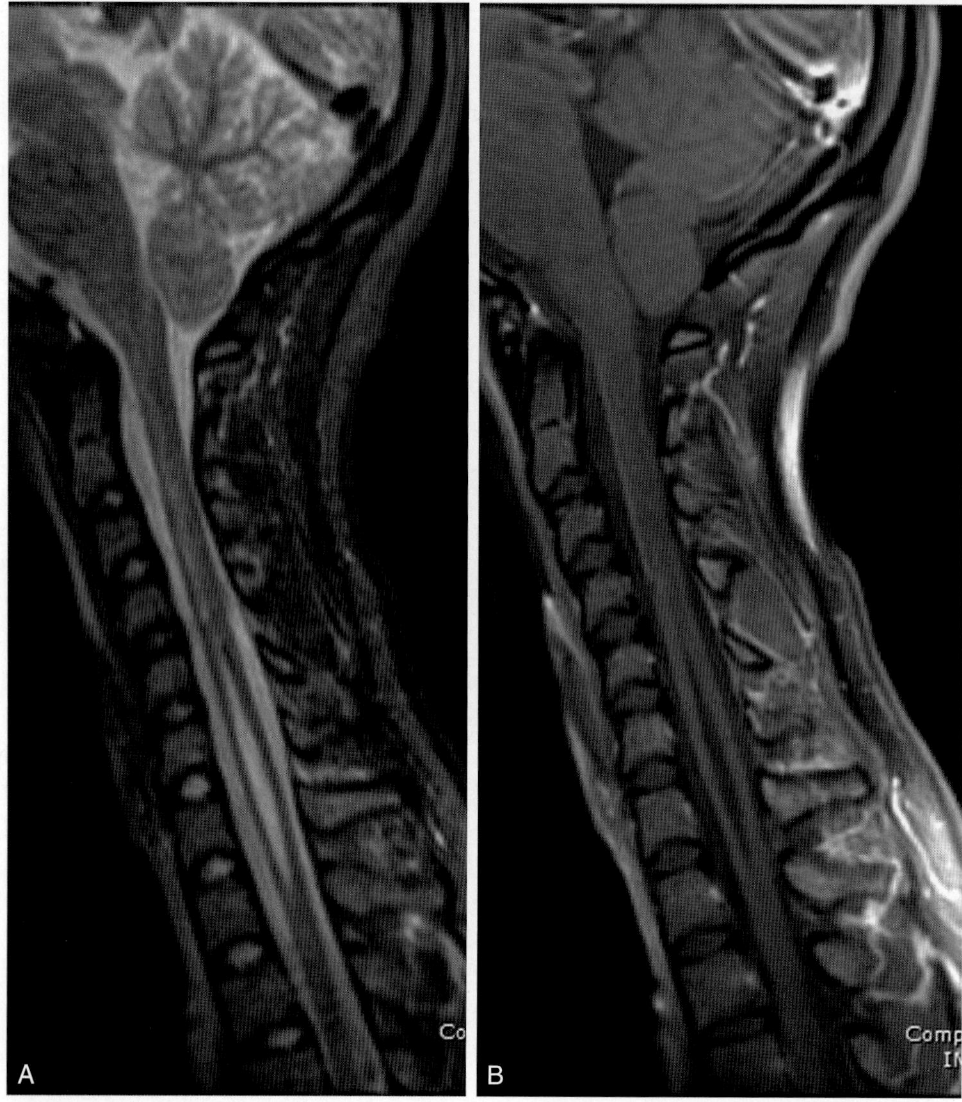

Fig. 16.39 Syringohydromyelia. (A) Sagittal T2W and (B) sagittal T1W+C images demonstrates a nonenhancing T2W hyperintense well defined intramedullary central spinal cord lesion.

Key Points

Background

- Clinical: Segmental weakness with atrophy, loss of tendon reflexes, and segmental loss of pain and temperature sense with preservation of the sense of touch, and dysesthesias.
- While hydromyelia refers to dilatation of the central spinal canal and syringomyelia refers to fluid-filled space in the spinal cord, the term "syringohydromyelia" is more frequently used because the two can be indistinguishable when centrally located.
- Etiology: The most common causes are Chiari 1 malformation, trauma, tumor, and tethered spinal cord, but a large number are idiopathic.

Imaging

- *Well-defined intramedullary central T2 hyperintense signal*
- Presyrinx terminology used when fluid is not well defined and presumed to be the precursor prior to becoming a syrinx or resolving if the cause for CSF flow alteration is removed
- Contrast typically administered for initial syrinx evaluation but more recent data suggest that T2W sequences have high sensitivity and high negative predictive value in detecting an associated mass

REFERENCE

1. Timpone VM, Patel SH. MRI of a syrinx: is contrast material always necessary?. *AJR Am J Roentgenol.* 2015 May;204(5):1082–1085.

17 Spine Masses

APPROACH TO SPINE MASSES

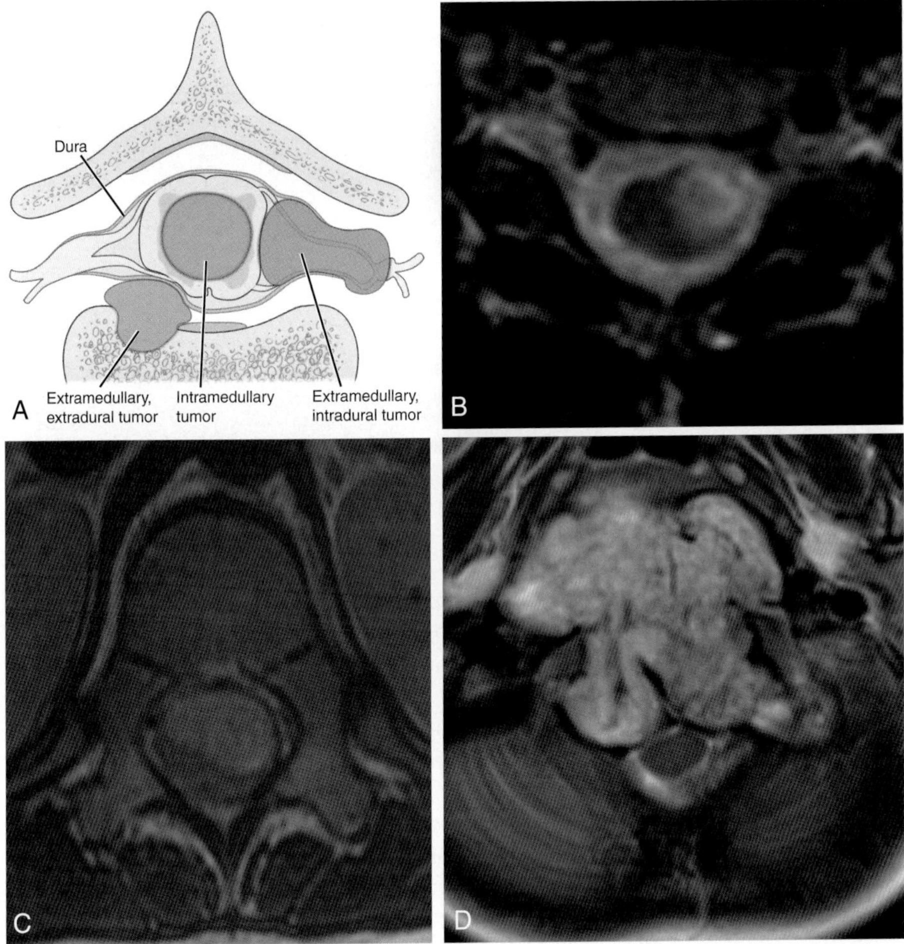

Fig. 17.1 Approach to Spinal Masses. (A) Diagram of the relationship of various tumors to the spine, nerve roots, and spinal cord. (B) Example of an intradural intramedullary mass expanding the left side of the spinal cord. (C) Example of an intradural extramedullary mass which is compressing the spinal cord. (D) Example of an extradural mass. (A from Kliegman RM, Nelson WE. *Nelson Textbook of Pediatrics*. 2nd ed. Philadelphia: Elsevier; 2020. Used with permission from Barrow Neurological Institute.)

Key Points

Background

- Spinal masses include those arising from the central nervous system, as well as those arising from other organ systems with either direct extension or systemic spread to the spine.
- It is important to remember that inflammatory processes such as transverse myelitis can present with mass-like features and congenital malformations such as lipomas or meningoceles can present as a mass. These entities should not be misdiagnosed as neoplastic.

Imaging

- An approach to a spinal mass starts with determination of whether the mass is intramedullary, intradural extramedullary, or extradural. Extradural masses can be additionally subdivided into those involving bone, bone and soft tissue, or soft tissue. This approach allows for a narrow differential diagnosis, which, in many instances, is the limitation of imaging and at which point a tissue diagnosis is required.
- This section will illustrate the common and uncommon spinal masses in children using this organizational approach.
- Spinal imaging modalities include radiographs, ultrasound, CT, and MRI. The majority of spinal masses are best evaluated with MRI, and consequently, the majority of diagnoses presented in this section will feature MRI images.

SPINAL CORD LOW-GRADE ASTROCYTOMA

Intramedullary

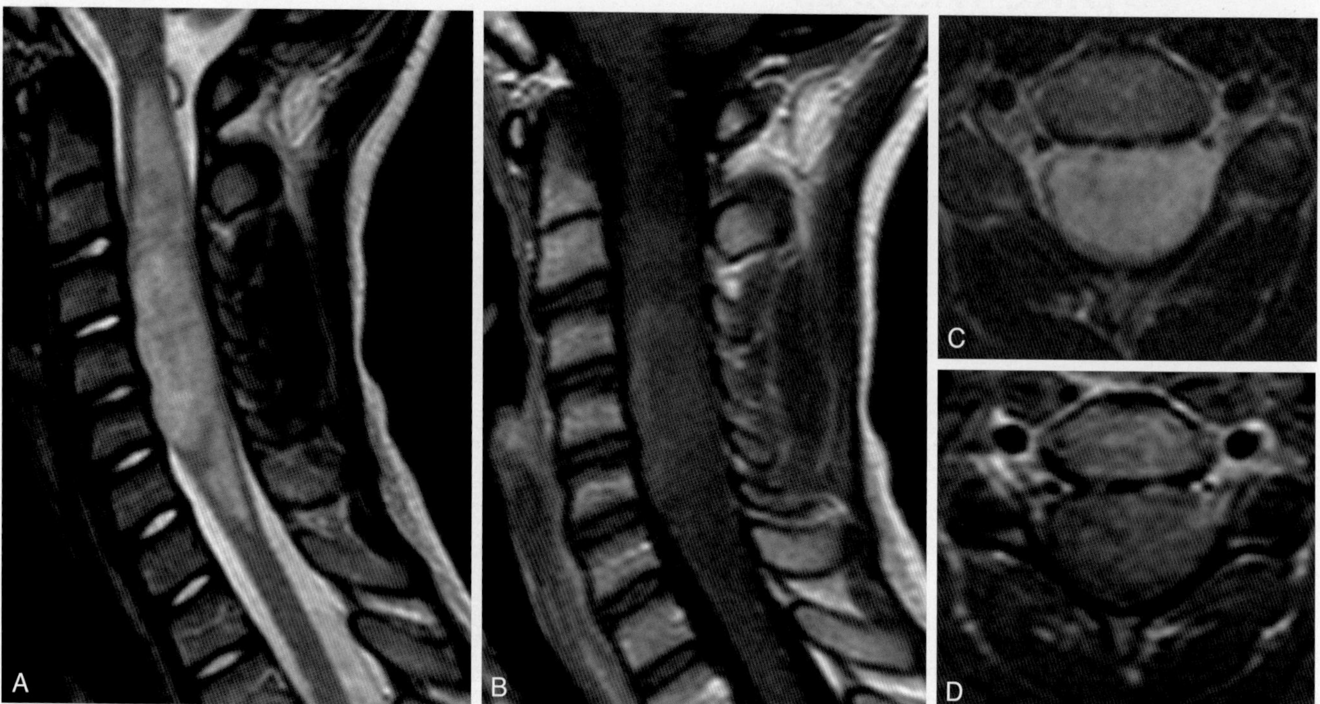

Fig. 17.2 Spinal Cord Low-Grade Astrocytoma. (A and C) Sagittal and axial T2W and (B and D) sagittal and axial T1W+C images demonstrate an intramedullary expansile, T2W hyperintense mass with small areas of ill-defined enhancement from C1 to C7. Cross-section images through the mass demonstrate the intramedullary location of the mass and the degree of expansion fills the thecal sac such that no CSF is visible.

Key Points

Background

- Astrocytomas are the *most common intramedullary tumor in children* (60%–80%).
- Majority (90%) are *low-grade* astrocytomas (pilocytic > fibrillary). Pilocytic astrocytomas typical occur in children ages 1 to 5 years; fibrillary astrocytomas typically occur in children ~10 years of age.
- Clinical symptoms include progressive scoliosis, torticollis, head tilt, dysphagia, dysphonia, back pain, and weakness.

Imaging

- Location: Intramedullary mass.
- MRI: Expansile T2W hyperintense. Variable enhancement. Usually no hemorrhage. May have a cyst and nodule pattern.
- Usually extend craniocaudally <4 vertebral body lengths.
- Tumor margins are usually indistinct.
- Pilocytic astrocytomas can have a necrosis/cystic degeneration, cyst and nodule, or solid appearance.
- Astrocytomas are more frequently located within the periphery of the spinal cord, but large size at presentation usually limits this as a helpful clue. Astrocytomas are typically ill defined and diffusively infiltrative without a clear cleavage plane.
- DTI may be helpful for determining margins/resectability.

REFERENCES

1. Rossi A, Gandolfo C, Morana G, et al. Tumors of the spine in children. *Neuroimaging Clin N Am*. 2007 Feb;17(1):17–35.
2. Haverkamp BT, Nizamuddin RA, Loskutov A, et al. Imaging spectrum of pediatric spinal neoplasms. *Neurographics*. 2017 May–June;7(3):151–162.

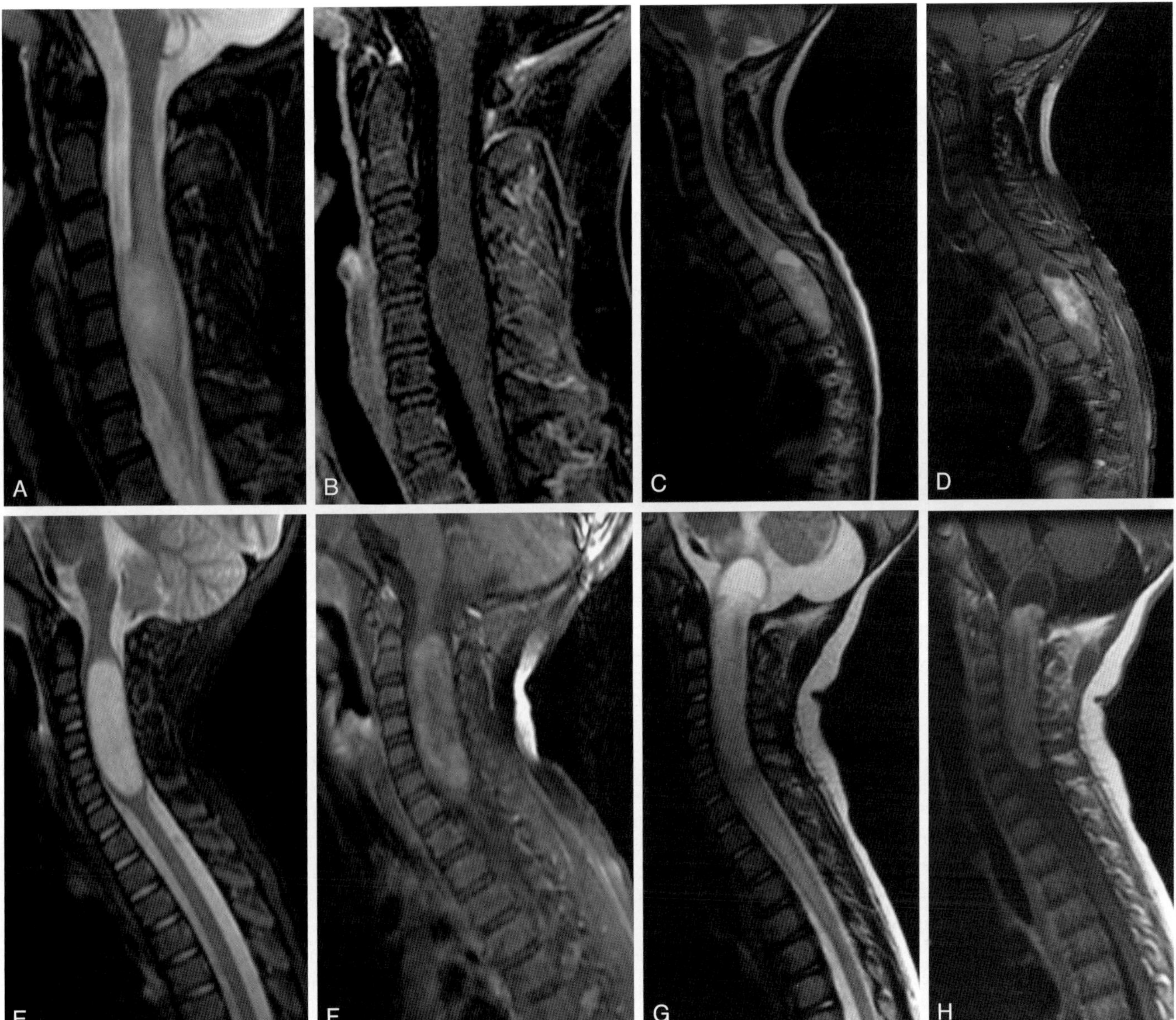

Fig. 17.3 Imaging Appearances of Spinal Cord Low-Grade Astrocytomas. (A and B) Sagittal T2W and sagittal T1W+C images demonstrate an intramedullary expansile, nonenhancing T2W hyperintense mass in the cervical spine with indistinct margins. (C and D) Sagittal T2W and sagittal T1W+C images demonstrate an intramedullary expansile, T2W hyperintense solid and cystic ovoid mass with heterogeneous enhancement in the thoracic cord from T3 to T6 with adjacent nonenhancing T2W hyperintensity superiorly. (E and F) Sagittal T2W and sagittal T1W+C images demonstrate an ovoid well-circumscribed intramedullary expansile, T2W hyperintense mass with mostly diffuse enhancement in the cervical cord from C2 to C7. (G and H) Sagittal T2W and sagittal T1W+C images demonstrate an intramedullary expansile, T2W hyperintense mass with cyst and nodule enhancement pattern in the cervical cord from the medulla to C7 and nonenhancing T2W hyperintense signal extending caudally to T5, which could be from edema or nonenhancing tumor.

SPINAL CORD EPENDYMOMA

Intramedullary

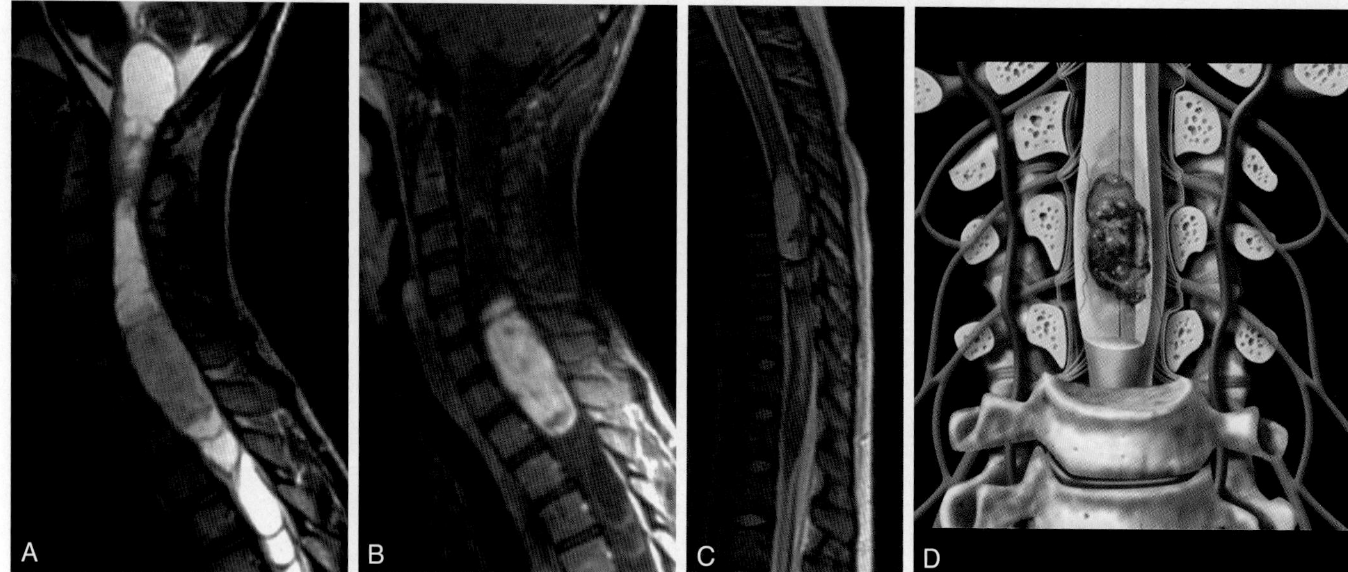

Fig. 17.4 Spinal Cord Ependymoma. (A) Sagittal T2W and (B) sagittal T1W+C images demonstrate an intramedullary expansile, T2W hyperintense solid and cystic mass with large nodular enhancement from C5 to T1 and adjacent nonenhancing cyst formation superiorly and inferiorly. (C) Sagittal T2W image demonstrating an intramedullary mass with T2W hypointense curvilinear areas due to hemorrhage, also known as the "cap sign." (D) Illustration of spinal cord ependymoma demonstrating the centrally located solid nodularity and peripheral cyst formation. (D, STATDx, Copyright © 2021 Elsevier.)

Key Points

Background

- Second most common intramedullary tumor in children; 30% of pediatric intramedullary tumors
- More centrally located than astrocytomas, therefore can present with sensory symptoms in addition to back pain and weakness
- Treated with surgical resection and radiotherapy for residual/recurrent tumor

Imaging

- Location: Intramedullary mass
- MRI: *Well-defined* nodular enhancement. Frequent *cyst formation* at the margins of the tumor. *Intratumoral hemorrhage* results in T2W hypointensity. "Cap sign" = hemosiderin at the cranial or caudal margin seen in 20% to 33%.
- Ependymomas are more frequently noted in a central location surrounding the central canal and are more often expansile rather than infiltrative with a better defined cleavage plane compared to astrocytomas.
- DTI fiber tracking demonstrating displaced tract rather than infiltration.
- *Neurofibromatosis Type-2*–associated ependymomas frequently small in size and multiple.
- Radiotherapy can result in pseudoprogression demonstrating new peripherally enhancing lesion that spontaneously regresses over time.

REFERENCES

1. Rossi A, Gandolfo C, Morana G, et al. Tumors of the spine in children. *Neuroimaging Clin N Am*. 2007 Feb;17(1):17–35.
2. Haverkamp BT, Nizamuddin RA, Loskutov A, et al. Imaging spectrum of pediatric spinal neoplasms. *Neurographics*. 2017 May–June;7(3):151–162.

SPINAL CORD GANGLIOGLIOMA

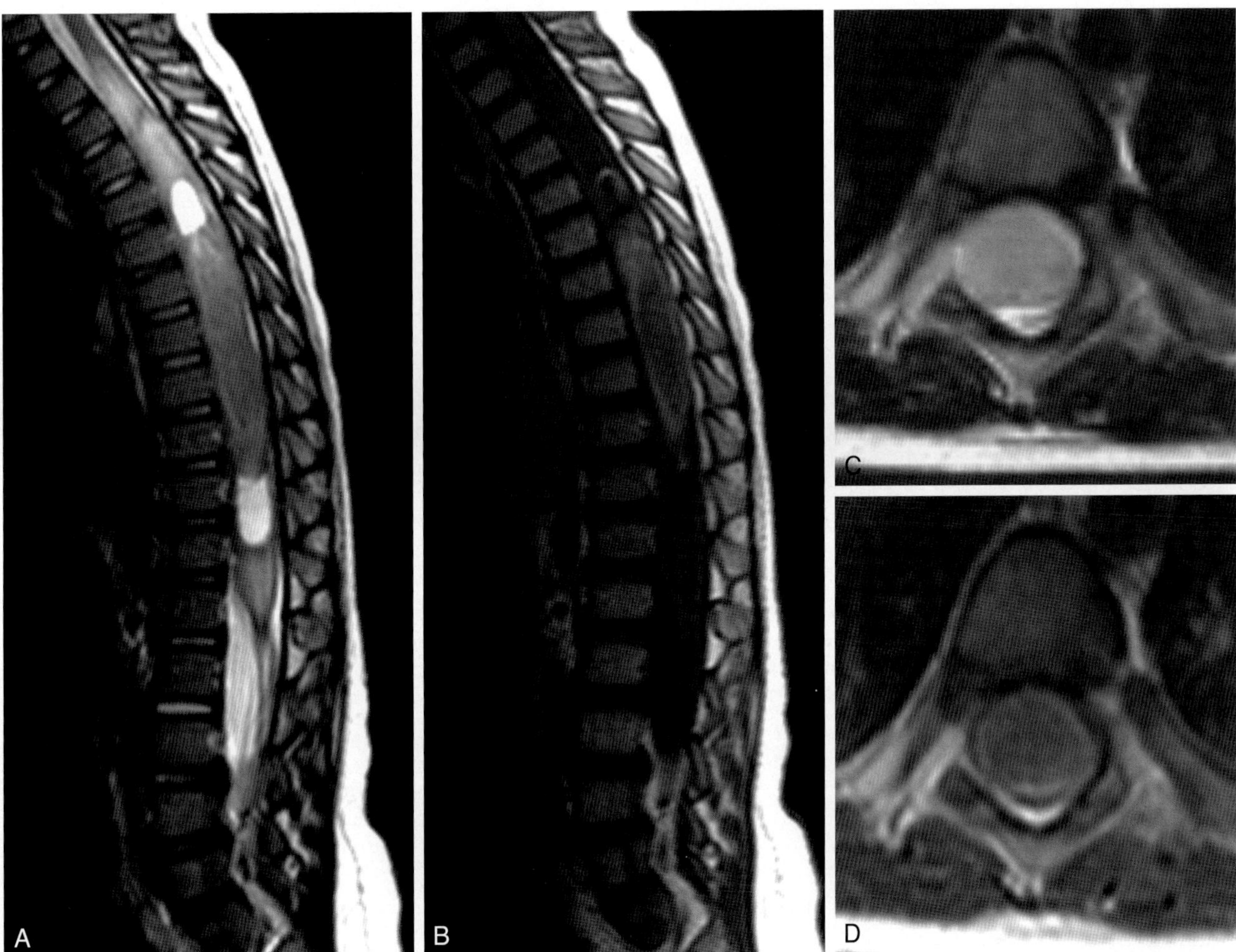

Fig. 17.5 Spinal Cord Ganglioglioma. (A and C) Sagittal and axial T2W and (B and D) sagittal and axial T1W+C images demonstrate an intramedullary expansile, T2W hyperintense mass with partial nodular enhancement and cysts in the thoracic and lumbar spinal cord. Cross-section images through the mass demonstrate the intramedullary location of the mass and the degree of expansion which fills the thecal sac such that no CSF is visible.

Key Points

Background

- Third most common intramedullary spinal cord tumor in children (15%)
- Low grade (WHO grade 1 and 2) with low potential for malignant degeneration
- Age 1–5 years. Typically present with slow progression of pain, myelopathic symptoms, and/or scoliosis
- Often centered in the cervical cord with extension to the medulla or upper thoracic cord

Imaging

- Location: Intramedullary mass
- MRI: May appear completely solid or have cyst formation. Variable enhancement. May contain calcification
- Currently not possible to distinguish from astrocytoma

REFERENCE

1. Rossi A, Gandolfo C, Morana G, et al. Tumors of the spine in children. *Neuroimaging Clin N Am.* 2007 Feb;17(1):17–35.

SPINAL CORD HIGH-GRADE MIDLINE GLIOMA

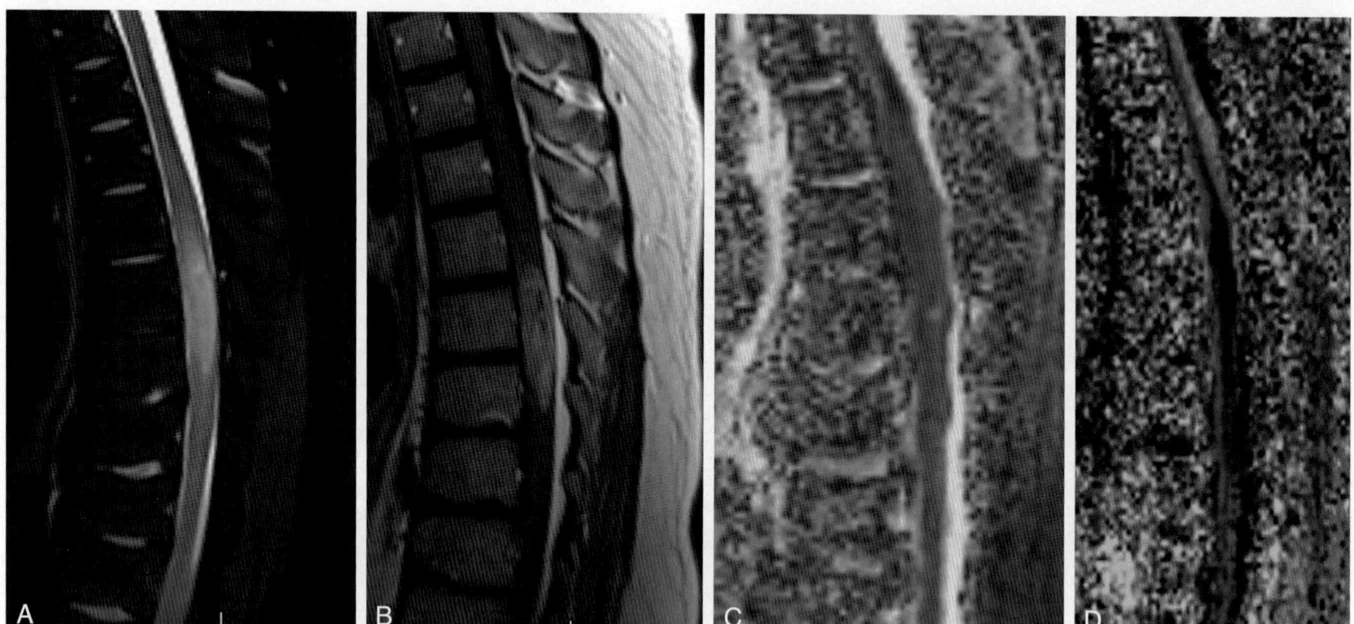

Fig. 17.6 Spinal Cord High-Grade Midline Glioma. (A) Sagittal T2W and (B) sagittal T1W+C images demonstrate an intramedullary expansile, T2W hyperintense mass with heterogeneous enhancement and ill-defined margins in the thoracic spinal cord. (C) Sagittal ADC and (D) sagittal color directional encoded images demonstrate isointense ADC signal and loss of directionality suggestive of an infiltrative glioma.

Key Points

Background

- Rare high-grade glioma of the spinal cord
- H3K27M mutation similar to high-grade thalamic and pontine gliomas
- Poor prognosis

Imaging

- Location: Intramedullary mass
- MRI: Difficult to distinguish from low-grade tumors at this time; usually poorly defined margins; high-grade tumors may result in greater infiltration and disruption of fiber tracts.

REFERENCE

1. Haverkamp BT, Nizamuddin RA, Loskutov A, et al. Imaging spectrum of pediatric spinal neoplasms. *Neurographics*. 2017 May–June;7(3):151–162.

HEMANGIOBLASTOMA

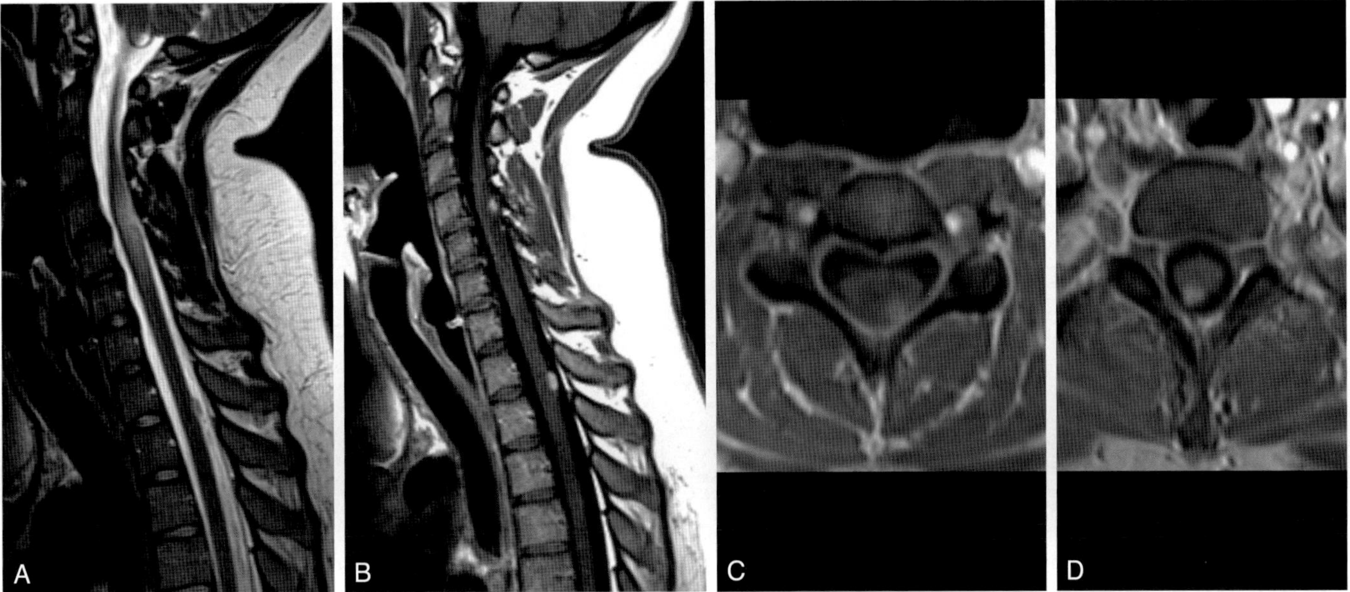

Fig. 17.7 Hemangioblastoma. (A) Sagittal T2W, (B) sagittal T1W+C, and (C and D) axial T1W+C images demonstrate intramedullary nodular foci of enhancement along the surface of the cervical and thoracic spinal cord associated with cervical spinal cord T2W hyperintense signal disproportionate to the size of the nodule.

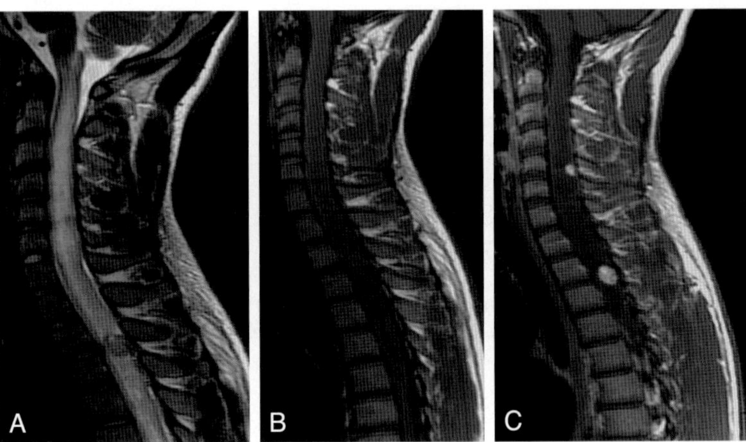

Fig. 17.8 Hemangioblastoma. (A) Sagittal T2W, (B) sagittal T1W, and (C) sagittal T1W+C images demonstrate intramedullary nodular foci of enhancement along the surface of the cervical and thoracic spinal cord associated with long segment cervical and thoracic spinal cord T2W hyperintense signal disproportionate to the size of the nodules.

Key Points

Background

- Benign vascular tumor
- Arise from the pial surface so may appear on the surface of the cord
- 25% to 40% associated with Von Hippel-Lindau disease

Imaging

- Location: Intramedullary mass along the *surface of the cord.*
- MRI: Typically small, circumscribed, *avidly enhancing*, and *disproportionate cord edema*. Larger tumors may have a cyst and nodule pattern.
- Dilated feeding and or draining subependymal or subpial vessels may be noted.
- Often multifocal and may be associated with von Hippel Lindau disease.
- Coexisting intracranial lesions must be excluded.
- Tendency to present with spontaneous intralesional hemorrhage including subarachnoid or intradural hemorrhage.

REFERENCE

1. Haverkamp BT, Nizamuddin RA, Loskutov A, et al. Imaging spectrum of pediatric spinal neoplasms. *Neurographics*. 2017 May–June;7(3):151–162.

MYXOPAPILLARY EPENDYMOMA

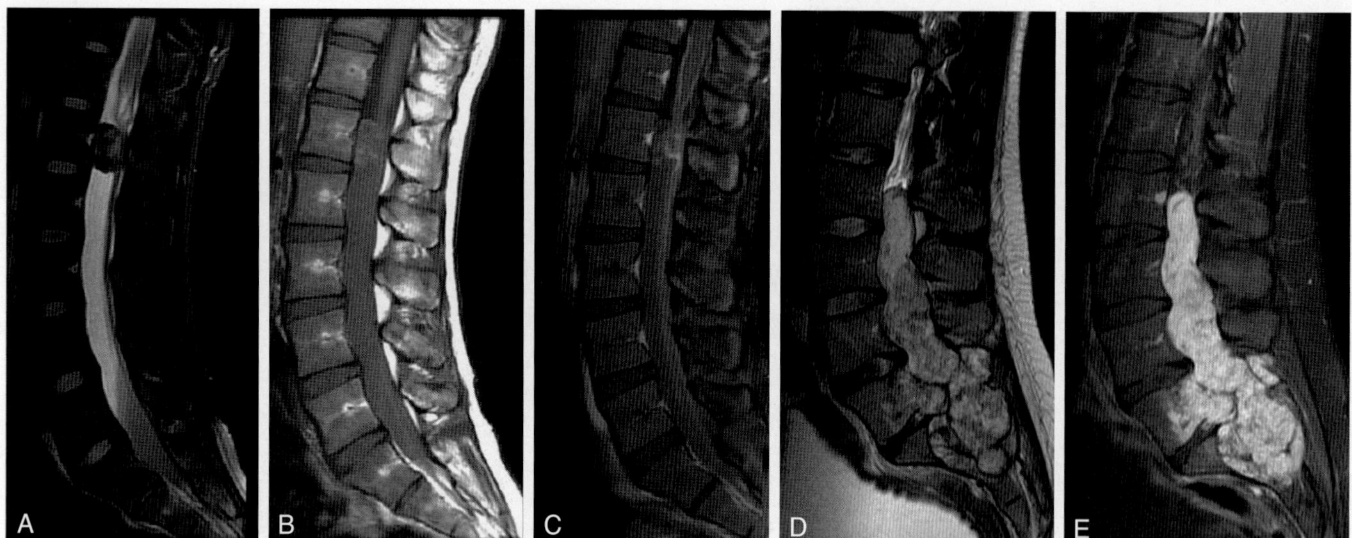

Fig. 17.9 Myxopapillary Ependymoma. (A) Sagittal T2W, (B) sagittal T1W, and (C) sagittal T1W+C images demonstrate an intradural extramedullary minimally enhancing nodule with heterogeneous T1W and T2W signal at the conus associated with layering fluid in the distal thecal sac. (D and E) Different patient with a myxopapillary ependymoma. (D) Sagittal T2W and (E) sagittal T1W+C images demonstrate a large intradural extramedullary and extradural mass with avid homogeneous enhancement that has invaded the L5 and S1 vertebrae. The origin of this mass is difficult to determine due to the large size. Location near the conus is a clue to the diagnosis.

Key Points

Background

- WHO grade 2
- Typically arise from ependymal glial cells of the conus/filum. Less commonly the vestiges of the neural tube in the sacrococcygeal region

Imaging

- Location: Intradural extramedullary mass.
- MRI: Variable T2 signal; variable but generally avid diffuse enhancement.
- *Located near the conus.* Can be very large, and subsequently the origin could be difficult to determine.
- *Propensity to spread in the CSF* despite low grade classification, requiring imaging of the entire spine and brain.
- Chronic pressure may result in dorsal scalloping or deformity of the adjacent vertebral bodies.

REFERENCE

1. Rossi A, Gandolfo C, Morana G, et al. Tumors of the spine in children. *Neuroimaging Clin N Am.* 2007 Feb;17(1):17–35.

MENINGIOMA

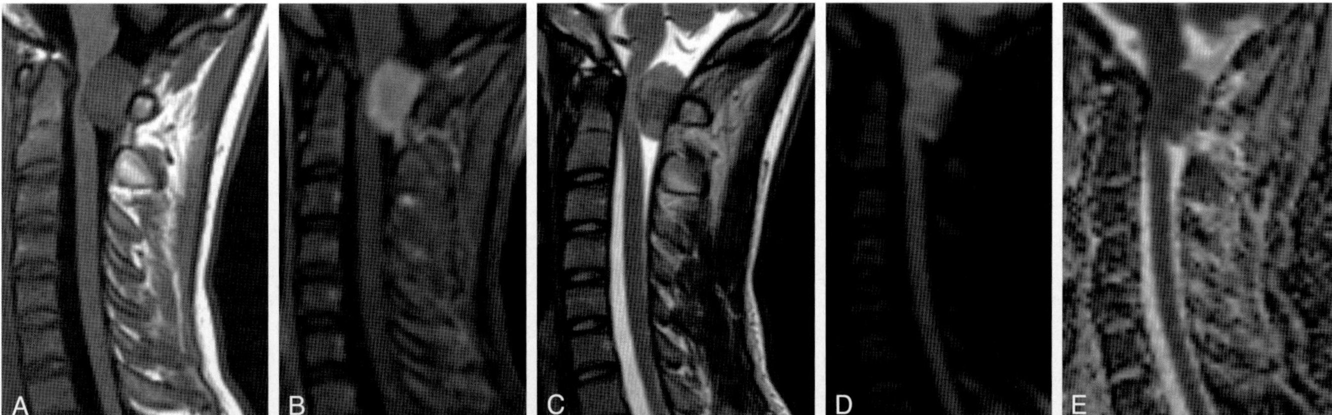

Fig. 17.10 Meningioma. (A) Sagittal T1W, (B) sagittal T1W+C, (C) sagittal T2W, (D) sagittal DWI, and (E) sagittal ADC map images demonstrate an intradural extramedullary homogeneously enhancing mass with mild diffusion hyperintensity and isointense ADC signal indicating cellularity consistent with a meningioma. There is compression of the dorsal medulla and cervical cord with small amount of cord T2W hyperintense signal which could reflect edema or myelomalacia that should be reassessed following removal of the mass.

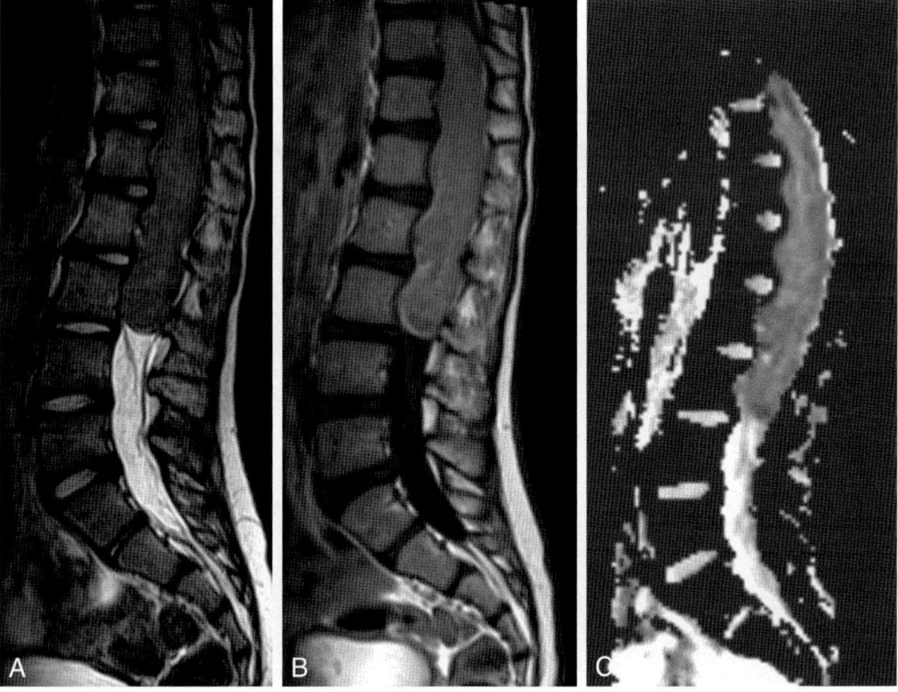

Fig. 17.11 Meningioma. (A) Sagittal T1W, (B) sagittal T1W+C, and (C) sagittal ADC map images demonstrate an intradural extramedullary homogeneously enhancing mass with mild mixed hyperintense and isointense ADC signal in the lower thoracic and upper lumbar spine mimicking a myxopapillary ependymoma.

Key Points

Background

- Uncommon in children
- Most commonly clear cell histopathology which has more aggressive behavior, higher recurrence rate, and potential for CSF spread
- Associated with NF-2

Imaging

- Location: Intradural extramedullary mass
- MRI: Homogeneous enhancement, circumscribed, dural tail
- Rare occurrence in children, and often *misdiagnosed as myxopapillary ependymoma* when located near the conus
- Significantly reduced diffusion due to high cellularity and, consequently, DWI-hyperintense with lowered ADC values

REFERENCE

1. Rossi A, Gandolfo C, Morana G, et al. Tumors of the spine in children. *Neuroimaging Clin N Am.* 2007 Feb;17(1):17–35.

CSF DROP METASTASES

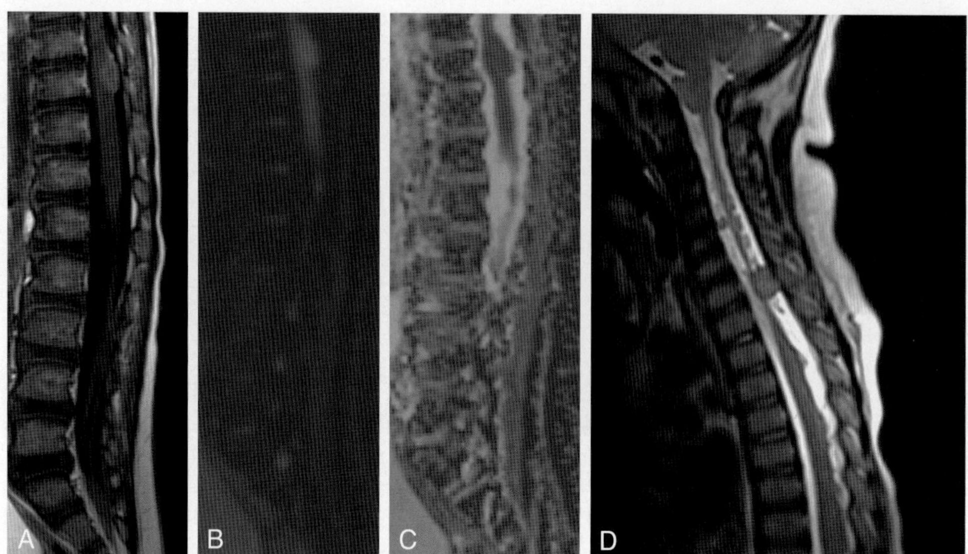

Fig. 17.12 CSF Metastases. (A) Sagittal T1W+C, (B) sagittal DWI, and (C) sagittal ADC map images demonstrate an intradural extramedullary homogeneously enhancing mass along the dorsal thoracic spinal cord with mild hyperintense DWI signal and isointense ADC signal indicative of a cellular tumor. (D) Sagittal 3D T2 image in a different patient with drop metastases demonstrates the utility of 3D T2W imaging for detection of intradural extramedullary masses due to the high contrast between the cord surface and CSF.

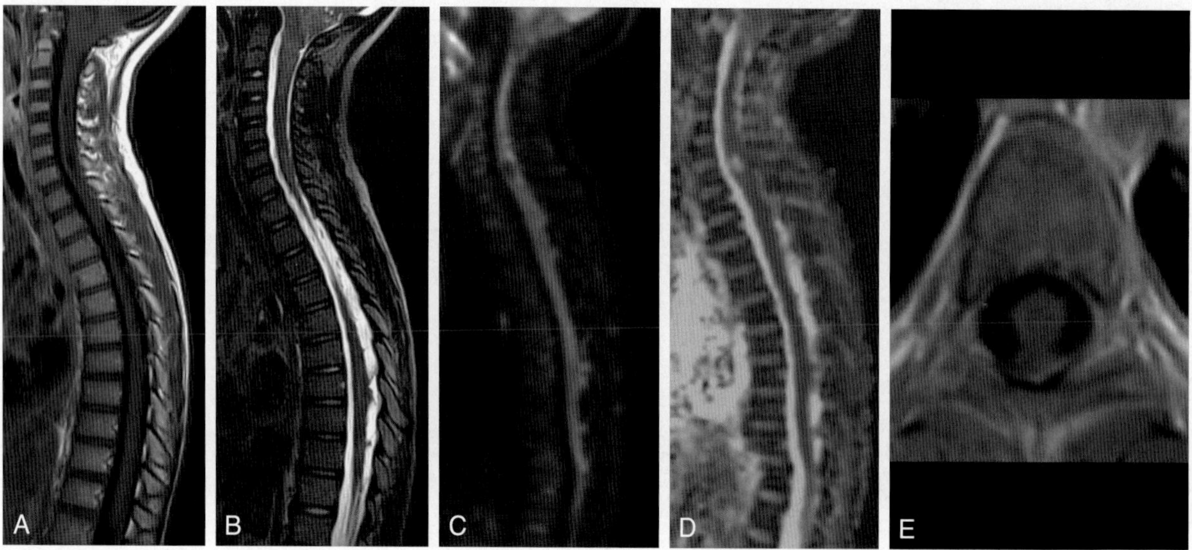

Fig. 17.13 CSF Metastases. (A) Sagittal T1W+C, (B) sagittal 3D T2, (C) sagittal DWI, (D) sagittal ADC map, and (E) axial T1W+C VIBE images demonstrate nonenhancing intradural extramedullary nodules along the dorsal thoracic spinal cord with mild hyperintense DWI signal and isointense ADC signal. The nodules are more readily detected using 3D T2 and DWI compared to T1W+C imaging.

Key Points

Background

- Both CSF cytology and MRI spine are used for detecting drop metastases; however, neither possesses 100% accuracy.
- Among patients with histological proof of leptomeningeal disease, no more than 59% demonstrate positive postmortem CSF cytology.
- Although most primary brain tumors have been reported with CSF metastases, medulloblastoma is the pediatric tumor most likely to have drop metastases.
- Accurate detection affects prognosis and management.

Imaging

- Location: Intradural extramedullary mass
- Homogenous enhancing discrete nodules or leptomeningeal thickening.
- Nonenhancing tumors can be seen with pilocytic/pilomyxoid astrocytomas, atypical teratoid rhabdoid tumor (ATRT), and medulloblastoma and require *DWI or 3D T2 imaging* for better conspicuity compared to T1W+C sequences.
    - DWI and 3D T2W imaging can be helpful in detecting nonenhancing tumors.
    - DWI is helpful in identifying high cellular tumors such as medulloblastoma or ATRT.
    - 3D T2 imaging (SPACE, FIESTA, CUBE) is helpful in identifying drop metastases due to the high contrast between CSF and spinal cord and the ability to acquire 1-mm slice thickness images in a short amount of time compared to fast spin echo T2W imaging.
- Important to *reduce MRI CSF flow artifacts* to provide a clear distinction between cord surface and CSF. This can be achieved using a T1 VIBE sequence or equivalent sequence depending on the MRI scanner.

REFERENCES

1. Haverkamp BT, Nizamuddin RA, Loskutov A, et al. Imaging spectrum of pediatric spinal neoplasms. *Neurographics*. 2017 May–June;7(3):151–162.
2. Kralik SF, O'Neill DP, Kamer AP, et al. Radiological diagnosis of drop metastases from paediatric brain tumours using combination of 2D and 3D MRI sequences. *Clin Radiol*. 2017 Oct;72(10):902.e13–902.e19.
3. Hayes LL, Jones RA, Palasis S, et al. Drop metastases to the pediatric spine revealed with diffusion-weighted MR imaging. *Pediatr Radiol*. 2012 Aug;42(8):1009–1013.

RARE INTRADURAL TUMORS

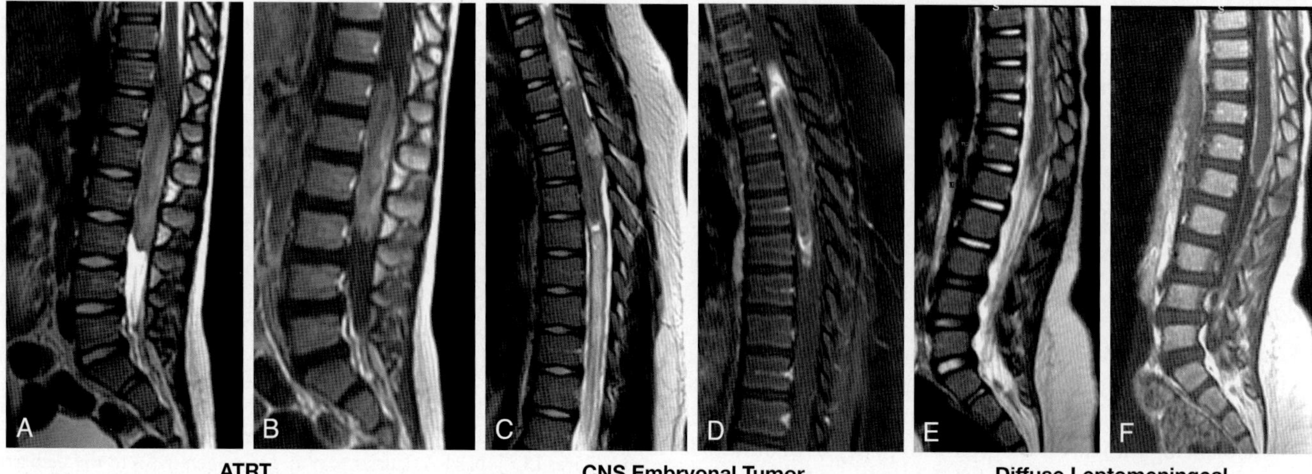

Fig. 17.14 Rare Intradural Tumors. ATRT: (A) Sagittal T2W and (B) sagittal T1W+C images demonstrate a T2W hyperintense homogeneously enhancing intradural extramedullary mass along the anterior thoracic spinal cord. CNS Embryonal tumor: (C) Sagittal T2W and (D) sagittal T1W+C demonstrate a T2W isointense and hypointense heterogeneously enhancing intramedullary mass in the thoracic spinal cord with adjacent long segment edema. Prospective diagnosis of both of these tumors would be difficult as the differential diagnoses would include more common tumors such as a myxopapillary ependymoma and a spinal cord astrocytoma, respectively. Diffuse leptomeningeal glioneuronal tumor: (E) Sagittal T2W and (F) sagittal T1W+C images demonstrate abnormal leptomeningeal enhancement diffusely along thoracic spinal cord as well as abnormal nodular enhancement of the cauda equina.

Key Points

- ATRT: Rarely occurs in the spinal canal. Intramedullary and intradural extramedullary locations are possible. Typically age <2 years. Heterogeneous T2W signal, often with necrosis and hemorrhage, and heterogeneous enhancement. May spread in the CSF
- CNS Embryonal Tumor: Rarely occur in the spinal canal. Can be intramedullary, intradural extramedullary or extradural; typically older children. Usually homogenous T2W signal and enhancement. May spread in the CSF
- Diffuse leptomeningeal glioneuronal tumor: Rare CNS neoplasm with oligodendrocyte-like cells, astrocytic cells, and neurons scattered in glial cells within desmoplastic or myxoid leptomeningeal stroma; mostly intradural extramedullary location involving the leptomeninges; T2W hyperintensity and areas of enhancing and nonenhancing tumor

REFERENCES

1. Rossi A, Gandolfo C, Morana G, et al. Tumors of the spine in children. *Neuroimaging Clin N Am*. 2007 Feb;17(1):17–35.
2. Kang JH, Buckley AF, Nagpal S, et al. A Diffuse leptomeningeal glioneuronal tumor without diffuse leptomeningeal involvement: detailed molecular and clinical characterization. *J Neuropathol Exp Neurol*. 2018;77(9):751–756.

SCHWANNOMA

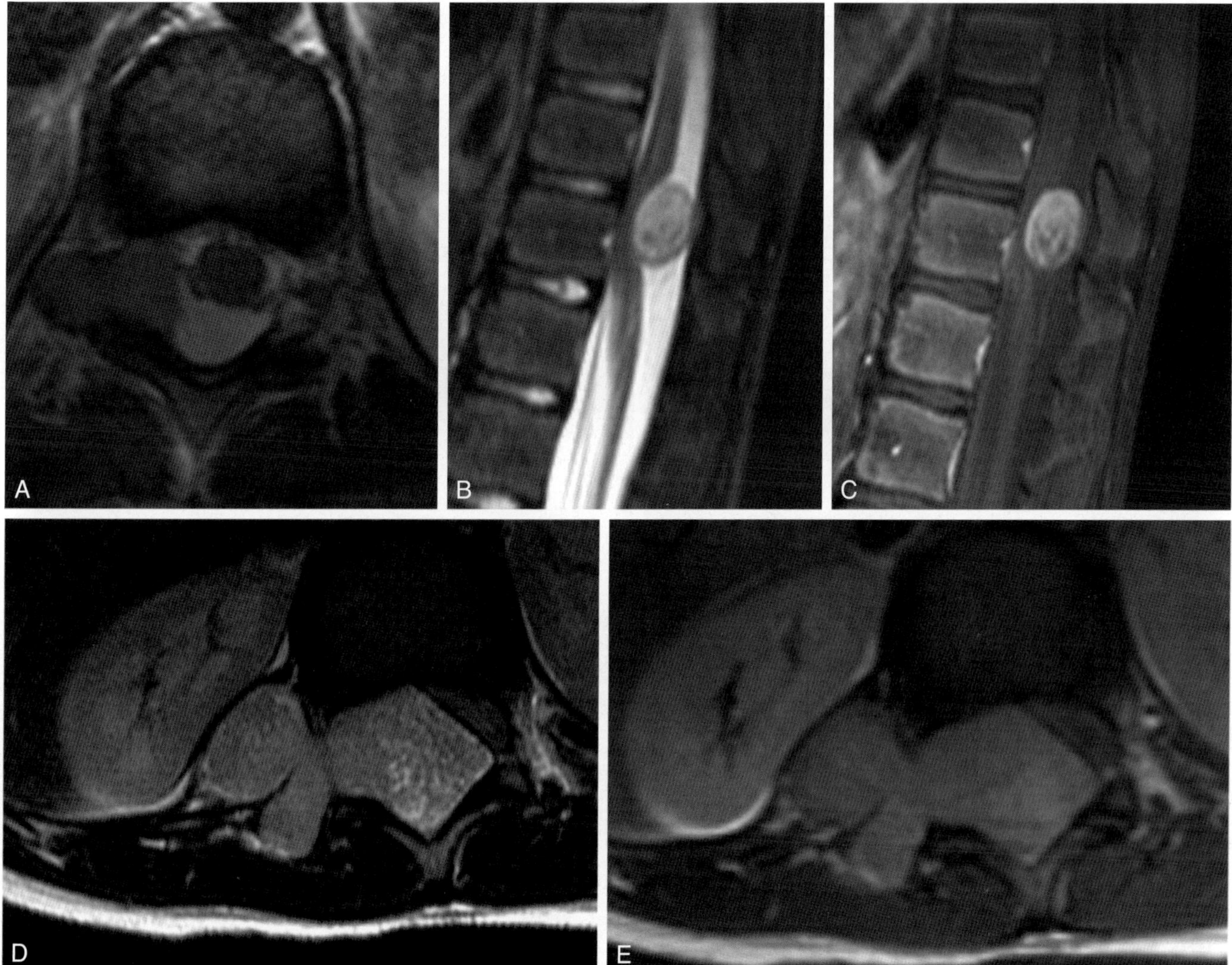

Fig. 17.15 Schwannoma. (A and B) Axial and sagittal T2W and (C) sagittal T1W+C images demonstrate a T2W hyperintense (relative to muscle) homogeneously enhancing dumbbell-shaped mass with both extradural and intradural extramedullary locations. (D) Axial T2W and (E) axial T1W+C images demonstrate a T2W hyperintense homogeneously enhancing dumbbell-shaped mass with both extradural location compressing the spinal cord.

Key Points

Background

- Benign tumor composed of Schwann cells.
- Schwannomas are the *most common intradural extramedullary mass.*
- Schwannomas can be completely resected due to growth on the surface of the nerve compared to neurofibroma which grows within the nerve.
- Associated with *NF-2.*

Imaging

- Location: Intradural extramedullary, extradural involving only soft tissue, or combined intradural extramedullary and extradural.
- MRI: Circumscribed, lobular, T2W hyperintense, homogeneous > heterogeneous enhancement.
- Large schwannomas *smoothly remodel the bone.*
- *Widening of the neuroforamina.*

REFERENCE

1. Rossi A, Gandolfo C, Morana G, et al. Tumors of the spine in children. *Neuroimaging Clin N Am.* 2007 Feb;17(1):17–35.

NEUROFIBROMA

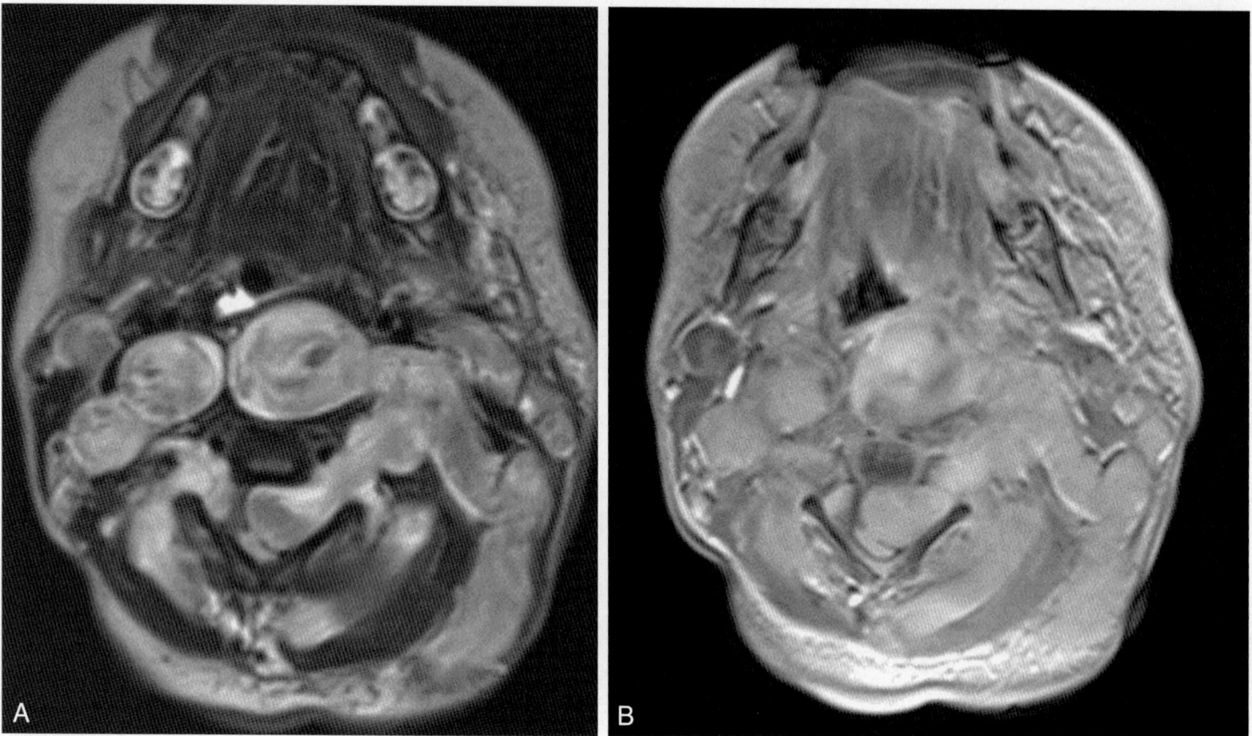

Fig. 17.16 Neurofibroma. (A) Axial T2W and (B) axial T1W+C images demonstrate multifocal T2W hyperintense homogeneously enhancing rounded and elongated masses involving extradural and intradural extramedullary locations with spinal cord compression.

Key Points

Background

- Benign neoplasm of the peripheral nerve
- Grows within the nerve, which limits ability to completely resect
- Associated with *NF-1*

Imaging

- Location: Intradural extramedullary, extradural involving soft tissue, or combined intradural extramedullary and extradural
- Localized, diffuse, and plexiform types
- Localized form is the most common and is seen as a solitary expansile mass not associated with NF-1. Difficult to distinguish from a schwannoma.
- MRI: T2W hyperintense with *target appearance* (peripheral T2W hyperintense, central T2W hypointense); generally homogenous enhancement
- *Necrosis or rapid growth can indicate malignant peripheral nerve sheath tumor* and would require biopsy.

REFERENCE

1. Rossi A, Gandolfo C, Morana G, et al. Tumors of the spine in children. *Neuroimaging Clin N Am.* 2007 Feb;17(1):17–35.

INFANTILE HEMANGIOMA

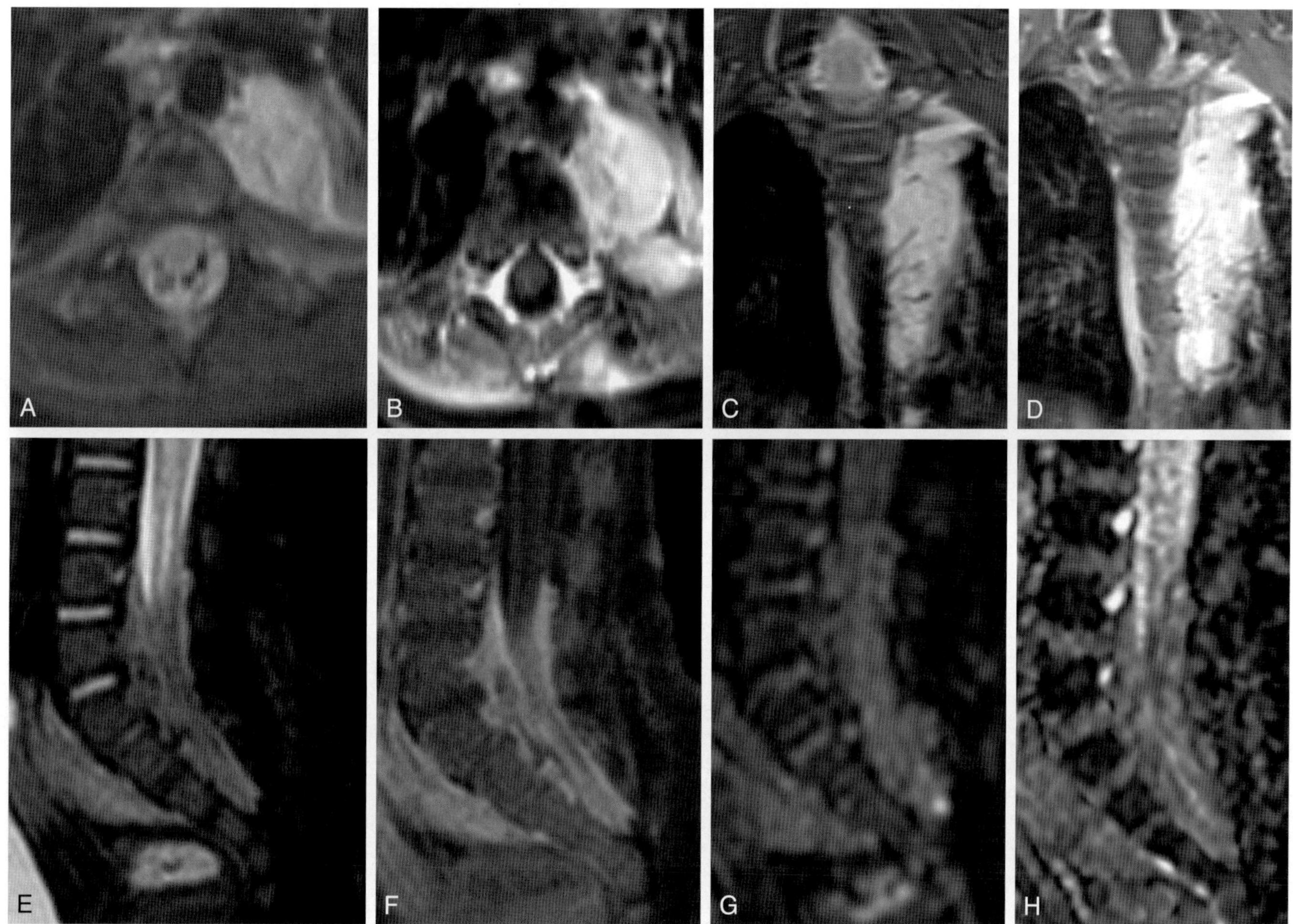

Fig. 17.17 Infantile Hemangioma. (A and C) Axial and coronal T2W and (B and D) axial and coronal T1W+C fat saturation images demonstrate an extradural circumscribed left thoracic paraspinal T2W hyperintense homogeneously enhancing mass with internal T2W hypointense linear flow voids. (E) Sagittal STIR, (F) sagittal T1W+C fat saturation, (G) sagittal DWI, and (H) sagittal ADC map images in a different patient demonstrate an infiltrative extradural T2W hyperintense homogeneously enhancing mass with internal T2W hypointense linear flow voids and mild ADC hyperintensity.

Key Points

Background

- *Most common benign tumor of infancy*
- 95% present before 6 months of age. Often involute spontaneously

Imaging

- Location: Extradural soft tissue. Most commonly paraspinal in location
- Circumscribed or infiltrative
- Ultrasound: Variable echogenicity with high flow velocity
- CT: Solid tissue density; homogenous enhancement; no gross Ca^{2+}
- MRI: Mild *T2W hyperintensity*; *flow voids*; *intense enhancement*; *ADC hyperintense*

REFERENCE

1. Baer AH, Parmar HA, McKnight CD, et al. Head and neck vascular anomalies in the pediatric population. *Neurographics*. 2014 March(4):2–19.

VASCULAR MALFORMATION

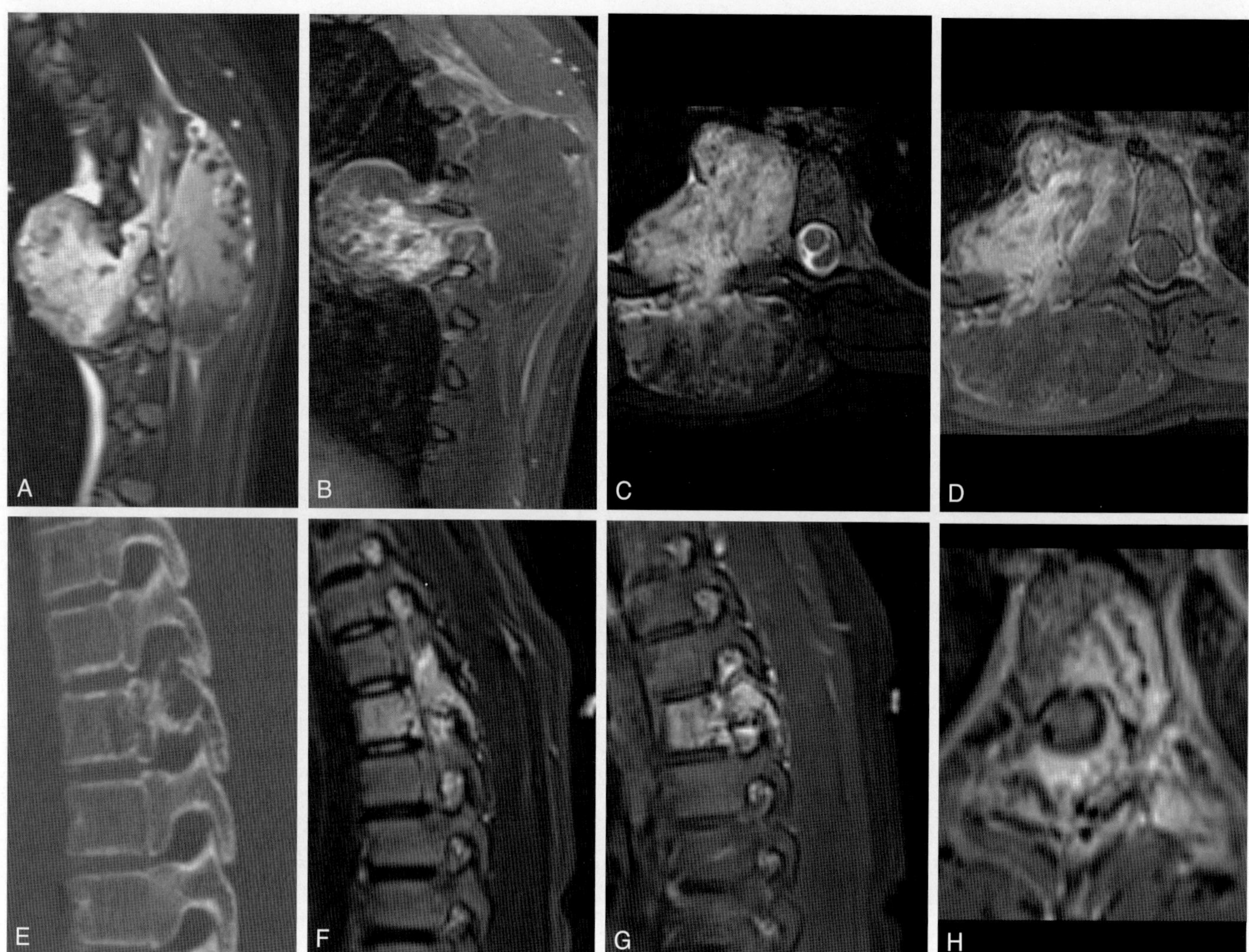

Fig. 17.18 Vascular Malformations. A 19-year-old with back pain. (A and C) Sagittal and axial STIR and (B and D) sagittal and axial T1W+C images demonstrate an extradural circumscribed thoracic paraspinal T2W hyperintense mass with rounded T2W hypointense foci due to phleboliths, heterogeneous enhancement, and fluid levels consistent with a mixed venous and lymphatic malformation. A 13-year-old with scapular pain. (E) Sagittal CT reformat image demonstrates mild expansion, lucency, and coarse trabeculae in the thoracic spine posterior vertebral body, pedicle, and facet. (F) Sagittal STIR and (G) sagittal and (H) axial T1W+C fat saturation images demonstrate a STIR hyperintense mass with homogeneous enhancement in the bone and adjacent soft tissue including the epidural space. Pathology from surgical resection confirmed a capillary malformation.

Key Points

Background

- Includes venous, venolymphatic, and capillary malformations

Imaging

- Location: Extradural. Located either in the bone marrow of the vertebrae and/or paraspinal extradural soft tissue
- MRI: T1W hyperintense, T2W hyperintense, homogeneous enhancement *versus progressive enhancement, especially well seen on delayed postcontrast injection imaging*
- CT: Osseous malformations demonstrate lucency with coarse trabeculae; soft tissue venous malformations demonstrate a low-density mass with coarse Ca^{2+} (*phleboliths*) with progressive enhancement.

REFERENCE

1. Rossi A, Gandolfo C, Morana G, et al. Tumors of the spine in children. *Neuroimaging Clin N Am.* 2007 Feb;17(1):17–35.

NEUROBLASTOMA

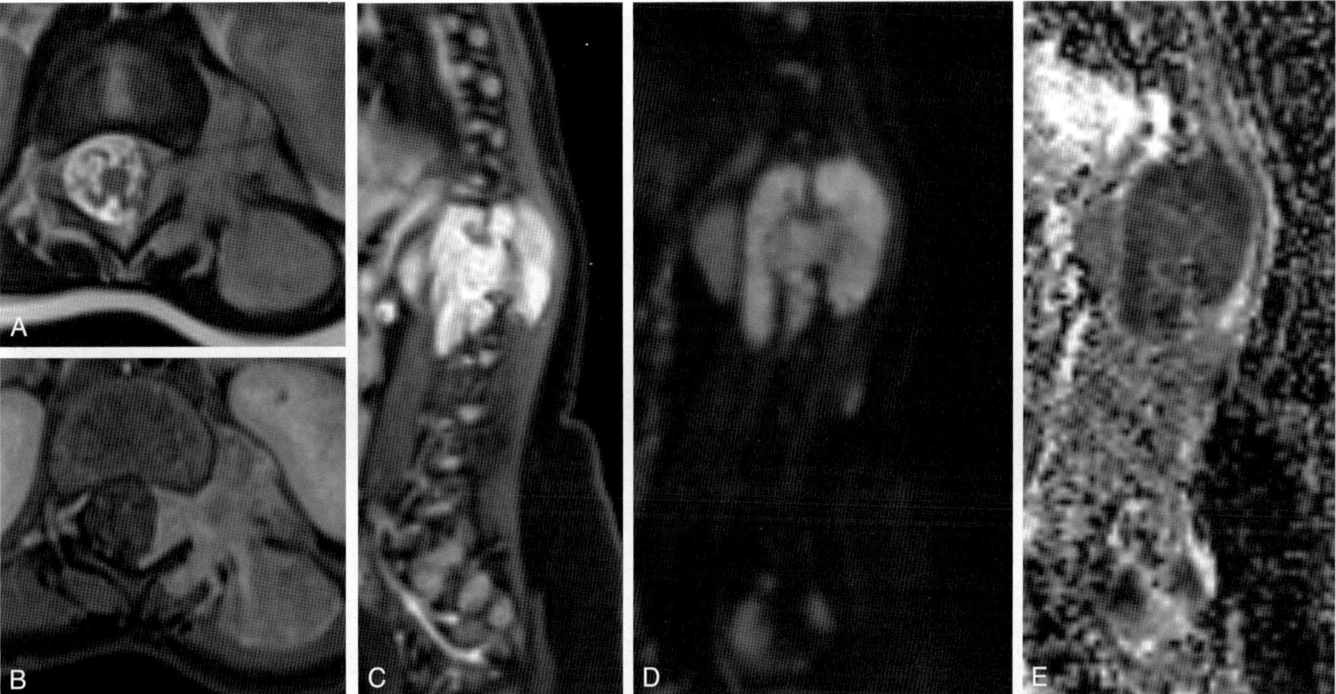

Fig. 17.19 Neuroblastoma. (A) Axial T2W, (B and C) axial and sagittal T1W+C fat saturation, (D) sagittal DWI, and (E) sagittal ADC map images demonstrate a multilobulated enhancing left paraspinal mass with extension into the left neural foramen and lateral epidural space. The mass has a relatively reduced diffusion consistent with a highly cellular tumor.

Key Points

Background

- Involves the spine from an adrenal or paravertebral primary tumor that extends into the spinal foramen
- Histologic spectrum from high grade (neuroblastoma), intermediate grade (ganglioneuroblastoma), and low grade (ganglioneuroma)

Imaging

- Location: Extradural soft tissues for the primary site of the tumor; metastatic disease will involve the bones
- MRI: Variable but typically homogenous enhancement; cellular tumor that may have *DWI restriction*; can demonstrate calcification, necrosis, and hemorrhage
- May show spontaneous involution over time
- Differential Diagnosis: Leukemia, and lymphoma

REFERENCE

1. Rossi A, Gandolfo C, Morana G, et al. Tumors of the spine in children. *Neuroimaging Clin N Am*. 2007 Feb;17(1):17–35.

SACROCOCCYGEAL TERATOMA

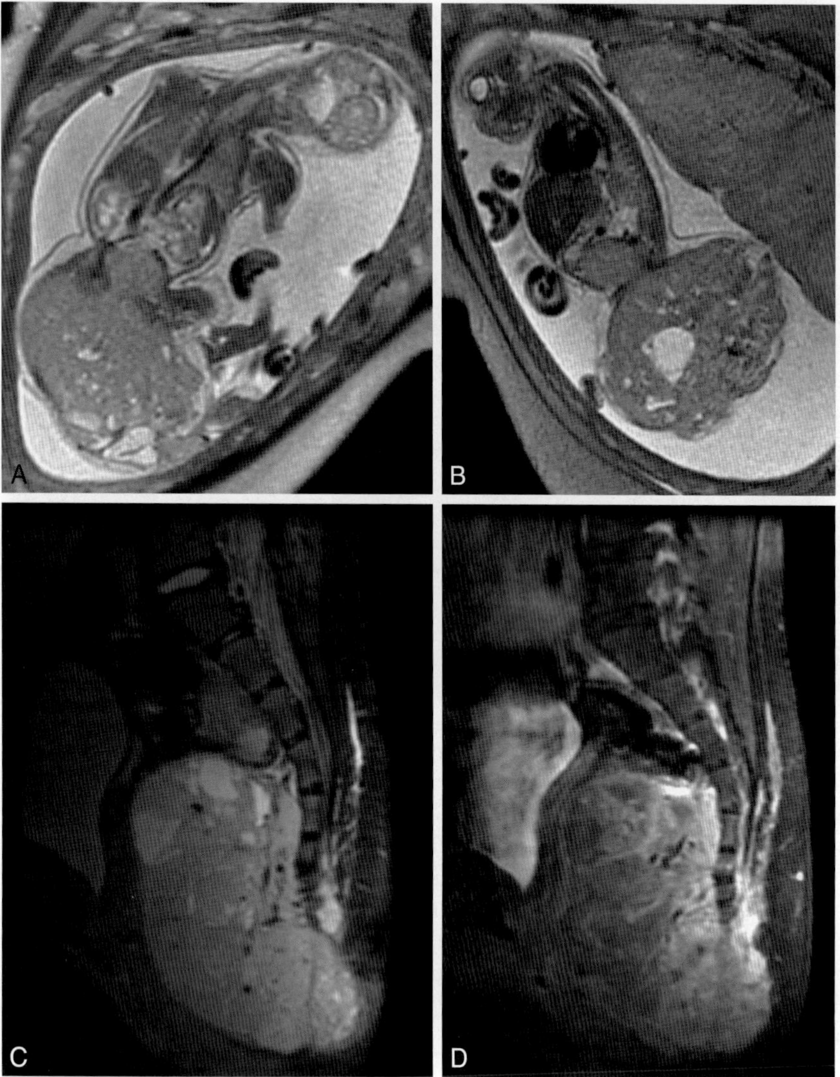

Fig. 17.20 Sacrococcygeal Teratoma. (A and B) Fetal MRI images demonstrate a solid and cystic type 2 sacrococcygeal teratoma with both extrafetal and internal components, which compresses the bladder and lower ureters, causing bilateral hydroureteronephrosis. The sacrum and coccyx are invaded with intraspinal/extraspinal tumor. Tumor fetal ratio (TFR) is 0.79. (C) Sagittal T2W and (D) sagittal T1W+C fat saturation images demonstrate a solid enhancing presacral mass with minor cystic component.

Key Points

Background

- Congenital tumor: Two-thirds are mature teratomas. Most are benign but with tendency for malignant transformation in older children. F:M ratio 4:1.
- Classification from the American Academy of Pediatric Surgery:
  - Type 1: External to the pelvis with small presacral component
  - Type 2: External to the pelvis with large intrapelvic extension
  - Type 3: External to the pelvis with majority within the pelvis and abdomen
  - Type 4: Entirely presacral
- *Currarino triad*:
  - Anorectal malformation (anal stenosis, anal extopia, and imperforate anus)
  - Presacral mass (anterior meningocele, teratoma, cyst)
  - Sacral bony anomaly (scimitar sacrum—crescentic bony defect and abnormal segmentation)

Imaging

- Location: Extradural soft tissue.
- MRI: Presacral solid, cystic or *solid and cystic mass*; 50% contain calcification; +/− macroscopic fat.
- Tumor fetal ratio: A cutoff of >0.12 before 24 weeks GA has been suggested as high risk for poor outcome.
- The coccyx is involved in nearly 100% of the cases and must be completely resected for cure.
- Typically diagnosed on prenatal ultrasound and/or fetal MRI. Depending on the size and degree of intralesional arteriovenous shunting, fetal hydrops and cardiac failure may be seen.

REFERENCES

1. Rossi A, Gandolfo C, Morana G, et al. Tumors of the spine in children. *Neuroimaging Clin N Am*. 2007 Feb;17(1):17–35.
2. Rodriguez MA, Cass DL, Lazar DA, et al. Tumor volume to fetal weight ratio as an early prognostic classification for fetal sacrococcygeal teratoma. *J Pediatr Surg*. 2011;46:1182–1185.

LEUKEMIA

Extradural: Bone and Soft Tissue

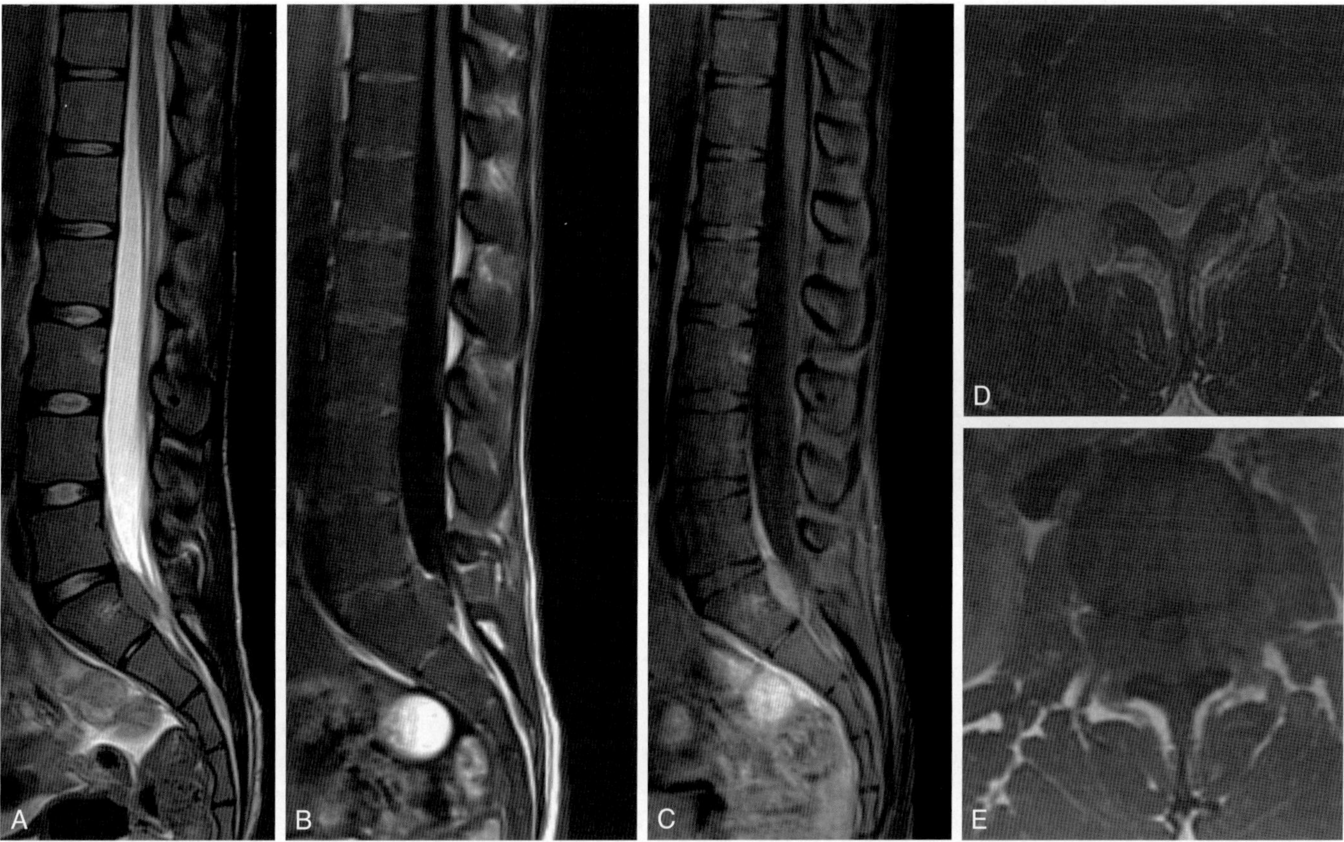

Fig. 17.21 Leukemia. A 17-year-old with acute lymphoctic leukemia and back pain. (A) Sagittal T2W and (B and C) sagittal T1W and T1W+C images demonstrate abnormal low T1W signal diffusely throughout the bone marrow and extradural soft tissue mass with mild T2W isointensity and homogeneous enhancement in the S1 epidural space. A 13-year-old with difficulty walking. (D) Axial T2W and (E) axial T1W images demonstrate a more extensive extradural infiltrative soft tissue mass with thecal sac compression.

Key Points

Background

- Granulocytic sarcomas/chloromas occur in acute myelogenous leukemia.

Imaging

- Location: Extradural bone with soft tissue extension
- MRI: Diffuse involvement of the bone marrow with low T1 signal intensity (darker than the disc space as an internal reference) with or without soft tissue extension, which demonstrates *homogeneous enhancement* and *diffusion restriction*
- Differential Diagnosis: Neuroblastoma, and lymphoma

REFERENCE

1. Rossi A, Gandolfo C, Morana G, et al. Tumors of the spine in children. *Neuroimaging Clin N Am*. 2007 Feb;17(1):17–35.

LYMPHOMA

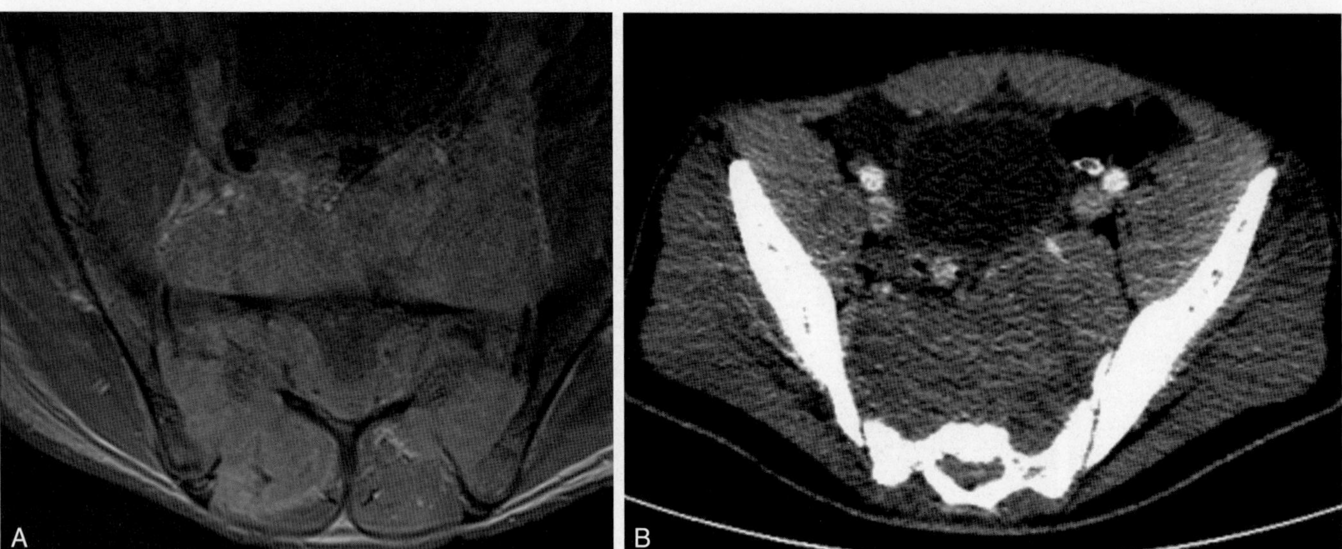

Fig. 17.22 Lymphoma. (A) Axial T1W+C and (B) axial CT with contrast images demonstrate infiltrative extradural soft tissue density mass with homogeneous enhancement in the spinal canal, neural foramen, and presacral space.

Key Points

Background

- Hodgkin lymphoma: ~50%; teenagers; primarily nodal; extranodal is uncommon.
- Non-Hodgkin lymphoma: Age 2 to 12; extranodal more common (Waldeyer ring).

Imaging

- Location: Extradural bone with soft tissue extension
- MRI: Homogeneous enhancement and diffusion restriction. May extend into the extradural space of the spinal canal from the bone or lymph nodes
- Differential Diagnosis: Neuroblastoma, and leukemia

REFERENCE

1. Rossi A, Gandolfo C, Morana G, et al. Tumors of the spine in children. *Neuroimaging Clin N Am*. 2007 Feb;17(1):17–35.

CHORDOMA

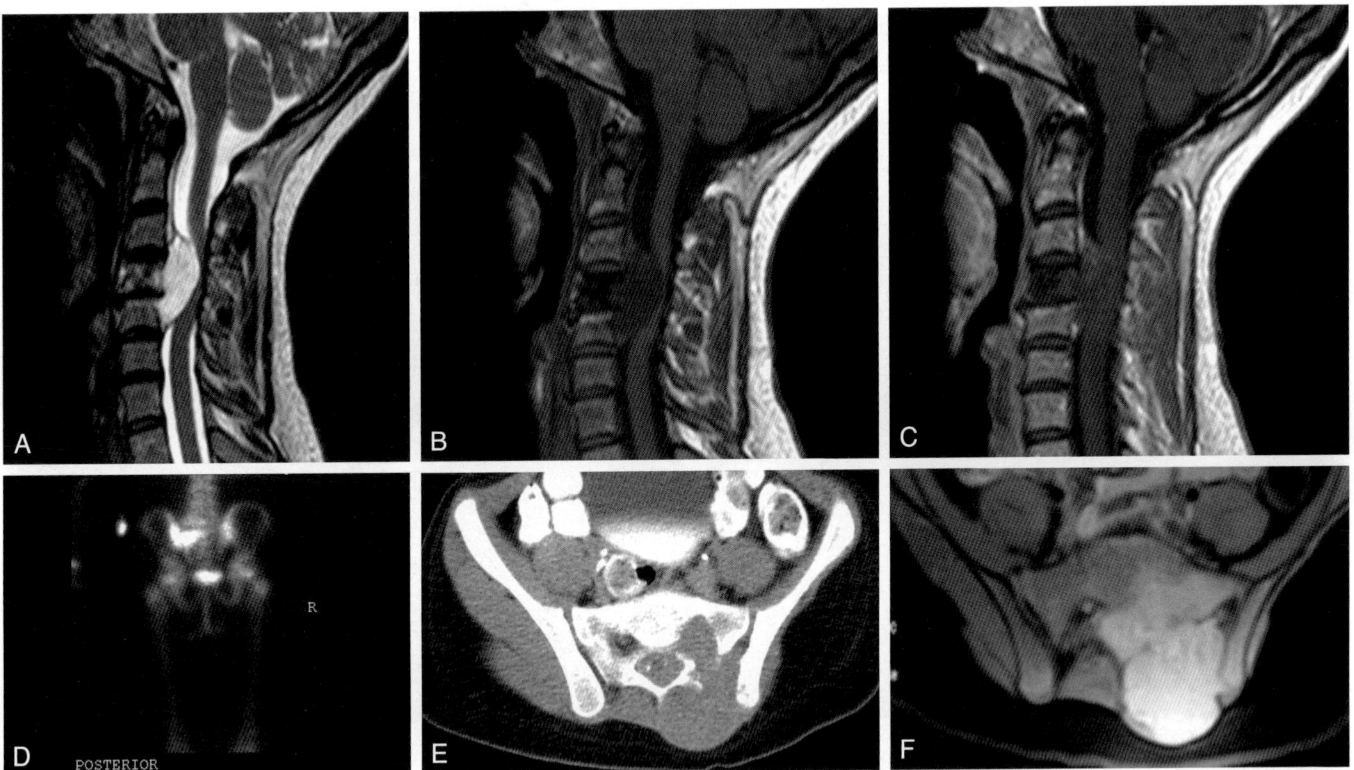

Fig. 17.23 Chordoma. (A) Sagittal T2W and (B and C) sagittal T1W and T1W+C images demonstrate a T2W hyperintense minimally enhancing mass arising from the C4 vertebral body with associated extradural soft tissue component resulting in spinal cord compression. (D) PA nuclear medicine Tc-MDP bone scan, (E) axial CT with contrast, and (F) axial T1W+C fat saturation images demonstrate a left sacral extradural bone and soft tissue mass with MDP uptake, bone destruction of the sacrum, and homogeneous enhancement.

Key Points

Background

- Rare tumor in patients younger than 30 years. Most common age: 30 to 50 years
- Originate in bone from remnant of notochord (fetal axial skeleton extending from spheno-occipital synchondrosis to coccyx).
- Presentation related to a mass effect on the spine, brainstem, and cranial nerves

Imaging

- Location: Extradural bone with soft tissue extension.
- Sacrococcygeal > clivus > spinal vertebrae.
- Destructive mass with prominent *T2W hyperintense* signal and heterogeneous or homogeneous enhancement.
- CT imaging demonstrates a lytic mass with aggressive margins and potentially ring and arc calcifications.
- Clival tumors indent the anterior pons typically without edema due to slow growth.

REFERENCE

1. Sen C, Triana AI, Berglind N, et al. Clival chordomas: clinical management, results, and complications in 71 patients. *J Neurosurg*. 2010 Nov;113(5):1059–1071.

LANGERHANS CELL HISTIOCYTOSIS

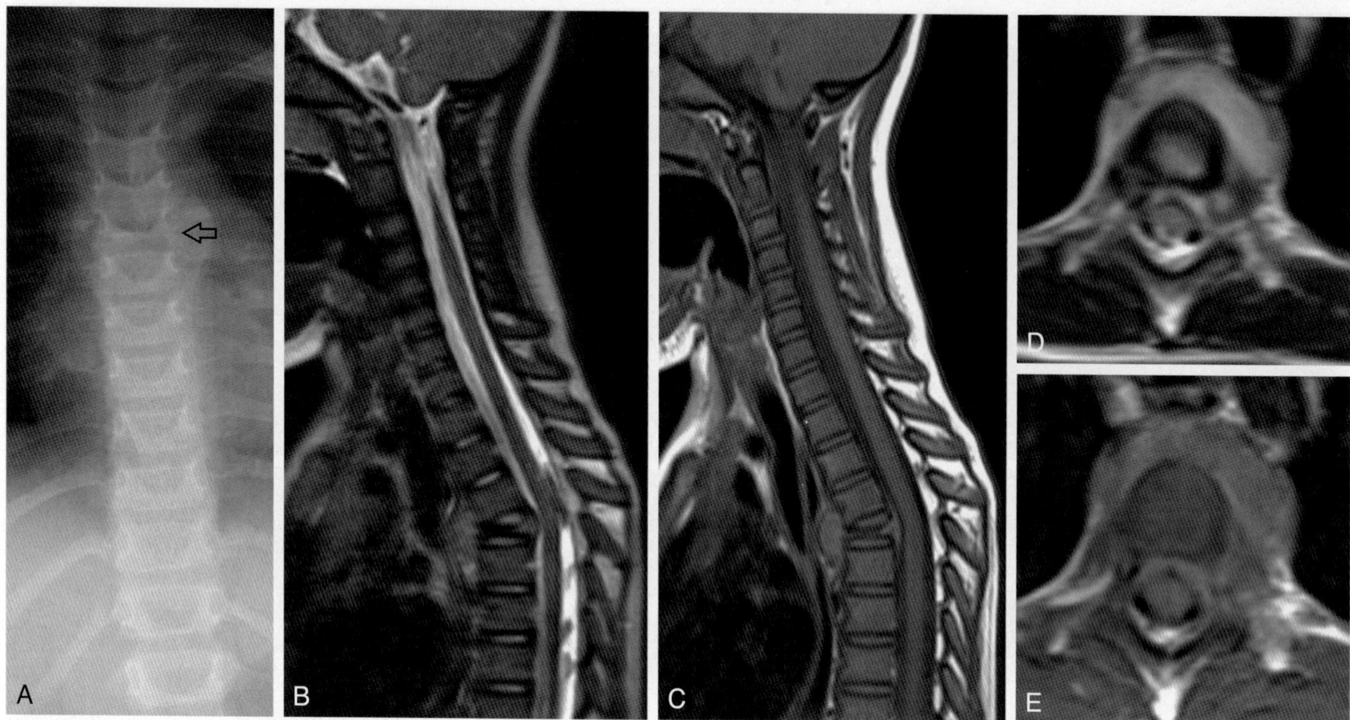

Fig. 17.24 Langerhans Cell Histiocytosis. (A) AP thoracic spine radiograph demonstrates vertebra plana of the T5 vertebral body. (B) Sagittal T2W, (C) sagittal T1, (D) axial T2W, and (E) axial T1W+C images demonstrate vertebra plana of the T5 vertebral body, T2W hyperintensity, and homogeneous enhancement in the bone and soft tissue extension is seen in the prevertebral and ventral epidural spaces.

Key Points

Background

- Infiltration by abnormal histiocytic cells.
- May be associated with systemic disease or isolated to the spine.
- Average age of onset is 1 to 3 years.

Imaging

- Location: Extradural bone with soft tissue extension
- *Lytic bone lesion* most commonly in the vertebral body rather than posterior elements, often resulting in pathologic fracture and *vertebra plana*
- Often a soft tissue component present
- Additional skull, skull base, or additional bone lesions must be excluded by total body scintigraphy or MRI.
- Differential Diagnosis: Aneurysmal bone cyst (ABC), Ewing sarcoma, and osteomyelitis.

REFERENCE

1. Rossi A, Gandolfo C, Morana G, et al. Tumors of the spine in children. *Neuroimaging Clin N Am.* 2007 Feb;17(1):17–35.

EWING SARCOMA

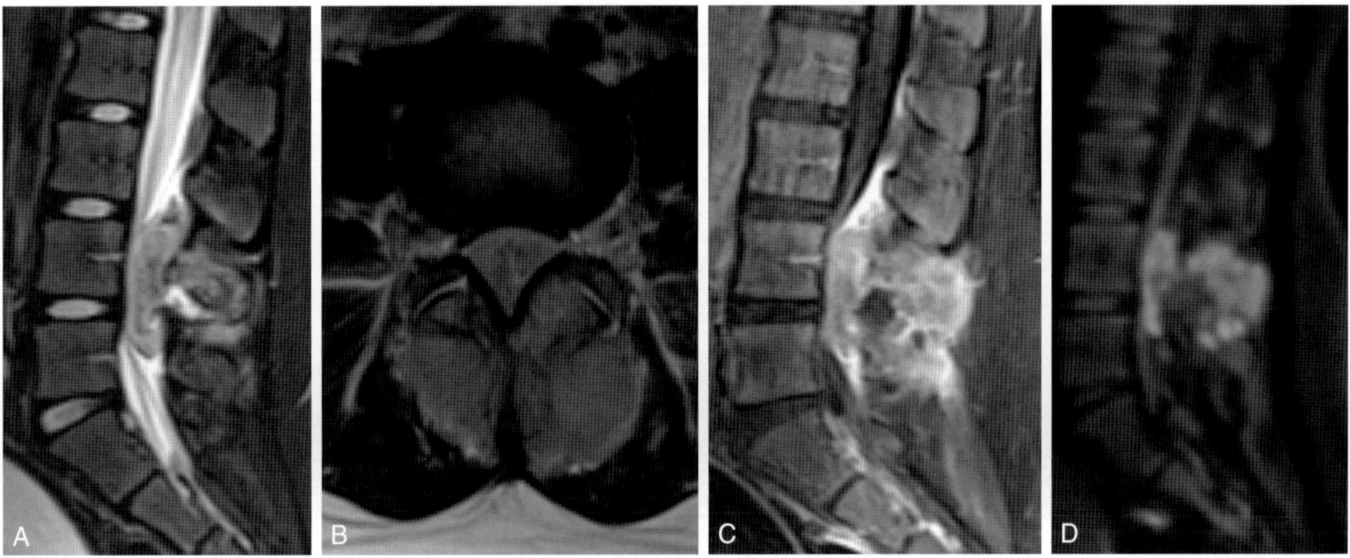

Fig. 17.25 Ewing Sarcoma. (A) Sagittal STIR and (B) axial T2W, (C) sagittal T1W+C, and (D) sagittal DWI images demonstrate a heterogeneously enhancing mass in the posterior lumbar spine involving the bone and soft tissues with diffusion restriction (ADC hypointense not shown) indicative of a hypercellular tumor and cauda equina compression.

Key Points

Background

- Most common primary bone tumor in children.
- Extraskeletal Ewing sarcoma has a similar histological appearance but originates in the meninges without bone involvement.
- Lumbosacral region is the most common spinal location.
- Usually present at age 10 years; pain, radiculopathy, cord, or nerve root compression symptoms.

Imaging

- Location: Extradural bone with soft tissue extension
- CT: Aggressive, *lytic*, *permeative* bone lesion, usually involving *the posterior elements* (lamina, spinous process), with associated soft tissue mass
- MRI: Homogeneous enhancement and restricted diffusion from high cellularity
- Differential Diagnosis: Langerhans cell histiocytosis (LCH), leukemia, and lymphoma

REFERENCE

1. Rossi A, Gandolfo C, Morana G, et al. Tumors of the spine in children. *Neuroimaging Clin N Am*. 2007 Feb;17(1):17–35.

OSTEOID OSTEOMA

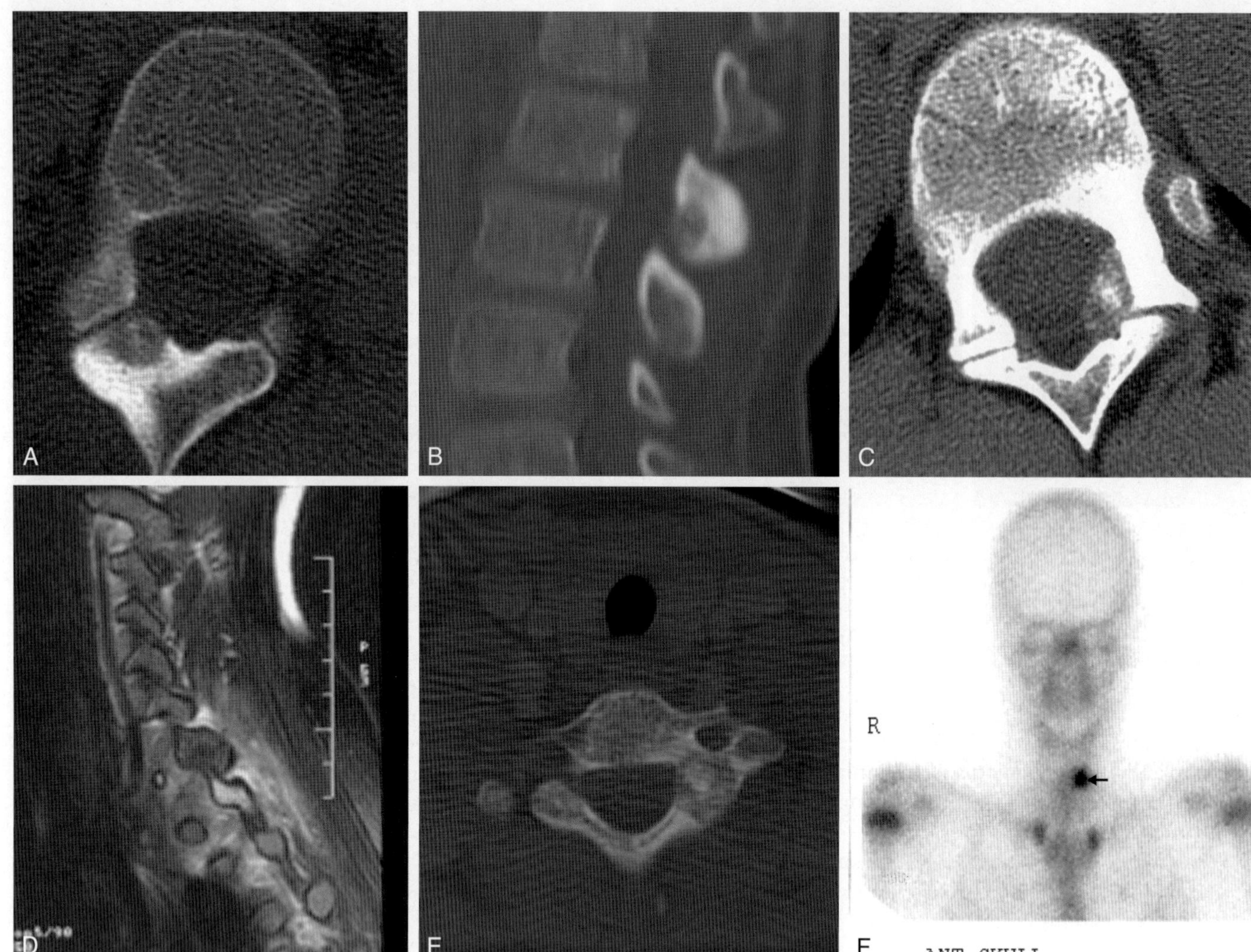

Fig. 17.26 Osteoid Osteoma. (A and B) Axial CT and sagittal reformat CT images demonstrating a lucent rounded bone lesion with central sclerotic nidus in the right lamina. (C) Axial CT image demonstrating an expansile lucent bone lesion with central sclerotic nidus along the left pedicle and lamina. (D) Sagittal STIR, (E) axial CT, and (F) AP Tc-MDP bone scan images in a different patient demonstrate a lesion in the left C7 facet, which is hypointense on STIR indicative of a bone or fibrous lesion, lucency with central sclerosis on CT, and MDP uptake (arrow) with a large amount of surrounding soft tissue enhancement.

Key Points

Background

- Presents with pain, which improves with antiinflammatory medication

Imaging

- Location: Extradural bone
- Usually located in the *posterior elements* of the lumbar and sacral spine, less commonly the cervical or thoracic spine
- CT: *Centrally sclerotic nidus with surrounding lucency*
- T2W hyperintensity and avid enhancement of the lesion on MRI with *soft tissue edema* indicative of inflammation
- Focal Tc-MDP accumulation on bone scan

REFERENCE

1. Rossi A, Gandolfo C, Morana G, et al. Tumors of the spine in children. *Neuroimaging Clin N Am*. 2007 Feb;17(1):17–35.

OSTEOBLASTOMA

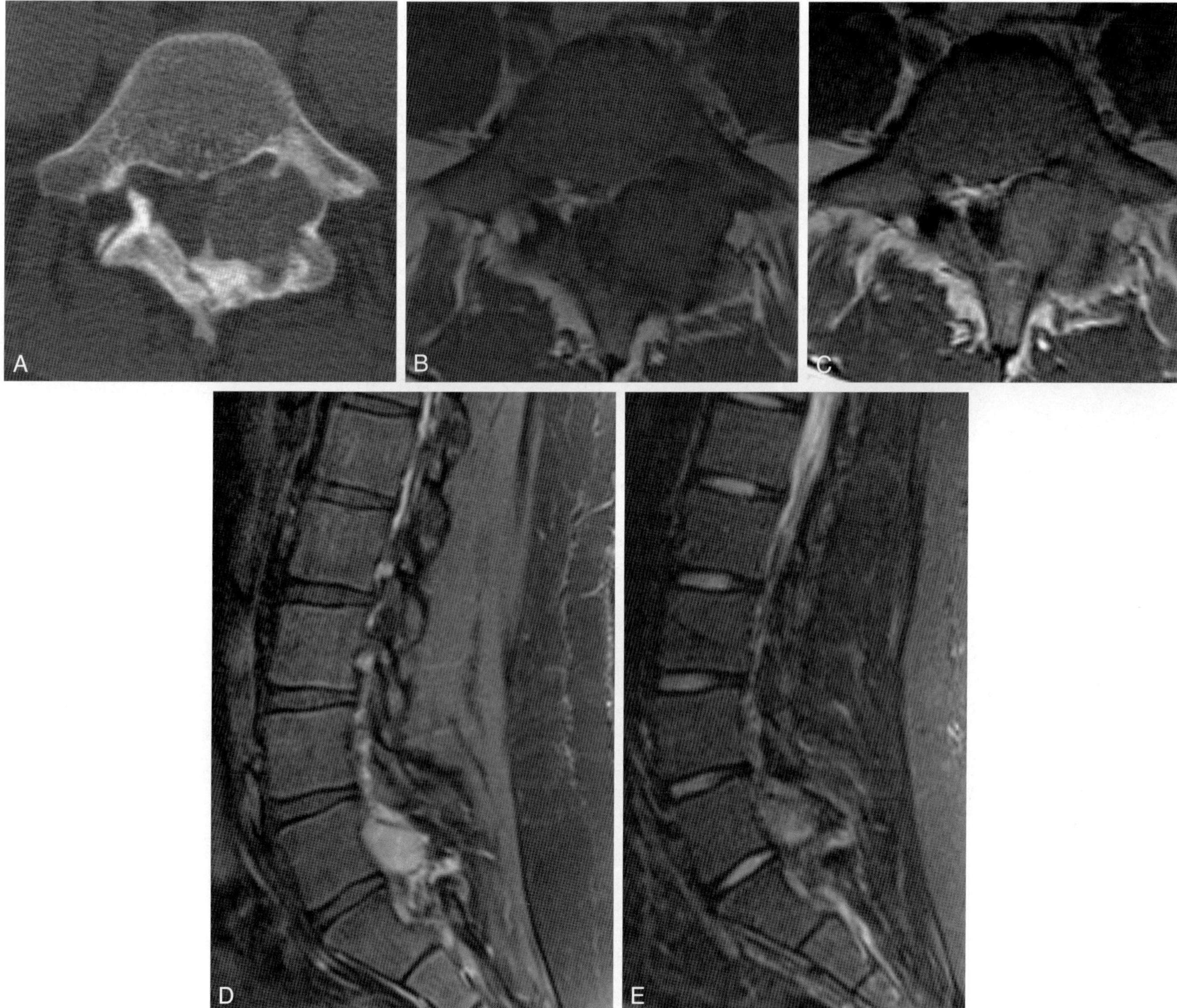

Fig. 17.27 Osteoblastoma. (A) Axial CT demonstrating a lytic expansile mass in the left pedicle and lamina of the L5 vertebrae. (B and C) Axial T1W and T1W+C, (D) sagittal T1W+C fat saturation, and (E) sagittal STIR images demonstrate homogenous enhancement of the bone tumor.

Key Points

Background

- Usually occur in the first decade of life.
- Osteoblastomas are *similar to osteoid osteomas* on histopathology but are defined as being *>2 cm in size.*

Imaging

- Location: Extradural bone with soft tissue extension
- *Lytic expansile bone lesion*; more aggressive than osteoid osteomas including *soft tissue extension*, bone destruction, hemorrhage, and spinal canal/cord compression

REFERENCE

1. Rossi A, Gandolfo C, Morana G, et al. Tumors of the spine in children. *Neuroimaging Clin N Am*. 2007 Feb;17(1):17–35.

ANEURYSMAL BONE CYST

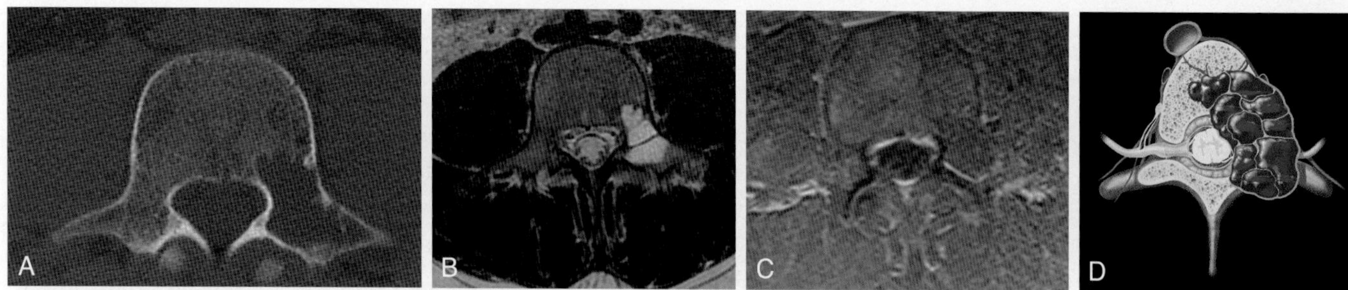

Fig. 17.28 Aneurysmal Bone Cyst (ABC). (A) Axial CT demonstrating a lytic expansile mass centered in the left pedicle. (B) Axial T2W and (C) axial T1W+C images demonstrate T2W hyperintense signal and no solid enhancement indicative of an ABC. (D) Illustration of an ABC showing the multiple loculations and expansile bone lesion. (D, from STATDx, Copyright © 2021, Elsevier Inc.)

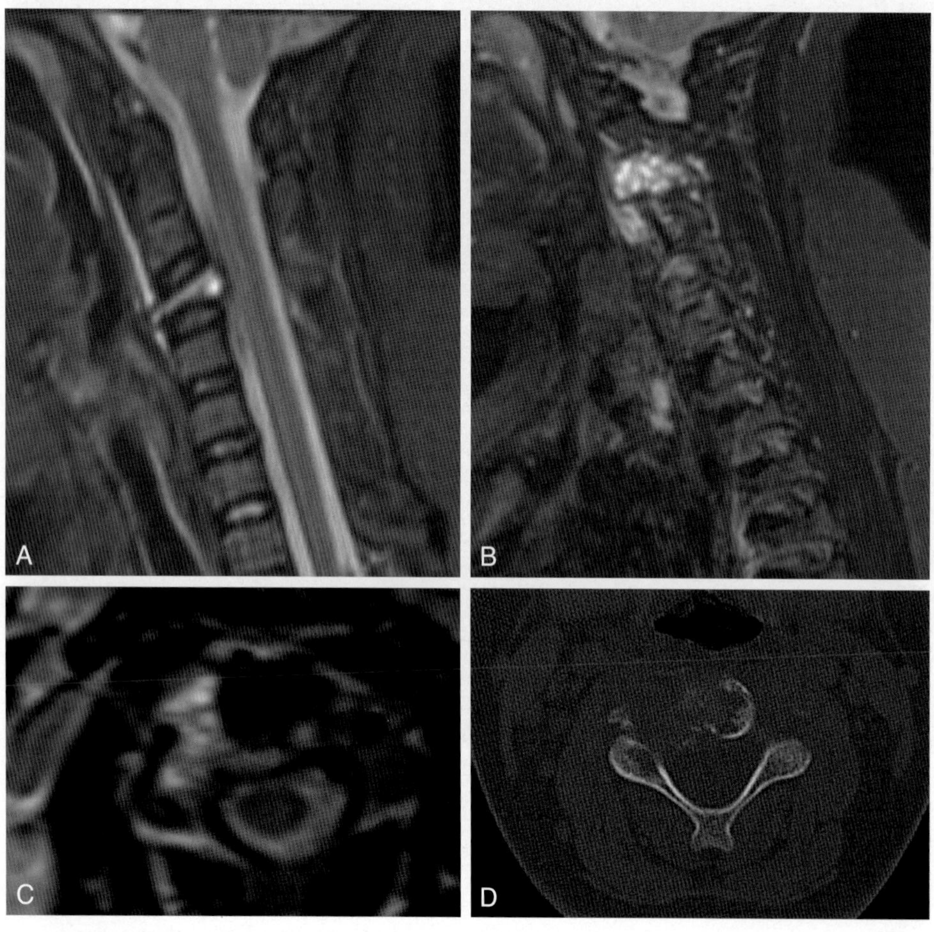

Fig. 17.29 Aneurysmal Bone Cyst (ABC). Challenging presentation mimicking LCH. (A and B) Sagittal STIR and (C) axial 3D T2W images demonstrate vertebra plana of the C3 vertebral body, which raised suspicion of LCH; however, internal fluid-fluid levels were present that suggests an ABC. (D) Axial CT demonstrates the lytic expansile mass involving the vertebral body. Pathology confirmed an ABC.

Key Points

Background

- Primary ABCs are benign bone lesions.
- Secondary ABCs associated with a bone tumor such as osteosarcoma or giant cell tumor are uncommon in the spine in children.

Imaging

- Location: Extradural bone
- *Lytic expansile bone lesion.*
- Fluid signal/*fluid-fluid levels. No solid enhancement* unless a secondary ABC. *No soft tissue component.* May be uniloculated or multiloculated
- Usually located in the *posterior elements*
- Differential Diagnosis: Langehans cell histiocytosis (LCH)

REFERENCE

1. Rossi A, Gandolfo C, Morana G, et al. Tumors of the spine in children. *Neuroimaging Clin N Am.* 2007 Feb;17(1):17–35.

18 Infection, Inflammatory, Demyelination, and Vascular Disorders

INTRODUCTION

Background

- Infectious, inflammatory, and demyelinating disorders of the spinal cord are commonly encountered in children. Children typically present with acute neurologic signs and symptoms, including sensory and motor deficits, hyporeflexia or hyperreflexia, and bowel or bladder incontinence.
- Lumbar puncture is often performed to confirm an infectious, inflammatory, or demyelinating process via demonstration of CSF pleocytosis or the presence of oligoclonal bands.
- Similar to adults, spinal vascular disorders including spinal cord infarcts and vascular malformations are rare in children. While spinal cord infarcts in adults are often attributable to atherosclerosis or aortic surgery, these are uncommon etiologies in children. Conversely, children are more likely to develop spinal cord infarcts from disc embolism compared to adults.

Imaging

- MRI is the primary modality for evaluating infectious, inflammatory, demyelinating, and vascular disorders of the spine because these disorders primarily affect the spinal cord and nerve roots.
- MRI is typically not able to provide a specific cause of spinal cord inflammation or demyelination due to the imaging overlap but can suggest greater likelihood of a specific process when additional findings from brain MRI and CSF are combined with clinical history.
- Spinal DWI has improved over time. Modern techniques such as RESOLVE or ZOOM sequences allow for reliable diffusion imaging of the spine. Usage of a spinal DWI sequence can add value to patient care when a spinal cord infarct, epidural abscess or phlegmon is encountered.
- This section will illustrate the common infectious, inflammatory, demyelinating, and vascular disorders affecting the spine in children.

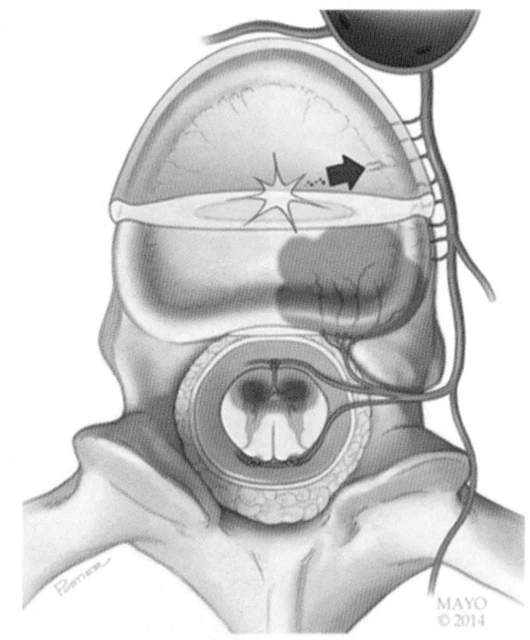

Reproduced from Mayo Foundation for Medical Education and Research.

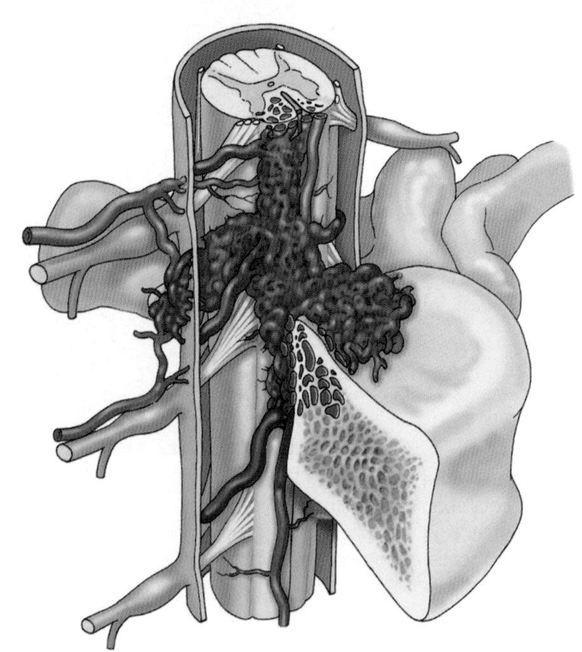

From McDougall CG, Deshmukh VR, Fiorella DJ, Albuquerque FC, Spetzler RF. Endovascular techniques for vascular malformations of the Spinal Axis. *Neurosurg Clin N Am*. 2005;16(2):395–410.

TRANSVERSE MYELITIS

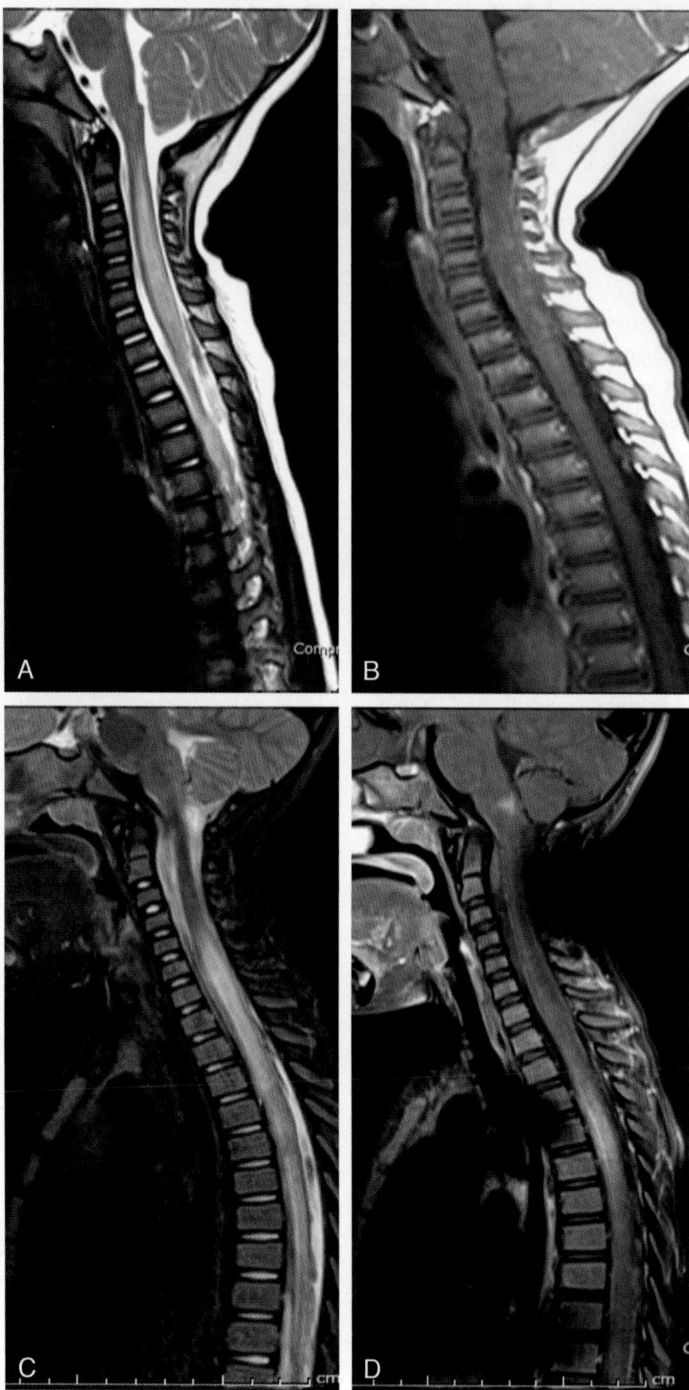

Fig. 18.1 Transverse Myelitis. (A) Sagittal T2W and (B) sagittal T1W+C images demonstrate a longitudinally extensive minimally expansile T2 hyperintense spinal cord abnormality with minimal mild patchy areas of enhancement. Different patient with (C) Sagittal STIR and (D) sagittal T1W+C fat saturation images demonstrating a longitudinally extensive minimally expansile STIR hyperintense spinal cord abnormality with incomplete enhancement. Imaging patterns of both patients demonstrate typical appearance of transverse myelitis with T2W hyperintensity extending more than 2 vertebral body lengths, mild expansion and variable enhancement.

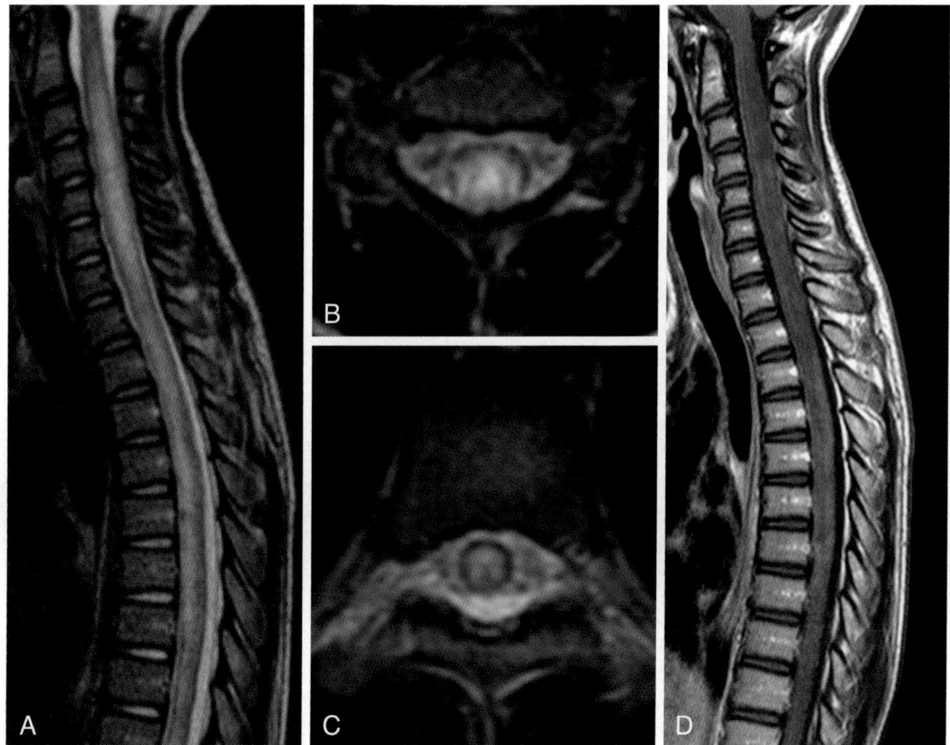

Fig. 18.2 Transverse Myelitis. A 10-year-old with lower extremity weakness, urinary retention, and T6 level decreased light touch and pinprick sensation but intact position and vibratory sensation. CSF demonstrated elevated white blood cell (WBC) count (124 cells/mm^3), normal glucose, and elevated total protein (171 mg/dL). (A to C) Sagittal and axial T2W and (D) sagittal T1W+C images demonstrate a longitudinally extensive minimally expansile T2W hyperintense spinal cord abnormality involving majority of the cross section of the spinal cord with mild patchy areas of enhancement.

Key Points

Background

- Inflammatory process resulting in acute onset of motor, sensory, and autonomic dysfunction with maximum symptoms ~24 hours (range 4 hours–21 days) after the onset of symptoms
- Criteria from the Transverse Myelitis Consortium Working Group: (1) Appropriate clinical picture; (2) evolution of symptoms to maximum severity between 4 hours and 21 days; and (3) CSF demonstrating cellular infiltrate and/or elevated protein or spinal cord enhancement on MRI
- Transverse myelitis can be divided into disease-associated and idiopathic transverse myelitis. Disease-associated causes include para-infectious, post-infectious, NMO, ant-MOG, autoimmune disorders, and multiple sclerosis (uncommon). Para-infectious transverse myelitis accounts for ~ 40% of cases and can be diagnosed when there is a history of an infectious prodrome within 4 weeks of clinical presentation and culture, serologic or PCR evidence of infection is present.
- Immune-mediated mechanisms include molecular mimcry which is damage to neuronal structures due to similarity between microbial antigens and neuronal components, microbial superantigen mediated infection in which microbial peptides bind to T-cell receptors causing polyclonal activation, and humoral derangement in which there is polyclonal B-cell activation or deposition of immunocomplexes in the spinal cord Approximately 30% of children with transverse myelitis have a recent history of vaccination
- Prognosis: One-third good/complete recovery, one-third fair recovery, and one-third poor outcome
- Poor outcome associated with cord signal abnormality involving >10 spinal levels
- Treated with high-dose steroids. Most often has a monophasic course.

Imaging

- Typically *longitudinally extensive* (more than two vertebral body lengths)
- T2W hyperintense, central cord involvement or *more than two-thirds cross-sectional area*
- *Nonenhancing or partially enhancing, minimal/mild expansion*
- Facilitated diffusion on DWI
- Improvements in spinal cord DWI and DTI may improve diagnosis and allow better determination of prognosis of transverse myelitis. Small studies have shown that a spinal cord DTI fractional anisotropy could detect additional lesions not seen on T2W images, and greater reduction of fractional anisotropy within the lesion and normal appearaing spinal cord distal to the lesion correlated with worse outcomes

REFERENCES

1. Rossi A.*Pediatric Neuroradiology*. 1st ed. Berlin/Heidelberg: Springer-Verlag.
2. Goh C, Phal PM, Desmond PM. Neuroimaging in acute transverse myelitis. *Neuroimag Clin N Am*. 2011;21:951–973.

NEUROMYELITIS OPTICA

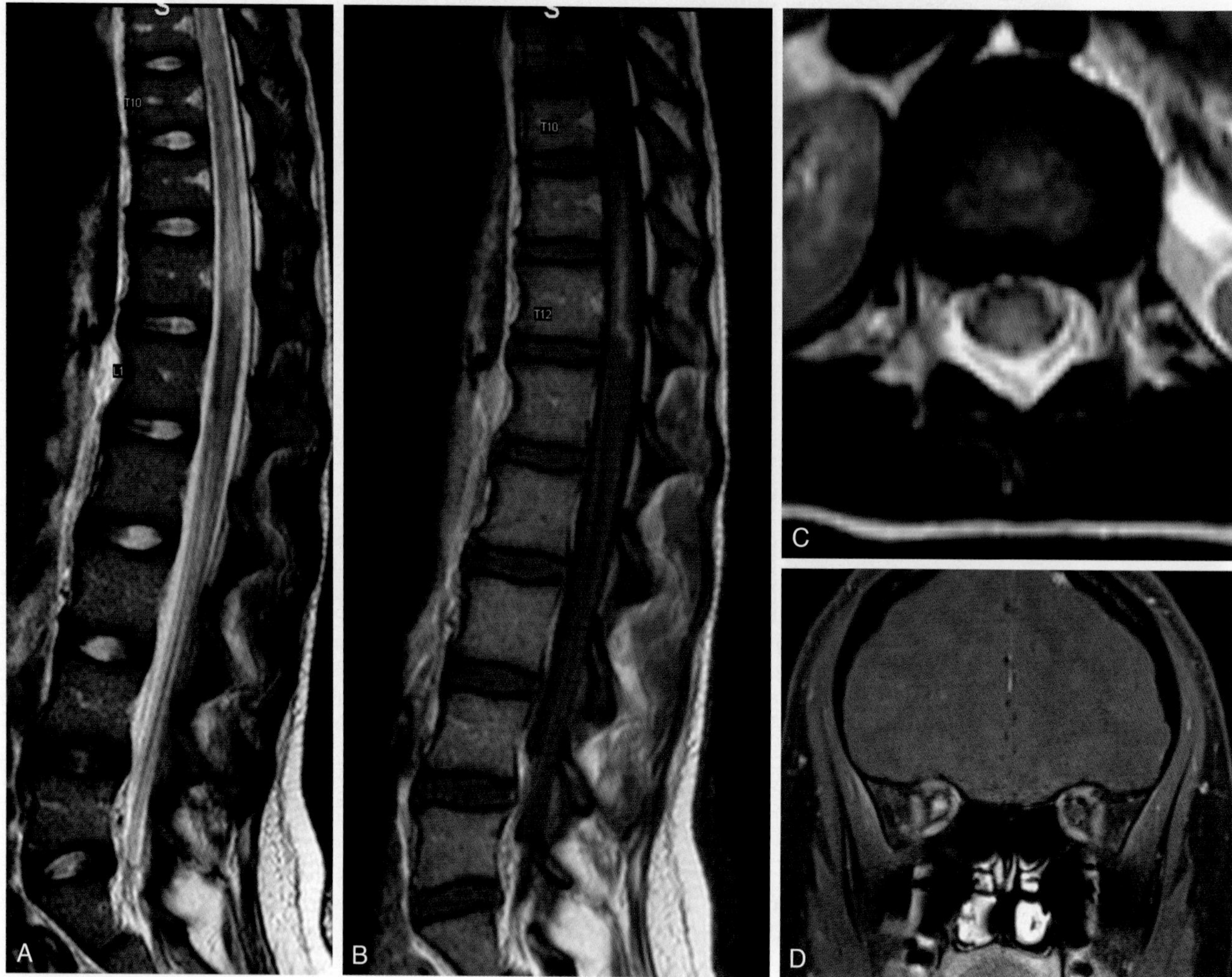

Fig. 18.3 Neuromyelitis Optica. (A and C) Sagittal and axial T2W and (B) sagittal T1W+C images demonstrate a longitudinally extensive nonexpansile T2W hyperintense spinal cord abnormality with incomplete enhancement. (D) Coronal T1W+C image of the orbits demonstrates abnormal homogeneous enhancement of the right optic nerve.

Key Points

Background

- An autoimmune disease targeting the aquaporin-4 protein on astrocytes.
- Aquaporin-4 IgG is positive in 60% to 80% of patients.
- Number of attacks and disability level at 2 years from diagnosis may be greater than with MS.

Imaging

- Longitudinally extensive myelitis: T2W hyperintensity involving two or more spinal segments typically with central gray predominance; enhancement is variable but present to some degree in 78% of patients; the entire cross-section of the cord may be involved.
- Intracranially involves *optic nerves*, hypothalamus, medial thalami, and dorsal brainstem. Minimal to no involvement of the cerebral white matter is present.

REFERENCE

1. Chitnis T, Ness J, Waubant E, et al. Clinical features of neuromyelitis optica in children: US Network of Pediatric MS Centers report. *Neurology*. 2016;86(3):245–252.

ANTI-MOG DEMYELINATION

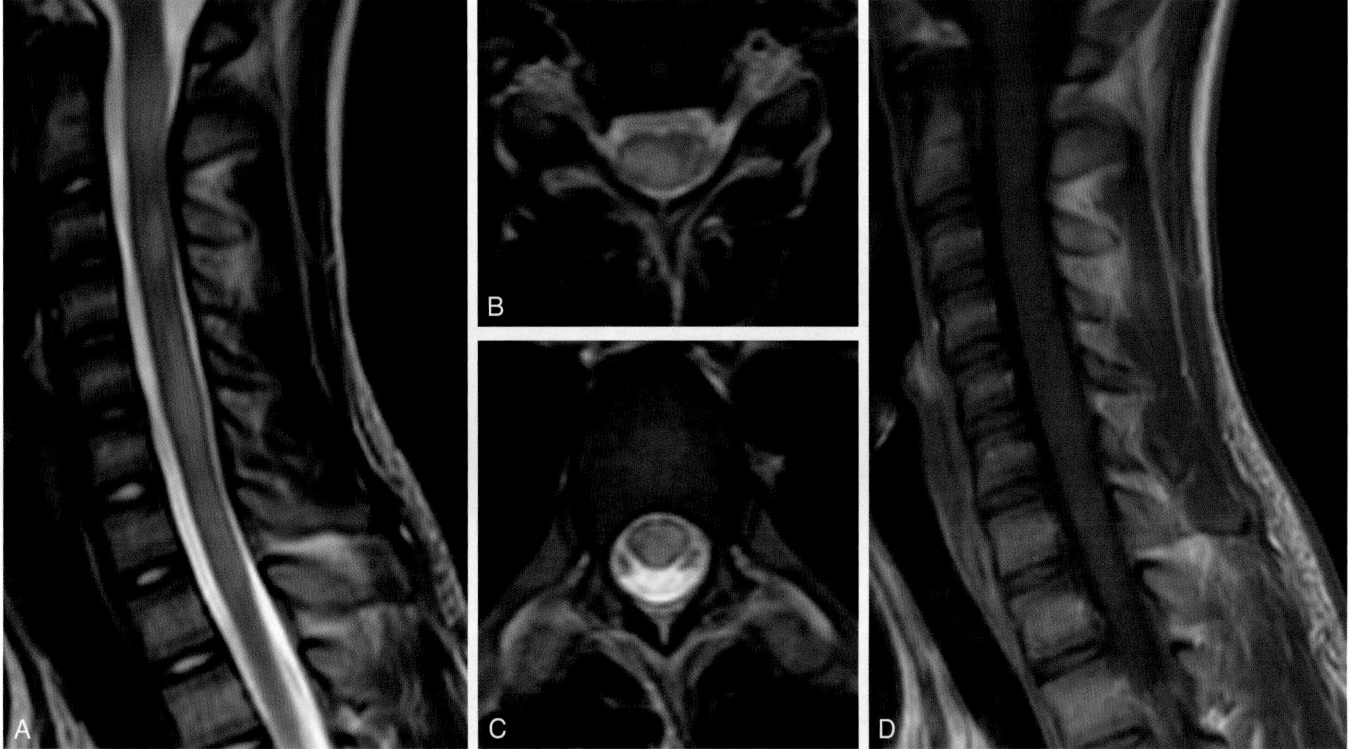

Fig. 18.4 Anti-MOG Myelitis. A 15-year-old with numbness in the toes and hands progressing to upper and lower extremity weakness. (A to C) Sagittal and axial T2W images demonstrate multiple short and a longitudinally extensive minimally expansile T2W hyperintense spinal cord lesions involving gray and white matter without enhancement.

Key Points

Background

- Inflammatory disorder associated with antibodies to myelin oligodendrocyte glycoprotein (MOG). Associated with a variety of demyelinating disorders including optic neuritis, ADEM, myelitis, and non-ADEM encephalitis
- Monophasic or relapsing-remitting course

Imaging

- *Longitudinally extensive transverse myelitis*: two or more vertebral body lengths with minimal expansion and patchy or no enhancement.
- Clinical and imaging criteria can result in a diagnosis of acute flaccid myelitis in 21%.
- No reliable imaging differentiators from ADEM and NMO. Involvement of the lower spinal cord and conus is more common in anti-MOG (11%–41%) than other CNS demyelinating diseases; one-third of cases have multifocal cord lesions; typically gray matter predominant.
- Differential Diagnosis:
  - MS—less severe, short craniocaudal cord involvement, and eccentric location.
  - NMO—worse outcome than anti-MOG, central cord involvement more often cervical and thoracic spinal cord, and more often enhancing (78% compared to 26% with anti-MOG).

REFERENCE

1. Parrotta E, Kister I. The expanding clinical spectrum of myelin oligodendrocyte glycoprotein (MOG) antibody associated disease in children and adults. *Front Neurol.* 2020;11:960.

ACUTE FLACCID MYELITIS

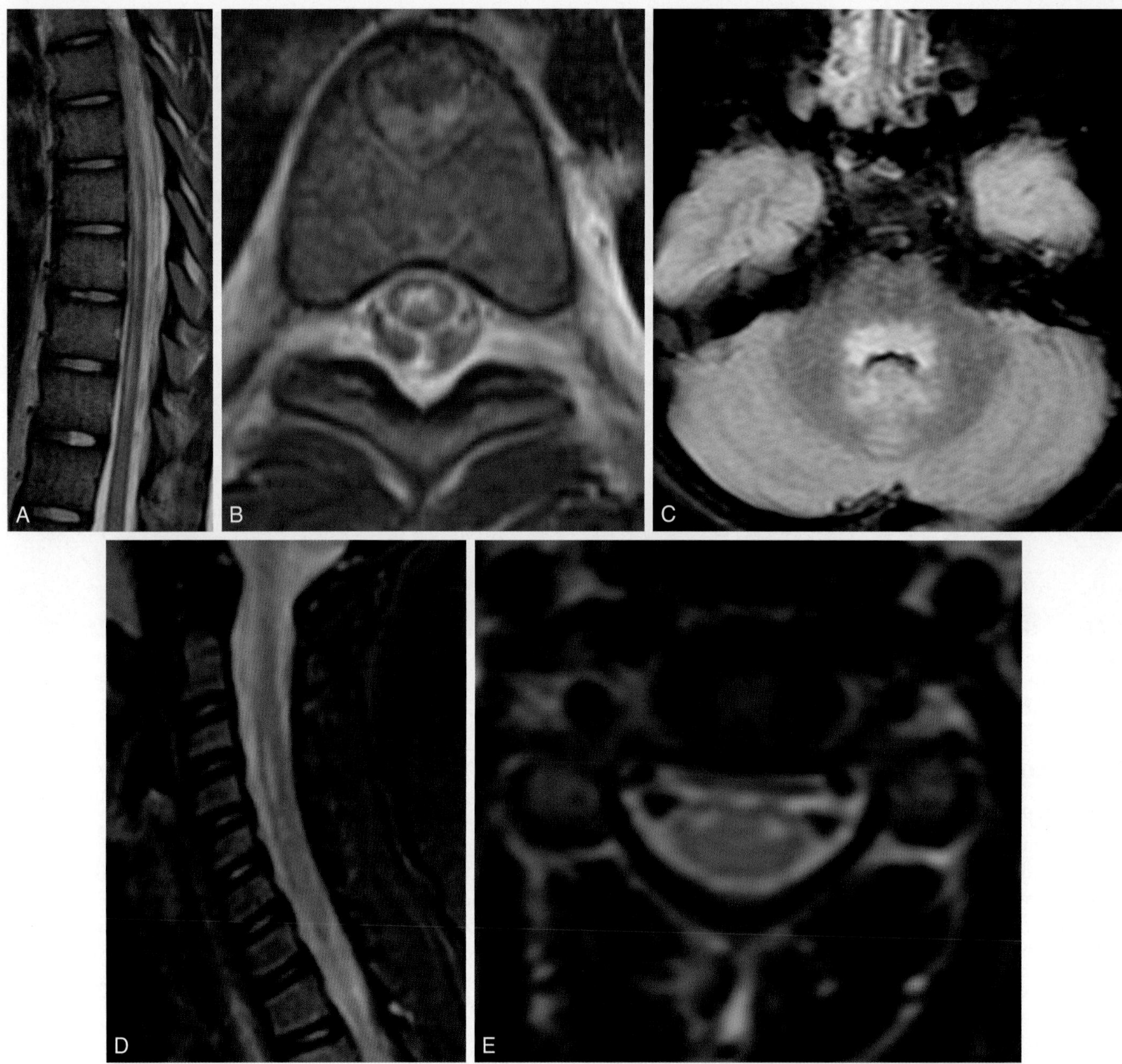

Fig. 18.5 Acute Flaccid Myelitis. (A to C) A 17-year-old with acute-onset flaccid lower extremity weakness. (A and B) Sagittal and axial T2W images demonstrate longitudinally extensive nonexpansile linear T2W hyperintense spinal cord abnormality in the central gray matter of the thoracic spinal cord without enhancement (not shown). (C) Axial FLAIR image demonstrates FLAIR hyperintense signal in the dorsal pons. (D and E) Acute onset of upper extremity weakness in a child. Sagittal and axial T2W images demonstrate short segment T2W hyperintensity limited to the anterior horns of the central gray matter.

Key Points

Background

- Etiology presumed to be secondary to a viral infection or postinfectious immune response. Enterovirus D68 implicated.

Imaging

- *Longitudinally extensive* T2W hyperintense signal predominantly involving the *central gray matter* or limited to the *anterior horns* of the central gray matter. Minimal to no enhancement.
- Brain findings can include T2W hyperintensity in the medulla, and dorsal pons. Less commonly the thalami may be involved.
- Cauda equina can enhance in the subacute phase.

REFERENCE

1. Messacar K, Schreiner TL, Van Haren K, et al. Acute flaccid myelitis: a clinical review of US cases 2012–2015. *Ann Neurol.* 2016 Sept;80(3):326–338.

MULTIPLE SCLEROSIS

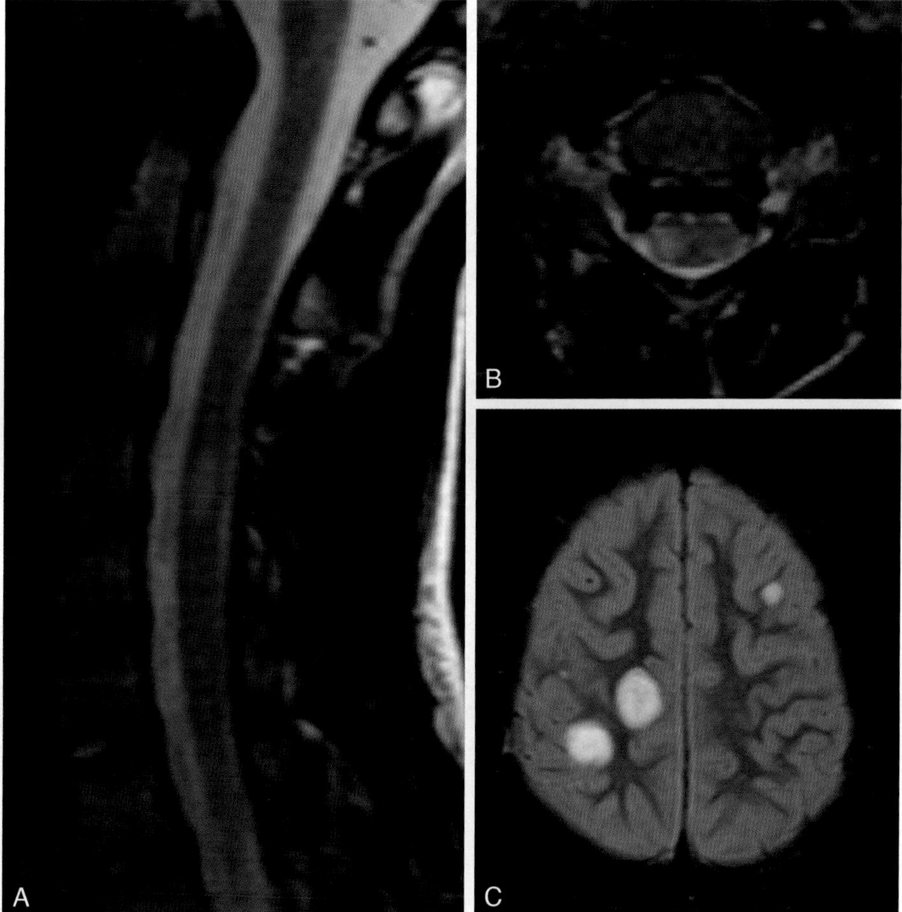

Fig. 18.6 Multiple Sclerosis. (A and B) Sagittal and axial T2W images demonstrate short segment nonexpansile T2W hyperintense right lateral spinal cord abnormality. (C) Axial FLAIR image demonstrates ovoid FLAIR hyperintensities in the juxtacortical white matter.

Key Points

Background

- A chronic autoimmune condition with genetic predisposition triggered by unknown factors affecting patients typically between the age of 20 and 40 years.
- Pediatric MS versus adult MS:
  - Male:female ratio is closer to 1 in children <10 to 12 years of age
  - Greater ADEM-like onset, more brainstem and cerebellar involvement, and less destructive lesions (less T1 hypointense supratentorial lesions) with pediatric MS
  - Children <12 years have a greater number of relapses, more severe clinical involvement, worse prognosis, and polysymptomatic onset
  - Oligoclonal bands are detected in 40% to 70% of pediatric patients with MS compared to 90% of adult patients with MS.

Imaging

- *Short craniocaudal length* (<2 vertebral bodies in length) spinal cord lesions that are T2W hyperintense and enhance in the acute phase.
- Cord lesions have *predilection for the white matter* areas of the spinal cord and are consequently seen within the periphery of the spinal cord more than the gray matter.

REFERENCE

1. Rossi A.*Pediatric Neuroradiology*. 1st ed. Berlin/Heidelberg: Springer-Verlag.

GUILLAIN-BARRE SYNDROME

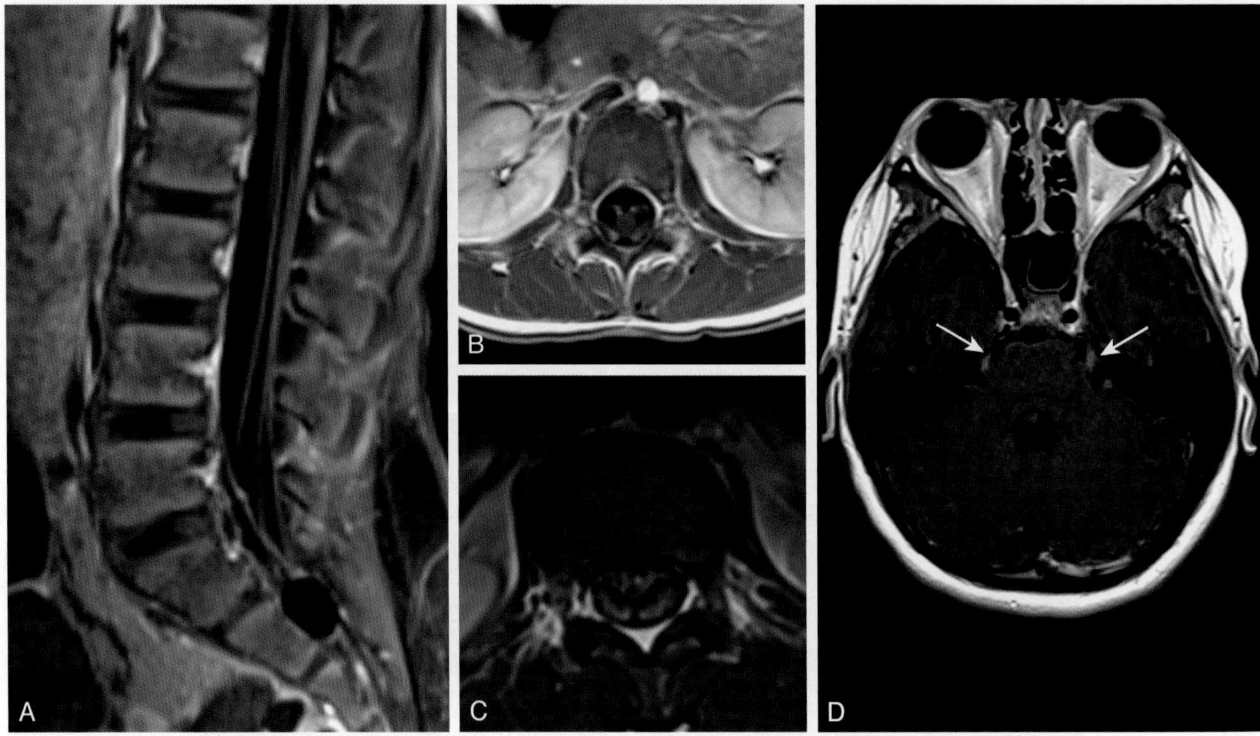

Fig. 18.7 Guillain-Barre Syndrome. (A to D) Sagittal and axial T1W+C images demonstrate enhancement of the cauda equina and the fifth cranial nerves.

Key Points

Background

- Acute inflammatory demyelinating disorder involving the spinal and peripheral nerves
- Typically affects children aged 4 to 12 years old
- Presents with *rapidly progressive ascending flaccid paralysis with hypotonia.*
- Occurs 1 to 3 weeks following URI or GI infection
- Rapidly progresses, plateaus, then improves over 2 to 18 months

Imaging

- *Enhancement of cauda equina nerve roots.* Anterior nerve roots are often more prominently enhancing than the posterior nerve roots.
- Normal appearance of the spinal cord.
- The Miller Fisher variant of Guillain-Barre syndrome (GBS) also demonstrates cranial nerve enhancement
- Differential Diagnosis: West Nile virus, leptomeningeal carcinomatosis, Lyme disease, and metabolic disorders including metachromatic leukodystrophy

REFERENCE

1. Rossi A.*Pediatric Neuroradiology*. 1st ed. Berlin/Heidelberg: Springer-Verlag.

LYME DISEASE

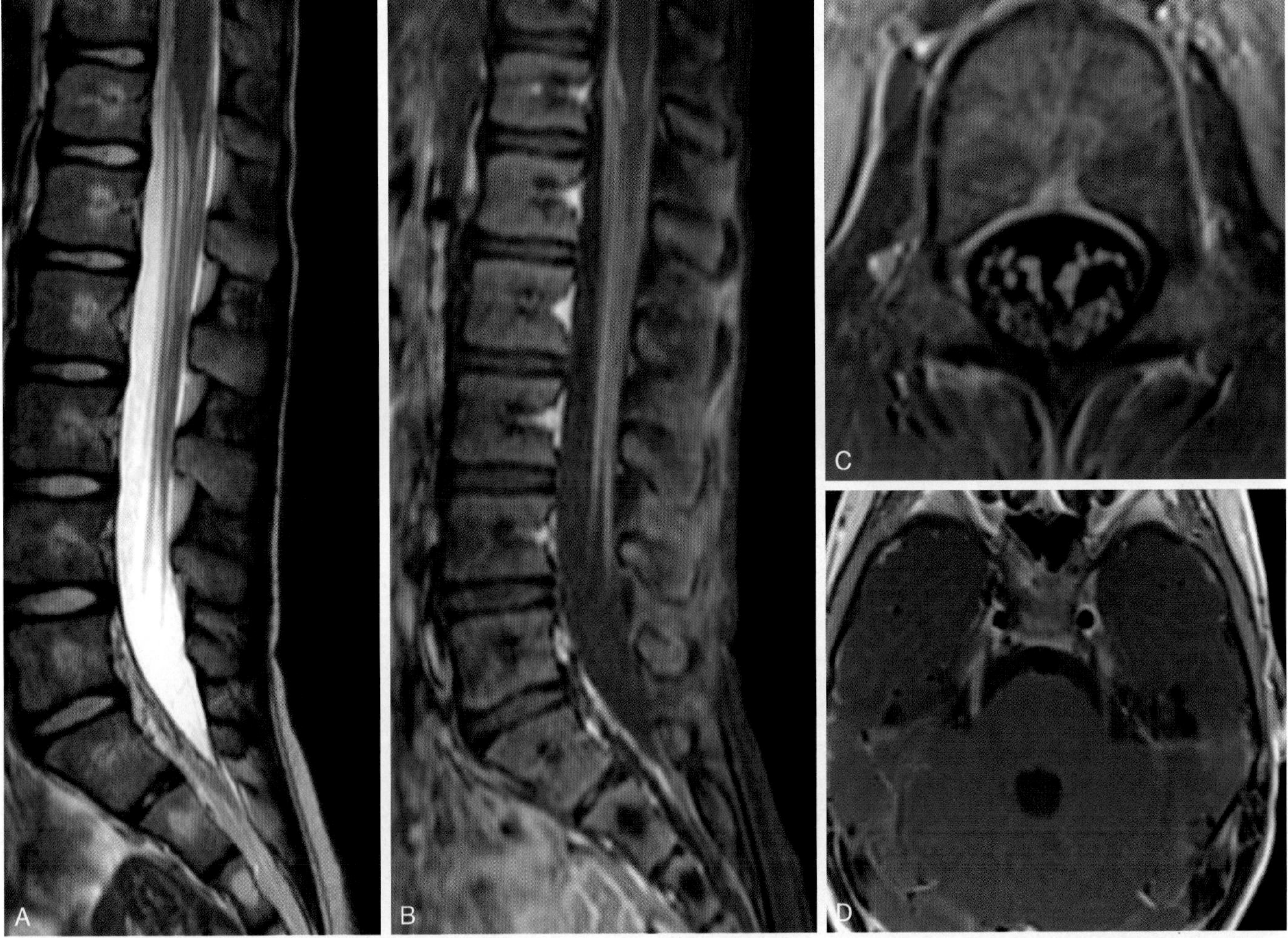

Fig. 18.8 Lyme Disease. An 11-year-old with a large target-like rash 3 months prior and new leg weakness. (A) Sagittal T2W and (B to D) sagittal and axial T1W+C images demonstrate normal lower spinal cord T2 signal but abnormal enhancement of the cauda equina and cranial nerve 5. CSF Borrelia burgdorferi IgM and IgG were positive confirming the diagnosis of Lyme disease.

Key Points

Background

- Infection from spirochete *Borrelia burgdorferi* in the United States
- Geographical and seasonal prevalence
- Clinical hallmark of *erythema migrans rash*; flulike symptoms; carditis; arthritis

Imaging

- *Enhancing cranial nerves and spinal nerve roots*, and leptomeningeal enhancement
- Cerebral white matter T2 FLAIR hyperintensities
- Diffuse or multifocal spinal cord T2 hyperintense lesions (rare)
- Ocular manifestations (rare)

REFERENCES

1. Hildebrand P, Craven DE, Jones R, et al. Lyme neuroborreliosis: manifestations of a rapidly emerging zoonosis. *Am J Neuroradiol.* 2009 Jun;30(6):1079–1087.
2. Kontzialis M, Poretti A, Michell H, Bosemani T, Tekes A, Huisman TA. Spinal nerve root enhancement on MRI scans in children: a review. *J Neuroimaging.* 2016 Mar–Apr;26(2):169–179.

OSTEOMYELITIS, DISCITIS, EPIDURAL ABSCESS/PHLEGMON

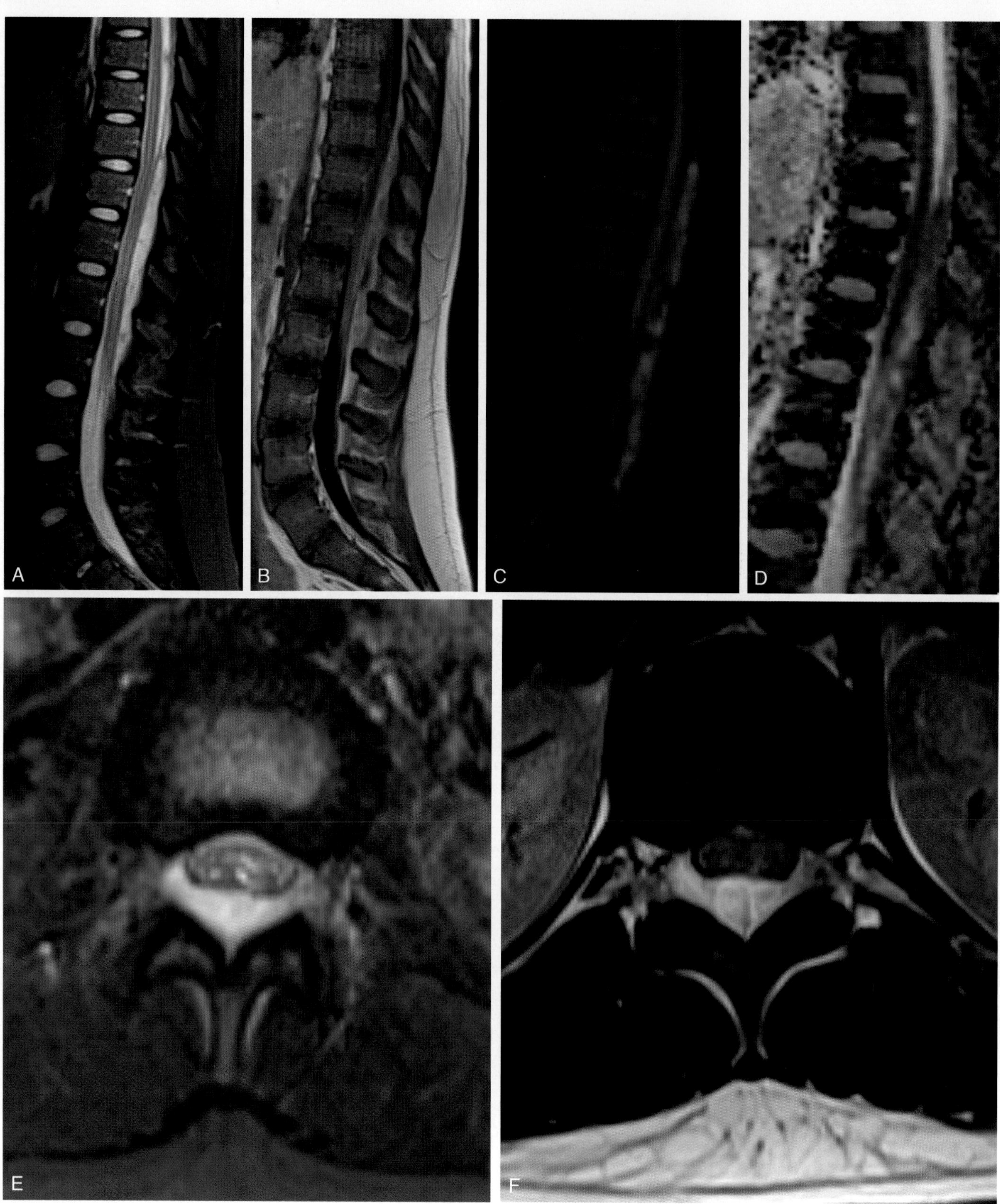

Fig. 18.9 Epidural Phlegmon and Abscess. (A and F) Sagittal and axial T2W, (B and E) sagittal and axial T1W+C, (C) sagittal DWI, and (D) sagittal ADC images demonstrate abnormal T2W hyperintense enhancing soft tissue in the thoracic and lumbar posterior epidural space with diffusion restriction.

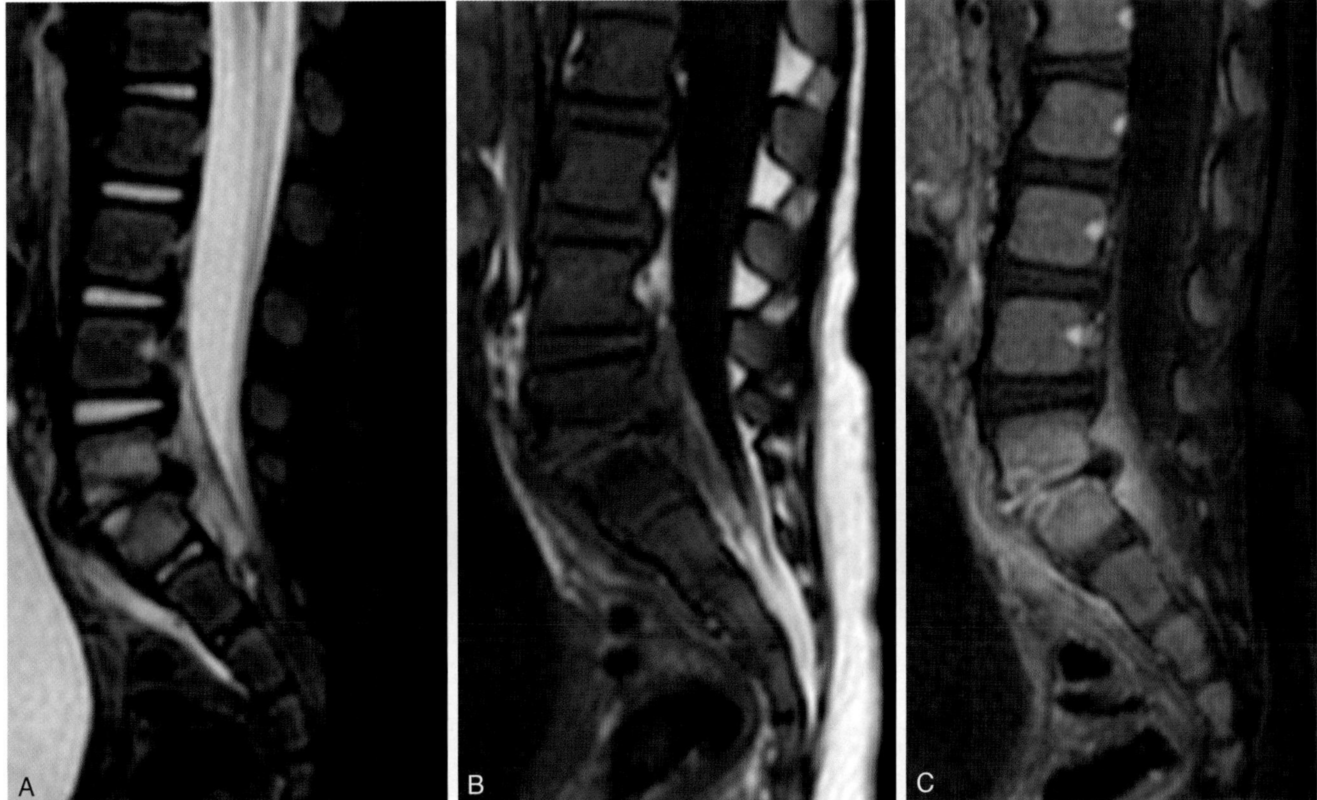

Fig. 18.10 Osteomyelitis, Discitis, and Phlegmon. (A) Sagittal STIR, (B) sagittal T1W, and (C) sagittal T1W+C fat saturation images demonstrate abnormal STIR hyperintensity and enhancement in the bone marrow of L5 and S1, severe L5–S1 disc space narrowing, and prevertebral and anterior epidural space soft tissue enhancement indicative of osteomyelitis, discitis, and phlegmon.

Key Points

Background

- The source of infection in children is usually hematogenous. Bacterial infection is more common than fungal or parasitic.
- Osteomyelitis and discitis affect the bone and intervertebral disc. Sixty percent of spondylodiscitis occurs in ages 6 months to 4 years and are sterile or grow *Kingella kinga*. Among children older than 4 years, the most common pathogen is *Staphylococcus aureus*. Sickle cell anemia patients can have *Salmonella* infections.
- Epidural phlegmon and abscess are caused by spinal infection with purulent material in the epidural space.
- Signs and symptoms in children include back pain, inability to walk, and fever.
- Biopsy yield for organism identification ranges from 36% to 91% depending on the preceding antibiotic administration and technique.
- Treatment with intravenous antibiotics and neurosurgical consultation for potential drainage of an epidural abscess.

Imaging

- Osteomyelitis demonstrates increased T2/STIR signal and enhancement in the vertebral body, and is associated with *paraspinal soft tissue T2/STIR hyperintense signal.*
- Phlegmon demonstrates homogeneous enhancement, while abscess demonstrates peripheral enhancement with central nonenhancement. Often, phlegmon, abscess, osteomyelitis, and discitis are simultaneously present.
- DWI helpful for evaluating epidural fluid. Diffusion restriction helps confirm the presence of purulent material.
- Differential Diagnosis: Leukemia, CRMO, and LCH.

REFERENCE

1. Tyagi R. Spinal infections in children: a review. *J Orthop.* 2016;13(4):254–258.

INTERVERTEBRAL DISC CALCIFICATION

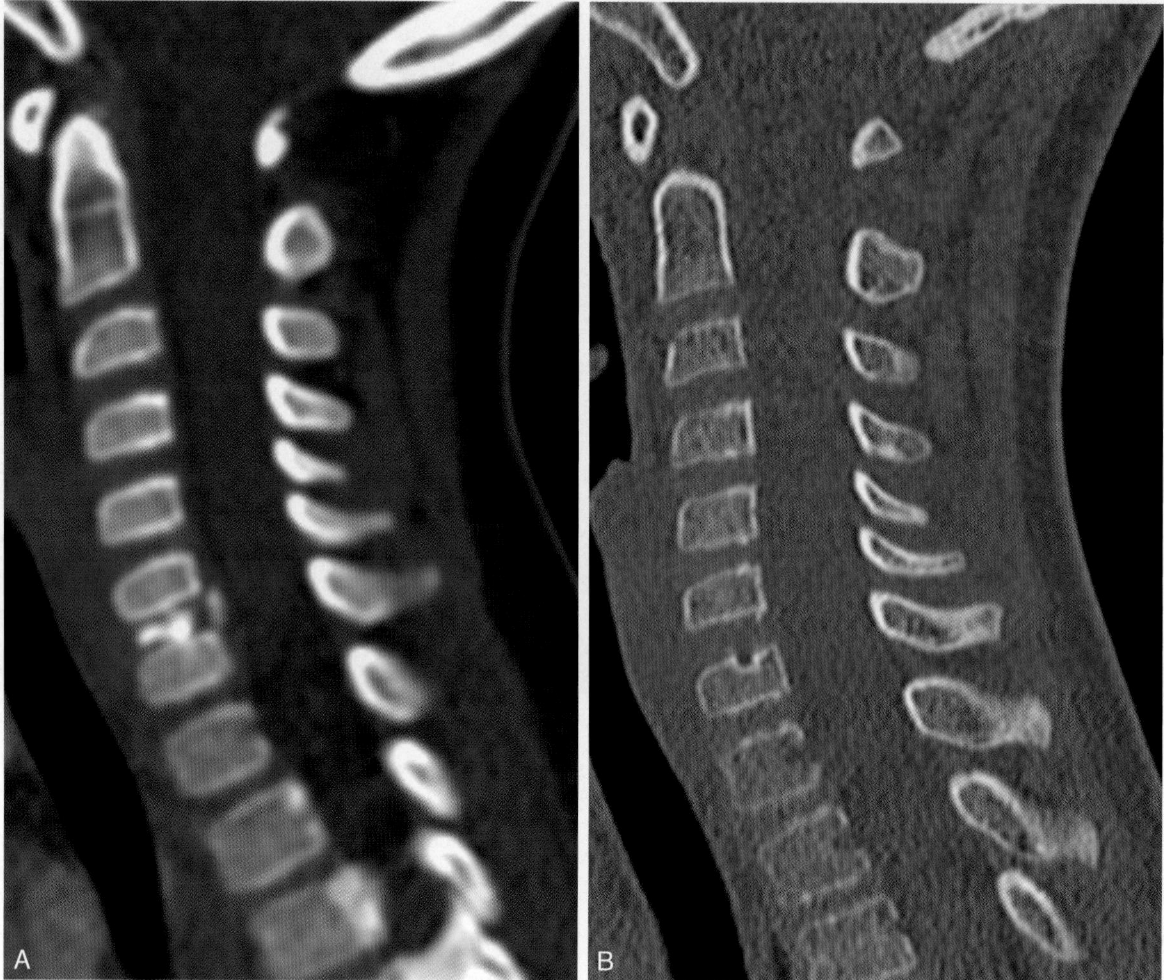

Fig. 18.11 Intervertebral Disc Calcification. (A) Sagittal reformat CT image demonstrates abnormal calcification in the C6–7 intervertebral disc space. (B) Sagittal reformat CT performed at follow-up demonstrates resolution of the calcification.

Key Points

Background

- Relatively rare phenomenon presumably due to inflammation. Most commonly involves the lower cervical spine.
- Most patients are asymptomatic; less commonly can present with neck pain and torticollis.
- Laboratory evaluation and lumbar puncture usually normal.
- Intervertebral disc calcification can also be seen in alkaptonuria.

Imaging

- Calcification usually involves the nucleus pulposus.
- ~30% have associated disc herniation.
- X-ray and CT demonstrate intervertebral disc calcification, while MRI demonstrates T1W and T2W hypointense signal.
- *Disc calcification can completely or partially resolve.*

REFERENCE

1. Dushnicky MJ, Okura H, Shroff M, et al. Pediatric idiopathic intervertebral disc calcification: single center series and review of the literature. *J Pediatr*. 2019 Mar;206:212–216.

SPINAL CORD INFARCT

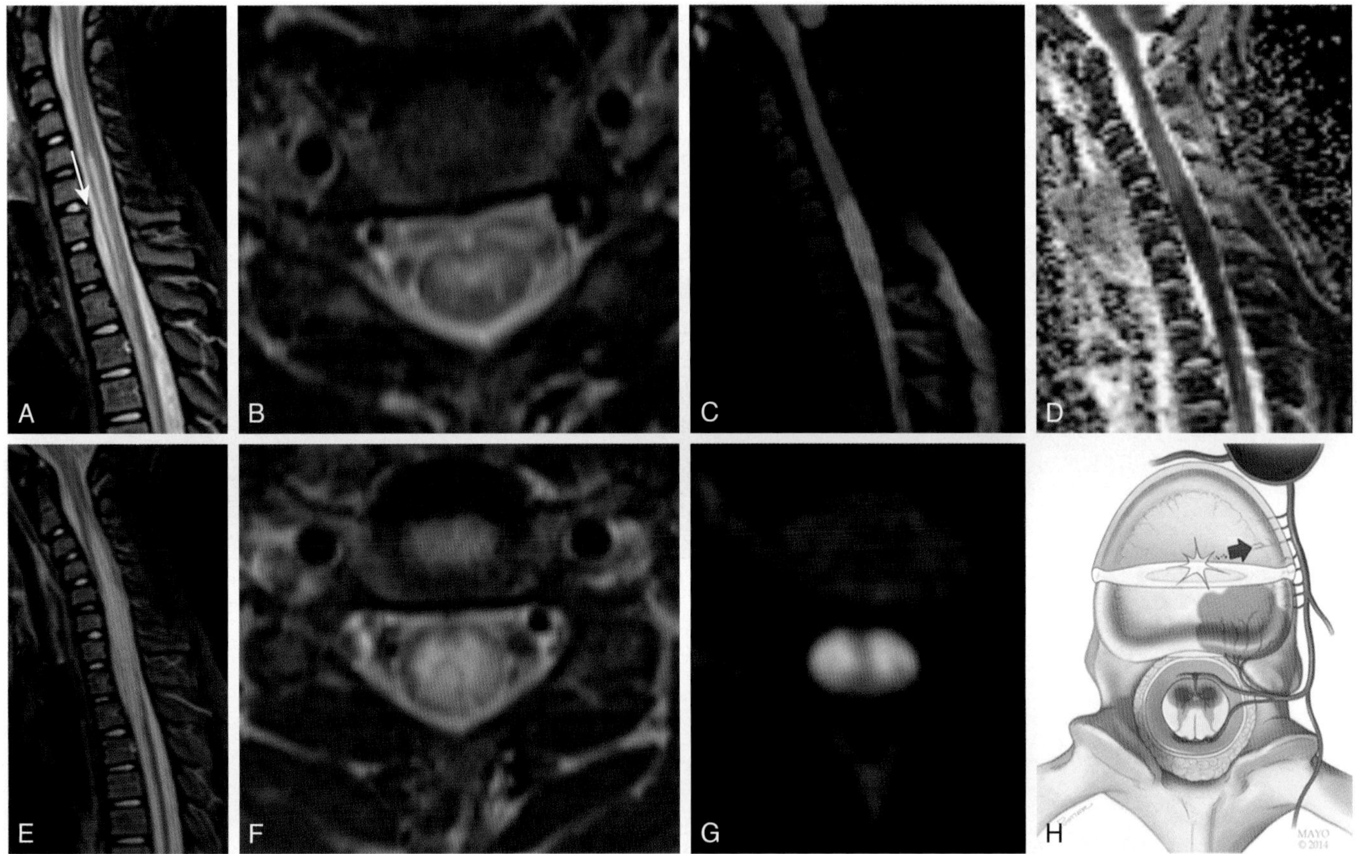

Fig. 18.12 Spinal Cord Infarct. An 11-year-old with acute-onset upper extremity weakness. (A and B) Sagittal T2W image demonstrates linear T2 hyperintense signal in the spinal cord from C5 to T5 levels that corresponds to abnormal T2W hyperintensity in the central gray matter on (B) axial T2W image. A subtle annular fissure is present at the C6–7 level (*arrow*). (C and D) Sagittal DWI and ADC map images demonstrate diffusion restriction from C5 through T3 levels greater in extent than the T2W hyperintensity. Follow-up MRI 3 days later with (E) sagittal STIR, (F) axial T2W, and (G) axial DWI images demonstrate more extensive T2W hyperintensity in the spinal cord involving majority of the entire spinal cord in lower cervical levels and diffusion restriction of the anterior two-thirds of the spinal cord. A disc embolism is the presumed etiology based on clinical history, spinal cord diffusion restriction, and annular tear at the C6–7 level. (H) Illustration of a mechanism of fibrocartilaginous embolism resulting in spinal cord infarct.
(H Reproduced from Mayo Foundation for Medical Education and Research.)

Key Points

Background

- Uncommon in children but may be underdiagnosed as the diagnosis often not considered in children and etiology can be difficult to confirm.
- Associated with trauma/dissection, thromboembolic disease (CNS infection, vasculitis, fibrocartilage embolism), cerebellar herniation, and cardiovascular disease.
- *Typically reaches nadir at 4 hours from onset.*
- Variable prognosis that depends on the level and extent of ischemia and rehabilitation.

Imaging

- MRI findings may be subtle in the early stages.
- *DWI restriction* may be slow to develop.
- Three common patterns on axial T2W imaging of a spinal cord infarct include T2 hyperintense signal involving central gray matter only, anterior 2/3 of the spine cross section, or the entire cross section of the spinal cord. Pattern on T2W imaging can change on short term follow up MRI.
- Close inspection of the spine in the region of the cord signal abnormality for an annular tear can help make the diagnosis.

REFERENCE

1. Sheikh A, Warren D, Childs AM, et al. Paediatric spinal cord infarction – a review of the literature and two case reports. *Childs Nerv Syst*. 2017;33(4):671–676.

ARTERIOVENOUS MALFORMATION

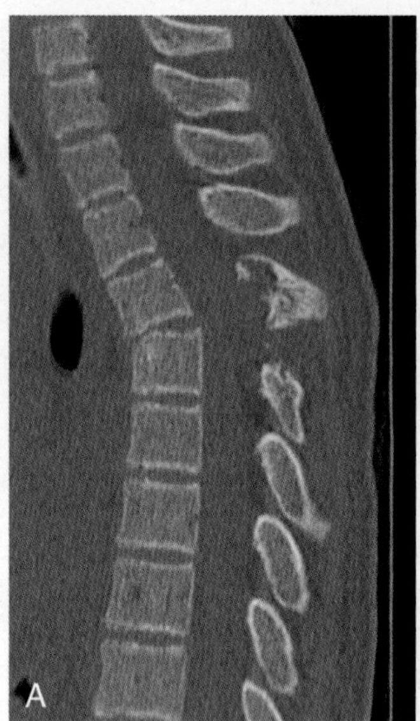

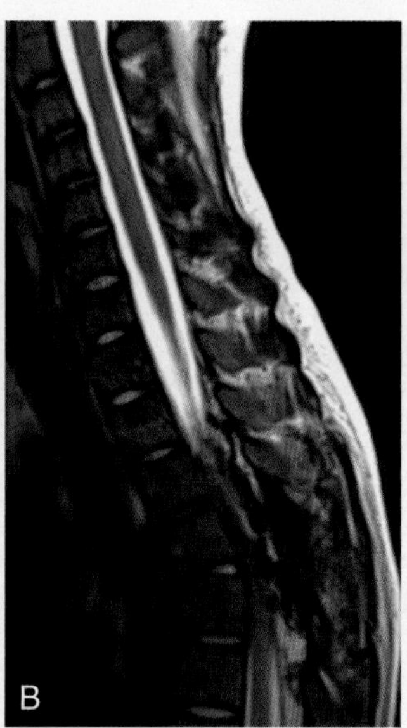

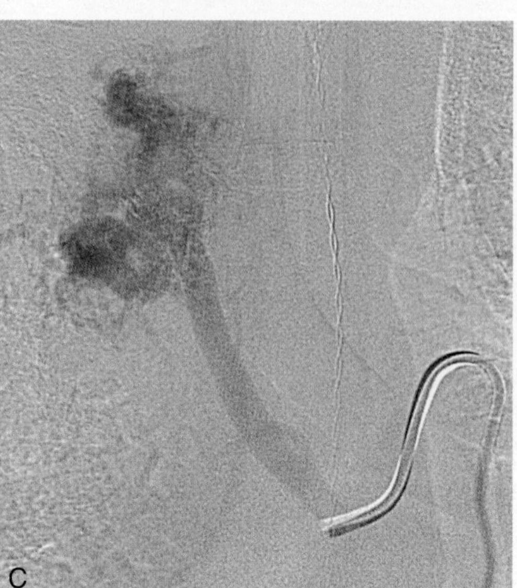

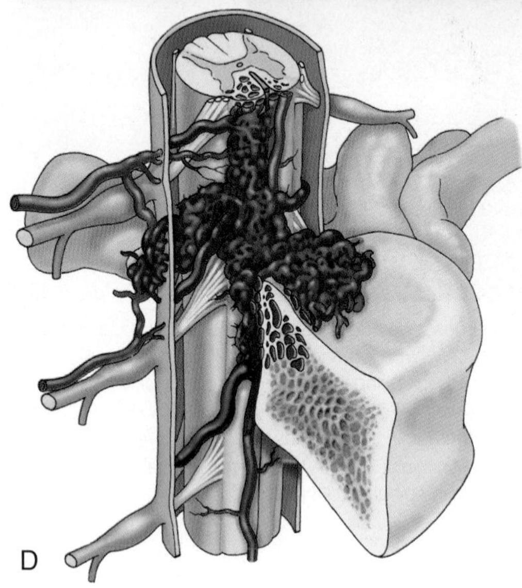

Fig. 18.13 Spinal Arteriovenous Malformation. A 13-year-old with bilateral lower extremity numbness and weakness. (A) Sagittal reformat CT of the thoracic spine demonstrates midthoracic kyphosis, loss of disc space height, and irregular lucency of the spinous process. (B) Sagittal T2W image demonstrates a tangle of vessels in the epidural space. (C) Spinal catheter angiogram following injection of a T5 intercostal artery demonstrates a tangle of vessels consistent with an AVM. (D) Illustration of extradural-intradural arteriovenous malformation involving neural and bony elements. (D From McDougall CG, Deshmukh VR, Fiorella DJ, Albuquerque FC, Spetzler RF. Endovascular techniques for vascular malformations of the Spinal Axis. *Neurosurg Clin N Am.* 2005;16(2):395–410.)

Key Points

Background

- Arteriovenous malformations (AVMs) are abnormal connections between spinal arteries and veins with a nidus.
- Pediatric spinal AVMs are usually the juvenile type rather than glomus.
- Pediatric spinal AVMs tend to present with more acute symptoms and have a higher hemorrhage rate compared to adult spinal AVMs.
- Angiographic obliteration, clinical cure, and clinical improvement rates are 12% to 90%, 11% to 45%, and 45% to 55%, respectively.
- Spinal vascular malformations are categorized as follows:
  - Type 1: Dural arteriovenous fistula
  - Type 2: Intradural-intramedullary AVM and conus AVM
  - Type 3: Juvenile spinal AVM, spinal metameric syndrome (Cobb syndrome)
  - Type 4: Intradural-perimedullary arteriovenous (AV) fistula
  - Spinal epidural AV fistula

Imaging

- MRI: *abnormal tangle of flow voids* on T2W imaging. May present with spontaneous spinal hemorrhage
- Catheter angiography performed for definitive diagnosis, mapping arterial and venous drainage, and potential treatment

REFERENCE

1. Cho WS, Wang KC, Phi JH, et al. Pediatric spinal arteriovenous malformations and fistulas: a single institute's experience. *Childs Nerv Syst.* 2016;32:811–818.

ARTERIOVENOUS FISTULA

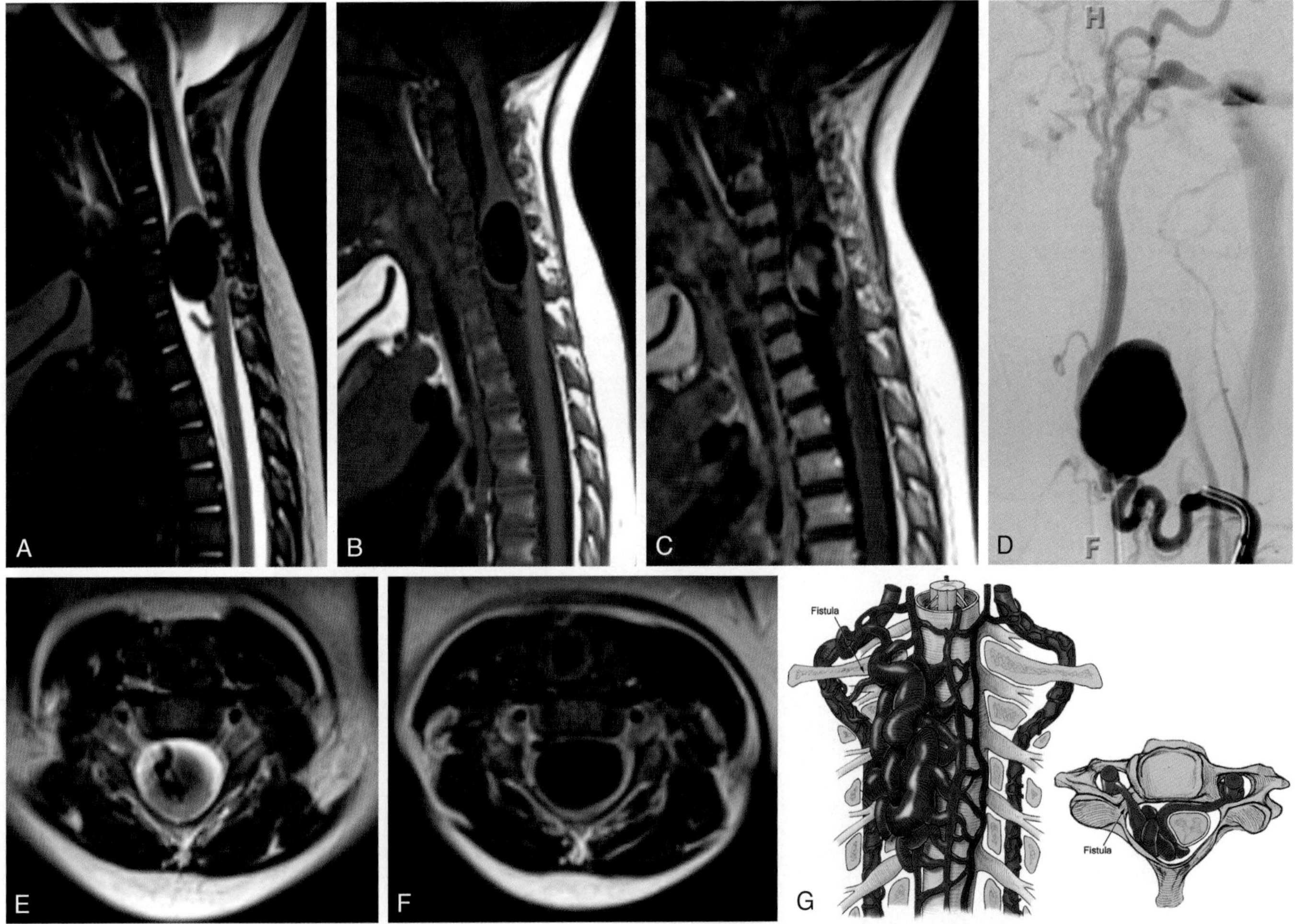

Fig. 18.14 Arteriovenous Fistula. (A) Sagittal T2W, (B) sagittal T1W, (C) sagittal T1W+C, and (D) catheter angiography confirms an arteriovenous fistula with large nidal aneurysm. (E and F) Axial T2W images. (G) Artist's rendering of an extradural arteriovenous fistula. (G from Riina HA, Spetzler RF. Classification of vascular lesions affecting the spinal cord. *Oper Tech Neurosurg*. 2003;6(3):106–115.)

Key Points

Background

- More common in adults than children
- Arteriovenous communication between spinal arteries and veins without a discrete nidus
- Can present with cord compression, steal phenomenon, hemorrhage, and/or venous hypertension
- Can be associated with cutaneous vascular malformation, spinal metameric syndrome (Cobb syndrome), hereditary hemorrhagic telangiectasia, or Klippel-Trenauny syndrome
- Treated with embolization and/or microsurgical disconnection

Imaging

- MRI: *Abnormal prominence of flow voids* on T2W imaging; non-masslike *spinal cord T2W hyperintensity*, and variable cord enhancement; cord signal abnormality typically lower spinal cord due to venous congestion; potentially reversible cord T2W hyperintensity following treatment
- Catheter angiography performed for definitive diagnosis, mapping arterial and venous drainage, and potential treatment

REFERENCE

1. Jingwei L, Zeng G, Zhi X, et al. Pediatric perimedullary arteriovenous fistula: clinical features and endovascular treatments. *J Neurointerv Surg*. 2019 Apr;11(4):411–415.

HIRAYAMA DISEASE

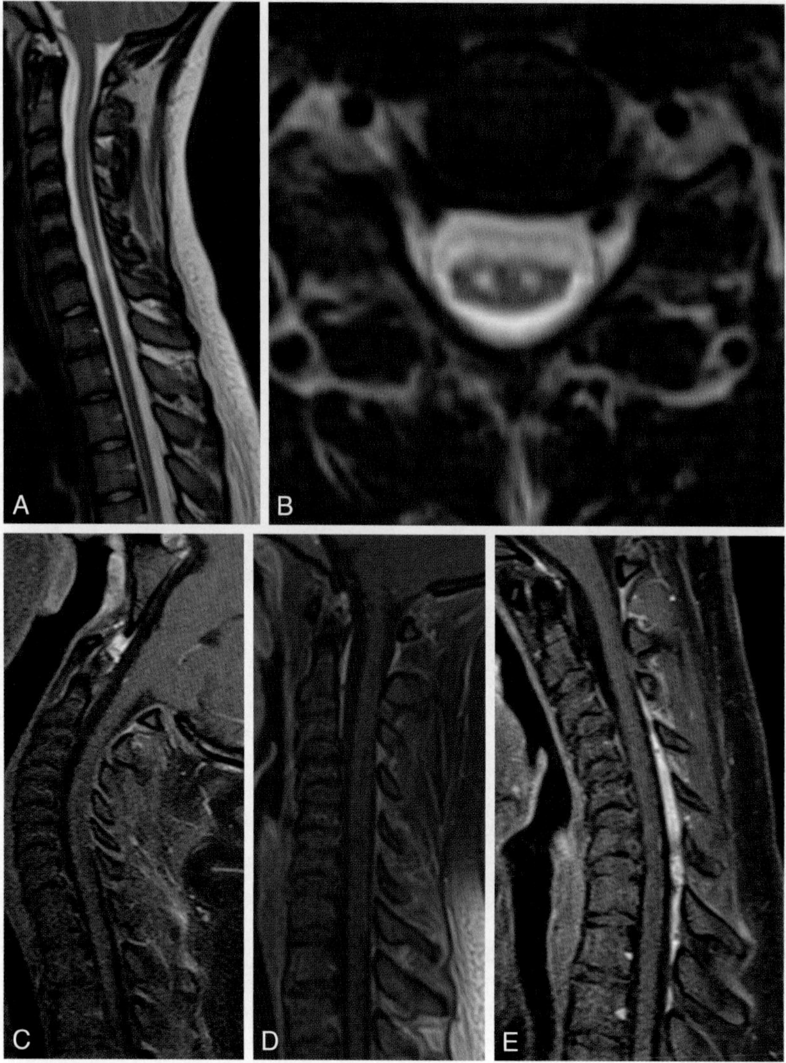

Fig. 18.15 Hirayama Disease. 16-year-old with hand weakness. (A and B) Sagittal and axial T2W images demonstrate loss of cervical lordosis in neutral position and abnormal T2W hyperintensity in the anterior horns of the spinal cord gray matter at the C6–7 level. (C to E) Sagittal T1W+C images in extension, neutral, and flexion demonstrate abnormal enlargement of the epidural venous plexus of the cervical spine associated with spinal canal narrowing in flexion that normalizes in the neutral and extension positions.

Key Points

Background

- Rare disease process that results in asymmetric weakness of the distal upper extremity muscles in the C8–T1 muscle distribution.
- Most commonly occurs in patients aged 15 to 25 years.
- The presumed etiology is abnormal spinal dura growth relative to the spine that allows forward displacement of the dura in flexion and compression of the spinal cord and potential ischemia.

Imaging

- Lower cervical spinal cord atrophy and T2W hyperintensity usually less than two vertebral segments in craniocaudal length and involves unilateral or bilateral anterior horns of the central gray matter
- Loss of attachment of the dura to the lamina
- Anterior displacement of the dura in flexion position with a decrease in the AP and transverse spinal diameter due to enlargement of the epidural venous plexus (useful for distinguishing from a forward shift that can occur in healthy subjects)
- Loss of cervical lordosis in neutral position

REFERENCE

1. Lehman VT, Luetmer PH, Sorenson EJ, et al. Cervical spine MR imaging findings of patients with Hirayama disease in North America: a multisite study. *AJNR Am J Neuroradiol.* 2013 Feb;34(2):451–456.

BONE INFARCTS

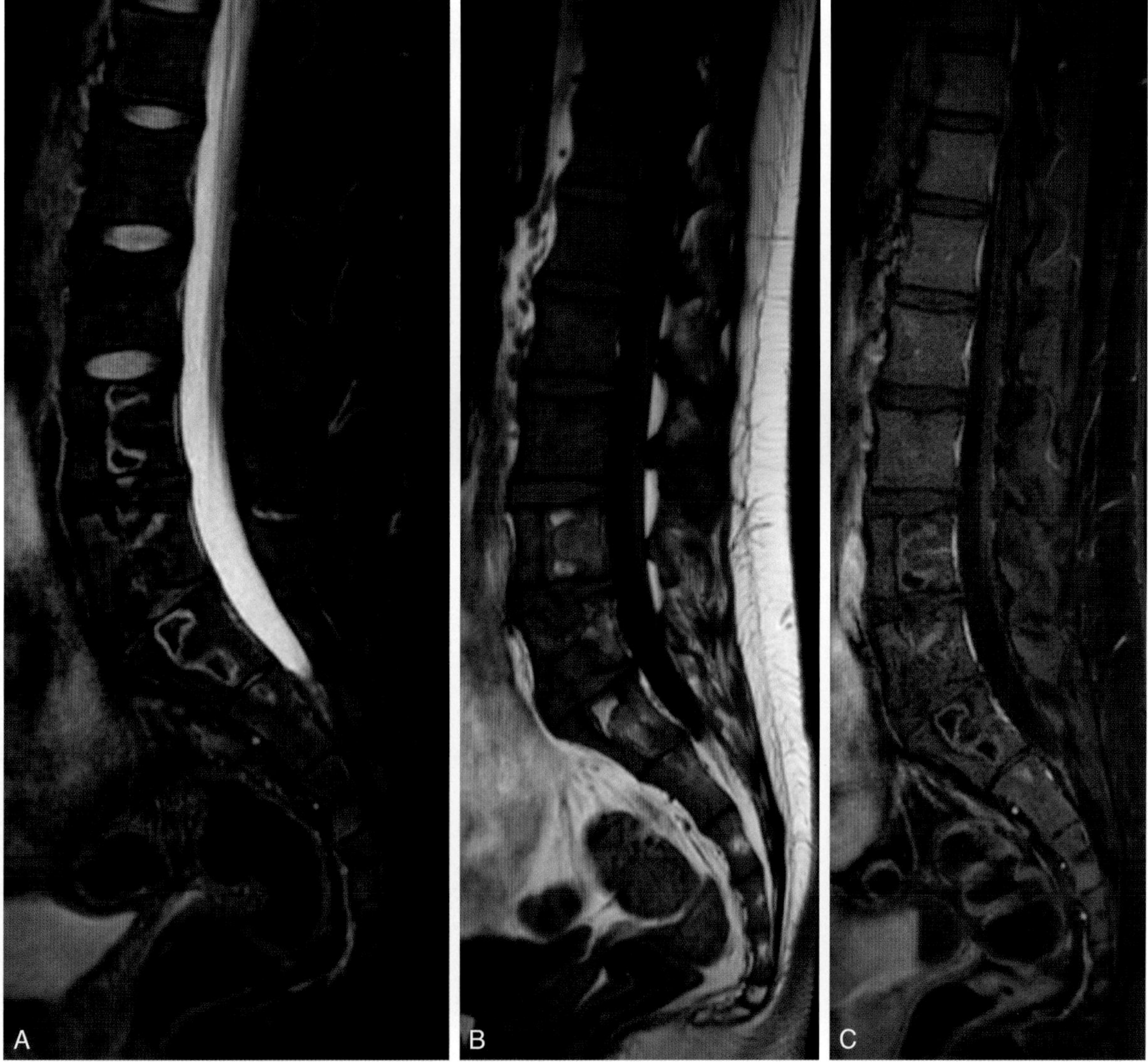

Fig. 18.16 Bone Infarcts. (A) Sagittal STIR, (B) Sagittal T1W, and (C) sagittal T1W+C fat saturation images sharply defined T1W and T2W hyperintense areas in the central vertebral bodies of L4–S2.

Key Points

Background

- Segmental arteries from the aorta supply the thoracic and lumbar bone marrow, paraspinal muscles, dura, and spinal cord.
- Most commonly associated with *sickle cell anemia and leukemia.*

Imaging

- Most commonly involve the thoracic, lumbar, and sacral spine.
- *Sharply defined linear/serpentine/geographic areas* of T2W hyperintensity and enhancement usually in the anterior or middle of the vertebral bodies.
- In sickle cell disease, this results in H-shaped vertebral bodies.
- Differentiate from osteomyelitis by lack of surrounding soft tissue enhancement, sharply defined pattern and normal adjacent disc space.

REFERENCE

1. Hanrahan CJ, Shah LM. MRI of spinal bone marrow: part 2, T1-weighted imaging-based differential diagnosis. *AJR Am J Roentgenol.* 2011 Dec;197(6):1309–1321.

19 Spine Trauma

INTRODUCTION

Background

- The majority (80%) of pediatric spine trauma occurs in the cervical spine and annual incidence is 1% to 2%. Pediatric spine trauma is most commonly secondary to motor vehicle accidents (52%), sports injury (27%), falls (15%), and nonaccidental trauma (3%). Spinal trauma from nonaccidental injury is more common in children younger than 2 years of age, while sports-related injuries are more common in older children and adolescents.
- The overall mortality of pediatric cervical spine injuries is 16% to 18%, with higher mortality associated with upper cervical spine injuries (particularly atlanto-occipital dislocation), younger age, and associated head injury.
- The pediatric age and associated spine maturity impacts the susceptibility to injury. The pediatric spine reaches a more adult configuration at ~8 years of age. In children younger than 8 years of age, the majority of injuries occur at C1–C3, while injuries are more common from C5 and below in children older than 8 years of age.
- Compared to adults, younger children have greater ligamentous laxity, greater head:torso ratio, weaker neck muscles, shallow occipital condyles, developing ossification centers, horizontal facets (upper cervical facet angulation of 30 degrees vs 60–70 degrees in adults; lower cervical spine angulation of 55 degrees vs 70 degrees in adults), absent uncinate processes in children under 10 years old allowing for greater rotational movement, and underdeveloped spinous processes allowing for greater flexion and extension.

Imaging

- The primary modalities for evaluating cervical spine trauma are radiography, CT, and MRI. Often, all these modalities are used in various combinations for accurately diagnosing spinal trauma.
- The National Emergency X-Radiography Utilization Study (NEXUS) trial established five high-risk criteria for cervical spine injury in children under 18 years of age: (1) midline cervical tenderness, (2) evidence of intoxication, (3) altered level of alertness, (4) focal neurologic deficit, and (5) painful distracting injury. The presence of any one of the five criteria placed a patient into the high-risk group; the absence of all criteria defined a patient as low risk. Among the low-risk group, no patient suffered a cervical spine injury, indicating that no imaging was necessary in this group. The high-risk group should first undergo AP and lateral spine radiographs. If a child has worsening symptoms and deficits despite negative radiographs, CT or MRI is recommended. However, many institutions bypass radiographs for children with major trauma or neurologic deficits or those who are unconscious.

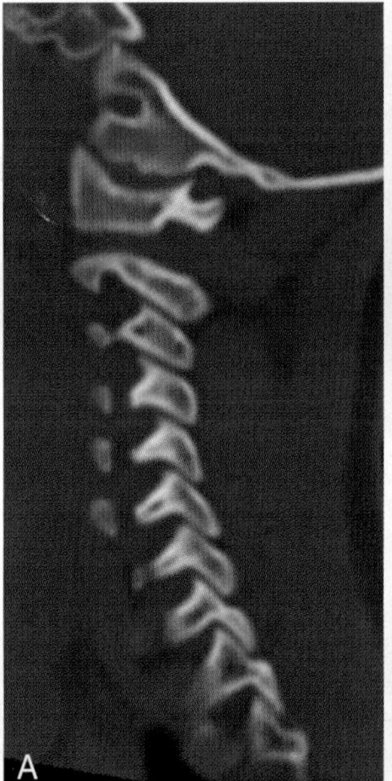

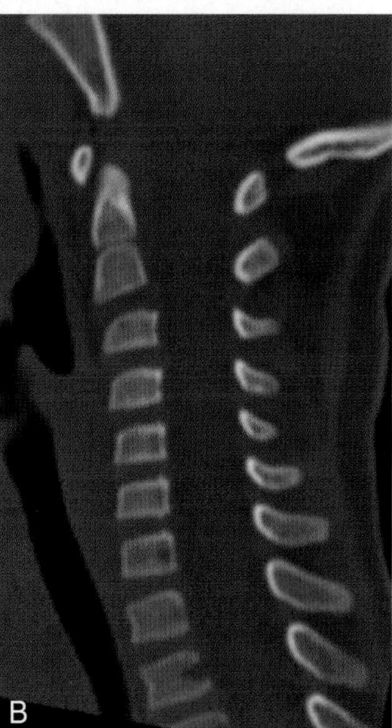

- Because there is a greater prevalence of ligamentous injury in children relative to adults, it is important for the radiologist to be knowledgeable of normative values for measurements that can indicate a ligamentous injury and require MRI for direct assessment of the ligaments. It is also important for radiologists to be familiar with the ossification centers and normal physiologic variants in the cervical spine that may be encountered.
- MRI is the most sensitive technique for identification of spine injury, particularly the spinal ligaments, spinal cord, and soft tissue of the spinal canal. Up to 24% of children with radiographically occult injury had injuries visible on MRI.
- This section will illustrate the imaging appearance of spinal trauma, with particular emphasis on CT and MRI findings that indicate spinal trauma, as well imaging of uncommon spinal trauma and normal anatomic variants.

REFERENCES

1. Traylor KS, Kralik SF, Radhakrishnan R. Pediatric spine emergencies. *Sem Ultrasound CT MR.* 2018 Dec;39(6):605–617.
2. Huisman TA, Wagner MW, Bosemani T, Tekes A, Poretti A. Pediatric spinal trauma. *J Neuroimaging.* 2015 May–Jun;25(3):337–353.

CRANIOCERVICAL JUNCTION CT MEASUREMENTS

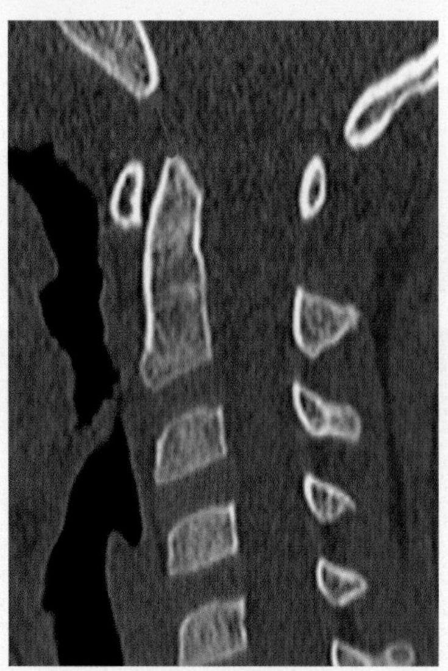

Basion-Dens Interval (BDI). Measured as the shortest distance between the basion and the tip of the ossified odontoid process of C2. Normal <10 mm. Alternatively, the basion-cartilaginous dens interval can be used in children with incomplete ossification.

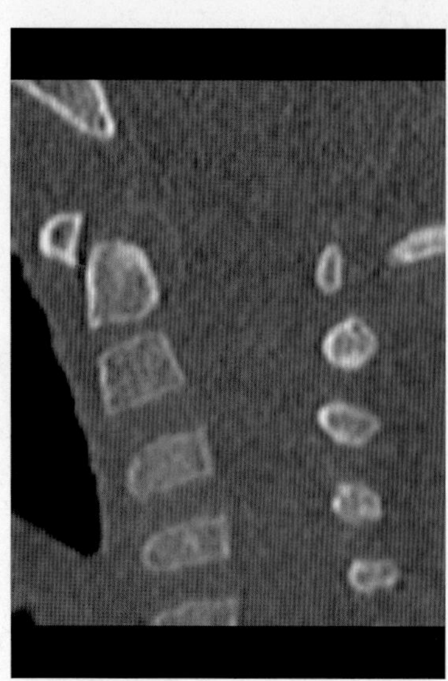

Anterior Atlantodental Interval (ADI). Measured as the distance between the inferior posterior margin of the anterior arch of C1 and the anterior margin of the odontoid process. Normal <2.5 mm.

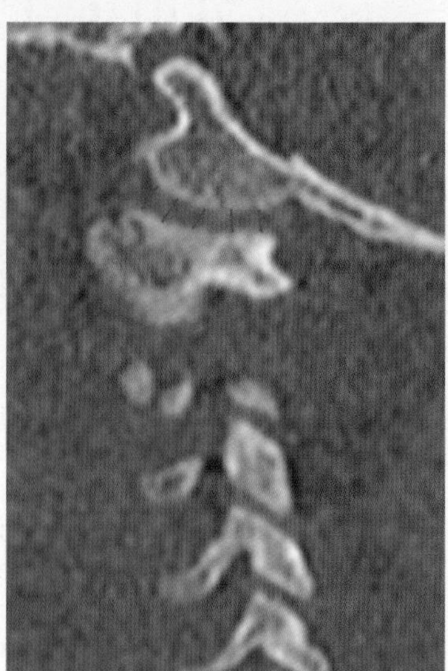

Atlantooccipital Interval. The largest of five perpendicular measurements between the occipital condyle and C1 on a lateral sagittal image on each side. The anterior intraoccipital synchondrosis should not be in the measurement. Normal < 2.5 mm.

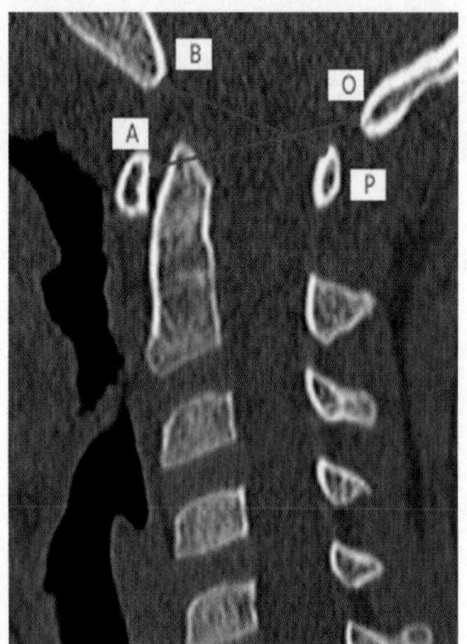

Powers Ratio. Measured as the distance between the basion and anterior margin of the posterior arch of C1, divided by the distance between the opisthion and the posterior margin of the anterior arch of C1. Normal <1

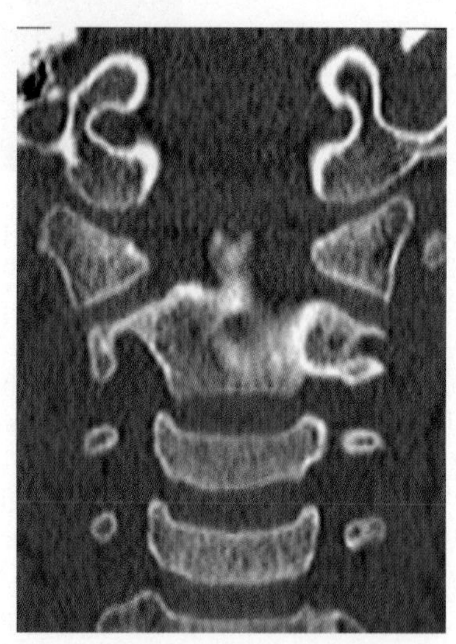

Atlantoaxial Interval. Measured as the shortest perpendicular distance between the lateral masses of C1 and C2 on each side. Normal <3.9 mm.

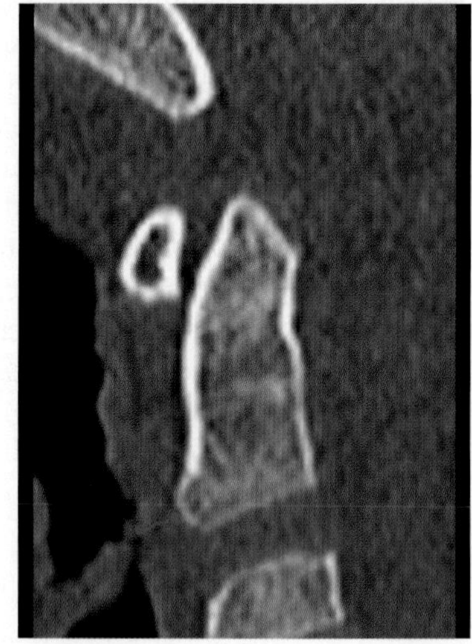

Prevertebral Soft Tissue Thickness. Measured at C2 as the narrowest distance between the posterior wall of the trachea and the anterior margin of the C2 vertebral body. Normal <6 mm.

■ TABLE 19.1 Normal Measurements of the Cervical Spine on CT

Measurement	Value
Basion-dens interval	<10 mm
Anterior atlantodental interval	<2.5 mm
Atlantooccipital interval	<2.5 mm
Powers ratio	<1
Atlantoaxial interval	<3.9 mm
Prevertebral soft tissue at C2	<6 mm

REFERENCES

1. Singh AK, Fulton Z, Tiwari R, et al. Basion-cartilaginous dens interval: an imaging parameter for craniovertebral junction assessment in children. *AJNR Am J Neuroradiol.* 2017 Dec;38(12):2380–2384.
2. Booth TN. Cervical spine evaluation in pediatric trauma. *AJR Am J Roentgenol.* 2012 May;198(5):W417–W4125.

NORMAL CRANIOCERVICAL JUNCTION LIGAMENTS

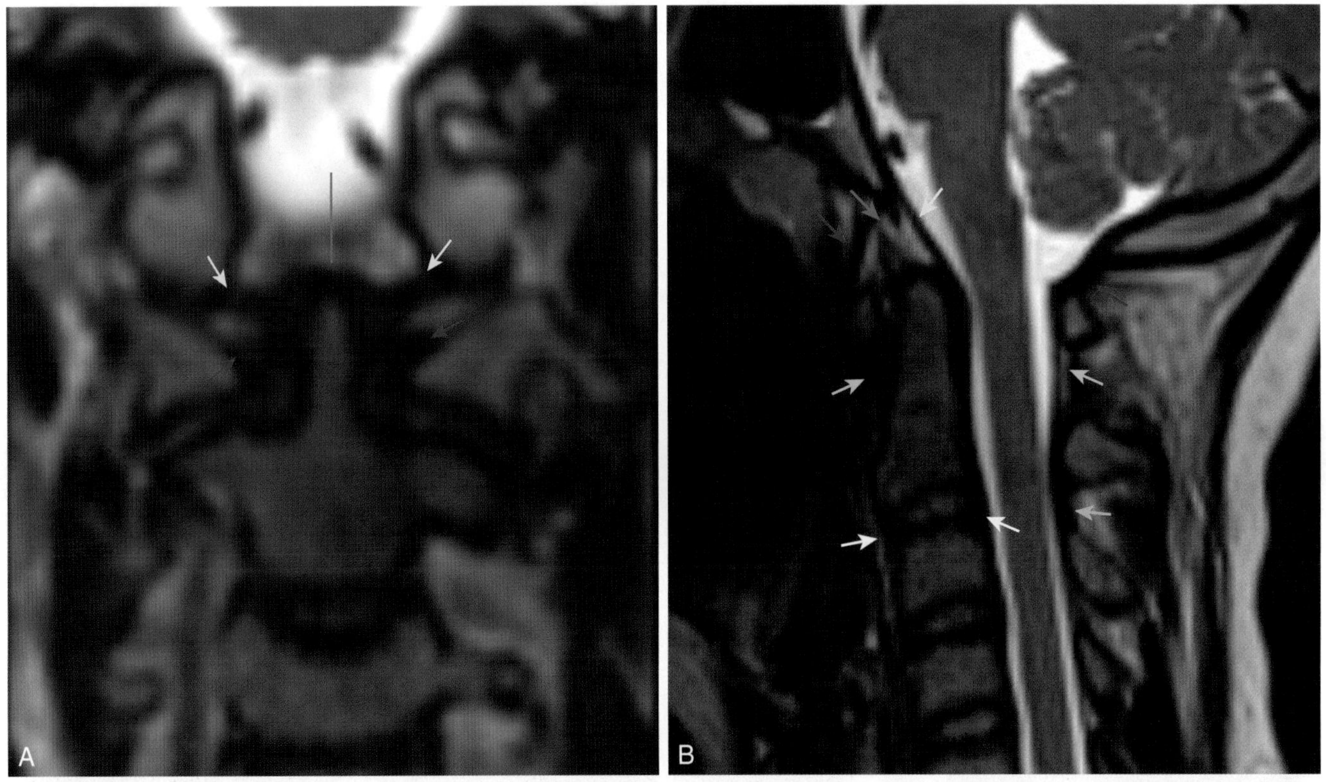

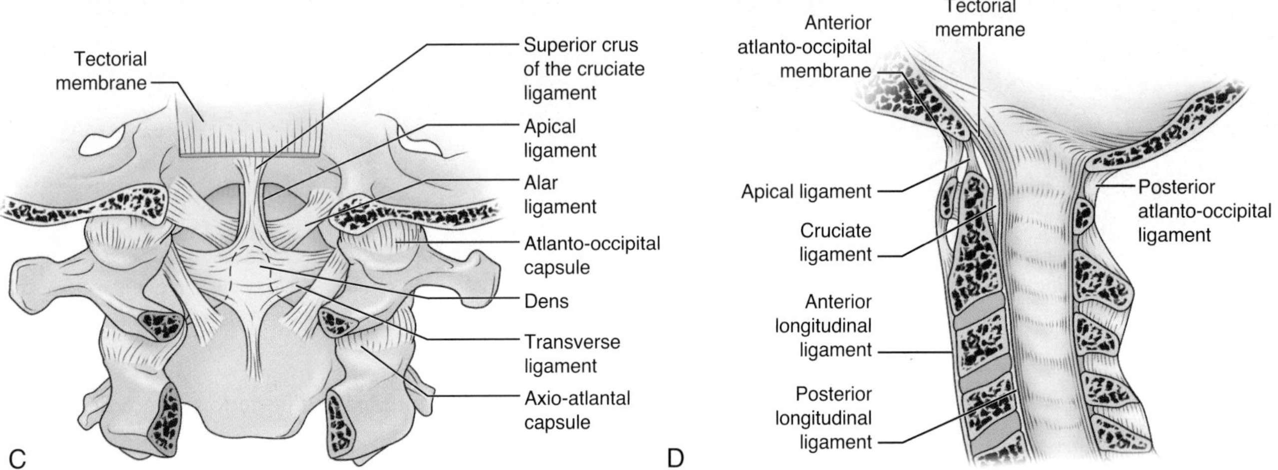

Craniocervical Junction Ligament Anatomy. (A) Coronal 3D T2W image demonstrating the alar ligaments *(yellow arrows)*, transverse ligaments *(red arrows)*, and expected location of the apical ligament *(blue line)*. (B) Sagittal 3D T2W image demonstrating the apical ligament *(blue arrow)*, tectorial membrane *(yellow arrow)*, anterior and posterior atlantooccipital ligaments *(red)*, anterior and posterior atlantoaxial ligaments *(light green arrows)*, anterior and posterior longitudinal ligaments *(white arrows)*, and ligamentum flavum and interspinous ligaments *(dark yellow arrow)*. Determination of intact versus disrupted status of these ligaments is important for determination of ligamentous injury. (C) Diagram of a posterior view of the CCJ; the posterior elements have been removed and ligaments are demonstrated. In the center of the image lies the cruciate ligament. (D) Diagram of a cross-sectional view of the craniocervical junction (CCJ) demonstrating the ligamentous anatomy. (C and D from Boll DT, Haaga JR: *CT and MRI of the whole body*, 6th ed, Philadelphia, 2017, Elsevier.)

CRANIOCERVICAL JUNCTION LIGAMENTOUS INJURY

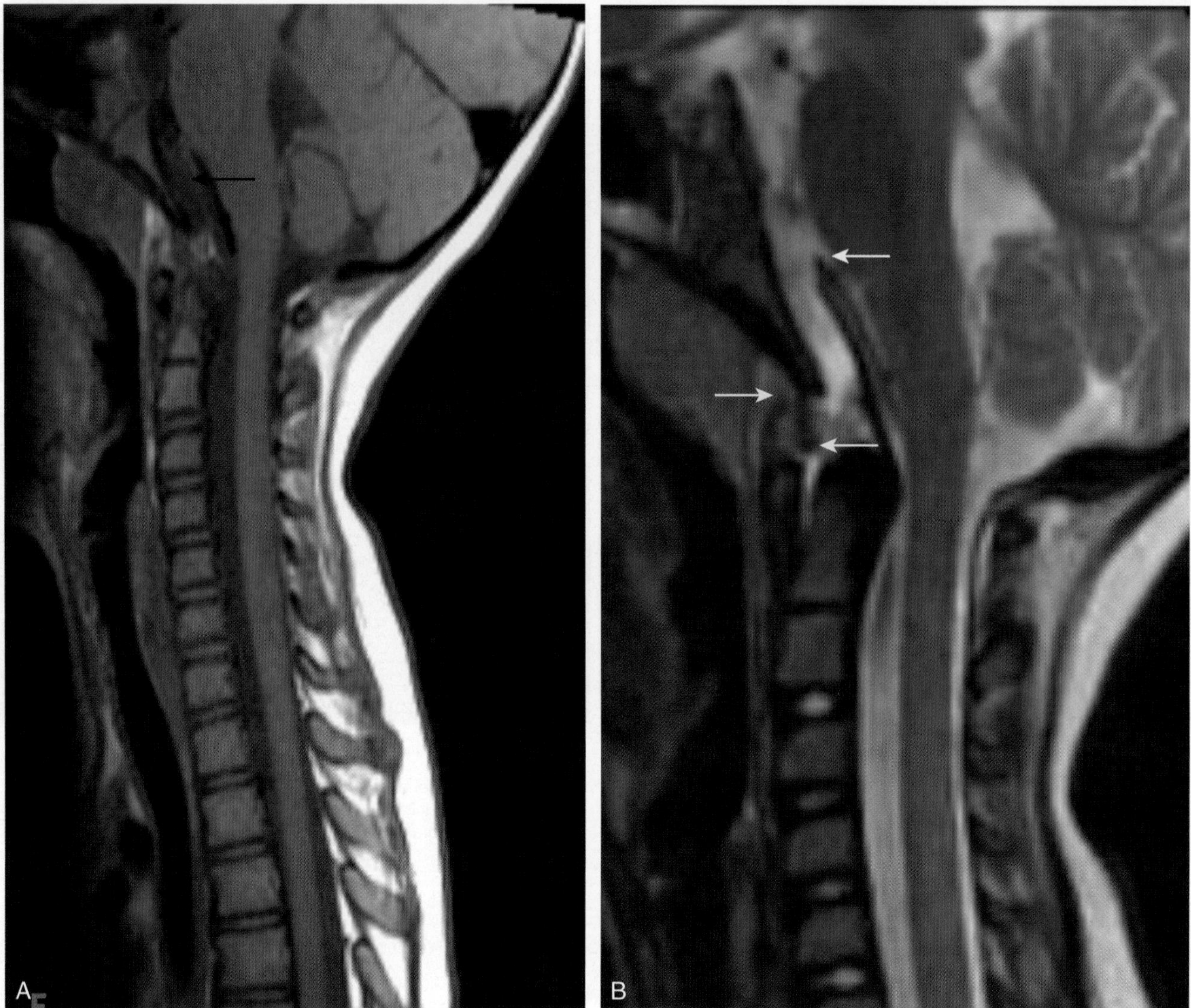

Fig. 19.1 Craniocervical Junction Ligamentous Injury. (A) Sagittal T1W and (B) sagittal T2W images demonstrate disruption of the tectorial membrane *(white arrow)*, apical ligament and anterior atlantooccipital ligament *(yellow arrows)*, and retroclival hematoma *(black arrow)*.

Key Points

Background

- Severe trauma resulting in ligamentous injury, instability, and potential spinal cord trauma
- Usually associated with significant intracranial traumatic injury

Imaging

- CT findings include basion dens interval >10 mm, prevertebral swelling, retroclival hematoma, widened atlantooccipital interval >2.5 mm, and widened anterior atlantodental interval >2.5 mm.
- MRI necessary to visualize the disrupted ligaments, including the transverse and alar ligaments, tectorial membrane, and anterior and posterior atlanto-occiptal and atlantoaxial ligaments.
- Important to perform high-resolution 3D T2W imaging to improve diagnostic accuracy.
- MRI may also reveal retroclival and prevertebral hematomas, as well as compression and/or injury to the lower brainstem or upper cervical spinal cord.

REFERENCES

1. Lustrin ES, Karakas SP, Ortiz AO, et al. Pediatric cervical spine: normal anatomy, variants, and trauma. *Radiographics*. 2003 May–Jun;23(3):539–560.
2. Meoded A, Singhi S, Poretti A, et al. Tectorial membrane injury: frequently overlooked in pediatric traumatic head injury. *AJNR Am J Neuroradiol*. 2011 Nov–Dec;32(10):1806–1811.

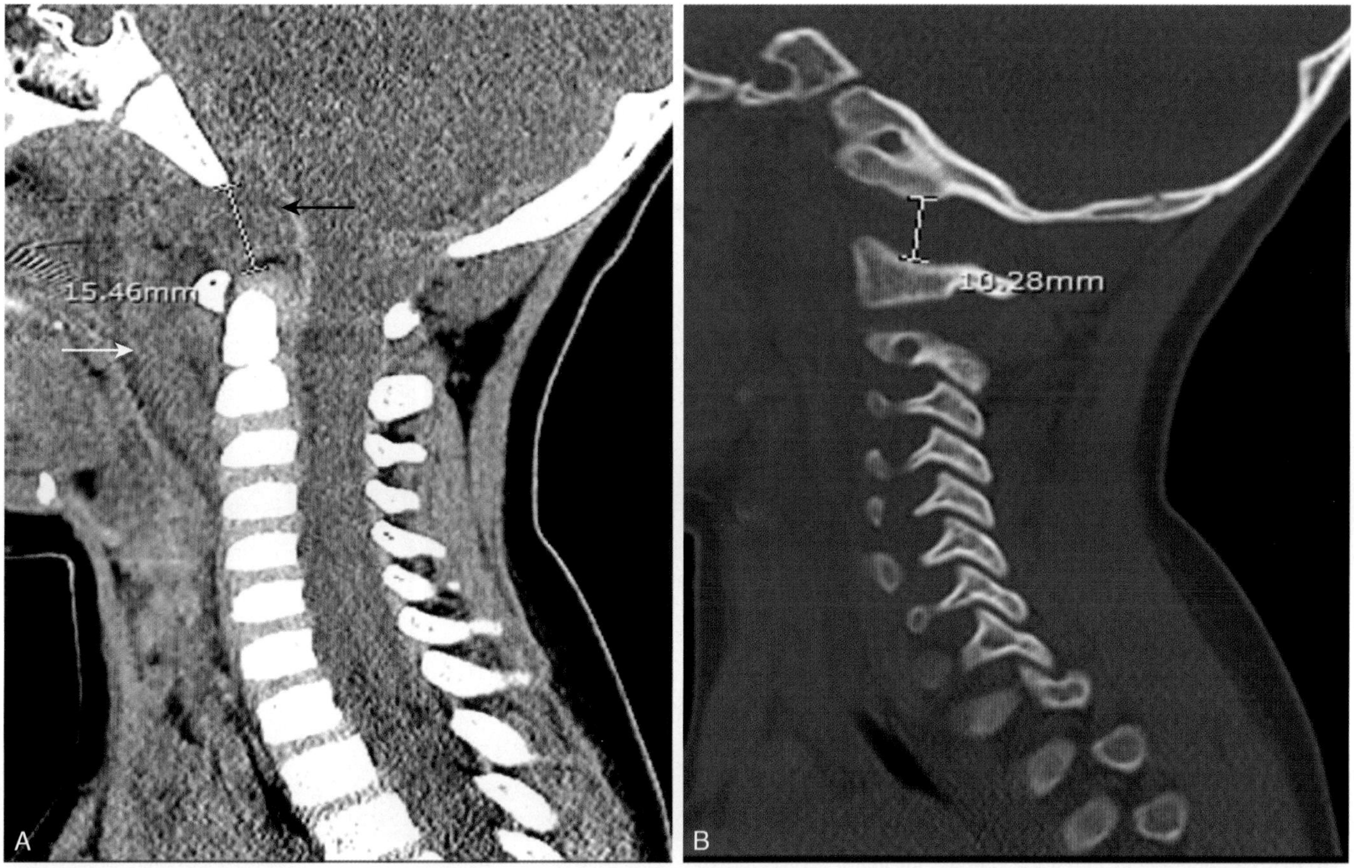

Fig. 19.2 Craniocervical Junction Ligamentous Injury. (A and B) Sagittal reformat CT images demonstrate abnormal basion-dens interval measuring 15 mm, widened condylar gap measuring 10 mm, prevertebral soft tissue swelling *(white arrow)*, and retroclival soft tissue swelling *(black arrow)*.

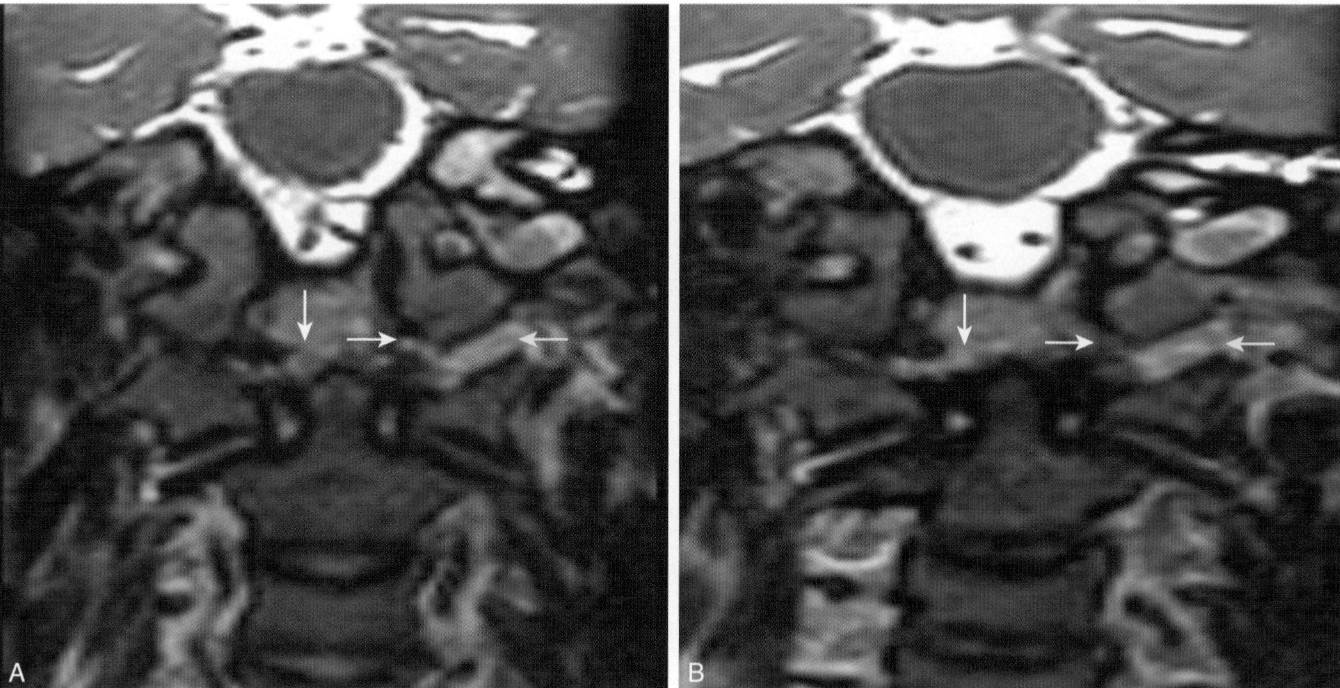

Fig. 19.3 Craniocervical Junction Ligamentous Injury. (A and B) Coronal T2W images demonstrate disruption of bilateral alar ligaments *(white arrows)* and a widened left condylar gap *(yellow arrow)*.

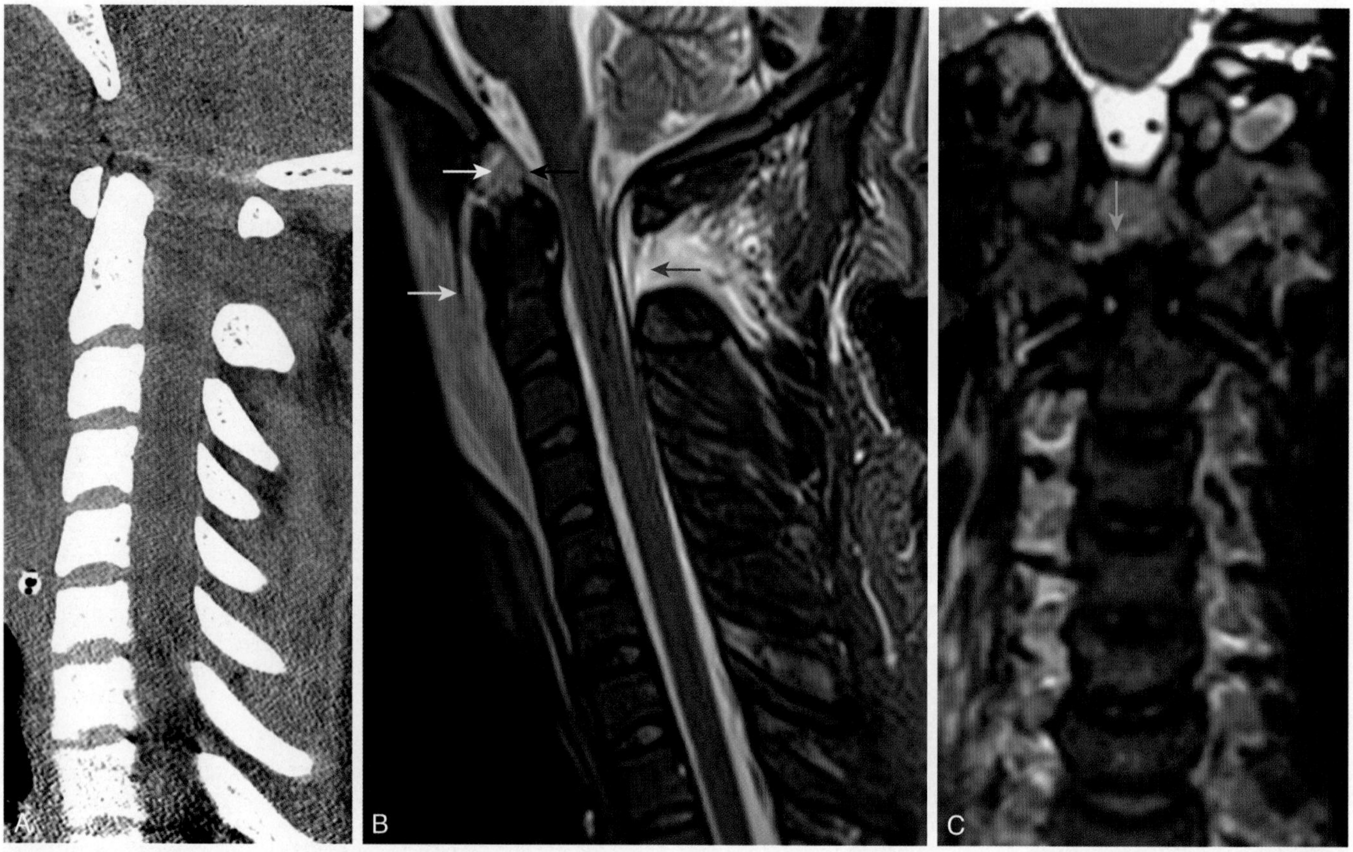

Fig. 19.4 Craniocervical Junction Ligamentous Injury. (A) sagittal reformat CT, (B) sagittal STIR, and (C) coronal 3D T2W images demonstrate prevertebral swelling, basion-dens interval greater than 10 mm, widened C1–C2 interspinous space, ligamentous injury of the anterior atlantooccipital ligament *(yellow arrow)*, apical ligament *(white arrow)*, tectorial membrane *(black arrow)*, posterior atlantoaxial ligament *(red arrow)*, and right alar ligament *(green arrow)*.

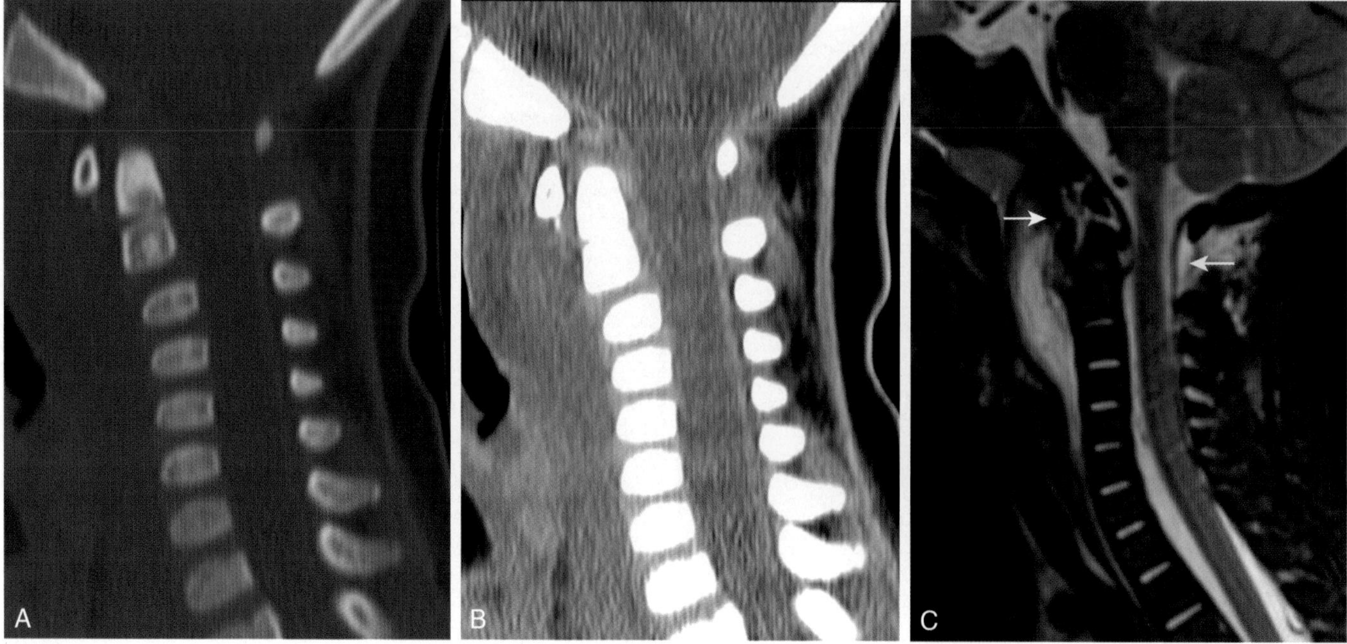

Fig. 19.5 Craniocervical Junction Ligamentous Injury. (A and B) Sagittal reformat CT images and (C) sagittal STIR image demonstrate prevertebral edema and ligamentous injury of the anterior longitudinal ligament, anterior atlantooccipital ligament *(white arrow)*, and posterior atlantoaxial ligament *(yellow arrow)*.

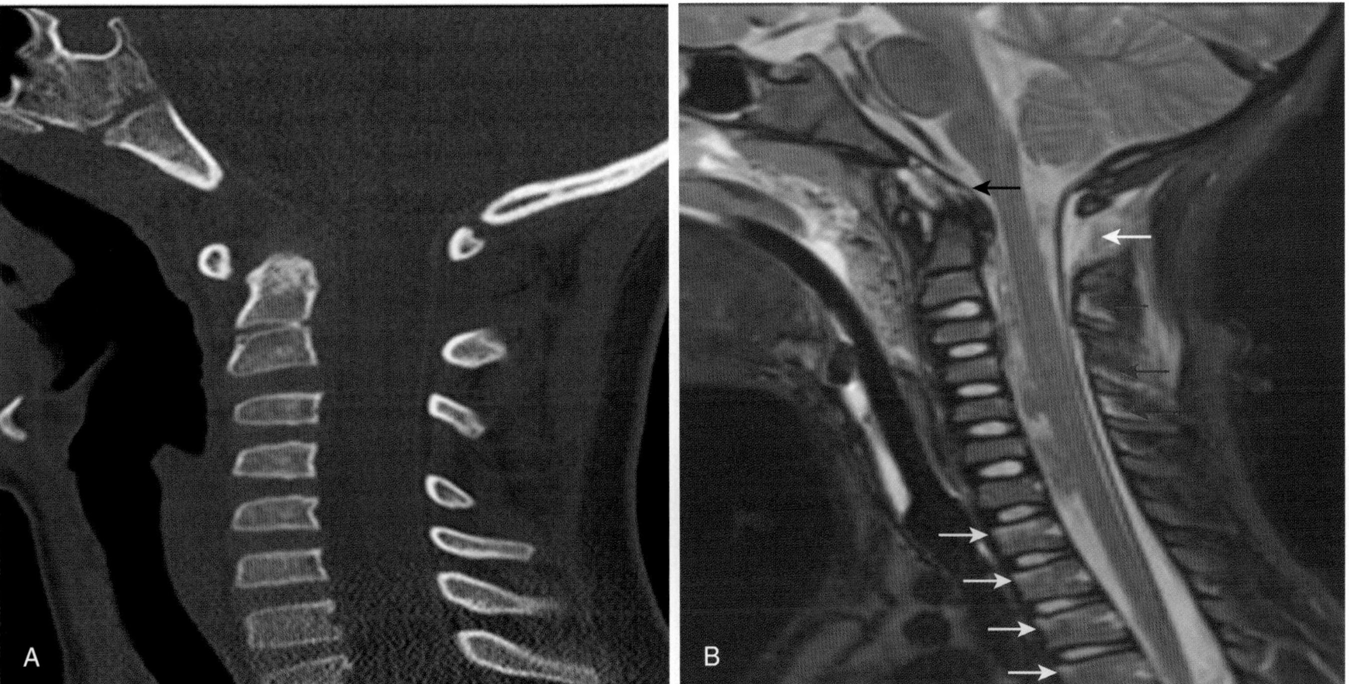

Fig. 19.6 Craniocervical Junction Ligamentous Injury. (A) Sagittal reformat CT and (B) sagittal T2W images demonstrate abnormal basion dens interval greater than 10 mm, widened C1–C2 and C3–C4 interspinous spaces, ligamentous injury of the posterior atlantoaxial ligament *(white arrow)*, tectorial membrane *(black arrow)*, probable apical ligament disruption, interspinous ligaments of C2–3, C3–4, and C4–5, and trabecular microfractures of thoracic vertebrae *(yellow arrows)*.

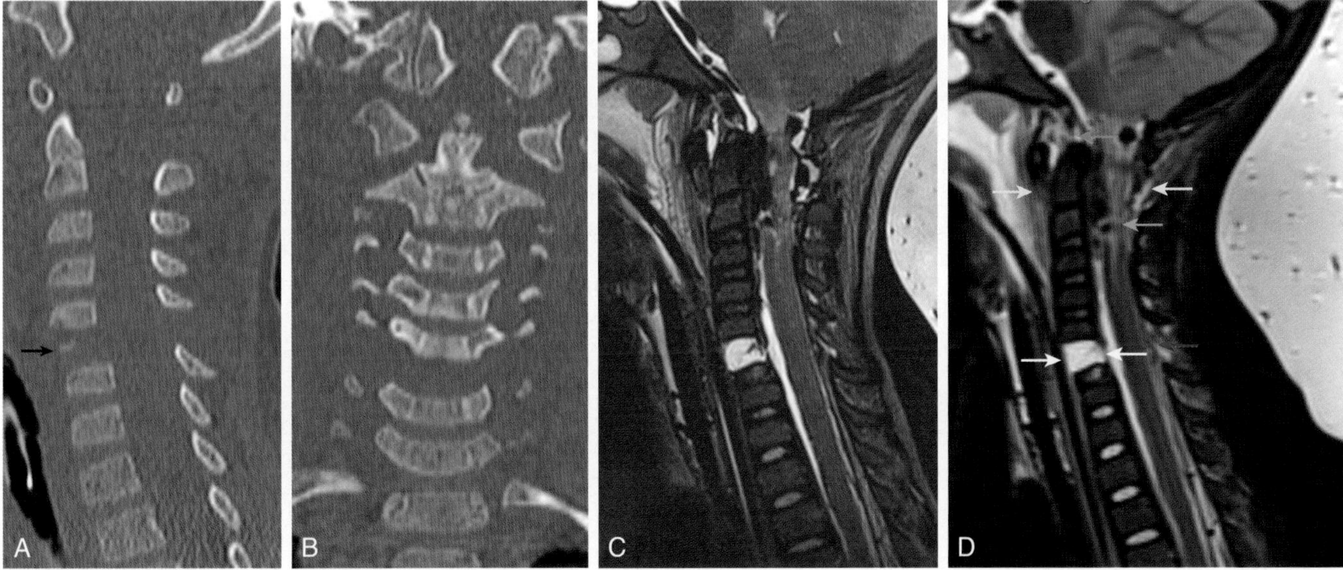

Fig. 19.7 Craniocervical Junction Ligamentous Injury. (A and B) Sagittal and coronal reformat CT and (C and D) sagittal T2W images demonstrate prevertebral edema, spinal cord injury with hemorrhage *(green arrow)*, ligamentous injury of the anterior atlantooccipital ligament, anterior and posterior atlantoaxial ligaments *(yellow arrows)*, apical ligament *(orange arrow)*, left alar ligament (not shown except for small avulsion fragment on coronal CT), widened facet joints indicative of facet capsular ligament tears at occipital–C1 and C1–C2, C5–6, anterior and posterior longitudinal ligament tear *(white arrows)*, widened interspinous space due to interspinous ligament and ligamentum flavum tears at C5–6 *(red arrow)*, and intervertebral disc transection and endplate avulsions at C5–6 *(black arrow)*.

C2 SYNCHONDROSIS FRACTURE

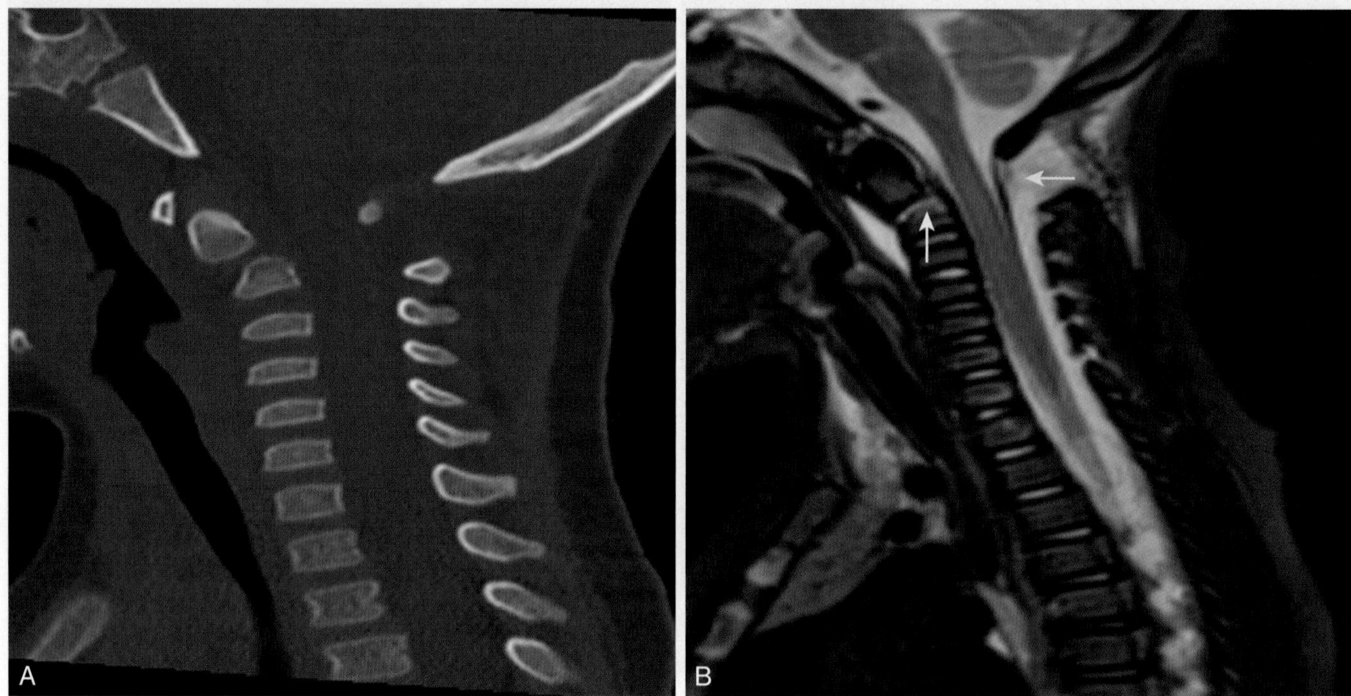

Fig. 19.8 C2 Synchondrosis Fracture. (A) Sagittal reformat CT and (B) sagittal T2W images demonstrate abnormal anterior tilt of the odontoid, abnormal edema along the C2 synchondrosis *(white arrow)*, prevertebral edema, and widening of the C1–C2 interspinous space from ligamentous injury of the posterior atlantoaxial ligament *(yellow arrow)*.

Key Points

Background

- Hyperflexion mechanism
- Spinal injury finding found in younger patients because the cartilage between the odontoid and body of C2 does not ossify until age 5 to 7 years.

Imaging

- Results in angulation of the dens with respect to the C2 body
- May have associated prevertebral soft tissue swelling, widened C1–C2 interspinous space, disruption of spinolaminar line, ligamentous injury of anterior longitudinal ligament (ALL), and posterior atlantoaxial ligament (PLL)

REFERENCE

1. Rusin JA, Ruess L, Daulton RS. New C2 synchondrosal fracture classification system. *Pediatr Radiol.* 2015 Jun;45(6):872–881.

FACET DISLOCATION

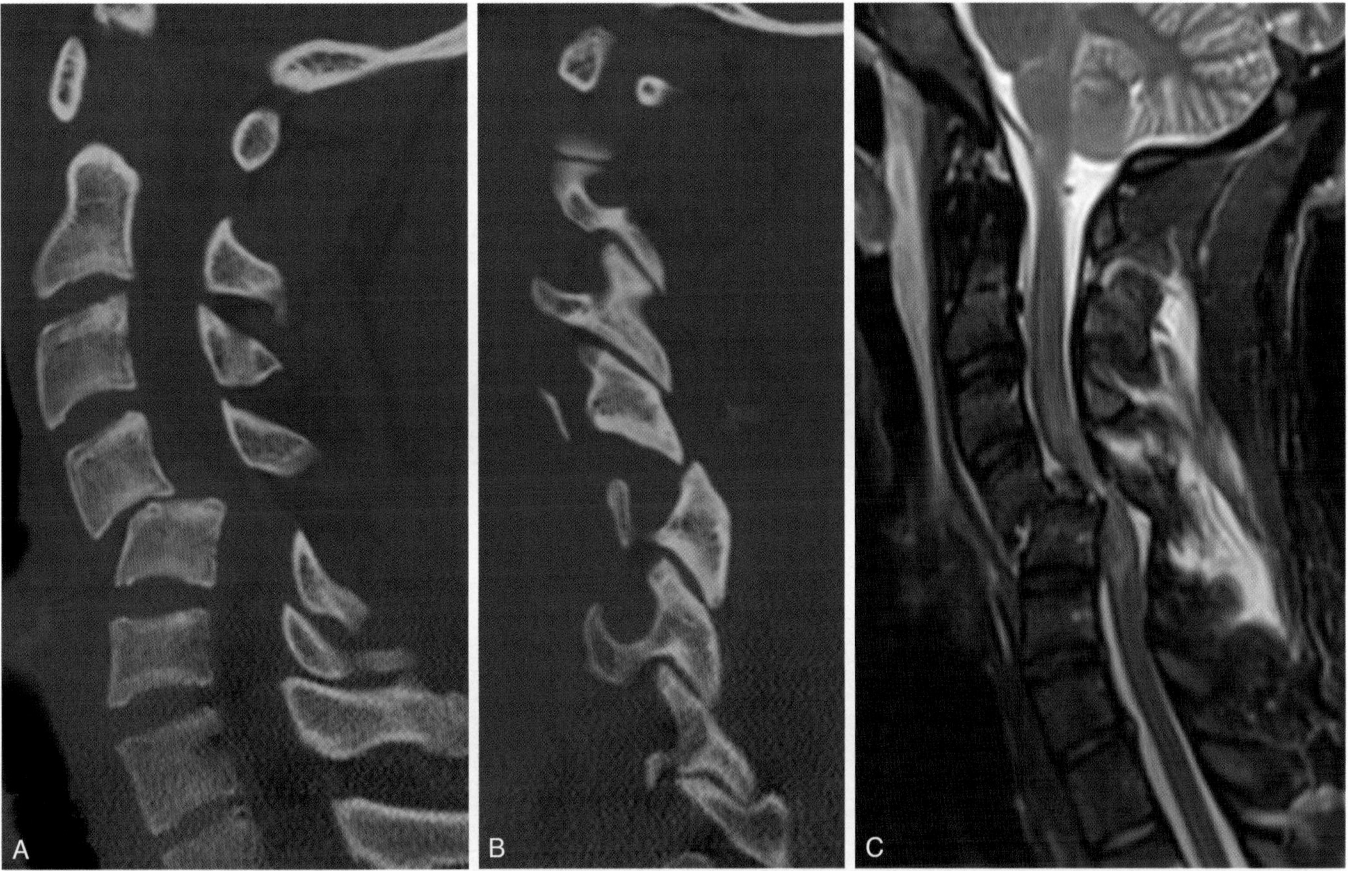

Fig. 19.9 Facet Dislocation. (A and B) Sagittal reformat CT and (C) sagittal T2W images demonstrate malalignment with C4–C5 anterolisthesis, narrowed C4–C5 disc space, prevertebral edema, ligamentous injury of the anterior and posterior longitudinal ligaments, C3–C4 and C4–C5 interspinous ligaments, disc herniation, spinal cord compression, and cord edema.

Key Points

Background

- Severe traumatic injury resulting in dislocation of the facets, ligamentous injury and usually spinal cord injury

Imaging

- Imaging findings often include malalignment of facet joints, spondylolisthesis, disc injury, disruption of anterior longitudinal ligament (ALL), posterior longitudinal ligament, interspinous ligaments, ligamentum flavum, and cord compression/injury

REFERENCE

1. Lustrin ES, Karakas SP, Ortiz AO, et al. Pediatric cervical spine: normal anatomy, variants, and trauma. *Radiographics*. 2003 May–Jun;23(3):539–560.

SPINE TRAUMA FROM ABUSIVE HEAD TRAUMA

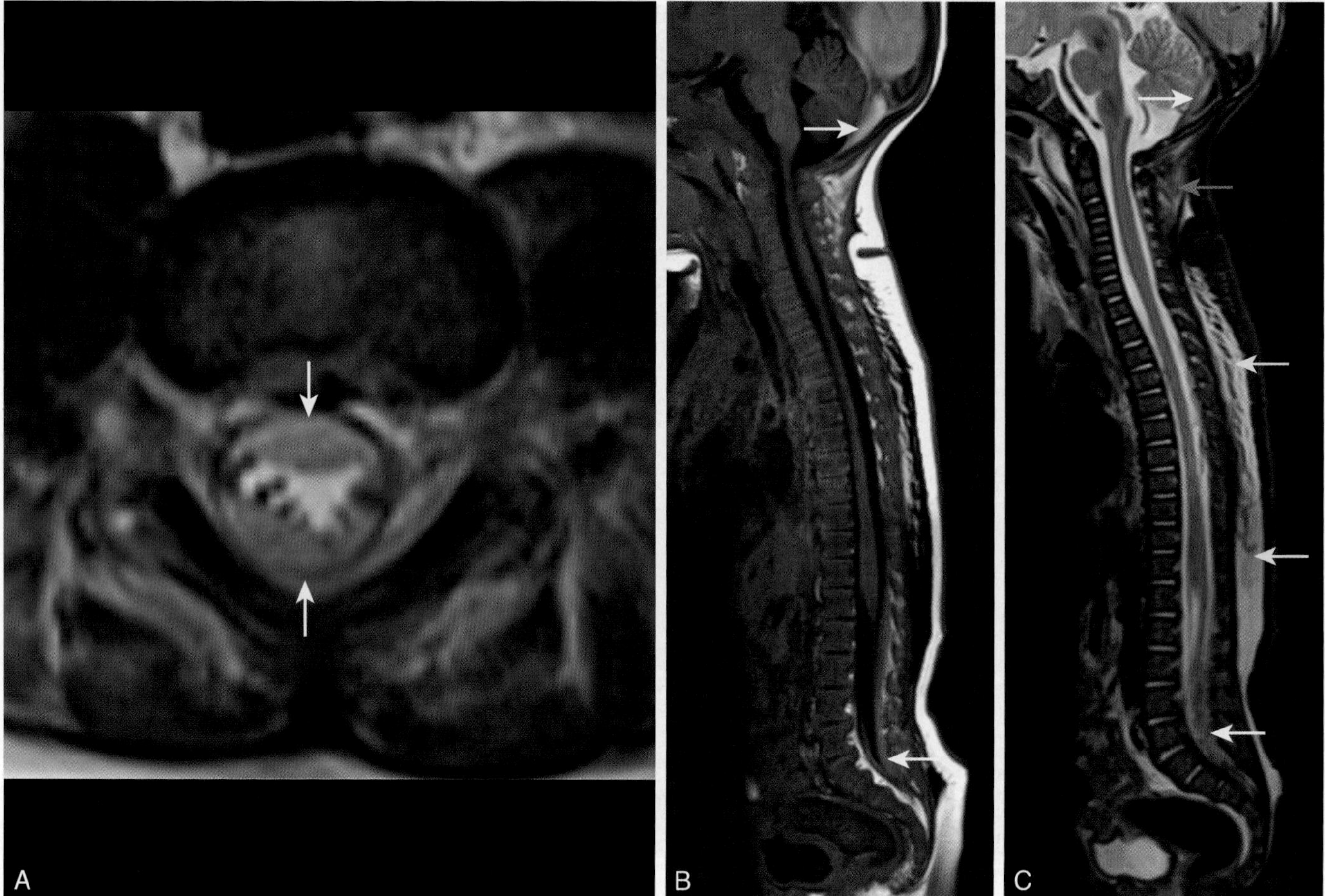

Fig. 19.10 Abusive Trauma: Spinal Trauma. (A) Axial T2W, (B) sagittal T1W, and (C) sagittal STIR images demonstrate abnormal T2W signal less than CSF and T1W signal greater than CSF along the periphery of the distal thecal sac in a configuration consistent with subdural hemorrhage (*white arrows*). Large region of subcutaneous edema along the vertebral column (*yellow arrows*), edema along the nuchal ligament (*orange arrow*), and posterior fossa subdural hemorrhage (*white arrow*) are also seen.

Key Points

Background

- Traumatic findings can include ligamentous injury, cord injury, muscular injury, and spinal hematoma.

Imaging

- Spinal subdural hemorrhage is suspected to be due to gravitational movement of intracranial subdural blood. Imaging demonstrates an intrathecal fluid collection with distinct boundary with sites of adherence, typically in a V shape configuration posteriorly.
- Retroclival hematoma found in 32% of abusive head trauma (AHT).
- Ligamentous injury typically from hyperflexion and include injury to the nuchal ligament, atlanto-occipital and atlantoaxial ligaments.

REFERENCES

1. Choudhary AK, Bradford RK, Dias MS, et al. Spinal subdural hemorrhage in abusive head trauma: a retrospective study. *Radiology*. 2012 Jan;262(1):216–223.
2. Choudhary AK, Ishak R, Zacharia TT, et al. Imaging of spinal injury in abusive head trauma: a retrospective study. *Pediatr Radiol*. 2014 Sep;44(9):1130–1140.

ENDPLATE AVULSION

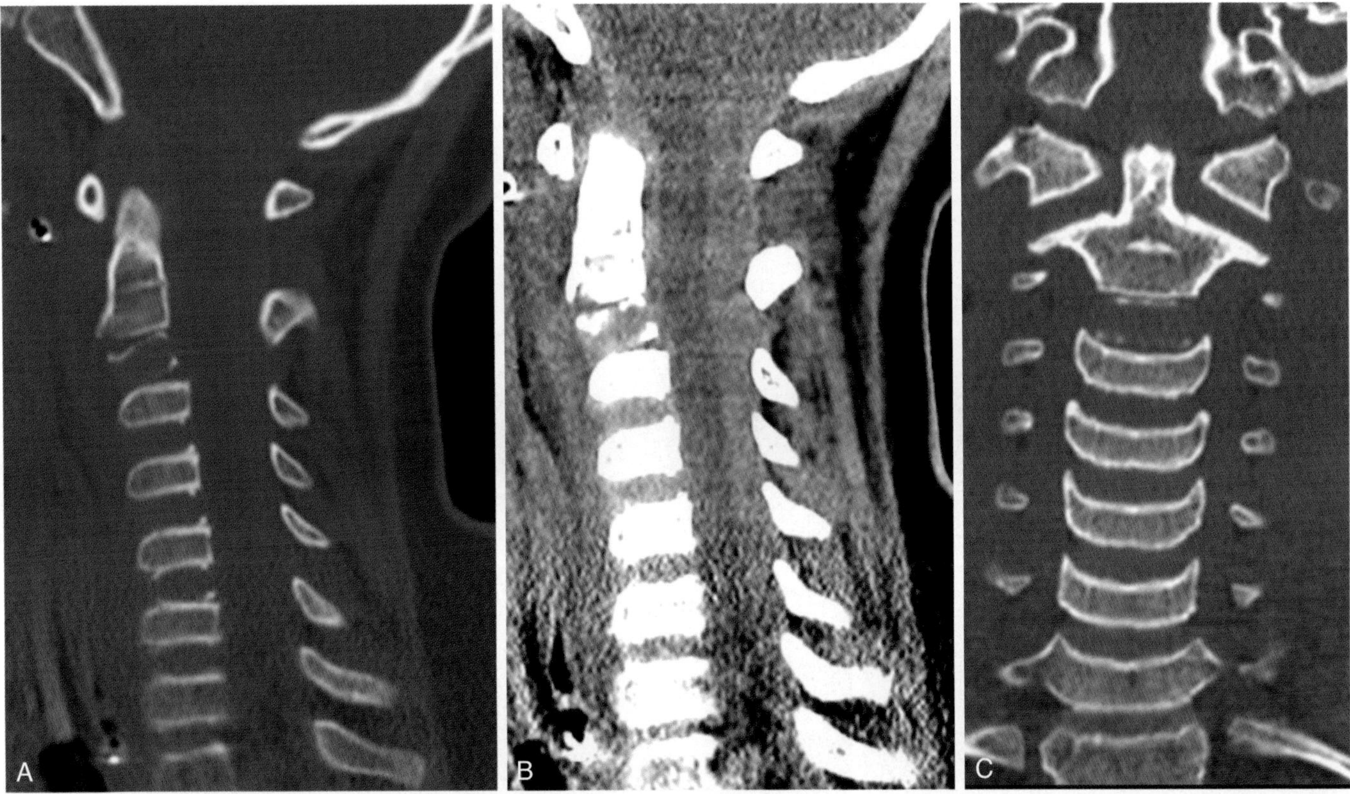

Fig. 19.11 Endplate Avulsion. (A to C) Sagittal and coronal reformat CT images demonstrate linear ossification in the C2–C3 disc space due to avulsion of the disc from the vertebral bodies.

Key Points

Background

- Rare traumatic injury of the spine resulting in separation of the endplate and disc from the vertebral body

Imaging

- Imaging findings of linear ossification adjacent to the endplates due to the avulsed endplates

POSTERIOR APOPHYSEAL RING FRACTURE

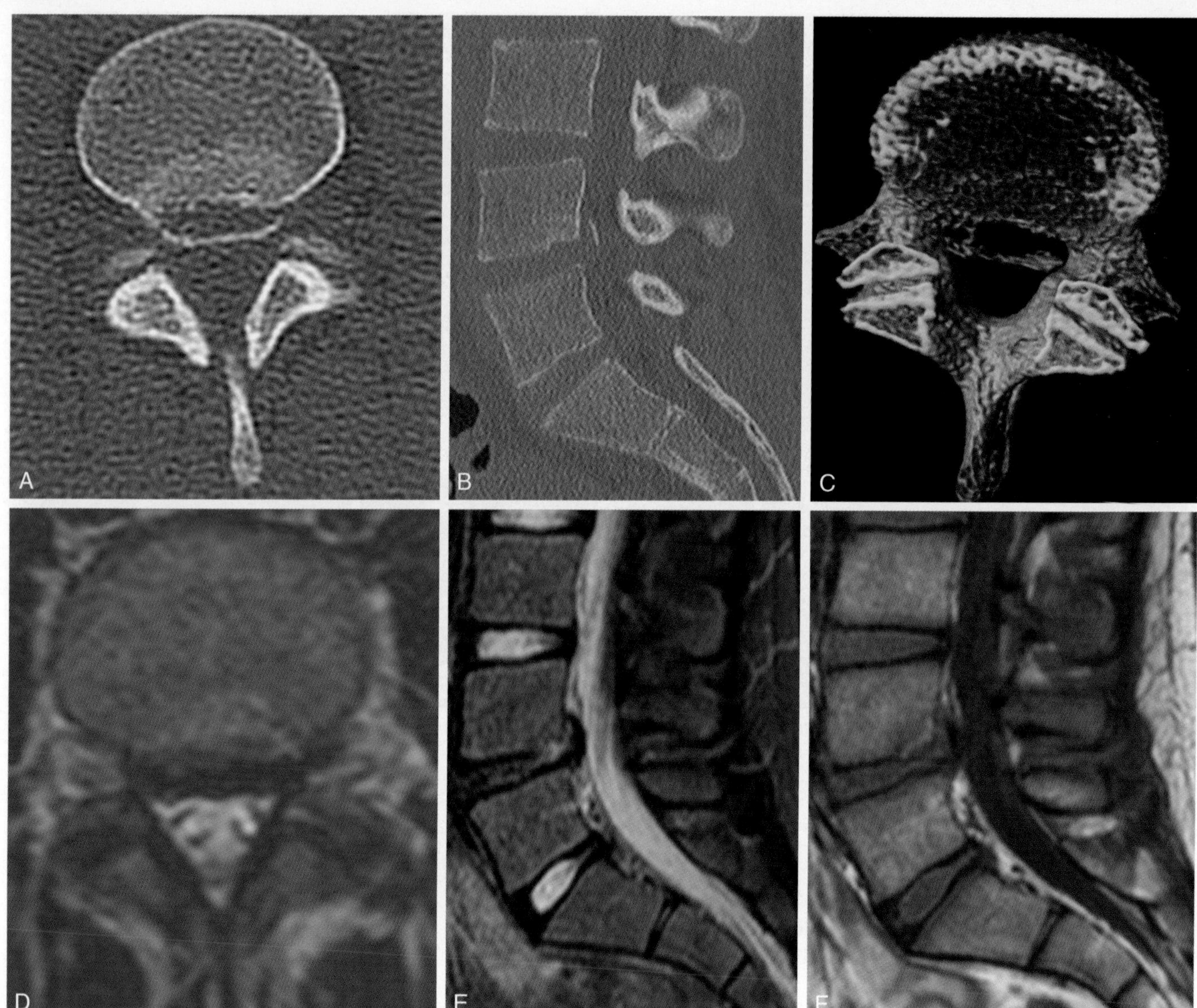

Fig. 19.12 Posterior Apophyseal Ring Fracture. (A) Axial CT, (B) sagittal reformat CT, and (C) volumetric reformat CT images demonstrate a linear ossification posterior to the L4–L5 disc space. (D) Axial T2W, (E) sagittal T2W, and (F) sagittal T1W images demonstrate posterior disc herniation, loss of normal T2W hypointense cortex along the posterior inferior L4 endplate, and hypointense thickening posterior to the L4–L5 disc space related to a posterior apophyseal ring fracture.

Key Points

Background

- Uncommon disorder seen in adolescents.
- Symptoms include back pain +/– radiculopathy.
- The epiphyseal ring ossifies between 4 and 6 years of age and fuses around 18 to 25 years. Sharpey fibers attach the apophyseal ring to the annulus fibrosis.
- Etiology unknown. Possibly sports injury, repetitive extension, degeneration of the disc and cartilage, and microtrauma and degeneration.

Imaging

- CT demonstrates separation of a bony fragment at the posterior endplate where the apophyseal ring and vertebral body were fused.
- Difficult to identify on X-ray and MRI.
- Marrow edema adjacent to the avulsion may be seen during the acute phase.
- May be mistakenly confused with calcified ligament or disc, or a degenerative osteophyte.

REFERENCE

1. Seo YN, Heo YJ, Lee SM. The characteristics and incidence of posterior apophyseal ring fracture in patients in their early twenties with herniated lumbar disc. *Neurospine*. 2018;15(2):138–143.

CHANCE FRACTURE

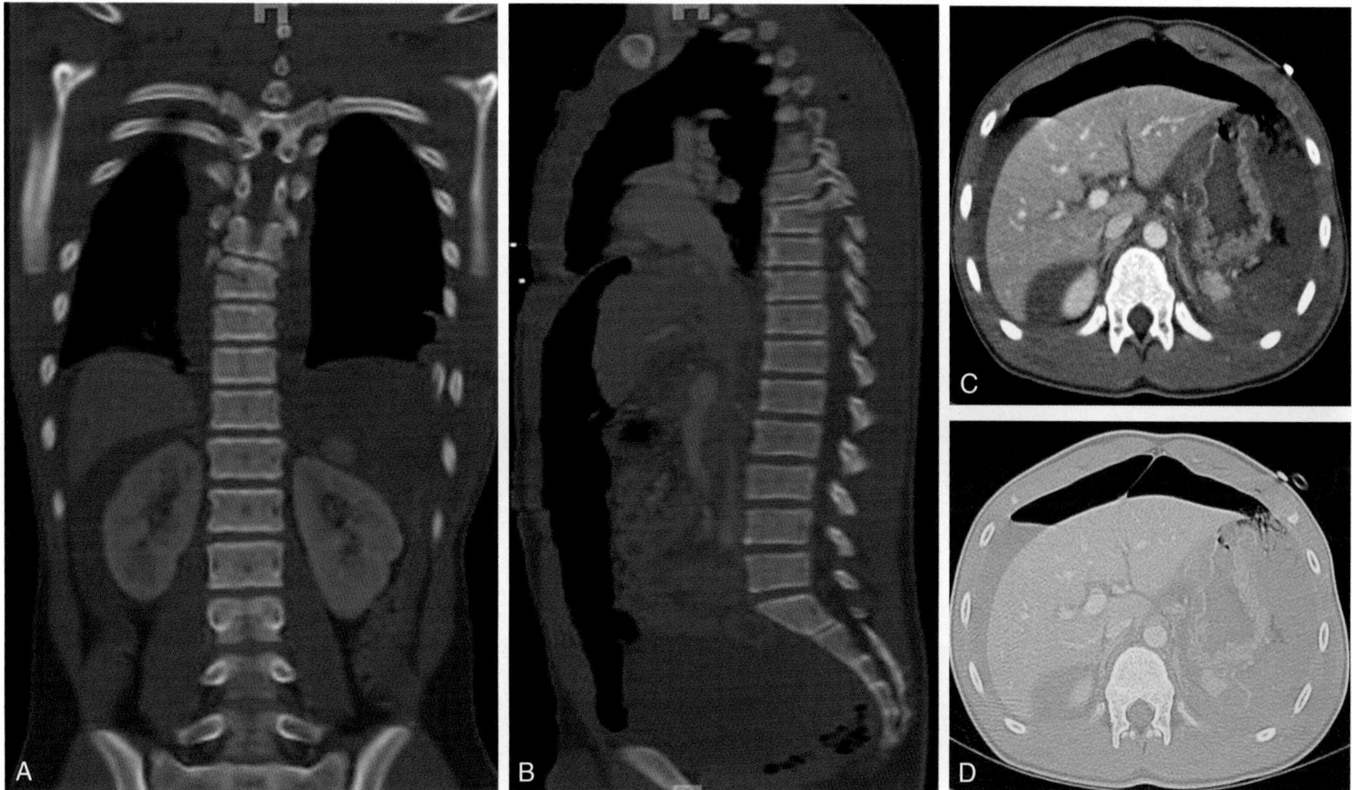

Fig. 19.13 Chance Fracture. (A to D) Multiplanar CT images demonstrate a linear fracture with widening through the posterior T8 vertebral body, pedicle, and par interarticularis and mild anterior compression of the T8 vertebral body. Additional laceration of the stomach with resultant hemato-pneumoperitoneum and retroperitoneal hematoma.

Key Points

Background

- Flexion-distraction mechanism of spinal injury.
- Unstable fracture pattern accounting for ~ 5% to 15% of thoracolumbar fractures; however, neurologic injury is rare.
- Often seen with motor vehicle accident and seat belt restraint (Fulcrum around seat belt).
- ~50% occur at the thoracolumbar junction due to anatomic transition from rigid thoracic spine to mobile lumbar spine, change from coronal facet orientation in thoracic spine to sagittal orientation in the lumbar spine, change from the thoracic kyphosis to lumbar lordosis, and change from stability from the rib-sternum articulation.
- Associated with intrabdominal trauma (~40% incidence), particularly in children, including duodenal and pancreatic injury.

Imaging

- Horizontal fracture through the vertebral body or through the disc space extending through the pedicles and facet joints resulting in widening and ligamentous disruption of the facet capsular ligaments and interspinous ligament while the anterior vertebral body shows a compression fracture appearance.

REFERENCE

1. Bernstein MP, Mirvis SE, Shanmuganathan K. Chance-type fractures of the thoracolumbar spine: imaging analysis in 53 patients. *AJR Am J Roentgenol.* 2006;187(4):859–868.

PSEUDOSUBLUXATION

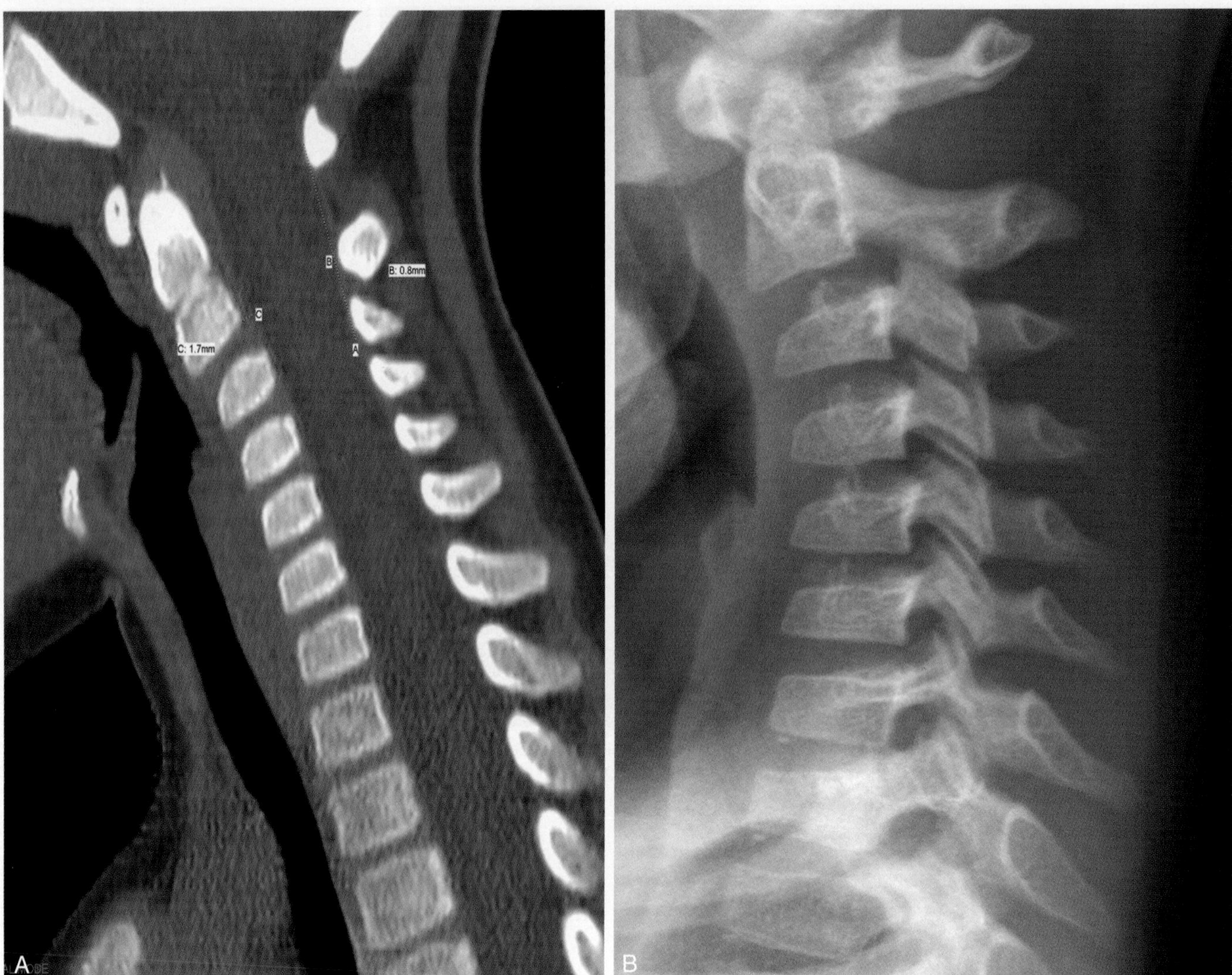

Fig. 19.14 Pseudosubluxation. (A) Sagittal reformat CT and (B) sagittal cervical spine radiograph demonstrate C2–C3 anterolisthesis; however, the distance of the offset from the spinolaminar line is 0.8 mm, indicating benign pseudosubluxation.

Key Points

Background

- Benign anatomic variant seen in young children due to ligamentous laxity

Imaging

- Most commonly at C2–C3 and less commonly at C3–C4
- The offset from the spinolaminar line drawn from C1 to C3 is within 1 to 2 mm.

REFERENCE

1. Lustrin ES, Karakas SP, Ortiz AO, et al. Pediatric cervical spine: normal anatomy, variants, and trauma. *Radiographics*. 2003 May–Jun;23(3):539–560.

OS ODONTOIDEUM

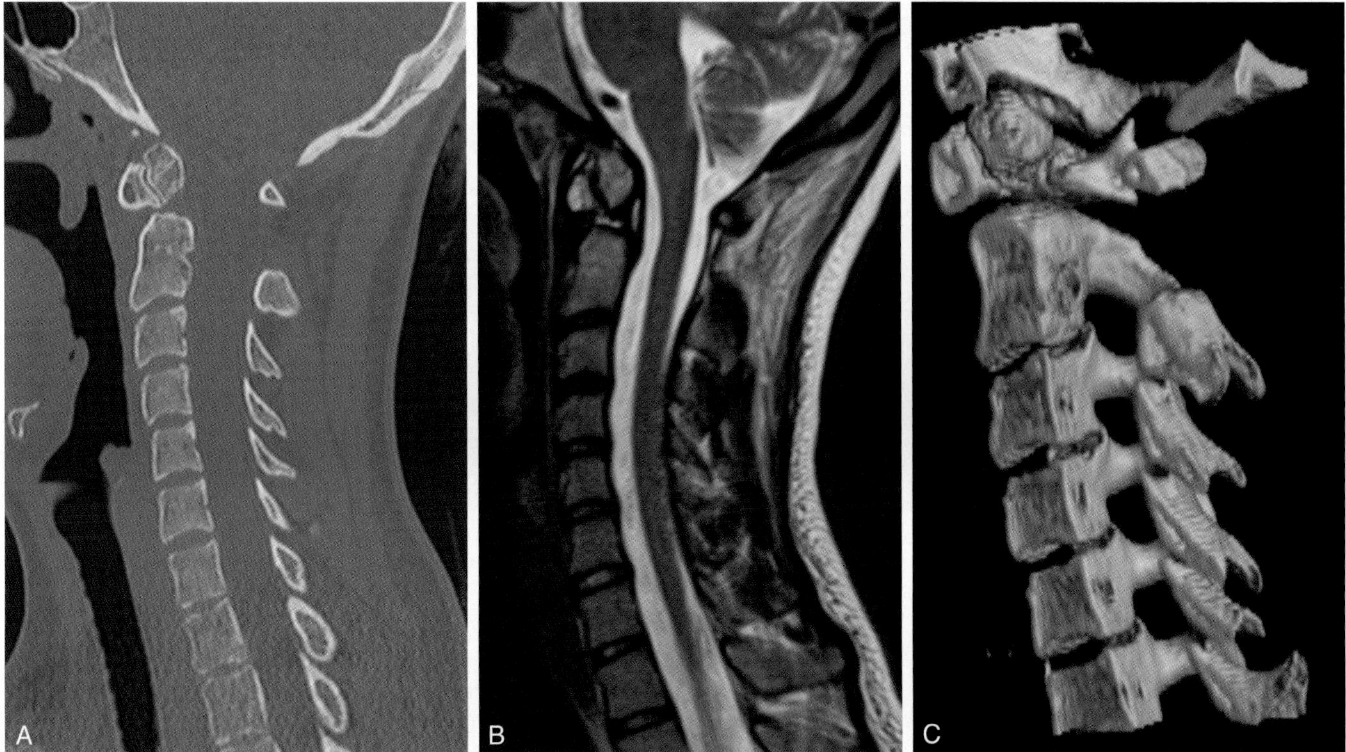

Fig. 19.15 Os Odontoideum. (A) Sagittal reformat CT, (B) Sagittal T2 W, and (C) 3D volumetric CT images demonstrate an os odontoideum seen as an ossification separated from the odontoid and an enlarged anterior arch of C1.

Key Points

Background

- Congenital versus traumatic etiology resulting in an ossicle with smooth corticated margins separated from the C2 body

Imaging

- The anterior arch of C1 is often enlarged, while the posterior arch may be hypoplastic or absent.
- Can be associated with atlantoaxial instability.
- Differential Diagnosis: Ossiculum terminale (small ossified fragment at the odontoid tip above the alar ligament) and type 2 odontoid fracture.

REFERENCE

1. Jumah F, Alkhdour S, Mansour S, et al. Os Odontoideum: a comprehensive clinical and surgical review. *Cureus*. 2017 Aug; 9(8):e1551.

SPONDYLOLYSIS

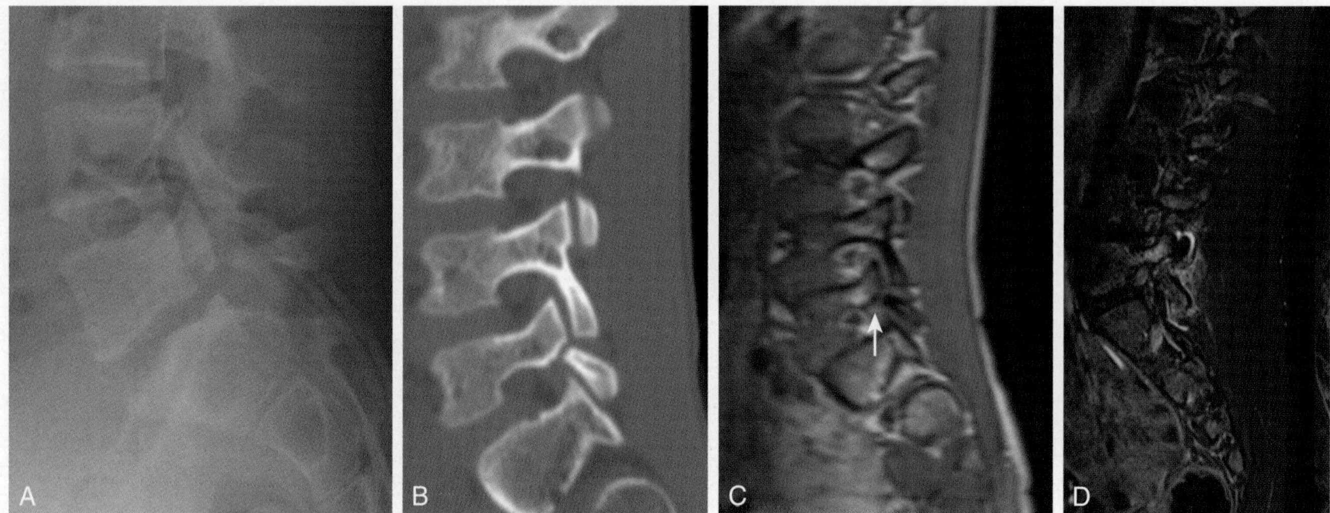

Fig. 19.16 Spondylolysis. (A) Sagittal lumbar spine radiograph, (B) Sagittal reformat CT, and (C) sagittal T1W images demonstrate a gap in the pars interarticularis at L5 indicative of spondylolysis. (D) Sagittal STIR image in a different patient demonstrating abnormal STIR hyperintensity in the L5 pedicle and discontinuity of the cortex of the pars interarticularis indicative of a pars defect.

Key Points

Background

- Refers to a defect in the pars interarticularis
- Presumed to be a result of repetitive microtrauma resulting in a stress fracture
- Biomechanical models demonstrate that the greatest stress is at the caudal-ventral aspect of the pars, and with extension, the stress on the ventral pars is double that of the dorsal pars
- Sacral and pelvic alignment may be risk factors as research has shown greater sacral slope and pelvic incidence in patients with pars defects and spondylolisthesis
- Most commonly involves the L5 pedicles (90%), and less commonly, L4 pedicles (10%)
- Present in ~5% of the population. Usually acquired. 25% will be symptomatic. 65% will develop a spondylolisthesis.

Imaging

- CT and high-quality MRI can demonstrate the pars defects. SPECT and MRI may also identify early-stage stress injury without fracture.
- MRI has a reported 81% sensitivity and 99% specificity for detection of spondylolysis and is generally preferred to CT when plain films demonstrate a pars defect or suspicion of a par defect remains in the setting of a negative radiograph. If MRI is indeterminate or questionable for pars defect, a limited-coverage CT can be performed for additional evaluation and reduce radiation exposure.
- MRI grading scale of pars defects:
  - Grade 0 (normal): normal marrow signal, intact cortical margins
  - Grade 1 (stress reaction): marrow edema, intact cortical margins
  - Grade 2 (incomplete fracture): marrow edema, cortical fracture incompletely extending through the pars
  - Grade 3 (complete active fracture): marrow edema, fracture completely extends through the pars
  - Grade 4 (fracture nonunion): no marrow edema, fracture completely extends through the pars
- Early identification when there is bone marrow edema (MRI grades 1–3) and conservative management can reduce the chance of progression to nonunion, which has an increased incidence of spondylolisthesis.

REFERENCES

1. Kobayashi A, Kobayashi T, Kato K, et al. Diagnosis of radiographically occult lumbar spondylolysis in young athletes by magnetic resonance imaging. *Am J Sports Med.* 2013 Jan;41(1):169–176.
2. Terai T, Sairyo K, Goel VK, et al. Spondylolysis origintates in the ventral aspect of the pars interarticularis: a clinical and biomechanical study. *J Bone Joint Surg Br.* 2010 Aug;92(8):1123–1127.
3. Dunn AJ, Campbell RSD, Mayor PE, et al. Radiological findings and healing patterns of incomplete stress fractures of the pars interarticularis. *Skeletal Radiol.* 2008 May;37(5):443–450.

BRACHIAL PLEXUS TRAUMA

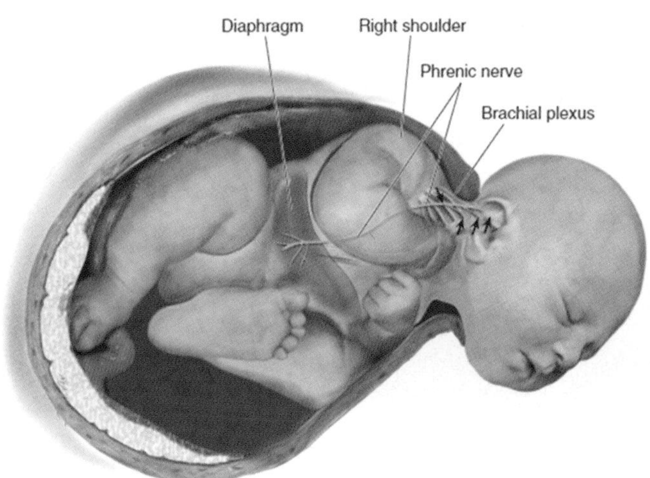

Fig. 19.17 Mechanism of Injury to Brachial Plexus and Phrenic Nerve due to Downward Lateral Traction of the Head and Neck During Delivery. (From Alvord EC, Austin EJ, Larson CP. Neuropathologic observations in congenital phrenic nerve palsy. *J Child Neurol* 1995;5:205. Used with permission from Elsevier.)

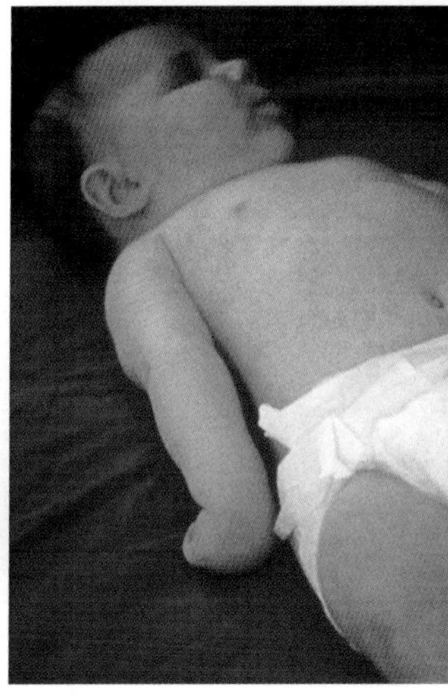

Fig. 19.18 The Classic "Waiter's Tip" Posture of Erb Palsy Following Brachial Plexus Injury at Birth. (From Rennie JM. *Rennie & Robertson's Textbook of Neonatology*. 5th ed. London: Churchill Livingstone/Elsevier; 2012.)

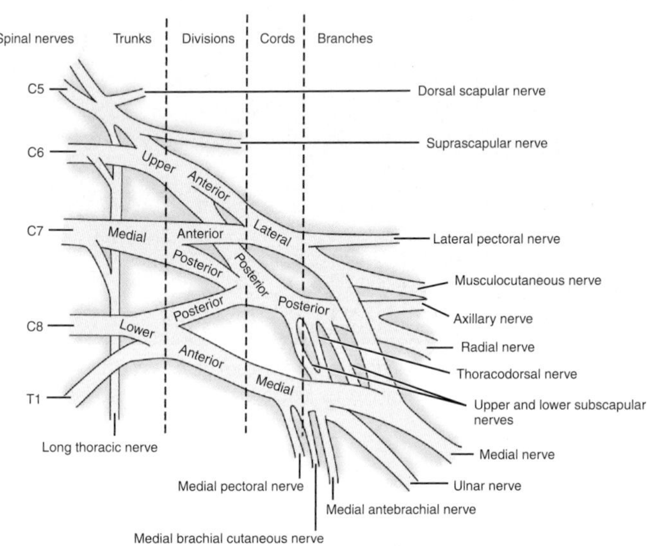

Fig. 19.19 The Brachial Plexus. Injury can occur at any point along the nerves as they branch off the spinal cord. (Redrawn from Waters PM. Obstetric brachial plexus palsy. *J Am Acad Orthop Surg*. 1997;5:205–214.)

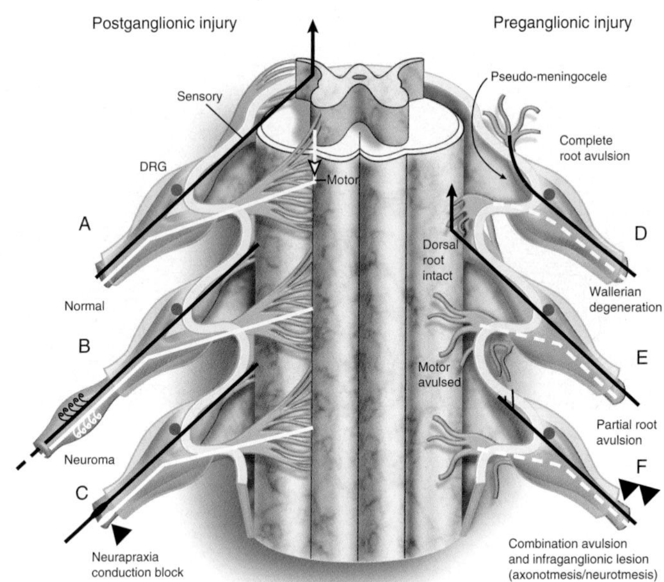

Fig. 19.20 Schematic representation of the normal anatomy of and injuries to the brachial plexus, demonstrating typical preganglionic and postganglionic abnormalities. (A) Normal ventral (motor) rootlets and dorsal (sensory) rootlets. (B) Postganglionic injury (axonotmesis or neurotmesis) with neuroma formation and partial or complete disconnection of neural elements. Continuity can be determined only by intraoperative neurophysiologic studies across damaged segments. (C) A neurapraxic lesion resulting in abnormal sensation and weakness. (D) Preganglionic injury with complete avulsion and traumatic pseudomeningocele. The cell body of the sensory neuron is intact in the dorsal root ganglion. (E) Partial root avulsion with dorsal root intact and ventral (motor) root avulsed. This produces weakness and normal sensation. (F) Combination of a preganglionic and postganglionic lesion, which often can be determined only intraoperatively and correlated with imaging. The roots (motor and sensory) have been avulsed, but the infraganglionic component is also abnormal (axonotmesis_neurotmesis), similar to B. (From Jones HR, Ryan MM, Levin KH. Radiculopathies and plexopathies. In: Darras BT, Jones HR, Ryan MM, De Vivo DC, eds. *Neuromuscular Disorders of Infancy, Childhood, and Adolescence*. 2nd ed. Elsevier; 2015, with permission.)

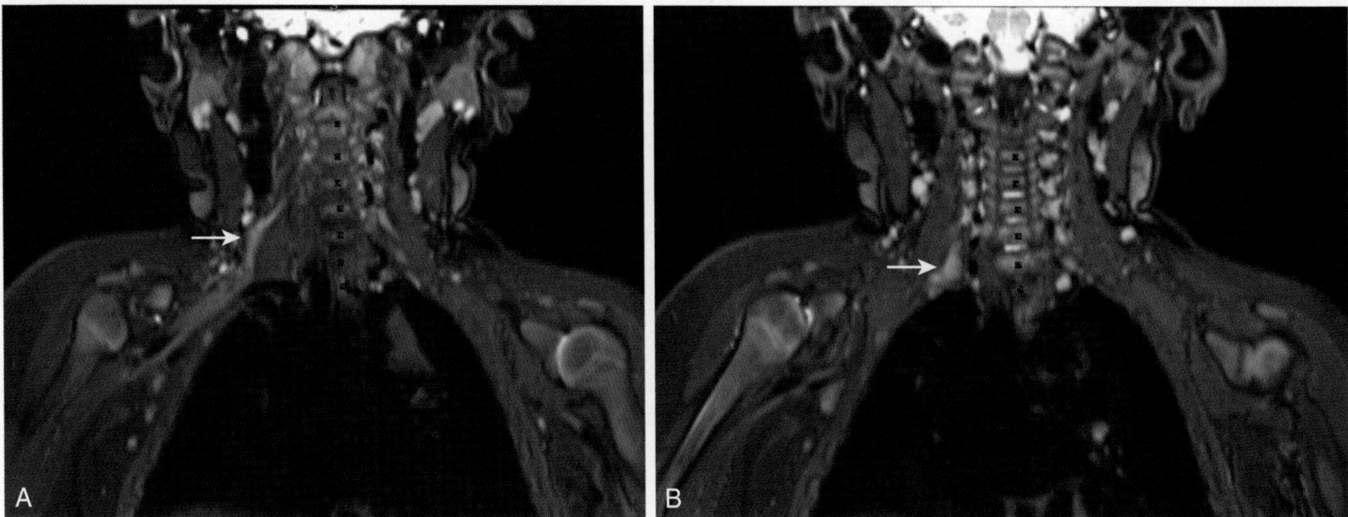

Fig. 19.21 Brachial Plexus Trauma. (A and B) Coronal STIR images demonstrate abnormal hyperintensity in the right brachial plexus, thickening, and abnormal contour of the upper truck *(arrow image A)* consistent with a birth-related traction injury to the brachial plexus and neuroma formation along the lower trunk *(arrow in image B)*.

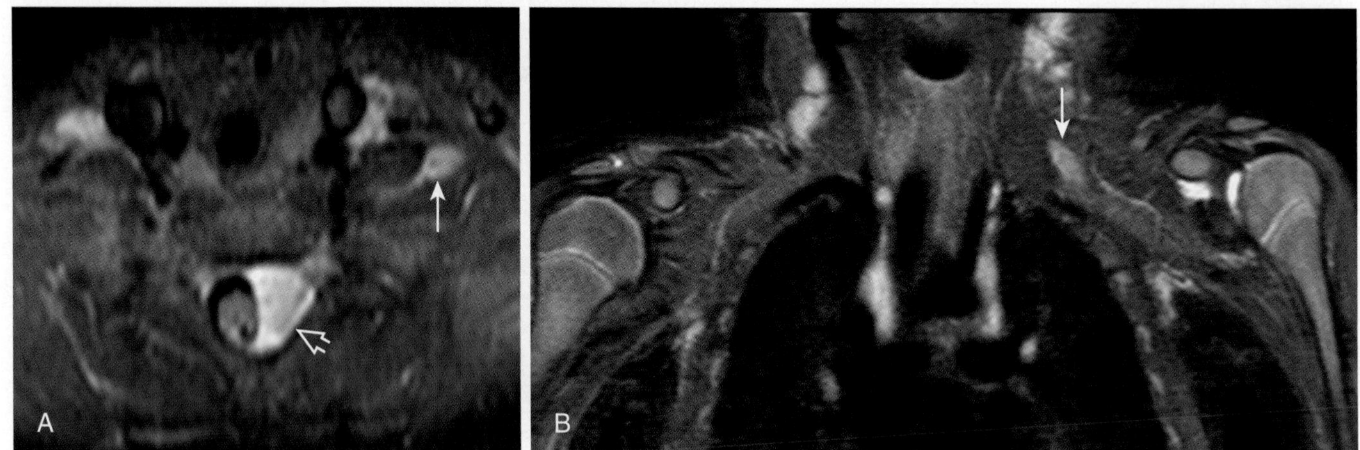

Fig. 19.22 Brachial Plexus Trauma. (A and B) Axial and coronal STIR images demonstrate a pseudomeningocele (*arrowhead*) of the left C8 root (C7–T1 foraminal level) and abnormal hyperintensity and thickening due to neuroma formation along the left brachial plexus just lateral to the interscalene space *(white arrow)*.

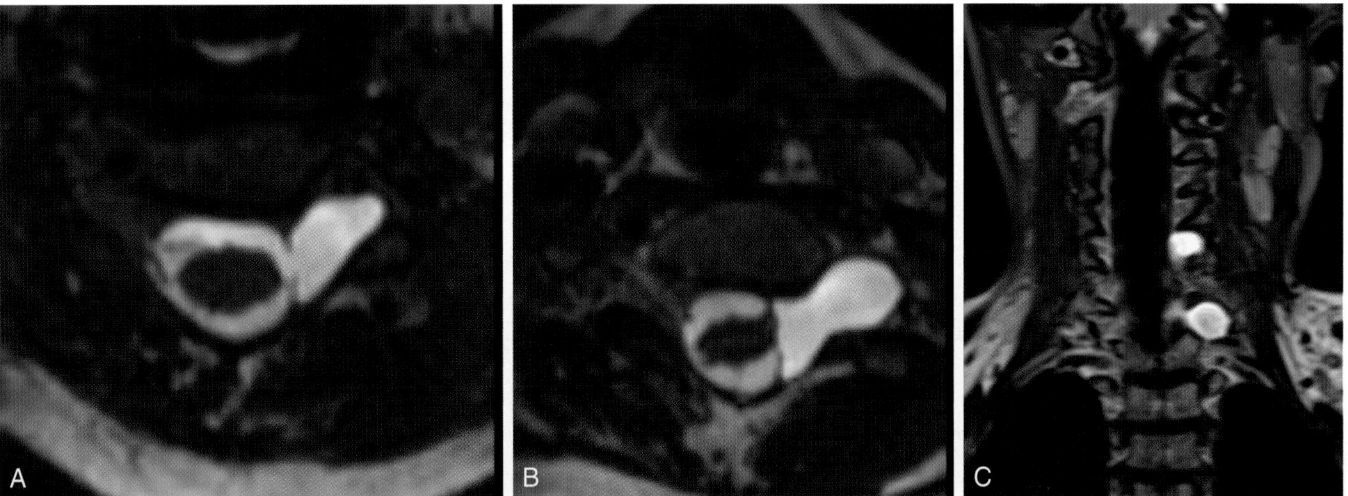

Fig. 19.23 Brachial Plexus Trauma. (A to C) Axial and coronal 3D T2W images demonstrate pseudomeningoceles of the left C6 and C8 roots indicative of preganglionic nerve injury.

Key Points

Background

- Traction injury on the brachial plexus.
- Relatively uncommon. Occurs in ~0.1% to 0.2% of births.
- Risk factors: Macrocephaly, shoulder dystocia, and instrumental delivery.
- Types of injury:
  - Upper plexus injury: Erb palsy. Most common injury pattern (90%). Injury of the C5–C7 nerve roots. Resulting in flaccid weakness, internally rotated and extended arm (waiter's tip sign), absent biceps reflex, absent Moro reflex
  - Lower plexus: Klumpke palsy. C8–T1 nerve root injury. About 1% of brachial plexus injuries. Weakness of intrinsic hand muscles and long flexors of the wrist and fingers. Absent grasp reflex. Ipsilateral Horner syndrome
  - Entire plexus: ~10% of cases. Flaccid upper extremity and absent reflexes
- 90% recover spontaneously.

Imaging

- Imaging technique should include coronal and axial sequences with high-resolution and thin slices, often accomplished well using 3D STIR sequence including a high-resolution 3D T2W CISS/SPACE sequence.
- MRI findings: Pseudomeningoceles due to preganglionic nerve root avulsion, brachial plexus edema, sagging contour of the brachial plexus, neuroma formation, muscle atrophy, and denervation edema.

REFERENCES

1. Smith AB, Gupta N, Strober J, et al. Magnetic resonance neurography in children with birth-related brachial plexus injury. *Pediatr Radiol.* 2008;38:159–163.
2. Tekes A, Pinto PS, Huisman TAGM. Birth-related injury to the head and cervical spine in neonates. *Magn Reson Imaging Clin N Am.* 2011 Nov;19(4):777–790.

20 Differential Diagnoses, Summaries, and Imaging Pitfalls

FETAL VENTRICULOMEGALY

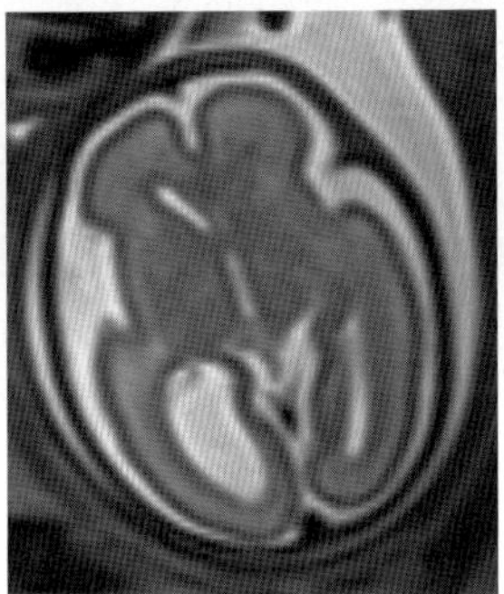

Isolated Mild Unilateral Ventriculomegaly
- Brain structurally normal
- Good prognosis

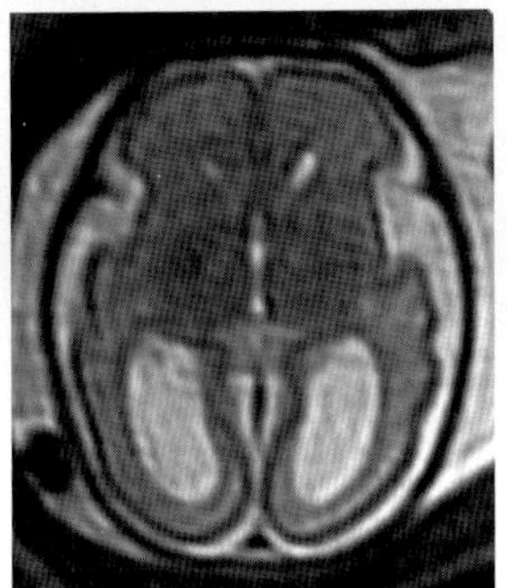

Isolated Bilateral Ventriculomegaly
- Brain structurally normal
- Often mild
- Good prognosis

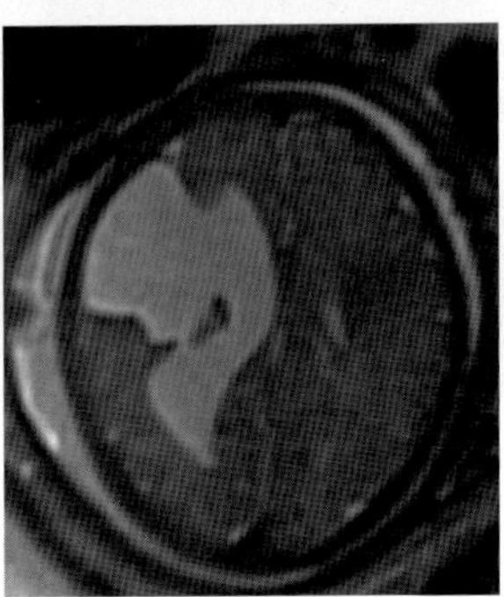

Porencephaly
- CSF-filled cavity
- Communicates (usually) with ventricle
- Ischemia and infection most common causes

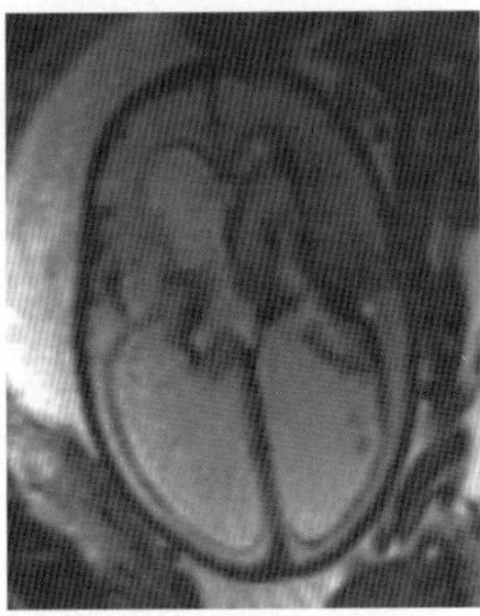

Hemorrhage
- Variety of maternal and fetal etiologies
- May cause hydrocephalus

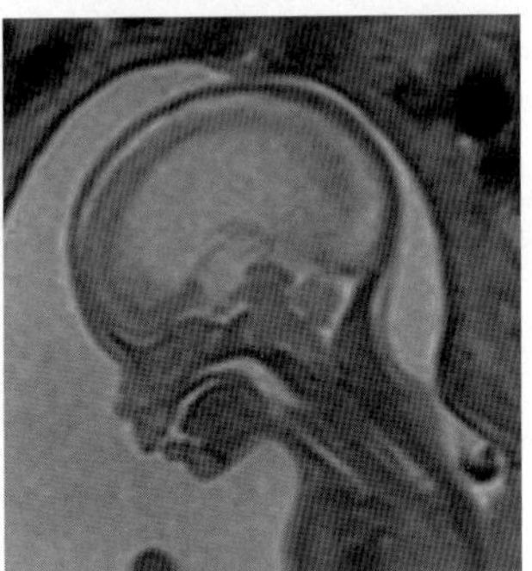

Aqueductal Stenosis
- Variety of acquired (hemorrhage, infection) and malformative etiologies
- Severe ventriculomegaly, including the third with normal fourth ventricle
- Ventricular diverticula
- Enlarged head circumference

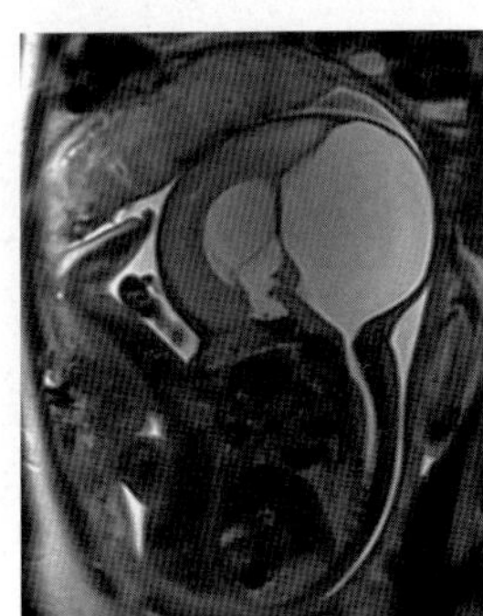

Dandy-Walker Malformation
- Hypoplastic and rotated vermis
- Fourth ventricle enlarged
- Large posterior fossa
- Hydrocephalus

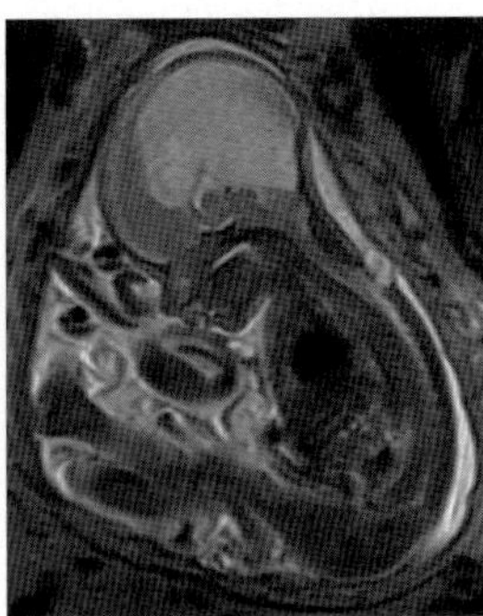

Chiari 2 Malformation
- Small posterior fossa with crowding ("banana sign")
- Hindbrain herniation
- Small head circumference
- "Lemon"-shaped calvarium
- Hydrocephalus
- Myelomeningocele

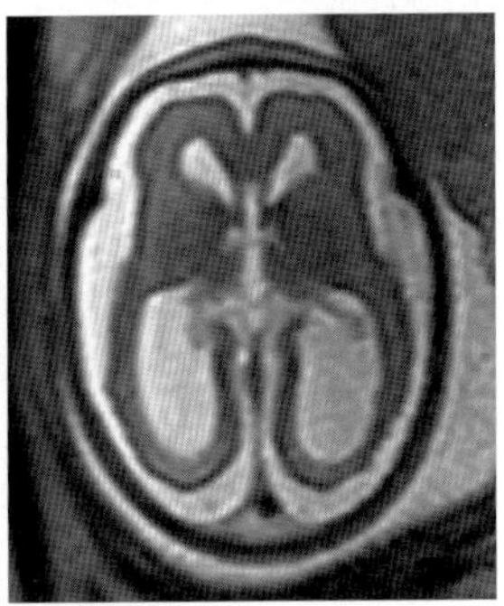

TORCH Infection
- Parenchymal calcification
- Volume loss and ventriculomegaly
- +/- malformations

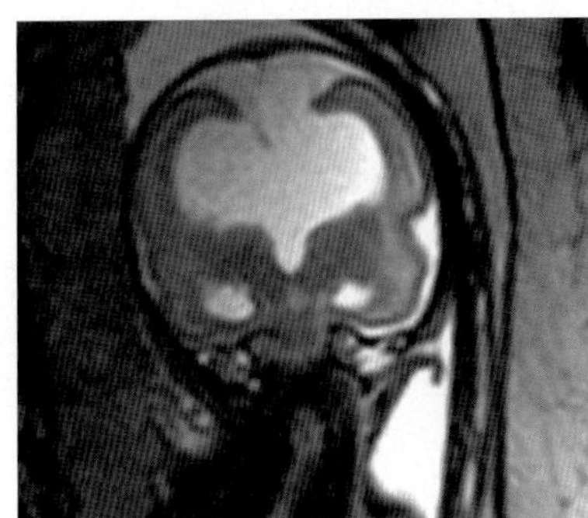

Callosal Dysgenesis/Agenesis
- May be isolated or occur with other malformations
- Colpocephalic ventriculomegaly
- Severe ventriculomegaly with coexisting aqueductal obstruction

NEONATAL ENCEPHALOPATHY

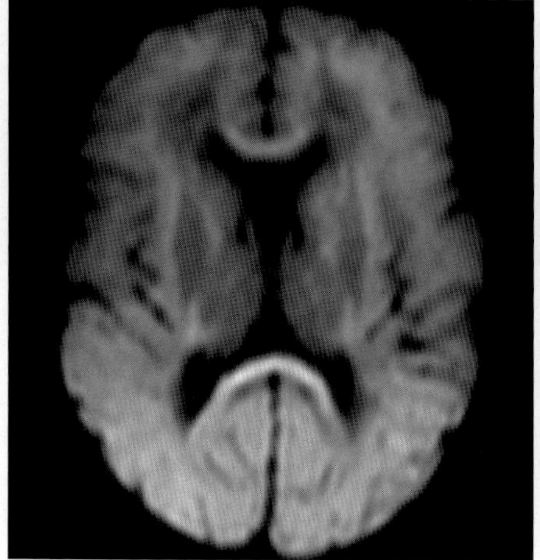

Hypoxic Ischemic Injury

- Variable pattern based on mild, moderate (watershed) versus severe insult (central gray or diffuse)
- Image at 3 to 5 days post insult

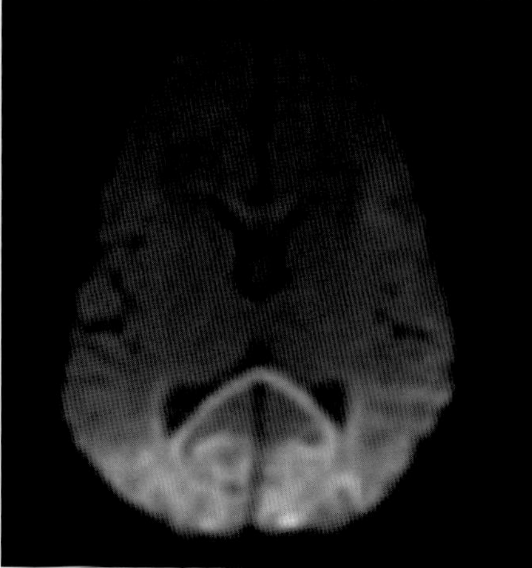

Hypoglycemia

- Posterior predilection
- Symmetric restricted diffusion in acute phase
- Atrophy in chronic phase

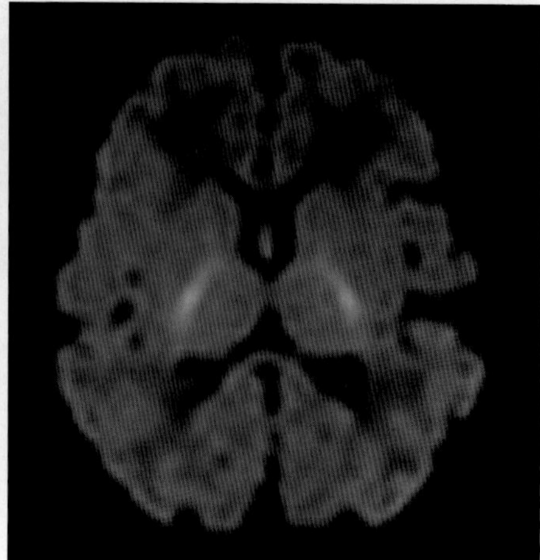

Metabolic Disorders

- Disorders presenting in the neonatal period and mimicking hypoxic ischemic injury (HII) include urea cycle disorders, nonketotic hyperglycinemia, maple syrup urine, and sulfite oxidase.

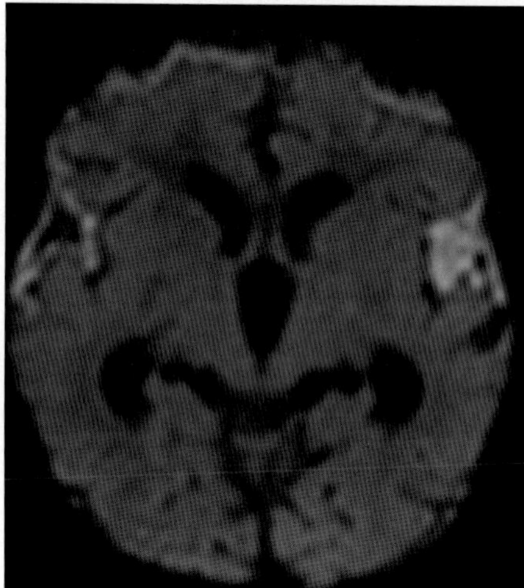

Meningoencephalitis

- Group B strep and Escherichia coli most common causes in neonates
- Leptomeningeal enhancement
- Purulent debris in the subarachnoid space and ventricles
- Cerebritis/central and peripheral infarcts
- Subdural empyema

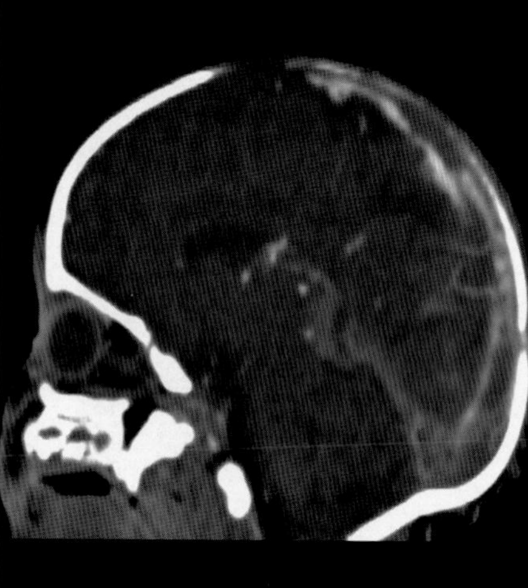

Dural Venous Sinus Thrombosis

- Etiology most commonly from dehydration or coagulopathy
- Peripheral, central, or combined venous
- Parenchymal venous edema, infarct, and/or hemorrhage

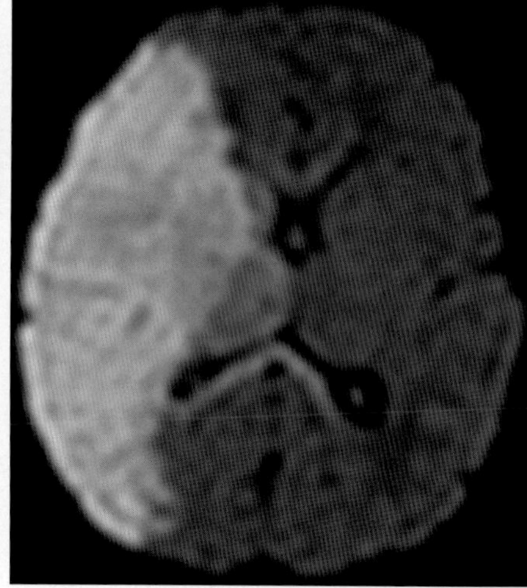

Arterial Stroke

- Variety of fetal and maternal causes (e.g., coagulopathy, arteriopathy, thromboembolic, etc.); often idiopathic
- Entire or partial singular or multiple arterial territories
- Middle cerebral artery distribution most common

HYPOXIC ISCHEMIC INJURY SEVERITY PATTERN ON MRI

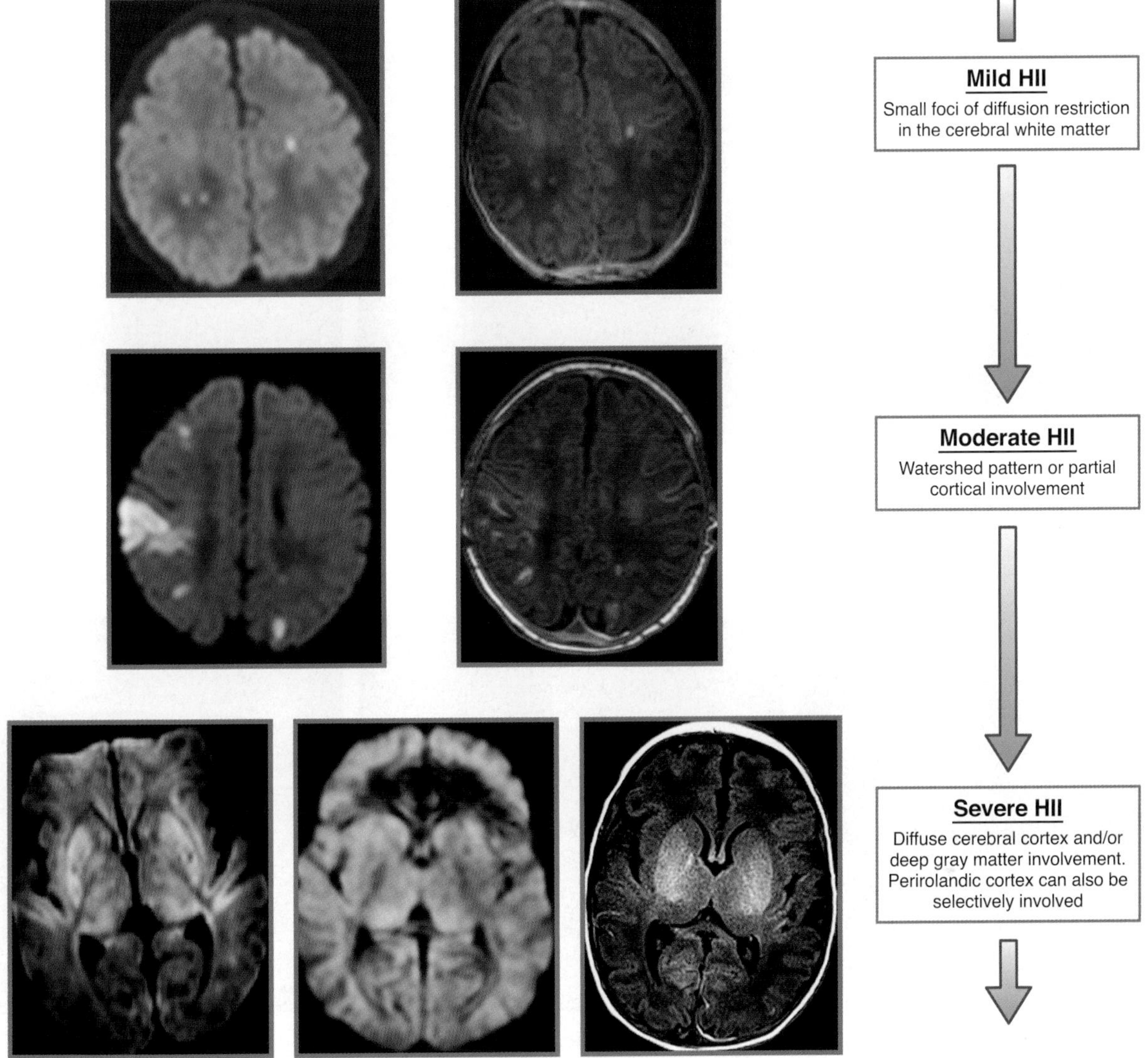

HEAD ULTRASOUND FINDINGS

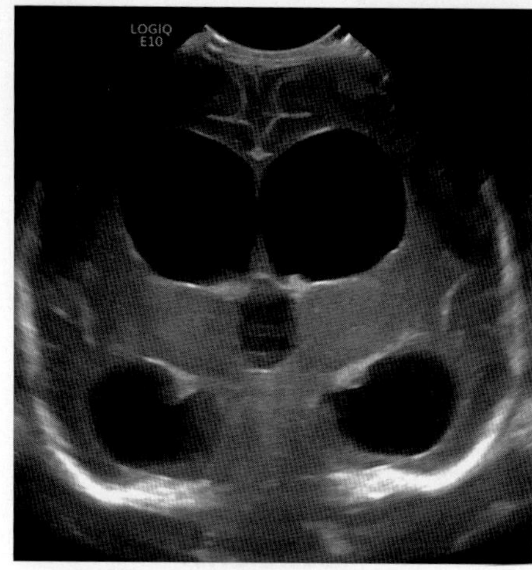

Hydrocephalus
- Disproportionate enlargement of the ventricles relative to the sulci

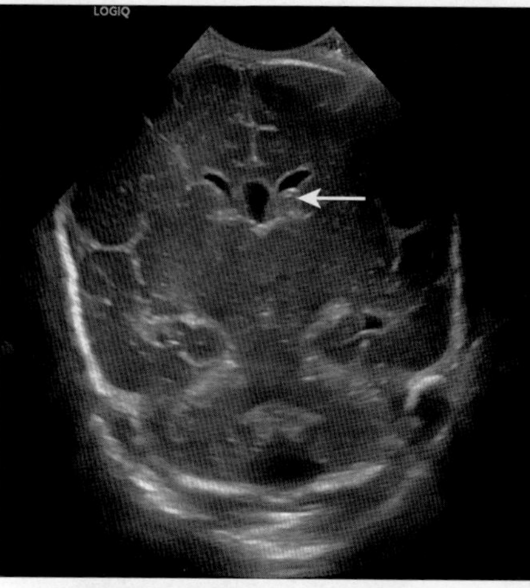

Germinal Matrix Hemorrhage
- Hyperechoic material at caudalthalmic groove

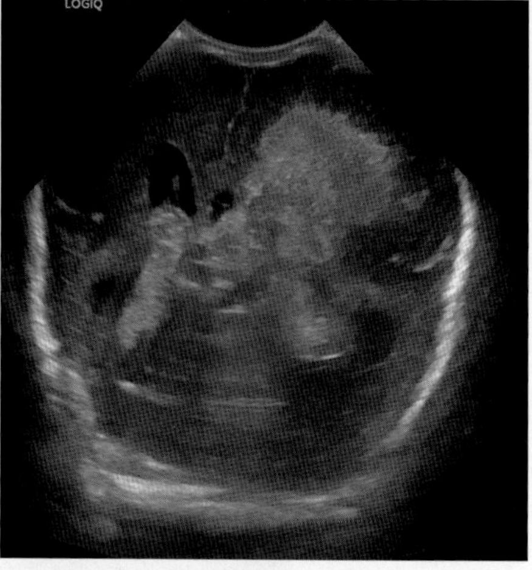

Periventricular Venous Hemorrhagic Infarct
- Complication of prematurity that results in a parenchymal hemorrhage

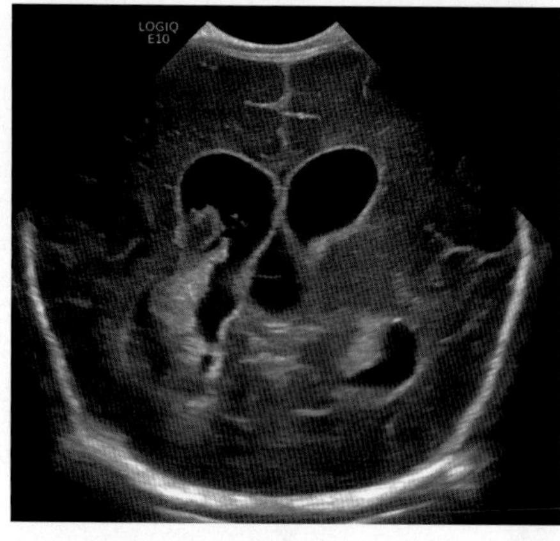

Intraventricular Hemorrhage
- Hyperechoic intraventricular material and hyperechogenic ependymal lining

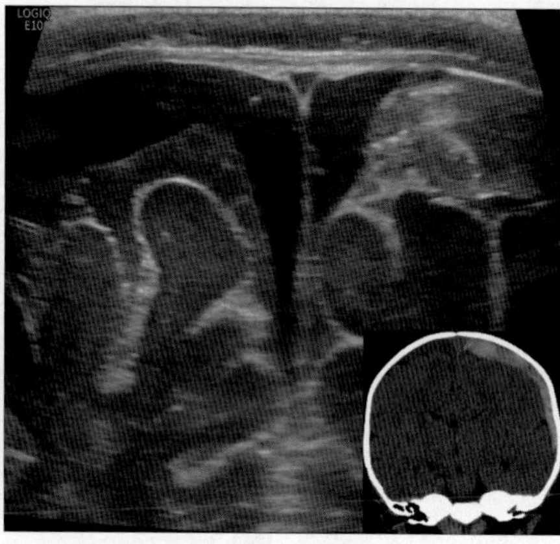

Subdural Hemorrhage
- Often seen with abusive head trauma and coagulopathy

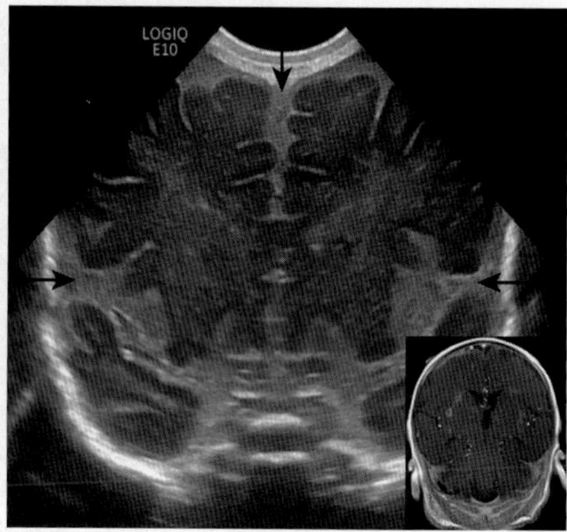

Meningitis
- Expanded hyperechoic subarachnoid spaces

HEAD ULTRASOUND FINDINGS

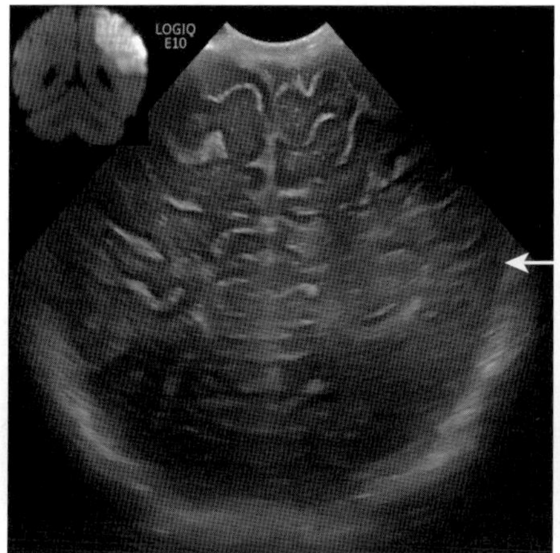

Stroke
- Wedge-shaped region of loss of gray-white matter differentiation
- Challenging diagnosis on ultrasound

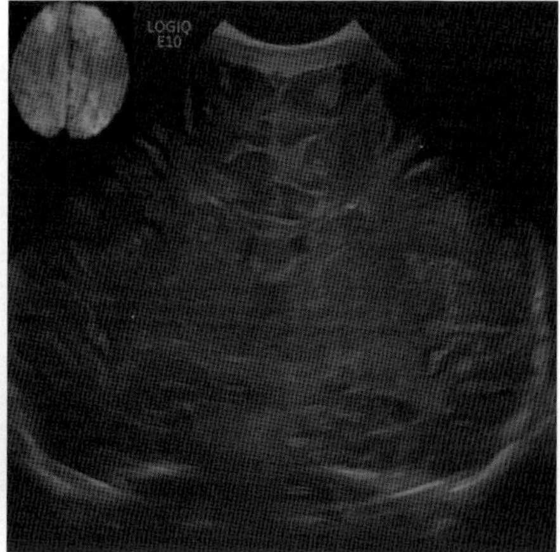

Hypoxic Ischemic Injury
- Effaced sulci and poor gray-white matter differentiation

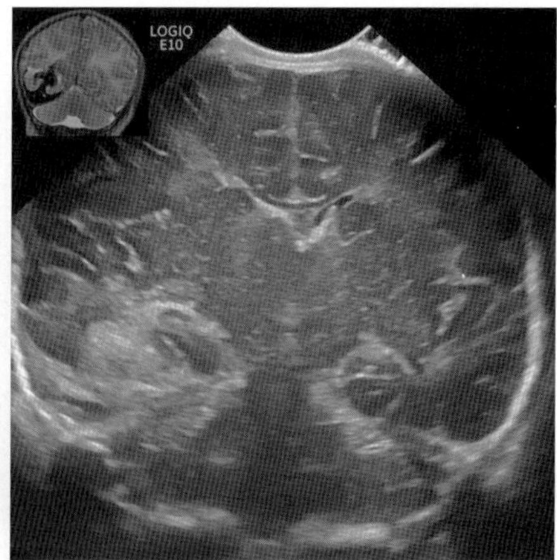

Subpial and Parenchymal Hemorrhage
- Hyperechoic region within the parenchyma and adjacent extra-axial space

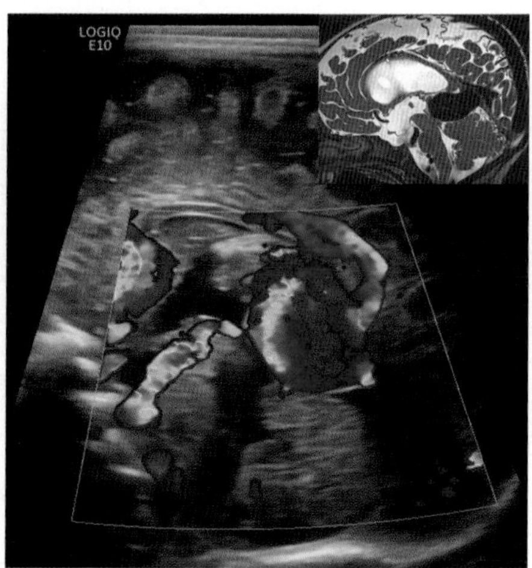

Vein of Galen Aneurysmal Malformation
- Hypoechoic structure in the pineal region with arterial and venous flow

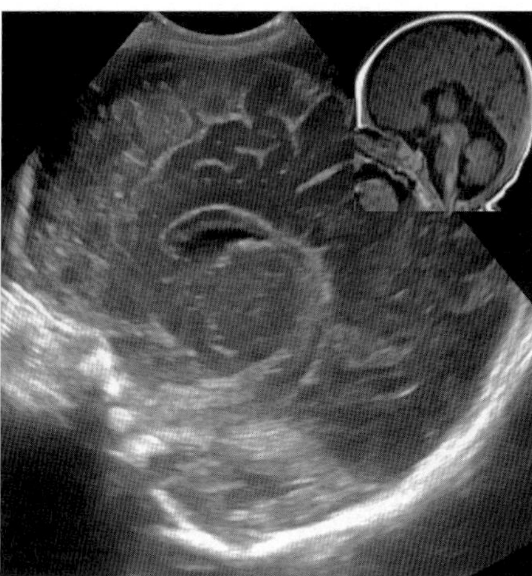

Callosal Malformation
- Common brain malformation

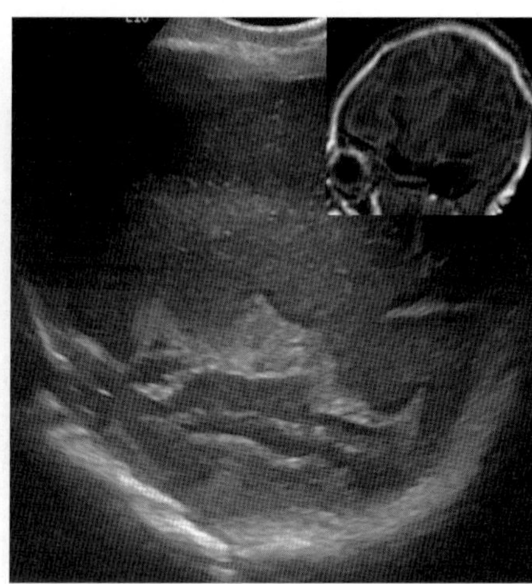

Simplified Gyral Pattern
- Undersulcation of the brain with respect to age

ABNORMAL CORTEX

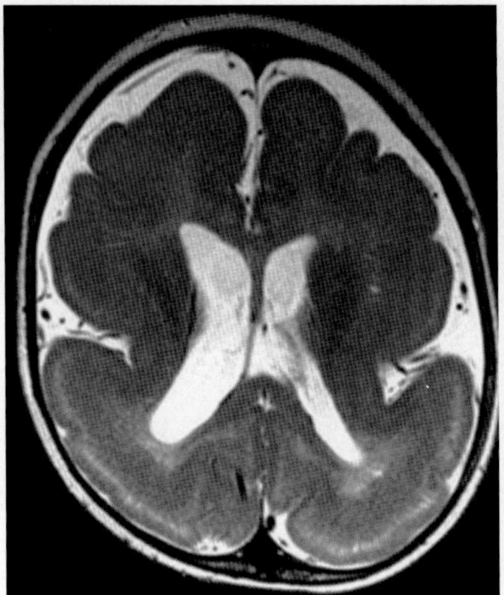

Classical Lissencephaly

- Agyria-pachygyria (broad thickened cortex); may be complete (diffuse) or incomplete with anteroposterior gradient

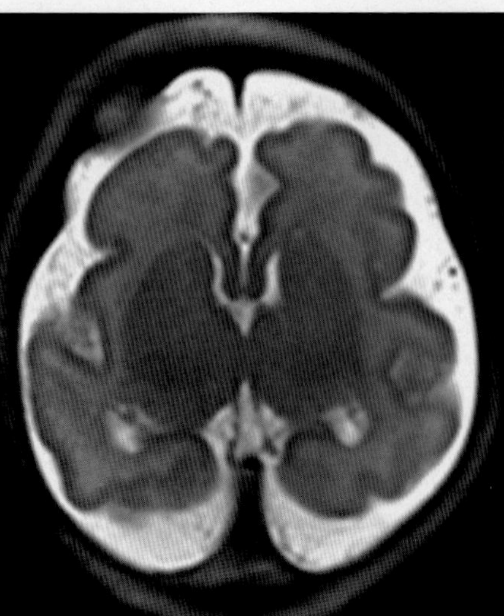

Simplified Gyral Pattern

- Diffuse undergyration of the brain parenchyma

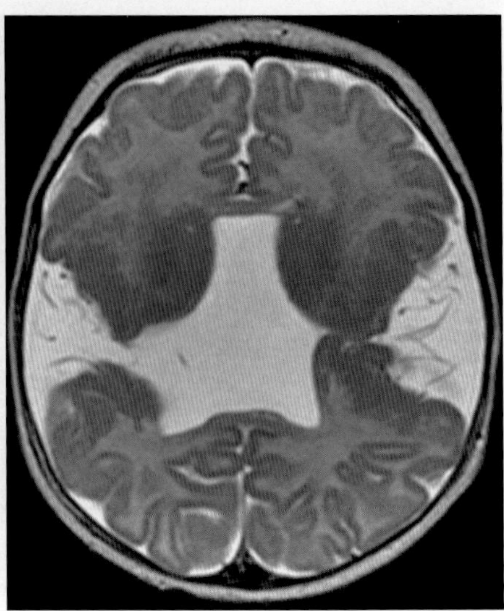

Schizencephaly

- Dysplastic gray matter lined open or closed CSF-filled clefts

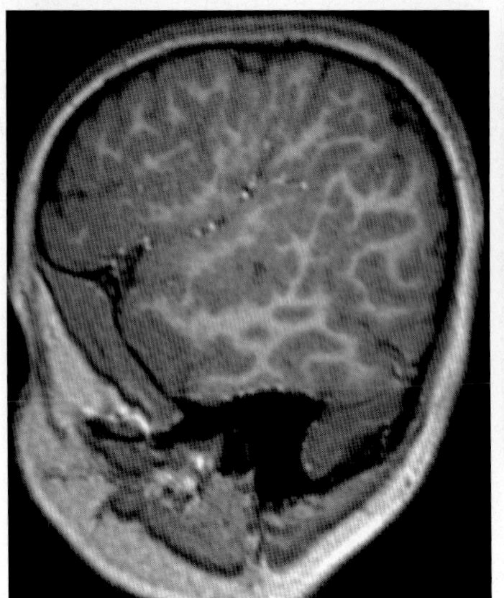

Polymicrogyria

- Excessive number of abnormally small gyri and sulci; may be unilateral or bilateral

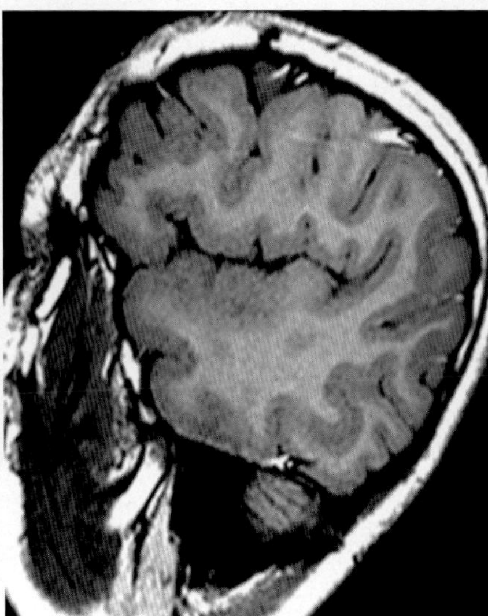

Pachygyria

- Thickened cortex with broad gyri

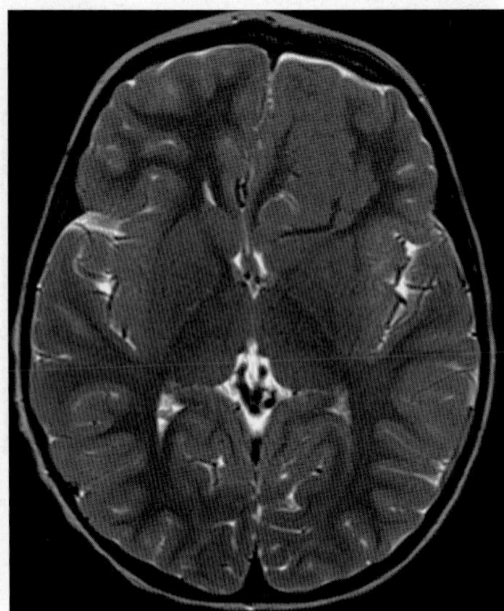

Heterotopia

- Anomalously located gray matter, which can be subependymal, subcortical, or transmantle

ABNORMAL CORTEX

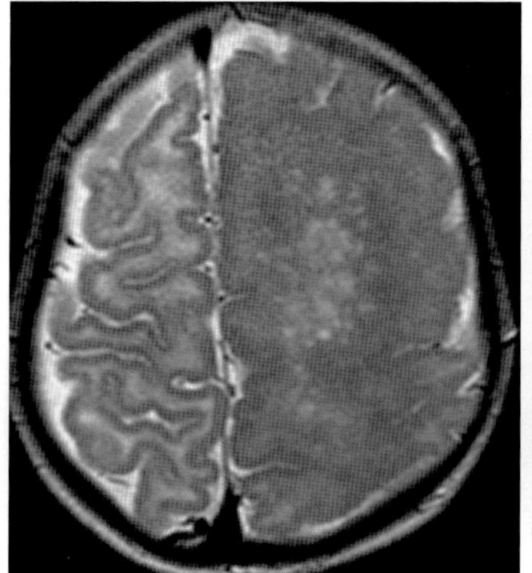

Hemimegalencephaly

- Enlarged dysplastic hemisphere with enlarged ventricle
- Can partially affect the cerebral hemisphere
- Can be isolated or syndromic

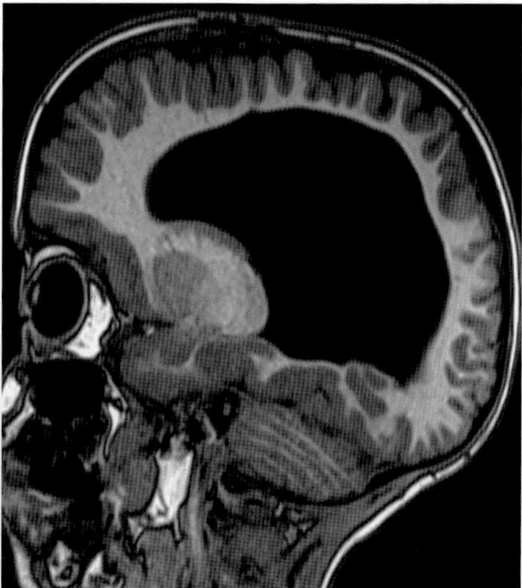

Stenogyria

- Apparent increase in number of gyri due to collapse of normal gyri without dysplasia
- Associated with Chiari 2 malformation

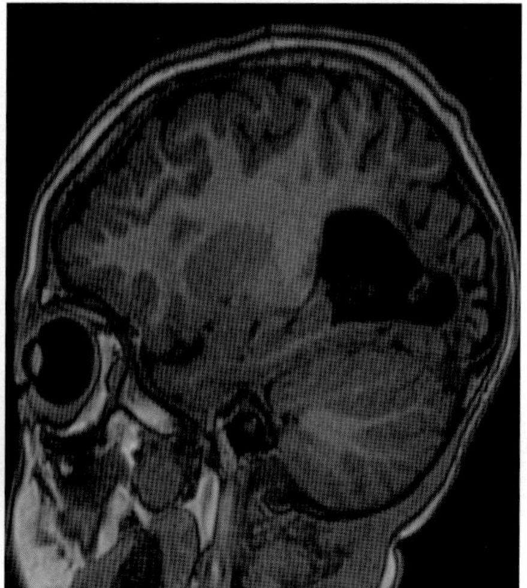

Ulegyria

- Ischemic cortical insult to the brain that preferentially involves the cortex within the depth of sulcus, creating "mushroom-shaped" gyri

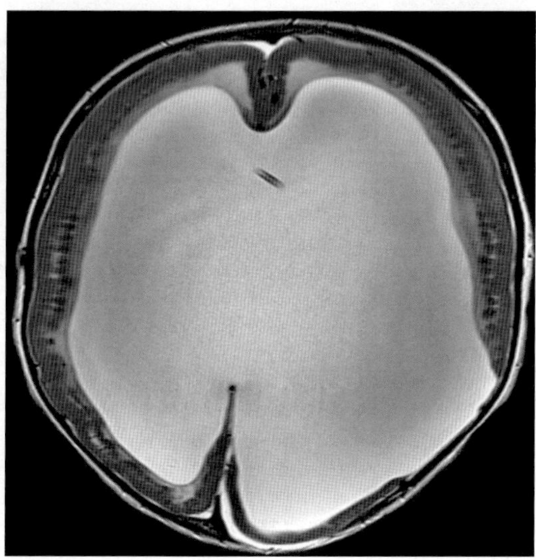

Cobblestone Lissencephaly

- Thickened cortex with nodules of gray matter deep to the cortex associated with congenital muscular dystrophies such as Walker-Warburg

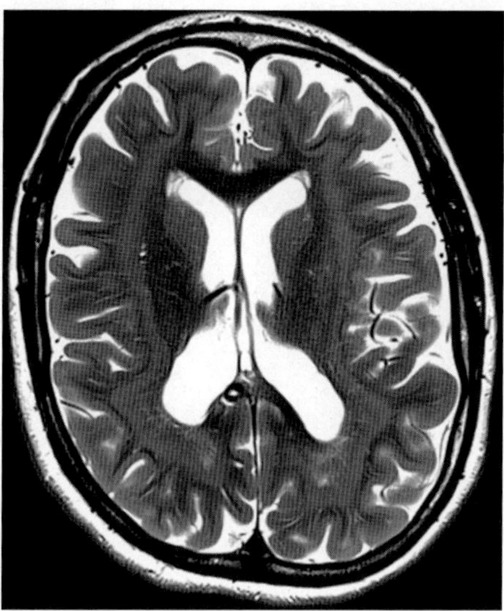

Band Heterotopia

- Band of gray matter deep to the cortex separated by subcortical white matter.
- Shallow sulci and ventriculomegaly may coexist.

ABNORMAL CORPUS CALLOSUM

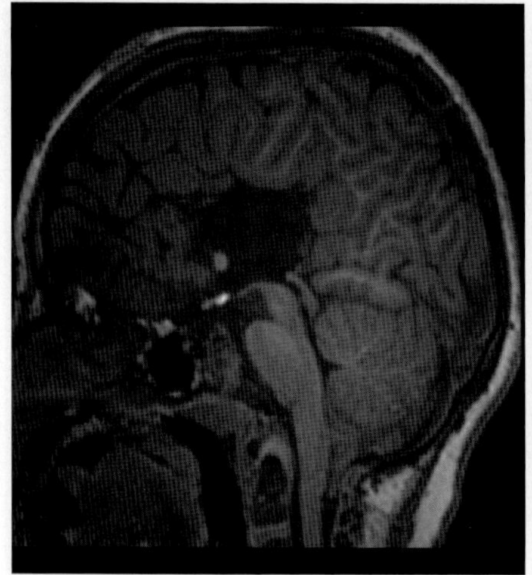

Callosal Agenesis

- Malformation resulting in complete absence of the corpus callosum.

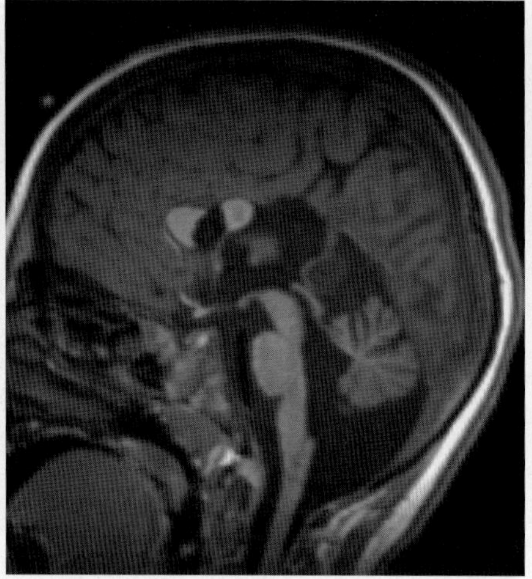

Callosal Hypogenesis and Dysgenesis

- Malformation resulting in incomplete (hypogenesis) or partial dysplastic (dysgenesis) formation of the corpus callosum.

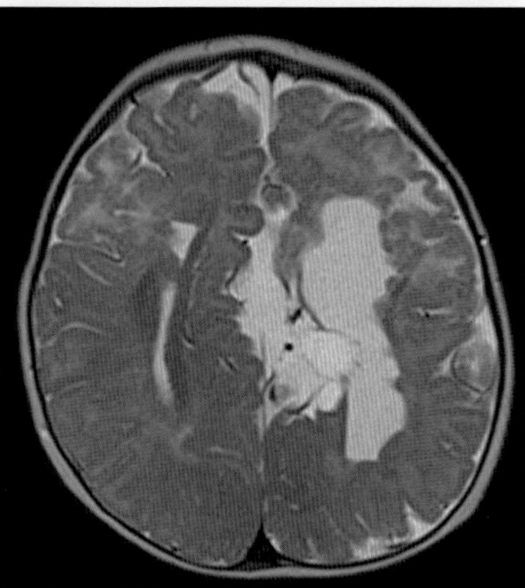

Callosal Agenesis with Interhemispheric Cyst

- Coexisting interhemispheric cysts may or may not communicate with the ventricle.

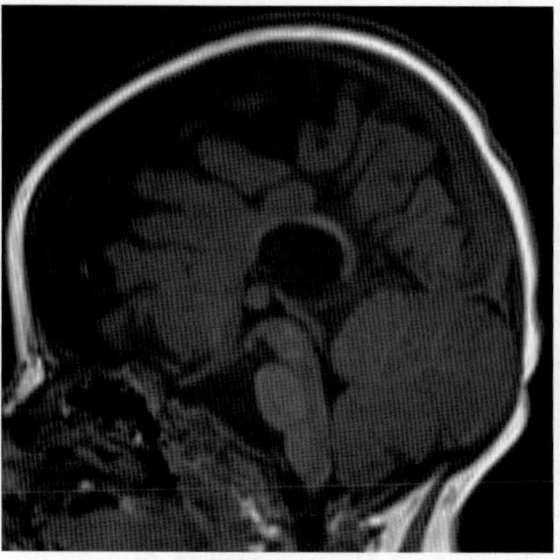

Holoprosencephaly

- Semilobar and lobar holoprosencephaly demonstrates greater posterior than anterior formation of the corpus callosum.

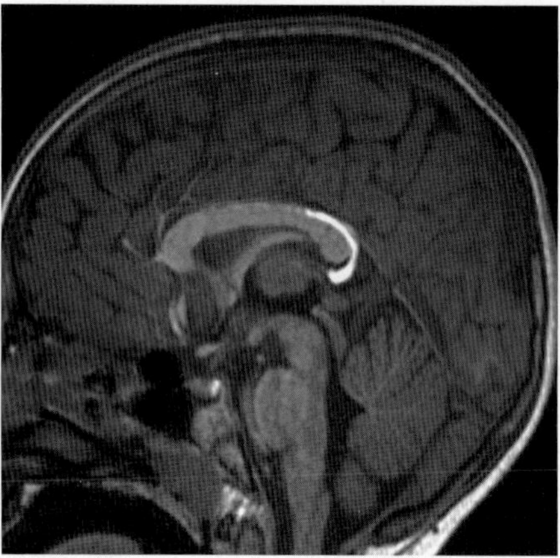

Callosal Lipoma

- Globular or curvilinear lipomas demonstrate T1W hyperintensity.

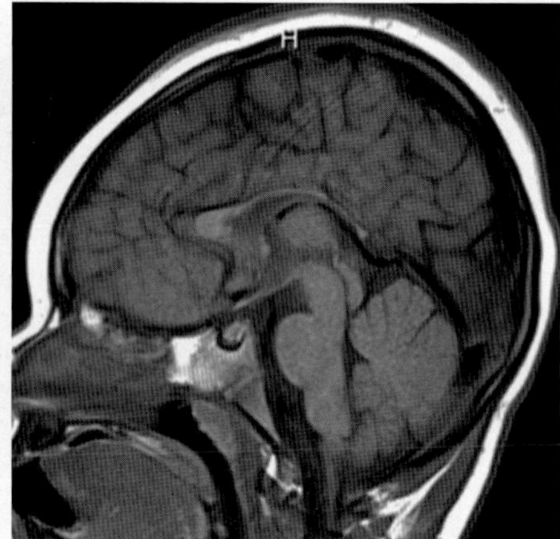

Callosal Thinning and Defects

- Callosal thinning and callosal defects can be secondary to white matter volume loss and injury due to HII, hemorrhage, or surgery.

HOLOPROSENCEPHALY SPECTRUM

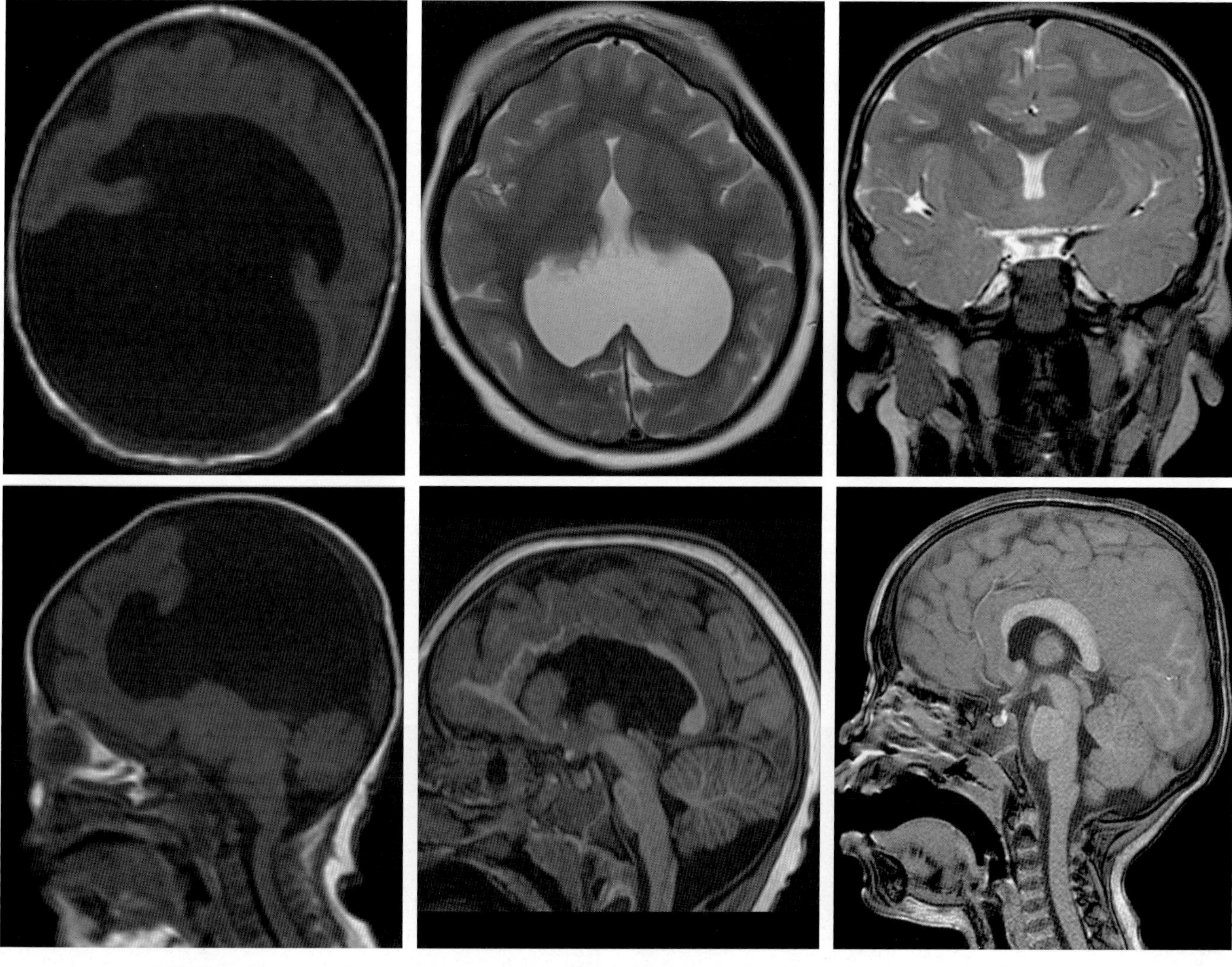

Alobar Semilobar Lobar

Finding	Alobar	Semilobar	Lobar
Craniofacial anomalies	Severe	Variable	Absent or mild
Ventricles	Monoventricle	Rudimentary occipital horns	Squared-off frontal horns
Septum pellucidum	Absent	Absent	Absent
Falx cerebri	Absent	Partial	Well-formed
Interhemispheric fissure	Absent	Partial	Present
Thalami, basal ganglia	Fused	Partial fusion	Separated

ASYMMERTRIC SIZE OF CEREBRAL HEMISPHERES

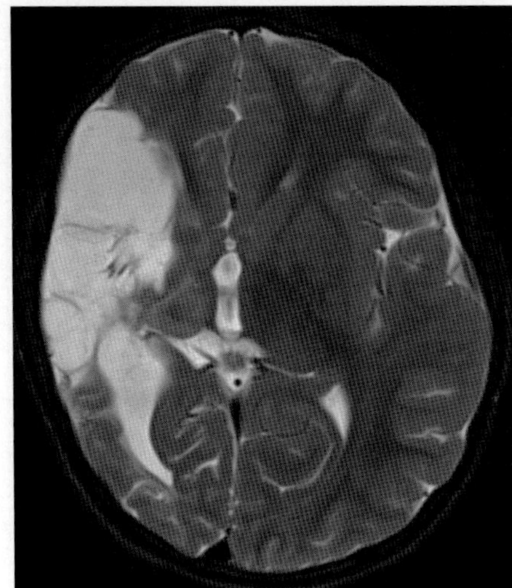

Encephalomalacia

- Old infarcts, trauma, and infections can result in encephalomalacia.

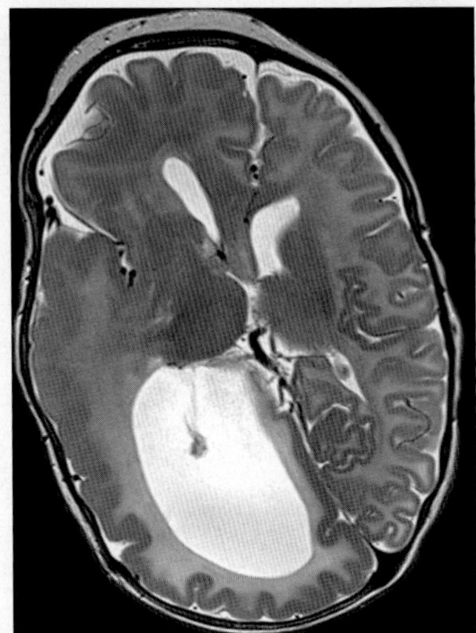

Hemimegalencephaly

- Hamartomatous overgrowth of a part or entire cerebral hemisphere characteristically demonstrating polymicrogyria and ipsilateral enlarged lateral ventricle.
- Caused by PIK3/Akt/mTOR pathway mutations.

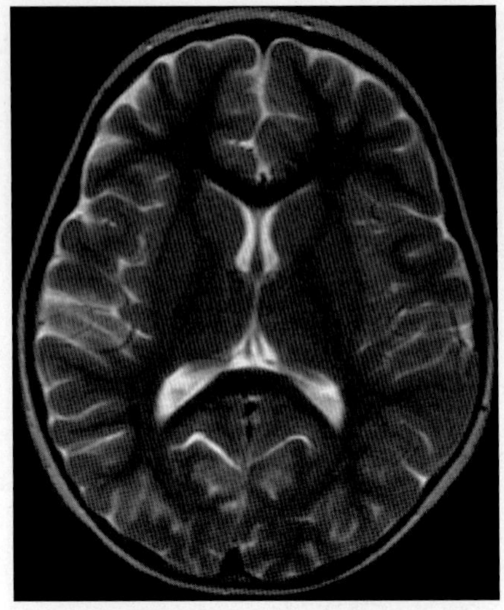

Rasmussen Encephalitis

- Refractory epilepsy caused by a viral, autoimmune, or inflammatory process.
- Progressive atrophy and subcortical T2 hyperintensity of a cerebral hemisphere.
- Typically involves the temporal, frontal, and insular lobes.

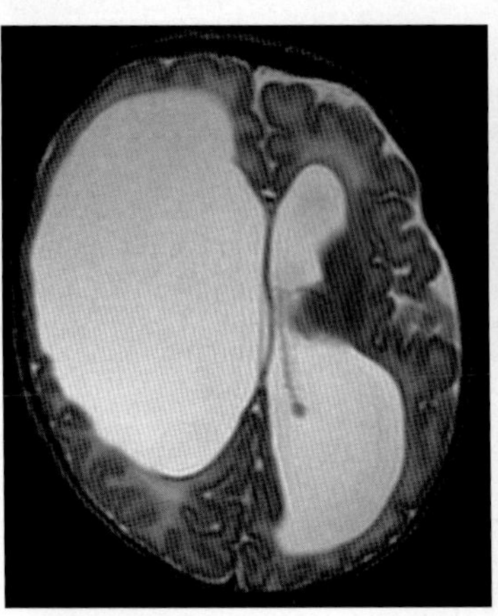

Porencephaly

- Prematurity-related periventricular hemorrhagic ischemia can result in focal parenchymal destruction and ventricular expansion, resulting in asymmetry.
- Following shunting, the brain will often collapse internally and become asymmetrically smaller.

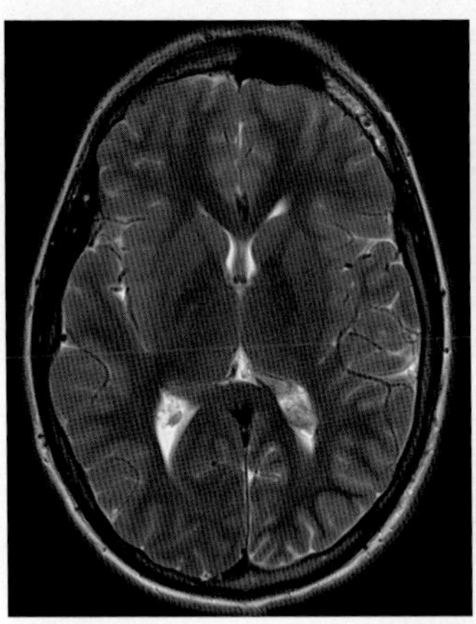

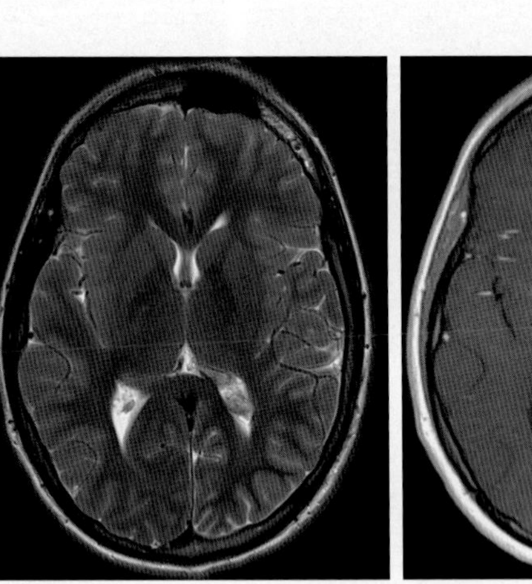

Sturge-Weber

- Chronic venous ischemia results in progressive parenchymal volume loss and cortical dystrophic calcification.
- Calvarial hypertrophy and paranasal sinus expansion.
- Enlarged ipsalateral choroid plexus.
- Glaucoma.

INTRACRANIAL CYST

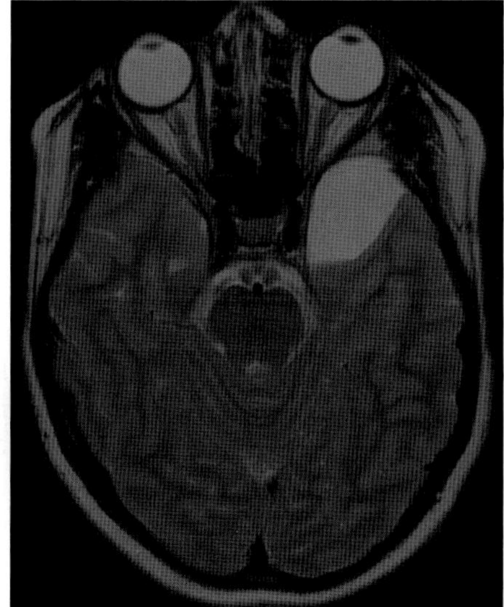

Arachnoid Cyst

- Arachnoid-lined extra axial CSF-filled cyst following simple fluid signal on all sequences most commonly found in the middle cranial fossa

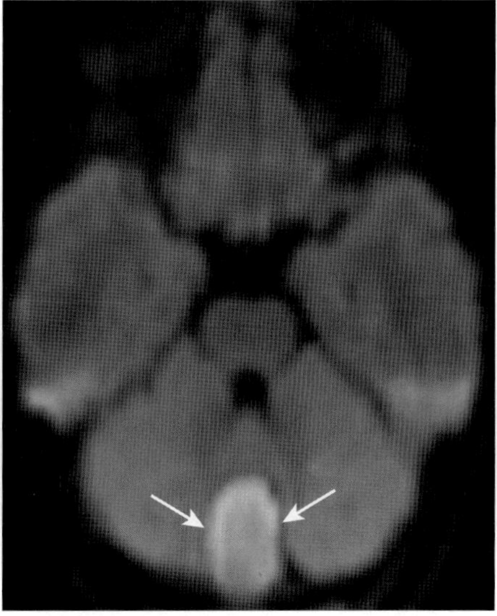

Epidermoid Cyst

- Ectoderm derived extra axial lesions with diffusion restriction

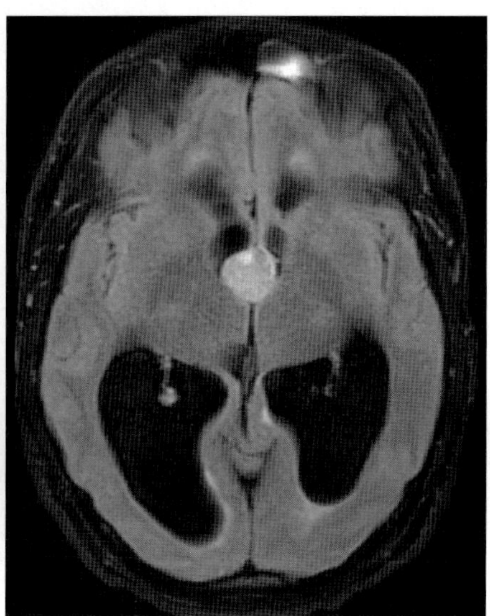

Colloid Cyst

- Anterior superior third ventricle cyst with variable signal intensity/density that may cause acute hydrocephalus

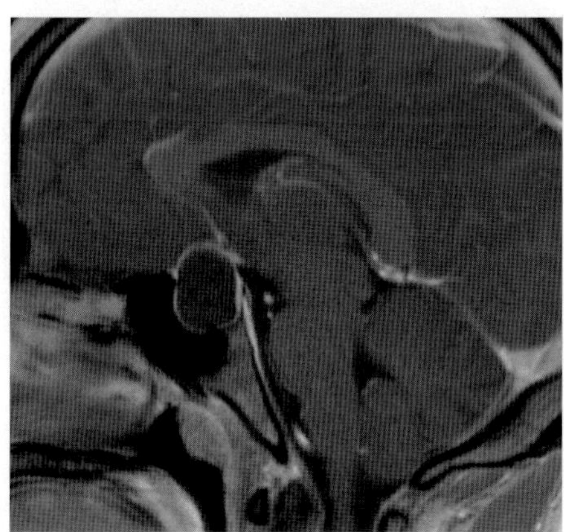

Rathke Cyst

- Congenital cyst centered in the sella

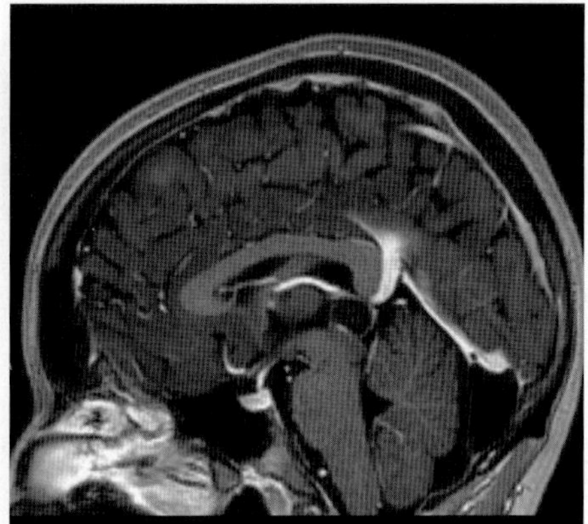

Pineal Cyst

- Usually an incidental finding.
- Follow-up imaging can be recommended if larger than 1 cm or wall thickening greater than 1–2 mm

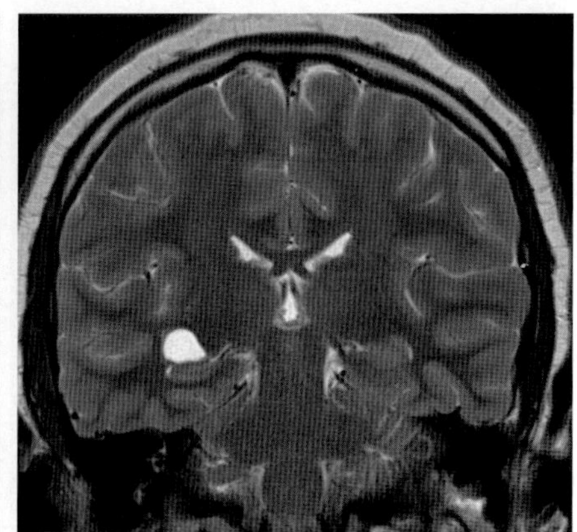

Choroidal Fissure Cyst

- Simple cyst in the medial temporal lobe above the fimbria/alveus

INTRACRANIAL CYST

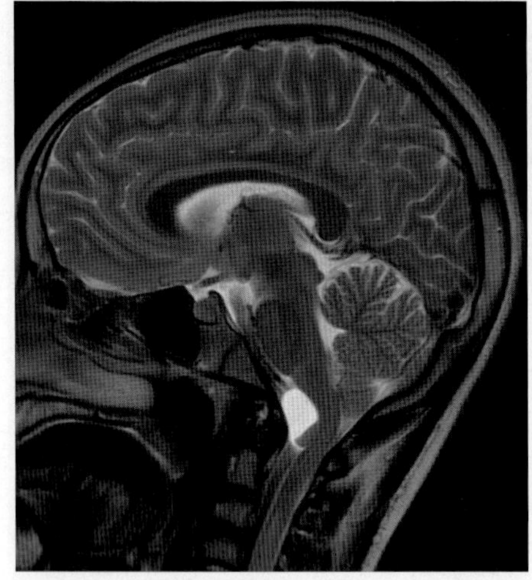

Neurenteric Cyst
- Cyst anterior to the pontomedullary junction
- Variable signal based on protein content

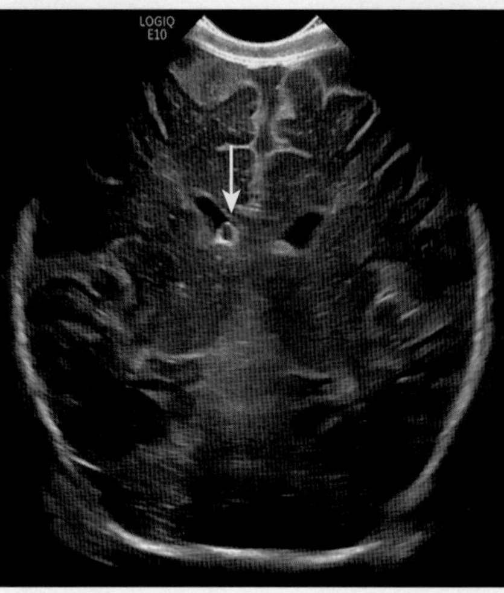

Choroid Plexus Cyst
- Simple cyst of choroid plexus typically not of clinical significance but can be seen with trimosies

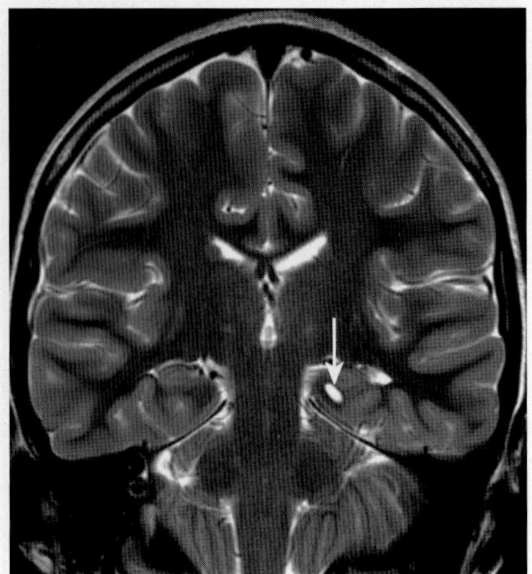

Neuroepithelial Cyst
- Also known as neuroglial cyst; congenital epithelial lined and can occur anywhere
- Typically simple fluid signal

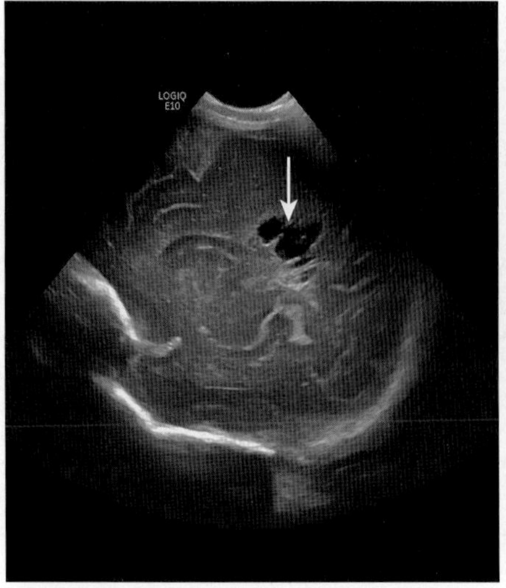

Cystic Periventricular Leukomalacia
- Irregular cystic spaces in periventricular white matter due to parenchymal insult in premature patients

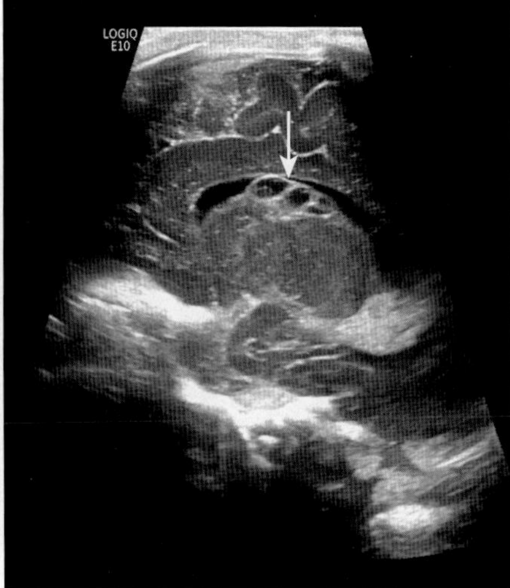

Germinolytic Cyst
- Congenital or acquired (e.g., posthemorrhagic) cyst(s) centered in the germinal matrix
- Classically seen with CMV infection and Zellweger syndrome

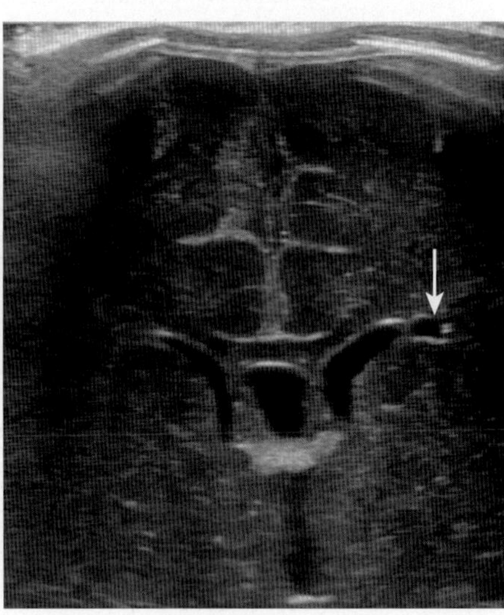

Connatal Cyst
- Normal variant small cysts superior and lateral to frontal horns

POSTERIOR FOSSA CYSTS

Differential Diagnosis of Posterior Fossa Cysts.

Malformation	Vermis	Fourth Ventricle	Posterior Fossa	Hydrocephalus	Occipital Scalloping
Dandy-Walker Malformation 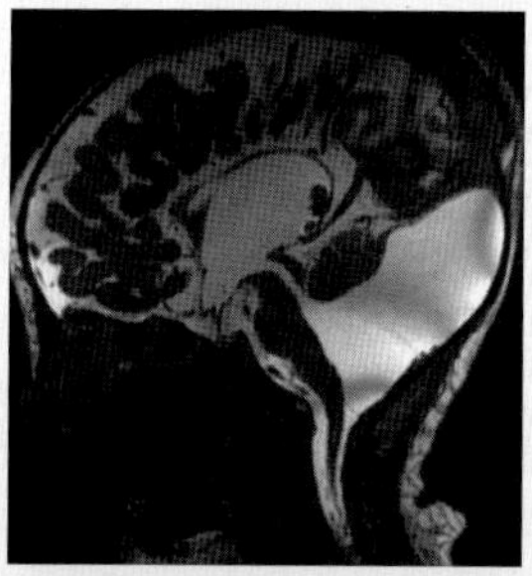	Hypoplastic, markedly rotated	Enlarged	Enlarged	Frequent	Yes
Inferior Vermian Hypogenesis 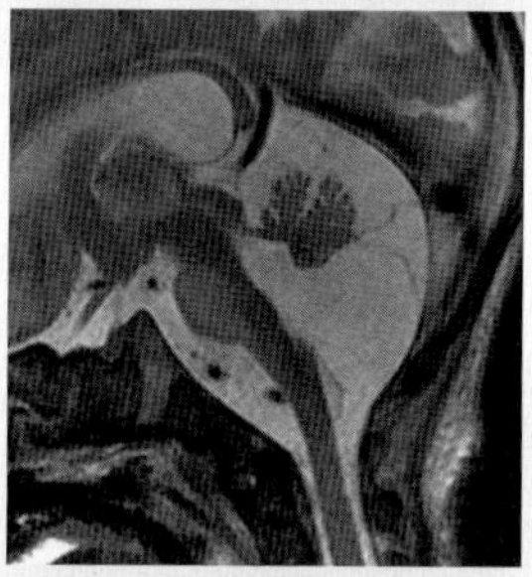	Inferior portion hypoplastic, and rotated to a lesser extent than Dandy-Walker	Enlarged	Normal or slightly enlarged	Usually absent	No
Blake Pouch Cyst 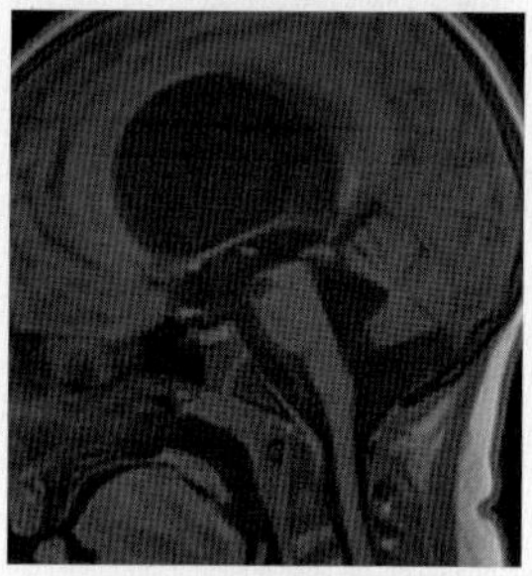	Normal, slightly upwardly rotated usually less than vermian hypoplasia	Often enlarged	Normal or slightly enlarged	Variable depending on whether the cyst perforates	Possible
Arachnoid Cyst 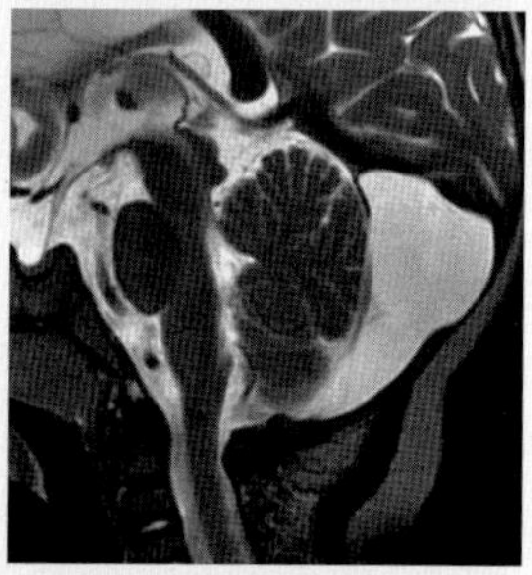	Normal, occasionally compressed, not rotated	Normal or reduced	Normal or slightly enlarged	Rare	Yes
Mega Cisterna Magna 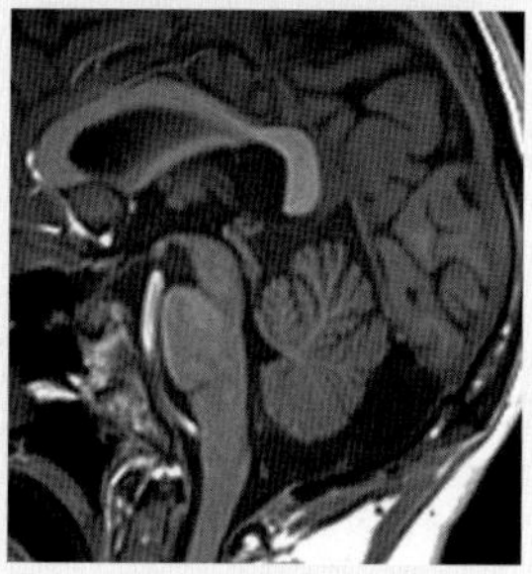	Normal and not rotated	Normal or slightly enlarged	Normal	Absent	No

LOW CEREBELLAR TONSILS

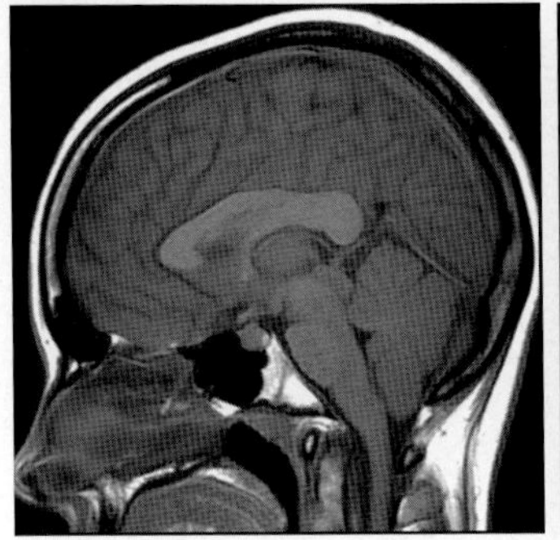
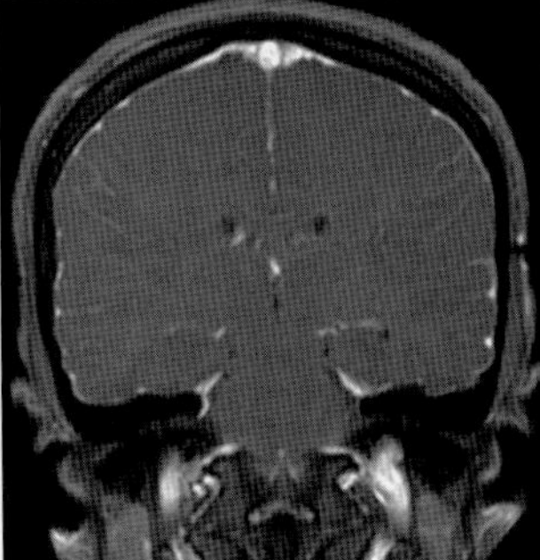

CSF Hypotension

- Pachymeningeal enhancement
- Enlarged pituitary
- Distended dural sinuses
- Subdural fluid collections
- Decreased mamillopontine distance

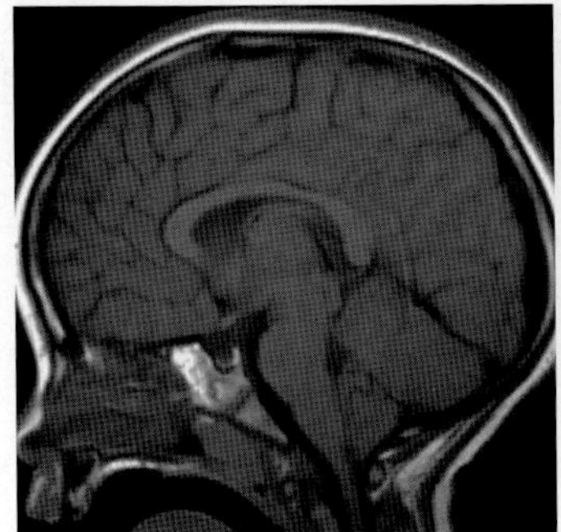
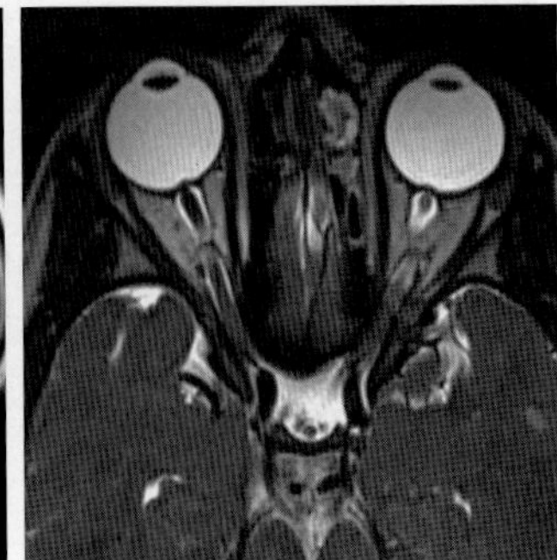

Idiopathic Intracranial Hypertension

- Papilledema
- Empty Sella
- Optic nerve tortuosity
- Optic nerve sheath dilatation
- Slit-like ventricles
- Transverse sinus compression

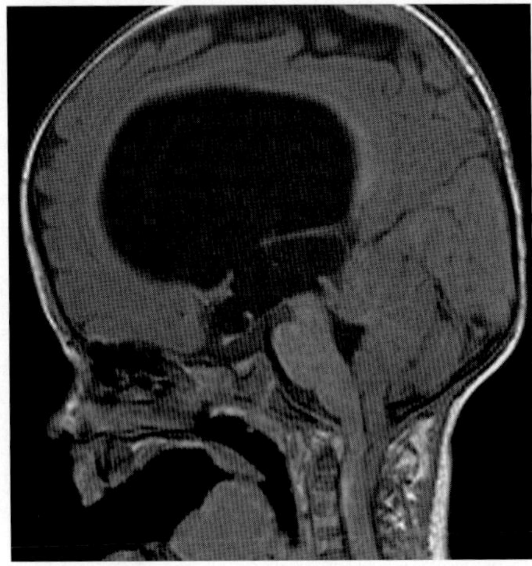

Chiari 1 and 2 Malformation

- Small posterior fossa.
- Chiari 2 has associated myelomeningocele.

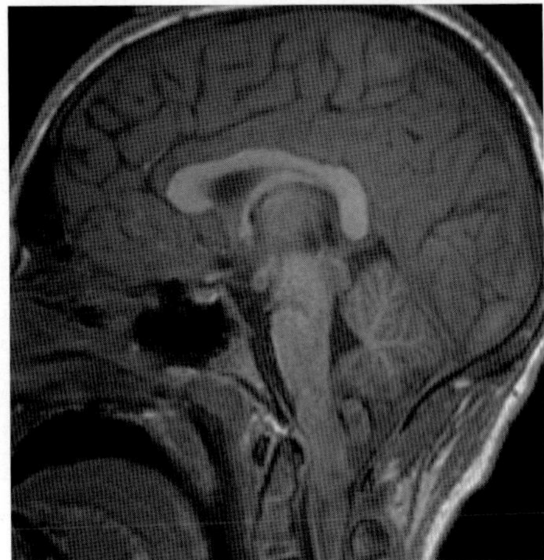

Elevated Intracranial Pressure

- Effaced sulci and cisterns
- Multiple causes: Hydrocephalus, cerebral edema, mass effect, meningitis, and trauma

DISORDERS WITH CEREBELLAR DYSPLASIA, HYPOPLASIA, OR ATROPHY

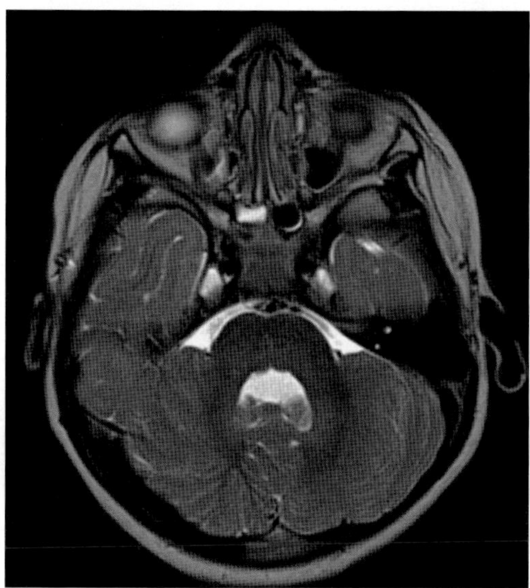

Unilateral Cerebellum Atrophy or Dysplasia

1. Prematurity—Germinal matrix hemorrhage can lead to symmetric or asymmetric hypoplasia.
2. Tubulinopathy—Malformation of basal ganglia.
3. PHACES—Hemangioma, arterial abnormality.
4. Tuberous sclerosis.

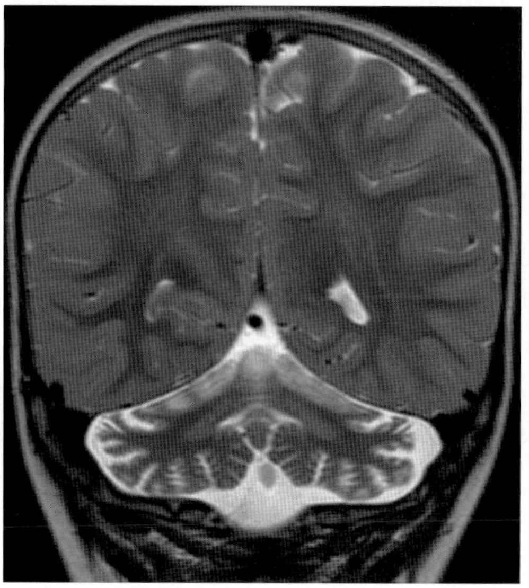

Bilateral Cerebellum with Progressive Atrophy

1. Neuronal ceroid lipofucinosis
2. Spinocerebellar ataxia
3. Congenital glycosylation disorder
4. Infantile neuroaxonal dystrophy
5. Ataxia telangiectasia
6. Medication toxicity

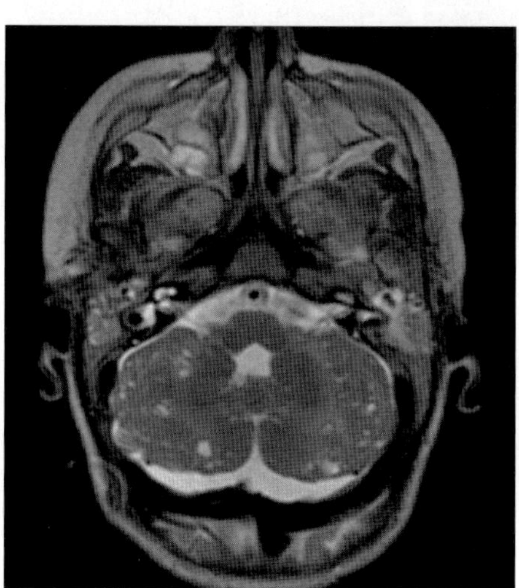

Bilateral Cerebellum with Cysts

1. Alpha-dystroglycanopathies (e.g., Walker-Warburg)—Supratentorial cortical malformation similar to PMG, brainstem kinking, muscle and eye involved
2. GPR56 & COL3A1—Bifrontal PMG
3. Poretti-Bolthauser (LAMA1)—Retinal abnormality

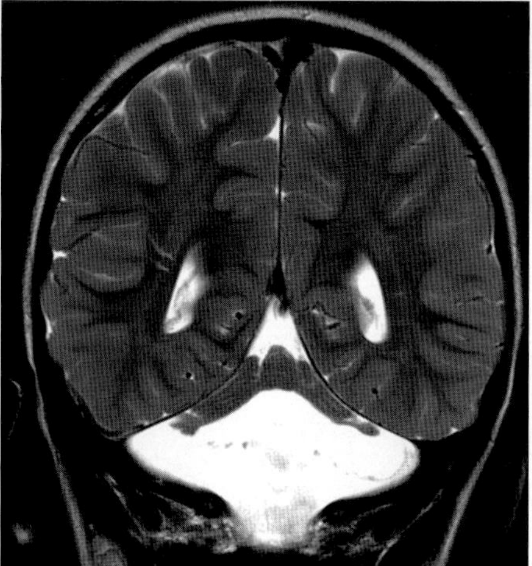

Bilateral Cerebellum without Progressive Atrophy

- Bilateral cerebellar germinal matrix hemorrhage

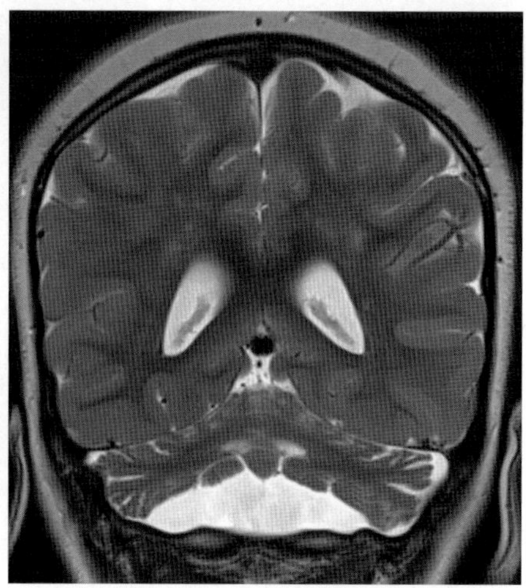

Bilateral Cerebellar Hypoplasia with Other Malformation

1. CASK—Simplified gyral pattern
2. VLDLR & Reelin-pachygyria/lissencephaly
3. Chudley-McCullough/GPSM2—Partial agenesis of corpus callosum, frontal PMG, heterotopia

DTI BRAIN MALFORMATIONS[1]

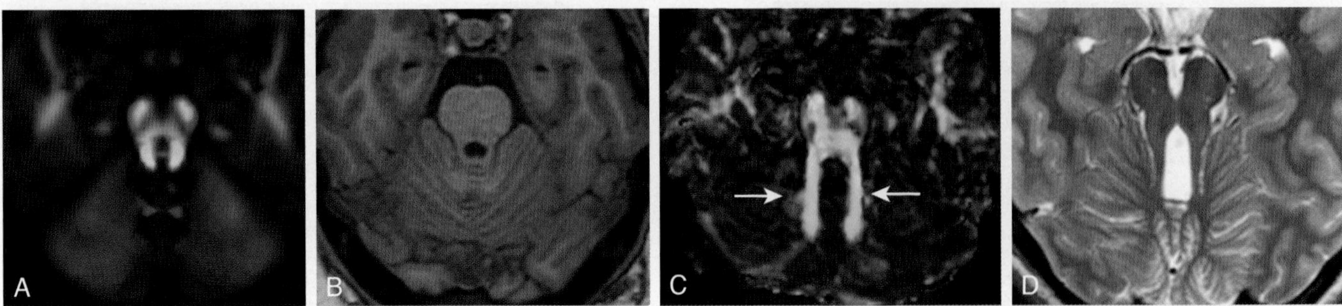

Joubert Syndrome (JS). (A and B) Normal axial diffusion tensor imaging (DTI) color-coded FA and T1W images for comparison. (C and D) Axial color-coded FA and T2W images of JS show the classic molar tooth sign including thickened, elongated, parallel, and horizontally orientated superior cerebellar peduncles (SCP) and a deepened interpeduncular fossa. Axial color-coded FA image at the level of the pontomesencephalic junction reveals the horizontal orientation of the SCP *(green color, white arrows)* and the absence of the red dot within the midbrain representing the failure of SCP to decussate. (C and D from Poretti A, Meoded A, Rossi A, Raybaud C, Huisman TA. Diffusion tensor imaging and fiber tractography in brain malformations. *Pediatr Radiol.* 2013 Jan;43(1):28–54.)

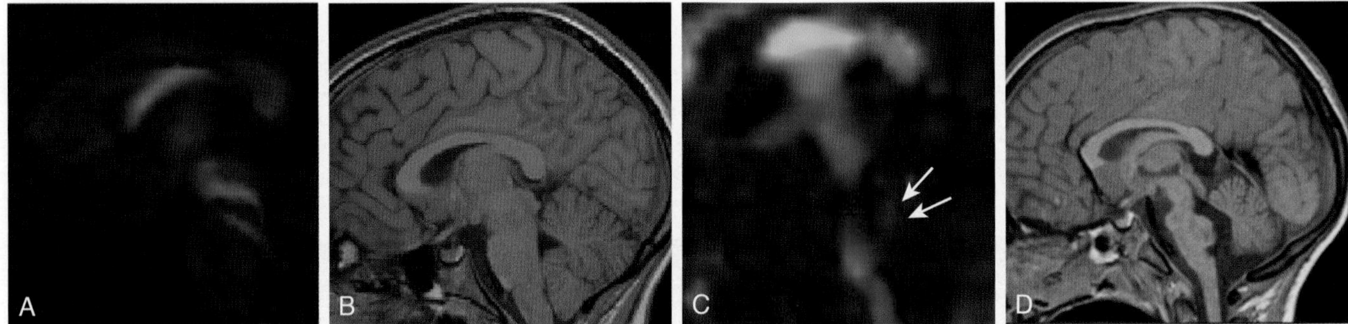

Pontine Tegmental Cap Dysplasia (PTCD). (A and B) Normal sagittal DTI color-coded FA and T1W images for comparison. (C and D) Sagittal DTI color-coded FA and T1W images of PTCD show the flat profile of the ventral side of the pons, the vaulted structure protruding into the fourth ventricle (the "cap"), and shortening of the pontomesencephalic isthmus. Midsagittal color-coded FA image shows the ectopic bundle of fibers ("cap") as a red tract at the dorsal aspect of the pons (*white arrows* in C). (D from Poretti A, Meoded A, Rossi A, Raybaud C, Huisman TA. Diffusion tensor imaging and fiber tractography in brain malformations. Pediatr Radiol. 2013 Jan;43(1):28–54.)

REFERENCE

1. Poretti A, Meoded A, Rossi A, Raybaud C, Huisman TA. Diffusion tensor imaging and fiber tractography in brain malformations. *Pediatr Radiol.* 2013;43(1):28–54.

[1]DTI data in this section were postprocessed by using DTIStudio software (Johns Hopkins University, Baltimore, Maryland).

DTI BRAIN MALFORMATIONS

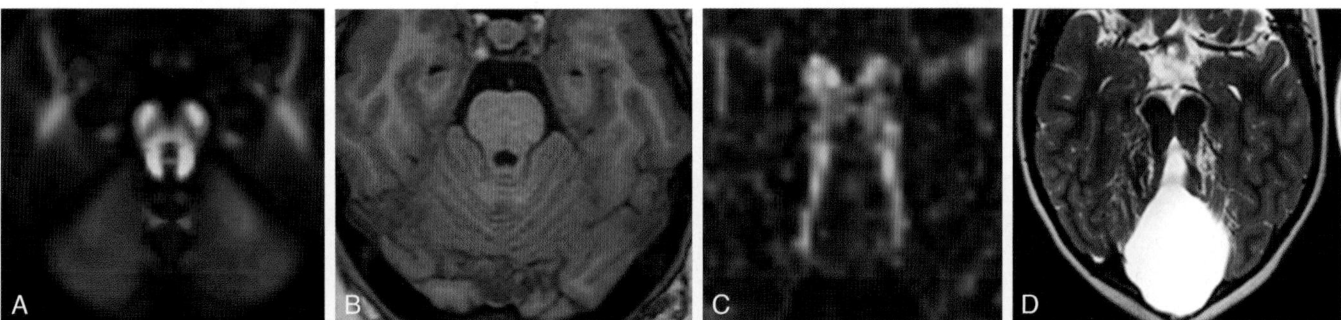

Tectocerebellar Dysraphism and Occipital Encephalocele (TCD-OE). (A and B) Normal axial DTI color-coded FA and T1W images for comparison. (C and D) Axial DTI color-coded FA and T2W images at the level of the pontomesencephalic junction show parallel orientation and elongation of the SCP, as well as a mildly deepened interpeduncular fossa, resulting in a molar tooth sign. Axial color-coded FA map at the level of the pontomesencephalic junction reveals the horizontal orientation of the SCP *(green color)* and the absence of the red dot within the midbrain representing the absence of decussation of the SCP. (C and D from Poretti A, Meoded A, Rossi A, Raybaud C, Huisman TA. Diffusion tensor imaging and fiber tractography in brain malformations. Pediatr Radiol. 2013 Jan;43(1):28–54.)

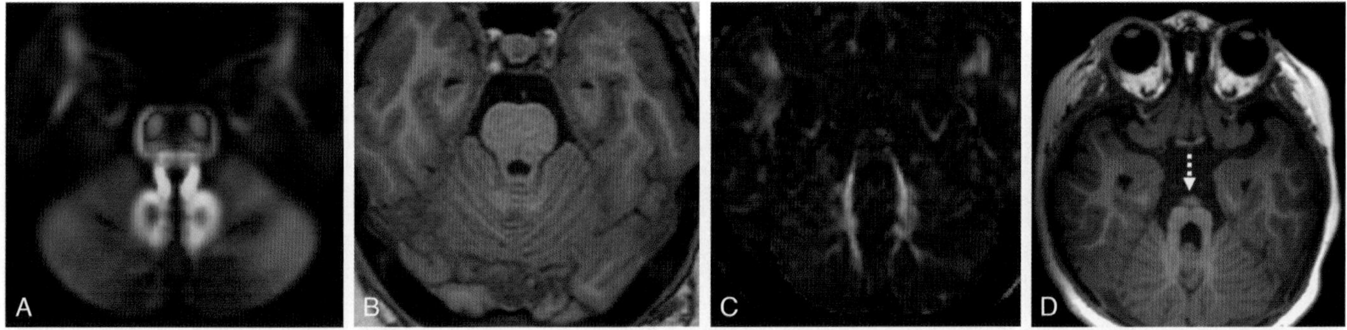

Anterior Mesencephalic Cap Dysplasia. (A and B) Normal axial DTI color-coded FA and T1W images for comparison. (C and D) Axial DTI color-coded FA and T1W images of anterior mesencephalic cap dysplasia show abnormal configuration of the brainstem with a molar tooth sign. An abnormal band-like structure is seen anterior to the midbrain with a gap between this formation and the adjacent midbrain *(dashed arrow)*.

REFERENCES

1. Poretti A, Meoded A, Rossi A, Raybaud C, Huisman TA. Diffusion tensor imaging and fiber tractography in brain malformations. *Pediatr Radiol.* 2013;43(1):28–54.
2. Meoded A, Poretti A, Dzirasa L, Izbudak I, Huisman TAGM. Aberrant course of the corticospinal tracts in the brain stem revealed by diffusion tensor imaging/tractography. *Neurographics.* 2012;2(3):139–143.

DTI BRAIN MALFORMATIONS

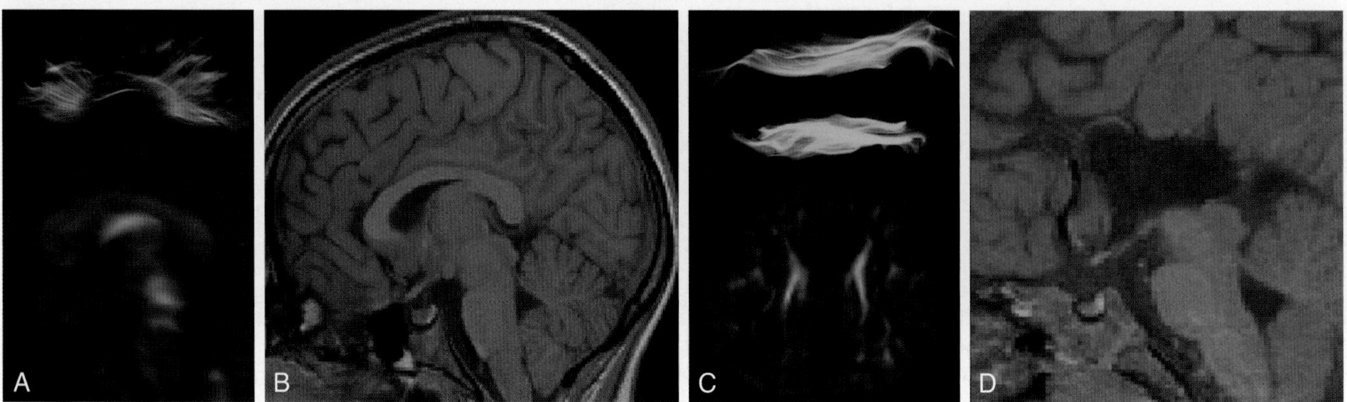

Corpus Callosum Agenesis. (A and B) Normal sagittal DTI color-coded FA, tractography, and T1W images for comparison. (C and D) Sagittal DTI color-coded FA, tractography, and T1W images demonstrate the absence of the corpus callosum. Axial DTI color-coded FA and tractography images show the bundles of Probst as large, longitudinally oriented (green on color-coded FA image) white matter tracts that run along the medial and superior wall of the lateral ventricles.

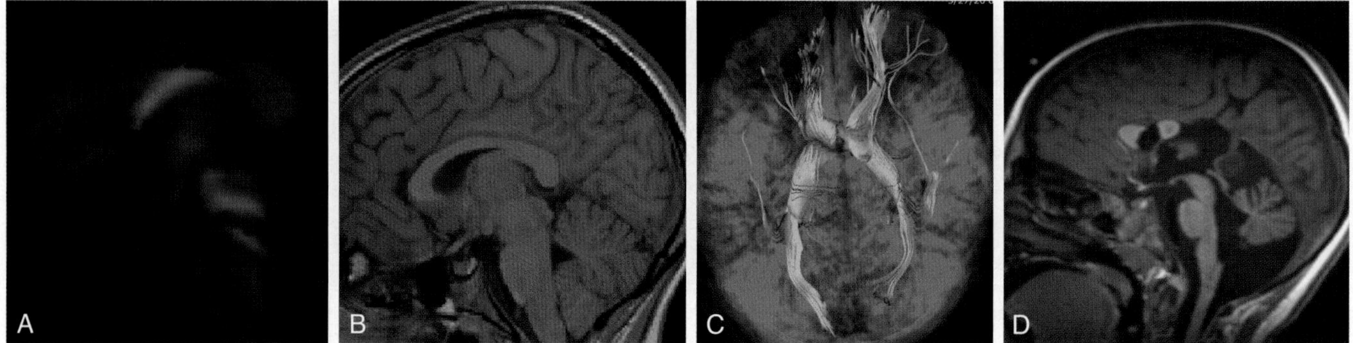

Corpus Callosum Dysgenesis. (A and B) Normal sagittal DTI color-coded FA and T1W images for comparison. (C and D) Axial DTI tractography and sagittal T1W images demonstrate the incomplete formation of the corpus callosum. Axial tractography of the callosal fibers shows unusual connections of aberrant crossing fibers that connect medial frontal lobe regions to medial contralateral parietal lobes.

DTI BRAIN MALFORMATIONS

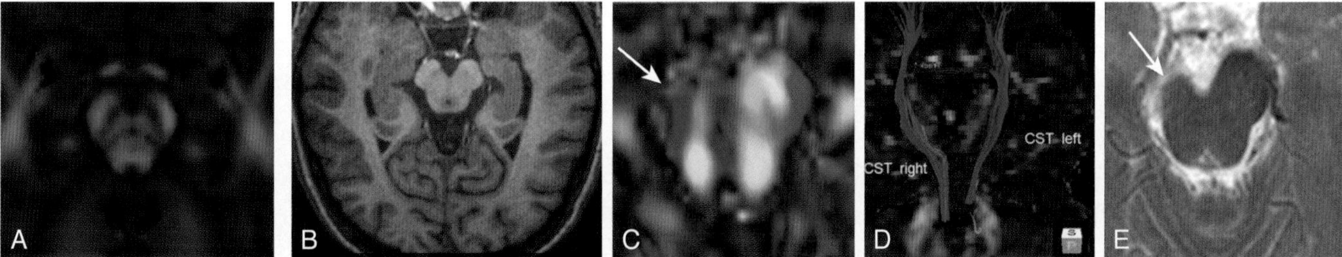

Aberrant Corticospinal tract (CST). A child with mild left-sided muscular hypotonia. (A and B) Normal axial DTI color-coded FA and T1W images for comparison. (C to E) Axial DTI color-coded FA, coronal DTI tractography, and axial T2W images show the reduced size of the right cerebral peduncle *(white arrows)* and absent violet color CST compared to the normal left CST. The coronal tractography image superimposed on the color-coded FA image shows the complete aberrant course of the right CST extending through the dorsal brainstem in the expected location of the medial lemniscus. (A, D, and E from Meoded A, Poretti A, Dimasa L, Izbudak I, Huisman TAGM. Aberrant course of the corticospinal tracts in the brain stem revealed by diffusion tensor imaging/tractography. *Neurographics*. 2012;2(3):139–143.)

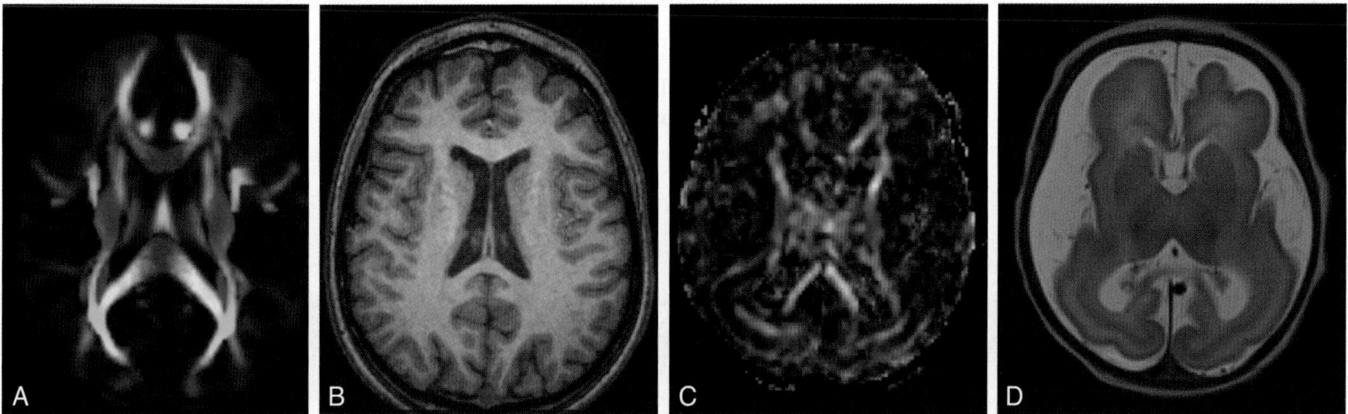

Lissencephaly. (A and B) Normal axial DTI color-coded FA and T1W images for comparison. (C and D) Axial DTI color-coded FA and axial T2W images show a diffuse thickening of the cortex with lack of gyration and thinned white matter. The axial DTI color-coded FA image shows bands of increased FA with different colors depending on their orientation. These bands correspond to the location of the thick, densely cellular fourth layer of neurons in arrested migration.

REFERENCES

1. Poretti A, Meoded A, Rossi A, Raybaud C, Huisman TA. Diffusion tensor imaging and fiber tractography in brain malformations. *Pediatr Radiol.* 2013;43(1):28–54.
2. Catania M, de Schotten MT. A diffusion tensor imaging tractography atlas for virtual in vivo dissections. *Cortex.* 2008;44(8):1105–1132.

CONGENITAL INFECTIONS "TORCHeZ"

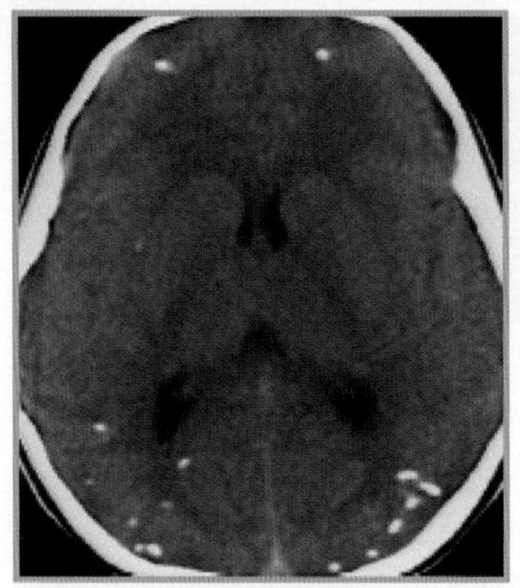

Toxoplasmosis

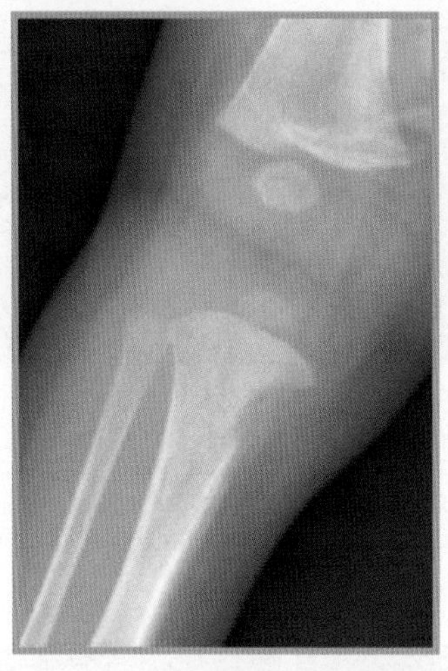

Other (Syphilis, Varicella Zoster Virus, Parvovirus B19)

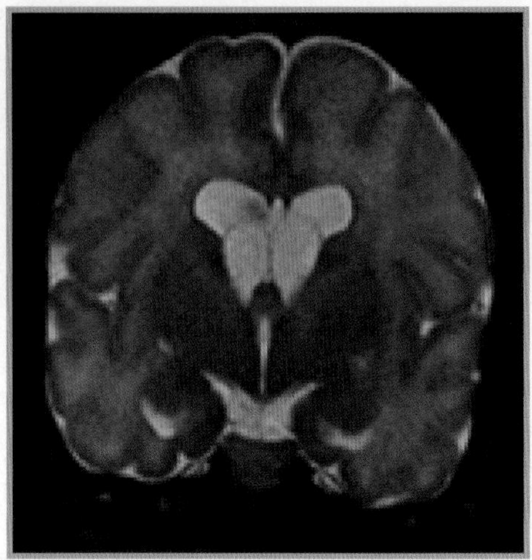

Rubella

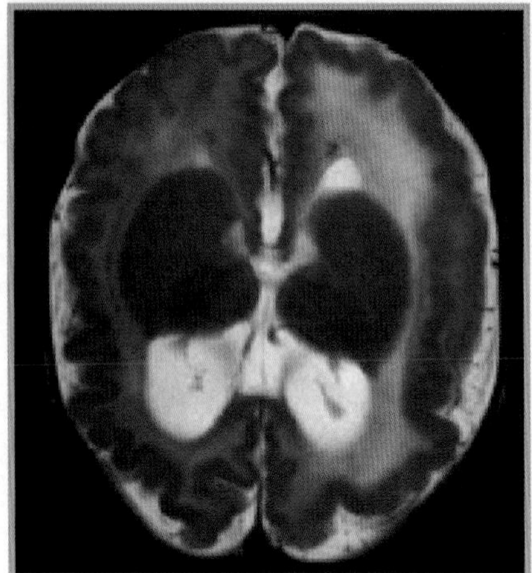

Cytomegalovirus

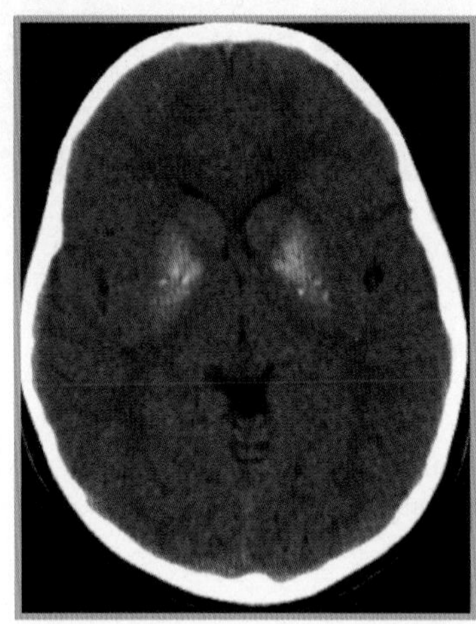

Herpes and Human Immunodeficiency Virus

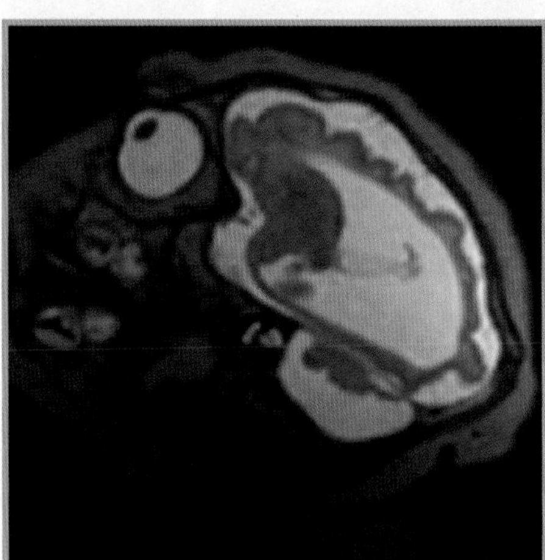

Zika

- Scattered intracranial Ca^{2+}
- Chorioretinitis and microphthalmia
- Ventriculomegaly
- Migration anomalies not a feature

BACTERIAL MENINGITIS IMAGING FINDINGS

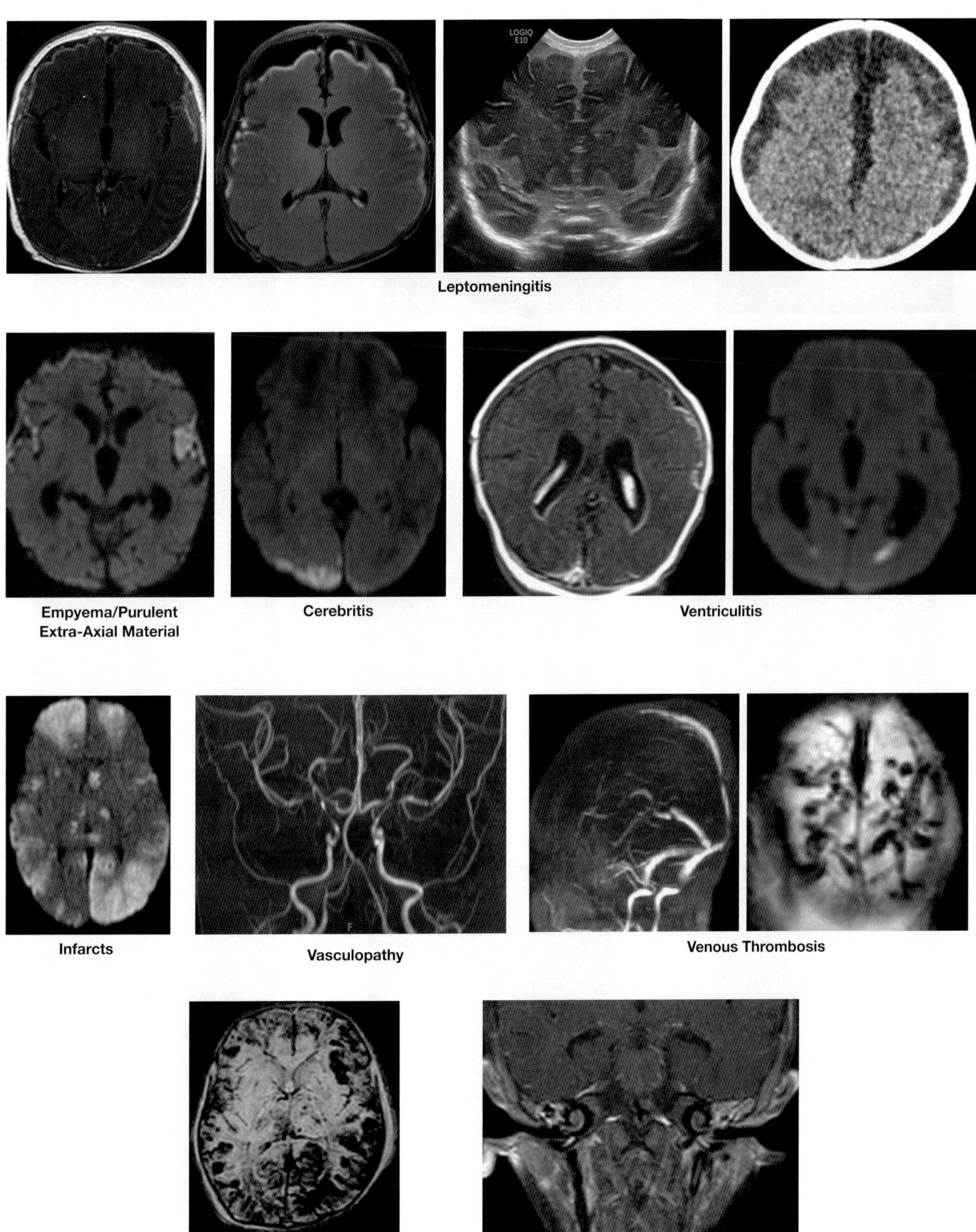

Leptomeningitis

Empyema/Purulent Extra-Axial Material

Cerebritis

Ventriculitis

Infarcts

Vasculopathy

Venous Thrombosis

Hemorrhage

Labyrinthitis

EPILEPTOGENIC LESIONS

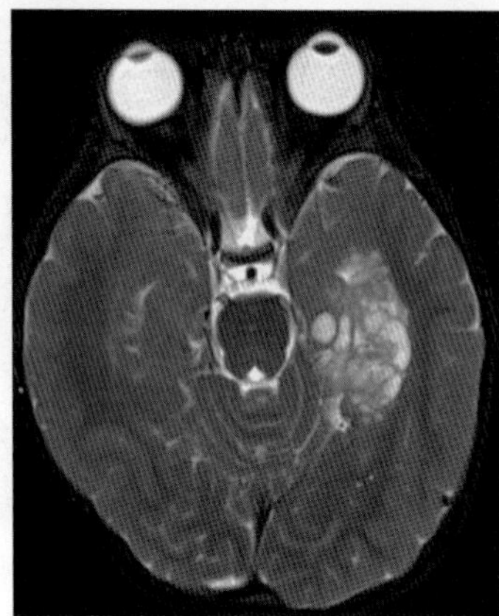

Tumors

- Cortical-subcortical variably enhancing masses including DNET, ganglioglioma, and PXA, among others

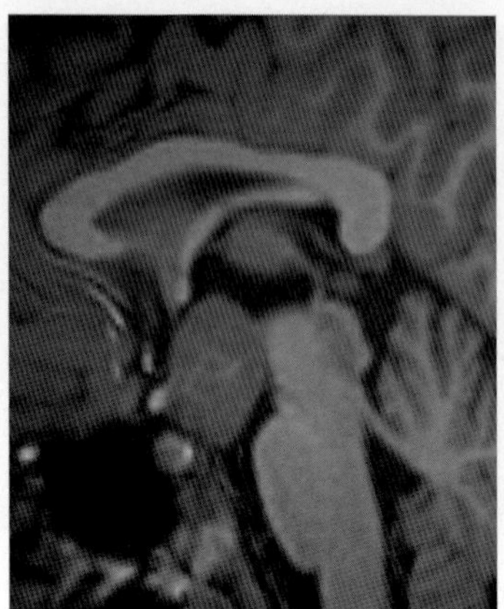

Hamartoma

- Sessile or pedunculated; large or small masses of the hypothalamus
- Follows gray matter signal on all sequences

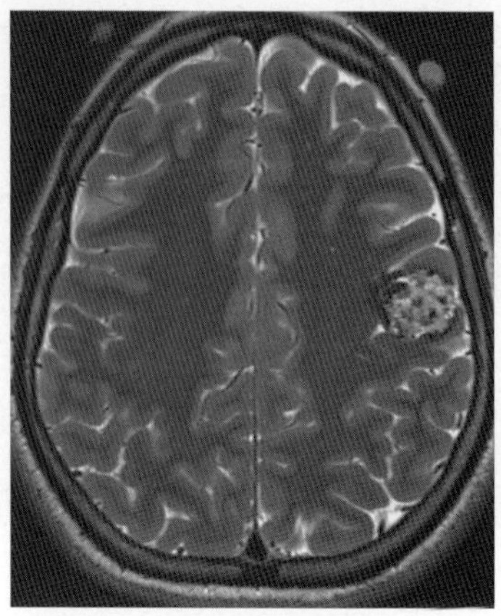

Cavernoma

- Heterogeneous T2W hypointense/T1W hyperintense
- Susceptibility with hemosiderin ring
- Associated with developmental venous anomaly in ~25% of patients

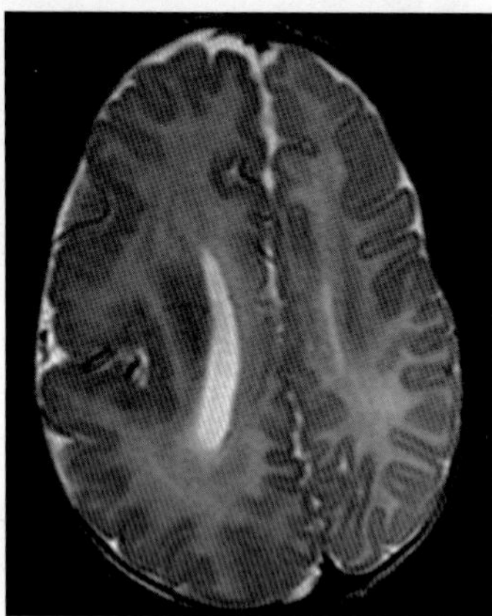

Cortical Malformation

- A wide variety of cortical malformations, including polymicrogyria, heteroropia, lissencephaly, hemimegalencephaly, etc., may cause epilepsy.

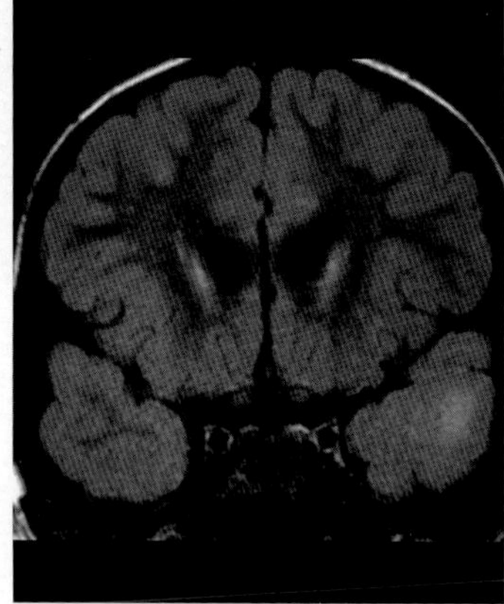

Focal Cortical Dysplasia

- Focal cortical dysplasia (FCD) type I, II and III.

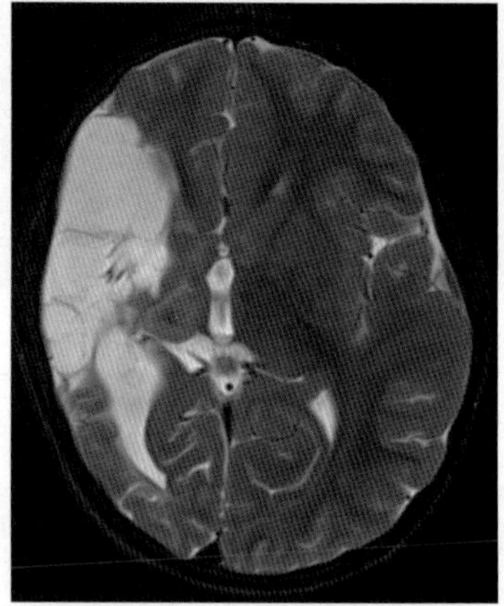

Encephalomalacia

- Cortical insults of any etiology may eventually cause epilepsy, including from prior infection or infarct.

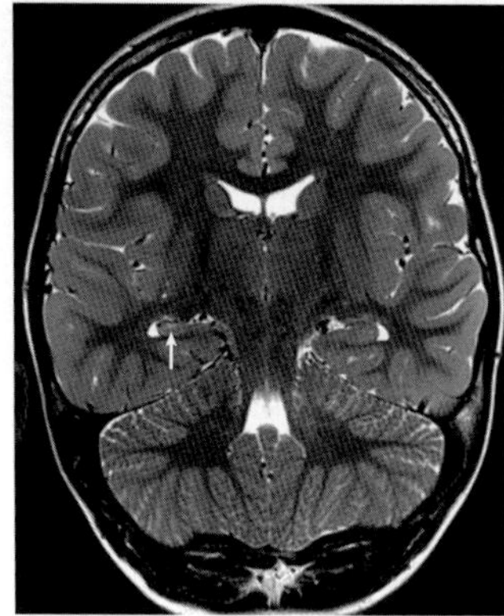

Mesial Temporal Sclerosis

- T2W hyperintensity, volume loss, and loss of internal architecture
- May be unilateral or bilateral
- Ipsilateral volume loss of the fornix and mamillary body can be seen
- Can occur in conjunction with cortical dysplasia

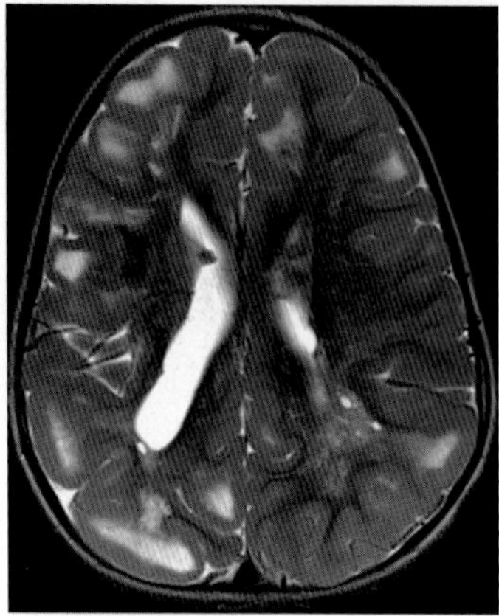

Tuberous Sclerosis

- Cortical tubers, subependymal nodules, giant cell astrocytoma, and retinal hamartomas

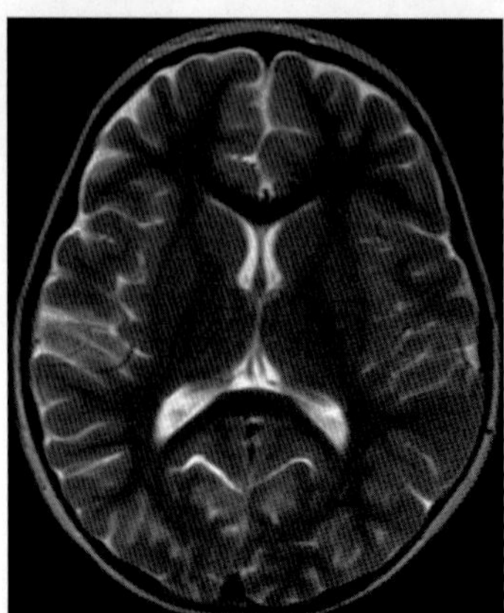

Rasmussen Encephalitis

- Progressive hemispheric volume loss typically involving frontal, temporal and insular lobes with T2 signal abnormality

STATUS EPILEPTICUS FINDINGS

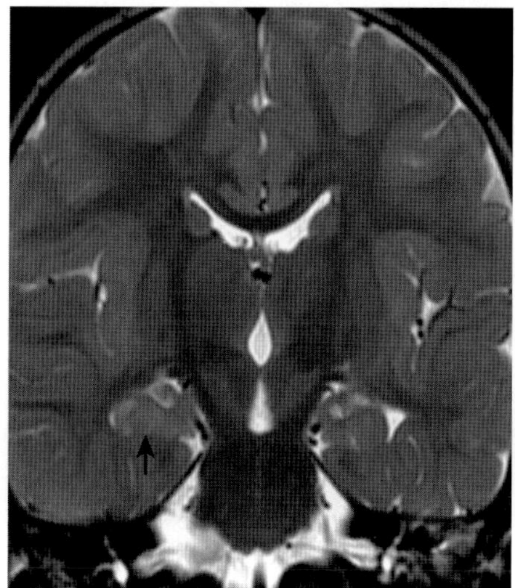

Hippocampal Edema

- T2W hyperintensity with or without restricted diffusion

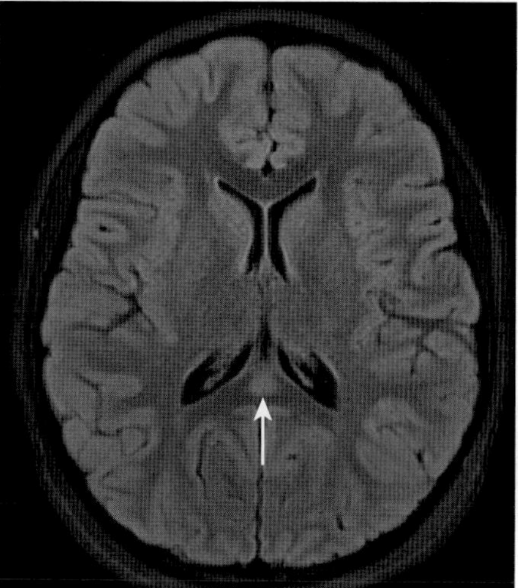

Transient Splenial Lesion

- Reversible T2W hyperintensity with or without restricted diffusion in central splenium

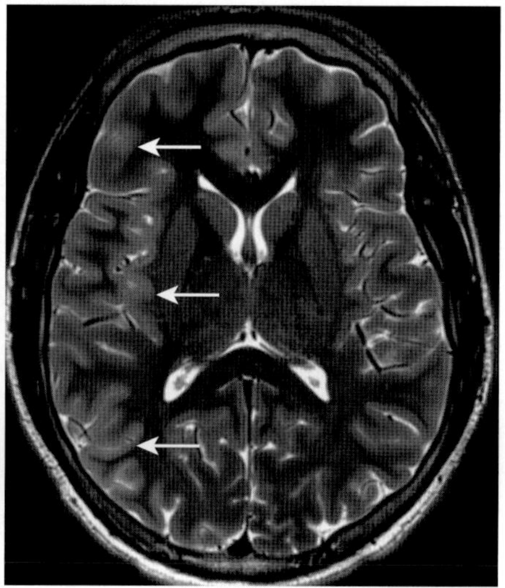

Cortical Edema

- Cortical T2W hyperintensity with regional sulcal effacement; may have restricted diffusion

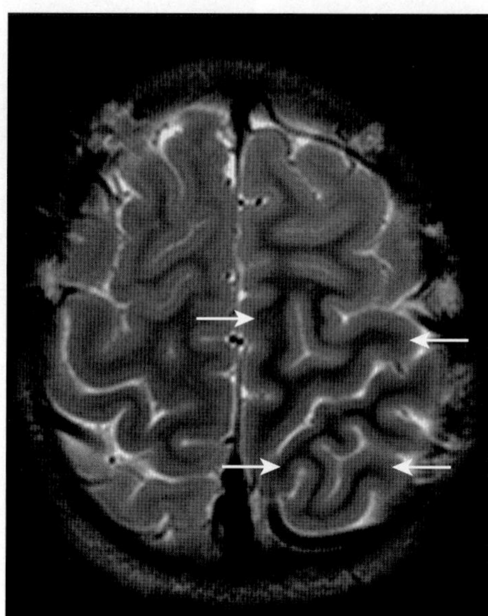

Juxtacortical T2W Hypointensity

- Subcortical T2W hypointensity in the epileptogenic zone; may have restricted diffusion

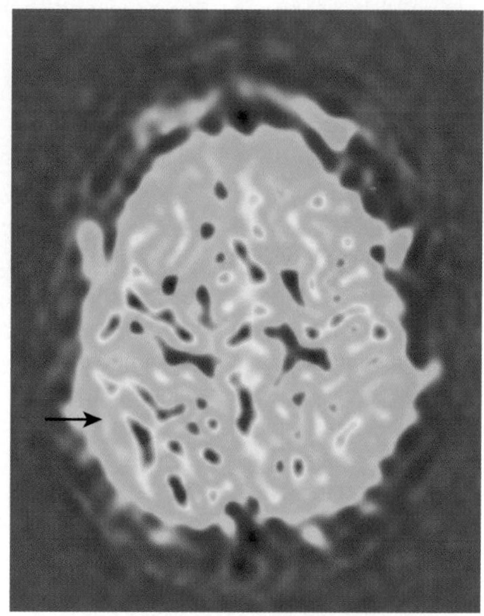

Altered Cerebral Blood Flow

- Increased CBF to the epileptogenic zone in the acute phase and decreased CBF in the subacute phase

PATTERNS OF DYSPLASIAS

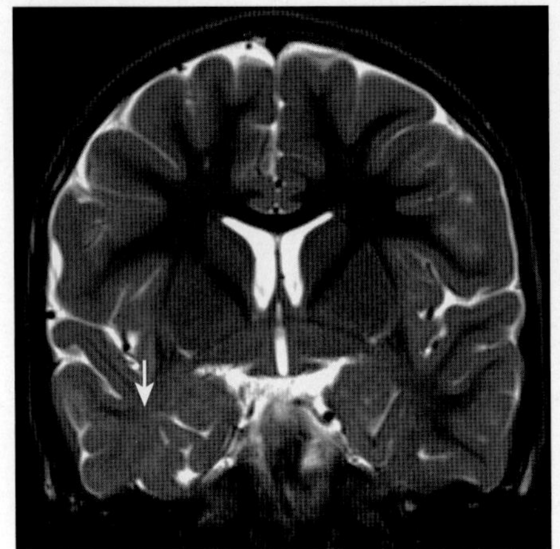

Asymmetric Volume Loss and Myelination

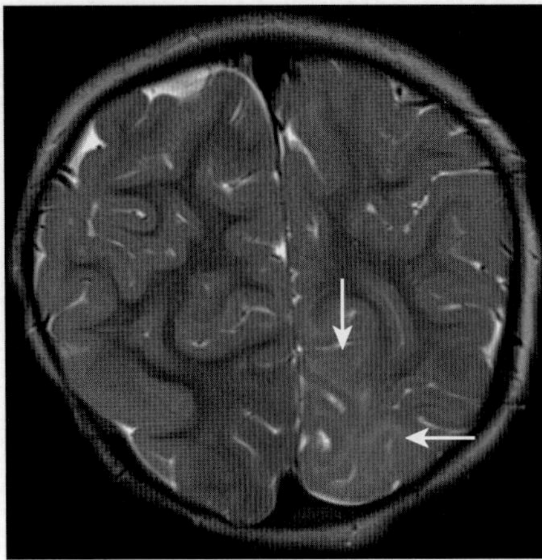

Juxtacortical T2/FLAIR Hyperintensity

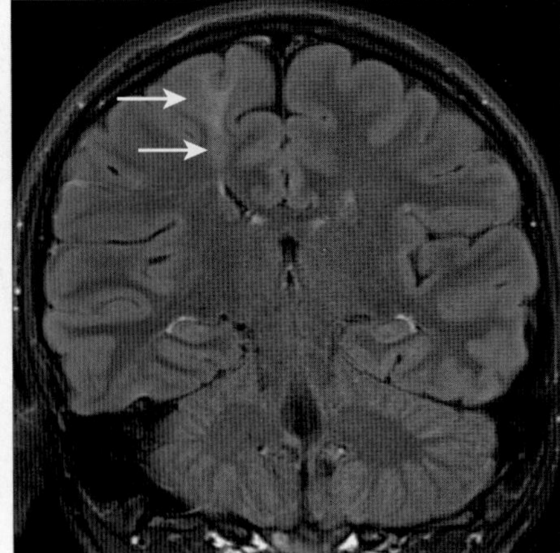

Transmantle FLAIR Hyperintensity

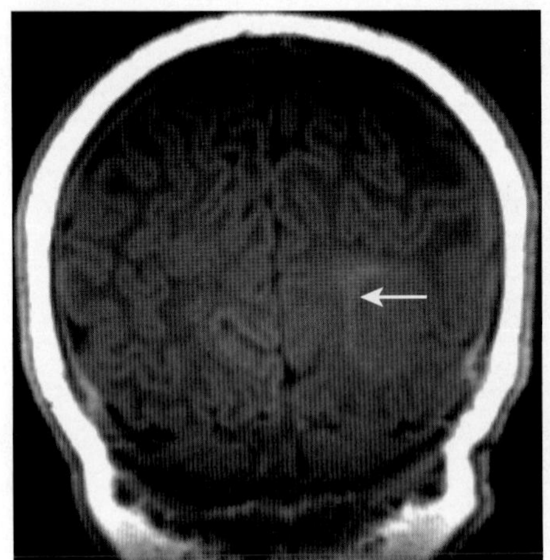

Accelerated Myelination

- Must be correlated with age

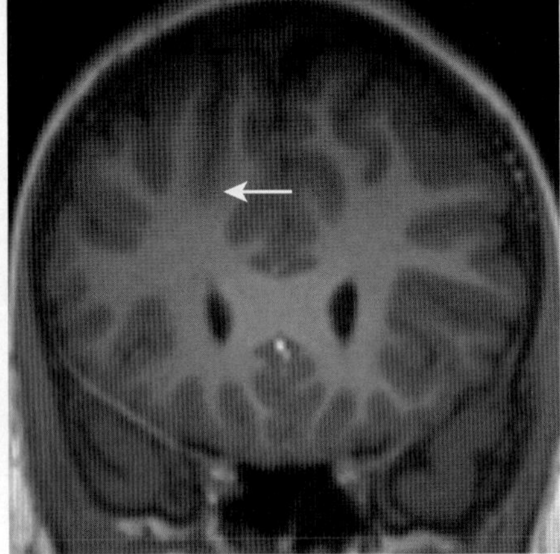

Blurring of Gray-White Matter Junction

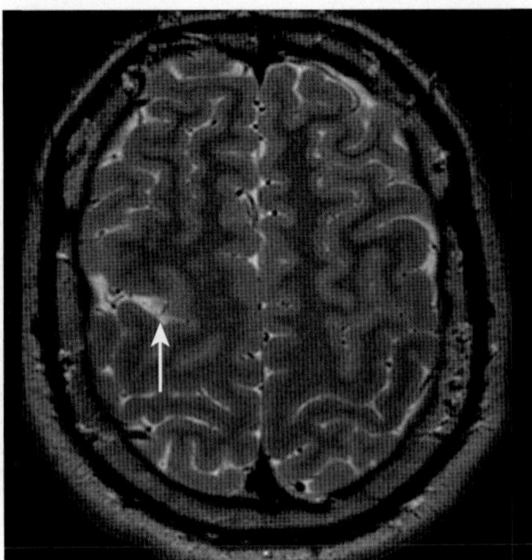

Abnormal Sulcation

ETIOLOGY OF INTRAPARENCHYMAL HEMORRHAGE

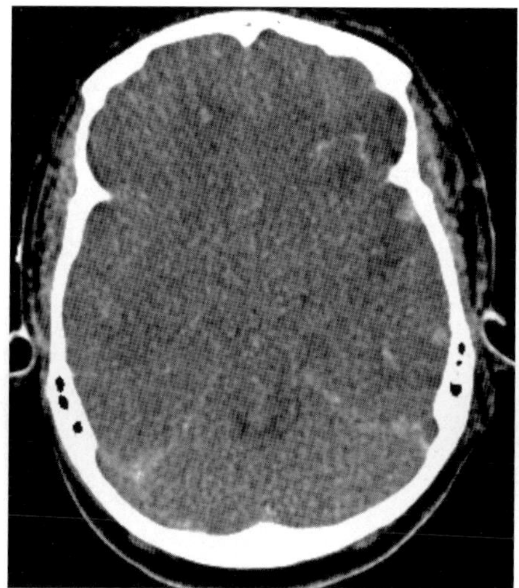

Trauma

- Parenchymal contusions commonly frontal and temporal
- Diffuse axonal injury commonly found in the corpus callosum, subcortical white matter and less commonly the basal ganglia and brainstem

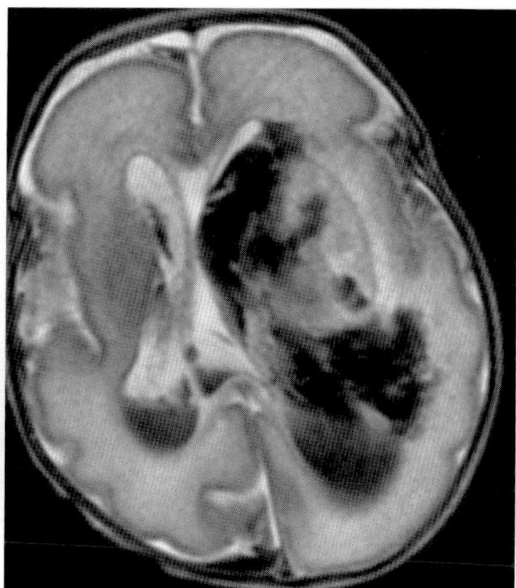

Germinal Matrix Hemorrhage

- Caudothalamic groove hemorrhage which can also lead to intraventricular hemorrhage and periventricular hemorrhagic venous infarcts

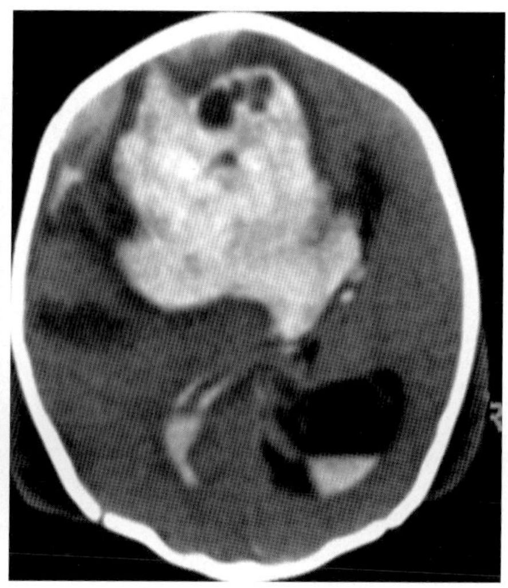

Coagulopathy

- Etiologies include anticoagulation, thrombocytopenia, and disseminated intravascular coaguloapthy.

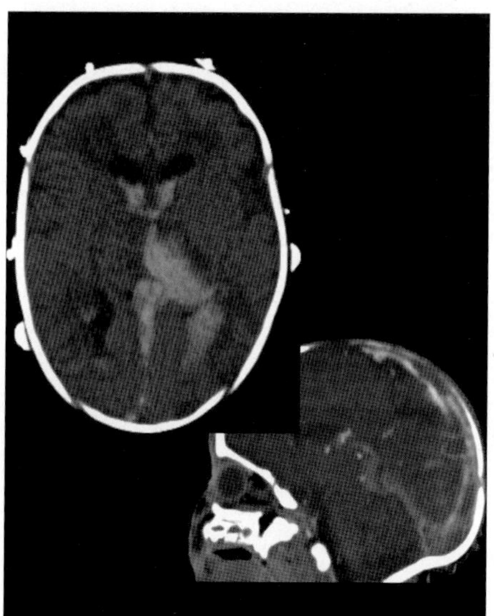

Venous Sinus Thrombosis

- Infection
- Fluid/electrolyte imbalance
- Autoimmune disorders
- Prothrombotic factor (e.g., protein C and S, factor V Leiden, etc.)
- L-asparaginase medication

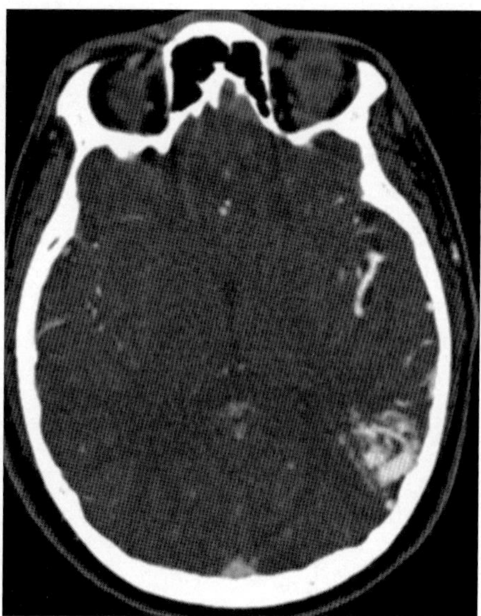

Vascular Malformation

- AVM
- AV fistula
- Cavernoma

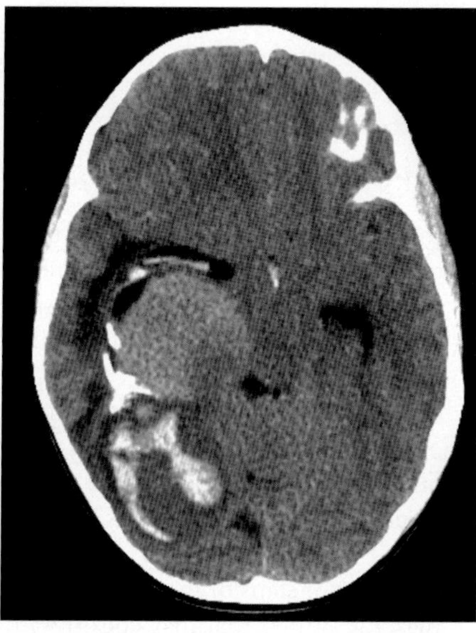

Tumor

- Usually high-grade gliomas but also some low-grade gliomas including JPA and PXA.

ENLARGED EXTRA-AXIAL SPACES

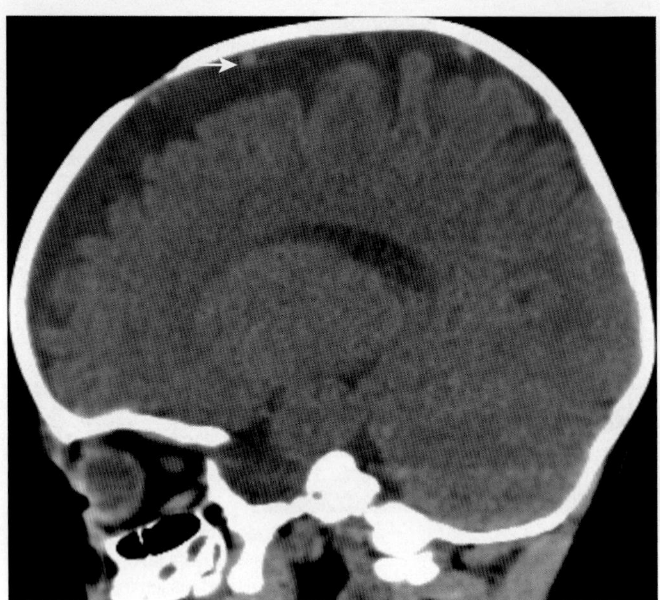

Benign Enlarged Subarachnoid Spaces of Infancy

- Macrocephaly
- Enlarged or normal sulci
- Vessels coursing thru subarachnoid space next to the inner table of the calvarium
- Normal neurodevelopment/neurologic state

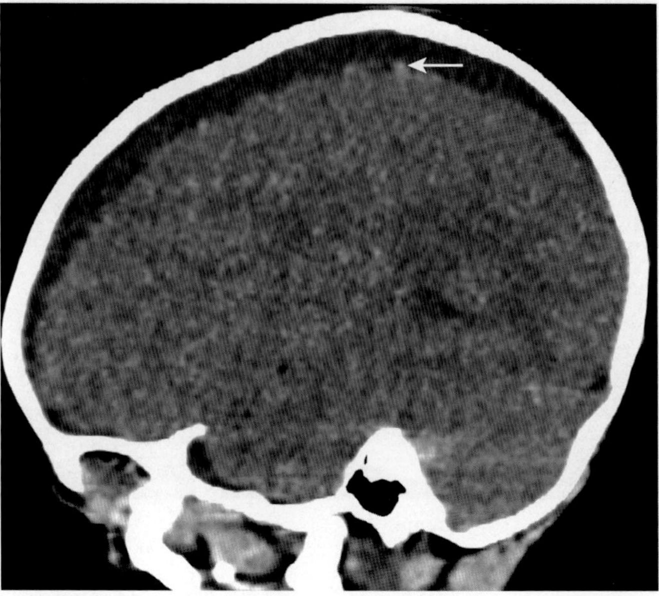

Abusive Head Trauma (AHT)

- +/– Macrocephaly
- Effaced sulci
- Vessels displaced away from the calvarium and onto the cortical surface except for bridging veins
- Variable density of subdural, will mimic BESSI when CSF isodense
- Normal or abnormal neurologic state

Key Points

- Important to determine whether the cortical vessels traverse closely opposed to the inner table of the calvarium, indicating enlarged subarachnoid spaces versus displaced onto the cortical surface of the brain by a subdural fluid collection.
  - Caution: Bridging veins will cross a subdural fluid collection.
- Subdural collections will efface the sulci while benign enlarged subarachnoid spaces of infancy will enlarge the sulci.
- Evaluate for signs of increased intracranial pressure such as diastatic sutures that may coexist with subdural collections.
- Evaluate for additional findings that may suggest trauma.

COMMON FINDINGS IN ABUSIVE HEAD TRAUMA

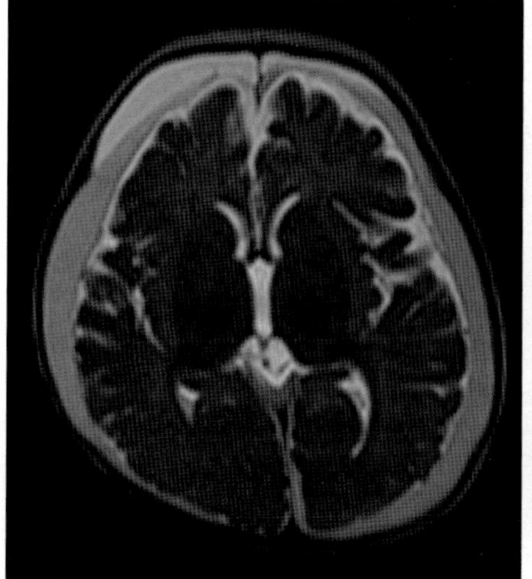

Subdural Hemorrhage

- Variable density/signal intensity; may have blood fluid layer
- Hemosiderin deposition
- Septations suggest chronicity

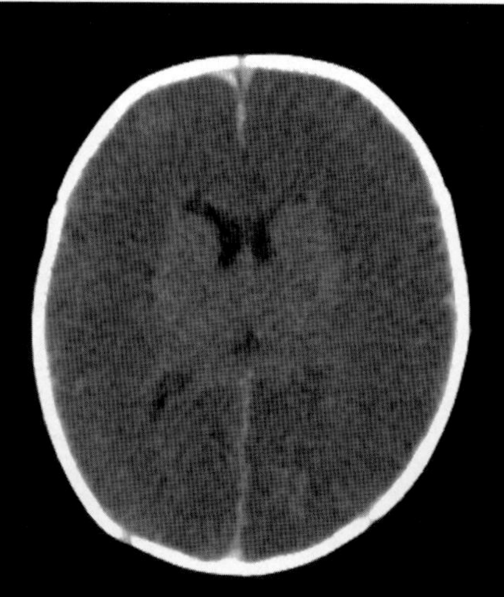

Ischemia

- Mild to moderate: Watershed pattern
- Severe: Cortical and/or central gray
- Posterior fossa uncommon

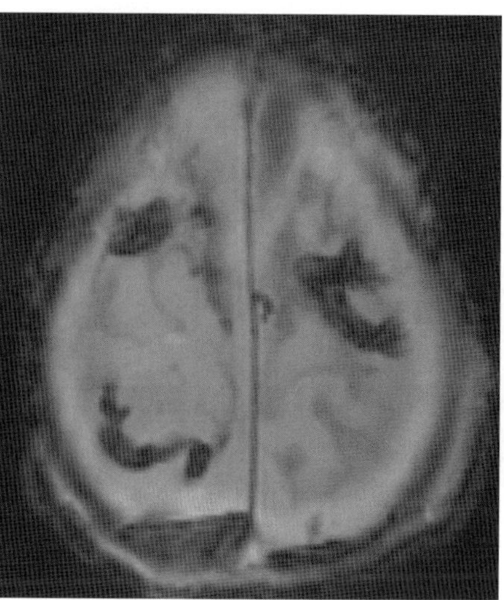

Venous Injury (Cortical Vein or Bridging Vein Thrombosis)

- "Tadpole" or "lollipop" sign
- Predominantly at the vertex
- Linear susceptibility along the veins

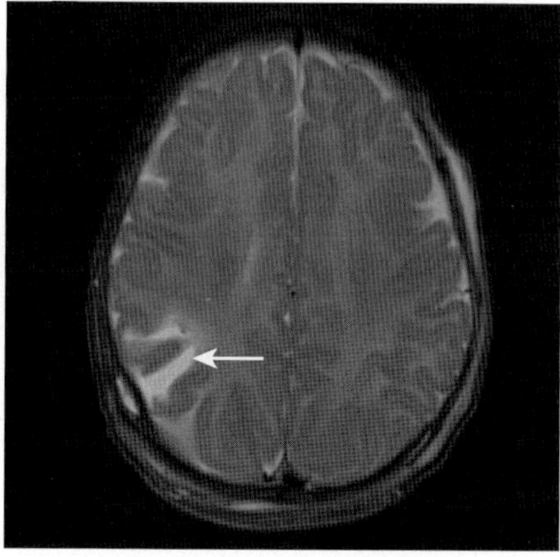

Parenchymal Laceration

- Cortical and subcortical tears of the white matter, often with hemorrhage
- Most common in young infants

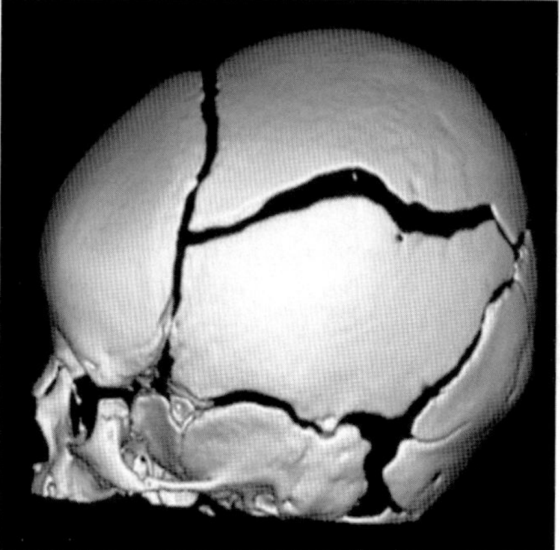

Skull Fracture

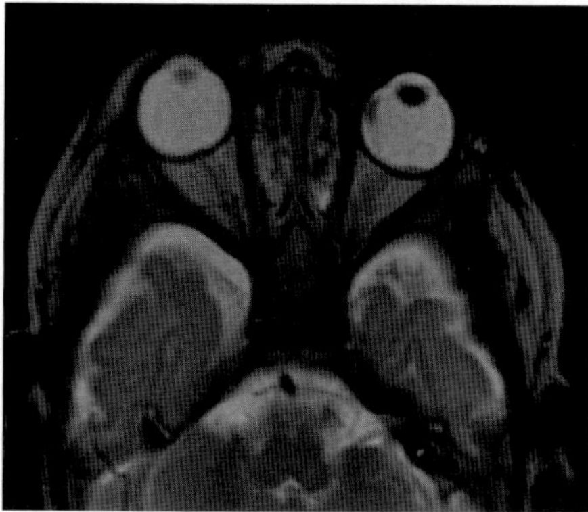

Retinal Hemorrhage

- Best seen on SWI
- Clinical exam more sensitive

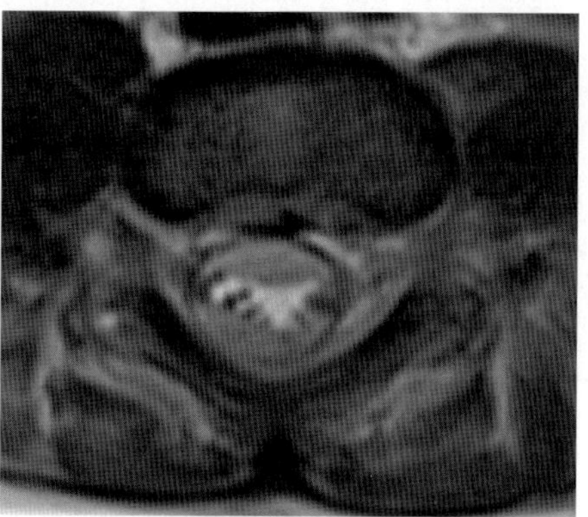

Spinal Subdural Hemorrhage

- Primary or secondary extension from intracranial subdural hemorrhage

ARTERIAL ABNORMALITY

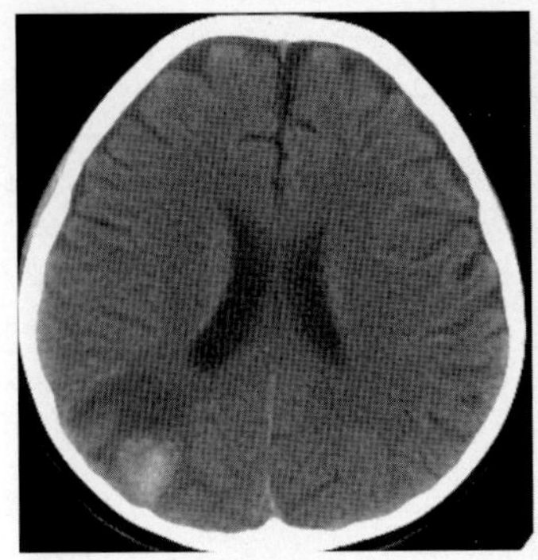
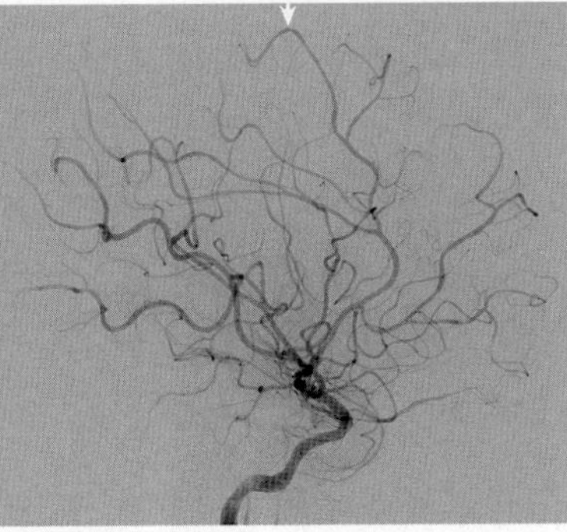

Vasculitis

- Primary: childhood primary angiitis of the central nervous system.
- Secondary: Infection, systemic vasculitides, autoimmune disorders.
- Cortical, central gray matter, and posterior fossa may be involved.
- Stenosis, or alternating stenosis and dilatation; often multifocal with anterior circulation predominance.

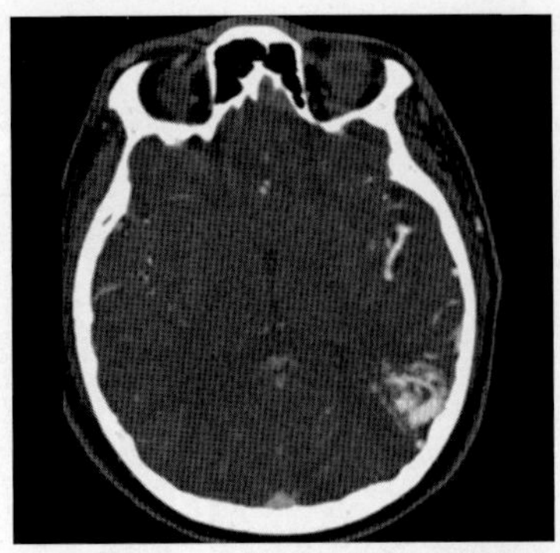

Arteriovenous Malformation (AVM)

- Arteriovenous communication with nidus
- Spetzler-Martin classification used for resectability risk potential

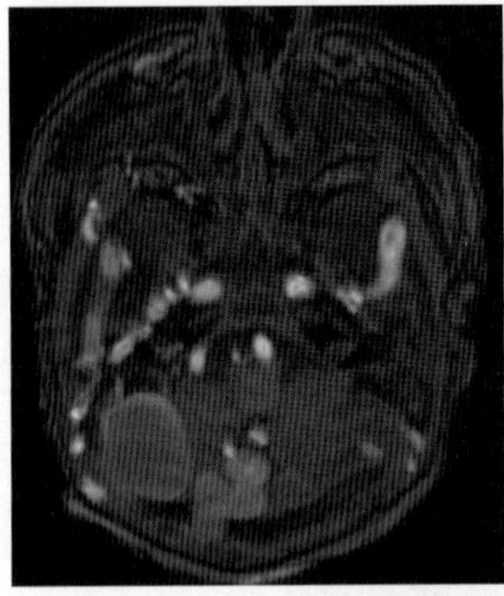
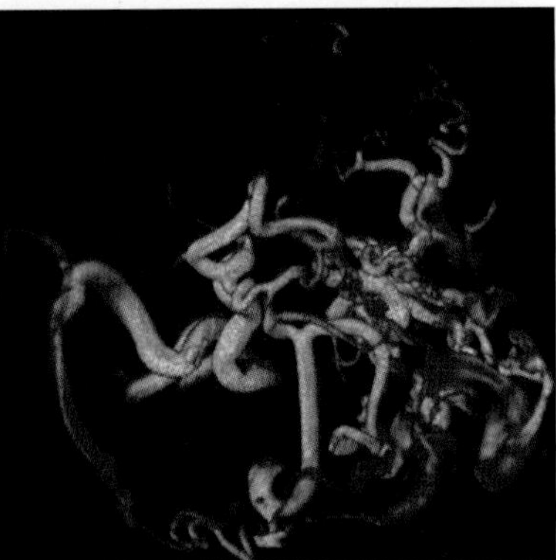

Arteriovenous Fistula

- Arteriovenous communication without nidus
- Most commonly dural and either congenital or acquired
- Enlarged arterial feeders and dural venous outflow

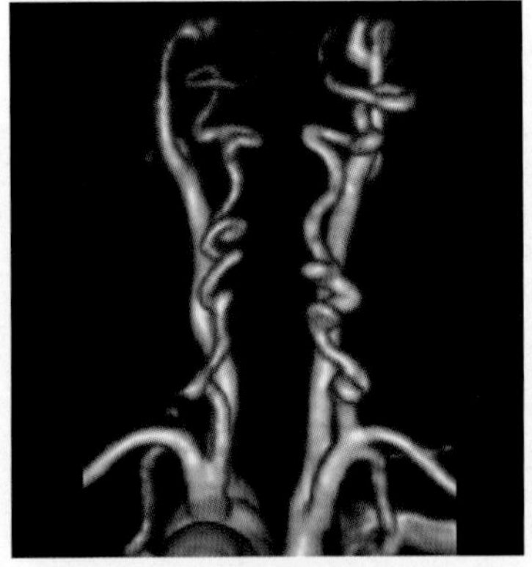

Genetic Disorder

- Tortuous vessels with predisposition for aneurysms and/or stenosis-occlusive disease
- Etiologies: Loeys-Dietz syndrome, sickle cell disease, fibromuscular dysplasia, Ehlers-Danlos syndrome, Marfan syndrome, morning glory syndrome, phakomatoses (NF-1, PHACES), ACTA-2 cerebral arteriopathy

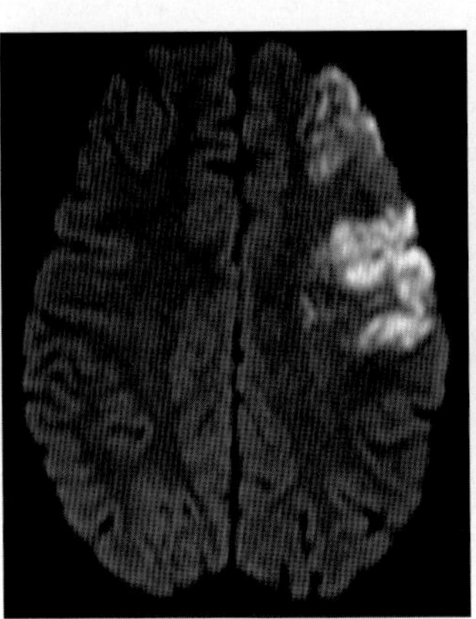
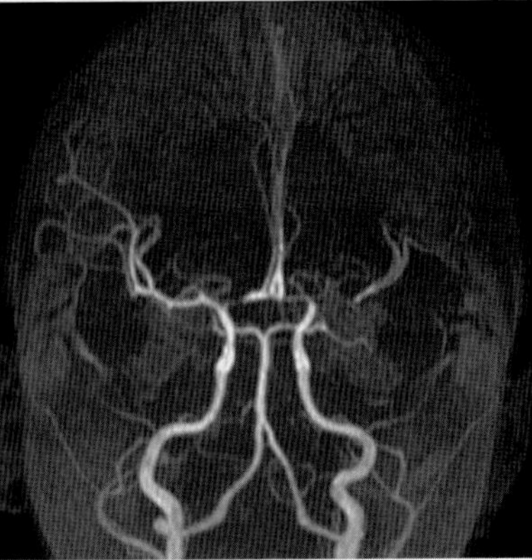

Moyamoya

- Progressive stenosis-occlusive arteriopathy with collateral formation.
- Moyamoya disease is idiopathic.
- Moyamoya syndrome is due to a known etiology, i.e., sickle cell disease, radiation, NF-1, and others.

STROKE ETIOLOGIES

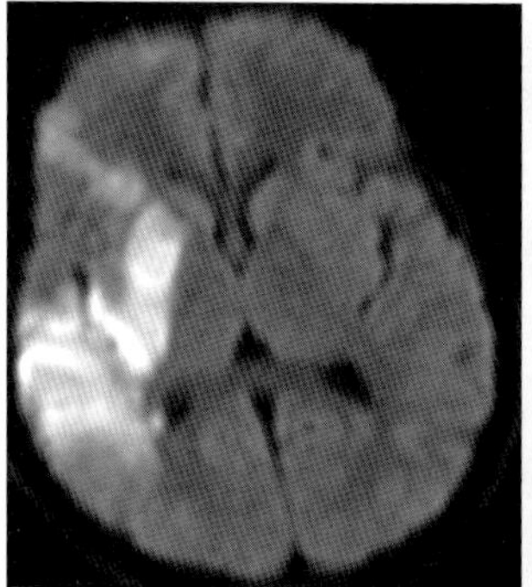
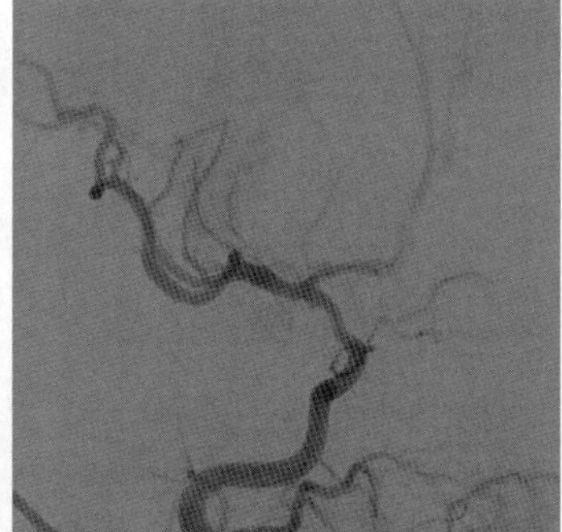

Transient/Focal Cerebral Arteriopathy of Childhood

- Usually involves the distal ICA and proximal MCA and lenticulostriate territory infarct.
- Presents with acute hemiplegia in a previously healthy child.
- Monophasic.
- Presumed inflammatory etiology. Varicella is one established cause.

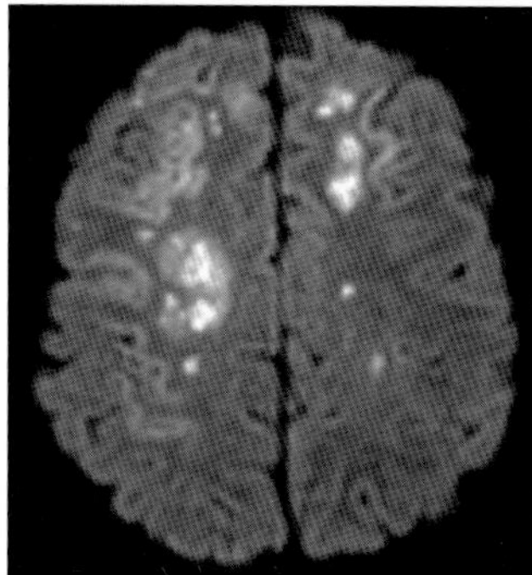
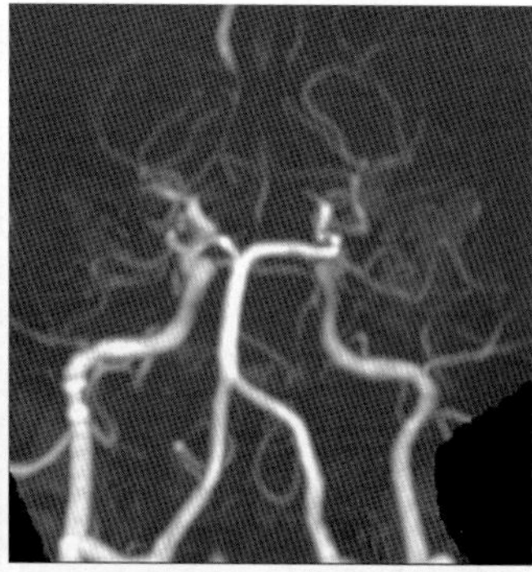

Moyamoya Vasculopathy

- Progressive stenosis-occlusive arteriopathy with collateral formation
- Moyamoya disease versus syndrome (sickle cell, radiation, etc.)

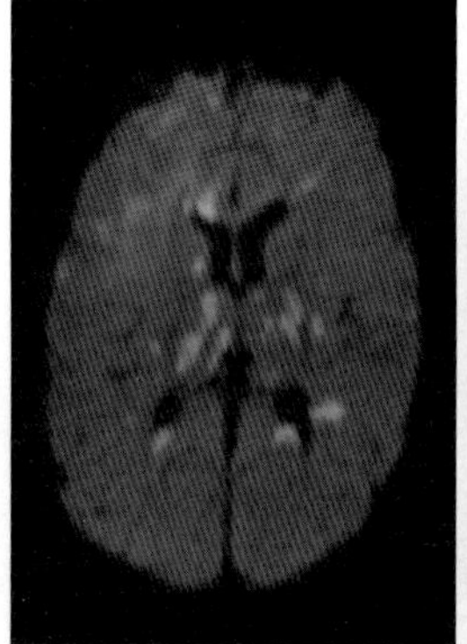
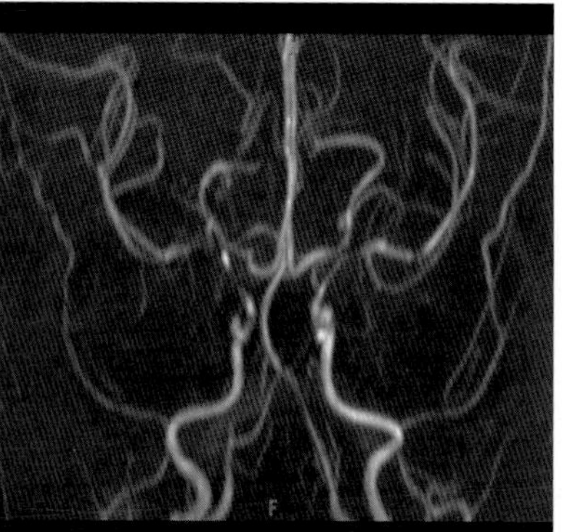

Vasculitis Secondary to Infection

- Causes: Bacterial, tuberculosis, viral, fungal

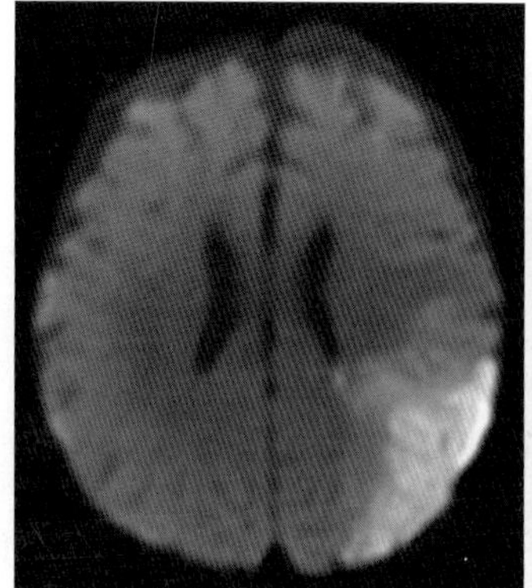
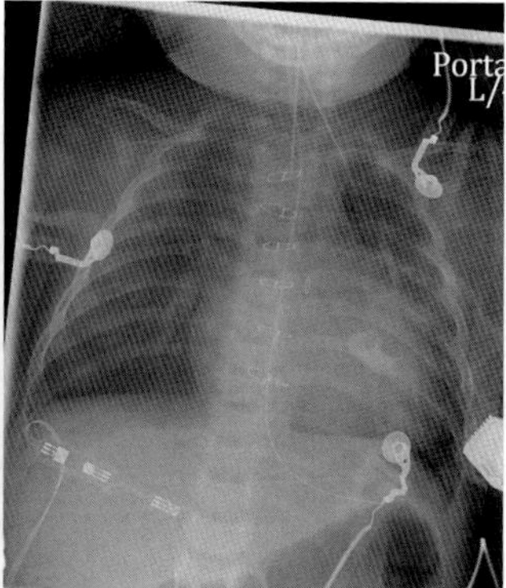

Thromboembolic Stroke

- Congenital heart disease
- Infection (e.g., endocarditis)

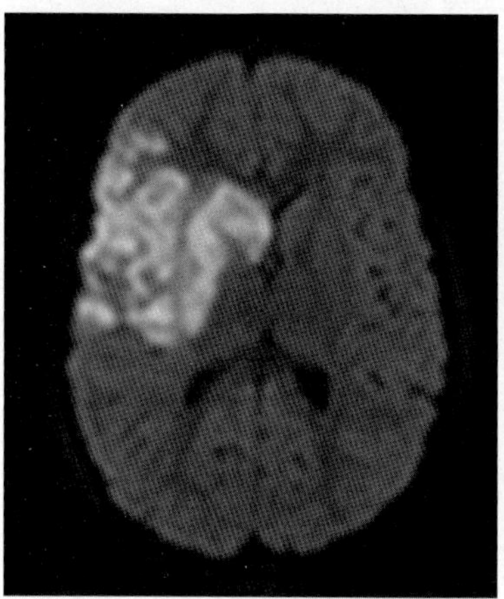
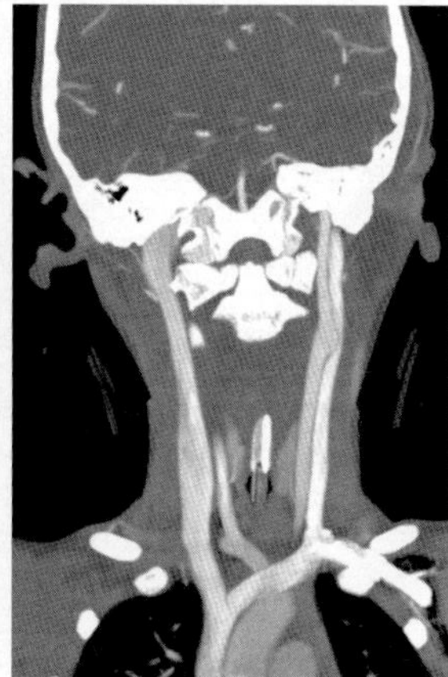

Arterial Dissection due to Trauma

- Penetrating versus blunt cerebrovascular injury

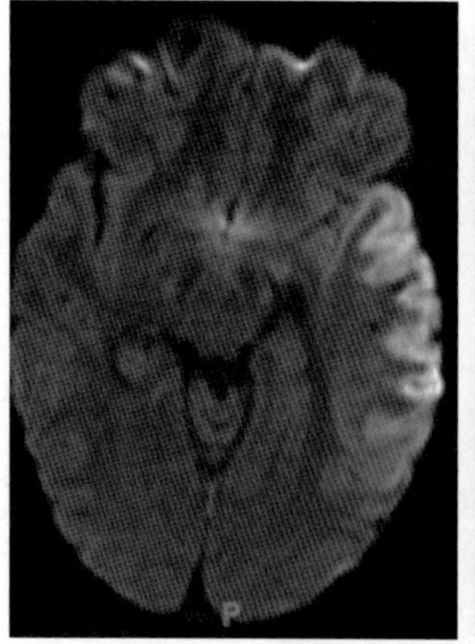
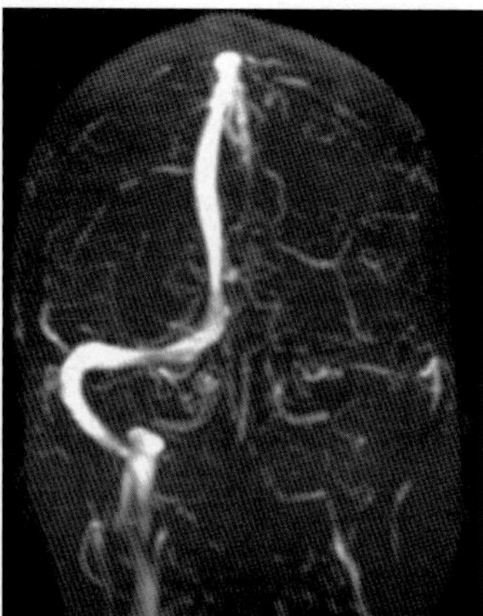

Venous Sinus Thrombosis

- Venous infarct from dural and/or cortical venous occlusion resulting in hemorrhage and/or ischemia.
- Superior medial frontal and parietal ischemia can occur from superior sagittal sinus thrombosis.
- Lateral temporal lobe ischemia can occur with vein of Labbe and/or transverse sinus thrombosis.
- Thalamic and basal ganglia ischemia can occur with internal cerebral vein thrombosis.

ASL PERFUSION ABNORMALITY

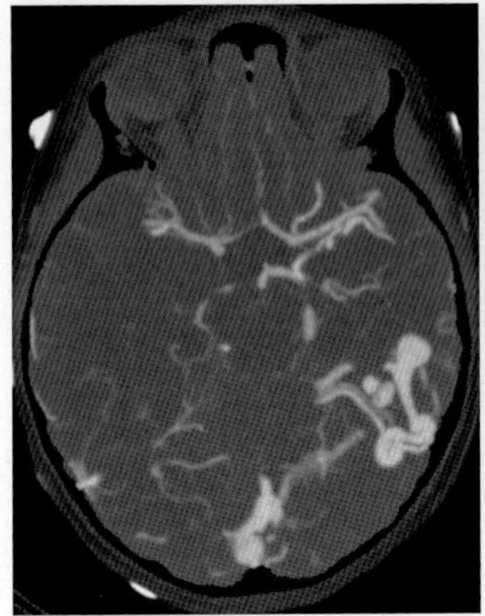
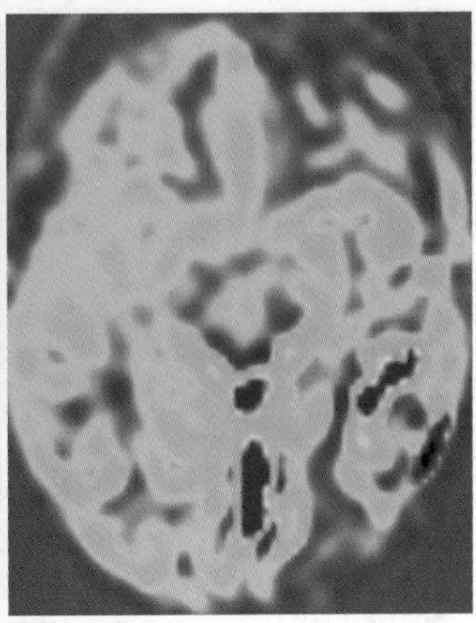

Vascular Malformation

- Increased flow is identified in the AVM or AVF, as well as the location of the early draining veins.

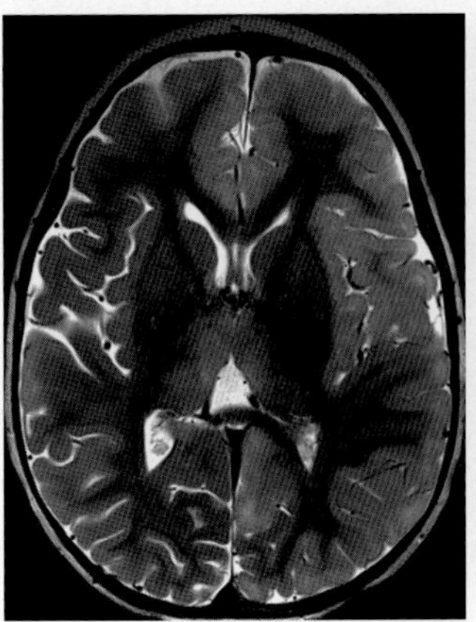
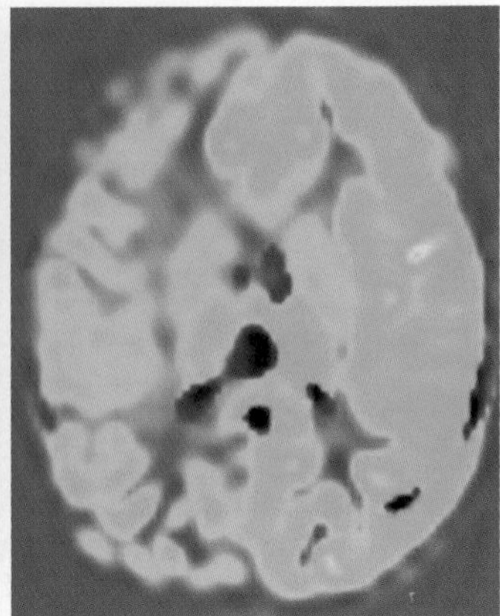

Seizure Activity

- Acute seizure activity can show increased CBF (as shown here in a patient with POLG mutation on the left side). Imaging ~24 hours after seizure activity can show reduced CBF to the seizure region.

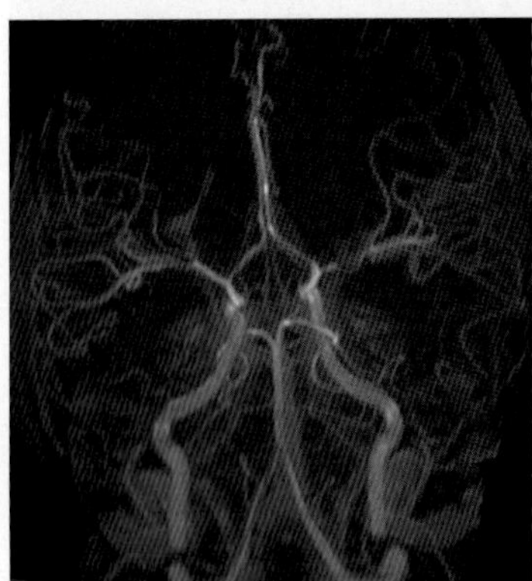
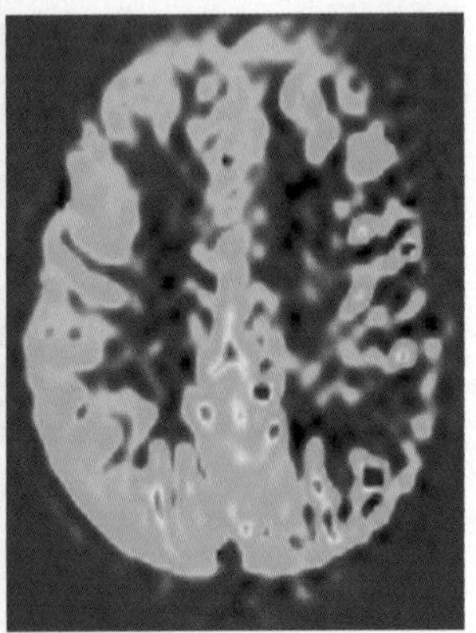

Ischemia

- Ischemic regions can show decreased CBF (shown here in the left lateral frontal and parietal lobes due to radiation vasculopathy of the left MCA). Acute infarcted areas can also show increased CBF due to reperfusion.

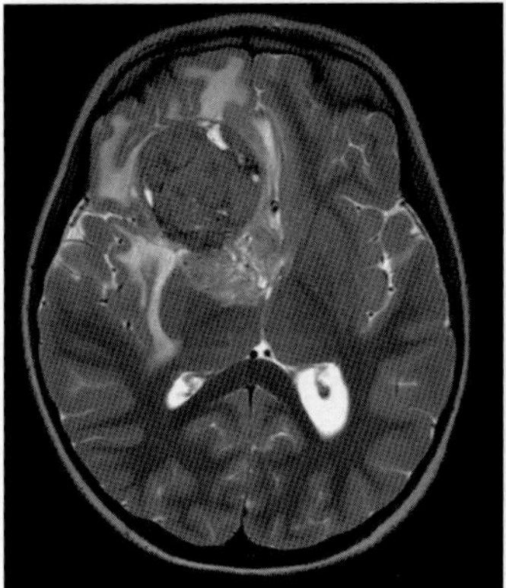
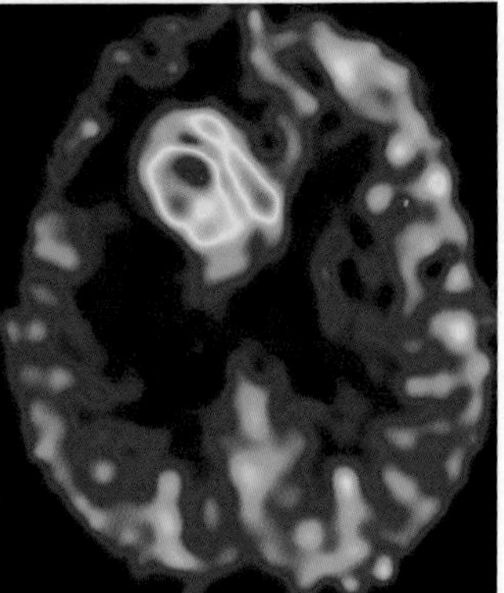

Brain Tumors

- In general, high-grade pediatric brain tumors have a trend of elevated CBF, while low-grade tumors demonstrate low CBF. Perfusion imaging in conjunction with conventional MRI sequences including DWI are helpful in differentiating low-grade and high-grade tumors.

BASAL GANGLIA ABNORMALITY

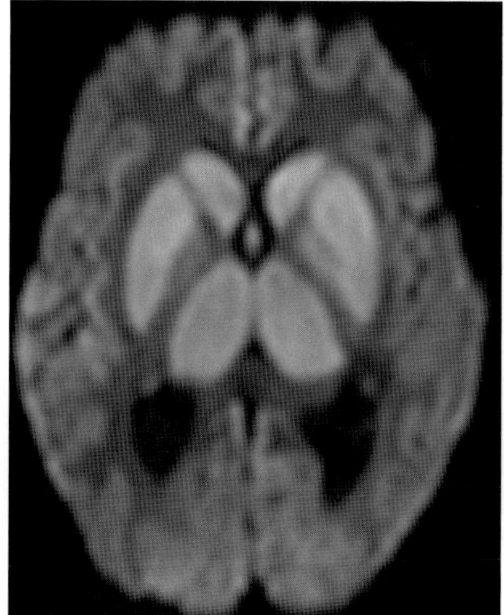

Hypoxic Ischemic

- Symmetric restricted diffusion usually with thalamic involvement
- Severe hypoxia and hypoperfusion

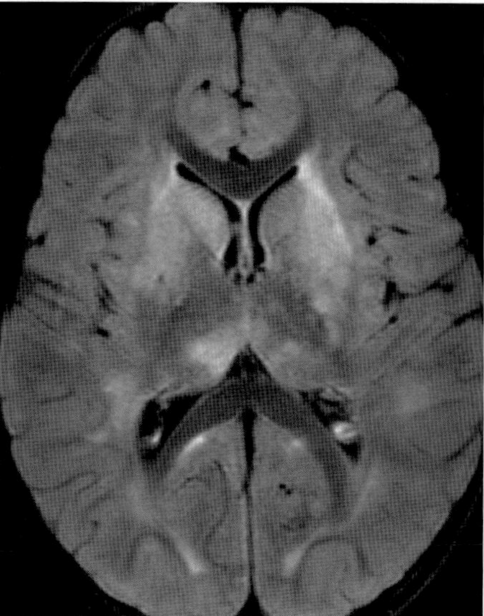

ADEM

- Symmetric or asymmetric involvement often without enhancement.
- White matter demyelinating lesions.
- The spinal cord may be involved.
- CSF helpful in identifying acute inflammation.

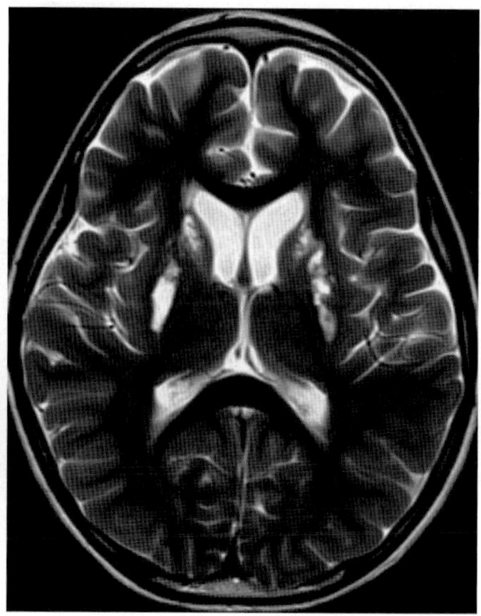

Metabolic Disorders

- Nonenhancing with or without restricted diffusion
- Symmetric
- Certain parts of the basal ganglia involved based on the disorder helps in diagnosis

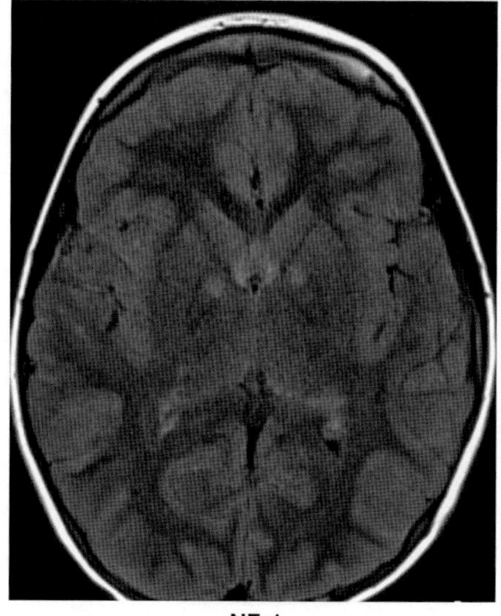

NF-1

- Myelin vacuolization

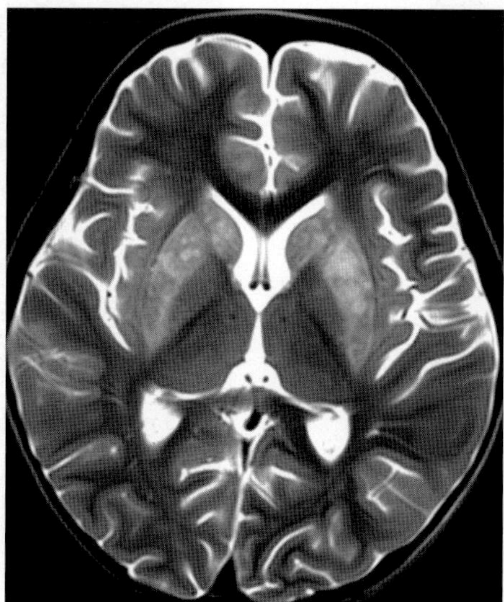

Encephalitis

- Viral or autoimmune
- Typically without restricted diffusion or enhancement

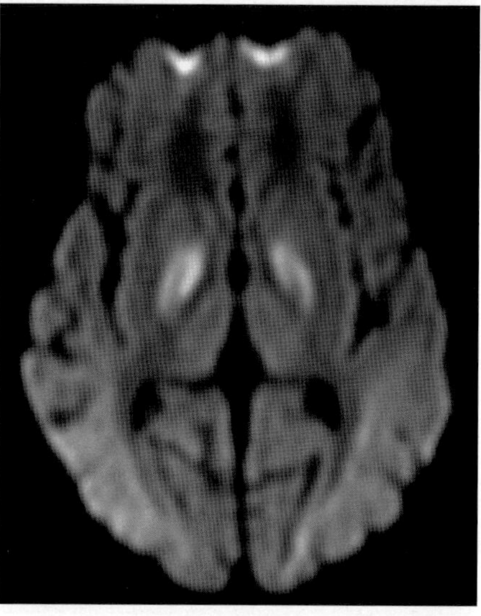

Mitochondrial

- Symmetric basal ganglia ischemia often sparing portions of the basal ganglia.

COMMON PHAKOMATOSES

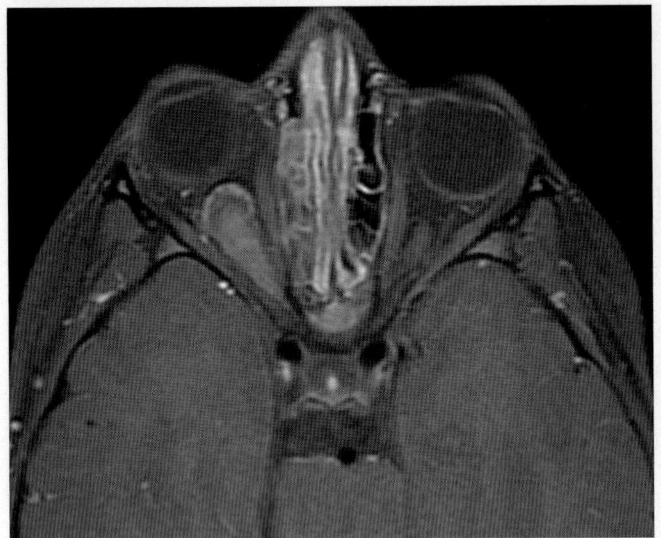

NF-1

- Optic pathway glioma
- Soft tissue neurofibromas and plexiform neurofibromas
- Myelin vacuolization
- Sphenoid wing dysplasia
- Moyamoya
- Buphthalmos

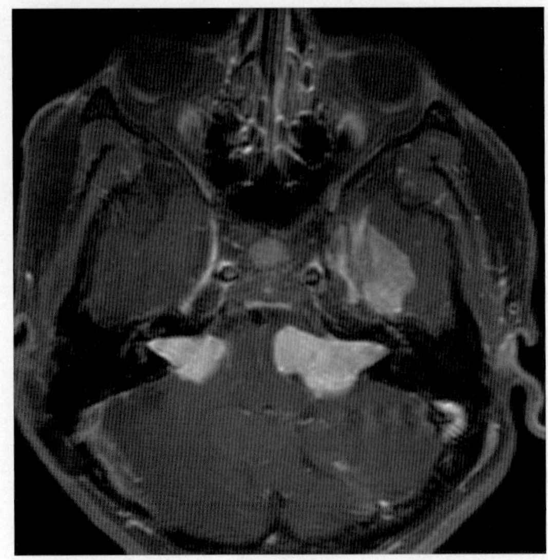

NF-2

- Meningiomas
- Schwannomas
- Ependymomas

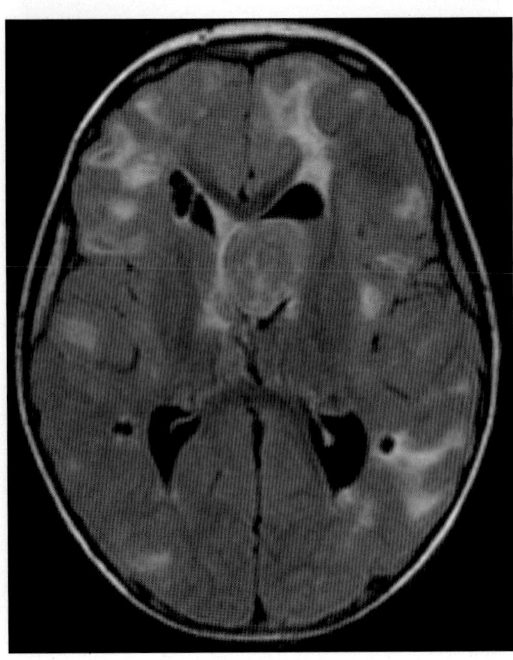

Tuberous Sclerosis

- Cortical tubers
- Subependymal nodules
- Retinal hamartoma
- Moyamoya
- Renal angiomyolipoma
- Lung cysts
- Cardiac rhabdomyoma

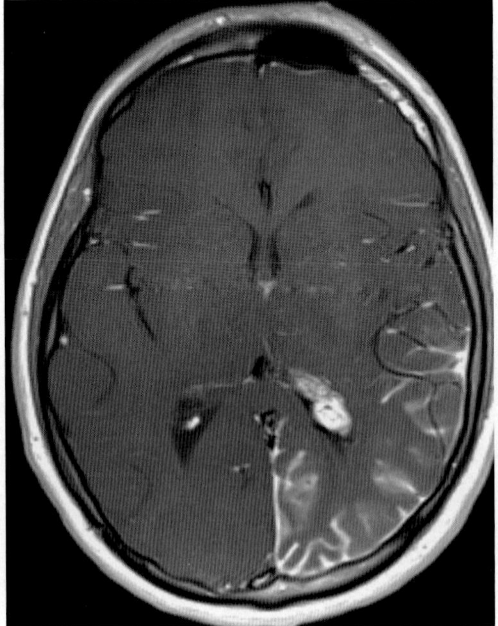

Sturge-Weber

- Port wine stain
- Pial angiomatosis
- Cortical atrophy
- Choroid plexus enlargement
- Calvarial thickening
- Choroidal angioma
- Glaucoma

POSTERIOR FOSSA INFECTION

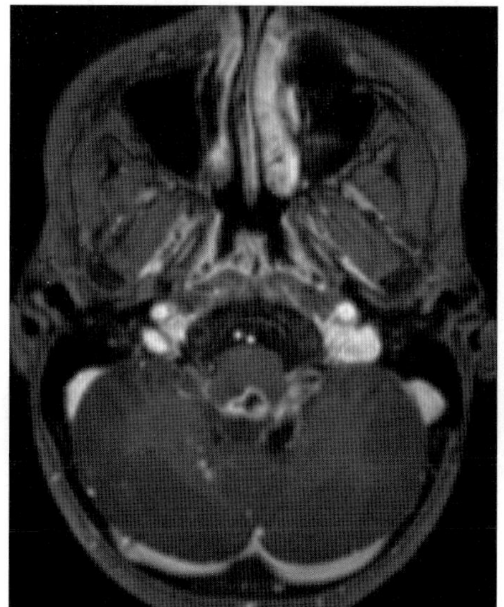

Fungal Infection

- Rare; typically immunocompromised
- Leptomeningitis
- Ring enhancing lesions
- Abscess
- May be invasive

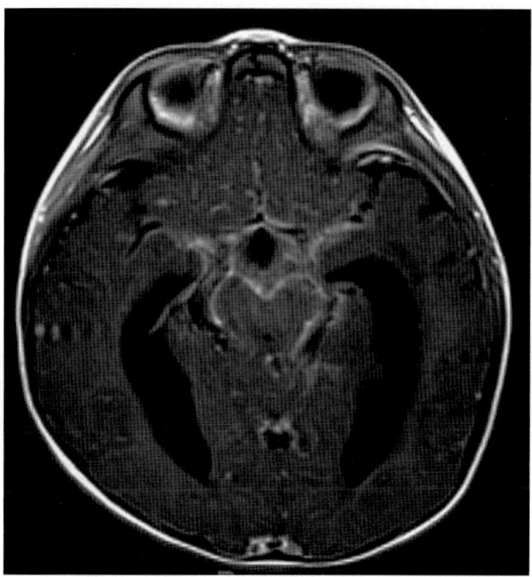

Tuberculosis

- Basal meningitis
- Tuberculomas (leptomeningeal, parenchymal)
- Vasculitis with secondary infarcts

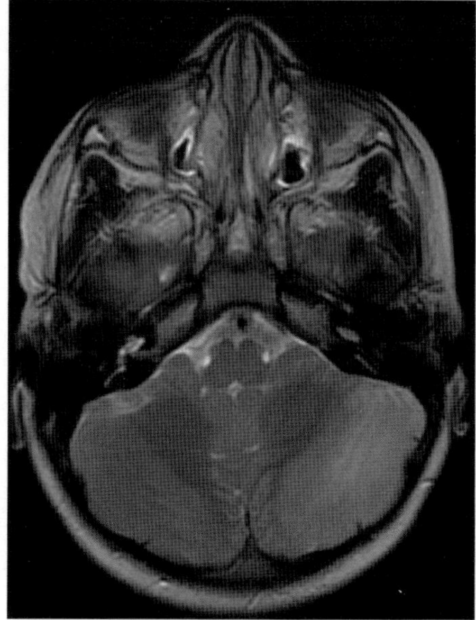

Cerebellitis

- Parainfectious, less commonly infectious
- T2W hyperintensity with or without restricted diffusion
- No enhancement is most common. May have regional mild leptomeningeal enhancement
- Bilateral or unilateral
- May cause acute hydrocephalus

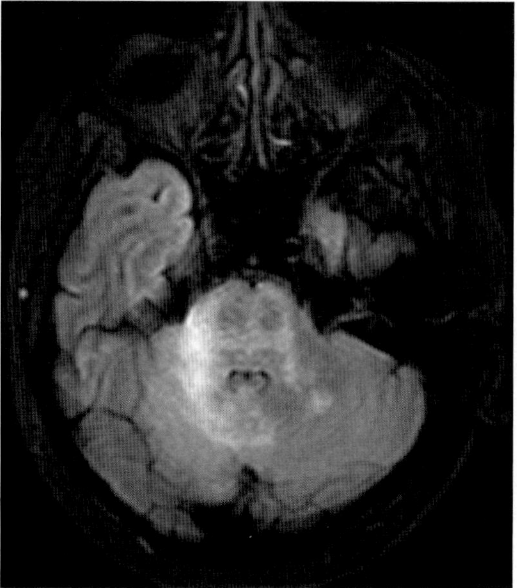

Rhombencephalitis

- Edema/inflammation of the brainstem and cerebellum
- Variety of infections including viral, classically listeria (rare)
- Autoimmune and paraneoplastic disorders

METABOLIC DISORDER WHITE MATTER PATTERN

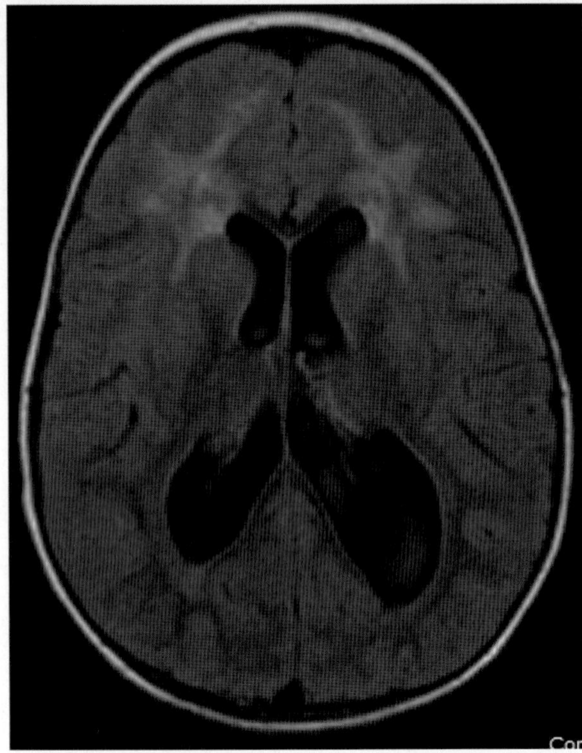

Anterior White Matter Predominant

- Alexander disease

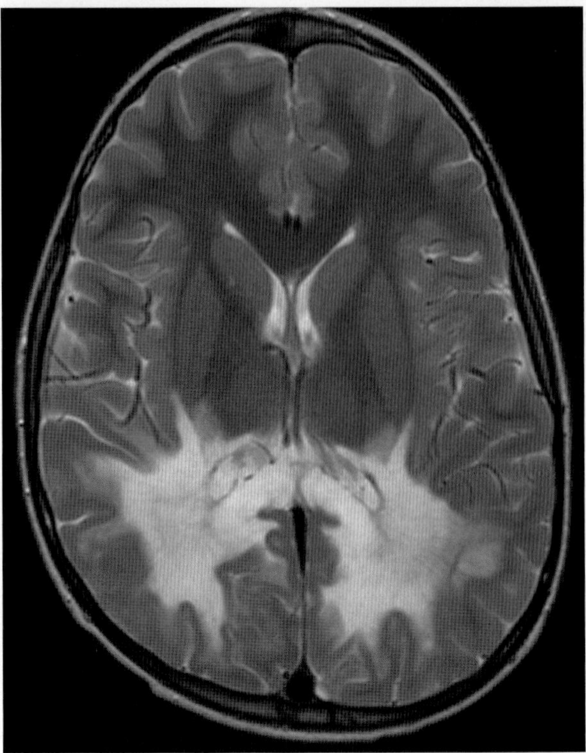

Posterior White Matter Predominant

- X-linked adrenoleukodystrophy

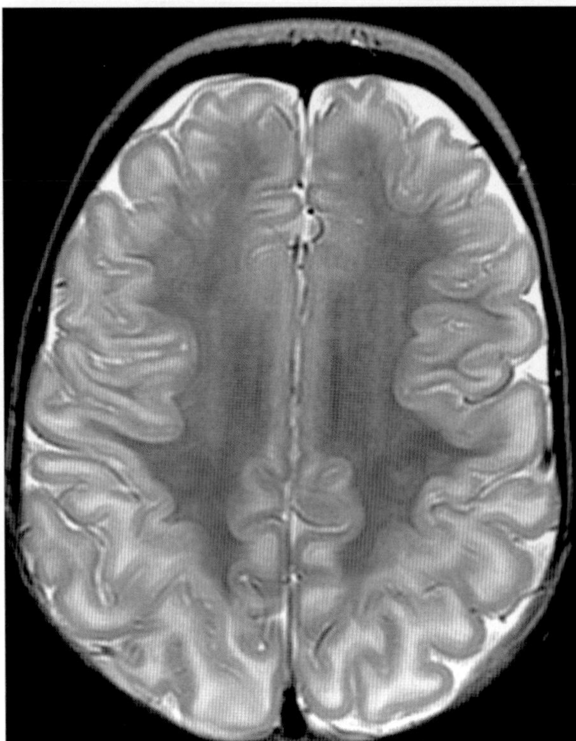

Peripheral White Matter Predominant

1. Canavan disease
2. L-2-hydroxy glutaric aciduria

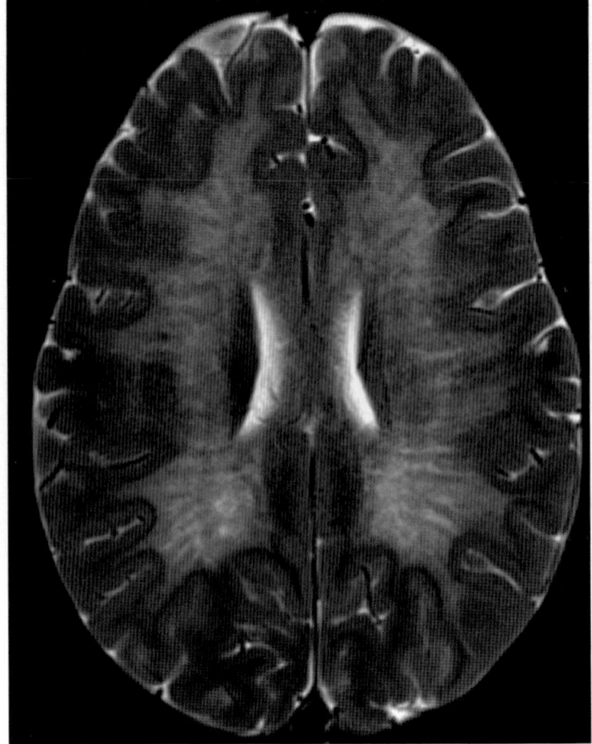

Deep White Matter Predominant

1. Krabbe
2. Metachromatic
3. Lowe
4. Mucopolysaccharidoses

METABOLIC DISORDER

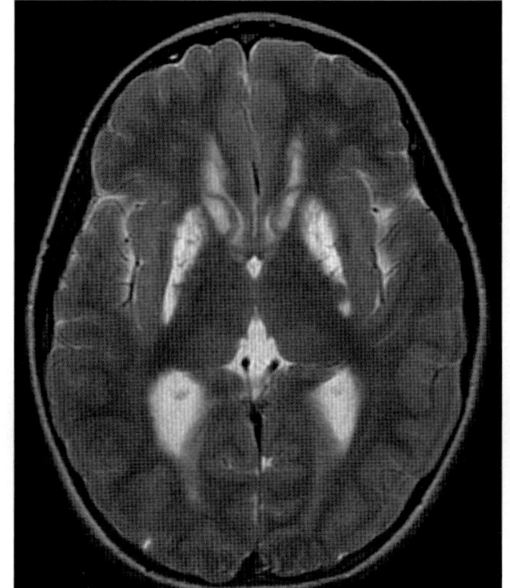

Basal Ganglia

1. Mitochondrial
2. Organic acidurias: Ethylmalonic, methylmalonic, and propionic aciduria

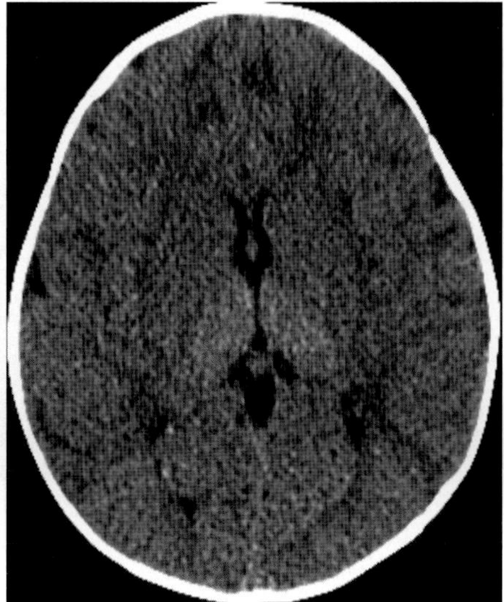

Thalamic

1. Krabbe
2. GM1 and GM2 gangliosidosis
3. Wilson disease
4. Thiamine deficiency

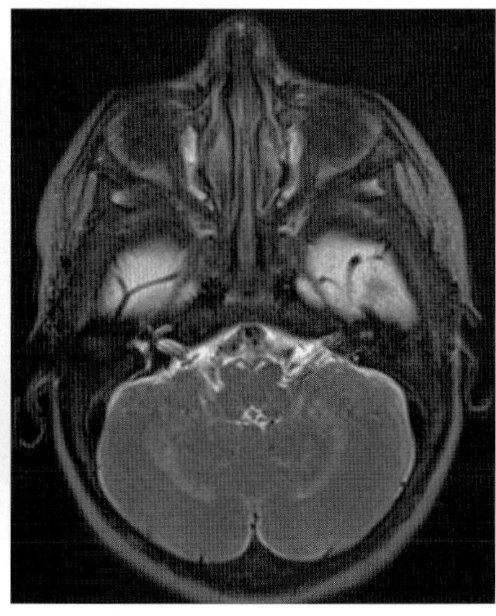

Cerebellar

1. Krabbe
2. X-linked adrenoleukodystrophy
3. Maple syrup urine disease
4. Nonketotic hyperglycinemia

SPECTROSCOPY PATTERNS OF METABOLIC DISORDERS

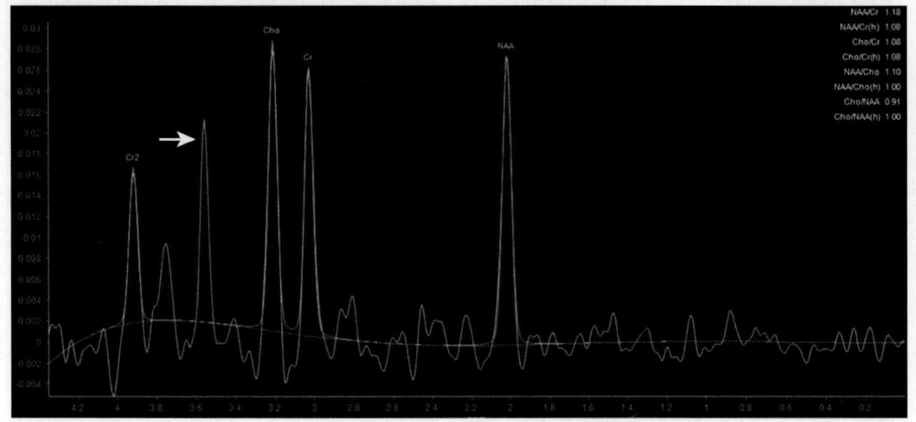

Nonketotic Hyperglycinemia

- Elevated peak at 3.6 ppm superimposed at myo-inositol peak at short TE.
- Elevated peak persistent at 3.6 ppm at long, or intermediate TE confirms glycine.

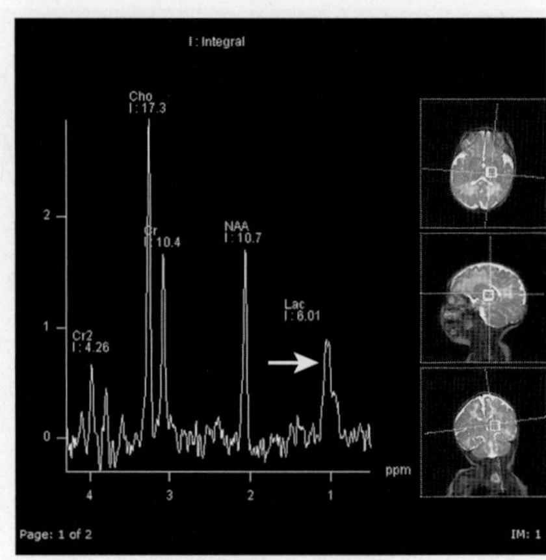

Maple Syrup Urine

- Branched chain amino acids at 0.9 ppm on short and long TEs

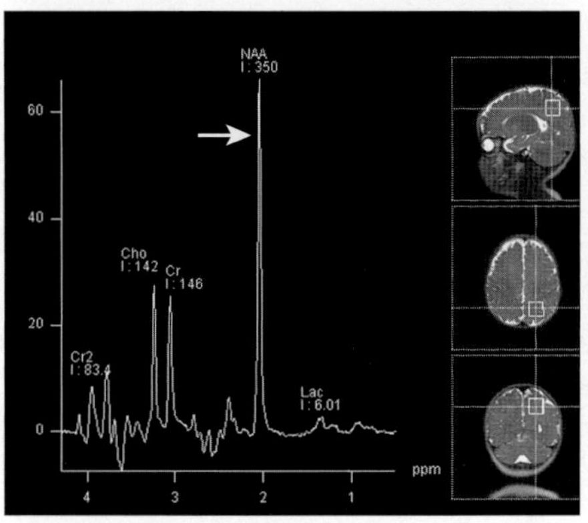

Canavans

- Elevated NAA

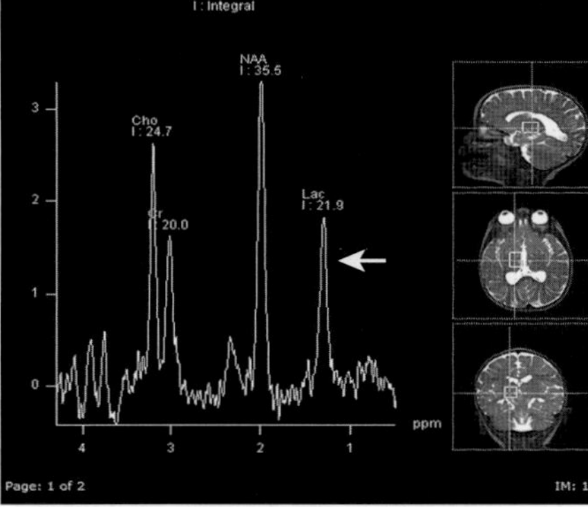

Mitochondrial

- Elevated lactate

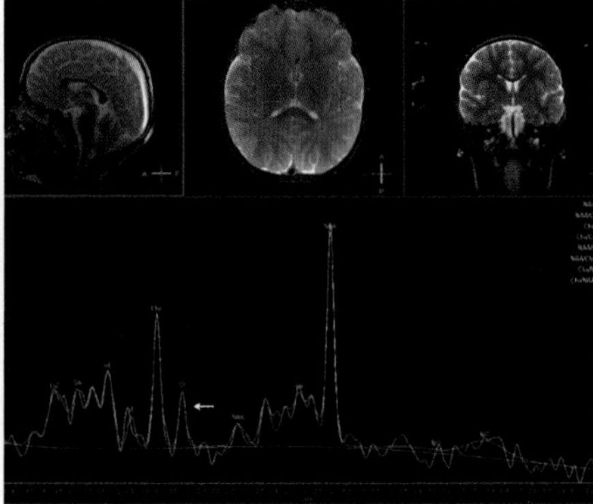

Creatine Deficiency

- Absent or decreased creatine peak

POSTERIOR FOSSA TUMOR ADC PATTERN

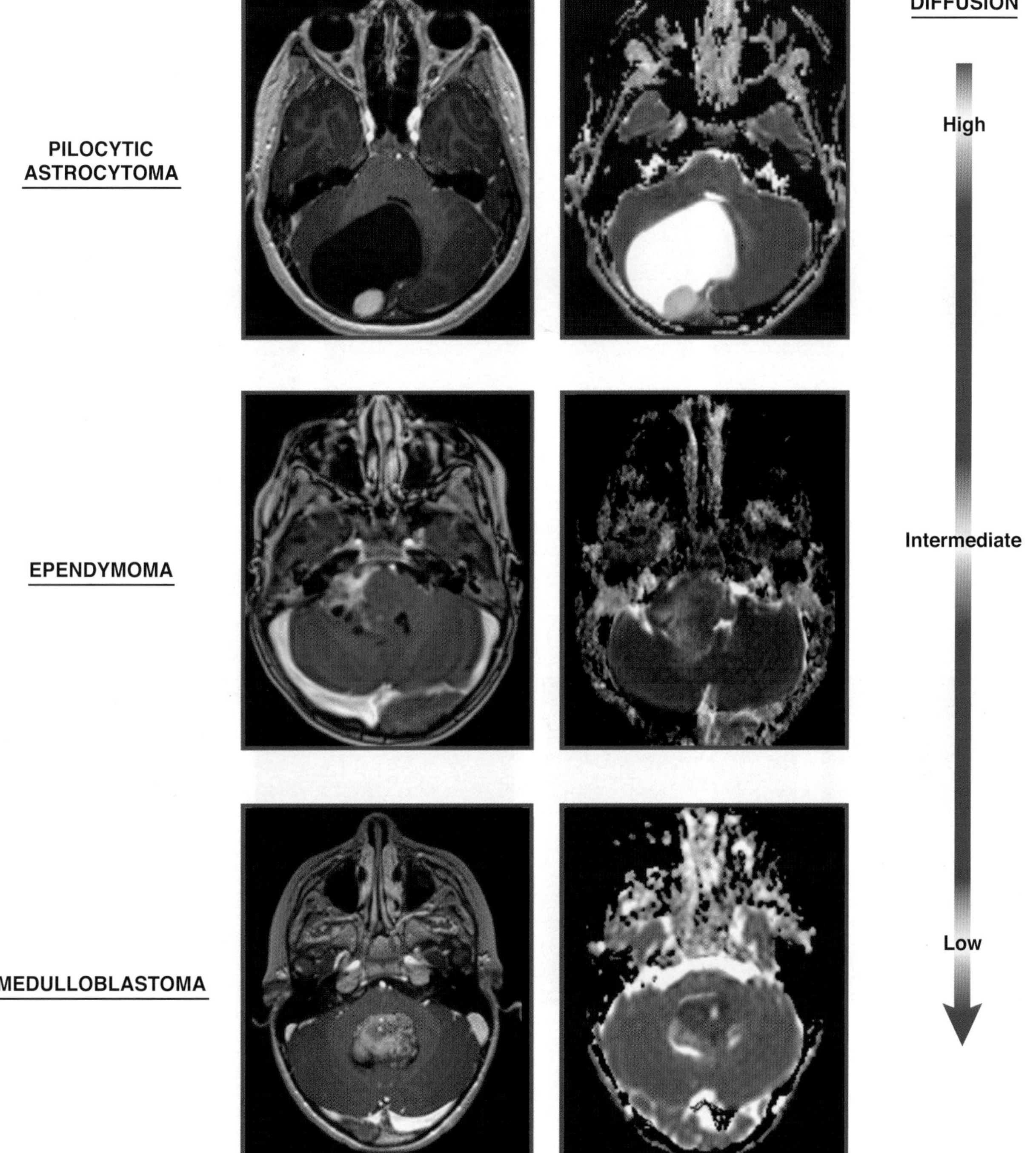

POSTERIOR FOSSA MASS

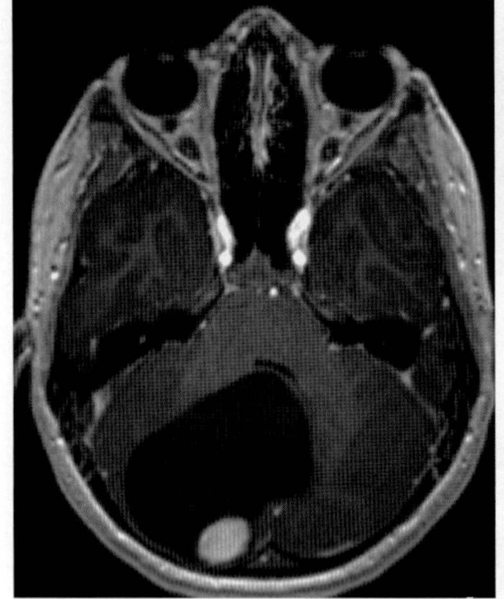

Pilocytic Astrocytoma

- Cerebellar hemisphere or vermis
- Solid and cystic vs solid
- Avidly enhancing T2W hyperintense solid components
- Increased ADC

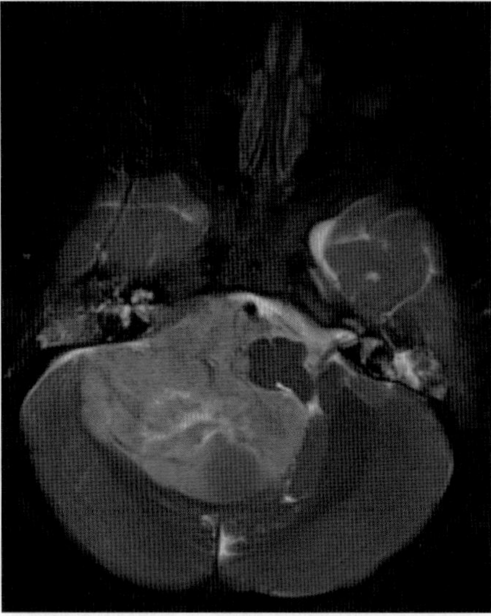

Ependymoma

- Foramen of Lushka; intraventricular
- Intermediate or hyperintense T2W signal
- Hetereogeneous enhancement
- Intermediate ADC

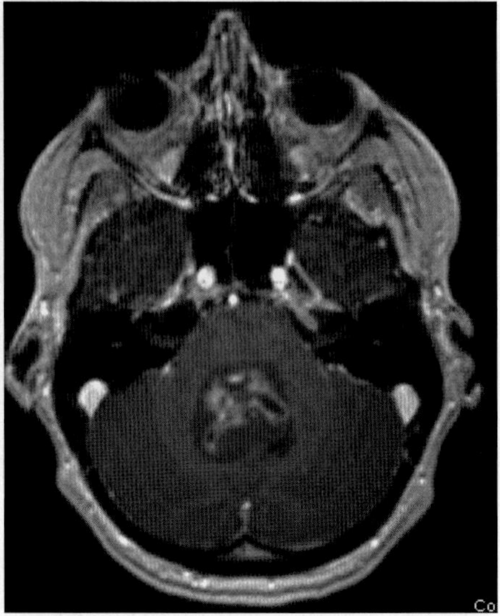

Medulloblastoma

- Midline or off midline
- Usually enhances heterogeneously or homogeneously but can be nonenhancing
- Low ADC

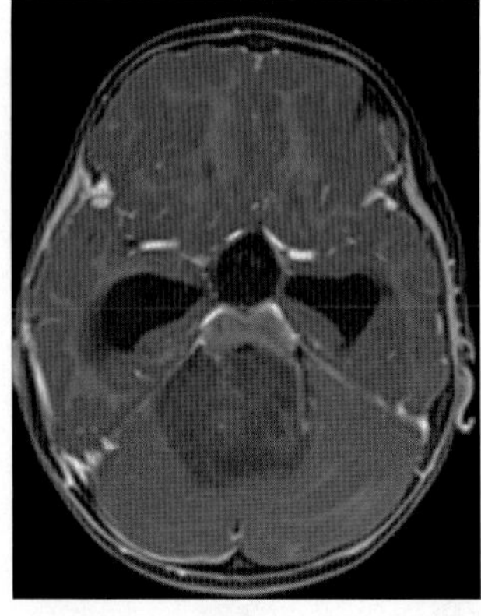

ATRT

- Similar to medulloblastoma
- Low ADC
- Often patients younger than 2 years

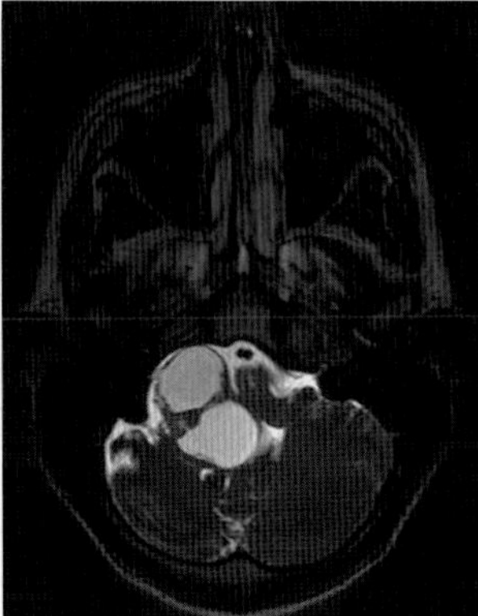

Ganglioglioma

- Uncommon location
- Slow growing
- Associated with ipsilateral cerebellar atrophy

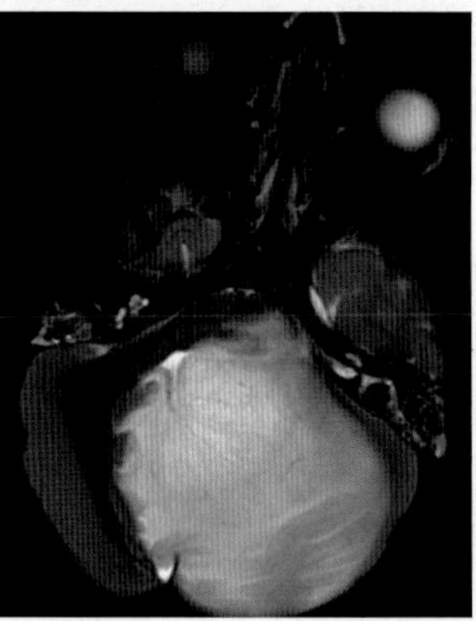

Lhermitte Duclos

- Sharply marginated
- Heterogeneous T2W hyperintensity with intervening cortical signal; nonenhancing
- "Corduroy" appearance

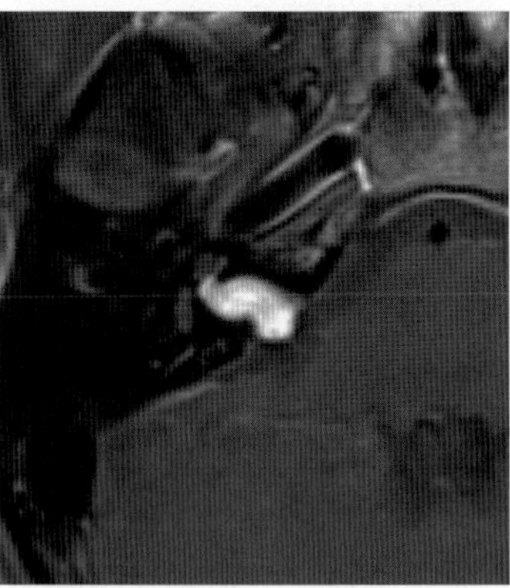

Schwannoma

- Uncommon in children compared to adults.
- Involves the cerebellopontine angle and/or internal auditory canal.
- Homogeneously enhancing. Large schwannomas may have internal necrosis and blood products.
- Bilateral vestibular schwannomas seen with NF-2.

POSTERIOR FOSSA MASS

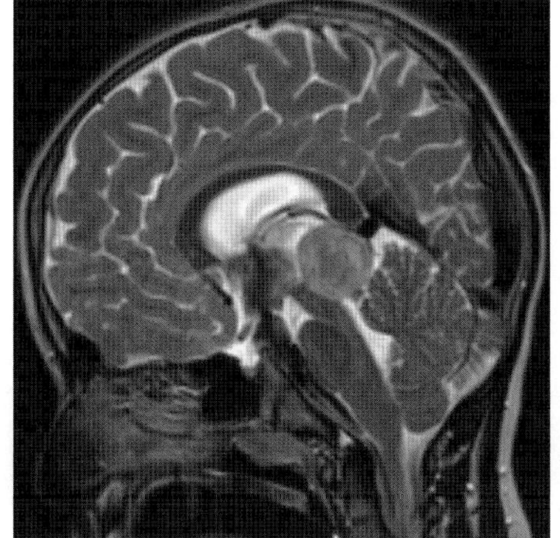

Tectal Glioma

- Low-grade astrocytoma
- Slow growing
- T2W hyperintensity
- Often no enhancement
- Hydrocephalus due to aqueductal obstruction

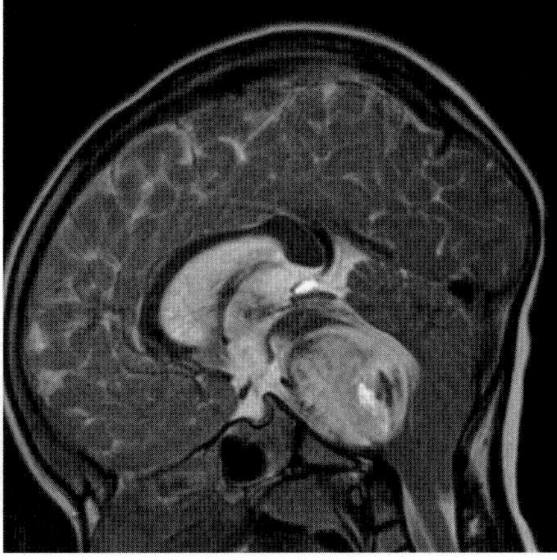

Pontine Glioma

- Diffuse midline glioma
- Majority are high grade and have poor prognosis
- Expansile T2W hyperintensity; nonenhancing but may have enhancing components

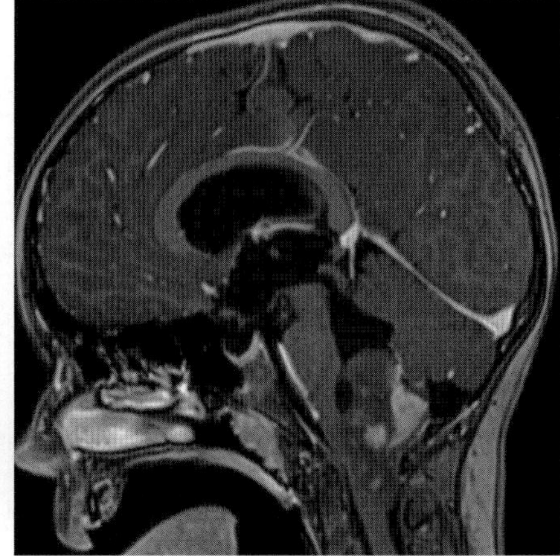

Medullary Glioma

- Dorsally exophytic
- Majority are low grade
- Expansile T2W hyperintensity
- Variable enhancement

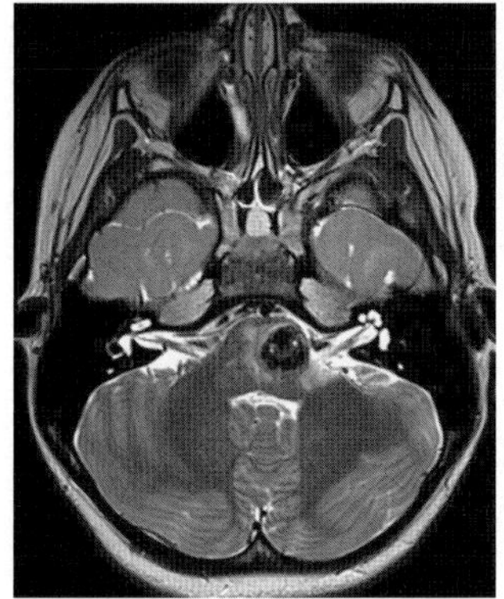

Cavernoma

- Heterogeneous T2W hypointense/T1W hyperintense
- Susceptibility with complete hemosidering ring
- Associated with developmental venous anomaly

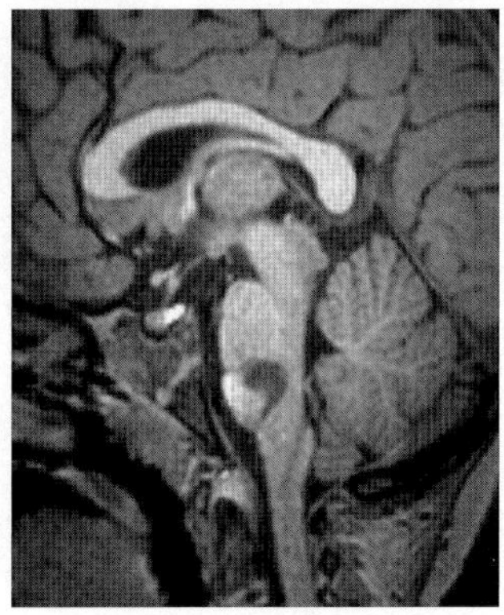

Neurenteric Cyst

- Prepontine, cerebellopontine
- Variable T1W and T2W signal; often T1W hyperintense due to proteinaceous contents

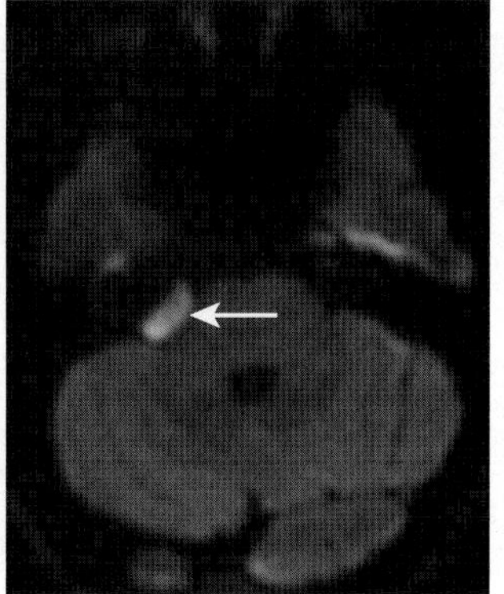

Epidermoid Cyst

- Cerebellopontine angle or midline posterior fossa
- T1W hypointense, T2W hyperintense
- Incomplete suppression on FLAIR
- Restricted diffusion
- No enhancement

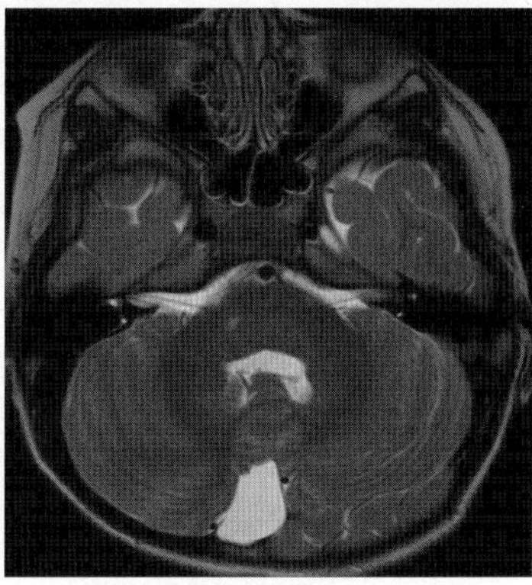

Arachnoid Cyst

- Very common
- Usually midline and posterior in location in the posterior fossa
- T2W hyperintense
- No enhancement
- No diffusion restriction

SELLAR/SUPRASELLAR MASS

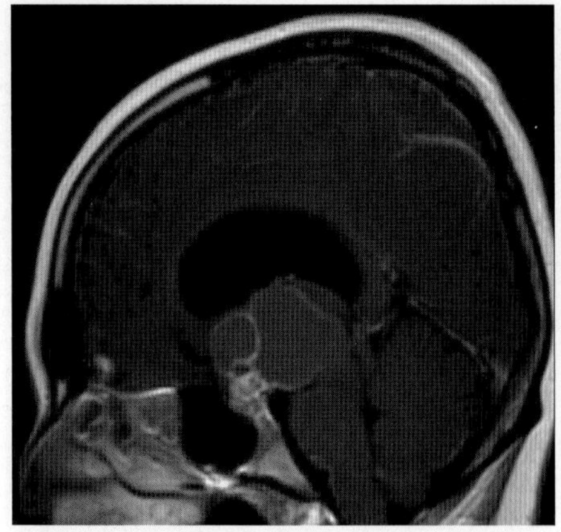

Craniopharyngioma

- Cystic >> solid
- 90% cystic, 90% Ca^{2+}
- Age 9 to 12 years
- Short stature

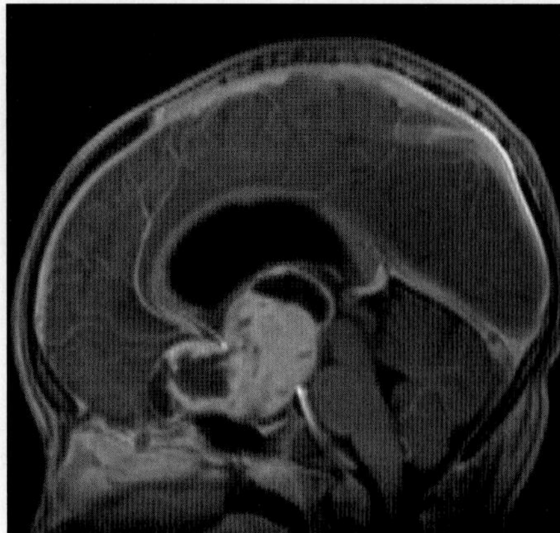

Hypothalamic Chiasmatic Glioma

- Solid and cystic
- NF-1
- Age 5 to 9 years
- Vision changes, diencephalon syndrome precocious puberty

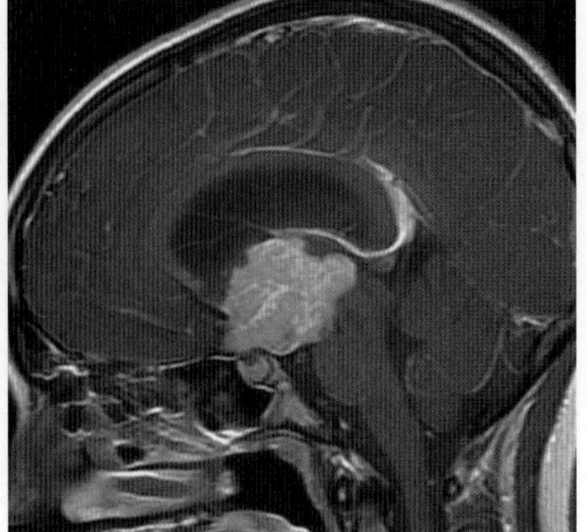

Germinoma

- Solid >> cystic
- Age 10 to 20 years
- Reduced DWI
- Diabetes insipidus
- Loss of normal pituitary bright spot

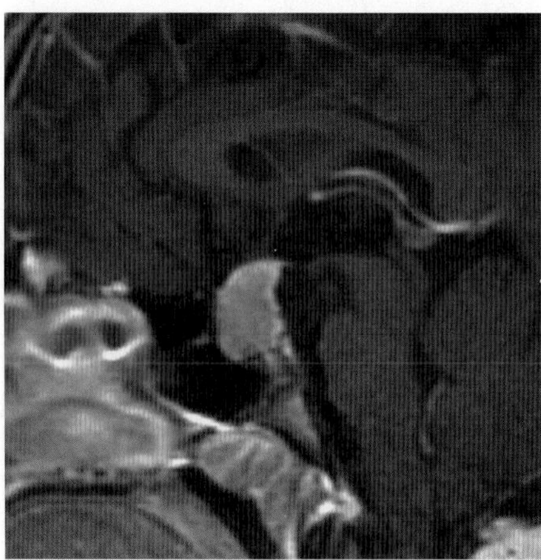

Pituitary Adenoma

- Endocrine abnormality
- Hypoenhancing compared to normal pituitary
- May invade cavernous sinuses

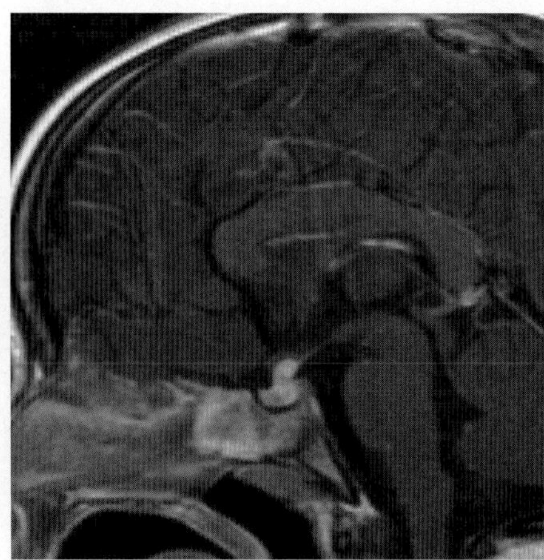

Langerhans Cell Histiocytosis (LCH)

- Homogeneous enhancement and thickening of the infundibulum
- Loss of normal pituitary bright spot

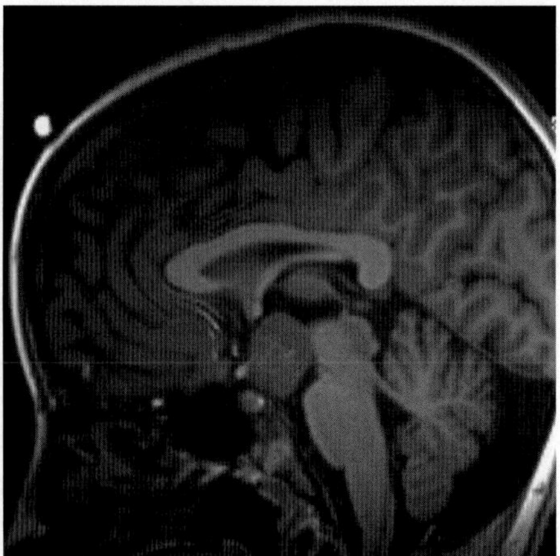

Hypothalamic Hamartoma

- Hypothalamic location
- Follows gray matter signal on all sequences
- No enhancement unless treated with radiotherapy or thermal ablation

SELLAR/SUPRASELLAR MASS

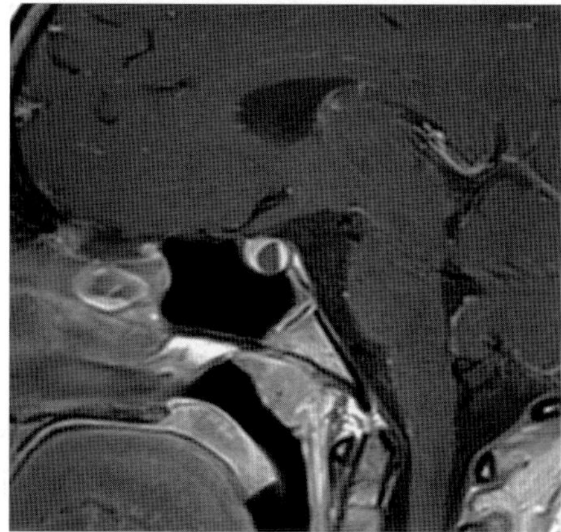

Rathke Cleft Cyst

- Sellar or suprasellar
- No enhancement

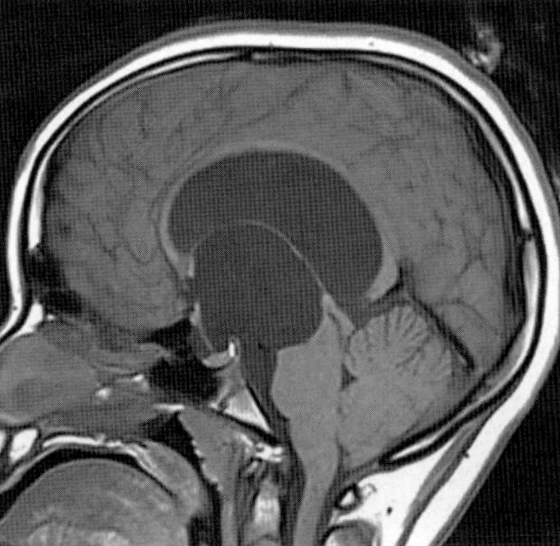

Arachnoid Cyst

- Suprasellar
- No enhancement

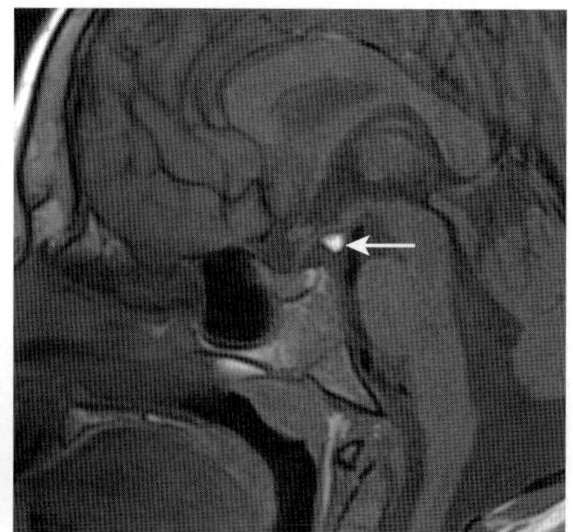

Lipoma

- Suprasellar
- Fat density/intensity

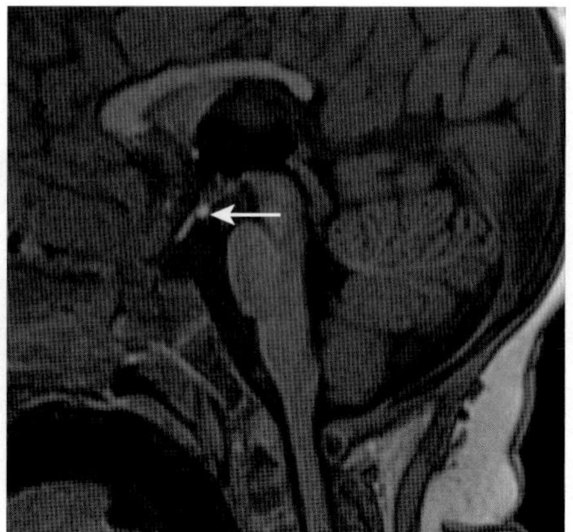

Ectopic Pituitary

- T1W hyperintensity located along the tuber cinereum.
- Normal T1 bright spot in the sella is absent.

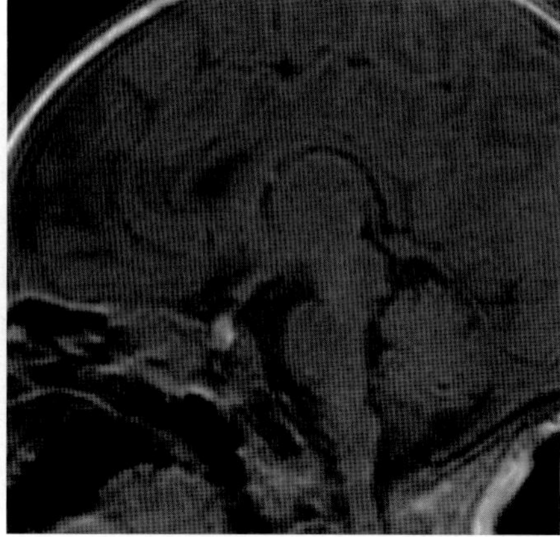

Physiologic Pituitary Hyperplasia

- Occurs in newborns and during puberty
- Enlarged gland that maintains normal morphology and signal

PINEAL REGION MASS

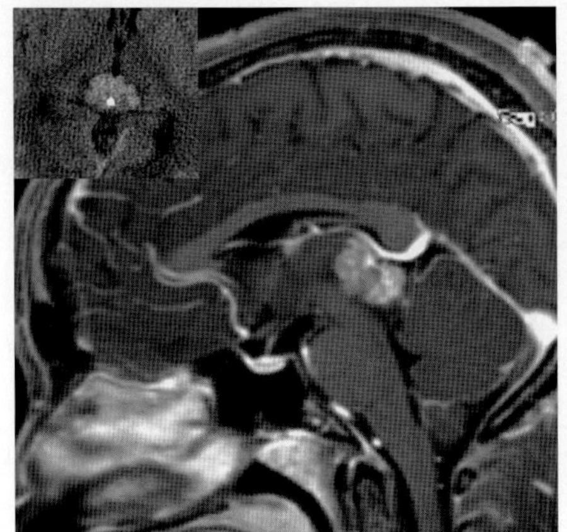

Germinoma

- Mostly solid
- Engulfed Ca^{2+}
- Age 10 to 20 years most commonly
- Reduced DWI

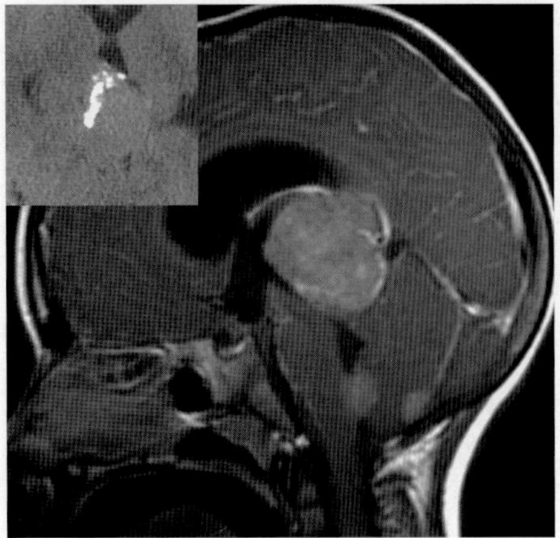

Pineoblastoma

- Mostly solid
- Diffuse or peripheral Ca^{2+}
- Age <5 years most commonly
- Reduced DWI

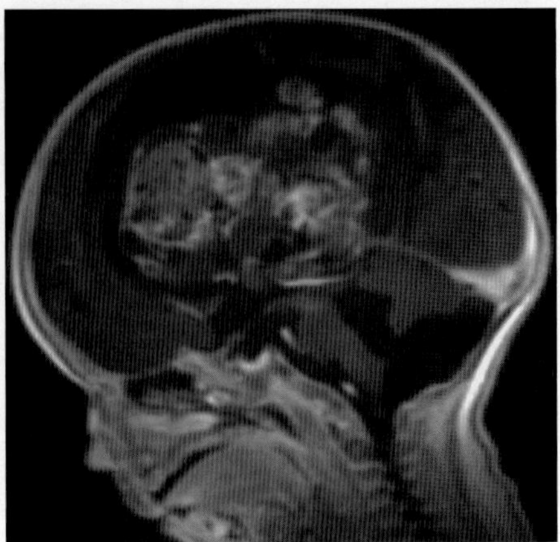

Teratoma

- Solid and cystic
- +/– macroscopic fat
- Often present in neonates

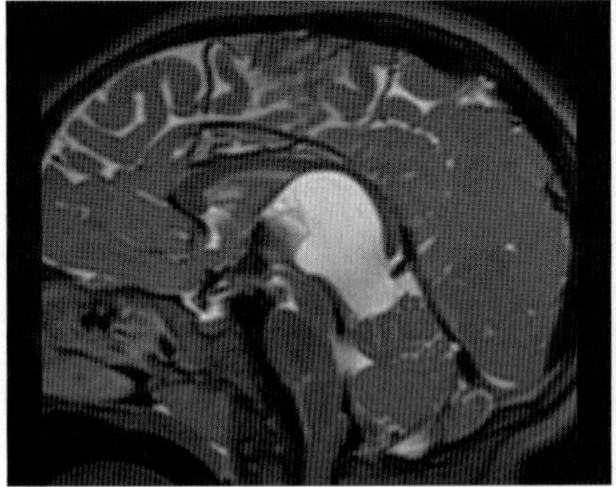

Cavum Velum Interpositum

- Benign anatomic variant
- CSF density/intensity

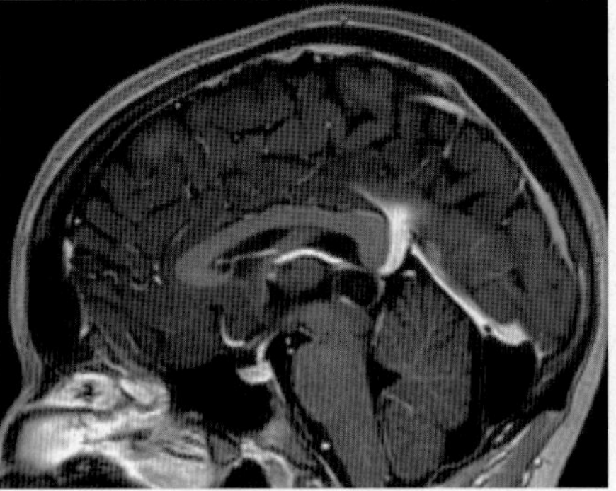

Pineal Cyst

- Thin walled (<2 mm)
- T2W hyperintensity
- No nodularity

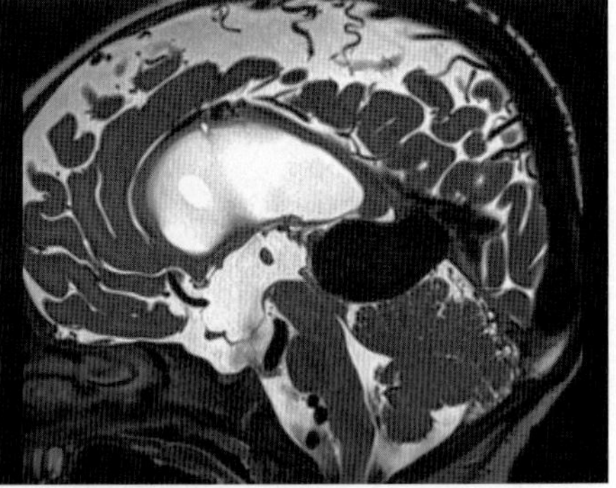

Vein of Galen Aneurysmal Malformation

- AV fistula
- T2W hypointensity flow void

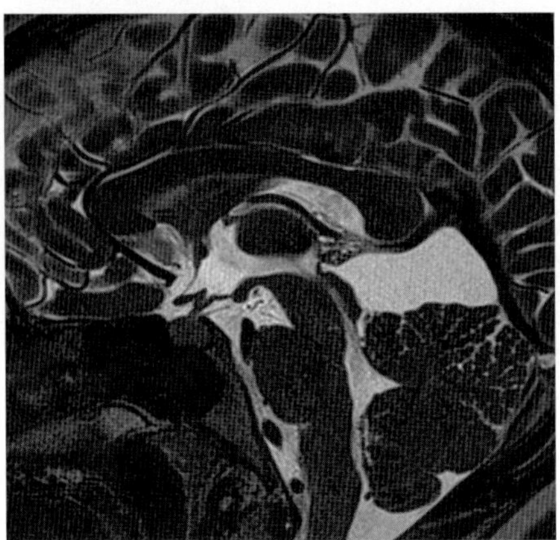

Arachnoid Cyst

- Benign
- CSF intensity space
- Mass effect

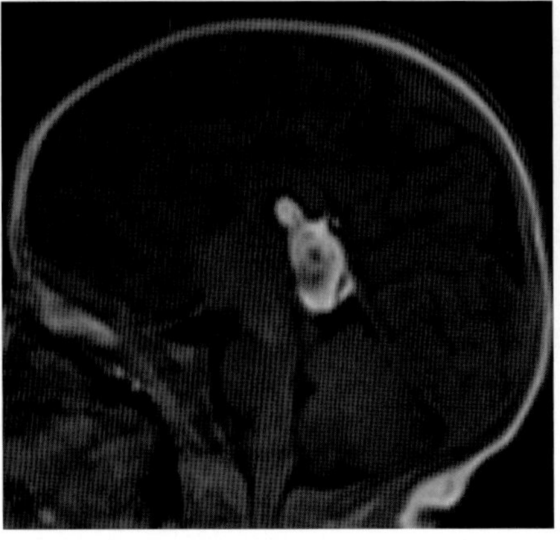

Lipoma

- T1W hyperintensity
- Loses signal with fat saturation
- May have associated callosal malformation

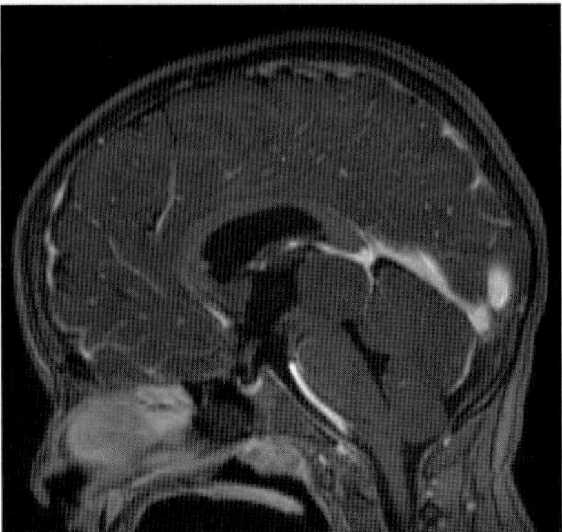

Tectal Glioma

- Expansile mass arising from the tectal plate
- Usually low-grade gliomas and nonenhancing

INTRAVENTRICULAR MASS

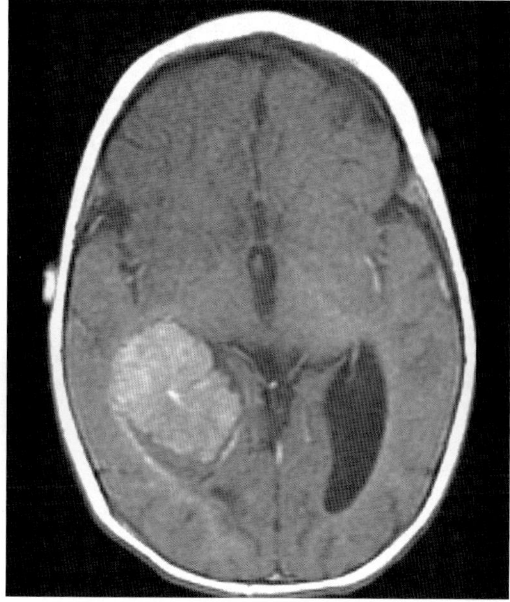

Choroid Plexus Papilloma

- Homogeneously enhancing
- Cauliflower/frond-like.
- Carcinomas are less common

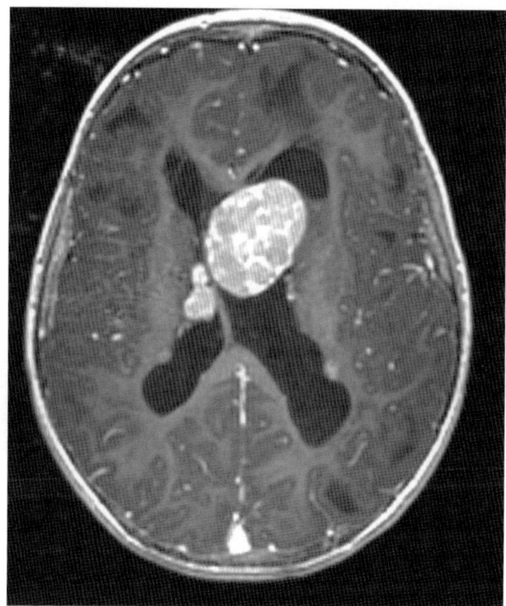

Subependymal Giant Cell Astrocytoma

- Tuberous sclerosis
- Foramen of Monroe

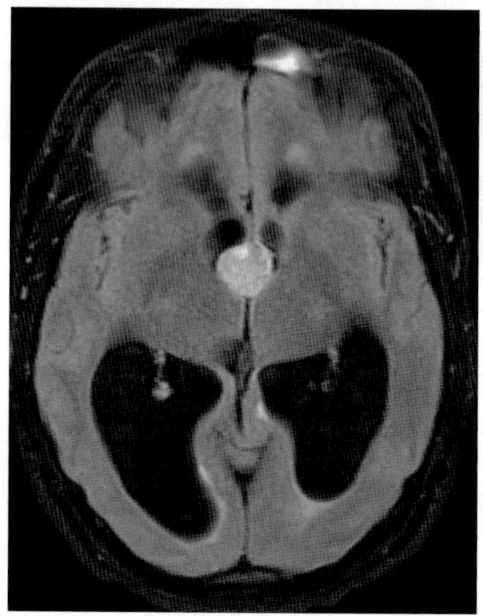

Colloid Cyst

- Nonenhancing
- Variable protein content
- Foramen of Monroe

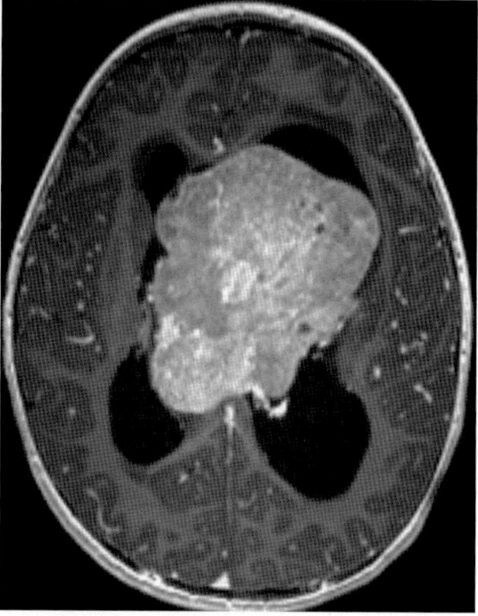

Meningioma

- Homogeneously enhancing
- Intermediate or low ADC
- Uncommon in children
- NF-2

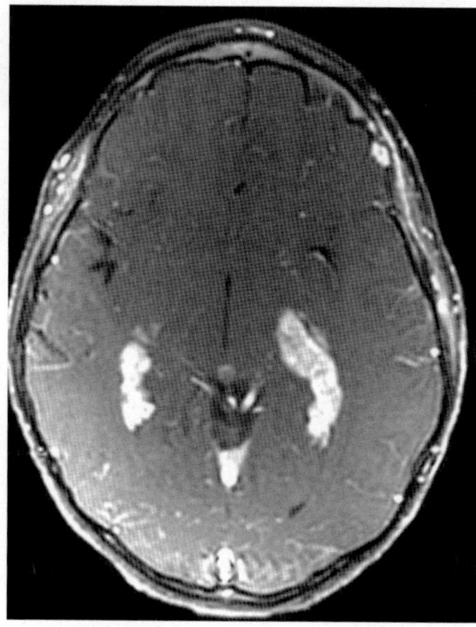

Langerhans Cell Histiocytosis

- Uncommonly involve the choroid plexus
- Associated with other LCH findings such as bone lesions or other systemic involvement

LOW-GRADE CEREBRAL HEMISPHERE TUMOR

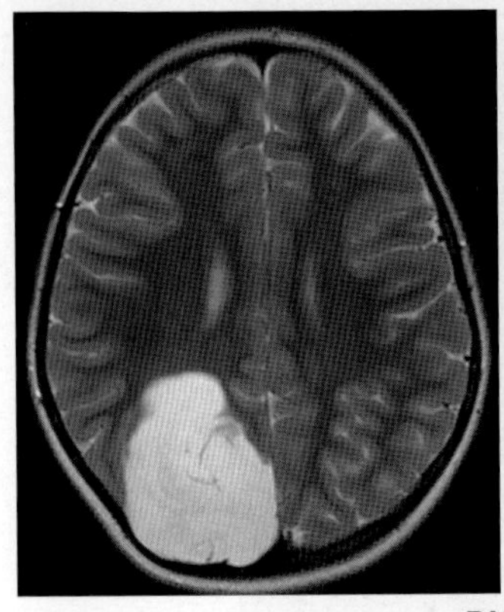
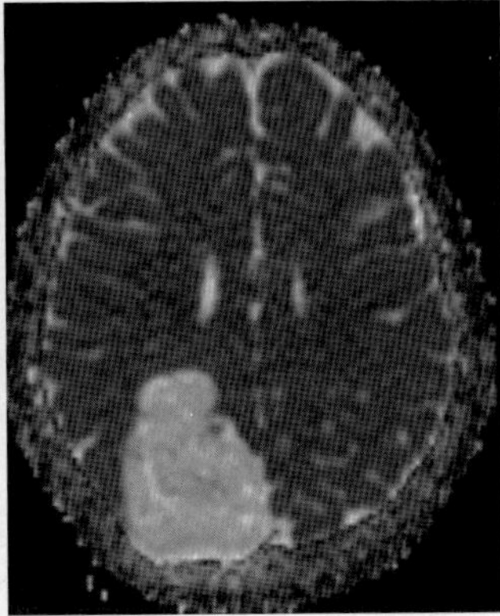

DNET

- Cortical or subcortical well defined
- T2W hyperintensity; usually nonenhancing
- Overlying bony remodeling
- ADC hyperintense

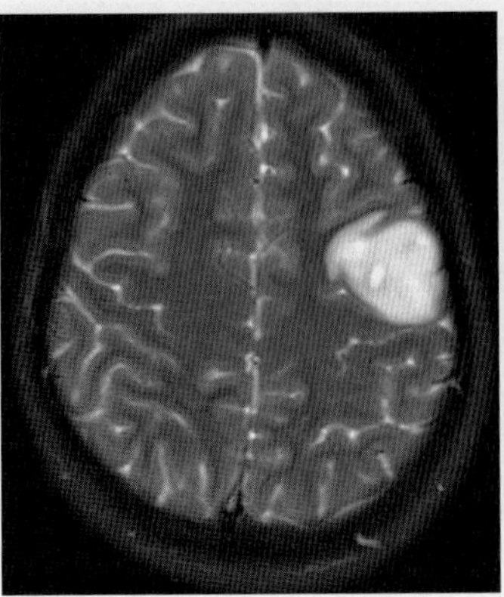
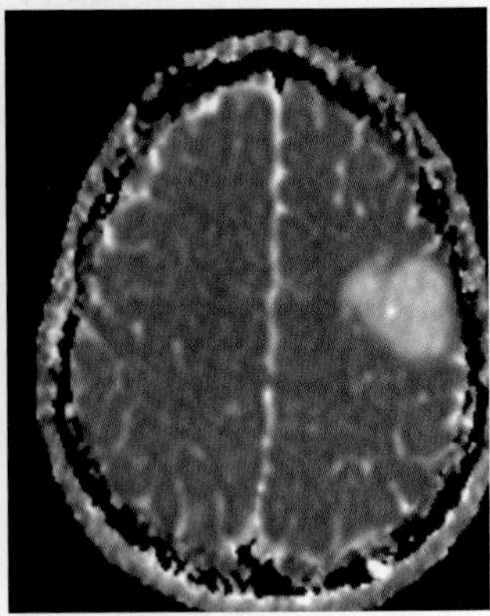

Oligodendroglioma

- Cortical or subcortical well defined
- T2W hyperintense, may enhance
- Calcification
- ADC hyperintense

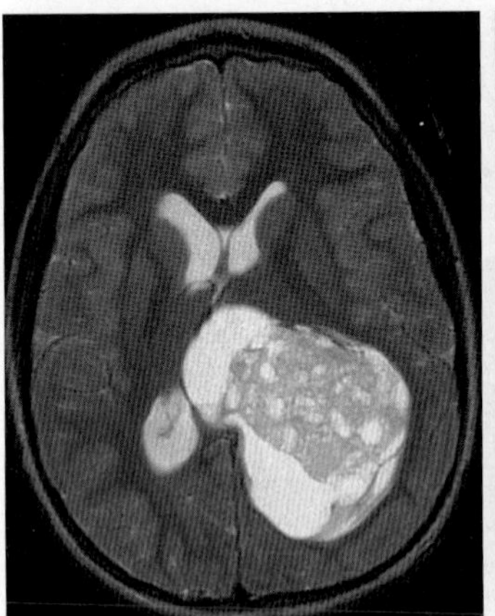
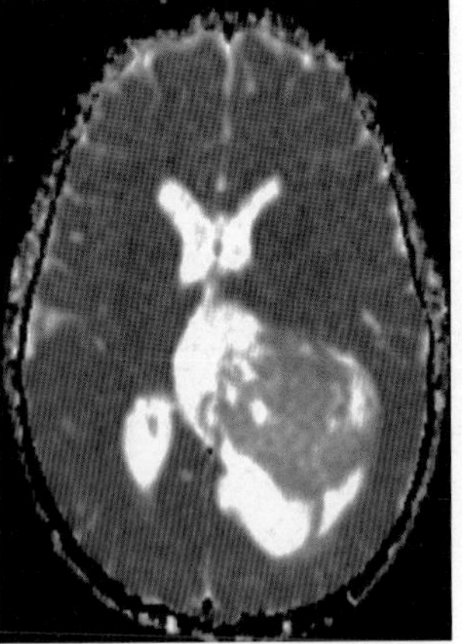

Pilocytic astrocytoma

- Solid and cystic vs solid
- Avidly enhancing T2W hyperintense solid components with facilitated diffusion
- ADC hyperintense

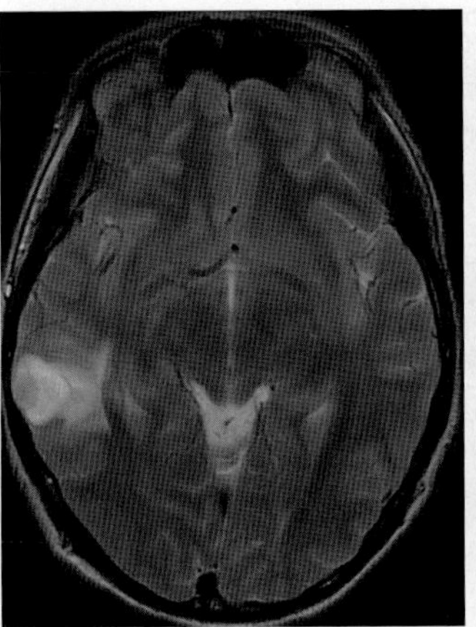
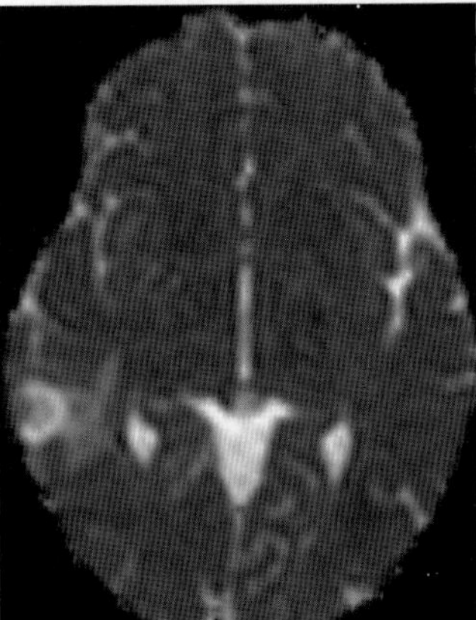

Ganglioglioma

- Cortical or subcortical well defined
- Solid and cystic vs solid
- Variably enhancing T2W hyperintense solid components
- ADC hyperintense

Low-grade tumors involving the cerebral cortex have high ADC. Further imaging differentiation is typically not possible.

HIGH-GRADE CEREBRAL HEMISPHERE TUMOR

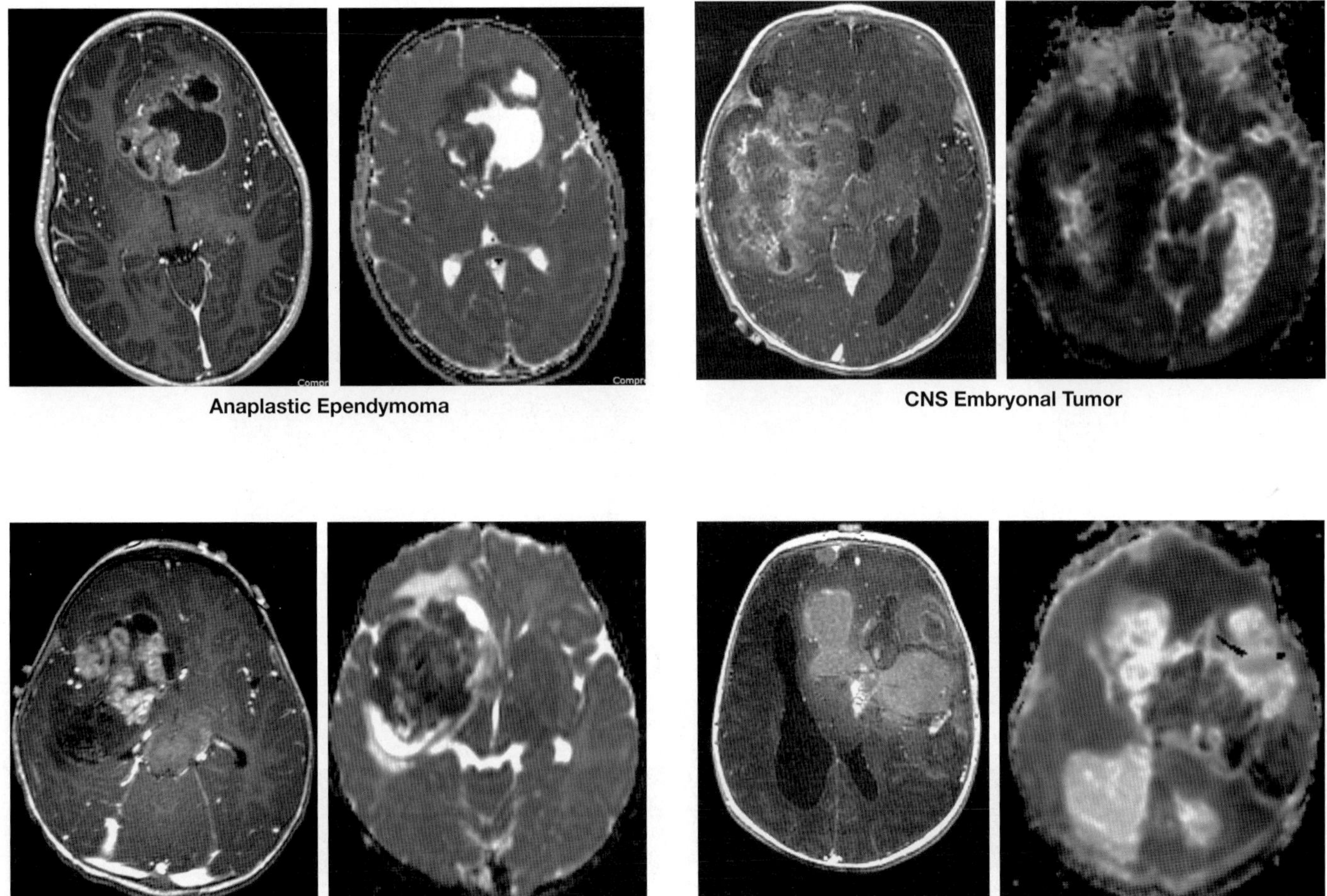

High-grade tumors involving the cerebral cortex have low ADC. Further imaging differentiation is typically not possible.

TUMOR CYST AND NODULE

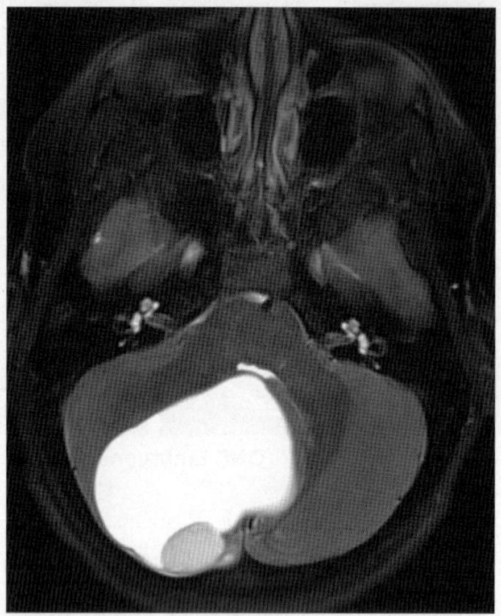

Pilocytic Astrocytoma
- Solid and cystic vs solid
- Avidly enhancing T2W hyperintense solid components with facilitated diffusion

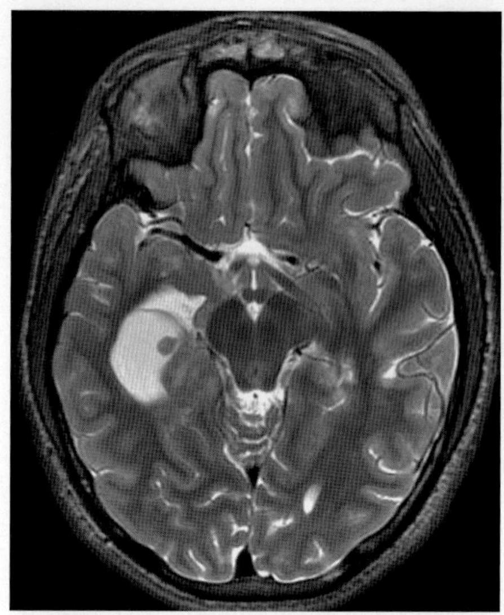

Ganglioglioma
- Cortical or subcortical, well defined
- Solid and cystic vs solid
- Variably enhancing T2W hyperintense solid components

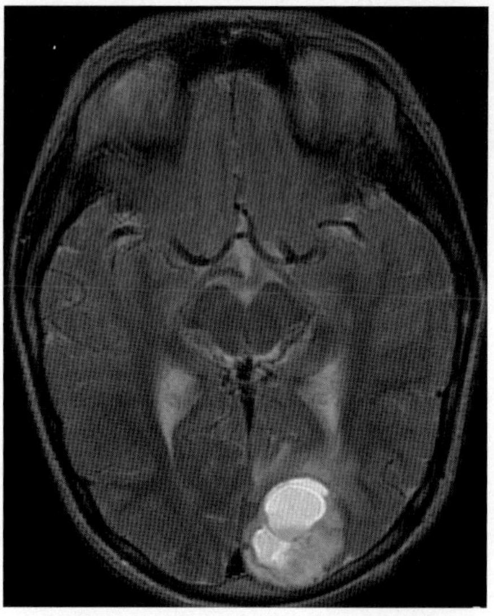

Pleomorphic Xanthoastrocytoma
- Cortical or subcortical mass that may have leptomeningeal invasion
- Solid and cystic
- Enhancing T2W isointense solid components
- Intermediate ADC

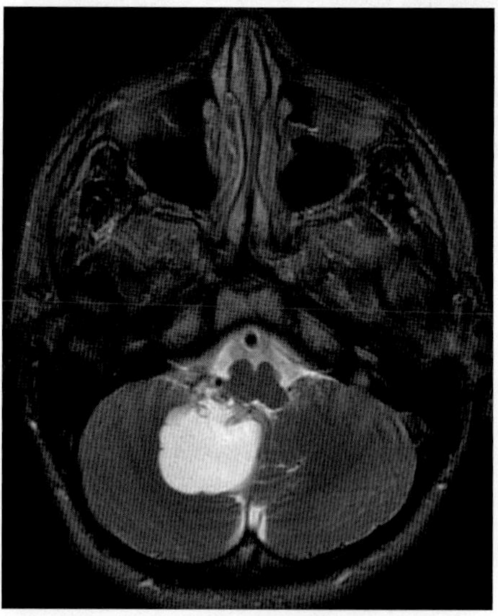

Hemangioblastoma
- Large cystic lesion with small mural nodule presenting to a pial surface or small avid enhancing nodule
- Von Hippel-Lindau

GRE/SWI ABNORMALITY

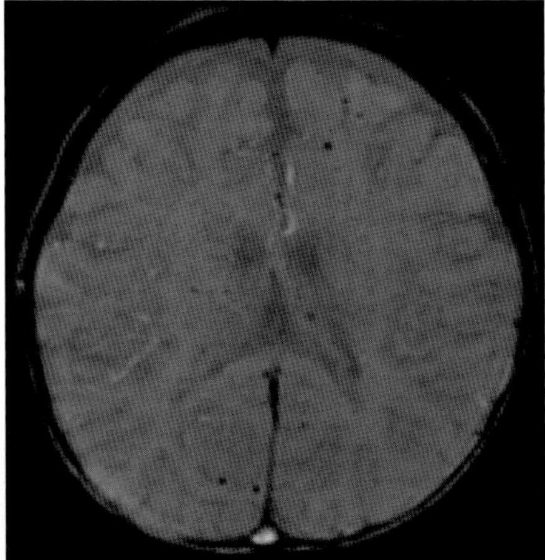

Congenital Heart Disease

- Small, scattered thromboembolic foci common post corrective surgery/bypass

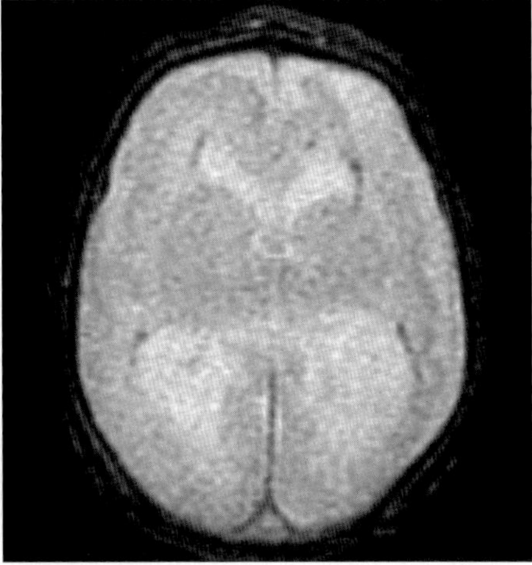

TORCH Infection

- Periventricular predominant or scattered foci of calcification

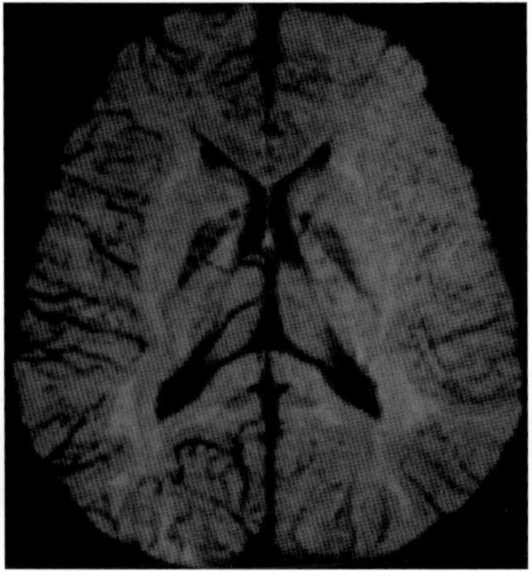

Seizure

- Asymmetric increased sulcal susceptibility

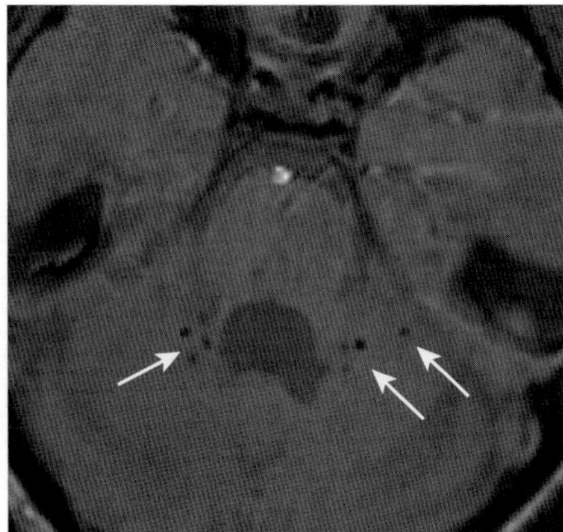

Radiotherapy Microhemorrhages

- Associated with younger age, higher doses, higher volume, and percentage of brain irradiated
- Seen with photon and proton therapy

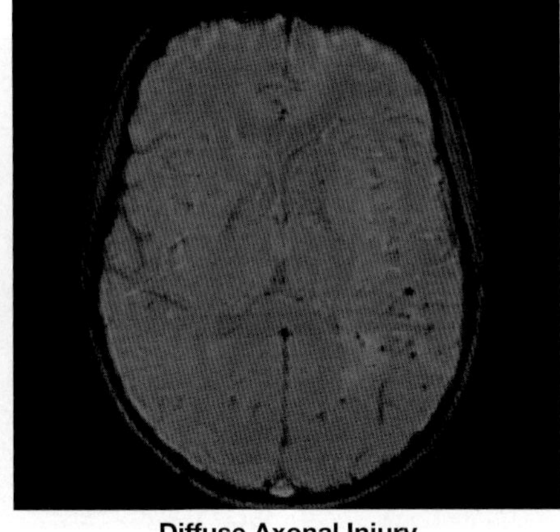

Diffuse Axonal Injury

- Acceleration and deceleration forces with hemorrhagic and nonhemorrhagic shearing injury at gray white junction, corpus callosum, central gray matter, and brainstem.

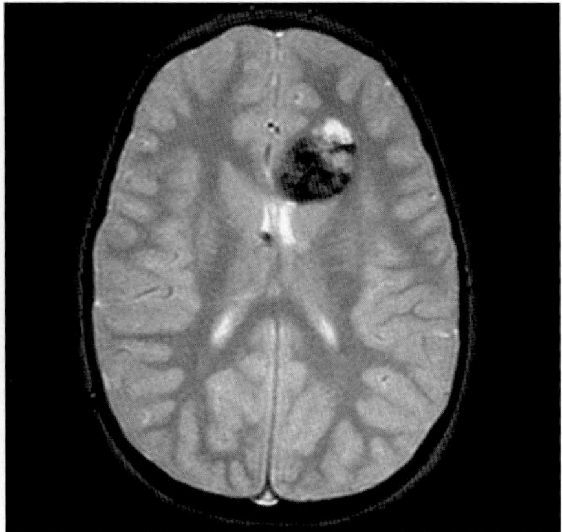

Cavernoma

- Heterogeneous T2W hypointense/T1W hyperintense
- Susceptibility with complete hemosidering ring
- Associated with developmental venous anomaly
- May be numerous when hereditary

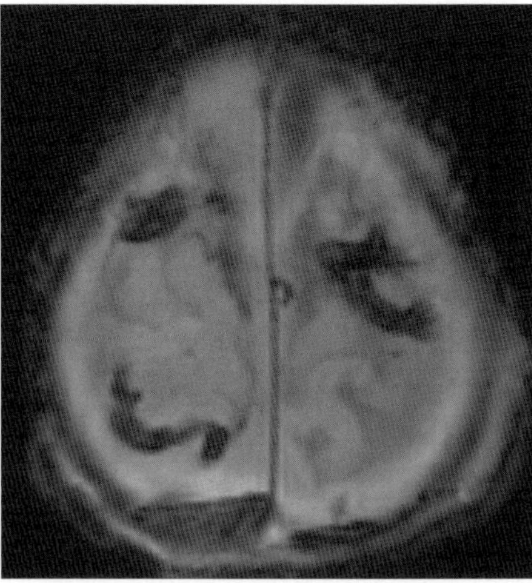

Venous Thrombosis From Abusive Head Trauma

- Linear areas that correspond to veins.

MACROCEPHALY

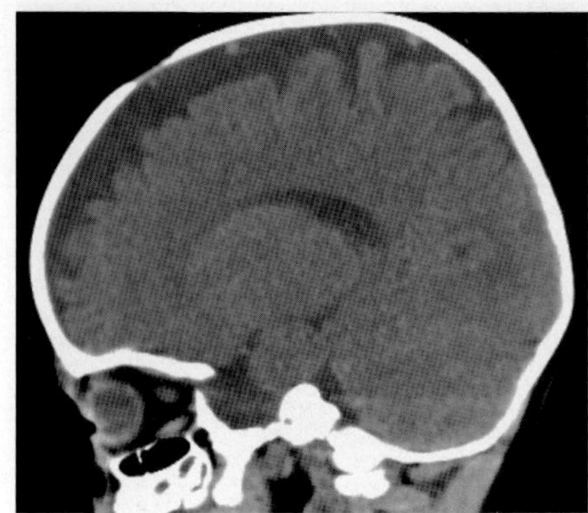

Benign Enlarged Subarachnoid Spaces of Infancy

- Enlarged subarachnoid spaces along the frontal lobes typically seen from 3 months to 2 years of age.

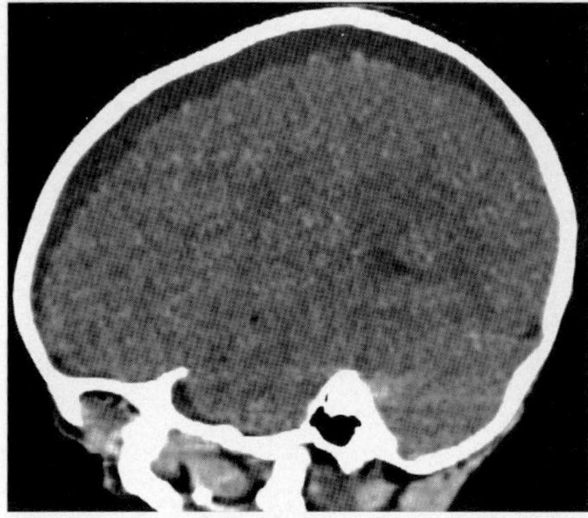

Subdural Hemorrhage/Abusive Head Trauma

- Uncommonly, subdural hemorrhages can present with macrocephaly.

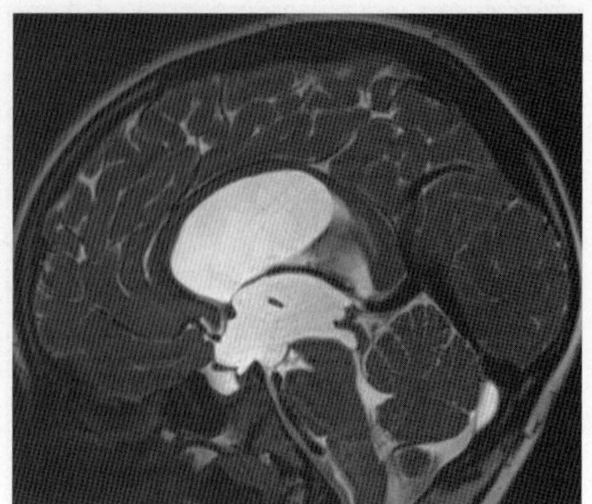

Hydrocephalus

- Ventricular enlargement due to communicating or noncommunicating hydrocephalus.

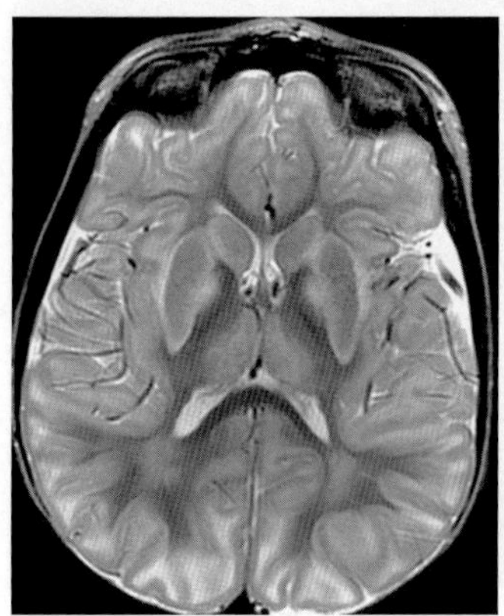

Metabolic Megalencephaly

1. Canavan disease
2. Alexander disease
3. Organic acid disorders (GA-1)
4. Megalencephalic leukoencephalopathy with cysts
5. Lysosomal storage disorders (mucopolysaccharidoses, gangliosidoses)

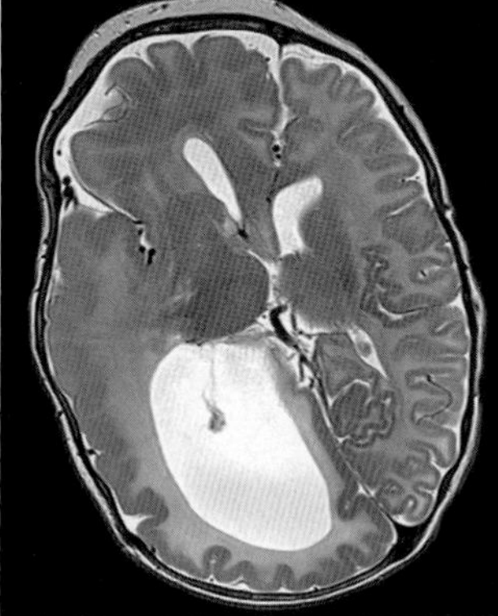

Dysplasia

- Hemimegalencephaly or megalencephaly seen with PIK3/Akt/mTOR pathway mutations.

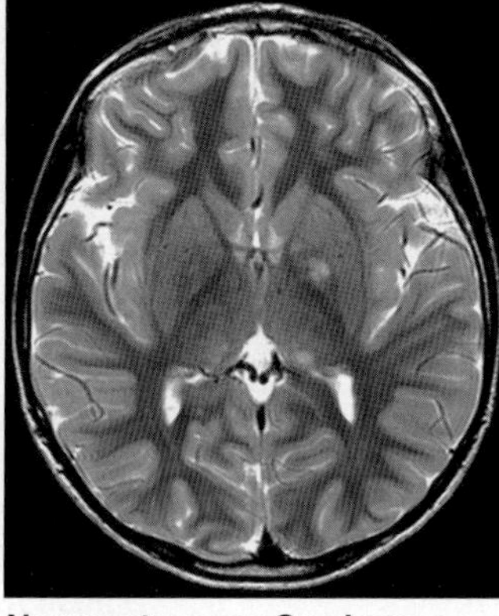

Neurocutaneous Syndromes

1. NF-1
2. Tuberous sclerosis
3. Hypomelanosis of Ito

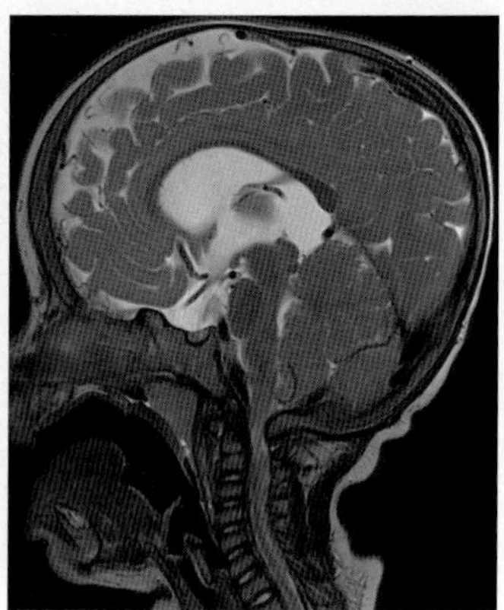

Achondroplasia

- Venous outflow stenosis and foramen magnum stenosis lead to ventriculomegaly and macrocephaly.

NORMAL ANATOMIC VARIANTS

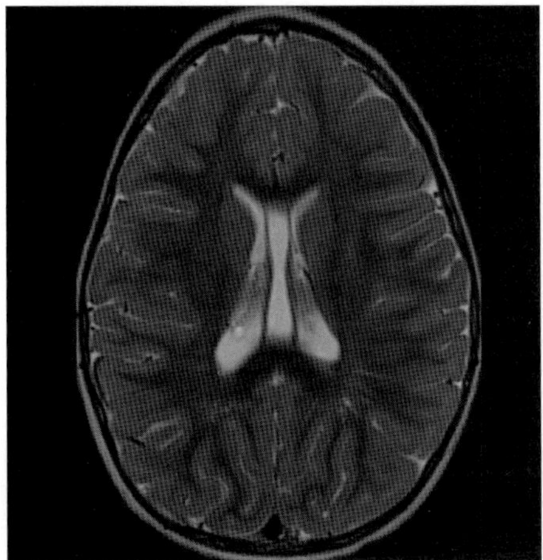

Persistent Cavum Septum Pellucidum

- Cavum septum pellucidum is often seen in neonates. Persistence beyond infant age is considered an anatomic variant.

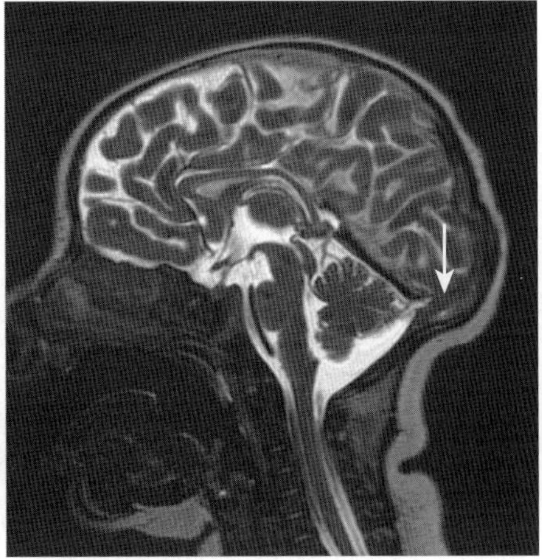

Neonatal Torcular Pseudomass

- Tissue posterior to the torcula seen in neonates and involutes over time. Should not be mistaken for thrombus or hemorrhage

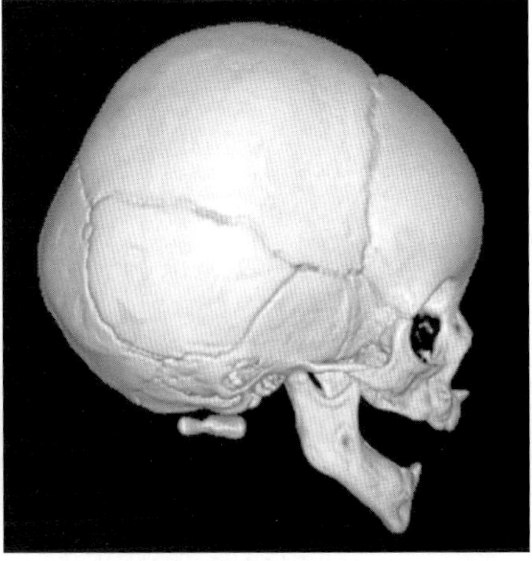

Accessory Parietal Suture

- 3D images are very helpful for distinguishing an accessory suture from a fracture. Sutures have a jagged appearance.

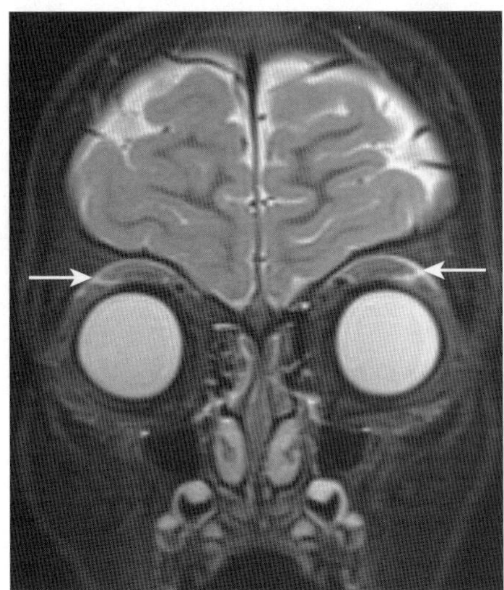

Orbital T2 Signal

- Increased T2 signal can be seen in the postseptal superior orbit. Etiology is unknown. Should not be mistaken for cellulitis.

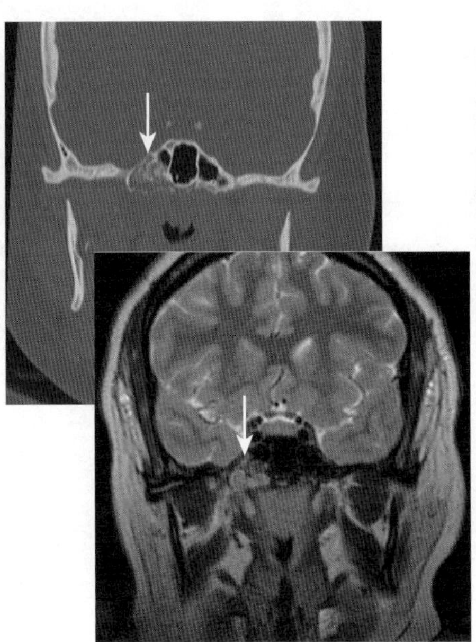

Arrested Pneumatization

- Non–mass-like and coarse ossification and areas of fat density located in the sphenoid sinus. Should not be mistaken for a primary bone tumor.

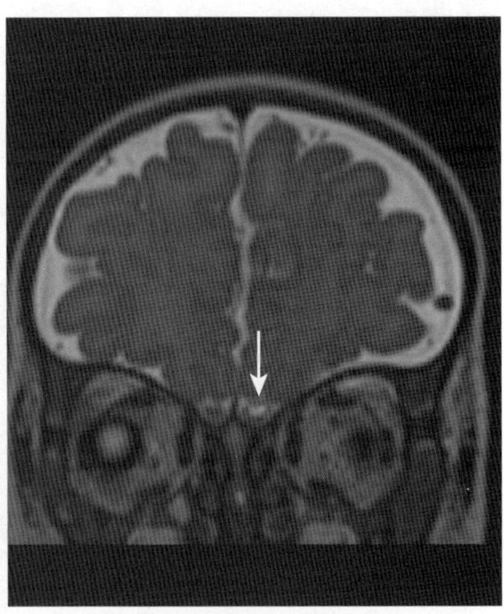

Olfactory Bulb T2 Signal From Maturation

- T2W signal changes can be seen in the olfactory bulbs with maturation.

REFERENCE

1. Schneider JF, Floemer F. Maturation of the olfactory bulbs: MR imaging findings. *AJNR Am J Neuroradiol.* 2009;30(6):1149–1152.

CHALLENGING HEAD CT DIAGNOSES

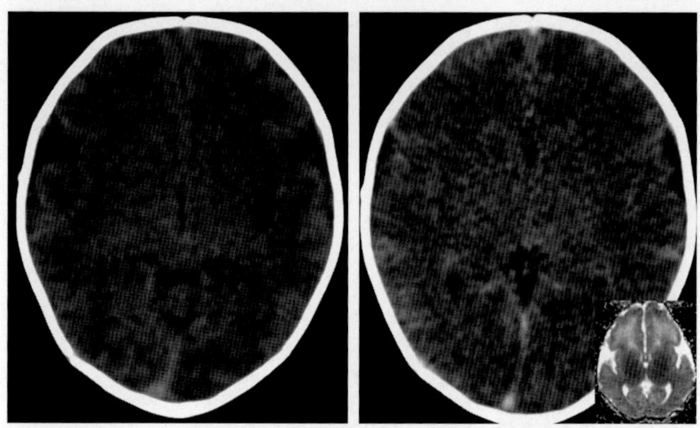

Hypoxic Ischemic Injury

- Basal ganglia and thalami should retain their gray matter density. Neonatal ischemia can be challenging due to the higher water content of the parenchyma.

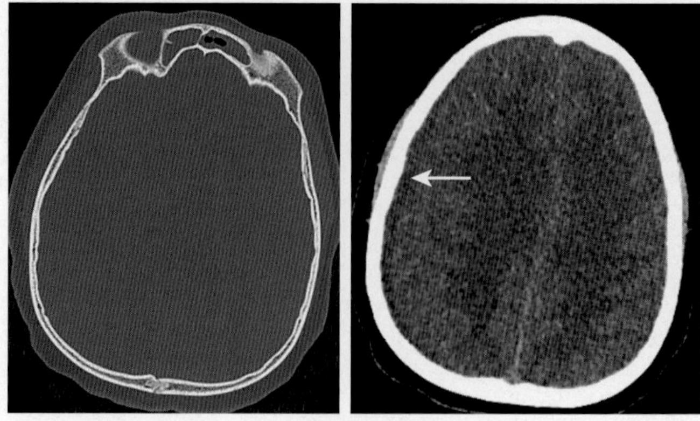

Empyema

- Extra-axial fluid collection in association with sinusitis should raise concern for empyema.

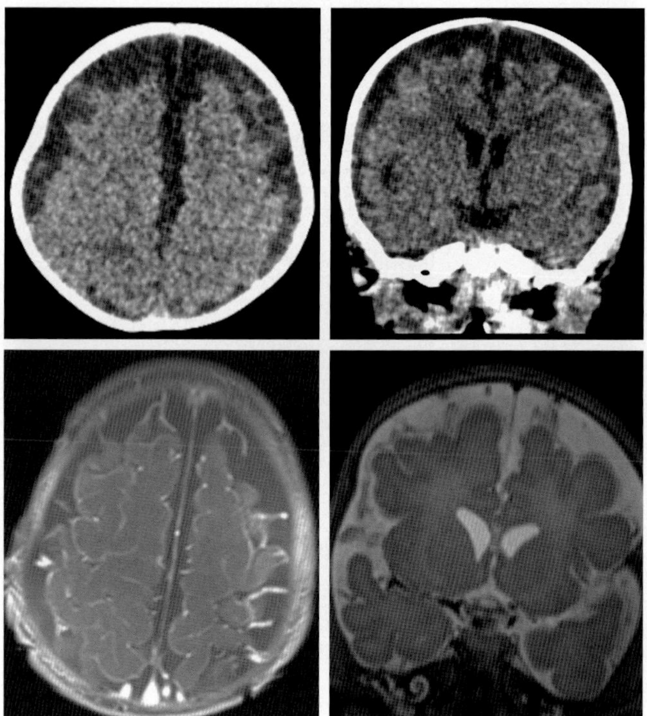

Meningitis

- Difficult to identify on CT but may have a "dirty CSF space" appearance and thick subarachnoid vessels.

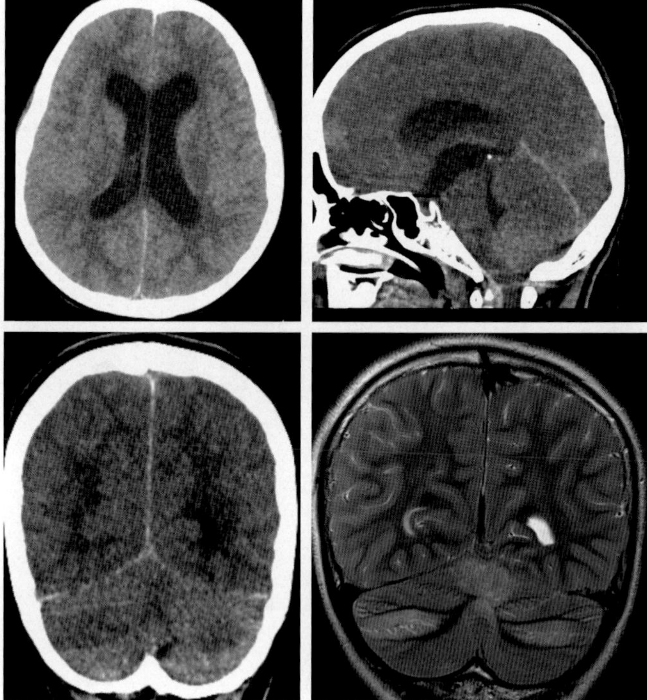

Acute Cerebellitis

- Acute cerebellitis can present with hydrocephalus, effaced sulci, and cisterns due to posterior fossa edema and mass effect.

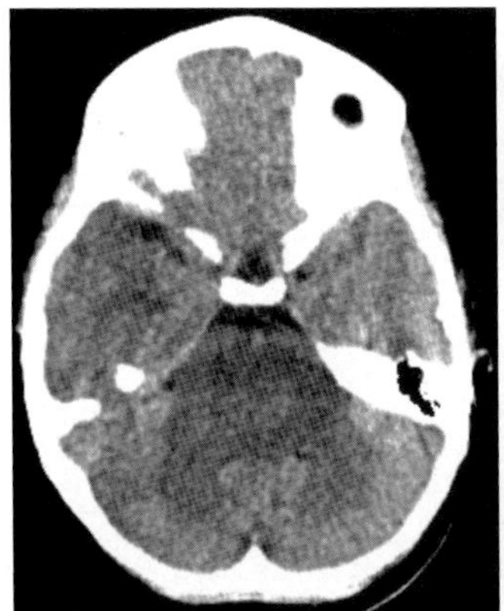
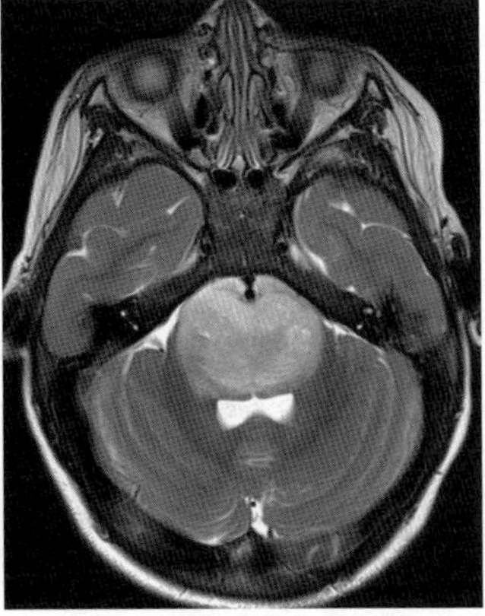

Diffuse Pontine Glioma

- Artifactual low density in the pons is common, but when accompanied by cerebellar pontine angle effacement and/or fourth ventricle effacement this should be identified and raise concern for a mass

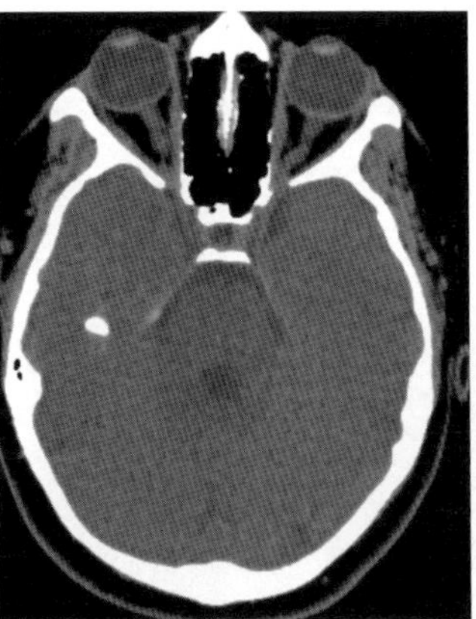

Papilledema

- Important not to overlook the globes, which can show bulging of optic discs indicating elevated intracranial pressure.

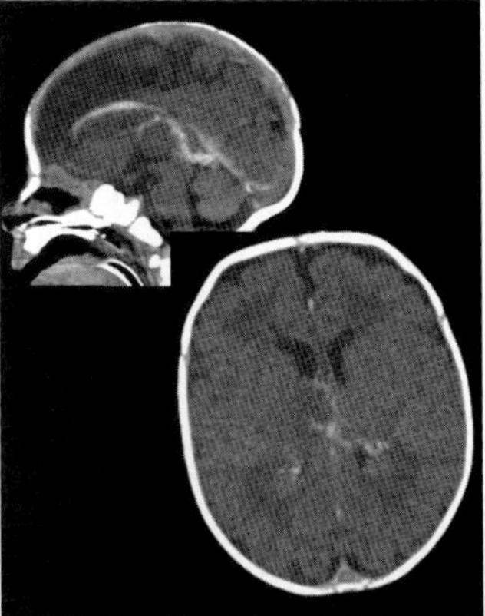

Internal Cerebral Vein Thrombosis

- Noncontrast head CT can show abnormal hyperdense veins and edema in the parenchyma. The deep venous thrombosis shown here has a high rate of mortality due to deep gray matter involvement.

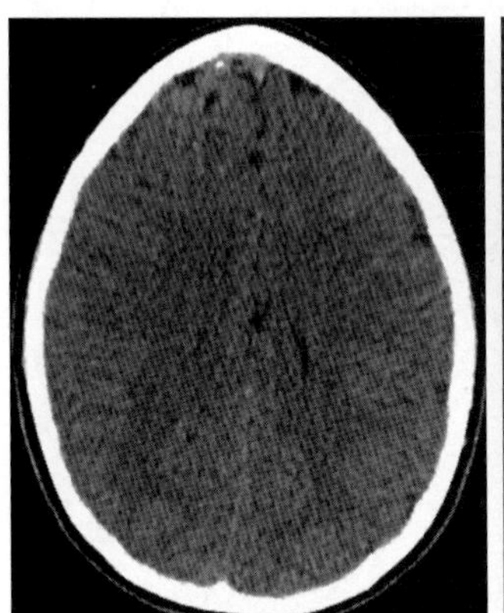
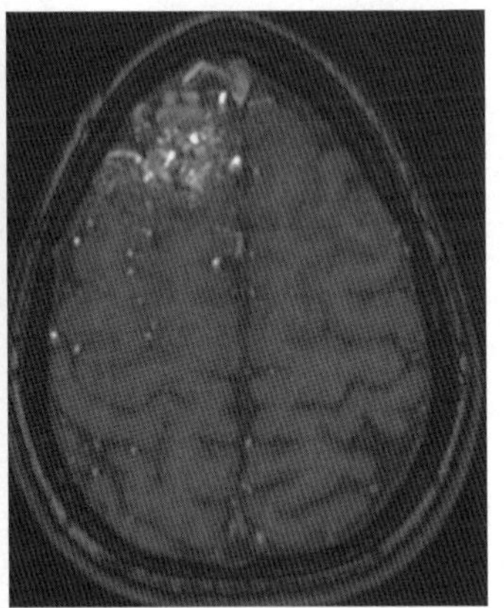

Arteriovenous Malformation

- Subtle rope-like parenchymal hyperdensity, enlarged veins, and/or linear calcifications can indicate an AVM.

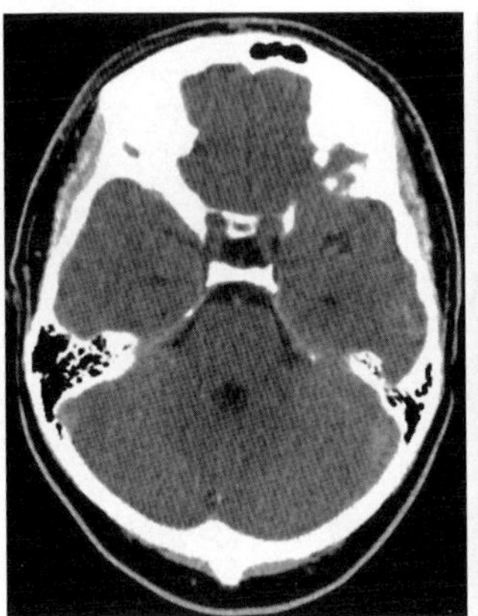
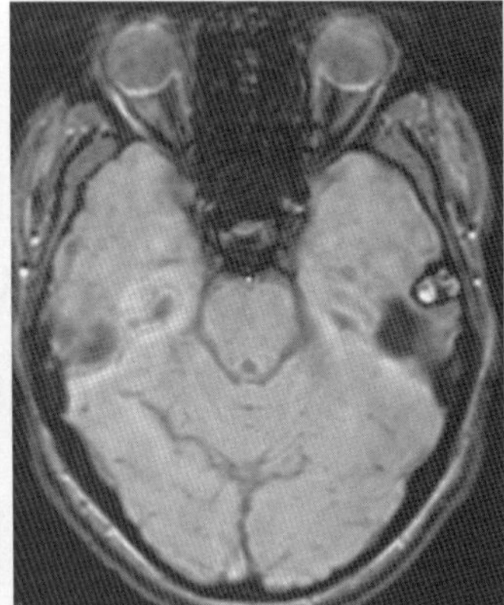

Cavernoma

- Parenchymal hyperdensity can be mistaken for acute hemorrhage or overlooked as artifact when peripheral or adjacent to the skull base.

CHALLENGING FETAL MRI DIAGNOSES

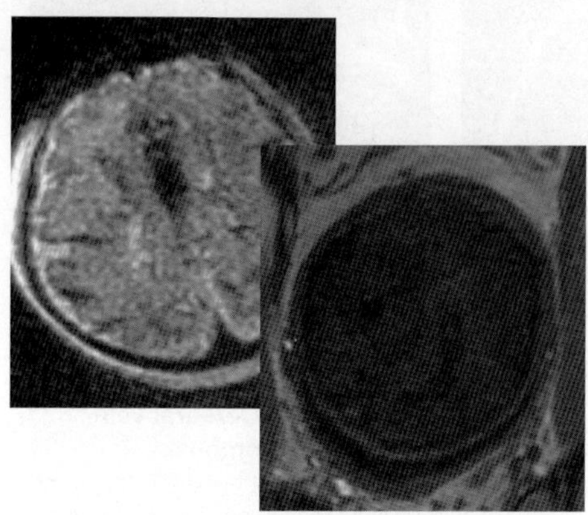

Callosal Lipoma Without T1 Hyperintensity

- Typical callosal lipomas demonstrate T1W hyperintensity; however, some fetal callosal lipomas may not be due to the immature fat cells.

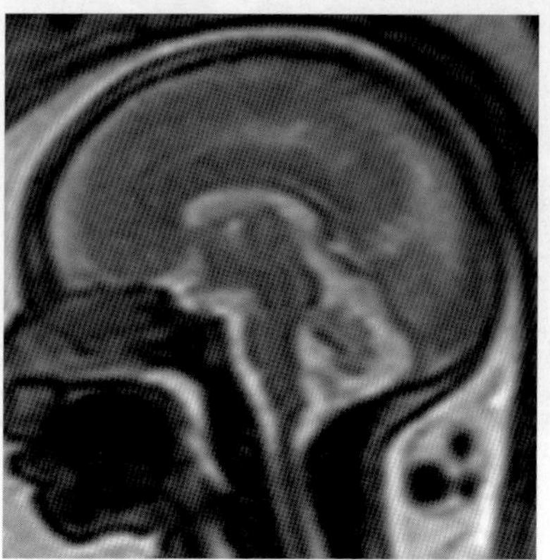

Delayed Rotation of the Vermis Mimicking a Malformation

- Early imaging of the fetal cerebellum may demonstrate an underrotated cerebellum, which in lateral gestational age becomes normal. Inferior vermian hypoplasia was overdiagnosed on fetal MRI in 32% in one series.

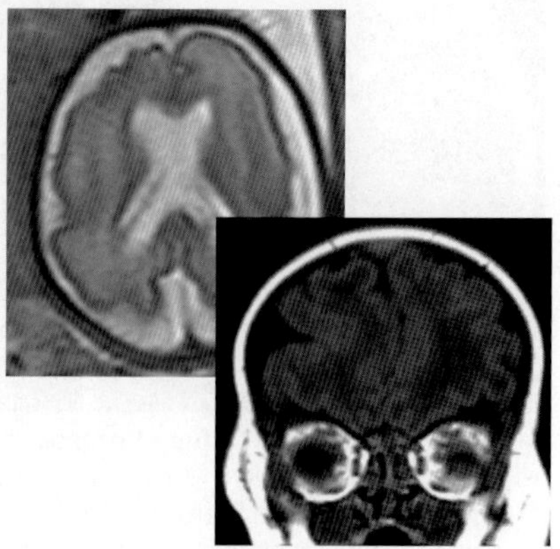

Polymicrogyria

- Detection of early appearance of sulci is an indicator of polymicrogyria. The sensitivity of fetal MRI for polymicrogyria is ~75% to 85% compared to postnatal MRI. Similarly, sensitivity for fetal MRI detection of gray matter heterotopia is ~44% to 75% depending on fetal age.

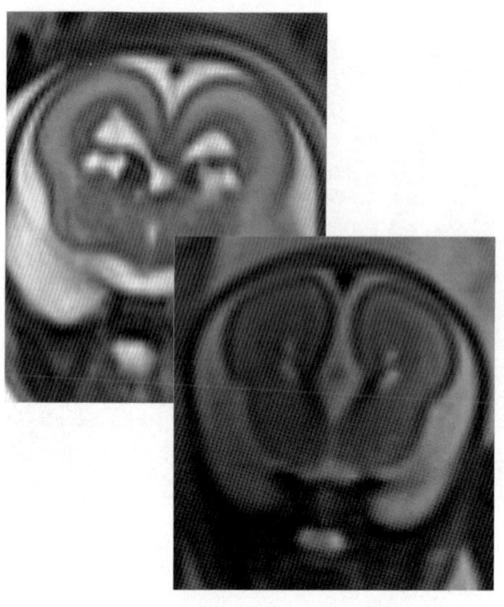

Ganglionic Eminence Cavitation

- Associated with cerebral anomalies. Should not be mistaken for choroid plexus or connatal cysts.

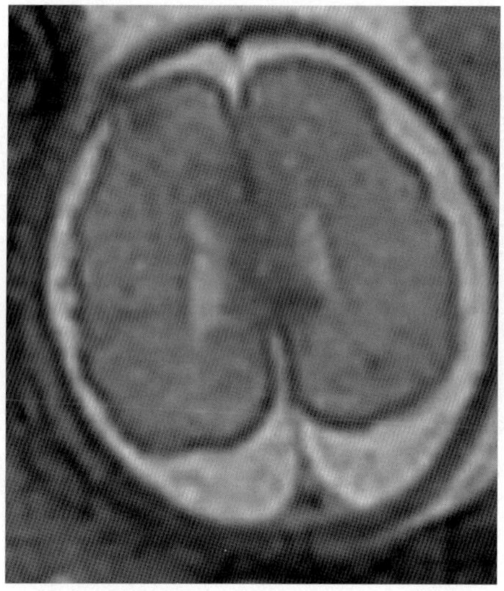

Tuberous Sclerosis

- Cortical tubers can be difficult to identify on fetal MRI, particularly in the 20 to 30 weeks' gestational age.
- Areas of T2W hypointense signal represent the cortical tubers.
- Often, fetal MRI is performed when a suspected cardiac rhadomyoma is identified on ultrasound.

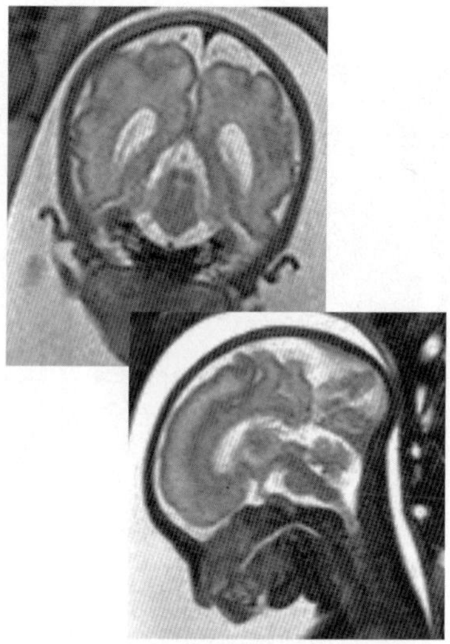

Rare and Lethal Anomalies: Agnathia Otocephaly

- The diagnoses are difficult due to the rarity and lethality
- Some examples include agnathia otocephaly (absent mandible and low-set ears fused below the mouth), acrania-exencephaly-anencephaly sequence, and iniencephaly.

REFERENCES

1. Chougar L, Blondiaux E, Moutard ML, et al. Variability of T1-weighted signal intensity of pericallosal lipomas in the fetus. *Pediatr Radiol.* 2018;48(3):383–391.
2. Limperopoulos C, Robertson RL, Estroff JA, et al. Diagnosis of inferior vermian hypoplasia by fetal magnetic resonance imaging: potential pitfalls and neurodevelopmental outcome. *Am J Obstet Gynecol.* 2006;194:1070–1076.
3. Pinto J, Paladini D, Severino M, et al. Delayed rotation of the cerebellar vermis: a pitfall in early second-trimester fetal magnetic resonance imaging. *Ultrasound Obstet Gynecol.* 2016;48(1):121–124.
4. Righini A, Frassoni C, Inverardi F, et al. Bilateral cavitations of ganglionic eminence: a fetal MR imaging sign of halted brain development. *AJNR Am J Neuroradiol.* 2013;34(9):1841–1845.

CHALLENGING MRI BRAIN DIAGNOSES

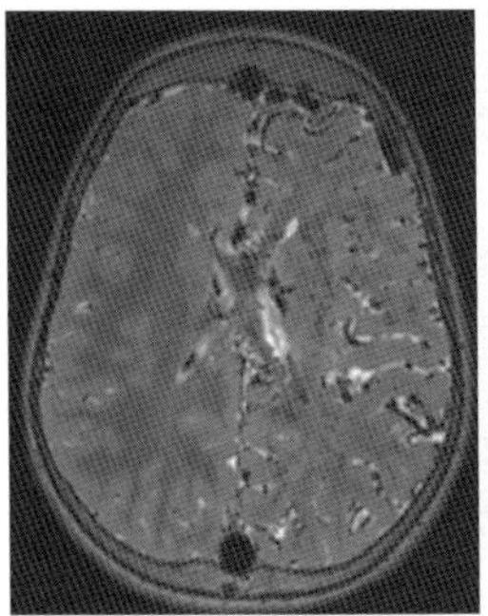
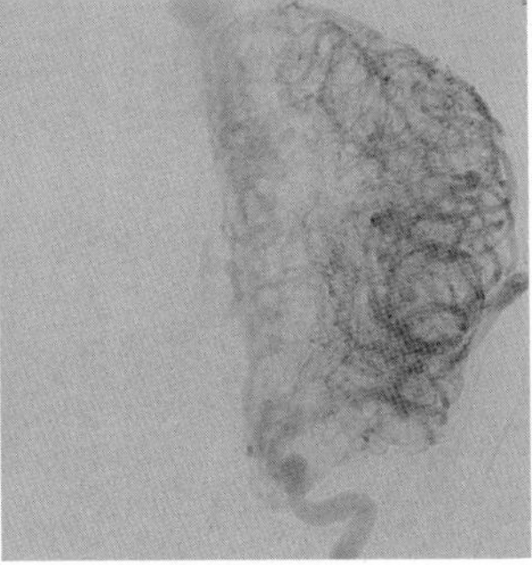

Diffuse Hemispheric AVM

- Rare type of AVM that diffusely involves the cerebral hemisphere.

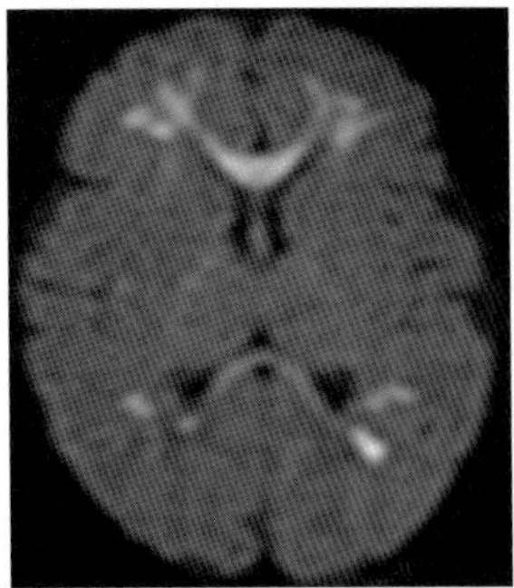

Parechovirus Mimicking HIE

- Parechovirus results in periventricular diffusion restriction and should be considered when clinical history does not support HIE.

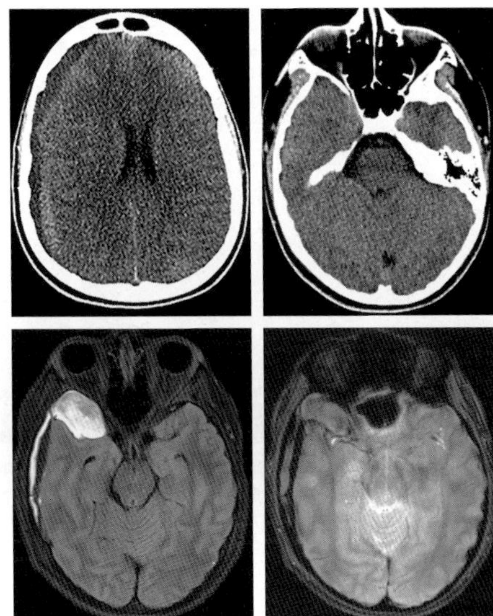

Ruptured and Hemorrhagic Arachnoid Cyst

- Arachnoid cysts may uncommonly rupture and hemorrhage, resulting in a subdural hemorrhage. Key to diagnosing this is the evidence of longstanding mass effect on the bone (seen in this example as a remodeled and anterior positioned right greater wing of the sphenoid).

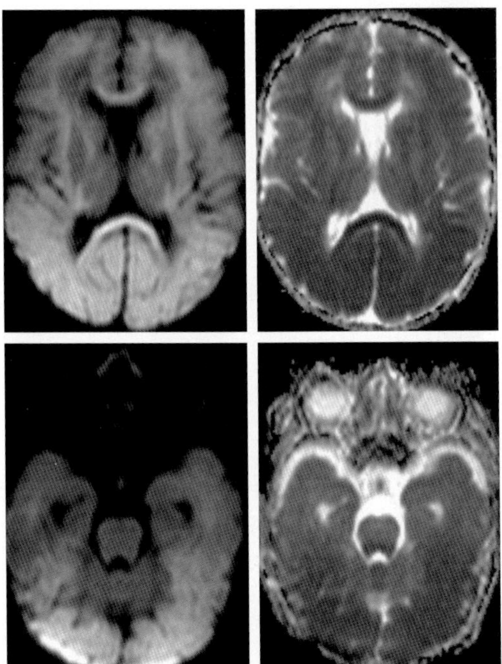

Diffuse Hypoxic Ischemic Injury

- The diffuse symmetric abnormality can be mistaken for normal. Keys to avoiding this pitfall is to use the cerebellum as an internal reference, measure ADC values, and remember that the unmyelinated white matter should allow greater diffusion and thus have ADC hyperintensity.

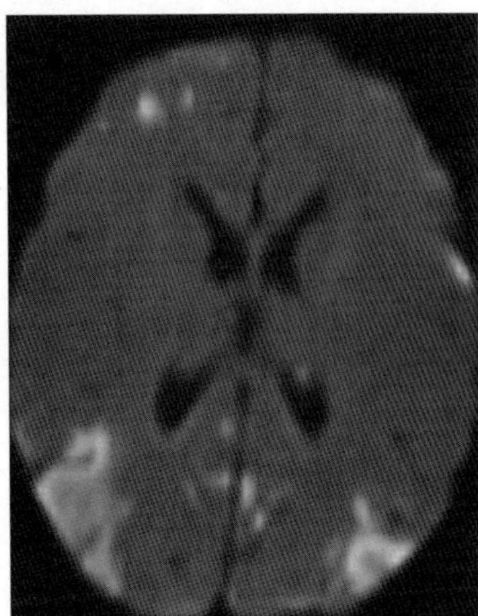

HSV-2 Mimicking Hypoxic Ischemic Injury/Perinatal Infarcts

- Consider HSV-2 in the neonatal period when there are multifocal infarcts and supportive clinical history such as fever and normal Apgar scores.

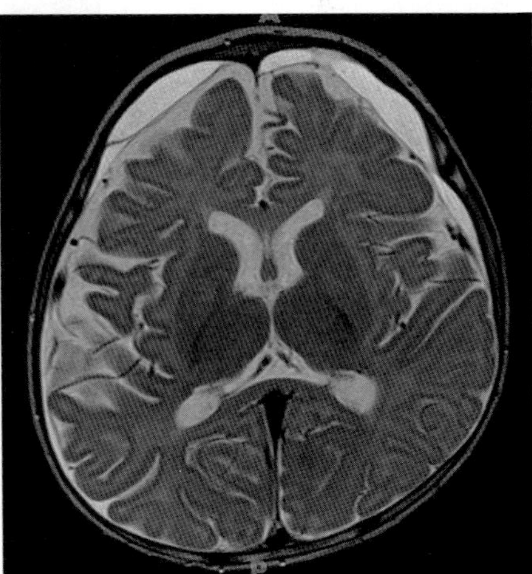

Glutaric Acidura Mimicking Abusive Head Trauma (AHT)

- Although subdurals are more common in AHT than glutaric aciduria, this diagnosis could be considered when the clinical history does not support AHT diagnosis and if there are other imaging features such as wide Sylvian fissures.

BRAIN TUMOR PITFALLS

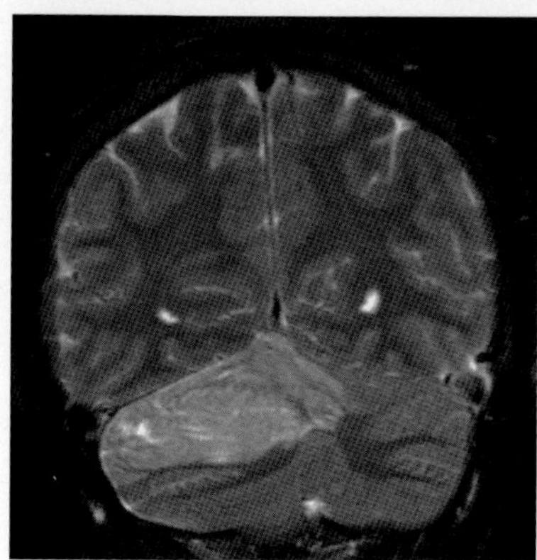
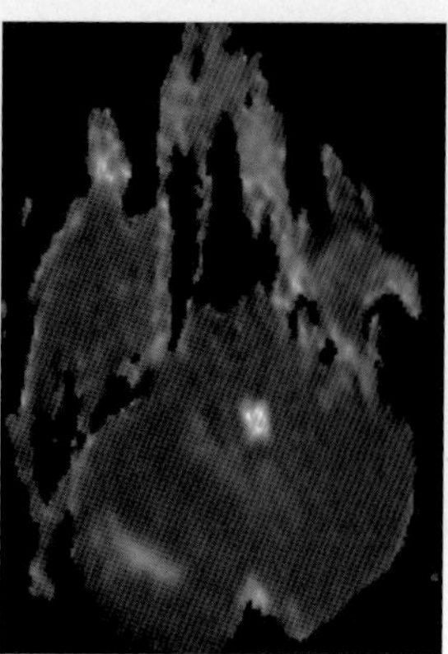

Medulloblastoma Mimicking Lhermitte Duclos

- ADC images are helpful in avoiding this pitfall. Medulloblastoma will have reduced ADC compared to Lhermitte Duclos with increased ADC.

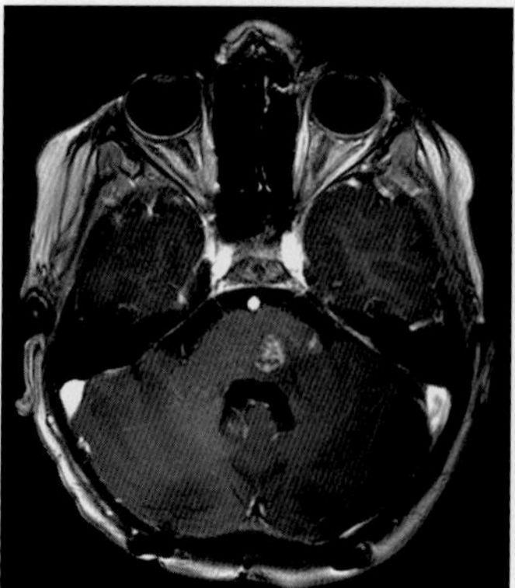
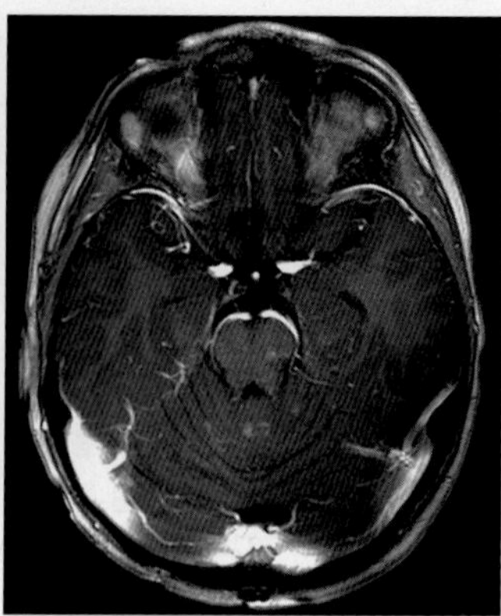

Radiation Necrosis

- Multiple scattered ring or nodular enhancing parenchymal lesions in the posterior fossa, a pattern that is uncommon for metastatic disease

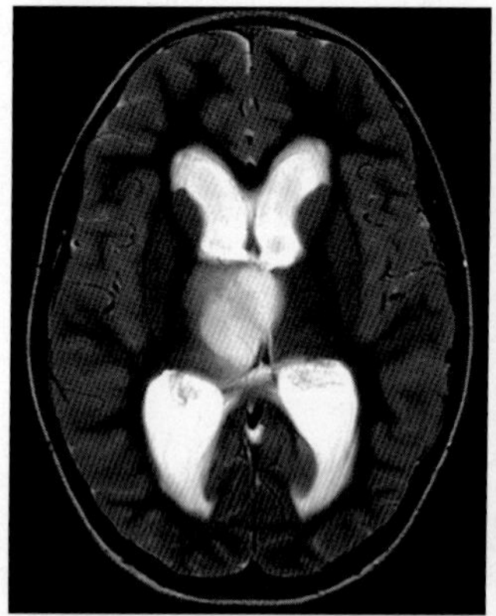
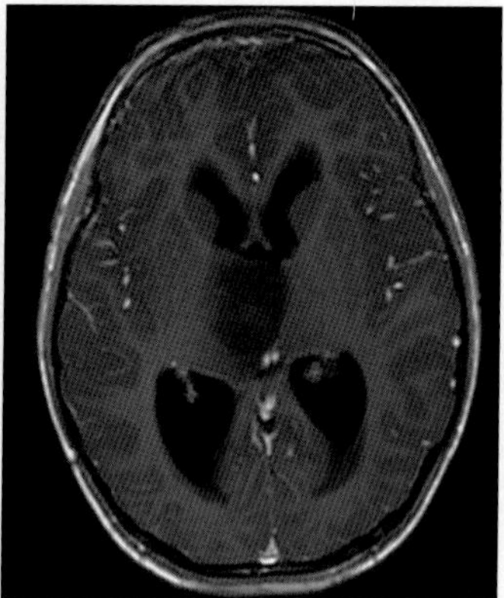

Thalamic High-Grade Glioma

- Such neoplasms may have the appearance of low-grade tumors. Pathology is needed to differentiate low- from high-grade tumors.

INNER EAR MALFORMATIONS

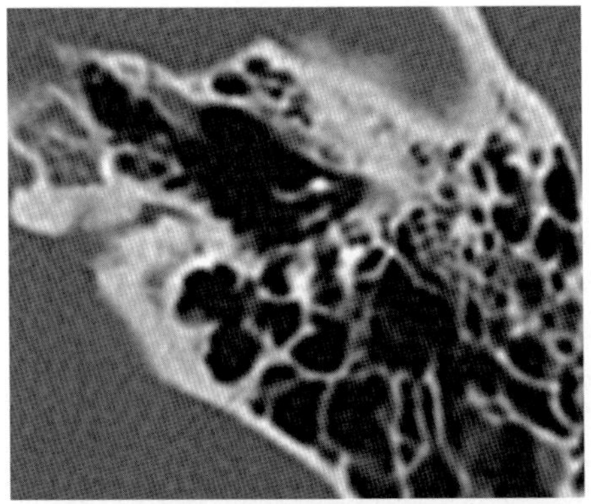

Labyrinthine Aplasia

- Findings: Absent inner ear structures, flat cochlear promontory, narrow petrous apex, and small or absent IAC.

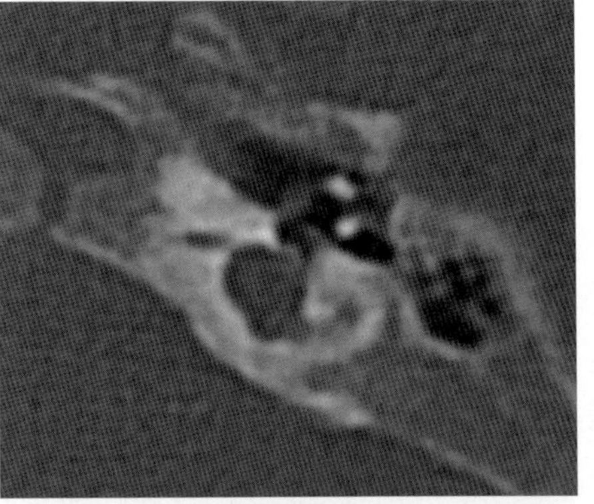

Cochlear Aplasia

- Findings: Absent cochlea, absent cochlear nerve, flat cochlear promontory, hypoplastic IAC, dysmorphic vestibule, semicircular canals, and anomalous facial nerve canal.

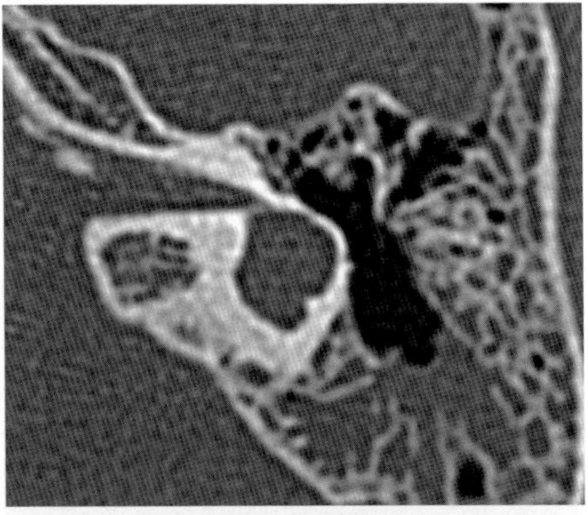

Common Cavity

- Findings: Single rounded/ovoid inner ear cavity comprised of the cochlea, vestibule, and semicircular canals, absent of hypoplastic cochlear nerve, IAC variable size and often opens at the center of the cavity.

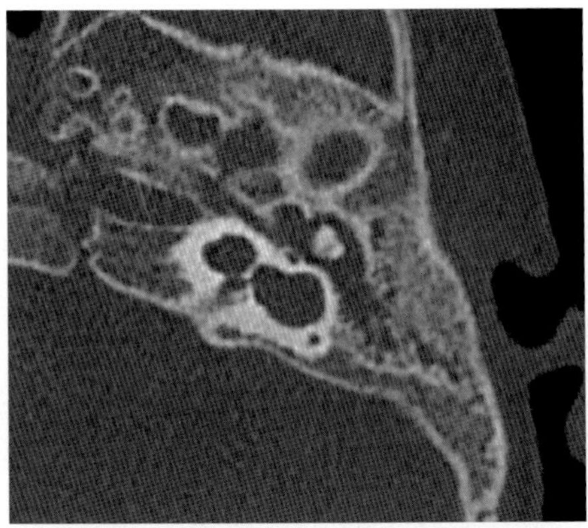

Incomplete Partition Anomaly Type 1 (IP-1)

- Also known as cystic cochleovestibular anomaly seen as a "figure of 8" appearance of the cochlea and vestibule.

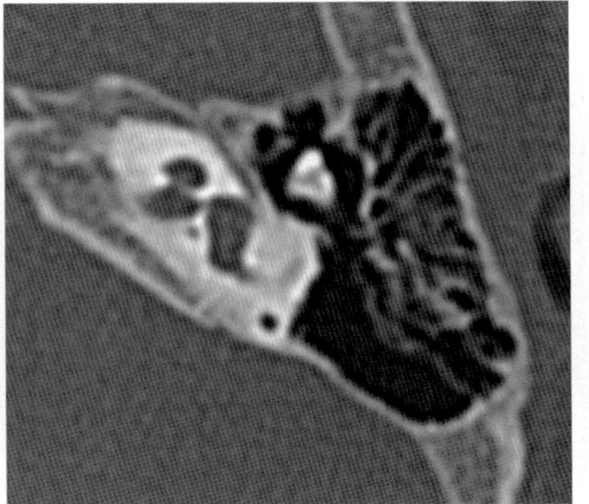

Cochlear Hypoplasia

- Findings: Incomplete formation of the cochlea with a single turn or bud-like appearance; IAC normal or narrow; cochlear aperture small; cochlear nerve absent or hypoplastic; vestibule and semicircular canals can be normal, dilated, or hypoplastic; aberrant facial nerve.

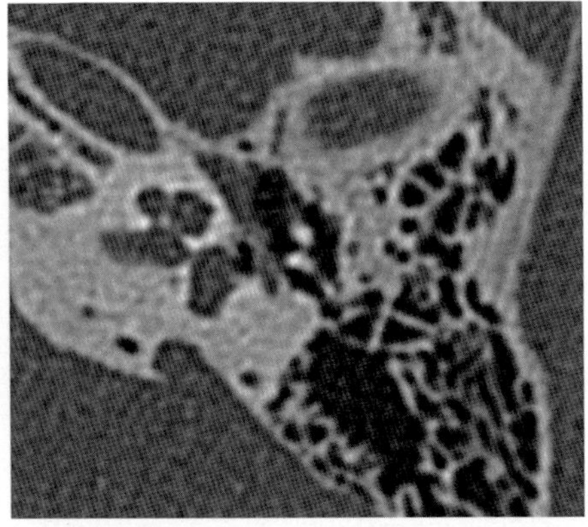

Incomplete Partition Anomaly Type 2 (IP-2)

- Findings: Malformation of the apical and middle turns of the cochlea with enlarged vestibular aqueduct.

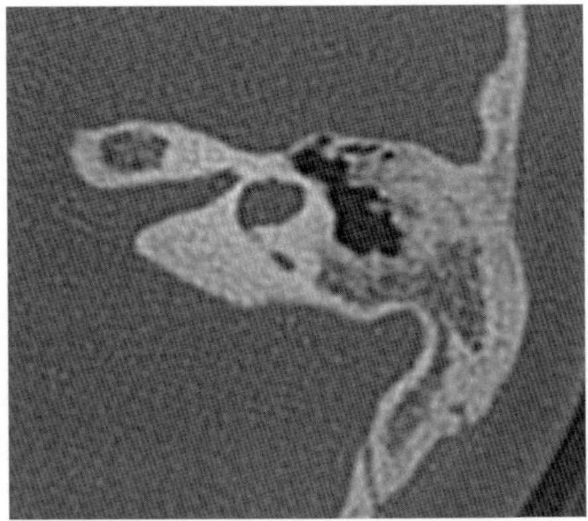

Lateral Semicircular Dysplasia

- The lateral semicircular canal is the last canal to form such that it is the most common canal to be malformed. The canal appears short and wide and either lacks or has a small bone in the center separating the canal from the vestibule.

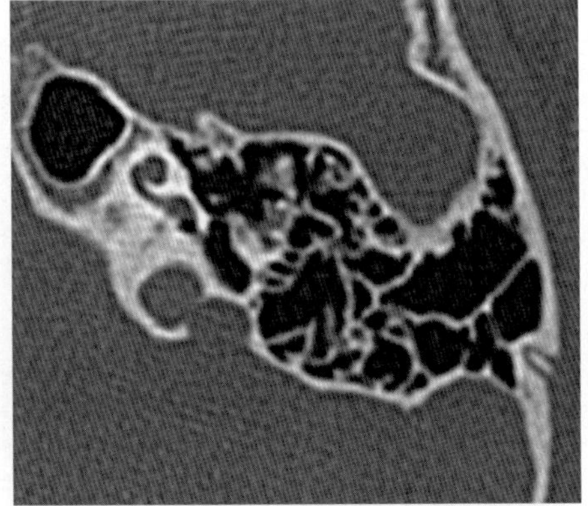

Branchio-Oto-Renal Syndrome

- Findings: Cochlea has an "unwound" appearance. Associated with branchial fistulas or cysts and renal anomalies.

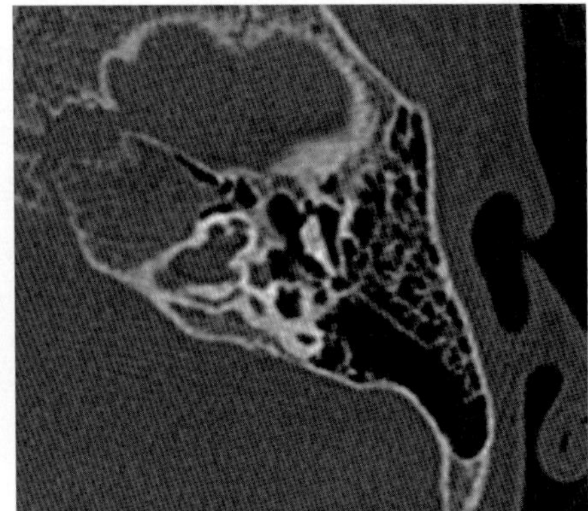

X-linked Deafness

- Findings: Absent modiolus and lamina cribosa allows for communication between perilymph and CSF and potential for CSF leak if stapes is removed.

HEARING LOSS FINDINGS

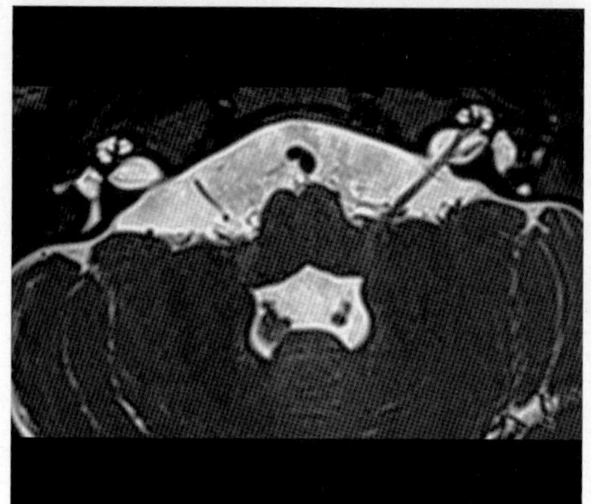

Absent Cochlear Nerve

- Ipsilateral small IAC
- Cochlear aperture atresia
- May be associated with inner ear malformations and other nerve deficiencies
- Unilateral or bilateral

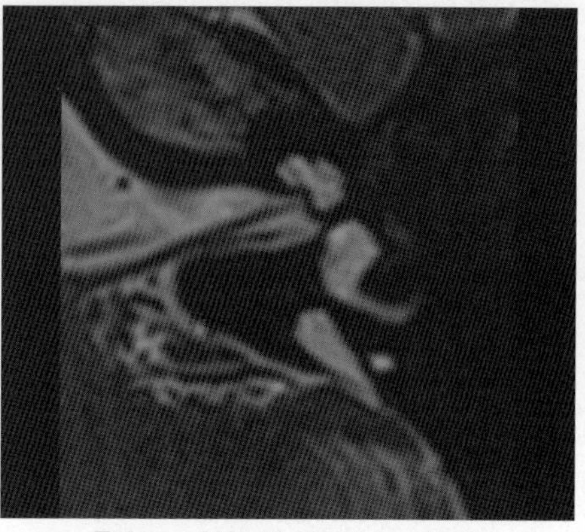

Enlarged Vestibular Aqueduct

- Common cause of SNHL
- Aqueduct measures >1.5 mm or larger than the adjacent semicircular canal
- Typically associated with incomplete partition type II
- Often bilateral

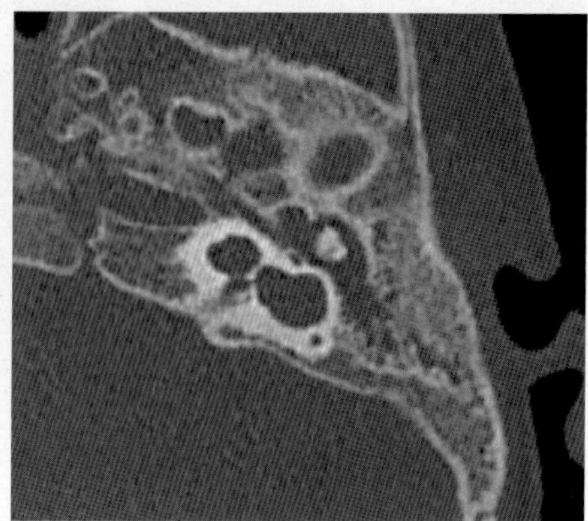

Inner Ear Malformation

- Includes labyrinthine aplasia, cochlear aplasia/hypoplasia, common cavity, IP-1, and IP-2.

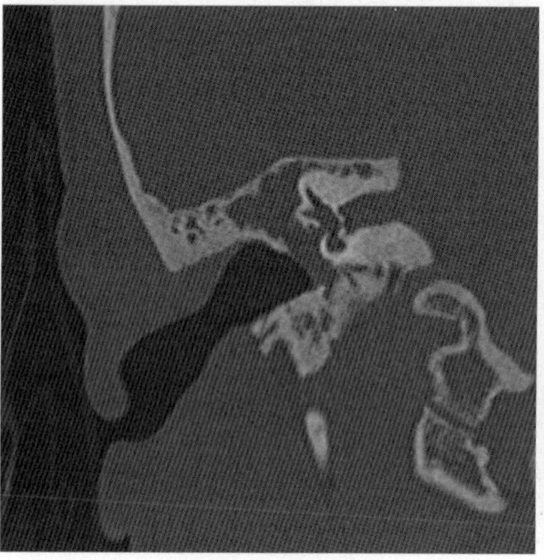

Cholesteatoma

- Growth of keratinizing squamous epithelium with aggressive bony and ossicular erosion
- Nonenhancing; restricted diffusion

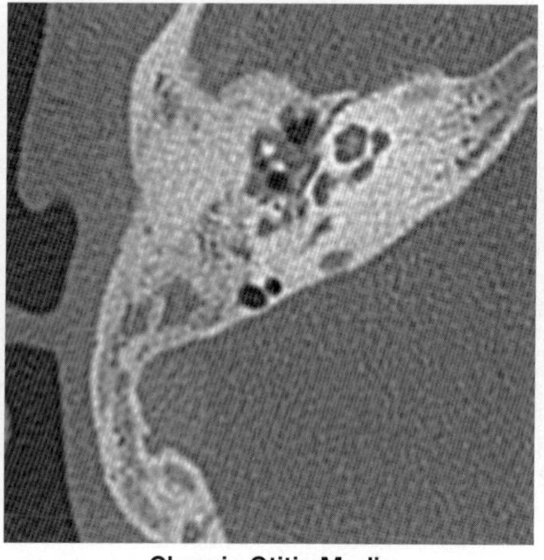

Chronic Otitis Media

- Associated with sensorineural hearing loss (SNHL) and conductive hearing loss (CHL).

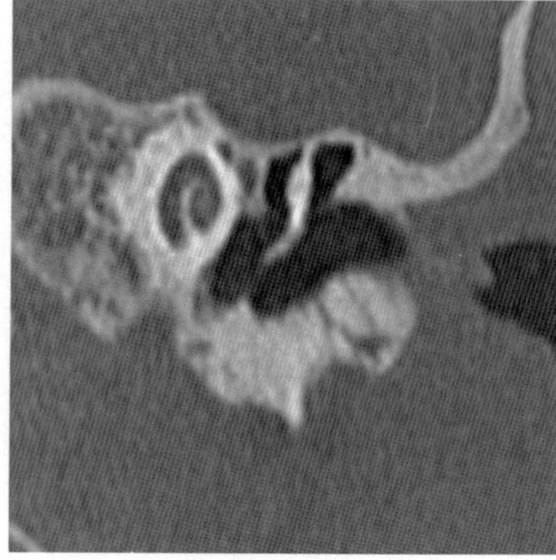

Malleus Fixation

- Congenital or sequelae of chronic otitis media (suspensory ligament ossification) or trauma.

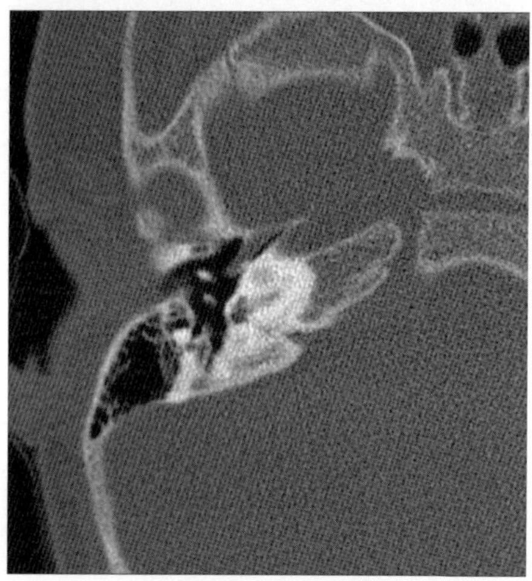

Labyrinthitis Ossificans

- Fibrous and/or ossific deposition of inner secondary to infection, trauma, or instrumentation.

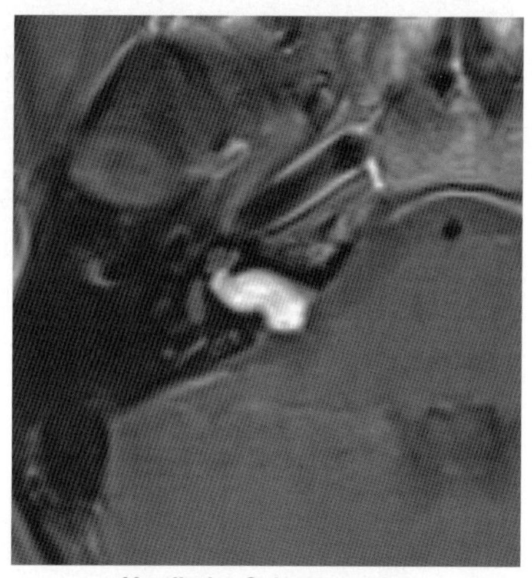

Vestibular Schwannoma

- Avidly enhancing sporadic or NF-2-associated mass centered within the IAC.

CRANIOSYNOSTOSIS

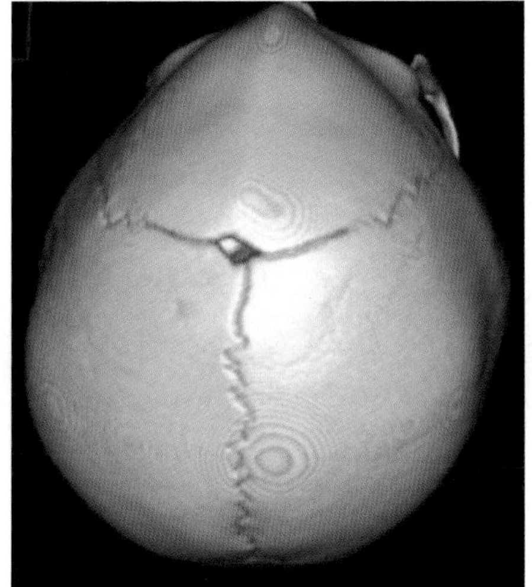

Metopic Craniosynostosis
- Trigonocephaly
- Hypotelorism

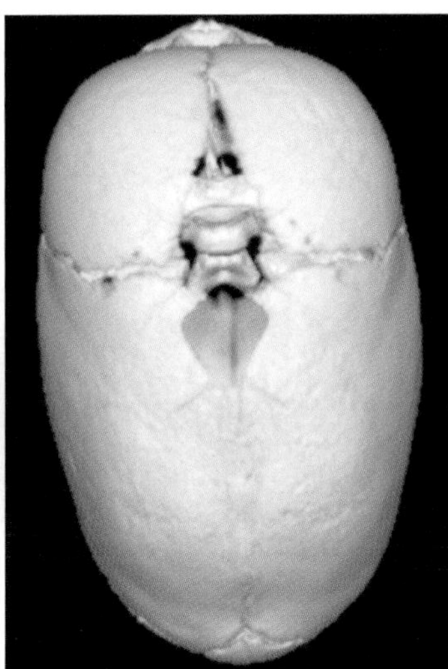

Sagittal Craniosynostosis
- Scaphocephaly
- Most common craniosynostosis

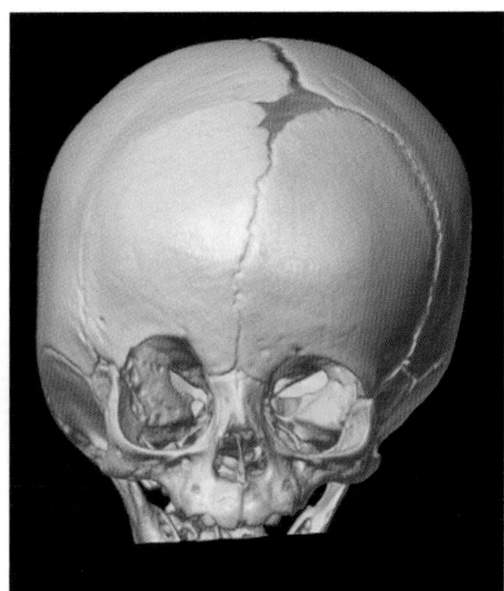

Unilateral Coronal Craniosynostosis
- Anterior plagiocephaly
- Harlequin eye

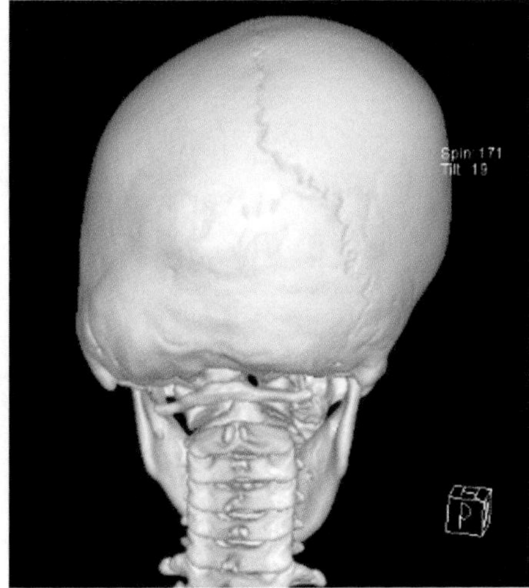

Lambdoid Craniosynostosis
- Posterior plagiocephaly

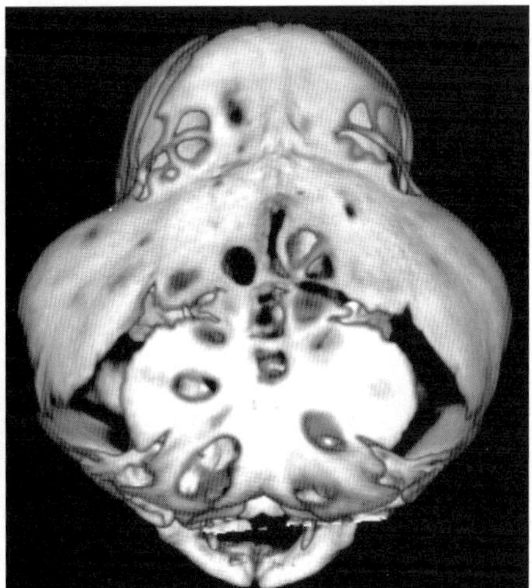

Multiple Craniosynostosis
- Cloverleaf calvarium or Kleeblattschadel deformity
- Associated with Crouzon syndrome, Pfeiffer syndrome, and Apert syndrome

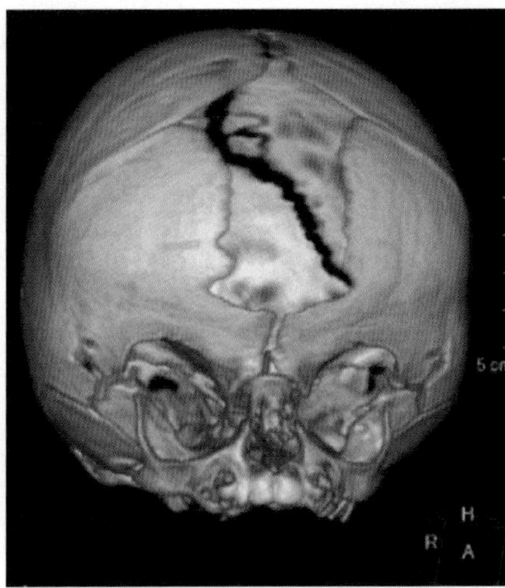

Bicoronal Craniosynostosis
- Brachycephaly

FACIAL MALFORMATION

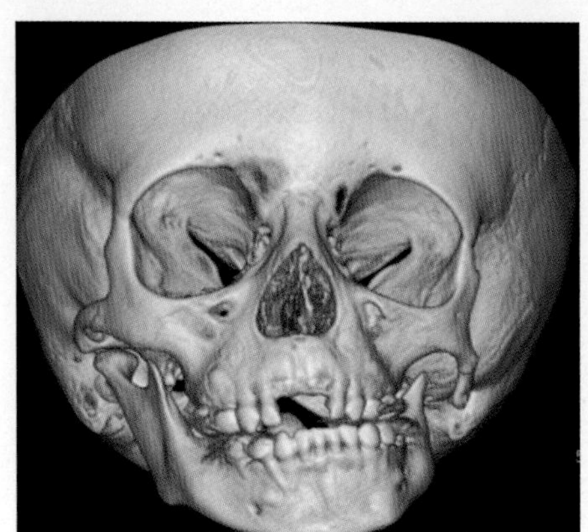

Hemifacial Microsomia

- Unilateral mandibular hypoplasia
- EAC atresia
- Vertebral anomalies

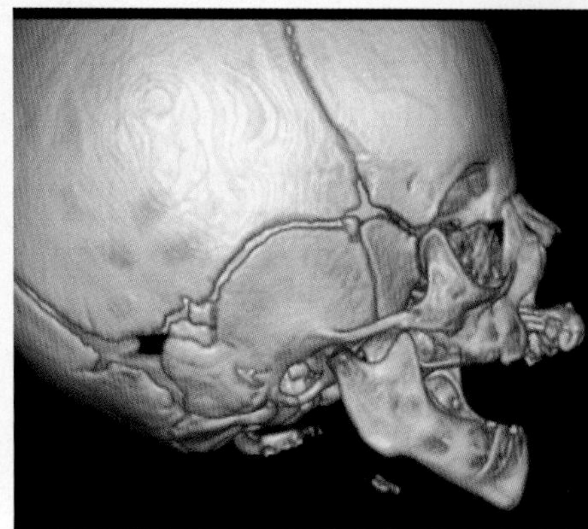

Pierre Robin Syndrome

- Micrognathia
- Glossoptosis
- Cleft palate

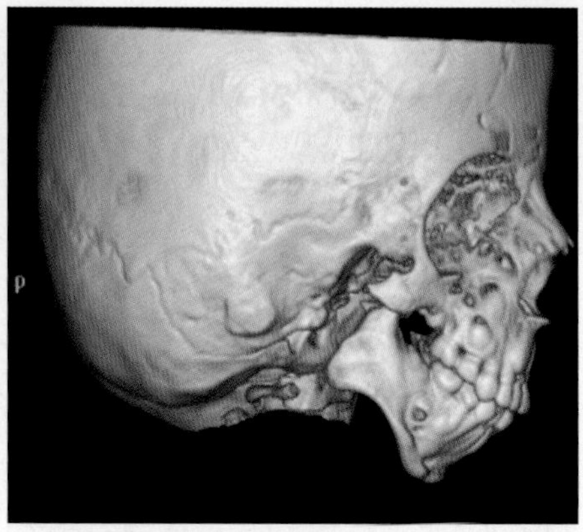

Treacher-Collins Syndrome

- Micrognathia
- Maxillary hypoplasia
- EAC atresia
- Cleft lip and palate

CYSTIC NECK MASS

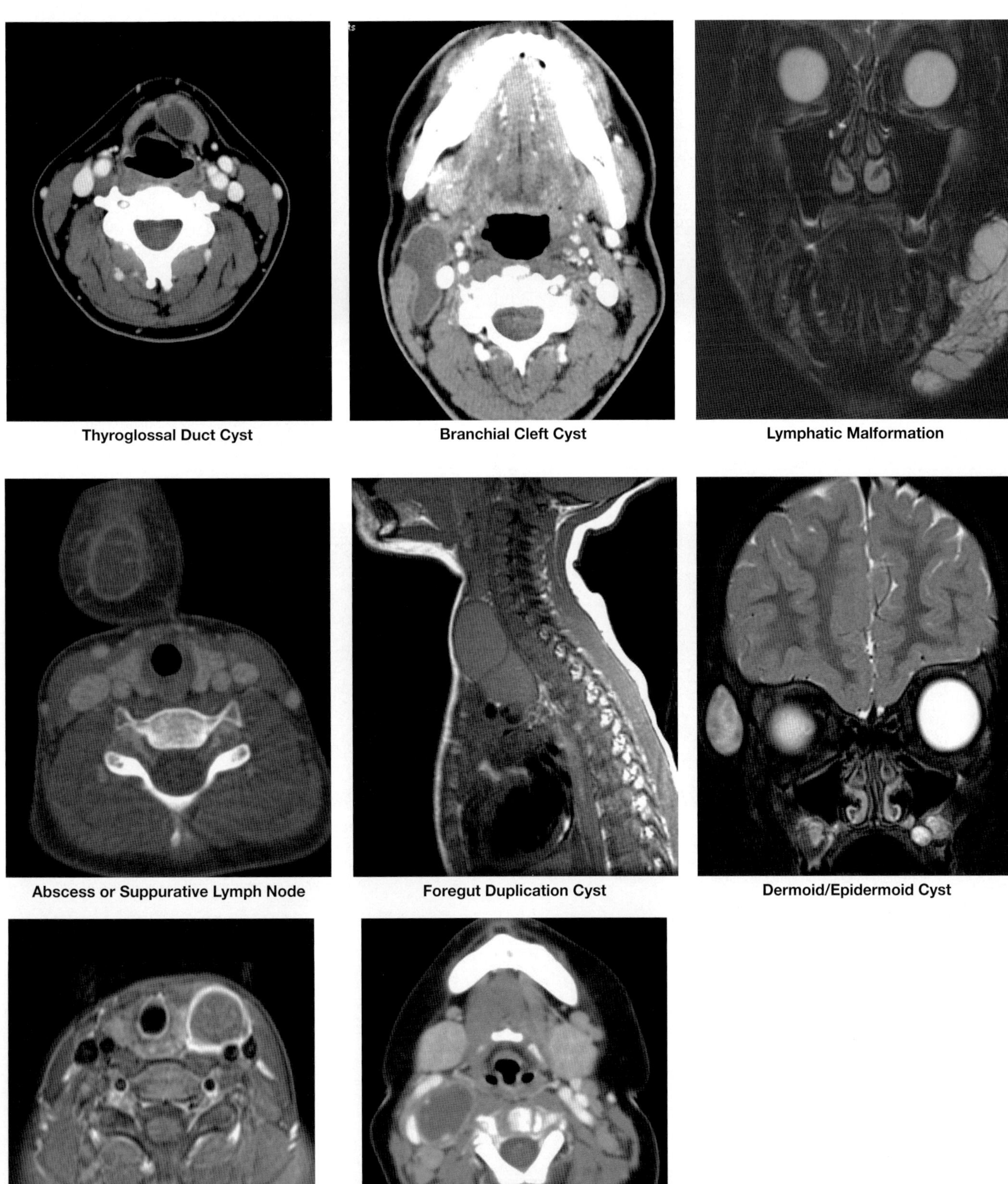

BRANCHIAL CLEFT ANOMALIES

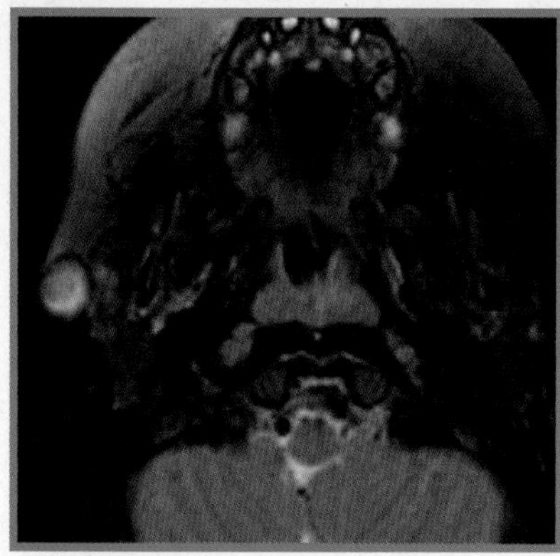

First BCC

Work type 1- preauricular
Work type 2- angle of mandible or submandibular

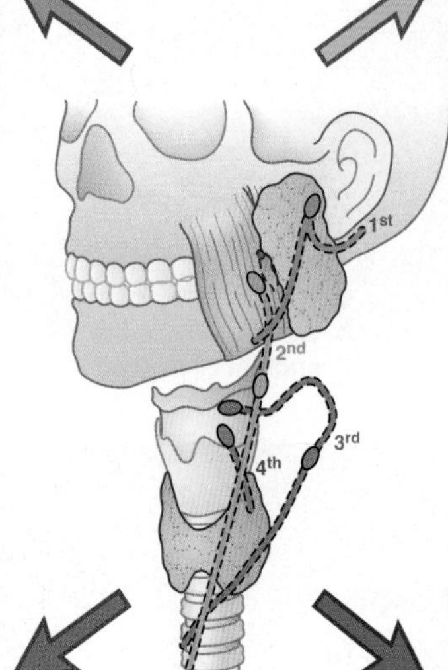

Second BCC

Commonly anterior to sternocleidomastoid, posterior to submandibular gland, and lateral to carotid space but can occur anywhere along the embryonic sinus from skin exit site at the level of the thyroid adjacent to the sternocleidomastoid muscle, between ECA and ICA to palatine tonsil.

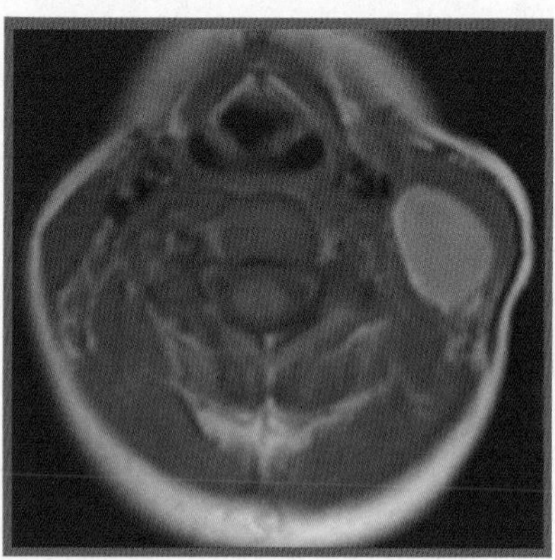

Third BCC

- Typically on left posterior to carotid space, deep or posterior to sternocleidomastoid occurring anywhere from piriform sinus, posterior to carotid space between CN IX and CN XII.
- Difficult to differentiate from 4th BCC.

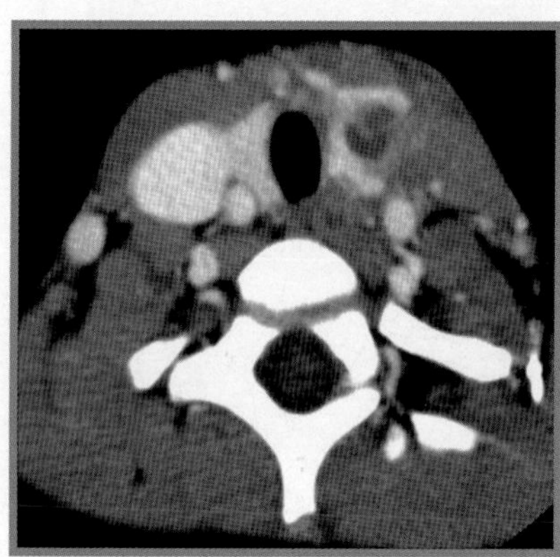

Fourth BCC

- Sinus extends from the left piriform sinus to the left thyroid lobe into the mediastinum.
- Commonly presents with left thyroiditis and/or thyroid abscess.

SOLID NECK MASS

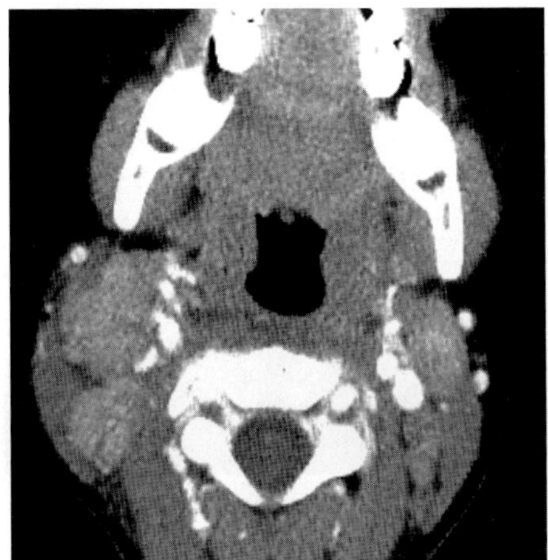

Nodal

- Lymphadenopathy and lymphadenitis
- Lymphoma
- Nasopharyngeal carcinoma
- Neuroblastoma

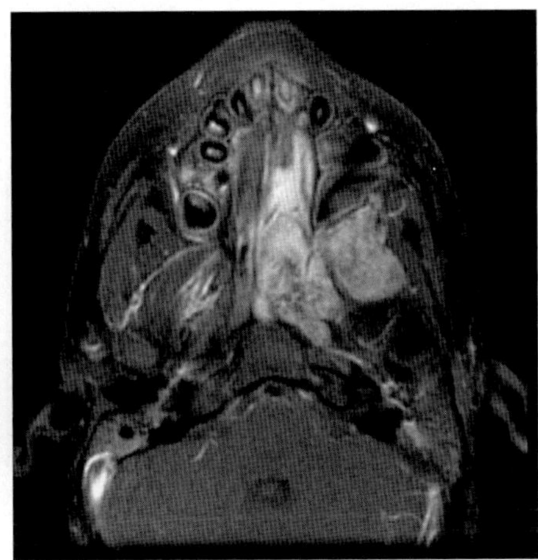

Nonnodal

- Rhabdomyosarcoma
- Juvenile angiofibroma
- Nerve sheath tumor

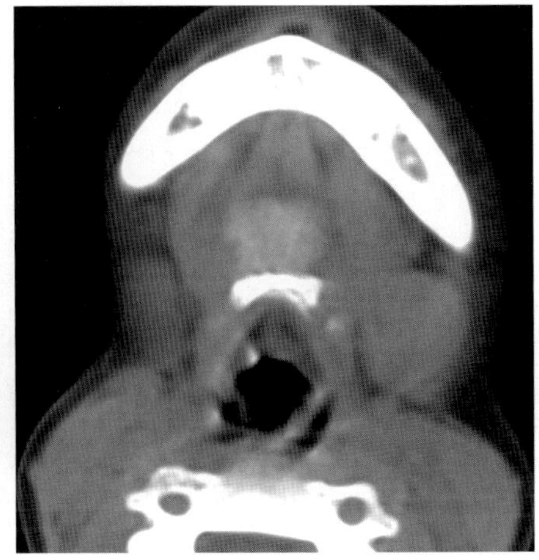

Congenital

- Ectopic thyroid
- Ectopic thymus
- Teratoma
- Nasal glial heterotopia

SCALP MASS

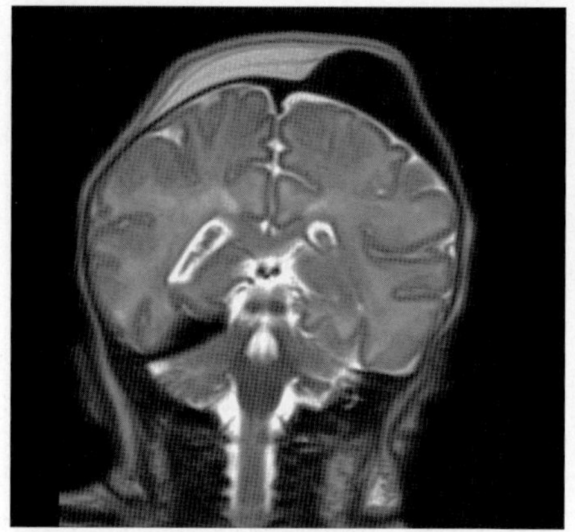

Hematoma

- Cephalohematoma crosses sutures.
- Subgaleal hematoma crosses sutures.
- Subperiosteal hematoma does not cross sutures.

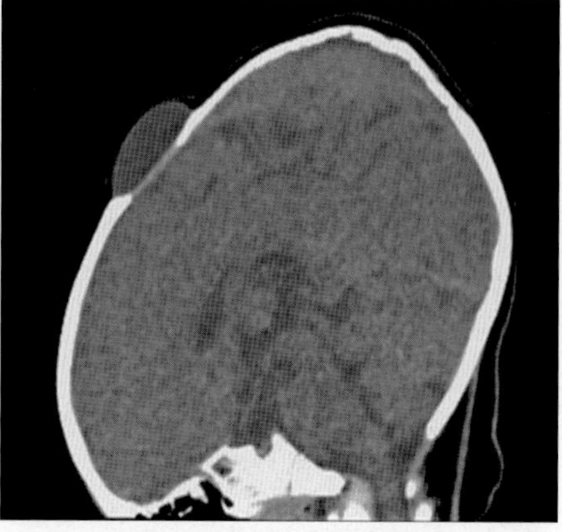

Dermoid/Epidermoid Cyst

- Associated with bregma and sutures
- Bony remodeling
- Restricted diffusion in epidermoids, often but not all dermoids
- No enhancement

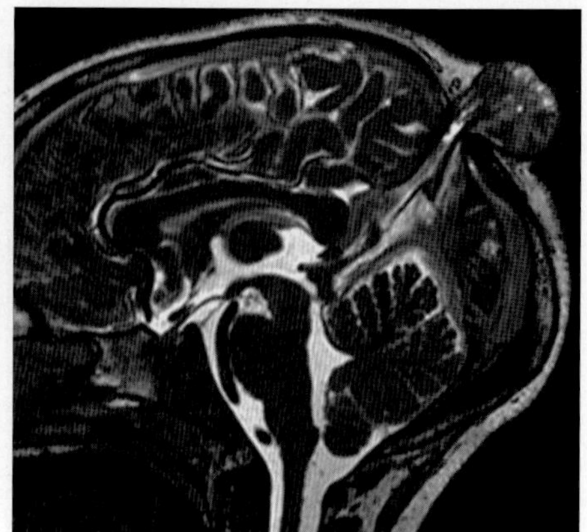

Atretic Encephalocele

- Involuted cephalocele containing dura, dysplastic brain with small bone defect.

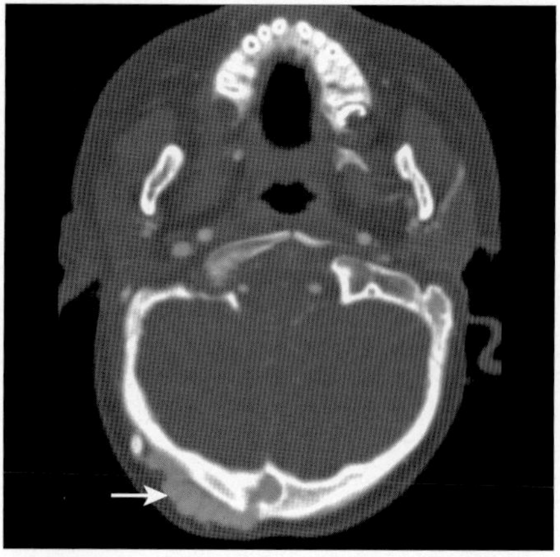

Sinus Pericranii

- Scalp vein(s) draining into dural venous sinus

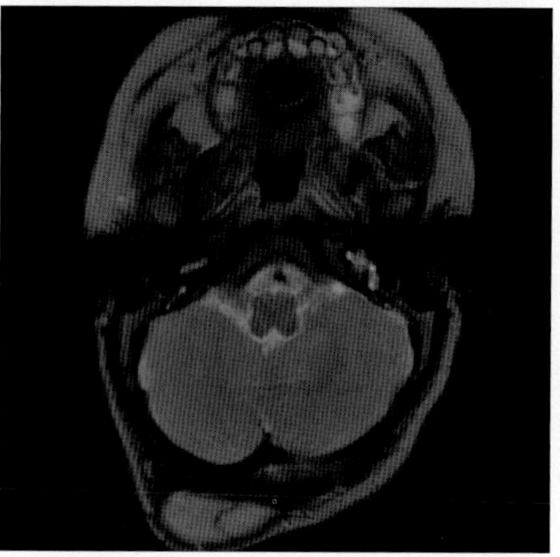

Infantile Hemangioma

- T2W hyperintense well-defined mass with homogenous avid enhancement and flow voids.

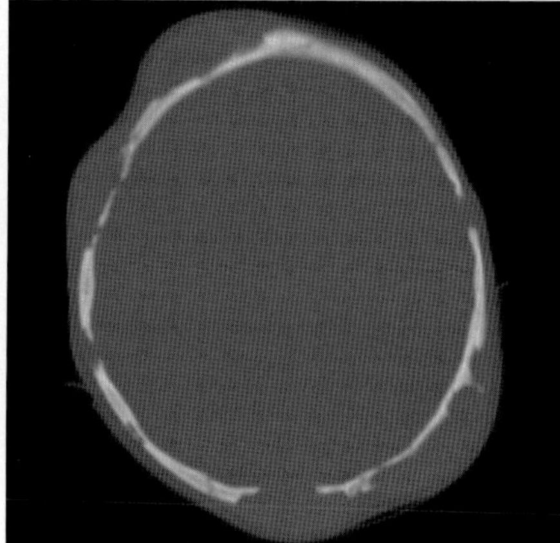

Langerhans Cell Histiocytosis

- Lytic mass lesions often multiple.

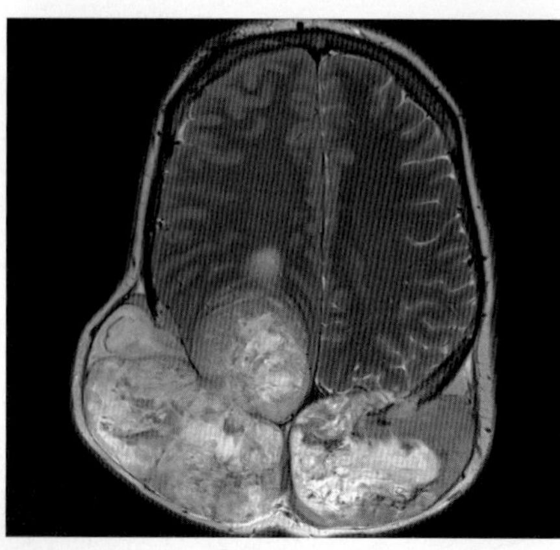

Sarcoma

- Small to large mass lesions often locally aggressive
- May have intracranial extension

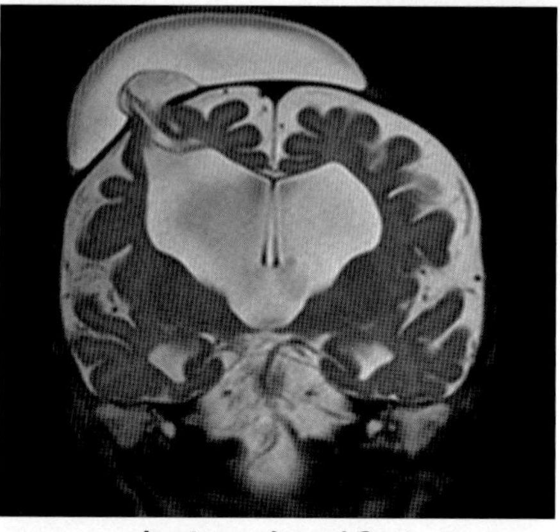

Leptomeningeal Cyst

- Dural tear associated with increasingly diastatic calvarial fracture/defect.

NEONATAL NECK MASS

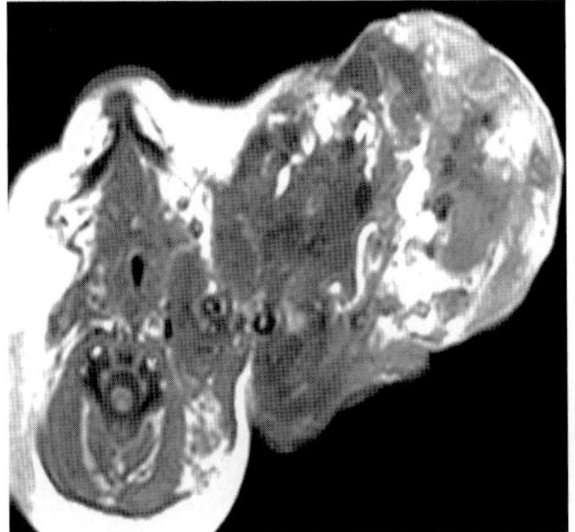

Teratoma

- Solid and cystic mass.
- May have Ca^{2+} and/or macroscopic fat.
- Usually encapsulated as a discrete mass; polyhydramnios can occur in utero due to fetal inability to swallow amniotic fluid
- Head and neck location accounts for only 5% of teratoma
- May result in respiratory distress or disfigurement
- Rarely become malignant in children

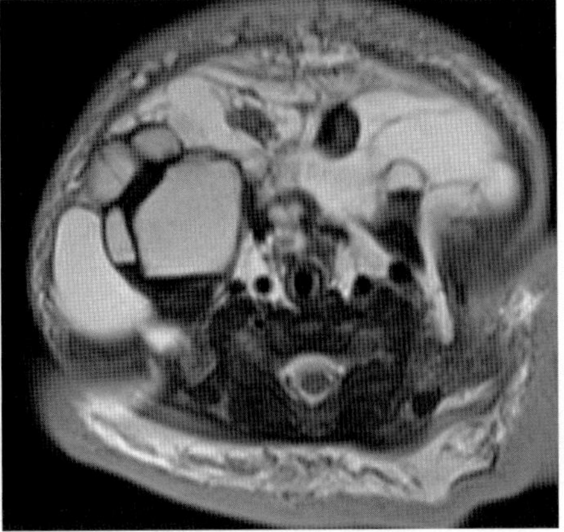

Lymphatic Malformation

- Complex multicystic transpatial hypovascular mass with fluid levels (containing blood products) and thin enhancing walls/septae
- May be enlarged due to hemorrhage or infection
- Associated with trisomy 21 and Turner syndrome

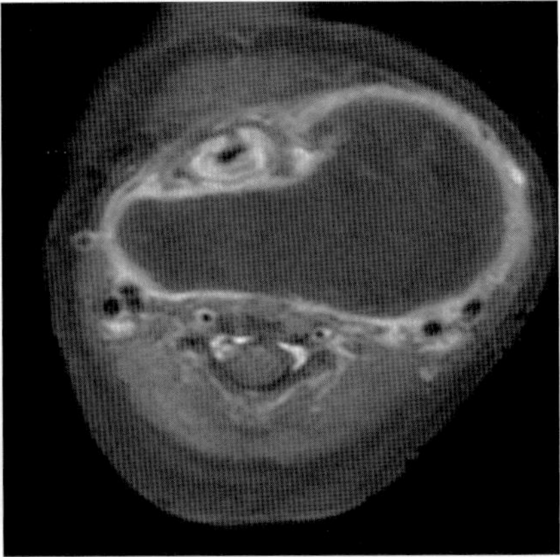

Infected Thymic Cyst

- Unilocular cyst in the lateral neck but extends into the retropharyngeal space when large
- Rapidly enlarging neck mass in a neonate due to superinfection from communication of the cyst with the GI tract

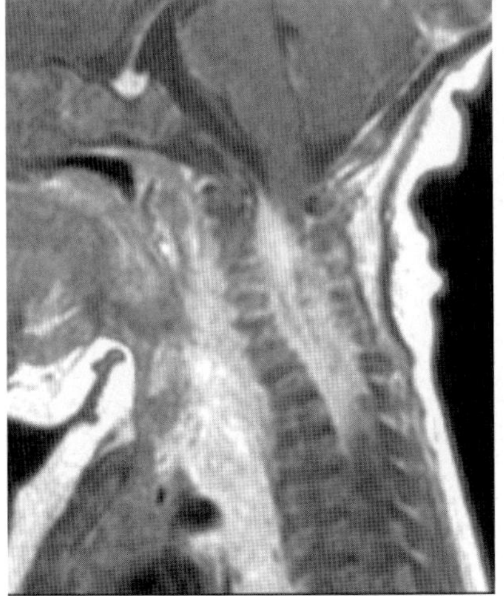

Infantile Myofibromatosis

- Infiltrative solid avidly enhancing mass with high cellularity that may mimic neuroblastoma
- Solitary or multicentric
- Despite benign clinical behavior, histopathology demonstrates vascularity, necrosis, local invasion, and increased cellularity

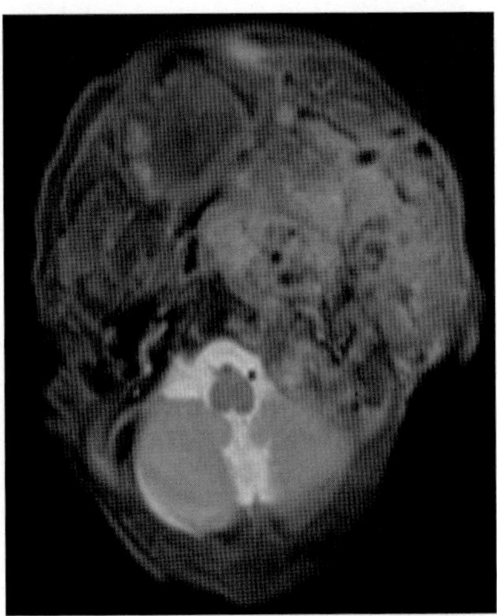

Kaposiform Hemangioblastoma

- Rare congenital vascular tumor
- Solitary or diffuse infiltrative solid mass with aggressive appearance, flow voids related to feeding and draining vessels, and hemorrhage
- T2W hyperintense relative to muscle. May have scattered areas of hemorrhage and diffusion restriction
- Hypervascular appearance on ultrasound
- May result in thrombocytopenia

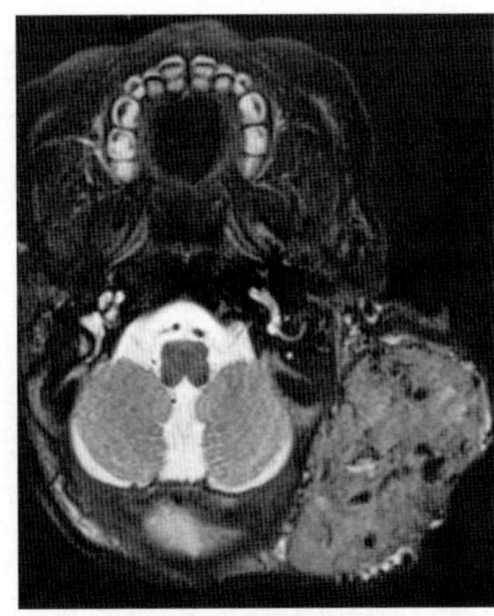

Congenital Hemangioma

- Benign vascular tumor present at birth. Avidly enhancing mass with flow voids and enlarged arterial feeding vessels
- May contain calcification and visible vessels on ultrasound to greater degree than infantile hemangiomas
- Types: Rapidly involuting congenital hemangioma (RICH) and noninvoluting congenital hemangioma (NICH). Neither expresses GLUT-1 transporter, which are present in infantile hemangiomas
- May result in vascular shunting or thrombocytopenia when large

NASOPHARYNGEAL MASS

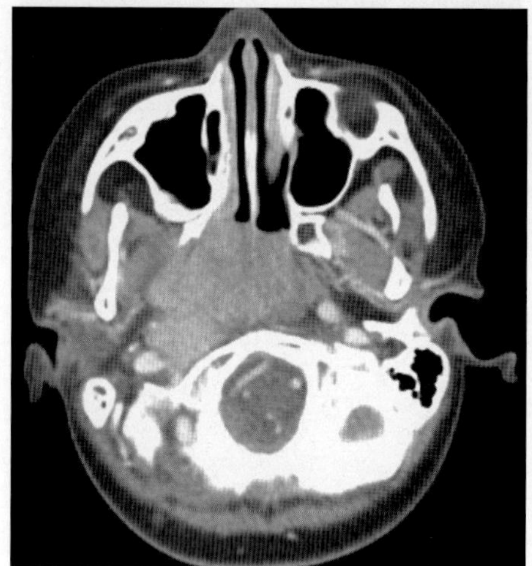

Nasopharyngeal Carcinoma

- Locally aggressive enhancing mass lesion
- May cause bony erosion, intracranial extension
- Lymphadenopathy in majority of patients at presentation
- Difficult to distinguish from lymphoma and rhabdomyosarcoma

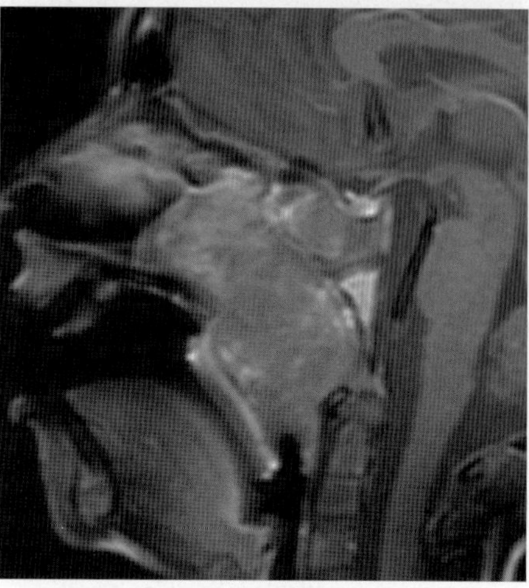

Lymphoma

- Waldeyer ring in sporadic form
- Endemic form involves facial bones
- Difficult to distinguish from nasopharyngeal and rhabdomyosarcoma

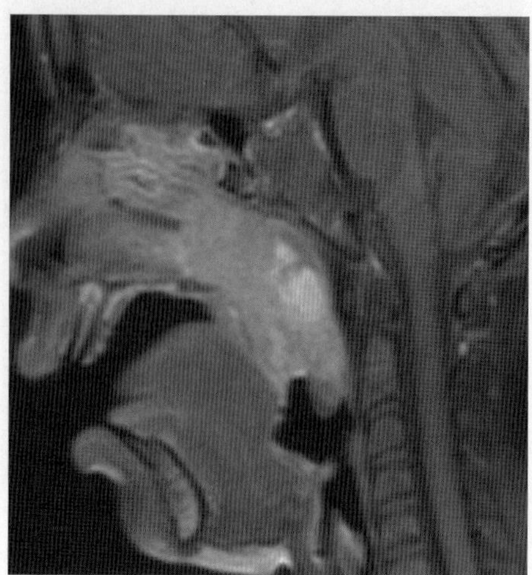

Rhabdomyosarcoma

- Locally aggressive enhancing mass lesion
- May cause bony erosion, intracranial extension
- Difficult to distinguish from nasopharyngeal and rhabdomyosarcoma

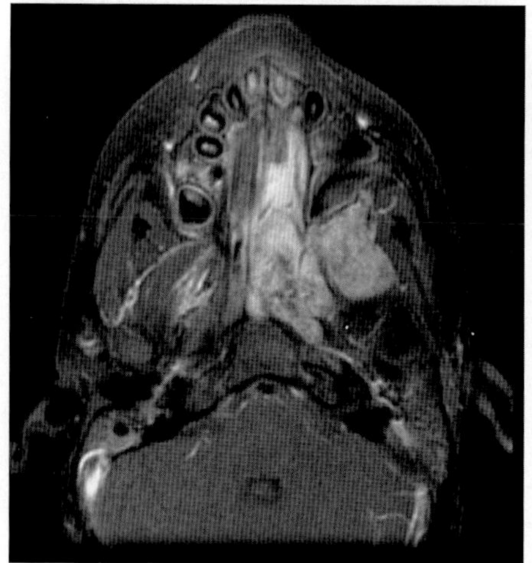

Juvenile Angiofibroma

- Benign but locally aggressive mass arising from sphenopalatine foramen widening pterygopalatine fossa with regional invasion
- Bony remodeling more than erosion
- Hypervascular, avidly enhancing, may have flow voids appearing
- M:F ratio 10:1
- Presents with epistaxis and/or nasal congestion

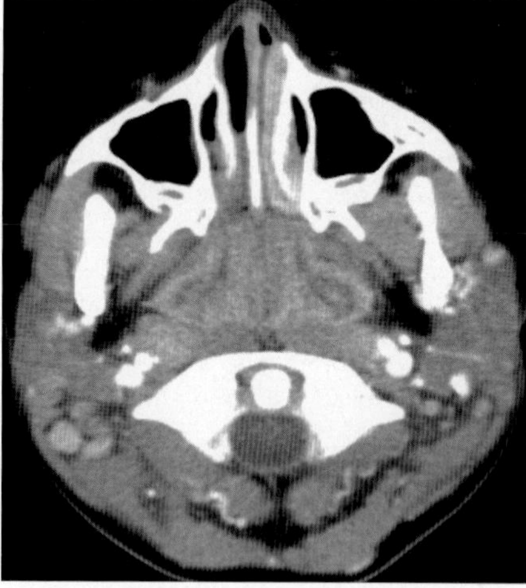

Adenoiditis/Pharyngitis

- Symmetric diffuse enlargement and striated enhancement

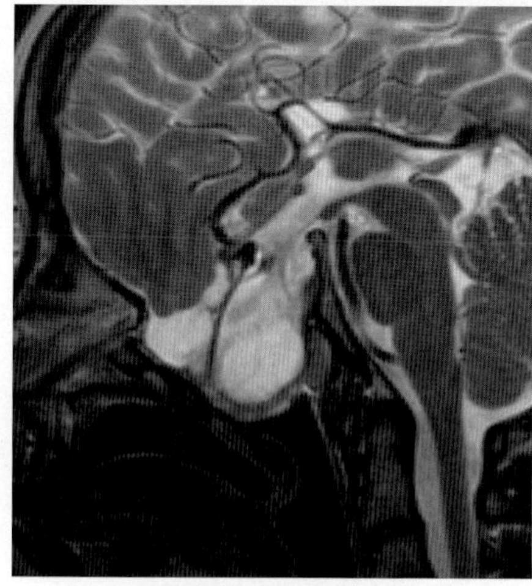

Meningoencephalocele

- Deficient central skull base with protrusion of the CSF sac containing variable brain parenchyma and/or optic apparatus, pituitary

ORBITAL MASS

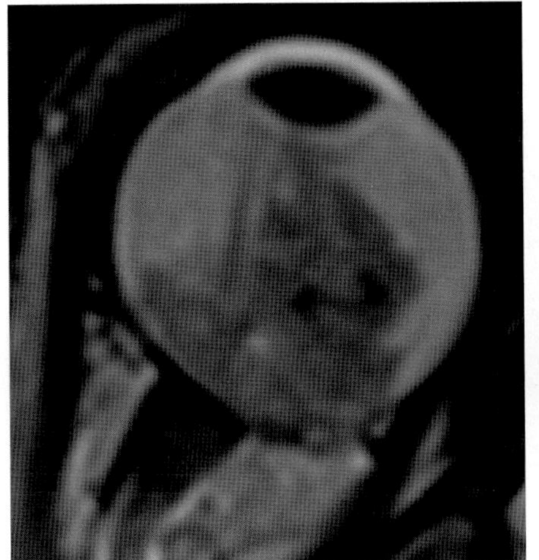

Retinoblastoma

- Most common intraocular neoplasm

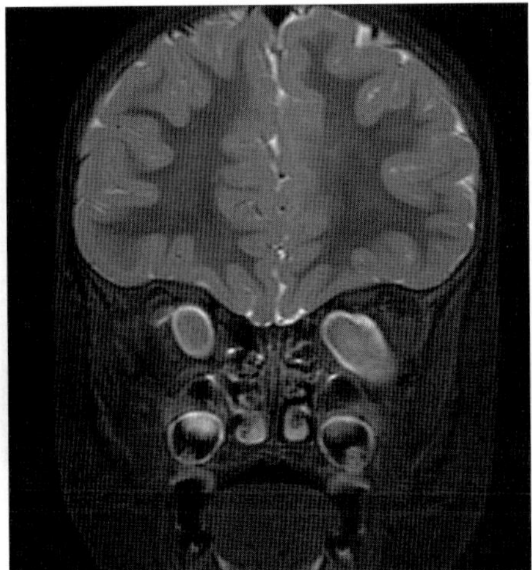

Optic Nerve Glioma

- Usually a low-grade glioma
- NF-1

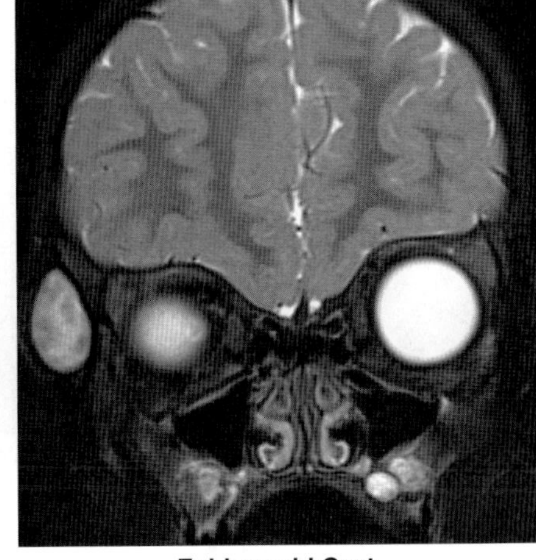

Epidermoid Cyst

- Cystic mass with diffusion restriction
- Usually along the suture lines, most commonly the superolateral orbit

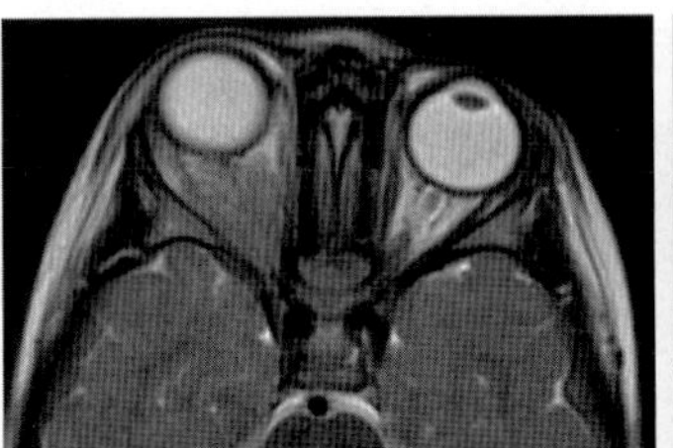

Rhabdomyosarcoma

- Orbital rhabdomyosarcomas may mimic infantile hemangioma except for reduced diffusion

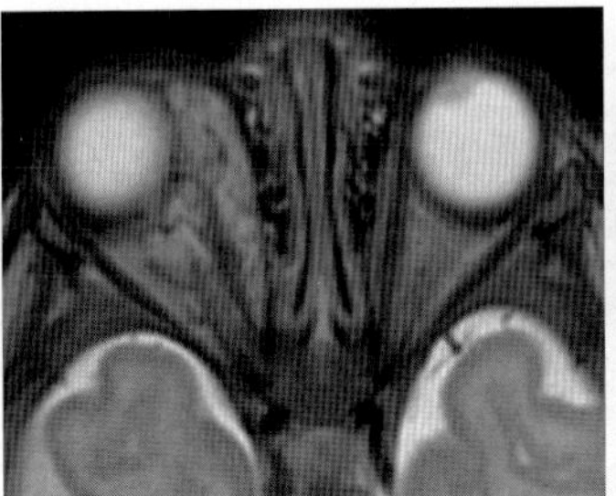

Infantile Hemangioma

- Vascular neoplasm
- Mild T2W hyperintensity, thin flow voids, and diffuse avid enhancement
- Facilitated diffusion is key to confirming diagnosis

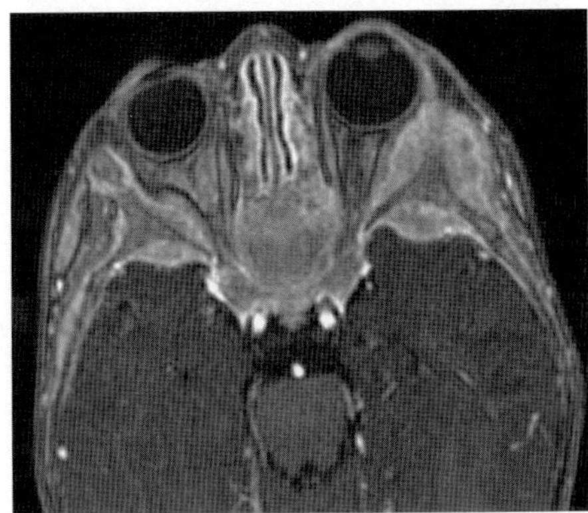

Neuroblastoma

- Usually bilateral involvement along the greater wings of the sphenoid bone
- CT imaging demonstrates aggressive periosteal reaction

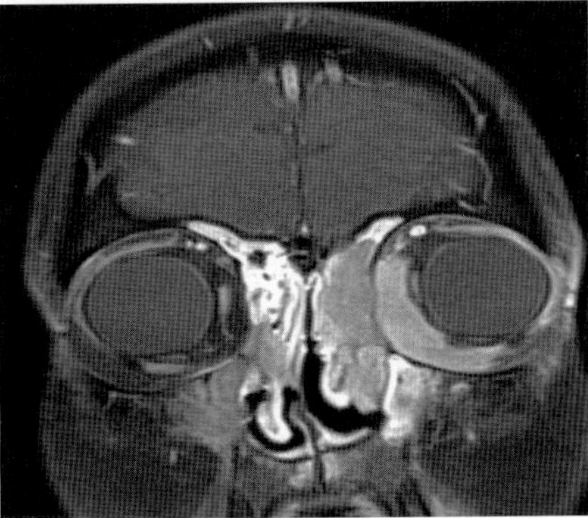

Leukemia and Lymphoma

- Homogeneous enhancing mass with reduced diffusion

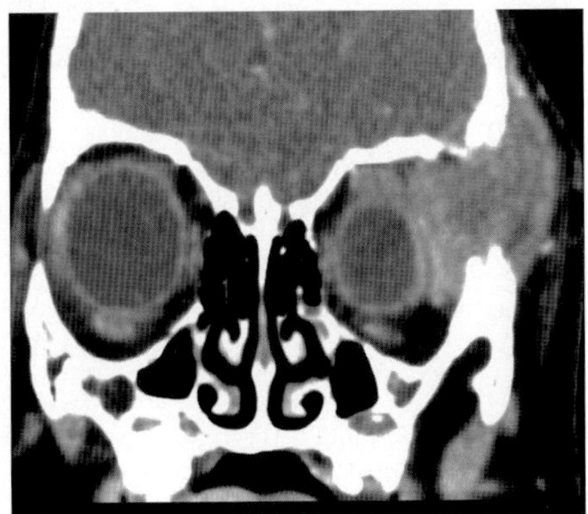

Langerhans Cell Histiocytosis

- Lytic bone lesion with associated soft tissue mass

BONE-ASSOCIATED MASS

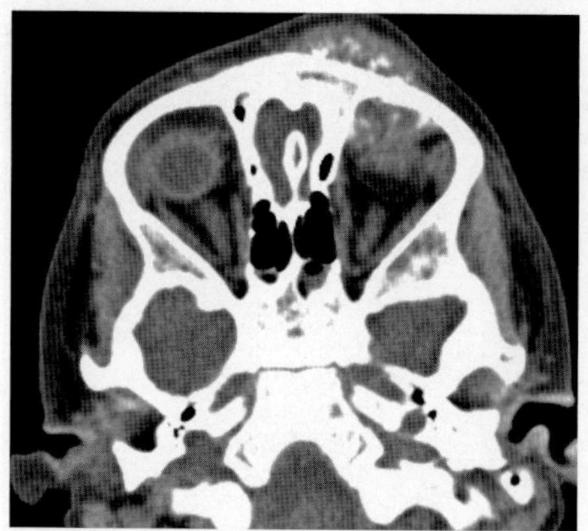

Neuroblastoma

- Aggressive bone lesions with periosteal reaction and soft tissue extension
- Predilection for the orbital bones

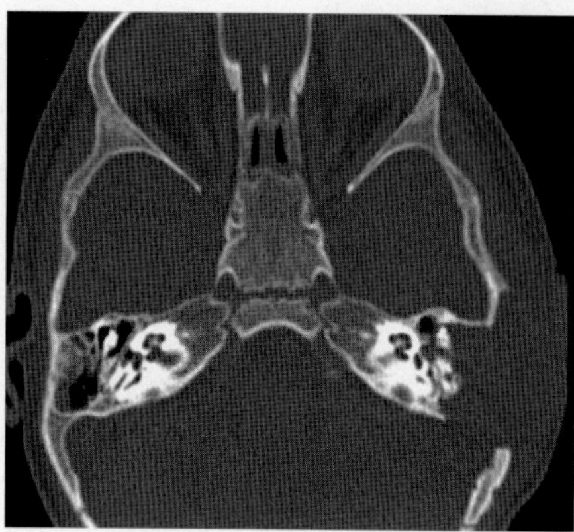

Langerhans Cell Histiocytosis

- Lytic bone lesion with sharp margins, often more outer than inner cortex involvement leading to a beveled edge appearance
- Often an associated soft tissue mass is present.

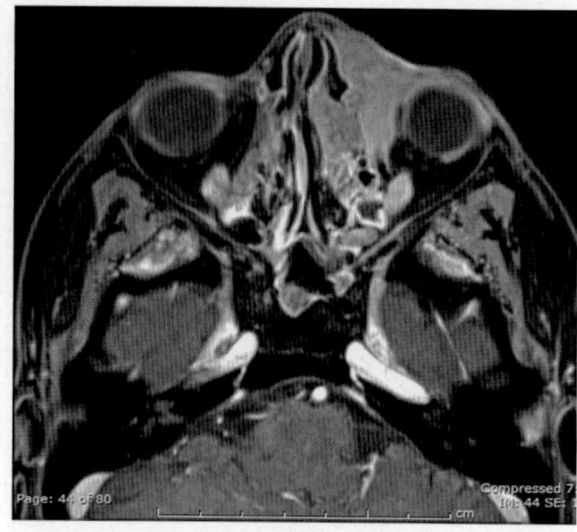

Leukemia

- Bone and soft tissue extension with predilection for the paranasal sinuses
- Occurs during leukemia relapse
- Homogeneous enhancement and bone changes usually subtle on CT

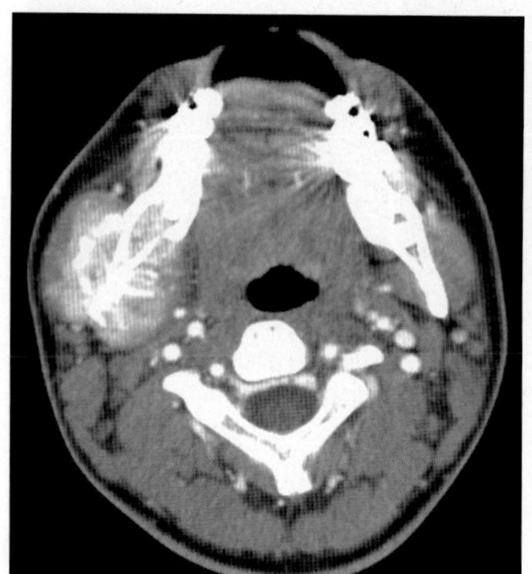

Ewing Sarcoma

- Aggressive solitary bone lesion with malignant periosteal reaction and an associated soft tissue mass

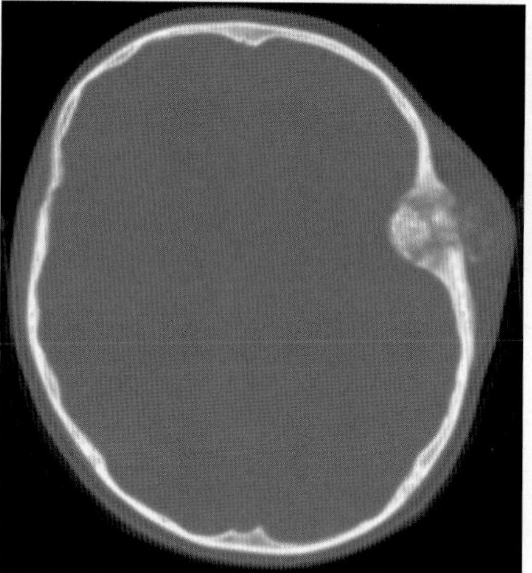

Osteosarcoma

- Aggressive solitary bone lesion with malignant periosteal reaction and ossified matrix

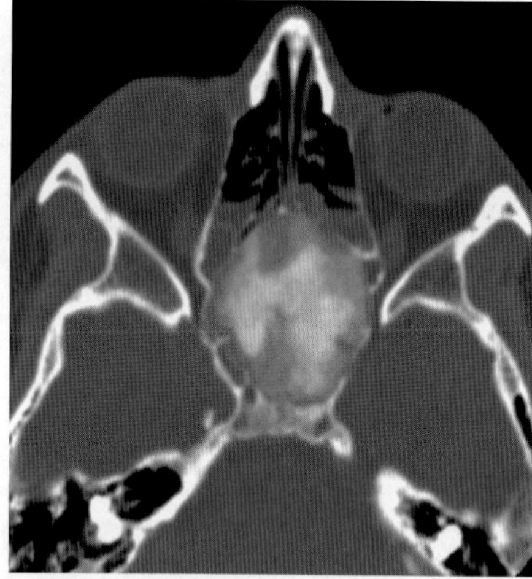

Fibroosseous lesions

- Expansile bone lesions with some component demonstrating ground glass fibroosseous matrix
- No associated soft tissue mass unless rare associated malignant sarcoma

TEMPORAL BONE MASS

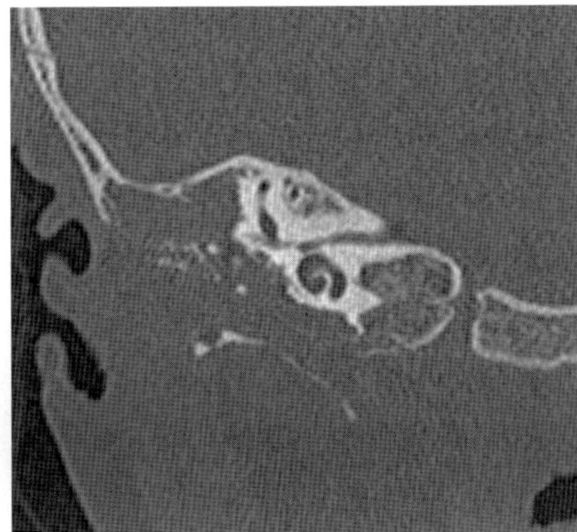

Rhabdomyosarcoma

- Locally aggressive enhancing mass lesion
- Advanced bony erosion
- Bloody chronic otitis media

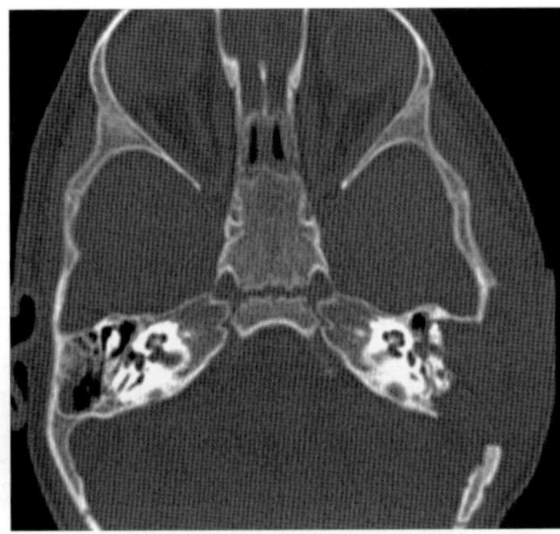

Langerhans Cell Histiocytosis

- Locally aggressive enhancing mass lesion
- Advanced bony erosion
- May coexist with external auditory canal disease
- Commonly multifocal

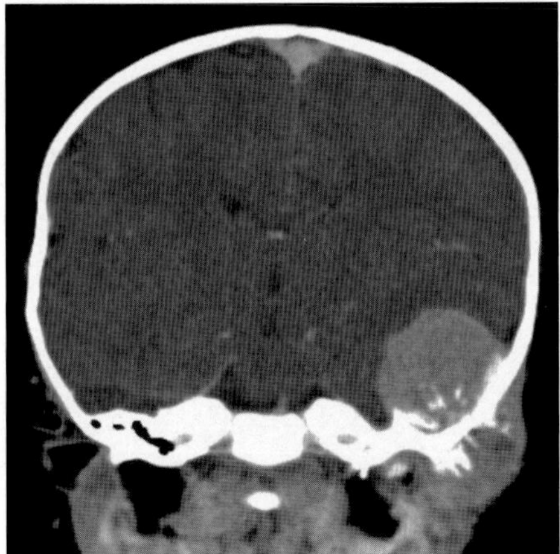

Ewing Sarcoma

- Locally aggressive enhancing mass lesion
- Difficult to distinguish from other sarcomas and mass lesions

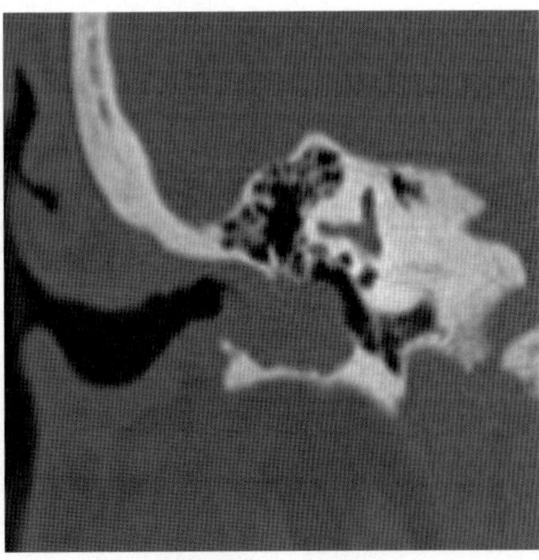

Cholesteatoma

- Growth of keratinizing squamous epithelium with aggressive bony and ossicular erosion
- Nonenhancing; restricted diffusion

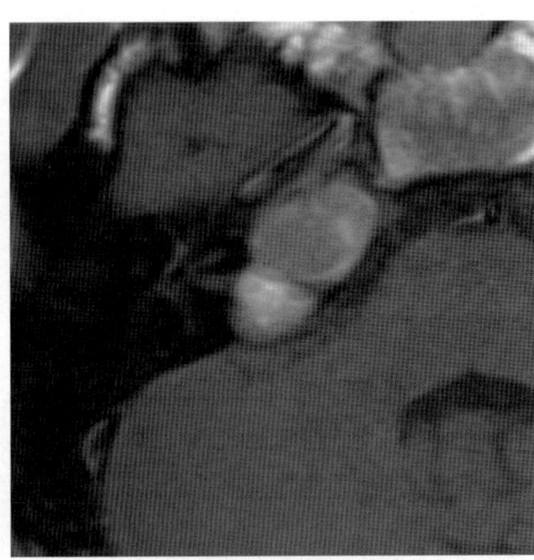

Cholesterol Granuloma

- Expansile lesion of middle ear cavity or mastoid temporal bone/petrous apex
- T1W and T2W hyperintense with peripheral hemosiderin
- Peripheral enhancement or no enhancement
- No restricted diffusion

VASCULAR NECK MASS

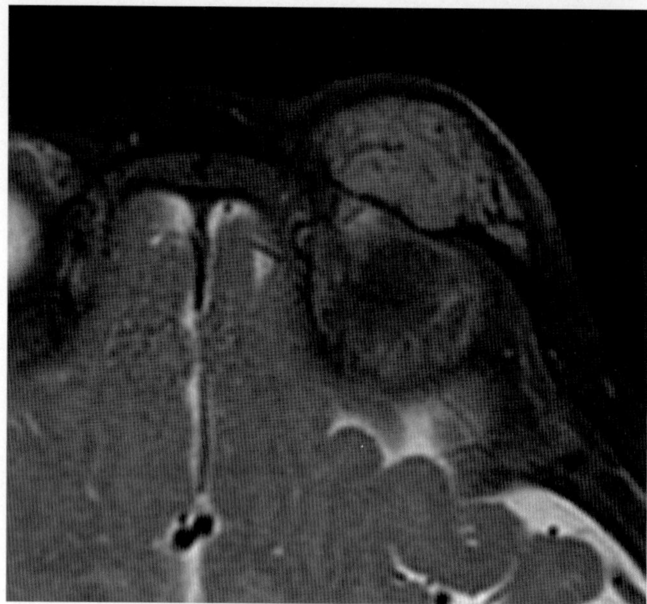

Infantile Hemangioma

- T2W hyperintense well-defined mass with homogenous avid enhancement and flow voids

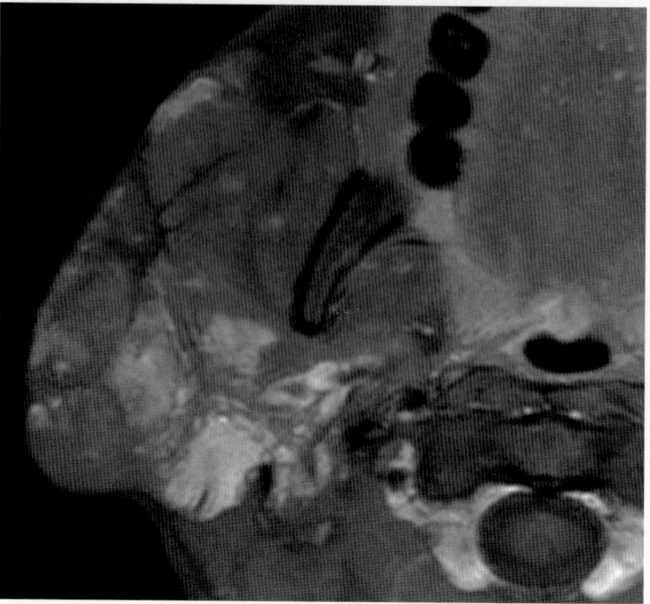

Venolymphatic Malformation

- Multiseptated multispatial or unispatial microcystic and macrocystic lesion
- T2W hyperintense with venous components enhancing and with potential phleboliths

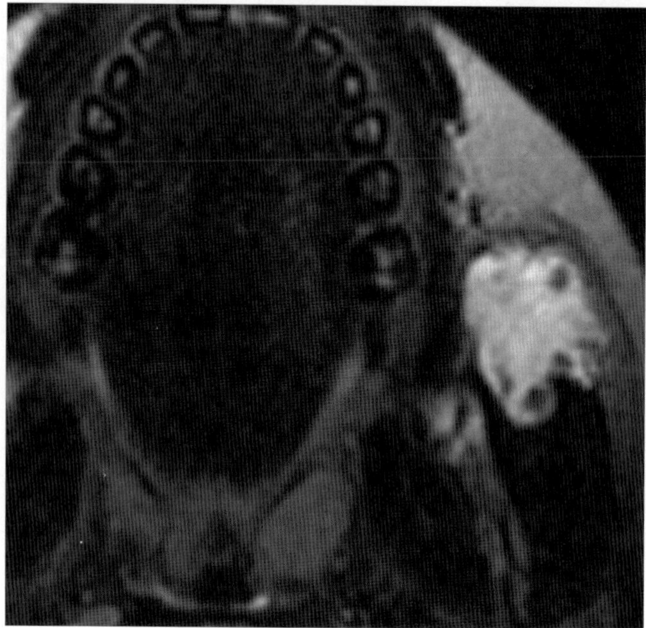

Venous Malformation

- T2W hyperintense multispatial or unispatial enhancing lesion. Enhancement occurs in venous phase, initially heterogeneous with progressive enhancement
- Phleboliths
- Lack of fluid-fluid levels and flow voids

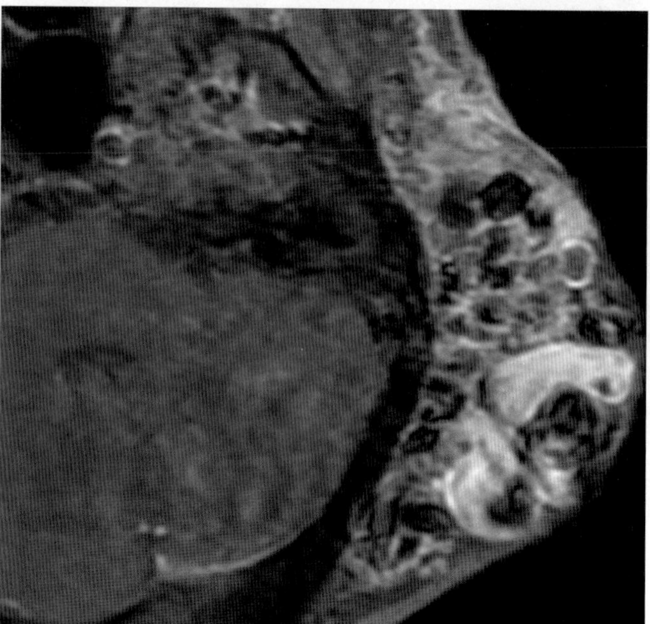

Arteriovenous Malformation

- Multispatial or unispatial tangle of vessels (flow voids); vessels may enhance.
- Regional bony erosion or overgrowth.
- Lack of phleboliths and fluid-fluid levels.
- May have variable T1W and T2W signal with fluid-fluid levels internal hemorrhage or infection.

CALCIFIED NECK MASS

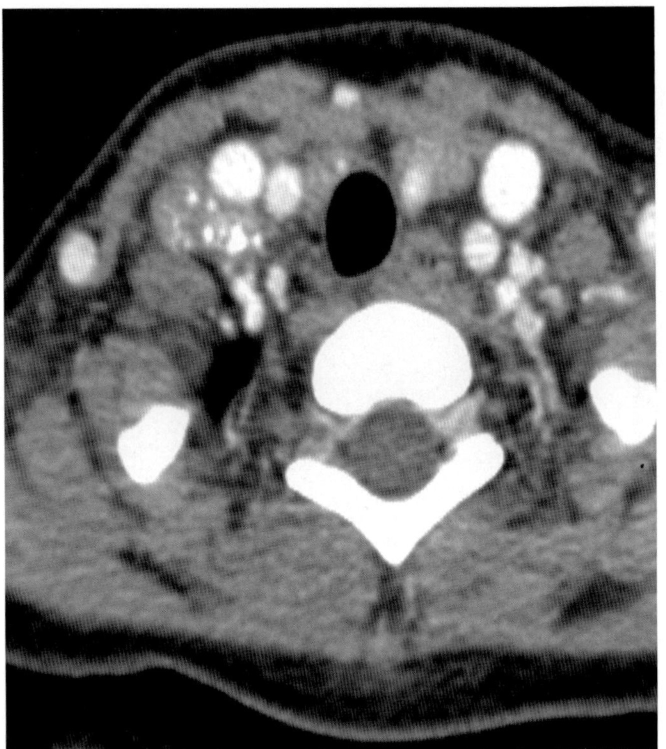

Granulomatous

- Infection—mycobacterial, cat scratch, and fungal causes

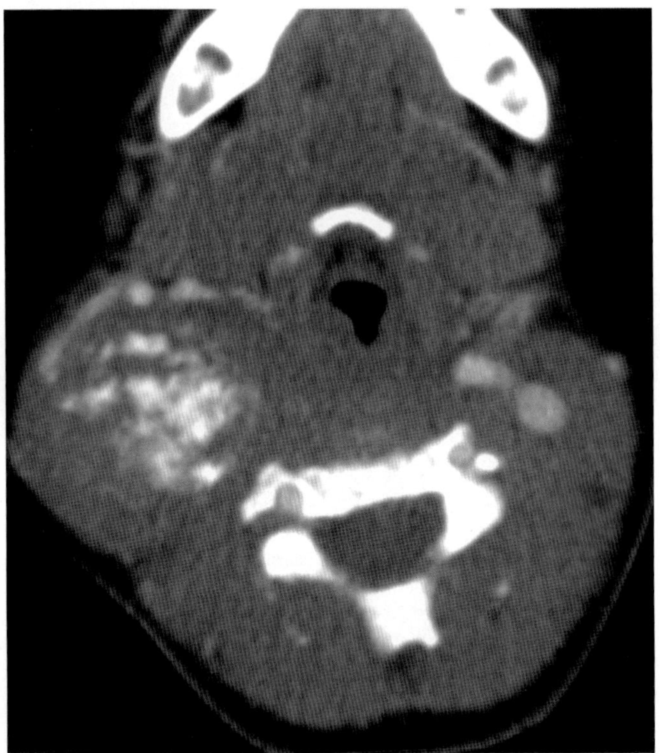

Neuroblastoma

- Primary or metastatic partially mass lesion

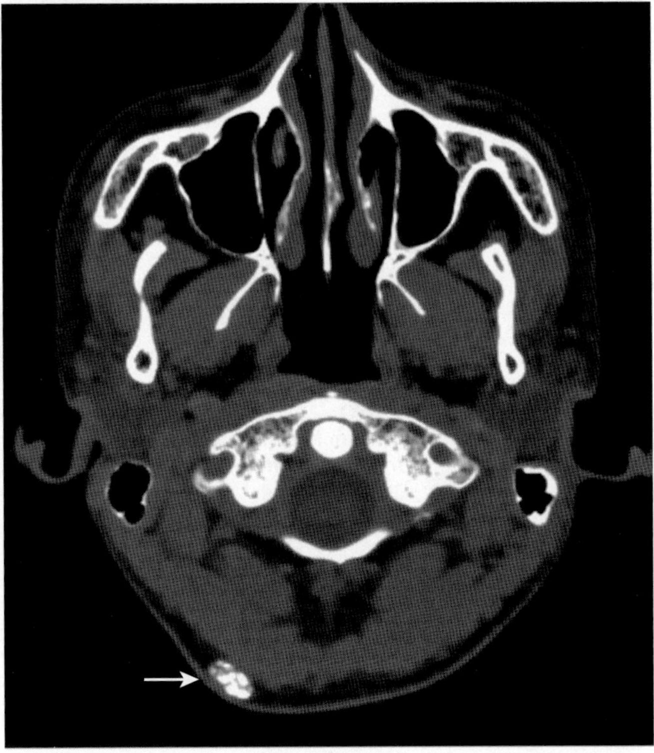

Pilomatrixoma

- Calcified subcutaneous lesion
- Enhancement; lack of restricted diffusion
- Hypointense to heterogeneous T2W signal

FACE AND NECK PITFALLS

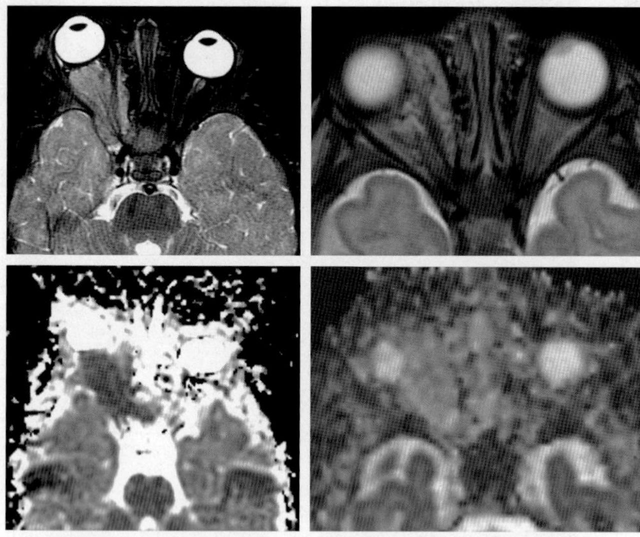

Rhabdomyosarcoma Mimicking Infantile Hemangioma

- Rhabdomyosarcoma (left-sided images) may mimic infantile hemangioma (right-sided images) except that the ADC will be low rather than high. Obtaining high-quality DWI/ADC is very helpful in avoiding this pitfall.

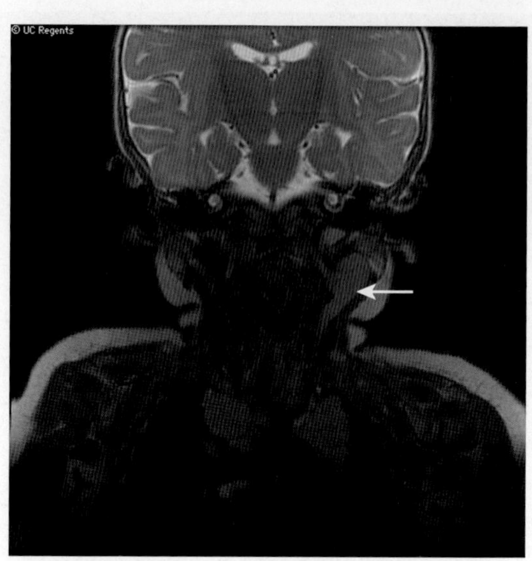

Ectopic Thymus Mimicking Lymphoma

- Look for a connection to the thymus or similar signal characteristics to avoid diagnosis of lymphoma

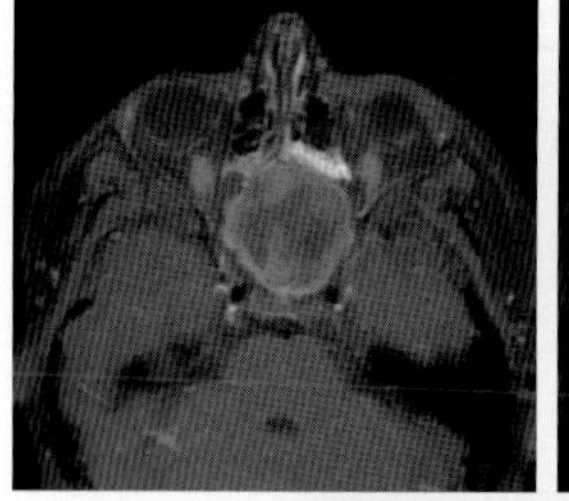

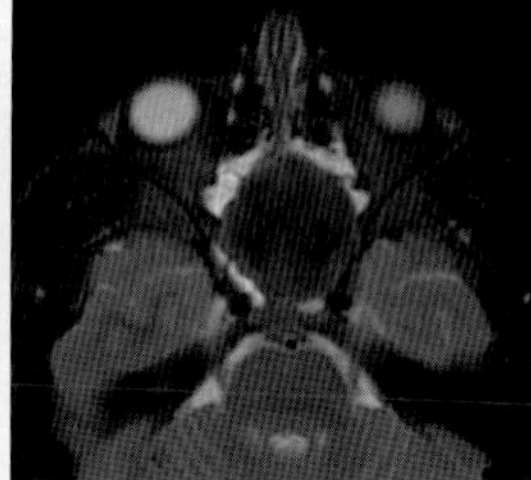

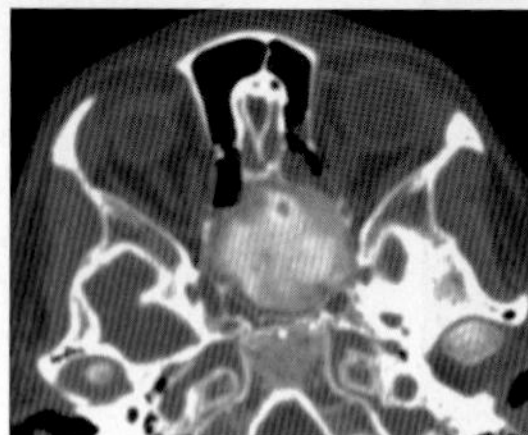

Fibrosseous Lesion

- Fibroosseous lesions first imaged with MRI may have an unusual and aggressive appearance, while CT imaging is more straightforward. A combination of both CT and MRI is helpful in reaching a diagnosis of a craniofacial bone lesion.

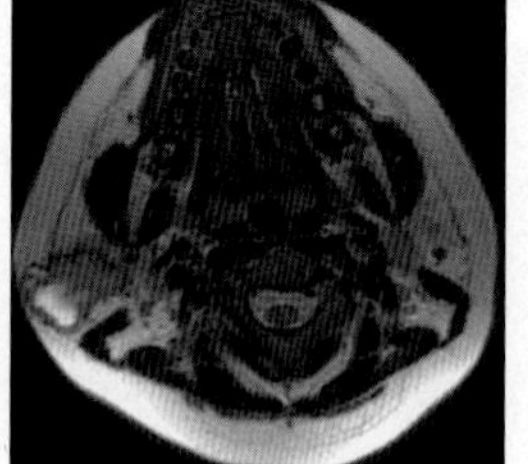

Neoplasm Mistaken for Branchial Cleft Cyst

- BCCs should be thin walled unless superinfected, in which case follow-up imaging should be obtained. This case was a mucoepidermoid carcinoma mistaken for a first BCC.

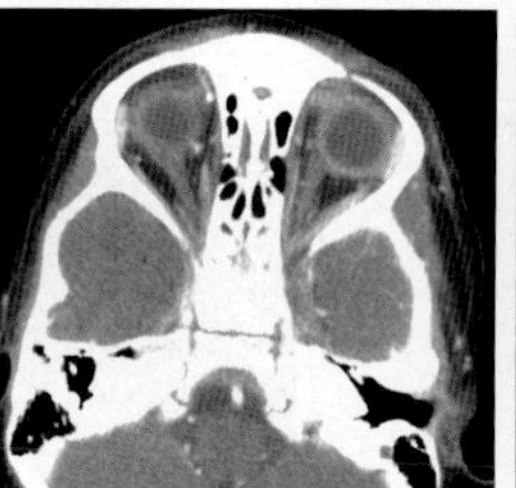

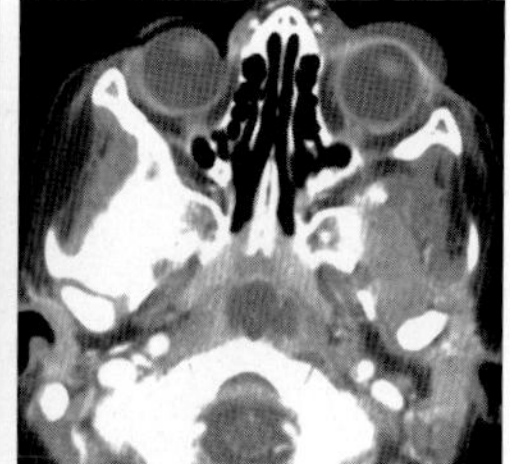

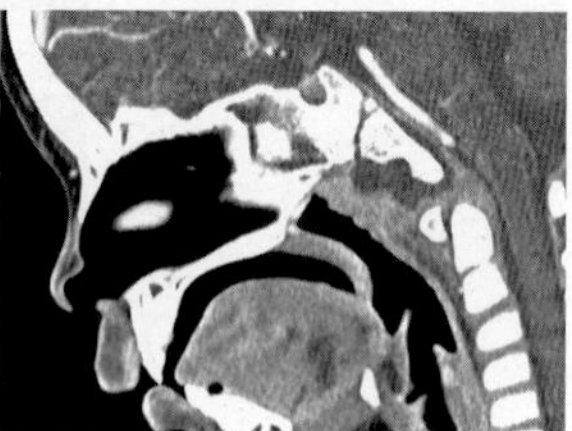

Retropharyngeal Abscess Spreading Intracranially and Presenting as Orbital Cellulitis

- Rarely, a retropharyngeal abscess may spread intracranially, and often has an associated fossa navicularis in the clivus as seen here. Intracranial extension resulted in cavernous sinus thrombosis, which appeared clinically as an orbital cellulitis, such that the clinicians ordered a CT of the face. This demonstrates the need to look at all the structures imaged and be aware of the potential for infection to spread to multiple compartments.

SPINAL MALFORMATION

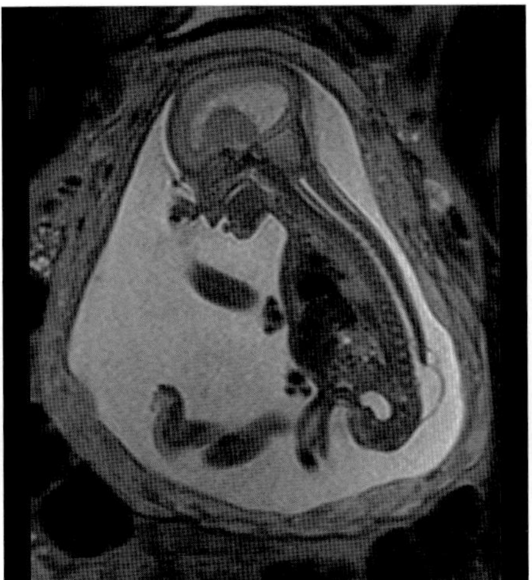

Myelomeningocele

- Open spinal dysraphism
- Low-lying exposed cord/neural placode with open defect in soft tissues and bone of affected levels
- Myelomeningocele sac
- Chiari II malformation

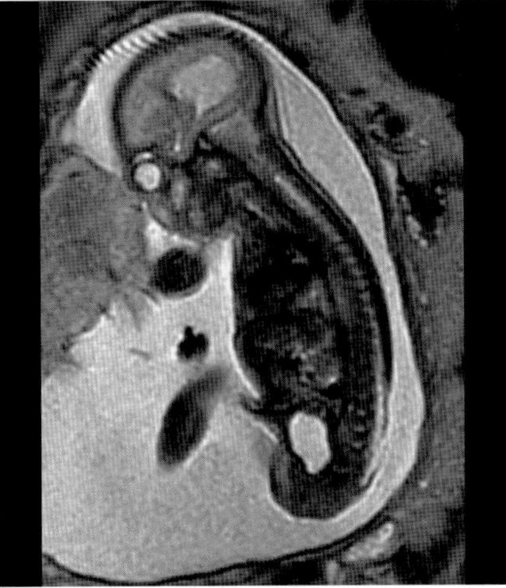

Myelocele

- Open spinal dysraphism
- Low lying exposed cord/neural placode with open defect in soft tissues and bone of affected levels
- Absent sac; neural placode flush with the adjacent skin
- Chiari II malformation

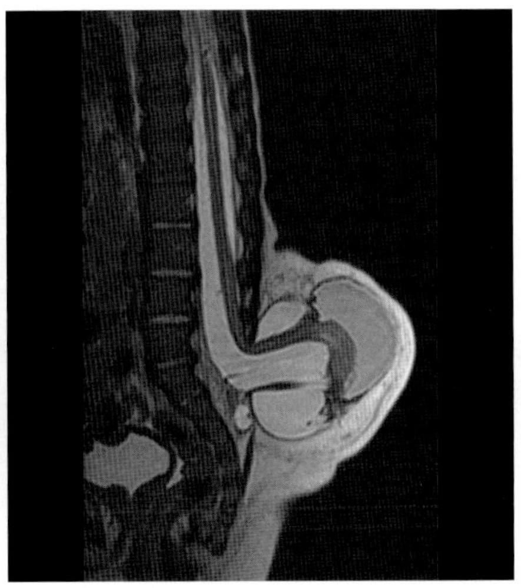

Myelocystocele

- Closed spinal dysraphism
- Posteriorly projecting cystic expansion of central canal of cord with defect in posterior elements

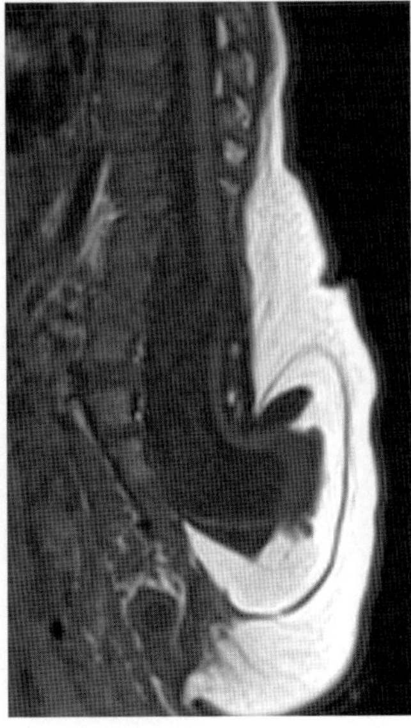

Lipomyelomeningocele

- Closed spinal dysraphism
- Low-lying cord/neural placode posteriorly herniating associated with fat contiguous with paraspinal/extradural fat

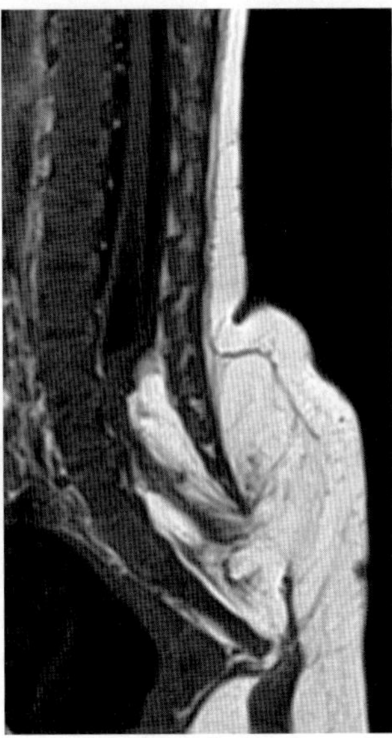

Lipomyelocele

- Closed spinal dysraphism
- Low-lying cord/neural placode associated with fat contiguous with paraspinal/extradural fat
- Absent sac with neural placode and lipoma are within the spinal canal

Differentiation made through determination of open versus closed malformation and position of the placode-lipoma interface

SPINE ULTRASOUND FINDINGS

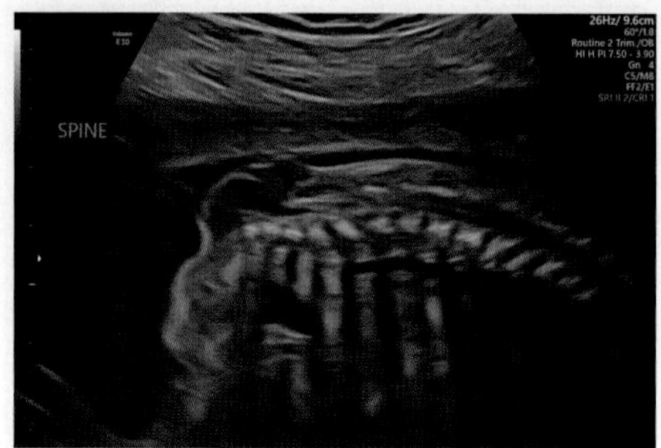

Myelomeningocele

- Open spinal dysraphism
- Low-lying exposed cord/neural placode with open defect in soft tissues and bone of affected levels
- Chiari II malformation

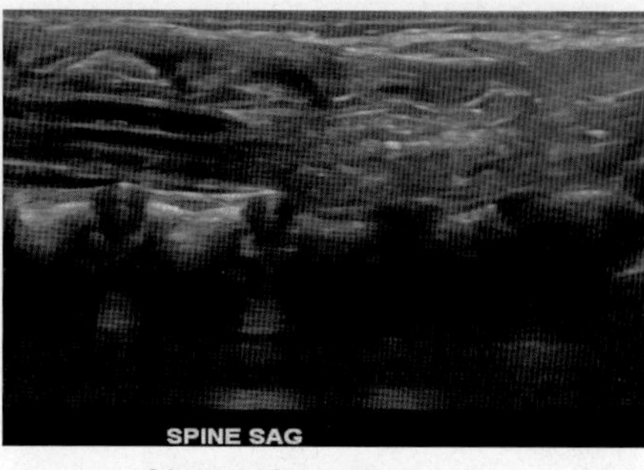

Lipomyelomeningocele

- Closed spinal dysraphism
- Low-lying cord/neural placode attached to fat outside the spinal canal that is contiguous with subcutaneous fat

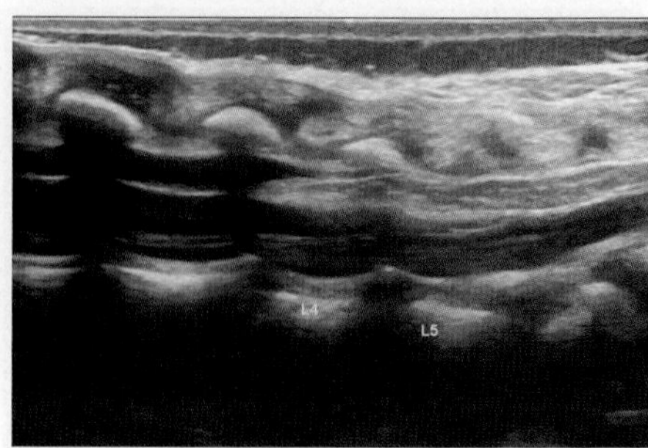

Intradural Lipoma

- Bony spinal canal and soft tissues intact
- Lipoma may be along the dorsal cord margin in cervical and thoracic spine or along the cauda equina/filum
- Cord may be tethered

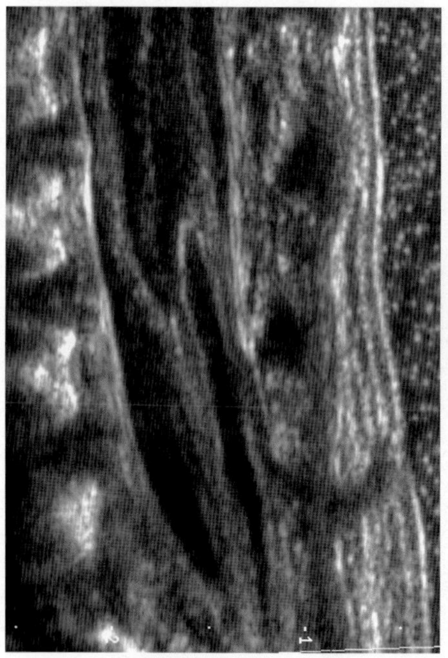

Dermal Sinus Tract

- May be associated with cutaneous nevus, hairy patch, or hemangioma
- Epithelium lined sinus tract to spinal canal
- Intraspinal dermoid may be present
- Most common in lumbar spine and occipital area
- Infection is a risk through communication from the skin to CSF

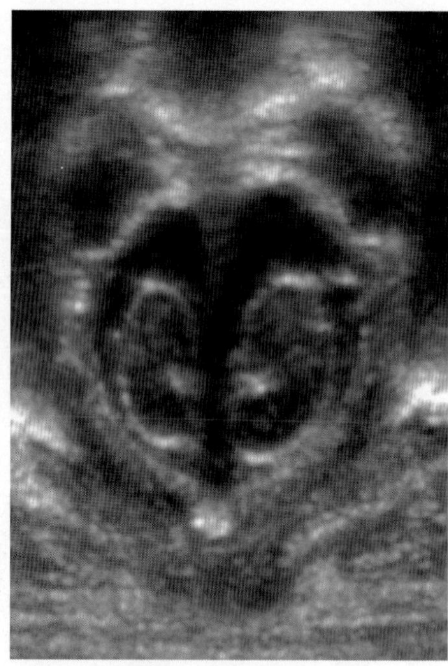

Diastematomyelia

- Split cord malformation types I and II
- Fibrous or bony septal spur
- Associated with other malformations, scoliosis

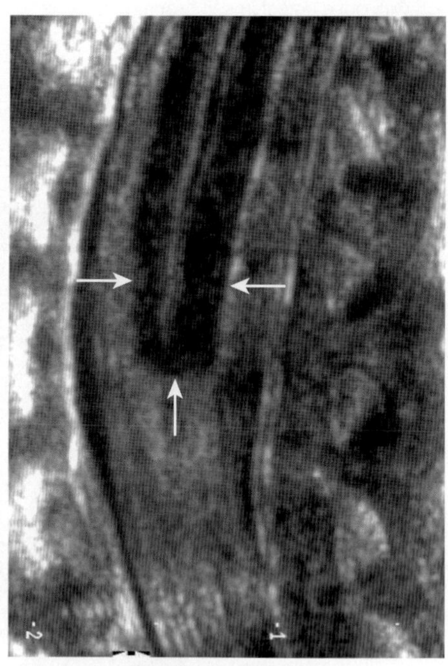

Caudal Regression

- Spinal column agenesis with truncation of the cord of variable severity
- Associated with a variety of systemic malformations

SPINAL CORD LESIONS

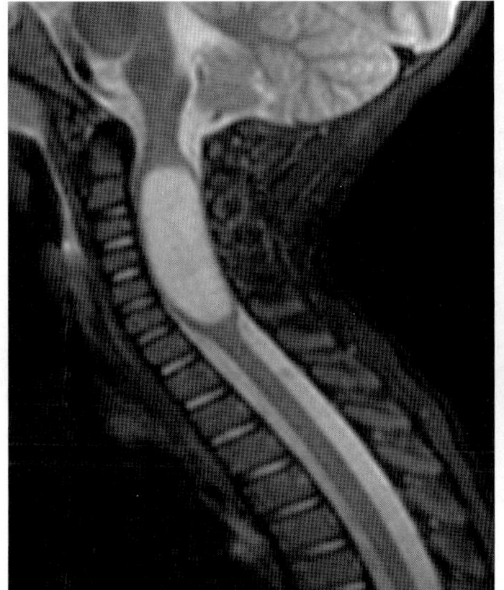

Tumor

- Subacute onset
- Expansion occupying majority of spinal canal

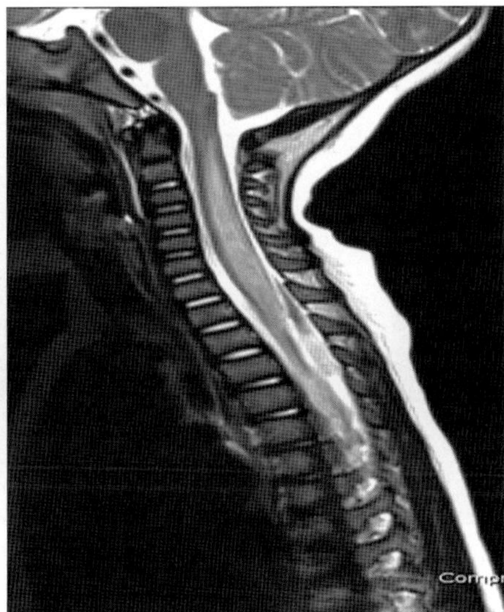

Inflammatory and Demyelination

- Acute onset
- Minimal to mild expansion
- Patchy enhancement
- CSF inflammatory findings

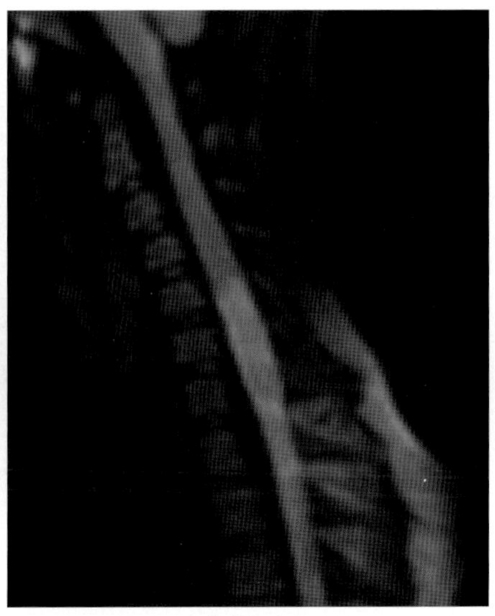

Infarct

- Acute onset
- Mild expansion
- Diffusion restriction

SPINAL CORD AXIAL PATTERN

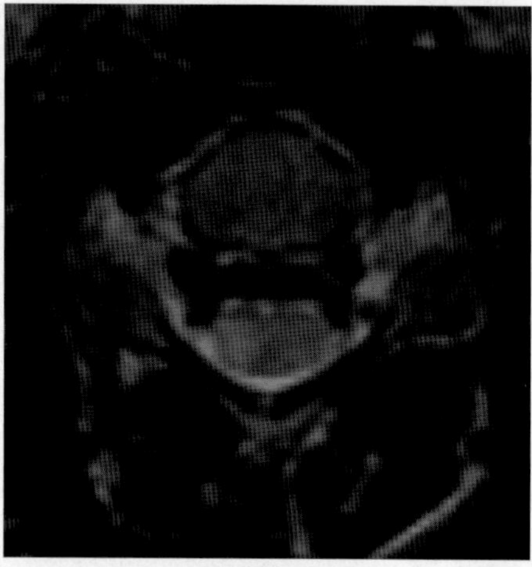

Peripheral

- Multiple sclerosis

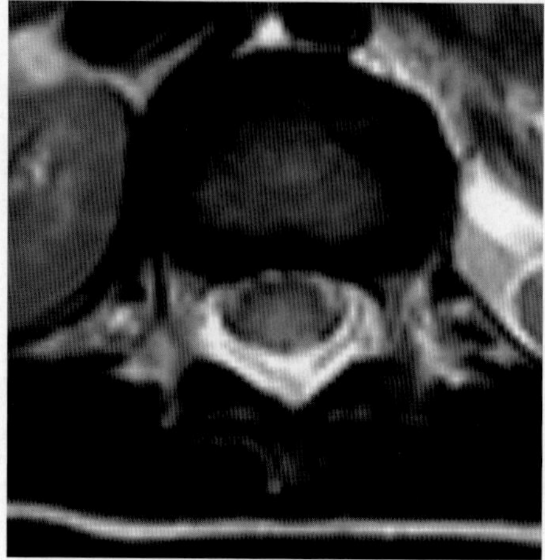

Central cord

1. Transverse myelitis
2. Neuromyelitis optica
3. Anti-MOG

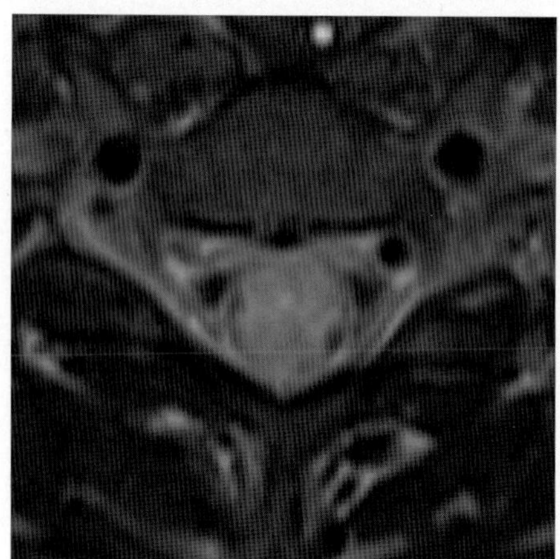

Diffuse Cross-Section

1. Transverse myelitis
2. Spinal cord infarct
3. Tumor
4. Anti-MOG
5. NMO
6. Multiple sclerosis

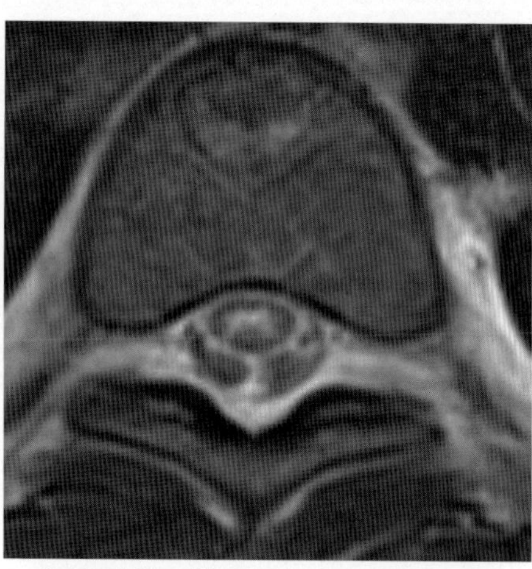

Central Gray Matter or Anterior Horns

1. Infarct
2. Anti-MOG
3. Acute flaccid myelitis
4. Hirayama
5. Polio

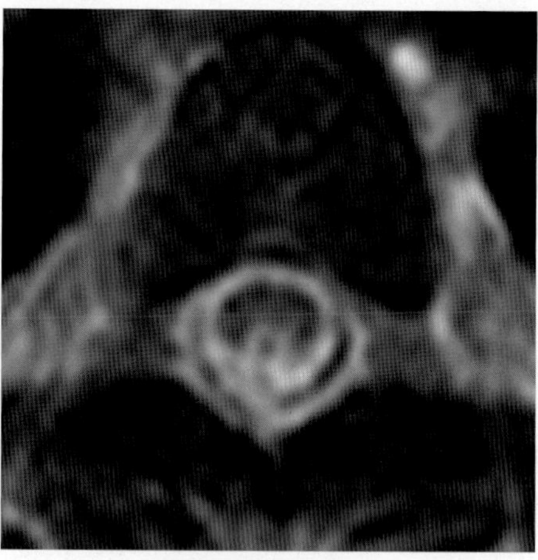

Posterior Medial

1. Vitamin B_{12} deficiency
2. Multiple sclerosis

COMPARISON OF SPINAL CORD DEMYELINATING AND INFLAMMATORY DISORDERS

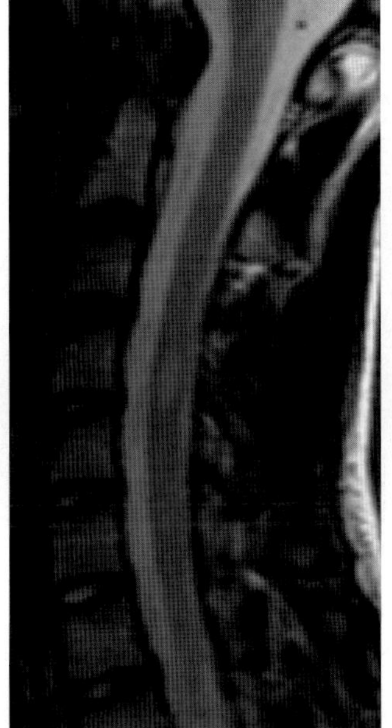

Multiple Sclerosis

1. Brain: White matter lesions; subcortical, callosum, and Dawson's fingers
2. Spine: short craniocaudal length cord lesions; white matter > gray matter
3. Optic neuritis
4. Oligoclonal bands

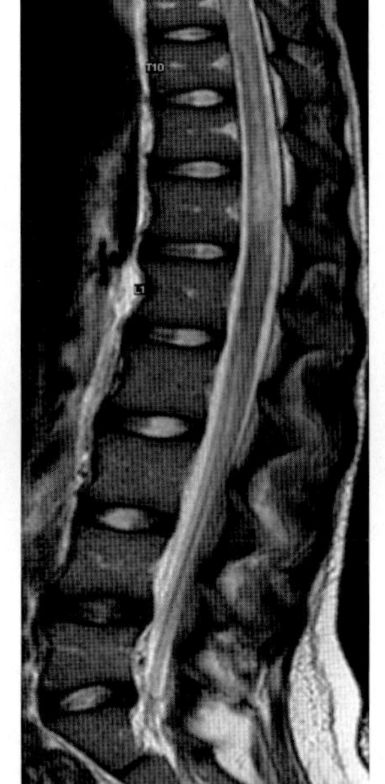

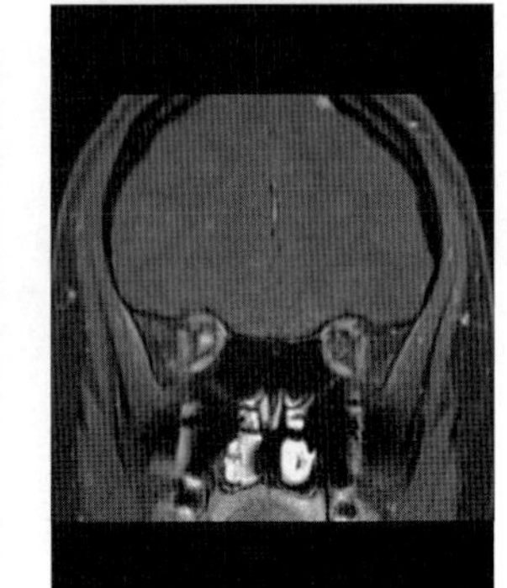

NMO

1. Brain: none or few white matter lesions; enhancement around the third ventricle, periqueductal gray, and dorsal medulla
2. Spine: longitudinally extensive cord lesions
3. Optic neuritis often bilateral
4. Aquaporin-4 antibody

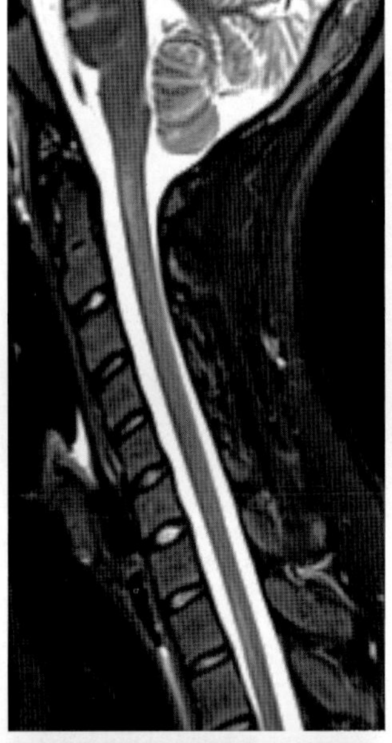

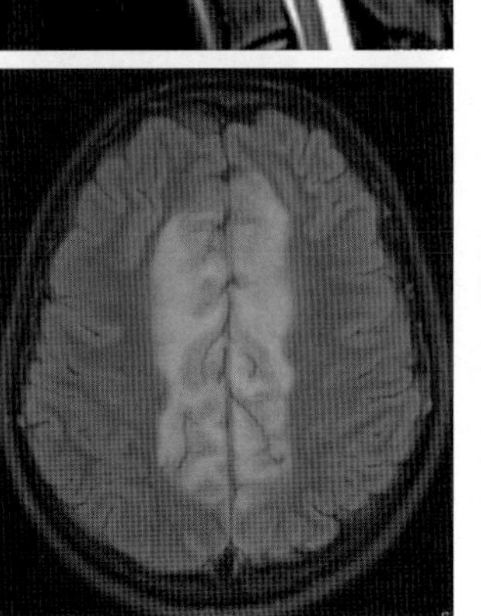

Anti-MOG

1. Brain: confluent white matter lesions similar to ADEM
2. Spine: longitudinally extensive and multiple cord lesions; gray matter > white matter
3. Optic neuritis: often recurrent
4. Anti-MOG antibody

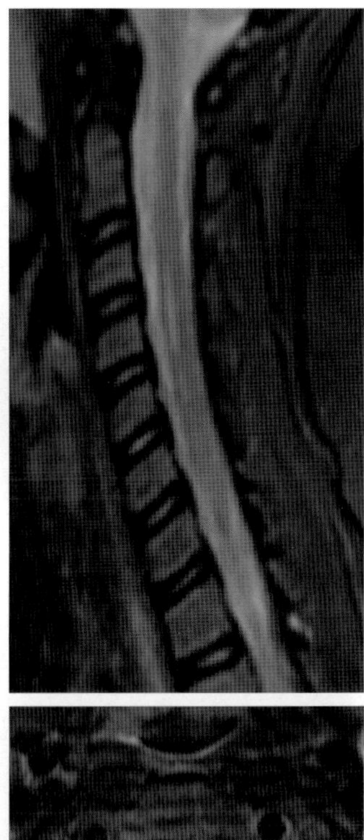

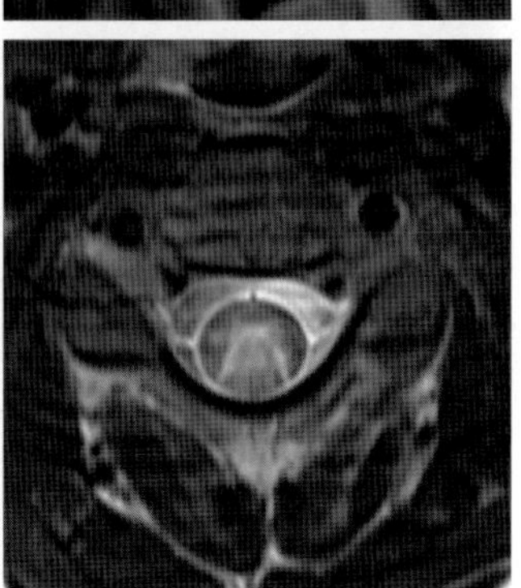

AFM

1. Brain: limited to dorsal pons
2. Spine: longitudinally extensive cord lesions; gray matter > white matter
3. No optic neuritis
4. Associated with enterovirus infection

SPINAL SOFT TISSUE LESIONS

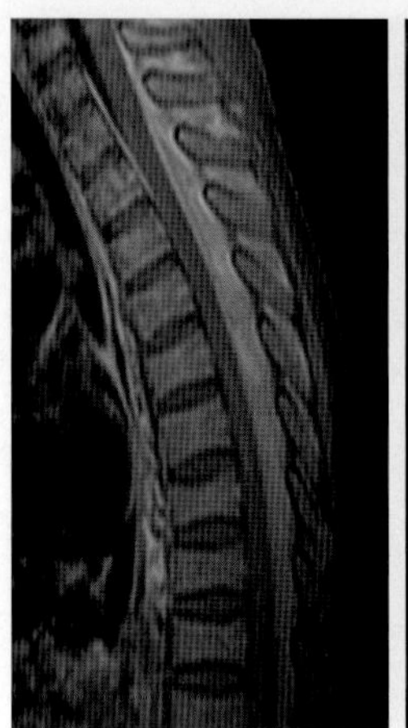
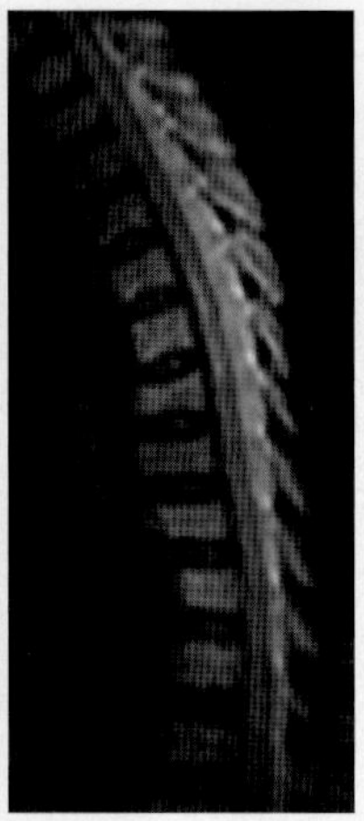

Leukemia

- Enhancing extradural +/– intradural mass lesion, may be extensive or multifocal
- Extradural disease may occur from extraosseous extension from the involved vertebrae
- Diffuse abnormal marrow
- Diffusion restricting

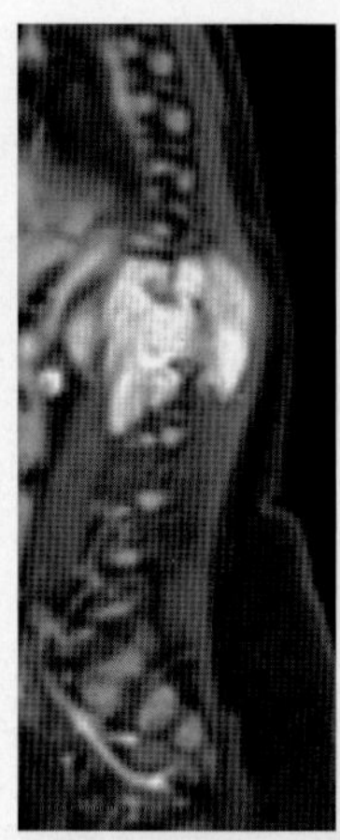
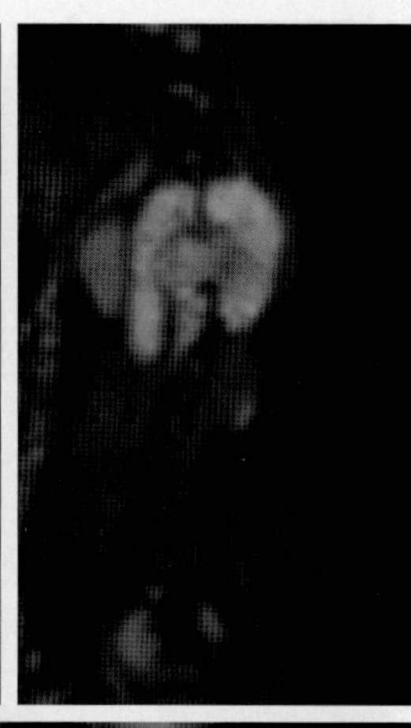

Neuroblastoma

- Enhancing; often large paraspinal mass that extends into and widen the neural foramen
- Diffusion restricting

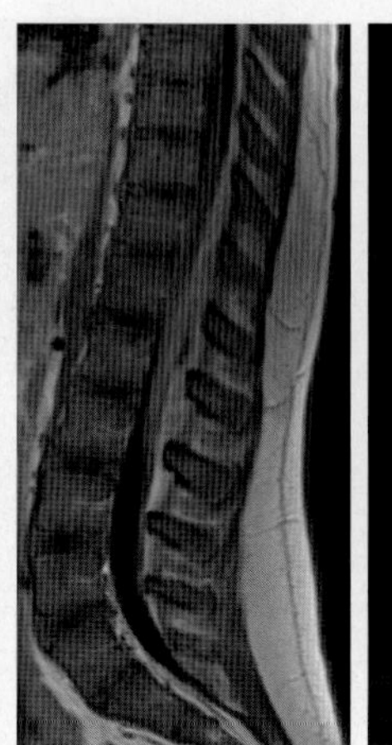
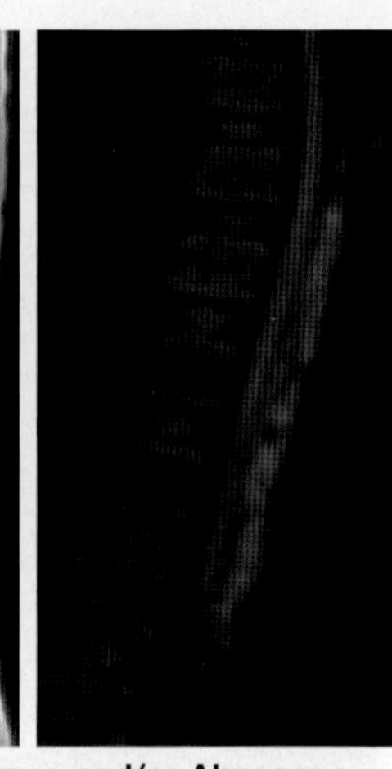

Epidural Phlegmon and/or Abscess

- Diffusion restricting
- Homogeneous enhancement (phlegmon) or peripherally enhancing (abscess) extradural collection commonly associated with discitis osteomyelitis

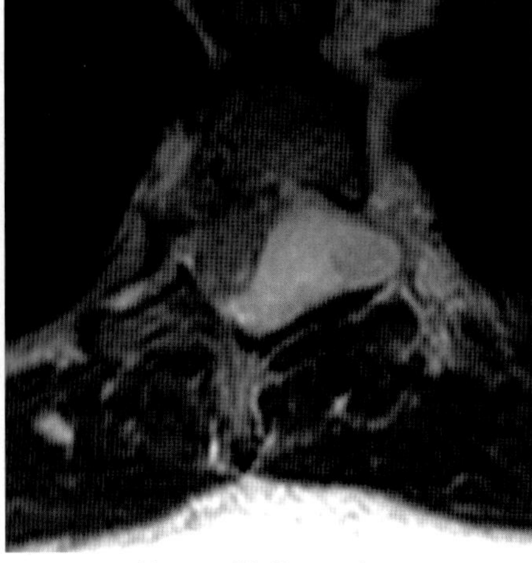

Venous Malformation

- T2W hyperintense multispatial or unispatial enhancing lesion. Enhancement occurs in the venous phase, initially heterogeneous with progressive enhancement
- Phleoboliths possible
- Lack of fluid-fluid levels and flow voids

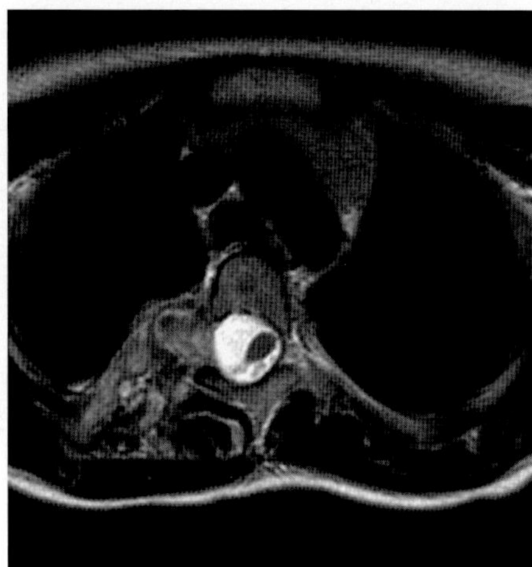

Plexiform Neurofibroma

- Enhancing T2W hyperintense infiltrative paraspinal mass lesions with target sign
- May extend into and widen the neural foramen

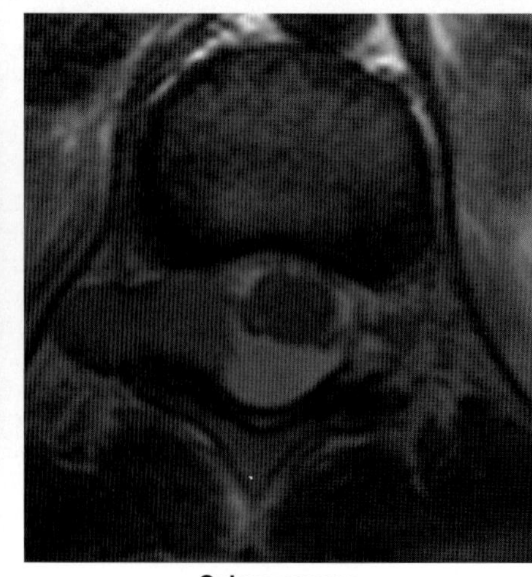

Schwannoma

- Well-defined enhancing extradural and/or intradural mass associated with nerve root
- May be numerous when associated with NF-2

SPINAL BONE LESIONS

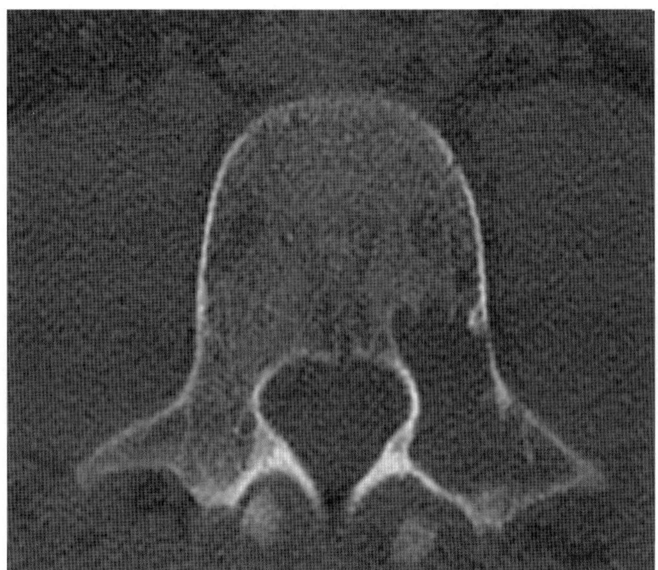

Aneurysmal Bone Cyst

- Lytic
- Well defined
- Posterior elements of the spine
- Fluid-fluid levels on MRI

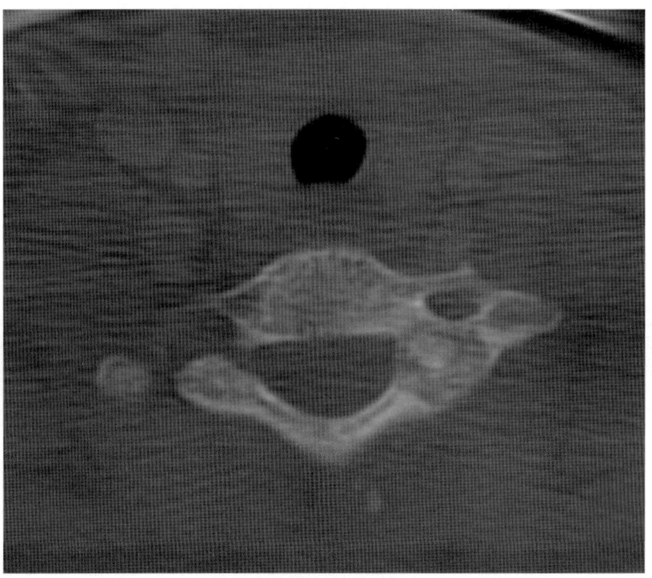

Osteoid Osteoma

- Lytic lesion with central sclerotic nidus
- Surrounding soft tissue inflammation

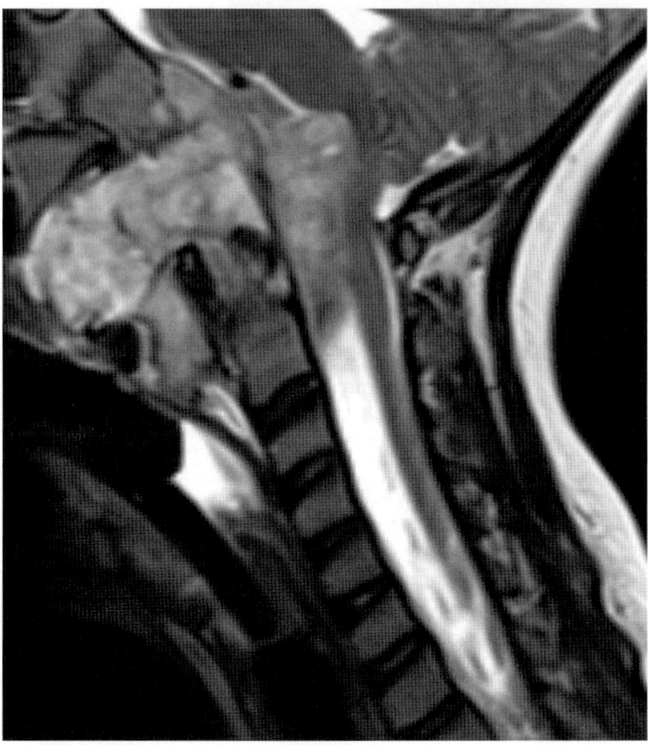

Chordoma

- Lytic bone lesion
- Dystrophic calcifications
- Clivus, upper cervical spine and sacrum
- T2W hyperintensity on MRI

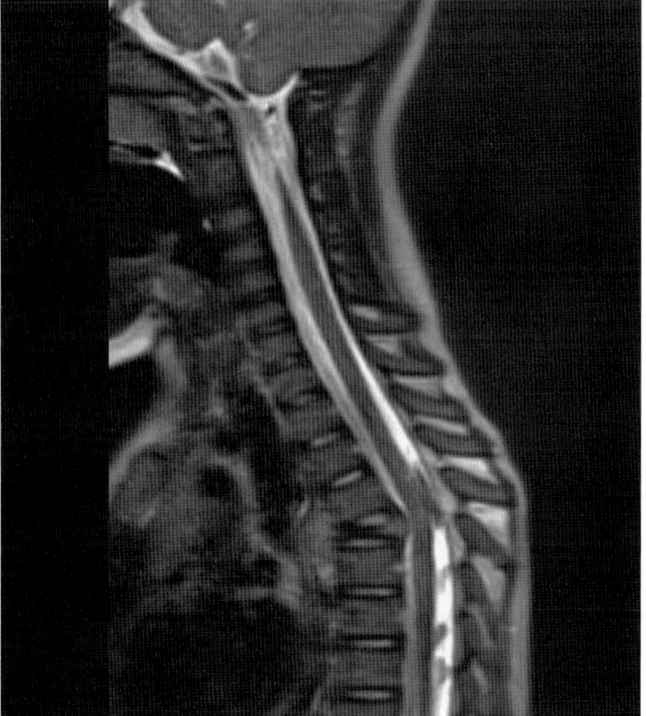

Langerhans Cell Histiocytosis

- Vertebra plana
- May have associated soft tissue mass

SPINE MASSES INVOLVING BONE AND SOFT TISSUE

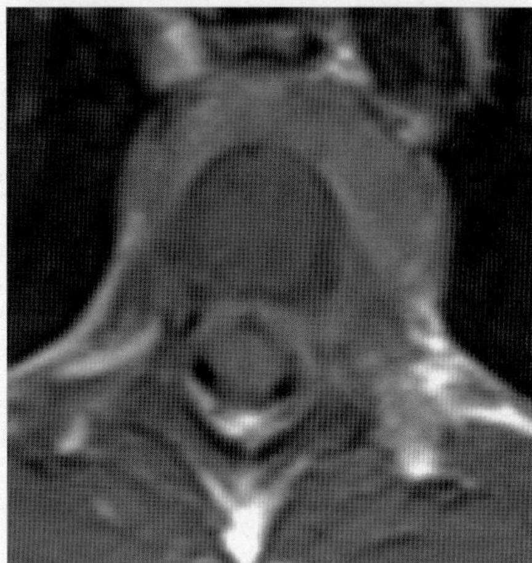

Langerhans Cell Histiocytosis

- Locally aggressive enhancing mass
- Bony erosion
- Commonly multifocal
- Vertebra plana

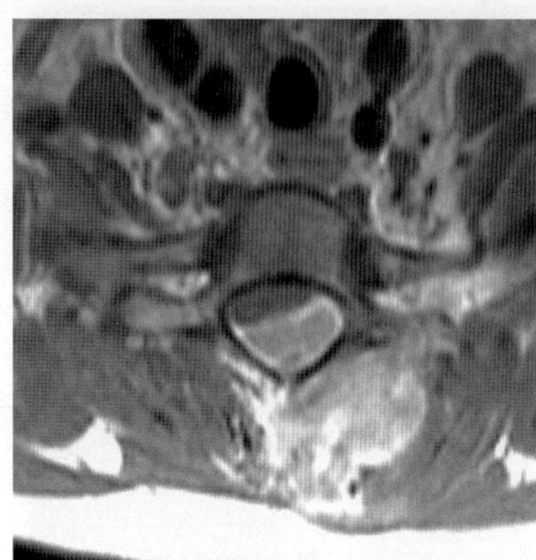

Ewing Sarcoma

- Locally aggressive enhancing mass lesion involving the bone (especially posterior elements), extradural, and paraspinal soft tissues

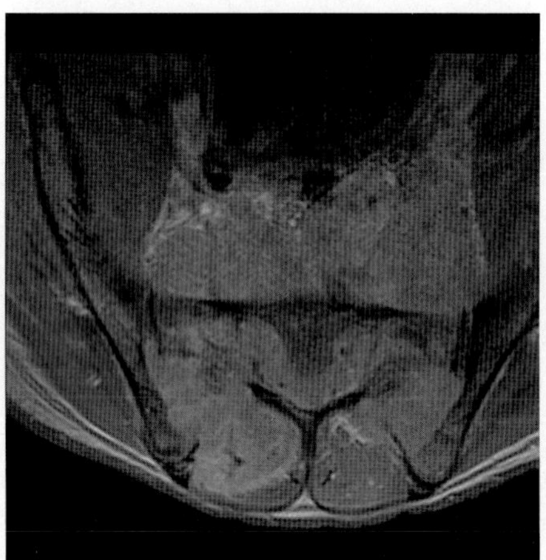

Lymphoma and Leukemia

- Enhancing extradural +/– intradural mass lesion
- Diffuse abnormal marrow
- Lymphoma often has bulky lymph nodes, which help differentiate from leukemia

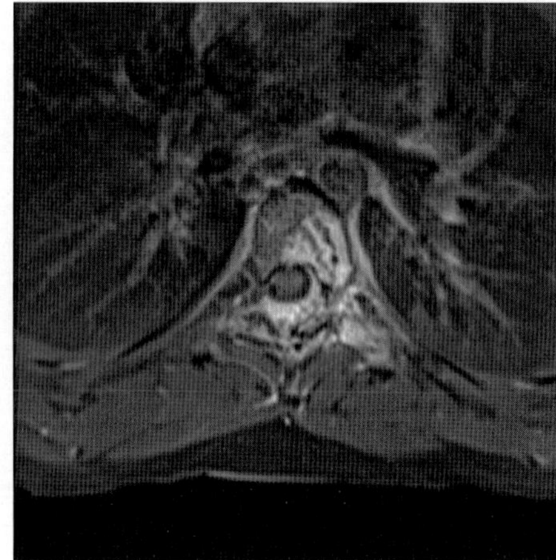

Giant Hemangioma

- Locally aggressive T2W hyperintense enhancing lesion involving bone, extradural, and paraspinal soft tissues
- Thickening of vertical trabeculae is classic best seen on CT

Potential further differentiation may or may not always be possible. LCH often has vertebra plana and does not diffusely involve all the bones. Leukemia will often involve all the bone marrow. Ewing sarcoma often limited to a single bone or a few bones and more often localized to the posterior elements.

NECK AND BACK PAIN

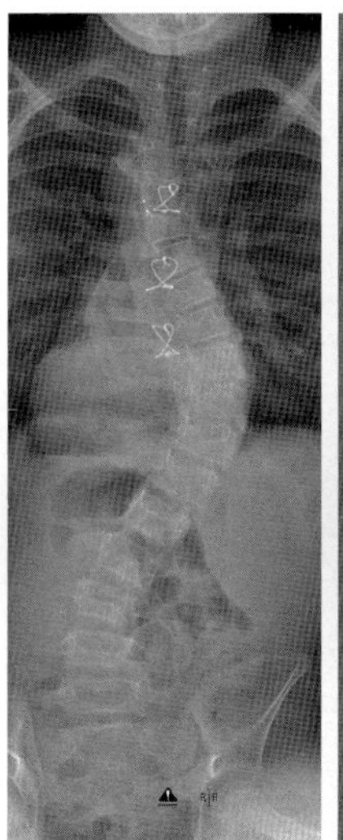
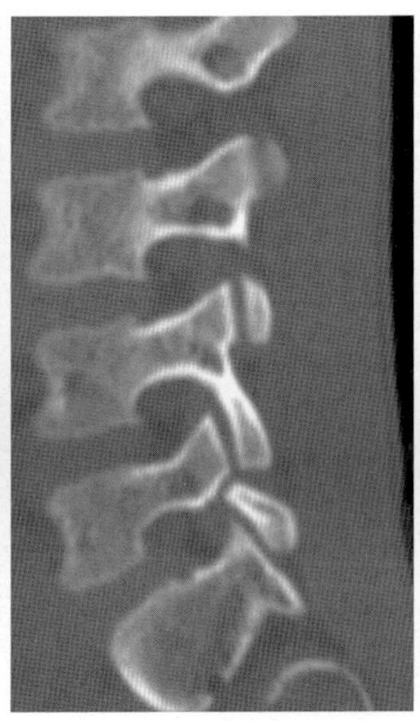
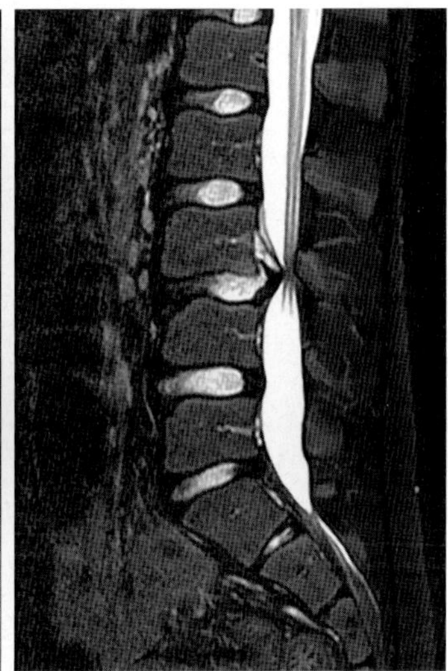

Biomechanical

1. Spondylolysis
2. Scoliosis
3. Scheuermann kyphosis
4. Disc herniation
5. Apophyseal ring fracture

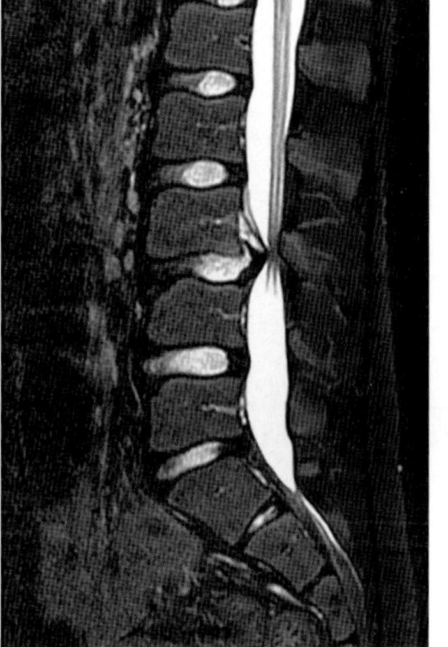

Infection

1. Discitis
2. Osteomyelitis
3. Epidural
4. Phlegmon
5. Myositis

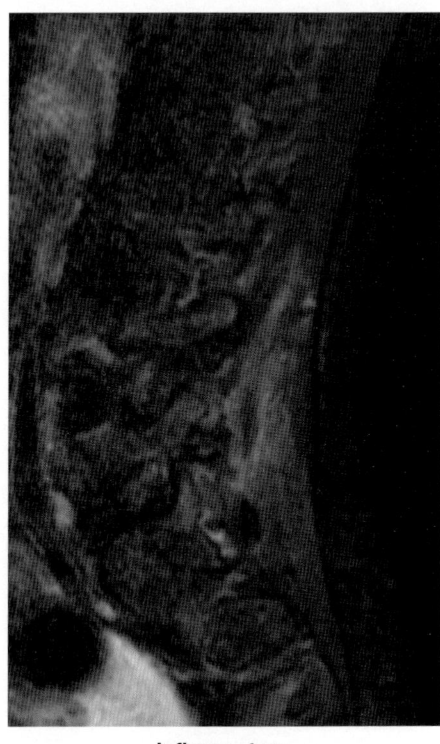

Inflammatory

1. Juvenile idiopathic arthritis
2. Chronic recurrent multifocal osteomyelitis
3. Disc calcification

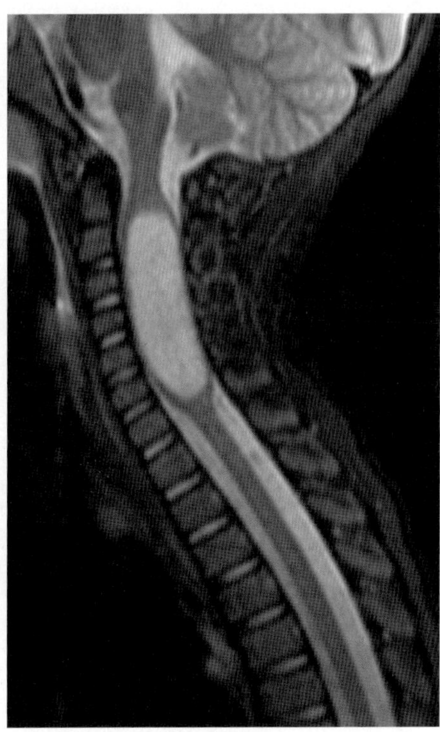

Tumor/Mass

1. Spinal cord tumors
2. Paraspinal tumors
3. Bone tumors
4. Arachnoid cysts

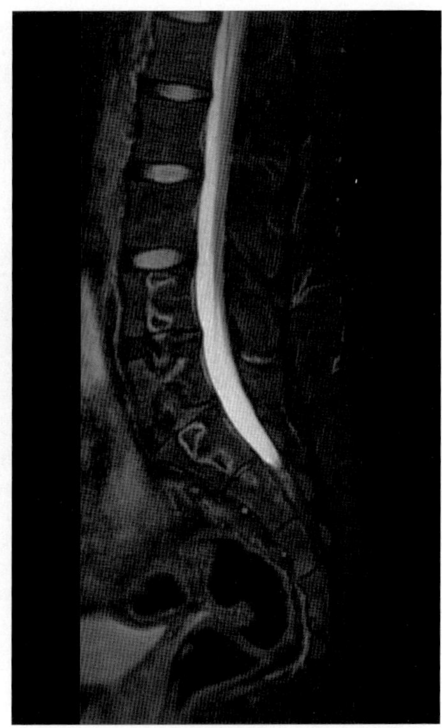

Vascular

1. Bone infarct
2. AVM and AVF
3. Hemorrhage

SPINE PITFALLS

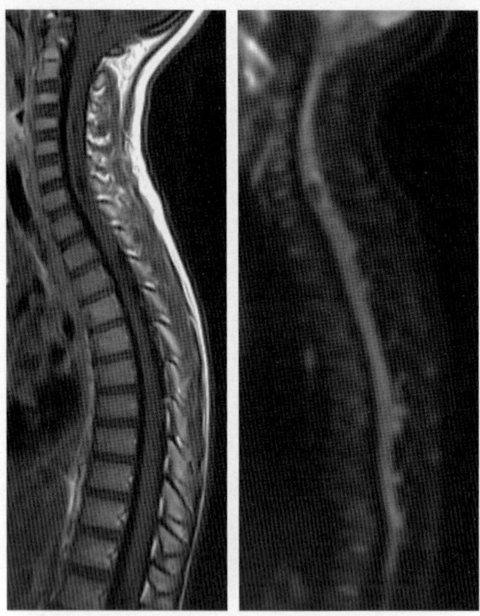

Pitfall: Nonenhancing CSF Metastases

- The addition of DWI or 3D T2W can help improve detection of spinal drop metastases.

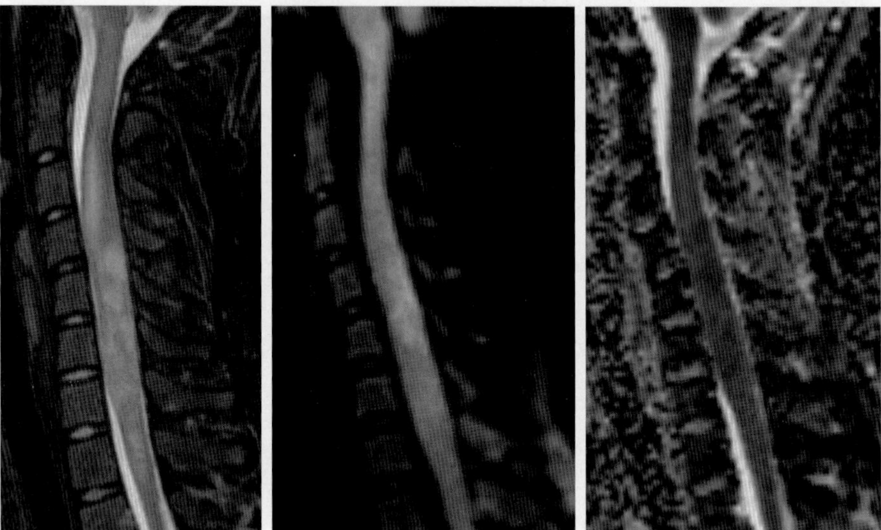

Pitfall: Spinal Cord Glioblastoma Multiforme

- Challenging diagnosis due to the rarity.

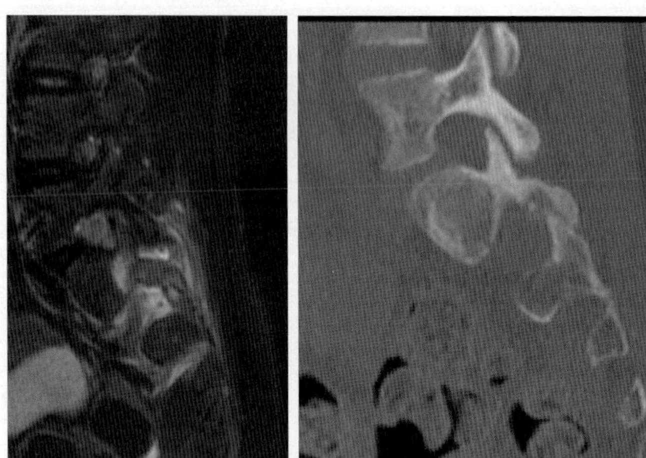

Pitfall: Osteoid Osteoma Presenting on MRI

- Detection of the bone lesion can be difficult on MRI. Consider the potential for an osteoid osteoma when there is a significant degree of bone marrow and soft tissue edema involving posterior elements. JIA and pars defects can also be considered when this finding is present and CT can help identify the osteoid osteoma.

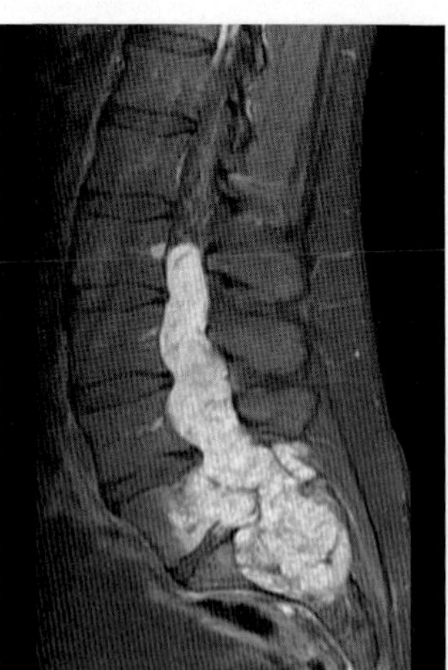

Pitfall: Large Myxopapillary Ependymoma

- Large myxopapillary ependymomas can have both intradural and extradural components, leading to difficulty in forming the correct diagnosis.

Index

Note: Page numbers followed by "*f*" indicate figures, "*b*" indicate boxes, "*t*" indicate tables, and "*e*" indicate online chapter pages.

C

D

I